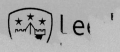 Le

OLYMPIC TEXTBOOK OF MEDICINE IN SPORT

OLYMPIC TEXTBOOK OF MEDICINE IN SPORT

VOLUME XIV OF THE ENCYCLOPAEDIA OF SPORTS MEDICINE

AN IOC MEDICAL COMMISSION PUBLICATION

EDITED BY

PROFESSOR MARTIN P. SCHWELLNUS, MBBCh, MSc, MD

WILEY-BLACKWELL

A John Wiley & Sons, Ltd., Publication

This edition first published 2008, © 2008 International Olympic Committee
Published by Blackwell Publishing Ltd

Blackwell Publishing was acquired by John Wiley & Sons in February 2007. Blackwell's publishing program
has been merged with Wiley's global Scientific, Technical and Medical business to form Wiley-Blackwell.

Registered office: John Wiley & Sons Ltd, The Atrium, Southern Gate, Chichester, West Sussex, PO19 8SQ, UK

Editorial offices: 9600 Garsington Road, Oxford, OX4 2DQ, UK
    The Atrium, Southern Gate, Chichester, West Sussex, PO19 8SQ, UK
    111 River Street, Hoboken, NJ 07030-5774, USA

For details of our global editorial offices, for customer services and for information about how to apply for
permission to reuse the copyright material in this book please see our website at www.wiley.com/wiley-
blackwell

Library of Congress Cataloging-in-Publication Data

The Olympic textbook of medicine in sport / edited by Martin Schwellnus.
    p. ; cm. – (Encyclopaedia of sports medicine ; v. 14)
  "An IOC Medical Commission publication in collaboration with the International Federation of Sports
Medicine."
  Includes bibliographical references.
  ISBN 978-1-4051-5637-0 (alk. paper)
  1. Sports medicine. I. Schwellnus, Martin. II. IOC Medical Commission. III. International Federation
of Sports Medicine. IV. Series.
  [DNLM: 1. Sports Medicine. 2. Athletic Injuries. 3. Athletic Performance. QT 13 E257 1988 v.14]

  RC1210.O46 2008
  617.1'027–dc22

                        2008005042

ISBNs: 978-1-4051-5637-0;
    978-1-4051-9077-0 (leather bound)

A catalogue record for this book is available from the British Library.

Set in 9/12 pt Palatino by Graphicraft Limited, Hong Kong
Printed and bound in Malaysia by Vivar Printing Sdn Bhd

1 2008

Contents

List of Contributors

BRIAN B. ADAMS MD, MPH, *Department of Dermatology, University of Cincinnati, Cincinnati, OH, USA, and Veterans Administration Medical Center, Cincinnati, OH, USA*

YUMNA ALBERTUS-KAJEE Bsc(Med), *UCT/MRC Research Unit for Exercise Science and Sports Medicine, Department of Human Biology, Faculty of Health Sciences, University of Cape Town, South Africa*

JEFFREY M. ANDERSON MD, *Division of Athletics, University of Connecticut, Storrs, CT, USA*

RAUL ARTAL MD, *Department of Obstetrics, Gynecology and Women's Health, St. Louis University, School of Medicine, St. Louis, MO, USA*

MATTEO BONINI MD, *IRCCS San Raffaelo, Rome, Italy*

SERGIO BONINI MD, *IRCCS San Raffaello, Rome, Italy*

ANDREW BOSCH PhD, *UCT/MRC Research Unit for Exercise Science and Sports Medicine, Department of Human Biology, University of Cape Town, South Africa*

VITO BRUSASCO MD, *Department of Internal Medicine, Genoa University, Genoa, Italy*

LOUISE M. BURKE PhD, APD, *Department of Sports Nutrition, Australian Institute of Sport, Bruce, ACT, Australia, and Deakin University, Melbourne, Victoria 3125, Australia*

WALTER CANONICA MD, *Department of Allergy and Respiratory Disease Clinic, Department of Internal Medicine, Genoa University, Genoa, Italy*

KAI-HÅKON CARLSEN MD, PhD, *University of Oslo, Norwegian University of Sport and Physical Education, Oslo, Norway*

DON H. CATLIN MD, *Department of Molecular and Medical Pharmacology, University of California, Los Angeles, Anti-Doping Research, Inc., Los Angeles, CA, USA*

JOSEPH CUMMISKEY MD, *The Blackrock Clinic, Blackrock, Dublin, Ireland*

STEFANO DEL GIACCO MD, *Policlinico Universitario, University of Cagliari, Monserrato, Italy*

WAYNE E. DERMAN MBChB, PhD, *UTC/MRC Research Unit for Exercise Science and Sports Medicine, Department of Human Biology, Faculty of Health Sciences, University of Cape Town, South Africa*

SIMON DOESSING MD, *Institute of Sports Medicine, Copenhagen University Hospital at Bispebjerg, Copenhagen, Denmark*

KYRIACOS I. ELEFTHERIOU MBBS, MRCS(Ed), *UCL Centre for Health and Human Performance, Royal Free and University College Medical School, London, UK*

CONLETH FEIGHERY MD, *Department of Immunology, St. James' Hospital and Trinity College Dublin, Dublin, Ireland*

ANDREW GREEN PhD, *National Centre for Medical Genetics, University College Dublin, Ireland*

GARY GREEN MD, *Division of Sports Medicine, University of California, Los Angeles, and Pacific Palisades Medical Group, Pacific Palisades, CA, USA*

SHONA HALSON PhD, *Department of Physiology, Australian Institute of Sport, Belconnen, ACT, Australia*

CHRIS HANNA MBChB, *Adidas Sport Medicine Center, St. Johns, Auckland, New Zealand*

CAROLINE K. HATTON PhD, *Anti-Doping Research, Inc., Los Angeles, CA, USA*

JOHN A. HAWLEY PhD, *Exercise Metabolism Group, School of Medical Sciences, RMIT University, Bundoora, Victoria, Australia*

TAMARA HEW-BUTLER PhD, *UCT/MRC Research Unit for Exercise Science and Sports Medicine, Department of Human Biology, Sports Science Institute of South Africa, South Africa*

SUSAN HOFFSTETTER PhD, *Department of Obstetrics, Gynecology and Women's Health, St. Louis University, School of Medicine, St. Louis, MO, USA*

LUCY-MAY HOLTZHAUSEN MBBCh, BSc, *Auckland Family Medical Center, Remuera, Auckland, New Zealand*

MIKEL IZQUIERDO PhD, *Studies, Research and Sport Medicine Center, Government of Navarra, Pamplona, Spain*

AUSTIN JEANS MBBCh, BSc, *Centre for Sport and Exercise Medicine, Harare, Zimbabwe*

PEKKA KANNUS MD, PhD, *Accident and Trauma Research Center, UKK Institute, Tampere, Finland*

CHRISTOS KASAPIS MD, *Department of Cardiovascular Medicine, University of Michigan, Ann Arbor, MI, USA*

KEUN-YOUL KIM MD, MPH, PhD, *Medical College of Seoul National University, Seoul, Korea*

MICHAEL KJÆR MD, PhD, *Institute of Sports Medicine, Copenhagen University Hospital at Bispebjerg, Copenhagen, Denmark*

CHRIS KLENCK MD, *University of Tennessee, Knoxville, TN, USA*

WILLIAM J. KRAEMER PhD, *Human Performance Laboratory, Department of Kinesiology, University of Connecticut, Storrs, CT, USA*

MICHAEL I. LAMBERT PhD, *UCT/MRC Research Unit for Exercise Science and Sports Medicine, Department of Human Biology, Faculty of Health Sciences, University of Cape Town, South Africa*

PAUL B. LAURSEN PhD, *School of Exercise, Biomedical and Health Sciences, Edith Cowan University, Joondalup, Western Australia, Australia*

PAUL MCCRORY MBBS, PhD, *Centre for Health, Exercise and Sports Medicine, University of Melbourne, Parkville, Victoria, Australia*

DOUGLAS B. MCKEAG MD, MS, *IU Center for Sports Medicine, Department of Family Medicine, School of Medicine, Indiana University, Indianapolis, IN, USA*

DONALD C. MCKENZIE MD, PhD, *Division of Sports Medicine, Faculty of Medicine, University of British Columbia, Vancouver, BC, Canada*

ROMAIN MEEUSEN PhD, *Vrije Universiteit Brussel, Faculteit LK – Department of Human Physiology & Sports Medicine, Brussels, Belgium*

KATJA PELTOLA MJØSUND MD, *Biomedicum – Helsinki, Helsinki University, Finland*

HUGH E. MONTGOMERY MBBS, MRCP, MD, *UCL Centre for Health and Human Performance, Royal Free and University College Medical School, London, UK*

SELLO MOTAUNG BSc, MBBCh, *Centre for Exercise Science and Sports Medicine, School of Therapeutic Sciences, Faculty of Health Sciences, University of the Witwatersrand, Johannesburg, South Africa*

IÑIGO MUJIKA PhD, *Department of Research and Development, Athletic Club Bilbao, Spain*

GUSTAVO A. NADER PhD, *Department of Clinical Neuroscience, Center for Molecular Medicine, Karolinska Institute, Stockholm, Sweden*

ROBERT U. NEWTON PhD, *School of Exercise, Biomedical and Health Sciences Edith Cowan University, Joondalup, Western Australia, Australia*

RIKU NIKANDER MD, PhD, *Accident and Trauma Research Center, UKK Institute, Tampere, Finland*

TIMOTHY D. NOAKES MBChB, MD, DSc, *UCT/MRC Research Unit for Exercise Science and Sports Medicine, Department of Human Biology, Sports Science Institute of South Africa, South Africa*

ALAN J. PEARCE PhD, *Centre for Aging, Rehabilitation, Exercise and Sport (CARES), School of Human Movement, Recreation and Performance, Victoria University, Melbourne, Victoria, Australia*

FABIO PIGOZZI MD, *Internal Medicine Unit, Department of Health Services, University of Rome (IUSM), Rome, Italy*

DALE E. RAE PhD, *UCT/MRC Research Unit for Exercise Science and Sports Medicine, Department of Human Biology, Faculty of Health Sciences, University of Cape Town, South Africa*

NICHOLAS A. RATAMESS PhD, *Department of Health and Exercise Science, The College of New Jersey, Ewing, NJ, USA*

BRIAN RAYNER MBChB, MMed, *Department of Medicine, Faculty of Health Sciences, University of Cape Town, South Africa*

MARK SAYERS PhD, *Centre for Healthy Activities, Sport and Exercise (CHASE), Faculty of Science, Health and Education, University of the Sunshine Coast, Maroochydore DC, Queensland, Australia*

MARTIN P. SCHWELLNUS MBBCh, MSc, MD, *UCT/MRC Research Unit for Exercise Science and Sports Medicine, Department of Human Biology, Faculty of Health Sciences, University of Cape Town, South Africa*

A. WILLIAM SHEEL PhD, *School of Human Kinetics, University of British Columbia, Osborne Centre, Vancouver, BC, Canada*

HARRI SIEVÄNEN MD, PhD, *Accident and Trauma Research Center, UKK Institute, Tampere, Finland*

JEROEN SWART MBChB, *UCT/MRC Research Unit for Exercise Science and Sports Medicine, Department of Human Biology, Sports Science Institute of South Africa, South Africa*

PAUL D. THOMPSON MD, *Preventive Cardiology & The Athletes' Heart Program, Division of Cardiology, Hartford Hospital, Hartford, CT, USA*

THOMAS H. TROJIAN MD, *Division of Athletics, University of Connecticut, Storrs, CT, USA*

ROSS TUCKER PhD, *UCT/MRC Research Unit for Exercise Science and Sports Medicine, Department of Human Biology, Sports Science Institute of South Africa, South Africa*

WAYNE VILJOEN PhD, *Sport Science Institute of South Africa, Newlands, Cape Town, South Africa*

DARREN E.R. WARBURTON PhD, *School of Human Kinetics, University of British Columbia, Vancouver, BC, Canada*

JOHN WRIGHT MBChB, PhD, *Fairfield Suites, Kingsbury Hospital, Claremont, South Africa*

WARREN YOUNG PhD, *School of Human Movement and Sport Sciences, University of Ballarat, Ballarat, Victoria, Australia*

Foreword

This Volume represents the XIVth volume of *The Encyclopaedia of Sports Medicine* series, scientific publications by the IOC Medical Commission which began in 1988 with Volume I, *The Olympic Book of Sports Medicine*. To produce each volume, the most respected clinicians and scientific investigators have collaborated to produce reference texts that are both comprehensive for the topic and representative of the leading edge of knowledge.

The positive impact of the Encyclopaedia on a central theme, the health and welfare of all persons participating in sport, has exceeded all expectations.

Volume XIV, *The Olympic Textbook of Medicine in Sport*, addresses the clinical issues that were included in the original Volume I and synthesizes the new research information that has been published during the intervening 20 years. I wish to congratulate Professor Martin Schwellnus and all of the Contributing Authors on the excellent quality of this publication.

Dr Jacques Rogge
President of the International Olympic Committee

Preface

Sports and Exercise Medicine can be defined as that scope of medical practice which focuses on (i) the prevention, diagnosis, treatment and rehabilitation of injuries that occur during physical activity, (ii) the prevention, diagnosis, and management of medical conditions that occur during or after physical activity, and (iii) the promotion and implementation of regular physical activity in the prevention, treatment and rehabilitation of chronic diseases of lifestyle. Over the past two to three decades, there has been an exponential increase in the number of published research articles, books and other publications that cover these areas of medical practice. In general, most publications (in particular textbooks) cover the first (injury prevention and treatment) and the third (chronic disease prevention and rehabilitation) areas of Sports and Exercise Medicine very well. However, the area in Sports and Exercise Medicine that has not received the same attention in the published literature is the prevention, diagnosis, and management of medical conditions that occur during or after physical activity. It is for that reason, that this new volume of *The Encyclopaedia of Sports Medicine* series has been compiled, specifically to provide sports medicine practitioners with a systematic approach to this very important aspect of sports medicine practice.

It is well recognized that the team physician, including the members of the medical team attending to Olympic athletes, commonly encounter medical problems that are non-injury related. It has been reported that about 50% of the 1804 athletes seen at the multipurpose medical facility at the 1996 Olympic Games were seen for treatment of non-injury related illnesses. A similar pattern has been observed in subsequent Olympic Games, and this is also a common observation by team physicians who travel with athletes in other sporting disciplines.

In compiling this volume, it was therefore decided to follow a systemic approach that will provide the sports medicine practitioner with a clinical approach to the prevention, diagnosis and treatment of common and less common medical problems encountered in athletes. This volume contains 20 chapters. The first three introductory chapters deal with the basic approach to training, monitoring training and the clinical implications of excessive training. The remaining 17 chapters systemically deal with all the major systems in the body, and focus on medical conditions that athletes may suffer from in each system. Special mention has to be made of three novel chapters that focus on medical conditions in athletes with disabilities, genetics and exercise and emergency sports medicine. Each chapter editor was selected on the basis of their expertise, and chapter editors were also encouraged to solicit contributing authors for specialized sections within chapters. This approach has led to a volume that has an impressive list of authors – all experts in their field.

It has been a privilege for me to work with these experts in compiling this volume, and I trust that you as the reader will find the volume inspiring, comprehensive and a truly novel resource that will be consulted regularly in your practice. I also trust that the use of this volume by sports practitioners will also ultimately improve the medical service to our athletes.

Acknowledgements

I would like to sincerely thank all the chapter editors and contributing authors for their hard work, dedication, and willingness to share their expertise. In particular, I would like to thank all of the contributors for giving up time amidst their very busy schedules. A special thanks has to go to Professor Howard Knuttgen, Coordinator of Scientific Publications for the IOC Medical Commission, for initiating this project, and for his constant support and encouragement. Also many thanks to the editorial and support staff at Blackwell for their support. Finally, thanks to the IOC Medical Commission and the International Sports Medicine Federation (FIMS) for allowing me to edit this volume in the Encyclopaedia series.

Martin P. Schwellnus, MBBCh, MSc, MD

Chapter 1

General Principles of Training

MICHAEL I. LAMBERT, WAYNE VILJOEN, ANDREW BOSCH,
ALAN J. PEARCE AND MARK SAYERS

Exercise training can be defined as a systematic process of preparing for a certain physical goal. This goal used to be synonymous with peak physical performance; however, exercise training is also used to achieve targets for health-related fitness. As society evolves and becomes more sedentary (Dollman *et al.* 2005) there is greater emphasis on habitual physical activity with the aim of reducing obesity, adult onset diabetes, hypertension and the risk of heart disease. Indeed, there are specific guidelines which have been have written for prescribing exercise for these conditions (American College of Sports Medicine 1998).

An understanding shared by coaches and athletes alike, all over the world, is the general concept that physical performance improves with training (Foster *et al.* 1996). The specific guidelines on how to achieve peak performance are not so clear, because of the diverse capabilities, goals and types of sport. For example, a sedentary person may have a goal of training to develop sufficient fitness for running 5 km without stopping. This can be compared to the goal of a professional athlete who trains according to a program with the aim of reducing his 5-km time by 3 s. However, irrespective of the goal, there are basic principles of training which can be applied to plan training programs.

Training for peak sporting performance includes training for physical development (general and sport-specific factors), and technical and tactical

The Olympic Textbook of Medicine in Sport, 1st edition. Edited by M. Schwellnus. Published 2008 by Blackwell Publishing, ISBN: 978-1-4051-5637-0.

training (Bompa 1999). Athletes also have to train psychologic aspects and in team sports athletes have to train for the development of team compatibility to ensure harmony within the team structure. To complete the requirements for achieving peak performance, athletes need to be healthy and free of injuries and have a theoretical knowledge of their training in preparation for their sport so that they can take some responsibility for their progress (Bompa 1999).

Long-term planning for the career of an elite athlete covers 10–15 years (Smith 2003). However, the age at which competitors reach their peak varies according to the sport. For example, in sports such as gymnastics, figure skating, and swimming competitors reach their peak in their late teens or early twenties, in contrast to other sports such as soccer, rugby, and distance running where competitors reach their peak success in their late twenties or early thirties (Bompa 1999). In sports such as golf and lawn bowls, in which the technical attributes are the most important factors determining success, the age of elite performers may be 40 or 50 years. Generally, the starting age of athletes in the more technical sports, which require the development of fine motor coordination skills, is younger than athletes competing in sports that are less technical but depend more on physical ability.

This chapter discusses the evolution of training principles with a contemporary view of the factors that need to be considered in devising a training program. Specifically, it discusses the principles of training programs that are designed to improve peak performance coinciding with competition.

This is followed by sections on specific training principles for strength, endurance, and skill acquisition.

History

Exercise training to improve performance can be traced back to early civilizations (Kontor 1988). There is evidence for both strength training and strength contests as early as 2040 BC with illustrations of weightlifting and strength movements on the tomb of the Egyptian Prince Baghti (Stone et al. 2006). Other forms of training are described in folklore. For example, there is the story of the Milo the Greek wrestler who won six titles at the Olympic Games, getting his first title in 540 BC. In preparation for his competition Milo supported a calf above his head daily. As the calf grew, Milo became stronger and was the credited with being the first person to practice the principle of overload (Kontor 1988). This principle was only studied systematically nearly 2500 years later (Hellenbrandt & Houtz 1956). Planning a training program for improving performance was documented by Flavius Philostratus (AD 170–245), a coach of Greek Olympians. He mentioned that a coach should "be a psychiatrist with considerable knowledge in anatomy and heritage" (Bompa 1999).

In Britain towards the end of the 18th century methods of training were discussed by trainers of athletes from different sports involving humans (runners, boxers) and animals (racehorses) (Radford 2000). The description of these training methods became more formal after Sir John Sinclair completed a national survey of coaching methods and published his findings in 1806. These guidelines for training were based on anecdotal evidence and personal experiences of coaches and were devoid of any scientific testing or scrutiny. During this era, success in high performance sport could be attributed mainly to two factors: (i) the athlete had a predisposition to the sport; (ii) a coach with a disciplined approach to training supervised the athlete (Lambert 2006). The first scientific investigation into sports training methods occurred in 1950 (Tipton 1997) and since then there has been an acceleration in the discussion and scientific evaluation of athletic training programs (Booth et al. 2000).

The "scientific approach" to training coincided with the application of the principles of sports physiology to training (Tipton 1997). This initiated a systematic application into training programs of interval training (Laursen & Jenkins 2002) and other types of training such as acceleration sprints, circuit training, continuous fast running, continuous slow running, fartlek training, jogging, and repetition running.

During the 1960s and 1970s the development of sports science coincided with the transition of amateur into professional sports (Booth et al. 2000). This also prompted creative thinking about improving performance through strategies other than training. Not all the methods were accepted. Indeed, the use of drugs to improve performance was banned by the International Olympic Committee (IOC) and implemented at the Olympic Games in Mexico City in 1968 (Papagelopoulos et al. 2004). Nearly 40 years later this problem is still rife in competitive sport, with athletes and their medical support staff becoming more elusive in their use of drugs. This is countered by the authorities who have to invest large amounts of money to use more sophisticated methods to detect athletes who have used any substance that appears on the IOC banned list.

Equipment has also improved over the years and contributed significantly to an improvement in performance in sports such as golf, soccer, kayaking, cycling, and javelin. This has resulted in legislation standardizing the equipment to prevent competitors from having an unfair advantage over their rivals with less sophisticated equipment. A specific example of equipment influencing performance is pole vaulting where at the 1896 Olympics a bamboo pole was used and the height achieved was 3.2 m. In modern times, with the use of poles made out of carbon-fiber composite material, the current world record is nearly double that at 6.14 m (2008).

Despite the refinement in the preparation for elite performances, the improvement in world records in the last 20 years has been moderate. For example, the World Record in the marathon has improved by 2 min 17 s (1.8%), the 10,000 m and 5000 m track race times by 56 s (3.4%) and 22 s (3.0%), respectively, and the shot put distance has increased by 50 cm (2.2%) during this time.

In summary, the factors associated with improvement in the performance of contemporary athletes compared with the top athletes several decades ago are:

- Improvements in coaching;
- Advances in nutrition;
- Perfection of athletic facilities;
- Refinement of equipment; and
- Contributions from sports medicine (Tipton 1997).

Biologic process of training

Exercise training can be explained according to the principles of biologic adaptation. In accordance with this explanation, each training session imposes a physiologic stress (Brooks *et al.* 2005). As with all forms of physiologic stress, there is a homeostatic reaction. This results in transient physiologic and metabolic changes (Coyle 2000) which return to their pre-exercise resting levels during the recovery period when the exercise session is over. Examples of these transient changes are as follow (Brooks *et al.* 2005):

- Altered blood flow to the active muscles;
- Increased heart rate;
- Increased breathing rate;
- Increased oxygen consumption;
- Increased rate of sweating;
- Increased body temperature;
- Secretion of stress hormones such as adrenocorticotropic hormone (ACTH), cortisol and catecholamines;
- Increased glycolytic flux; and
- Altered recruitment of muscles.

If these acute bouts of exercise are repeated over time they induce chronic adaptations that are also known as training adaptations (Coyle 2000). Most of these changes involve remodeling of protein tissue as a consequence of changes between protein synthesis and degradation (Mader 1988). These changes are semi-permanent and do not disappear after the bout of exercise or training session. However, they do regress if regular exposure to the stress of training ceases, as occurs during periods of detraining (Mujika *et al.* 2004). Training adaptations result in altered metabolism (Coyle 2000), changes in neuromuscular recruitment patterns during exercise, and remodeling of tissue (Hakkinen *et al.* 2003).

The specific type of changes that occur after training depend on the type of stimulus, defined by the mode of exercise, intensity, and volume of training (Brooks *et al.* 2005; Coyle 2000). For example, the outcome of a resistance training program can increase either muscular endurance, hypertrophy, strength, or power. This depends on the manipulation of the training variables: (i) muscle action; (ii) loading and volume; (iii) selection of exercises and the order in which they are performed; (iv) rest periods; (v) repetition velocity; and (vi) frequency (Bird *et al.* 2005). The choice of the application of the training load (free weight vs. machine weights) can also influence the type of adaptation (Stone *et al.* 2000a).

The overt symptoms of training adaptations are shown by well-defined muscles, low body fat, and skilful movements. The covert symptoms of training are increased mitochondria in skeletal muscles (Irrcher *et al.* 2003), increased capillarization (Henriksson 1992), cardiac hypertrophy (Urhausen & Kindermann 1992), and increased density of bones (Chilibeck *et al.* 1995). The first signs of increased capillarization occur about 4 weeks after starting a training program (Jensen *et al.* 2004), while it takes at least 4 weeks for the mitochondrial mass in the skeletal muscle to increase (Lambert & Noakes 1989). A few days after starting an endurance training program there is an increase in plasma volume (Green *et al.* 1990), while an altered muscle recruitment is the earliest adaptation that occurs after resistance training (Carroll *et al.* 2001; Gabriel *et al.* 2006). This is followed by muscle hypertrophy which occurs after about 8 weeks, depending on the training status of the athlete.

Training adaptations can be classified either as those changes that increase performance (through either an increased muscle power, increased ability to resist fatigue, or increased motor coordination) or those changes that reduce the risk of injury. There is generally a positive relationship between training load and the physiologic adaptations resulting in improvements in performance. However, if a critical training load is exceeded there will be diminishing returns. For competitors at the elite level there is a fine line between insufficient training or too much training (Kuipers & Keizer 1988; Lehmann *et al.* 1993; Meeusen *et al.* 2006; Morton 1997).

Insufficient training does not induce adequate adaptations and results in suboptimal performance. In contrast, too much training results in maladaptations or the failure to adapt, causing symptoms of fatigue and poor performance (Budgett 1990; Derman *et al*. 1997). A more scientific approach to training with a systematic approach to monitoring training increases the chances of the athlete peaking at the correct time coinciding with important competition (Lambert 2006; Lambert & Borresen 2006).

Factors affecting physical performance

The many factors that have the potential to affect physical performance are shown in Table 1.1 (Lambert 2006). Exercise training is the overriding factor in the list and can account for an improvement in performance of over 400% in an untrained person who undergoes a systematic training program (Noakes 2001). The magnitude of this improvement is in stark contrast to the magnitude of improvement (1–30%) caused by the other factors shown in Table 1.1. All these factors are discussed in detail in various sections in this book.

Fitness components associated with sport

Performance in most sports requires integrated functioning of the different systems in the body.

Table 1.1 Factors that have the potential to affect performance.

Exercise training and preparation, including tapering
Health
Nutrition
Nutritional ergogenic aids
Drugs (positive and negative)
Inherited characteristics
Opposition
Tactics
Equipment
Home ground advantage
Environmental conditions (heat, cold, wind, altitude, allergens)
Mental readiness
Sleep (and circadian rhythms)

However, it is useful to compartmentalize these systems in order to gain a better understanding of how the athlete has developed and which aspects of their fitness need to be further developed. Accordingly, the systems can be compartmentalized into the following categories.

Strength

Muscle strength is defined as the ability to produce force. While a minimal amount of strength is needed for normal daily activities, the demands of certain sports require well-developed strength. In some sports strength is needed just as a basic component of fitness, while in other sports (e.g., weightlifting) strength is the main outcome variable which determines success or failure in competition. Strength can be increased by systematic resistance training using either specially designed machines or free weights (Stone *et al*. 2000a). The manifestation of an athlete's strength depends on muscle morphology and the motor system (Enoka 1988). Strength can be increased without any change in muscle size, but it is always dependent on changes in the neural system (Carroll *et al*. 2001). Increases in strength are transferred to sporting performances in varying amounts. For example, a weight-training program increased squat one-repetition maximum (1 RM) by 21% and this increase in strength was accompanied by improvements in vertical jump performance (21%) and sprinting speed (2.3%) (Young 2006).

Power

Muscle power, which is a function of the interaction between force of contraction and the speed of contraction, is associated with the explosiveness of the muscle. The relationship between force and speed of contraction and the subsequent point at which peak power occurs varies between athletes (Jennings *et al*. 2005). For example, peak power occurs at 50–70% of the maximum weight that can be lifted for one repetition for the squat and at 40–60% of 1 RM for the bench press (Siegel *et al*. 2002). A fundamental way of increasing muscle power is to increase maximal strength, particularly in untrained athletes (Stone *et al*. 2000a).

Muscle endurance

Muscle endurance is dependent on the muscle being able to contract repetitively without developing fatigue. A combination of muscle strength, metabolic characteristics, and local circulation in the muscle influence the endurance characteristics. Several tests have been developed to measure muscle endurance. A feature of these tests is that they all monitor the ability of a specific muscle, or group of muscles, to contract repetitively. Examples of these tests are the number of push-ups and abdominal curls in 1 min (Getchell 1985; Semenick 1994). Muscular endurance can also be measured with repeated static contractions (isometric) (Coetzer *et al*. 1993).

Repeat sprint

The ability to resist fatigue after repeated short duration, high intensity sprints is a fitness characteristic that is important for team sports such as soccer, rugby, football, basketball, and netball. Repeat sprint performance and, by implication, fatigue resistance during intermittent, short duration, high intensity activities, can be improved by decreasing body mass, specifically body fat, and by increasing strength and muscular endurance, providing this does not result in an increase in body mass (Durandt *et al*. 2006). Training that results in improvements in agility and/or aerobic power may also improve the ability to resist fatigue during repeat sprint activities (Durandt *et al*. 2006).

Speed

Speed consists of a number of components (Cronin & Hansen 2005; Delecluse *et al*. 1995), all of which are independent qualities: acceleration speed, maximum speed, and speed endurance. Performance in the 10-m sprint is influenced by acceleration speed, while performance in the 40-m sprint is dependent on both acceleration speed and maximum speed (Delecluse *et al*. 1995). Speed can be improved by increasing the power to weigh ratio. Plyometric training (i.e., counter-movement jumps or loaded squat jumps) is effective for improving speed (Cronin & Hansen 2005).

Motor coordination (skill)

Performance in sport often has a component of skill. This depends on the combined interaction of agility, balance, coordination, power, speed, and reaction time. Another aspect of skill, which is difficult to define or measure, is the ability of a sports person to make a strategic decision very quickly. The accuracy of this decision-making contributes to the success of the team. There are examples in different sporting codes of players who seem gifted and on most occasions make the correct decision during competition compared to their less "talented" team mates. While motor coordination can be trained, the superior decision-making ability that some players have, making them appear more skilled, is probably an intrinsic characteristic rather than being acquired by training.

Flexibility

Flexibility represents the range of motion specific to a joint. Flexibility can be dynamic or static. Dynamic flexibility involves the range of motion during movement of muscles around a joint whereas static flexibility defines the degree to which a joint can be passively moved through its full range of motion. Changes in flexibility occur after stretching exercises. Flexibility training is used in the warm-up before training or competition (Shellock & Prentice 1985) and also with the goal of preventing injuries. Although there is theoretical evidence to support the positive link between stretching and lowered risk of musculoskeletal injuries during exercise, the clinical evidence is not so strong (Gleim & McHugh 1997). Specific joint angle can be measured as a marker of flexibility for various joints with a goniometer, or a Leighton flexometer (Leighton 1966). A sit-and-reach field test has also been developed to measure the range of motion of the lower back and hamstring muscles.

Cardiovascular fitness

Cardiovascular fitness, also referred to as cardiovascular endurance or aerobic fitness, refers to the collective ability of the cardiovascular system to adjust to the physiologic stress of exercise. Cardiovascular fitness is usually measured in the laboratory during a high intensity exercise test to exhaustion with a mode of exercise that recruits a large muscle mass and with rhythmic muscle contractions (e.g., cycling, running, rowing). A feature of the test is that it should have a progressively increasing intensity which continues until the athlete is exhausted. Oxygen consumption and carbon dioxide produced are measured continuously during the test. The oxygen consumption coinciding with exhaustion is called the maximum oxygen consumption ($\dot{V}o_{2max}$). An athlete who excels in an endurance sport generally has a high $\dot{V}o_{2max}$. Although endurance training increases the $\dot{V}o_{2max}$, and by implication the cardiovascular fitness, the increases are generally moderate (about 15%; Zavorsky 2000) and are dependent on the level of fitness of the person at the start of the training program.

A 20-m shuttle test has also been developed to predict cardiovascular fitness in a field setting (Léger & Lambert 1982). In this field test athletes run backwards and forwards between two beacons 20 m apart, maintaining a prescribed pace which gets faster and faster until the athlete is unable to maintain the pace. The stage coinciding with fatigue is directly proportional to $\dot{V}o_{2max}$.

Body composition

Body composition is defined by the proportions of fat, muscle, and bone. Fat occurs beneath the skin and around the internal organs and is also found within tissues such as bone and muscle. Fat can be divided into non-essential and essential compartments. Fat tissue insulates and protects organs and is a storage form of energy and substrates for metabolism. Fat mass may vary from about 6% to 40% of body mass. Endurance athletes who perform at a high level have low levels of fat. Sumo wrestlers are examples of elite athletes who have a high fat content. Many sports have weight categories (e.g., boxing, judo, wrestling, rowing), and therefore the manipulation of body mass, in particular fat mass, becomes an important part of the athlete's preparation for competition (Fleck 1983).

Muscle mass can vary from about 40% (anorexic person) to 65% of body mass (e.g., a body builder with hypertrophied muscle) (Martin et al. 1990). The main function of muscle, from a sport and exercise perspective, is to contract and generate force. Depending on the sport and the type of training, some muscle is adapted to contract several thousand times per training session without developing fatigue (e.g., endurance activity), whereas other muscle is adapted to generate high levels of power with only a few contractions (e.g., powerlifting, shot put, weightlifting). This type of muscle fatigues rapidly.

Bone is a specialized type of connective tissue which is also dynamic and responds to stimuli by changing its shape and density, albeit at a much slower rate than fat and muscle tissue (Chilibeck et al. 1995). Bone mass varies from 10% to 20% of total body mass.

The diversity of body composition among elite athletes is dramatic and can be observed during a visit to the Olympic village. The smallest men competing at this level are the endurance athletes. Indeed, the winner of the marathon at the Atlanta Olympics in 1996 was Josiah Thugwane of South Africa who weighed 43 kg (Noakes 2001). The larger men who compete in the sports requiring strength and power weigh about 130 kg. The body mass of the champion women athletes competing at the Olympic Games range from about 35 to 110 kg. The body composition can be regarded as an inherited trait, although it can be manipulated to a certain extent by training and nutritional intervention.

Basic principles of training

In planning a training program there are some basic principles that need to be considered. They are discussed under the following headings.

Overload

An athlete has to be exposed to an overload stimulus at regular intervals for the induction of training adaptations. An overload stimulus can be manipulated by changing the mode of exercise, duration, frequency, intensity, and recovery period between training sessions (Bompa 1999). An overload training stimulus can also be imposed by altering nutrition and influencing the intracellular milieu before the training session. For example, to mimic the metabolic stress in the muscles towards the end of a marathon an athlete could start the training session with a low muscle glycogen concentration. This can be achieved by reducing carbohydrate intake about 24 hours before the training session. The athlete then begins the training session with lower than usual glycogen levels in the liver and muscles. After about 20–30 km of the training run the metabolic flux will be similar to the metabolism that occurs towards the end of a marathon. An advantage of this strategy is that a metabolic overload can be imposed without the same mechanical muscle stress and damage that occurs towards the end of a marathon.

Frequency

Training frequency refers to the number of training sessions in a defined period. For example, training frequency may vary between 5 and 14 sessions per week depending on the sport, level of performance of the athlete, and stage of training cycle (Smith 2003).

Duration

This refers to the time or amount of the exercise session. This is sometimes confused with the volume of training, which quantifies training over a period of time and combines duration and frequency (Smith 2003). Athletes competing at the international level need to train for approximately 1000 hours per year (Bompa 1999).

Intensity

Exercise intensity is a measure of "how hard is the exercise?" and is related to the power output. The exercise intensity lies somewhere on a continuum between rest (basal metabolic rate) and maximal effort, which coincides with the maximal oxygen uptake for that activity. Exercise intensity can be monitored by measuring submaximal oxygen consumption (Daniels 1985), heart rate (Lambert et al. 1998), blood lactate (Swart & Jennings 2004), the weight lifted during the exercise (Sweet et al. 2004), or the perception of effort (Foster et al. 2001). Training intensity is the major training stimulus that influences adaptation and performance. Athletes are only advised to incorporate high intensity training into their training programs after they have developed a sufficient base (Laursen & Jenkins 2002). If too much high intensity training is carried out the athlete will be at risk of developing symptoms of fatigue associated with overreaching (Meeusen et al. 2006) and overtraining or will increase the risk of getting injured (Noakes 2001).

Rest and recovery

Rest and recovery are important, often neglected principles of training. Factors that need to be considered during the recovery process after a training session are as follow:
1 *Age* Athletes older than 25 years need longer recovery periods than younger athletes (Bompa 1999).
2 *Environmental conditions* Training and competing in the heat imposes more physiologic stress on the athlete and requires a longer recovery period (Noakes 2001).
3 *Type of activity* Training and competition that induces muscle damage requires longer recovery periods than activities that cause fatigue but no muscle damage or soreness.

Even within a specific sport the demands on the players varies depending on their playing position (Takarada 2003). Ideally, the recovery for each player should be customized. It is recommended that players are monitored using subjective and objective strategies to ensure that the recovery period is customized (Lambert & Borresen 2006). Decisions about the different recovery strategies have to be made considering the team as a whole. A study of rugby players (Gill et al. 2006) showed that recovery was accelerated if the players performed low impact exercise immediately after competition, wore compression garments (Kraemer et al. 2001), or had contrast water therapy (Higgins & Kaminski 1998) compared with a situation where they recovered without any intervention.

A practical tool has been developed to assist coaches and athletes with monitoring recovery (Kenttä & Hassmen 1998). This is a simple questionnaire which the athletes complete on a daily basis. The questions probe aspects of recovery such as: (i) nutrition and hydration; (ii) sleep and rest; (iii) relaxation and emotional support; and (iv) stretching and active rest.

PSYCHOLOGIC STRESS

If the psychologic side of training and competing is not considered in the recovery process the athlete may develop symptoms of staleness or overtraining (Morgan *et al.* 1987). The Profile of Mood States (POMS) questionnaire, which was developed in 1971, is a useful tool for this purpose (McNair *et al.* 1971). The test was initially designed for patients undergoing counseling or therapy but has subsequently evolved to be used in sport. The POMS is a self-report test designed to measure the psychology of mood state, mood changes, and emotion (McNair *et al.* 1971). The test has 65 items which measures six identifiable moods or feelings: Tension-Anxiety, Depression-Dejection, Anger-Hostility, Vigor-Activity, Fatigue-Inertia, and Confusion-Bewilderment. The respondents answer according to a scale (0 = not at all, 1 = a little, 2 = moderately, 3 = quite a bit, 4 = extremely).

The Daily Analysis of Life Demands for Athletes (DALDA) questionnaire can also be used to monitor stress that high performance athletes have to encounter (Rushall 1990). This test monitors the physiologic stress of training in addition to the stresses that may exist outside the training environment but which may contribute significantly to the total stress exposure. The DALDA can be administered throughout a training season and can easily be incorporated into a training logbook. The scoring can be done by the athlete or coach. The test is widely used by coaches and is also sufficiently robust to be used in research (Halson *et al.* 2002).

Specificity

The principle of specificity states that adaptations are specific to the type of training stress. It follows that the type of training must be structured and planned in accordance with the requirements of the competition. However, this principle can be applied inappropriately if it is assumed that all training should simply mimic the demands of competition (Young 2006). In certain sports the physical demands of competition can induce muscle imbalances and the risk of injury is also higher in many types of competition compared to training for the competition. Therefore, it is necessary to vary training and structure it so that the athlete develops a good base of fitness before attempting the more high risk, competition-specific fitness. This concept of varying training volume at various stages of the season is explained by the principle of periodization.

Periodization

Periodization is the process of systematic planning of a short- and long-term training program by varying training loads and incorporating adequate rest and recovery. The plan serves as a template for the athlete and coach (Smith 2003). While it is important to have a plan, the day-to-day implementation of the plan should not be rigid, but rather should be modifiable based on the symptoms of the athlete (Lambert & Borresen 2006; Noakes 2001).

The classic approach of periodized training has been to distinguish between high volume, low intensity training designed to develop aerobic capacity, usually in the early part of the season, and high intensity training designed to develop qualities linked to performance, as the season progresses (Hellard *et al.* 2005). This approach to training reduces the risk of overtraining, while the athlete is more likely to peak at a predictable time, usually coinciding with important competition (Hellard *et al.* 2005; Stone *et al.* 1999). Another reason for this systematic approach to training is that different physiological systems vary in their retention rate after training (Hellard *et al.* 2005). Therefore, by varying the training loads as the season progresses, the desired adaptations, which are associated with peak performance, are achieved.

An advantage of periodization is that it provides a structure for controlling the stress and recovery for inducing training adaptations (Smith 2003). The success of the plan can also be tested regularly to confirm that specific goals have been met in preparation for the main competition (Lambert 2006).

A study of Olympic swimmers showed that the relationship between training load and performance varied according to the different phases of training. Low intensity training had a positive effect on performance in the long term, suggesting that this type of training is necessary to induce the adaptation of various physiologic mechanisms necessary for the subsequent high intensity training (Hellard *et al.* 2005). This study also concluded that the swimmers' response to a given training volume may vary between seasons and even between training sessions. They found that at the elite level training variables only accounted for 30% of the variation in performance (Hellard *et al.* 2005). This supports the concept that training programs need to be highly individualized for elite athletes (Hellard *et al.* 2005). Monitoring the training load–response relationship is important for elite athletes to ensure that the training program is individualized and accommodates the needs of each athlete (Lambert 2006).

There are several different models for periodizing training (Bompa 1999). These models differ depending on the sport, but they all share a common principle in having phases of general preparation, specific preparation, competition preparation and competition, transition or active rest. The terminology for dividing the cycles is referred to as follows:
- *macrocycles:* long plan, usually 1 year;
- *mesocycles:* shorter plan from about 2 weeks to several months; and
- *microcycles:* short plan of about 7 days (Stone *et al.* 1999).

Basic errors in training

The principles of training are guidelines that can be used to customize a training program. A deviation from, or inappropriate application of these guidelines, has consequences that can negatively affect performance. Common basic errors in training that detract from achieving peak performances include the following (Smith 2003):
- Recovery is neglected;
- Demands on the athletes are made too quickly;

- After a break in training because of illness or injury, the training load is increased too quickly;
- High volume of maximal and submaximal training;
- Overall volume of intense training is too high when the athlete is training for endurance events;
- Excessive time is devoted to technical or mental aspects, without adequate recovery;
- Excessive number of competitions – this includes frequent disturbances of the daily routine and insufficient training time that accompanies competition;
- Bias of training methodology; and
- The athlete has a lack of trust of the coach because of inaccurate goal setting.

Conclusions

This section attempts to discuss the basic principles of training. These principles have evolved from practical experience, but are also based on biologic principles of stress and adaptation. The next sections in this chapter discuss more specific examples of the basic principles of training, focusing on resistance training, endurance training, and skill acquisition.

TRAINING TO INCREASE MUSCLE STRENGTH AND POWER

The primary focus of research in the physical conditioning field has been on the promotion of physical activity and aerobic type exercise regimes (Winett & Carpinelli 2001). Strength or resistance training has generally taken a back seat in comparison. However, to perform activities of daily living efficiently and to maximize sporting performance capabilities one needs the muscles and joints of the body to function optimally. To ensure that this happens, one needs to strengthen and condition these structures sufficiently. One way of accomplishing this is by regular resistance training.

Program design

"The act of resistance training, itself, does not ensure optimal gains in muscle strength and performance" (Kraemer & Ratamess 2004). The key to successful resistance training is an appropriate program design. To obtain the best results, one has to consider the science behind exercise prescription and also take a practical approach. To perform this process efficiently one has to consider the following training variables: the exercise and workout structure, mode of resistance training, exercise intensity, rest intervals and frequency of training, volume of training, speed of movement, and progression. It is the correct manipulation of these training variables that optimize the resistance training outcomes.

Exercise and workout structure

There are three main types of strength training programs: total body workouts, upper body/lower body split programs, and muscle group split programs (American College of Sports Medicine 2002; Kraemer & Ratamess 2004). The *total body workout* is a commonly used approach that incorporates 1–2 exercises for each main muscle group covering the whole body in one session. The *upper body/lower body split* program is also a favored program design that focuses on training either the upper body or lower body on alternate days. The *muscle group split* approach is mainly used for people who wish to maximize hypertrophy of selected muscle groups. The choice of program depends on individual requirements and objectives (Kraemer & Ratamess 2004). The advantage of training using a split-program routine is that one can select a wider range of exercises which allows more focus on specific muscle groups than with the total body workout approach (American College of Sports Medicine 2002; Kraemer & Ratamess 2004). The split-program approach also allows a higher frequency of resistance training, but still provides adequate recovery periods for specific muscle groups during a training cycle (Pearson *et al.* 2000).

EXERCISE ORDER

It is important to maximize the benefits obtained from each exercise and to train at maximum effort for optimal results. Therefore, multi-joint exercises should be performed earlier on in the workout while the person is less fatigued (Kraemer & Ratamess 2004). Because multi-joint exercises involve more muscle groups, require lifting heavier weights, and necessitate enhanced balance and control, they also demand more physical effort to perform. If fatigue is present by the time these exercises are performed, the athlete will not be able to gain the maximum benefit from the exercise. Furthermore, there is a risk of losing good form and technique, which predisposes one to an increased risk of injury.

The general recommendations for sequencing of resistance training exercises for strength and power are as follows (American College of Sports Medicine 2002; Kraemer & Ratamess 2004):
- Large muscle groups before small muscle groups (all programs)
- Multi-joint exercises before single-joint exercises (all programs)
- Most complex exercises before least complex exercises (all programs)
- Rotate upper body and lower body exercises (total body programs) *or*
- Rotate opposing muscle groups; for example, push then pull movements, biceps then triceps (total body or upper body/lower body split programs)
- Higher intensity before lower intensity exercises (muscle group split programs)

These recommendations are primarily focused on maximizing the effort and strength gains via performance of the exercises in combination and minimizing the effects of fatigue in the execution of the more difficult multi-joint exercises.

VARIATION WITHIN A PROGRAM

There is sufficient evidence to support the concept that varying the exercises trained on a specific body part (e.g., the chest musculature) improves strength and power gains (Pearson *et al.* 2000). There are a few ways of doing this. One can either change the exercises trained every 2–3 weeks, or one can use two program variations on alternate training days (Pearson *et al.* 2000). However, one should be cautious not to vary core exercises too much, as this might hinder progression.

Mode of resistance training

MACHINE VS. FREE WEIGHTS

There is little evidence to suggest that one type of resistance training (e.g., machines vs. free weights) is superior to the other in terms of results, as long as the training prescription is correctly designed (Feigenbaum & Pollock 1999; Haff 2000; Winett & Carpinelli 2001). Training with free weights requires more functionality such as dynamic proprioception, stabilization, balance, and control, allows more variation and mimics activities of daily living and athletic movements more closely (American College of Sports Medicine 2002; Cronin *et al.* 2003; Field 1988; Haff 2000; Hass *et al.* 2001). It is better to train movements rather than muscles. The shift in resistance training has moved towards functional training, because of its strong neuromuscular contribution to muscle function (Santana 2001). The more specific the movement trained, the greater the transfer of training adaptations to performance of the intended skill or activity (Pearson *et al.* 2000), and free weight exercises have a greater degree of mechanical specificity (Haff 2000). One should therefore preferentially include exercises that mimic activities, as human movement and adaptation is very task-specific (Kraemer & Ratamess 2004). However, training on resistance training machines can still be advantageous, as certain movements are difficult to perform using free weights and can be simulated using machine apparatus. Examples of these exercises are leg extensions and seated cable pulls (for tibialis anterior; American College of Sports Medicine 2002; Haff 2000). For sports conditioning there are advantages for using free weight exercises for functional acceleration, speed, and power (Field 1988). However, most strength and conditioning coaches seldom train their athletes exclusively with machines or free weights but usually combine the two modes of training (Haff 2000).

MULTI-JOINT VS. SINGLE-JOINT EXERCISES

Multi-joint exercises involve more than one joint or major muscle group and are favored as being more effective than single-joint exercises for improving strength and power (American College of Sports Medicine 2002; Kraemer & Ratamess 2004). Examples of single-joint exercises are bicep curls and leg extensions; examples of multi-joint exercises are bench press and leg press. Multi-joint exercises generally involve more muscle mass and include integrated movement with more balance, coordination, and neuromuscular control than single-joint exercises (Kraemer & Ratamess 2004). However, for beginners, single-joint exercises might be more advantageous in that they require less skill and pose less risk of injury than the more complex multi-joint exercises (American College of Sports Medicine 2002; Kraemer & Ratamess 2004). When learning multi-joint exercises one should start with very light resistance such as a bar or even a long wooden stick, and not add any weights until the technique is adequate (Pearson *et al.* 2000).

SPECIFICITY OF RESISTANCE TRAINING

Specificity is one of the main principles of resistance training in preparation for sports performance. This principle is not as important for general health and well-being, as most resistance training programs will lead to improved strength and muscle mass. Specificity in resistance training for sport is designed to train the body to react in a similar way to that required during competition (Field 1988). As an example, it is inappropriate for a power athlete who needs explosiveness to train exclusively for maximum 1 RM strength. Becoming stronger at slow velocities will not ensure that strength necessarily improves at the same rate for ballistic movements such as jumping. To develop strength at faster velocities an athlete would need to include high-speed resistance training activities to address this component of strength development.

Exercise intensity

When prescribing the load used during resistance training, one usually uses a reference load to gauge the relative intensity of the exercise. For multi-joint, core, and power exercises with larger muscle mass involvement, this reference point would normally be in the form of a 1 RM load (Feigenbaum & Pollock 1997) or the maximum load that can be lifted only once with correct form and technique (Cronin & Henderson 2004; Evans 1999). The intensity of training would then be described as a percentage of this measured maximum or 1 RM (Baker 2001b,c; Campos et al. 2002; Feigenbaum & Pollock 1997; Fry 2004; Goto *et al.* 2004; Haff 2004a; Hass *et al.* 2001; Izquierdo *et al.* 2002; Robinson *et al.* 1995). This is a useful method of quantifying the training load and prescribing a similar training stimulus relative to the individual strength capabilities (Fry 2004).

Another method of gauging the relative intensity is that of the *multiple-RM* method (Baker 2001b; Feigenbaum & Pollock 1997; Fleck & Kraemer 1997; Haff 2004a). This is probably the easiest method of resistance prescription and functions on a load-repetition continuum (Fleck 1999; Fleck & Kraemer 1997). It is also a convenient method of gauging the physiologic stress of the exercise session (Fry 2004). An example of this would be selecting a 6 RM load. What the 6 RM effectively means is that a training load should be selected that only allows six repetitions to be performed. If six repetitions cannot be performed, then the load is too heavy, and if more than six repetitions can be performed then the load is too light. This technique is easy to understand and is usually determined in practice by trial and error, as it becomes logistically very time-consuming and impractical to test directly for every exercise prescribed (Haff 2004a).

EFFORT AND EFFECTIVE STRENGTH GAINS

Resistance training should generally be performed with moderate to high effort levels, where effort is defined as the relative amount of exertion that one has to employ to perform the exercise (Winett & Carpinelli 2001). A high level of exertion can be equated to a situation where one terminates the set because one is unable to perform another repetition with good technique or proper form. High effort levels do not necessarily equate to heavy loads! For example, if one aims for 15 repetitions in a set and the athlete manages to complete the 15th repetition yet cannot perform a 16th repetition, then they are exercising at a high level of exertion or relative intensity. For optimal strength development, the greater level of exertion (i.e., training to failure vs. discomfort), the greater the outcome (Fleck & Kraemer 1997).

Frequency of training and rest intervals

FREQUENCY OF TRAINING

Ideally, each major muscle group should be trained twice a week (Feigenbaum & Pollock 1999; Winett & Carpinelli 2001). Those athletes who have more time and want to improve further can increase their frequency of resistance training per muscle group to three times per week (Feigenbaum & Pollock 1999; Hass *et al.* 2001). For adequate recovery, resistance training days for specific muscle groups should be separated by at least 48–72 hours (Feigenbaum & Pollock 1999; Winett & Carpinelli 2001) and a minimum of 24 h should normally separate training sessions (Pearson *et al.* 2000). The recovery period is important for muscle recovery and adaptation, and also to prevent overtraining (Feigenbaum & Pollock 1997; Hass *et al.* 2001; Pearson *et al.* 2000). Based on an extensive literature review in this regard, there seems to be no optimal frequency of training as various muscle groups respond differently to frequency overload (Feigenbaum & Pollock 1997). The chest, arms, and leg muscle groups may respond better on ≥3 days per week; however, the lumbar extensors and smaller trunk muscles respond favorably to less training sessions per week (Feigenbaum & Pollock 1997). Generally, lesser trained athletes need more recovery time than their more highly trained counterparts (Kraemer & Ratamess 2004). Two to 3 days per week has been shown to be effective during the initial phases of resistance training, but the number of training days can be increased as one becomes more experienced and conditioned (American College of Sports Medicine 2002). Advanced training and increased training frequency leads to variations in program design such as split routines such as upper body/lower body and muscle group split programs, where more specialized and focused training is prescribed (American College of Sports Medicine 2002; Kraemer & Ratamess 2004).

REST INTERVALS

Rest intervals are extremely important in program design (Rhea *et al.* 2002b), as they do not only effect hormonal, metabolic, and muscular adaptations, but also effect acute force and muscle power generation, and their rates of improvement (American College of Sports Medicine 2002; Kraemer & Ratamess 2004). With shorter rest intervals the rate of strength gain will be limited (American College of Sports Medicine 2002; Kraemer & Ratamess 2004; Willardson & Burkett 2005). If the rest interval is too short, it will compromise the ability of the muscle to perform and lift the weight (American College of Sports Medicine 2002; Robinson *et al.* 1995; Willardson & Burkett 2005). It has been shown that by increasing the rest interval between sets with the same load, more repetitions can be performed in the subsequent sets and that this leads to improved strength gains (Robinson *et al.* 1995; Willardson & Burkett 2005). This is extremely pertinent when training specifically for strength and/or power.

Not every exercise requires the same rest interval (American College of Sports Medicine 2002). For the more complex core exercises rest periods should be longer (e.g., 3–5 min) between sets and exercises for optimal recovery (González-Badillo *et al.* 2005) and gains in strength and/or power (Kraemer & Ratamess 2004). A general guideline is to gauge the complexity of the exercise, the number of muscle groups involved, and the actual weight lifted to determine the rest period. For example, in a heavier strength program design, an exercise such as the power clean or back squat (multi-joint, complex, large muscle group involvement) would require 3–5 min rest, an exercise like the Lat pulldowns (multi-joint, less complex, moderate muscle group involvement) 2–3 min and a bicep curl (single-joint, simple, small muscle group involvement) 1–2 min between sets. All programs will lead to improvements in strength regardless of the length of the rest interval, but the design should be such that it

optimizes the time utilized during training in relation to the expected training outcomes.

Volume of training

Underprescription of training volume may lead to not achieving the desired improvements in strength and muscle performance, and overprescription of training volume may lead to overtraining and overuse injuries (Rhea *et al.* 2003). As a result, the optimal number of sets still remains an extremely controversial topic (American College of Sports Medicine 2002; Carpinelli & Otto 1998; Feigenbaum & Pollock 1997; Kraemer & Ratamess 2004; Pearson *et al.* 2000; Wolfe *et al.* 2004). Of all the training variables, most of the research around resistance training has focused on volume, and more particularly single vs. multiple set training (Rhea *et al.* 2003).

SINGLE SETS

Most research shows no difference between single and multiple set training in terms of superiority in strength gains in the *untrained, non-athletic* population. It would therefore seem as if within the first 3–4 months of training single set programs are equally efficient in developing strength (American College of Sports Medicine 2002; Carpinelli & Otto 1998; Feigenbaum & Pollock 1997, 1999; Fleck 1999; Hass *et al.* 2000). Eighty to 90% of the strength gains of a multiple set protocol are achieved during this initial period of resistance training using a single set approach (Hass *et al.* 2001). The increased gains in strength using a multiple set program do not seem to justify the time spent in performing additional sets in healthy, untrained adults (Carpinelli & Otto 1998; Hass *et al.* 2000, 2001). It has been proposed that once a basic level of fitness is acquired multiple sets are superior to single set programs in muscle development (Fleck & Kraemer 1997; Wolfe *et al.* 2004).

MULTIPLE SETS

Many meta-analyses on this topic have shown significant support that multiple sets are superior to single set programs in developing strength (Peterson *et al.* 2004; Rhea *et al.* 2002a, 2003; Wolfe *et al.* 2004). These superior strength gains were more noticeable in trained vs. untrained individuals (Rhea *et al.* 2002a), and were especially significant over longer duration programs (Wolfe *et al.* 2004). Rhea *et al.* (2003) determined the optimal dose–response relationship for strength gains in *untrained* individuals to be an average load of 60% of 1 RM (± 12 RM), training a muscle group three times per week, and performing four sets per muscle group (not per exercise!). For *trained* individuals, an average load of 80% of 1 RM (± 8 RM), training a muscle group twice a week, and performing four sets per muscle group was indicated for maximal strength gains (Rhea *et al.* 2003). For *athletic* individuals, the optimal dose–response relationship for maximizing strength in this population group lies at an average intensity of 85% of 1 RM, training a muscle group twice a week, and performing eight sets per muscle group per session (Peterson *et al.* 2004). Because of the limited data available above this training load, interpretation within this range is difficult. Additionally, strength benefits were minimal training with 1–3 sets at 50–70% of 1 RM training loads (Peterson *et al.* 2004), which strongly supports the conclusion that higher volume training with heavier loads is necessary for maximizing strength development in athletic and highly trained individuals. It has been shown that there might be a threshold or optimal volume of training to maximize strength gains, whereafter increases in volume add no further benefit (González-Badillo *et al.* 2005; Peterson *et al.* 2004; Rhea *et al.* 2003) and might even lead to decrements in muscle performance (González-Badillo *et al.* 2005).

Kraemer and Ratamess (2004) highlight some key issues to consider:
1 In the short term, untrained individuals respond equally well to single and multiple sets;
2 In the long term, higher volumes (i.e., more sets) are required to increase the rate of progression;
3 No studies have shown single set approaches to be superior to multiple set programs; and
4 Not all exercises need to be performed with the same number of sets.

This latter point is paramount to understanding program prescription. Depending on which muscle groups need more attention, the number of sets can be increased or decreased for the respective exercises or muscle groups accordingly.

Speed of movement

Winett and Carpinelli (2001) recommend using 4 s for lifting and 4 s for lowering in concentric and eccentric muscle actions, respectively, as it decreases momentum, creates a higher training stimulus for the working muscles, and reduces the injury risk. Many researchers and trainers recommend using approximately 2 s and 4 s when lifting and lowering weights, respectively (Evans 1999; Hass *et al.* 2000; Pollock & Graves 1994; Pollock *et al.* 2000). However, movement speeds requiring less than 1–2 s for completion of concentric muscle actions and 1–2 s for completion of eccentric muscle actions have been shown to be the most effective movement velocities during resistance training for enhancing muscle performance (American College of Sports Medicine 2002; Kraemer & Ratamess 2004). Force equals the product of mass and acceleration. By performing the lifts too slowly the muscles are exposed to less force generation and therefore have lesser strength gains in the long term (American College of Sports Medicine 2002). It is therefore important to train at moderate to higher velocities and at moderate to higher loads for effective strength development (Kraemer & Ratamess 2004). From a practical perspective, novice trainers would initially train more conservatively because of the possible risk of injury and muscle damage, and progress the velocity of muscle action accordingly as they become stronger, more trained, and proficient in resistance training.

Progression

Progressive overload is an essential component of any resistance training program whether it may be for improving muscle size, strength, or power (Pearson *et al.* 2000; Winett & Carpinelli 2001). To sustain increases in muscle development and performance one constantly needs to progress the program by gradually increasing the demands placed on the body (American College of Sports Medicine 1998, 2002; Evans 1999; Kraemer & Ratamess 2004; Pearson *et al.* 2000; Rhea *et al.* 2003; Winett & Carpinelli 2001). This can be incorporated into a training program by manipulating any of the following training variables appropriately: increasing the frequency of training; increasing the repetitions in each set; increasing the number of exercises; decreasing the rest periods between sets and/or exercises; increasing the load utilized; or changing the speed of movement (American College of Sports Medicine 2002; Fleck 1999; Haff 2004a; Hass *et al.* 2001; Kraemer & Ratamess 2004; Pearson *et al.* 2000).

Resistance training for sport

Training for strength

The best results for strength and power gain are achieved when heavier loads are utilized during resistance training (Hass *et al.* 2001). Strength and power will be developed to a certain extent regardless of whether one trains with heavy weights or light weights. However, within the light–heavy weight continuum, the load utilized will favor a specific component, either strength or power (American College of Sports Medicine 1998; Campos *et al.* 2002; Fry 2004; Hass *et al.* 2001). Heavier loads, which are maximal or near to maximal, elicit the greatest gains in absolute strength (American College of Sports Medicine 1998; Campos *et al.* 2002; Fry 2004), and regular exposure to this loading range will ensure improvement (Fry 2004). Heavy training is not a prerequisite for strength gains in untrained individuals as almost any form of resistance training increases strength initially (Cronin & Henderson 2004). During this phase the emphasis should be on form and technique. However, loads in excess of 80–85% of 1 RM, or alternatively in the range of 1–6 RM loads (preferentially 5–6 RM; American College of Sports Medicine 2002), are required to maximize the increase in strength (American College of Sports Medicine 2002; Campos *et al.* 2002; Fry 2004; Kraemer & Ratamess 2004).

Maximizing strength is only possible if more muscle is recruited during the exercise, and for this to happen one needs to lift heavier loads (Kraemer & Ratamess 2004). Additionally, it seems that using a variety of training loads within this 80–100% of 1 RM or ±1–8 RM range in a periodized fashion is the most effective way to maximize strength in advanced trainers (American College of Sports Medicine 2002).

A key factor to consider in strength training is that everyone does not need to develop maximal strength. Depending on individual requirements or training goals, strength training may be prescribed differently (i.e., using lesser loads, e.g., 70–80% of 1 RM or ±8–12 RM loads), and sufficient strength gains, albeit not maximal, may be incurred specific to each individual and their respective training goals. However, it is recommended that even distance runners should occasionally train within the loading range of ≥80% of 1 RM for other performance and physical benefits such as maintained or improved strength and muscle power. Another reason is to counteract the catabolic effects that occur during repetitive exercise such as long distance running (Fry 2004). Even though a specific training zone on the load–repetition continuum favors a specific type of muscle development, it is not recommended to spend all the time training in one zone as it can lead to overtraining or stagnation in performance benefits (Kraemer & Ratamess 2004).

Training for power

The ability to effectively generate muscle power is believed to be an essential component of athletic and sporting performance and as a result has been extensively researched (Cronin & Slievert 2005). To maximize power through resistance training one first has to understand what is meant by muscle power. Power is a product of force and velocity (Baker *et al.* 2001a; Cronin & Henderson 2004; Cronin & Slievert 2005; Hedrick 2002; Kawamori & Haff 2004; Kawamori *et al.* 2005; Stone *et al.* 2003b), and is generally defined as the amount of work that can be performed in a specific time period (Cronin & Slievert 2005; Fry 2004; Kawamori & Haff 2004;

Kawamori *et al.* 2005; Stone *et al.* 2003a). Work in this case is defined as the amount of force produced to move a weight over a distance traveled (force × distance). Generally, during weight training, the distance that the weight moves is determined by the length of the arms, legs, and torso, and remains constant for each individual. Bearing this in mind, the main effectors that can be manipulated in power training are the load lifted and the speed of the movement. So, practically, there are two ways of intervening for developing muscle power (American College of Sports Medicine 2002; Baker 2001c; Baker *et al.* 2001a; Field 1988; Hedrick 2002; Kawamori & Haff 2004; Kraemer & Ratamess 2004; Stone *et al.* 2003a):

1 by training to develop the force component (i.e., strength); and
2 by training the speed component, which reduces the time period over which the work is performed.

For the strength component of muscle power one trains specifically using the method mentioned above, and in novice athletes this form of training should predominate (Baker 2001a,c). The strength component is extremely important because it forms the basis of powerful movements (American College of Sports Medicine 2002; Baker 2001c). One should not underestimate the importance of strength training in this role (Baker 2001a), as it is strongly related to both peak power output and sports performance (Stone *et al.* 2003b). Maximum strength contributes significantly to power production in moving both light and heavy resistances (Baker 2001b; Stone *et al.* 2003b). However, strength training only forms half of the equation (Hedrick 2002) and the highest power outputs in a movement come at a compromise between force and velocity components (Kawamori *et al.* 2005). Training the velocity component for developing muscle power appears to be vital in highly trained individuals who have already developed a base level of maximal strength. The focus of resistance training should then shift to primarily accommodate this component (i.e., train to lift large loads at higher speeds rather than merely lifting larger loads; Baker 2001c; Cronin & Slievert 2005).

To develop high-speed movement ability optimally, one should train specifically using high-speed movements (Hedrick 2002; McBride *et al.* 2002). Therefore, one should utilize relatively lighter loads than for strength training and perform the movement explosively (Kawamori & Haff 2004). This form of training will more likely induce high-velocity adaptations within the muscle (Cronin *et al.* 2003). For developing this velocity component for optimal muscle power development one should generally train at moderate to light loads ranging 30–60% of 1 RM performed at high velocity (American College of Sports Medicine 2002; Baker 2001c; Baker *et al.* 2001a,b; Cronin & Slievert 2005; Izquierdo *et al.* 2002; Kraemer & Ratamess 2004; Newton *et al.* 1997; Wilson *et al.* 1993).

Single-joint and upper body exercises, and untrained individuals might respond better to power training at a lower range of loads (30–45% of 1 RM), while multi-joint and lower body exercises, and trained individuals might respond better to a higher range of loads (30–70% of 1 RM; Kawamori & Haff 2004). The optimal relative load for developing maximal power is yet to be determined as there is conflicting evidence as a result of different assessment techniques and protocols (Baker *et al.* 2001b; Cronin & Slievert 2005; Dugan *et al.* 2004; Kawamori & Haff 2004; Stone *et al.* 2003a). Therefore, it is pragmatic to train for power within the full range of loads specified above (American College of Sports Medicine 2002; Baker 2001b,c; Baker *et al.* 2001b; Cronin & Slievert 2005; Kraemer & Ratamess 2004; Wilson *et al.* 1993), as each force–velocity relationship will develop a different component of muscle power (Baker 2001b; Cronin & Slievert 2005). To illustrate this point more effectively it has previously been shown that there is a velocity-specific adaptation when training for muscle power and using different loading strategies (McBride *et al.* 2002). Training with lighter loads significantly improves the velocity of movement over a range of loads, and training with heavier loads significantly improves the force capabilities of the involved muscles over the same range of loads. However, the one aspect of muscle power that the one training strategy develops, the other does not (McBride *et al.* 2002). This reinforces the need to develop both the strength and velocity aspects that affect muscle power, as they both contribute in different ways to functional capacity and ability.

TRADITIONAL WEIGHT TRAINING

One problem with utilizing traditional high-speed weight training exercises for power is that of deceleration (American College of Sports Medicine 2002; Baker *et al.* 2001a; Kawamori & Haff 2004; Siegel *et al.* 2002). During traditional weight training exercises, the initial part of the movement involves acceleration and a considerable part of the remainder of the movement is spent on deceleration (American College of Sports Medicine 2002; Kraemer & Ratamess 2004). The reason for this is that they are closed-loop movements. The movement has to stop at the end-range before joint or muscle injury occurs. Therefore, the acceleration part of the movement is limited. For effective development of power using traditional resistance training exercises, one needs to increase acceleration and limit deceleration (American College of Sports Medicine 2002). The only way of doing this is to slightly increase the loads utilized (McBride *et al.* 2002), compared to open-loop movements such as ballistic resistance exercise where, for example, the weight is released or the body is projected off the ground (Kraemer & Ratamess 2004; Pearson *et al.* 2000). Siegel *et al.* (2002) demonstrated peak power outputs in traditional exercises such as the Smith machine squat and barbell bench press within slightly higher ranges of 50–70% 1 RM and 40–60% 1 RM, respectively, which supports this rationale.

BALLISTIC RESISTANCE EXERCISE

Ballistic resistance exercise is a popular form of training used in the development of explosive power, as the movement is open ended and acceleration continues into the release of the weight, bar, or object (American College of Sports Medicine 2002). This technique offers far greater movement specificity than traditional strength training (Cronin & Henderson 2004; Cronin & Slievert 2005; Cronin *et al.* 2003). It also allows for greater force, velocity, acceleration, and power output (Baker 2001c; Cronin & Slievert 2005; Cronin *et al.* 2003; Hedrick 2002)

and relatively less weight is required compared to the closed-loop traditional resistance exercises, as the deceleration component is significantly reduced (Baker *et al.* 2001b; Cronin & Slievert 2005; Kraemer & Ratamess 2004; Siegel *et al.* 2002). Examples of these types of exercises are jump squats, bench throws, and medicine ball toss. The potentiating effect of ballistic resistance exercise compared to traditional resistance exercises, however, becomes insignificant when using heavier loads (≥70% 1 RM), as the ability to release the bar or object or project the body off the ground becomes compromised (Cronin *et al.* 2003).

OLYMPIC LIFTS

Apart from ballistic resistance exercise, predominantly multi-joint exercises, such as power cleans, hang snatches and so forth are used in resistance training for power (Hedrick 2002; Tricoli *et al.* 2005). A well-balanced resistance training program for advanced trainers and athletes incorporates the use of these Olympic lifts, multi-joint and single-joint exercises (Pearson *et al.* 2000). Olympic lifts and their derivatives are considered to be the best resistance training exercises for maximizing dynamic muscle power, as they incorporate multi-joint movement patterns that are highly specific, have significantly less deceleration, and generate extremely high power outputs (Kawamori & Haff 2004; Kawamori *et al.* 2005). A key concern in using these types of exercises, especially the Olympic lifts, is the skill required to perform them correctly. A significant amount of time is spent in developing the correct technique of execution and form, and for novice and intermediate trainers it is highly recommended to focus primarily on this aspect (American College of Sports Medicine 2002). Even though teaching and learning these exercises can take a long time, once the correct technique and skill has been acquired, the benefits and transfer to functional performance are substantial (Tricoli *et al.* 2005). Because of the already ballistic nature, heavier loads may additionally be required to maximize power output in these exercises (i.e., 70–90% of 1 RM) depending on the sporting requirements and training status of the athletes (Baechle *et al.* 2000;

Baker *et al.* 2001a,b; Kawamori & Haff 2004; Kawamori *et al.* 2005). Power training over the range of lesser intensities (30–70% of 1 RM) will nonetheless provide sufficient benefits for a variety of sporting events.

PRACTICAL CONSIDERATIONS

No studies have focused on each individual training at their respective optimal loads for developing power output (Cronin & Slievert 2005), so it is not known how effective it is in maximizing power output in comparison to training at the immediate range of loads surrounding it. Depending on individual needs analysis, heavier resistances may be required to improve the force component, and lighter resistances may be required to maximize speed of movement (Baker 2001b; Baker *et al.* 2001a; Hedrick 2002; Kawamori & Haff 2004). One should also consider sport specificity when selecting appropriate loads. For example, in rugby union, which is an explosive, high intensity, full contact sport with high external resistances encountered during tackling, mauling, at a loose ruck (Duthie *et al.* 2003), training for power at higher loads with greater external resistance might be more beneficial (Baker 2001a; Kawamori & Haff 2004). The ability to generate maximal power against large resistances has been shown to be a significant predictor of performance level in rugby league players (Baker 2001a). However, a volleyball player might benefit more from training with lighter loads and focusing more on velocity training, as they do not move heavy loads.

Because athletic performance is so diverse and characterized by many different force–velocity qualities, it seems prudent to vary constantly the load used for power training (Cronin & Slievert 2005). Employment of this strategy may induce improved power output over the entire force–velocity spectrum (Baker 2001b). It is generally recommended for novice and intermediate athletes to train initially for power using the lower range of the loads specified earlier on. For competitive athletes a similar approach is used except that they should progress towards the higher range of loads, especially for the last few weeks in the training

block to peak at the right time (Baker 2001a). Practically, it is also recommended to reduce the resistance used for power training during hard training sessions and/or hard training weeks to avoid inducing excessive fatigue (Baker 2001a).

It is also recommended that one does not train to fatigue, especially in novice and intermediate trainers. Power exercises incorporated into a resistance training program are usually performed first (i.e., before fatigue develops). Also, power exercises should generally not be performed for more than six repetitions in a set (Fry 2004; Haff 2004a), as the focus should be on quality or maximal velocity of movement (Haff 2004a; Hedrick 2002). One should also try to maximize power output during a training set. One technique that can improve the quality of the exercise in power training is the cluster set (Kawamori *et al.* 2005). This incorporates adding an interval of 10–30 s rest between repetitions in lieu of performing all the repetitions continuously. This minimizes fatigue and maintains power output within the set (Kawamori *et al.* 2005). For advanced power training, the program design should also follow a periodized approach to ensure appropriate progression and avoid overtraining (American College of Sports Medicine 2002).

It is of utmost importance that different components of muscle power are trained at different times within the training cycle to avoid stagnation and optimize muscle performance. For example, the strength components should be trained early on in the season, with the focus gradually shifting towards the speed and power components closer to the competition season, when performance needs to be at a peak (Kawamori & Haff 2004).

Periodization

Periodization is not a rigid entity, but is rather an adaptable concept for a more pragmatic and effective approach to resistance training (Haff 2004a). This may take the form of a systematic and planned variation of training volume and load within a defined training period (Pearson *et al.* 2000) to bring about optimal gains in muscle performance (Fleck 1999). The main objective of periodization is to avoid stagnation and overtraining, and to promote peaking of athletic performance (Pearson *et al.* 2000; Stone *et al.* 2000b). Periodization also caters for long-term improvements in muscle strength and power (Fleck 1999). Significant gains in strength can be achieved through systematic variation of the program. Variation is the key principle used in resistance training programs (Field 1988) to optimize training by constantly shifting the training stimulus (Haff 2004a) and thereby changing the demands placed on the body (Fleck 1999). Periodization incorporates this principle of variation as the core component in its application (American College of Sports Medicine 2002). However, periodized training is not necessary until some form of base fitness has been obtained (Fleck 1999; Haff 2004b).

There are two main models of periodization (American College of Sports Medicine 2002; Haff 2004a; Kraemer & Ratamess 2004; Pearson *et al.* 2000; Wathen *et al.* 2000):

1 Linear or classic model of periodization; and
2 Non-linear or undulating model of periodization.

CLASSIC OR LINEAR MODEL OF PERIODIZATION

The classic or linear model is subdivided into different training phases, each with a specific training focus (e.g., hypertrophy, strength, power) and usually starts with high volume, low intensity workouts and progresses to low volume, high intensity workouts with the main aim to maximize the development of strength and/or muscle power (American College of Sports Medicine 2002; Haff 2004a; Kraemer & Ratamess 2004; Stone *et al.* 2000b). Sequenced progression from one type of training such as strength training can boost the gains obtained by another type of training such as power training (Haff 2004a), and this is where a periodized program is so effective. An adequately designed and periodized training program in the off-season lays the broader foundations to a successful competitive season (Haff 2004b). Generally, classic periodization plans are divided into different training epochs: a macrocycle (e.g., a 4–6 month period), which is subdivided into smaller epochs called mesocycles (e.g., 4–6 week blocks), which is further subdivided into even smaller units called microcycles (e.g., 1 week blocks; Haff 2004a). The time periods of these training blocks can vary significantly between sports. Each mesocycle has a very specific training focus and these all build up to preparing athletes to reach their peak athletic ability during competition (Pearson *et al.* 2000). Examples of these mesocycles are:

1 A preparatory period (which is predominantly in the off-season), which is subdivided into microcycles focusing on hypertrophy/strength endurance, basic strength, and strength/power in that order;
2 A first transition phase, which indicates a shift in focus from a high volume to high intensity training; followed by
3 The competition phase, where the focus can either be peak performance for a specific tournament or tournaments, or maintenance of strength/power throughout the in-season; and finally
4 An active rest or second transition phase, where a period of downtime/cross-training is allocated for recovery and regeneration (Haff 2004a; Stone *et al.* 2000b; Wathen *et al.* 2000).

Various combinations of these phases can be applied depending on the sport and/or individual's training goals, and each phase requires different levels of variation in training prescription (Stone *et al.* 2000b). The off-season period is where the most resistance training is performed and therefore also has the greatest application and manipulation of periodization (Haff 2004b).

It is important to note that one does not train at maximal effort (i.e., repetition maximum for every session). Day-to-day variation of intensity and/or volume across the various microcycles is also very important (especially for advanced trainers) in avoiding overtraining or stagnation (Stone *et al.* 2000b). In the linear periodization model, the volume (i.e., the number of repetitions within a weekly microcycle) remains the same, but the intensity fluctuates. For example, on Monday the athlete trains 8–12 repetitions using 8–12 RM loads, on Wednesday 8–12 repetitions with 5–10% less weight, and on Friday 8–12 repetitions with 10–30% less weight than the Monday's session (Pearson *et al.* 2000). Training blocks usually last ± 4 weeks (Haff 2004a). Variation in strength and power training is key for continuous improvement in muscle performance, especially during long-term resistance training. Therefore, it is common practice to repeat a macrocycle, such as indicated in the example above, 2–3 times within a 1-year period (Haff 2004a; Pearson *et al.* 2000).

UNDULATING OR NON-LINEAR MODEL OF PERIODIZATION

Because it has been shown that variation in training allows for greater gains in muscle development, conditioning specialists have begun to use a less traditional model of periodization called the non-linear or undulating model (Haff 2004a; Pearson *et al.* 2000). The key difference is that the non-linear variation is more dramatic during the individual microcycles than the more traditional linear model (Haff 2004a). The non-linear or undulating model allows for random variation in training focus (i.e., changes in volume and intensity within a smaller time-period, e.g., a 10-day training cycle; American College of Sports Medicine 2002; Fleck 1999; Kraemer & Ratamess 2004; Pearson *et al.* 2000). As with the linear model, it is recommended that the athlete performs some form of base training before embarking on this undulating periodized training model. As an example of the non-linear model, if one resistance trained on Mondays, Wednesdays and Fridays, one could train on the first Monday using 2–4 RM loads, on Wednesday at 12–15 RM loads, on Friday at 6–10 RM loads, and the following Monday using 15–20 RM loads where the cycle is repeated, this time starting on the Wednesday. Each day has a specific training focus (Rhea *et al.* 2002a). One can also add a power day where necessary; this design remains flexible according to the sport and individual requirements involved. This cycling of training continues for a predetermined time period (e.g., 16 weeks) and then progresses either into an in-season variation of this form of periodization, or an active rest period ranging 1–3 weeks.

Astute variation and combination of high intensity and low intensity resistance training can optimize strength development (Goto *et al.* 2004). The non-linear model appears to benefit sports that have a long competitive season (e.g., rugby union and hockey); in other words, there is not a specific build-up towards one specific event where they have to peak (Pearson *et al.* 2000). Also with long-season sports, there is not always sufficient time to focus on a big off-season build-up, as the off-season is sometimes too short in duration. This form of training allows these athletes to continue training throughout the season, except the volume and frequency of resistance training is reduced substantially and adjusted according to matches, tournaments, and sports practice (Pearson *et al.* 2000). This is where the undulating model has been used with great success (Haff 2004b). The non-linear model of periodization allows for great design flexibility and should be tailored specifically for individual needs.

PRACTICAL CONSIDERATIONS IN PERIODIZATION

Monitoring exercise tolerance and controlling recovery are important aspects in resistance training (Pearson *et al.* 2000). After individual training phases (mesocycles or microcycles), it is also common practice to allow a transition week, where a variation of active rest is incorporated before advancing onto the next phase; this is usually achieved by reducing the training volume and intensity within the week's training schedule (Haff 2004a). Incorporating this transition or recovery week is usually left to the discretion of the strength and conditioning specialist and can be very effective in avoiding overtraining and increasing performance levels in the following cycle.

Maintenance training is a popular form of resistance training which is frequently utilized by athletes during the competitive season (Allerheiligen 2003; Stone *et al.* 2000b) and by people who are not competitive but who train for health and fitness (Kraemer & Ratamess 2004). If the training is prescribed at too low an intensity to create some sort of training overload, one can actually stagnate and/or detrain. This can be detrimental for both general fitness and sports performance. Therefore, a structured and periodized approach to maintenance programs where smaller subprograms are prescribed in a cyclic fashion as part of the bigger training goal is recommended (Kraemer & Ratamess 2004). To prevent this detraining effect and/or stagnation it has been suggested that one applies a periodized approach using 2-week cycles within the in-season using primarily the core or complex multi-joint exercises such as squats, bench press, and power cleans (Allerheiligen 2003). This creates enough variation to challenge the body in different ways so that stagnation does not occur. Furthermore, it retains the strength, power, and muscle mass developed in the off- and preseason training programs (Allerheiligen 2003).

Programming of periodization and/or specific resistance training within the competitive season should also be micromanaged according to the weekly match or competition schedule. It has been suggested that one should schedule higher intensity training earlier on in the week, preferably at the beginning of the training week, and taper towards the matches or competition by lowering the intensity of training (Haff 2004b). With multiple matches or competitions, it is also recommended to shift the higher intensity strength and power training sessions to that period of the week, which allows maximum recovery before the following match or competition (Haff 2004b). An example of this form of manipulation is the "heavy/light" day system, resistance training 2 days per week (Haff 2004b). For example, training on the Monday would use RM loads (e.g., 3–5 RM, heavy day) and on the Thursday the loads utilized would be reduced by 15% (light day) using the same number of repetitions (Stone *et al.* 2000b). This method of training has been shown to be effective in developing muscle power (Baker 2001b). A major goal of the in-season program is to maintain as much of the athlete's strength and power developed in the off- and pre-season as possible (Haff 2004b).

The value of periodized versus non-periodized resistance training programs becomes noticeable in programs of longer duration where the risk of overtraining is prevented through variations in training and systematic progression (Kraemer & Ratamess 2004). Untrained individuals do not appear to be sensitive to volume, and sometimes even intensity during initial resistance training exposure, so a general strength program will accommodate their needs quite sufficiently (Kraemer & Ratamess 2004).

However, advanced resistance training programs are much more complex and require great variation with specific training goals in mind to maintain progression (Kraemer & Ratamess 2004).

Conclusions

Strength and power training forms an integral part of many sports conditioning programs. The appropriate development of strength and power can complement an athlete's sports-specific training and significantly enhance sports performance. The correct manipulation of resistance training variables and programs to develop these components requires a systematic and varied approach combining both science and practical experience. Strength training forms the basis of muscle power and also forms the basis of most sporting abilities to a large extent. The early training focus during the off- and early pre-season is to progressively develop this component. Thereafter the training focus shifts towards maintenance of muscle strength in combination with the development of functional muscle power. One cannot sustain high-level strength and power training for long periods of time, because of the risk of overtraining and injury, and therefore programs need to be structured and planned accordingly. To optimize an athlete's strength and power development and to gain the maximum advantage from this form of training one needs to follow a periodized training approach, which allows for maximizing strength and power at the appropriate times for peak performance capabilities.

TRAINING TO IMPROVE ENDURANCE

This section aims to provide information on the practical application of the theoretical information already covered on training, with particular reference to endurance training. The goal is to provide sufficient information to the clinician or sports medicine practitioner for an understanding of the contribution that the training regimen may have in influencing various clinical conditions. Specifically, this section should aid in determining whether the reason for the problem or concern of the athlete presenting to the clinician has its source in errors in training, or whether some other cause for the problem needs to be sought and investigated. Thus, this section does not provide specific information for training prescription as might be used by a coach, but rather sufficient information to identify errors in an existing training program as used by someone participating in an endurance sport such as running, cycling, swimming, or canoeing. Running has been used for most of the specific examples, as this is a major mass participation sport and is also the endurance sport that is least forgiving when training errors are committed, with a concomitant high incidence of injury.

Goal setting

Initially, no training program is easy, and indeed, seldom pleasurable because of the state of relative unfitness when the training commences. It takes time for someone to gain sufficient fitness for the activity to be truly enjoyable, be it running, cycling, or one of the other endurance sports. It may therefore help a beginner with motivation problems to set an achievable short-term goal, as well as long-term goals. A short-term goal may simply be to train a certain minimum number of times per week, whereas a long-term goal may be to complete a particular running or cycling race. To help with motivation it is often useful to keep a logbook of training progress. It could be suggested to write down the training that has been completed each day and to keep a weekly total of training distance or time. In this way the beginner can easily see the progress being made as fitness improves.

Limitations to training

Genetic ability

It is important to realize that everybody has some genetically determined limit that will ultimately dictate how well they will perform in their chosen sport, be that performance at an elite level of competition to win races and break world records, at a level of simply achieving one's own individual best possible performance or, at the other end of the spectrum, completing a specific event within a given time to simply be classified as an official finisher of an event. By training according to a scientifically designed and constructed training program that incorporates the various features necessary for optimal physiologic adaptation, it is possible for someone to achieve the best that they are capable of within the limitations imposed by their individual genetic capabilities. This is achieved by finding the right blend of volume of training undertaken, intensity of that training, and mix of specific types of training sessions that comprise a physiologically balanced training program. To achieve this requires a combination of both sound scientific principles and the "art" of coaching.

The significant part played by genetics in determining how much someone will improve once a training program is started has already been alluded to. Particularly, there are "adaptors" and "non-adaptors" to a training stimulus. In essence, even elite athletes have a genetically determined "ceiling" as to how much adaptation can occur in response to training. Similarly, some people possess a naturally high aerobic capacity without having participated in a training program, while others have to train very scientifically to elicit as much training adaptation as possible. Thus, we sometimes hear of athletes who appear to train very hard in order to excel, and at other times we find someone who has performed at a very high level on surprisingly little training. For example, if an elite athlete had to train very little, that individual will quite likely out-perform the genetically non-gifted person who has trained very hard according to systematic program. It is important to understand that not everyone can become an Olympic champion by hard training and adhering to a good training regimen. Thus, it is important to set goals based on improving individual performance.

Effect of gender

Gender differences exist only in the maximal volume and intensity of training that can be sustained. Specifically, women generally cannot tolerate as much training as men. Even at the elite level, top male athletes can tolerate a greater training load in terms of both volume and intensity than the top females. This can probably be attributed primarily to the fact that, generally, women do not have as much muscle mass and muscle cross-sectional area as men. Thus, men can generate more force and power. However, if normalized for cross-sectional area (i.e., if a male and female are matched for exactly the same amount of muscle) then gender differences are reduced. Therefore, in terms of the intrinsic ability of the muscle to generate force and power, there are few gender-related differences. However, the elite female athlete will have a higher percentage of body fat than an elite male athlete. Thus, in two elite athletes of similar body size and mass, the female will have more fat mass and less muscle mass than her male counterpart. This is probably one of the primary reasons that the performance of female endurance athletes is approximately 10% slower than that of men for most events. This is particularly so in sports in which the upper body is involved, because men have relatively more muscle in the upper body. It is interesting to note that when male and female runners with equal 10 km or marathon times are compared over a much longer race distance of 90 km, the female runners have been found to outperform their male counterparts (Bam *et al.* 1997). This is accomplished physiologically by the female runners maintaining a relatively higher percentage of $\dot{V}o_{2max}$ and for longer, without slowing their pace as much as the men. Thus, in the sample of "average" runners in this particular analysis, females appear to be more "fatigue resistant" than men. However, it is likely that at the extremes of the population from which the very best performers come, these differences become much less. Noakes (2001) theorized that while the average male marathon runners are likely to be taller and heavier with less body fat than the average female marathon runners, these differences are likely to be much less when the world's best male and female runners are compared. Noakes postulates that the world's best male and female marathon and ultramarathon runners are all equally small and light with a low percentage of body fat, although the percentage of body fat would be marginally greater in the female runners. When considering average runners, the

generally smaller women are at an advantage which becomes increasingly apparent as the race distance increases, hence their apparent greater fatigue resistance. However, because the size differences are much smaller in the world's best marathon and ultramarathon runners of both genders, it is expected that the relative advantage of the average female runner over the average male runner will disappear when the performances of the elite athletes of both genders (whose body sizes are more similar) are compared. Noakes (2001) concludes that the fatigue resistance of the very best male and female ultramarathon runners is probably not different.

Although the absolute training load that can be tolerated is less in females than males, the physiologic response to training does not differ between males and females. This is true for all the different elements of training that comprise a balanced endurance training program, such as long duration training performed at a moderate percentage of $\dot{V}o_{2max}$, high intensity interval training of short duration, longer duration intervals at lower intensity, "tempo" and "threshold" training sessions, and other specific types of training. Thus, females and males respond in the same way from a physiologic perspective to both endurance and interval training, although the upper limits of training load will be reached at a lower overall level in females.

Specificity

In all types of training a number of established physiologic principles apply. Most important of these is specificity. A swimmer will not gain much benefit by cycling or running. Similarly, a long distance runner should spend almost all training time running to gain the most benefit. Although impossible to run a marathon every day in training, the distance runner will maintain a high weekly training distance and in different training sessions include runs at slower than marathon speed, runs at marathon speed but over a shorter distance, and even shorter runs at a speed faster than marathon race speed. This is true also for other disciplines such as cycling, canoeing, and swimming. It is important to appreciate that training is absolutely specific and that the athlete is only fit for the sport for which they train. Thus, while runners may be capable of running effortlessly for hours, they are often unable to swim comfortably even for a few minutes. The reason is that running and swimming train different muscle groups. When a runner exercises the untrained upper body in swimming, for example, the body responds as if it were essentially untrained. Whereas running principally exercises the legs, leaving the upper body musculature relatively untrained, canoeing and swimming mainly train the upper body, leaving the legs untrained or less trained. This distinction becomes even more subtle: runners who do little running on hills will find hill running difficult. This is because uphill running stresses, in particular, the quadriceps – a muscle that is much less important during running on the flat and is therefore undertrained in people who run exclusively on flat terrain.

Training specificity also includes speed training, hot weather training, and altitude acclimatization. Because the speed of training determines which muscle fibers will be active in the particular muscle groups being exercised, training slowly and then racing at a faster pace utilizes muscle fibers that are relatively untrained. Similarly, to race effectively in the heat or at altitude, it is necessary to train under these conditions to allow the body to adapt. Therefore, the more closely the training simulates the specific demands of the sport for which one is training, and the environment in which competition will occur, the better the performance will be.

Start easily

When someone has decided to begin a training program, it is probably only human nature that they want to do as much as they possibly can within the first weeks of training. While this enthusiasm is laudable, it is definitely not the best way to start a new training program. The reason for this is that it takes time for the bones, tendons, muscles, and cardiovascular system to adapt to the cumulative stress of regular training. This is particularly so in the case of running where the stress on bone and tendon is high. With non-weight-bearing sports such

as cycling and canoeing, the problem is somewhat reduced, but nevertheless progress should be at a slow, consistent rate. Typically, when someone embarks on a new training program, the tendency is to try and train a little bit faster or harder than in the previous training session. This approach is not sustainable.

Training intensity

It is only ever necessary and possible to train at a high intensity for 5–10% of the total training time (Daniels 1998). For example, most of the best marathon runners do most of their training at a speed of 30–50 $s\cdot km^{-1}$ slower than their race pace. While training, the effort should be perceived as "comfortable." A good way of testing this is the "talk test." It should be possible to maintain a conversation with training companions. If it is not possible to talk, then the training intensity is too high and the session should be continued at an easier pace. Training intensity will be addressed in more detail subsequently.

Training structure

All training should follow some well-established principles. The first principle is to train initially to increase weekly training duration. Once the appropriate weekly training duration has been reached, then specific training sessions of high intensity can be introduced.

An athlete should gradually and systematically increase training distance until the maximum training load that the athlete can tolerate has been reached. Signs that the maximum training load has been reached is a failure to adapt to a new, higher training load, an increase in muscle fatigue, a feeling of "tired, heavy legs," an increase in the time taken to complete a given training session (i.e., getting slower, rather than faster), or the appearance of a mild injury or illness (Noakes 2001). The total training load that can be tolerated depends on genetic factors and careful increase in the training distance, and takes years to develop fully. Ignoring signs that the body is failing to adapt to the training load can result in overtraining.

The first step in increasing the total training load is to increase the duration of all the training sessions, followed by the frequency of those sessions (i.e., the number sessions per week). All of this training should be at an intensity that is significantly slower than race speed, correlating to an intensity of 60–70% of maximum oxygen uptake ($\dot{V}O_{2max}$). Closely coupled to the increase in weekly training distance is the introduction of one or two single, long duration training sessions; the so-called "long weekend" run or training run. This prepares the muscles of the athlete to resist fatigue during races of long duration. However, this training session should only be included in the training program after the muscles have adapted to the initial stress of the training program.

Regularity of training

Training regularly through the season is an important concept that has been emphasized by many of the great coaches of endurance sportsmen and women. While this concept may have been derived from experience gained over many years of prescribing training, there is now supporting physiologic evidence. Therefore, even if the training load is modest, such as when an athlete starts a training program for the first time, the training sessions should be undertaken regularly to achieve the best possible increase in fitness. In the case of the elite performer, training regularly is an obvious element of the training schedule, and in this case regularity of training is synonymous with consistency. Specifically, the training schedule should be consistent in terms of the nature of the various training sessions undertaken. Thus, in any given 1–2 week cycle of training, a similar training structure should be followed, including the nature of the high intensity sessions. The "pattern" and the type of workouts should be retained for some time before any change is made to the fundamental components of the sessions. It is inappropriate to have an inconsistent approach as this will produce unpredictable results and also increase the risk of injury.

Although training should be consistent, it should not be followed blindly based on the assumption that any program will guarantee success. Rather, the effects of the program on the individual's performance must be constantly assessed and appropriate modifications made where necessary. Such an approach allows for varying rate of change and adaptations which are attributed to the genetic variance between athletes. Therefore, every training program must be tailored and continuously adjusted to the individual who will be following it.

Frequency of training

When someone starts a training program for the first time, training should only be on every second day. In high impact sports such as running, this ensures adequate time for adaptation and repair between training sessions, specifically to the load-bearing bones of the legs. Bone adaptation is particularly slow. In fact, for approximately 3 months after the start of a weight-bearing training program, bone loses strength. Thereafter, the osteoblasts become very active and new bone is laid down (Scully & Besterman 1982). Thus, until this time, the risk of developing a bone stress injury if the training load becomes too high, too rapidly, is greatly increased. The number of training sessions each week should be increased only once the duration of each training session performed every second day has reached an appropriate time. This depends on the sport type and training time available. For example, in the case of a running program in which weight-bearing stress is high, a more cautious increase in training frequency should be followed than in a sport such as cycling. In cycling, limitations are more likely to be related to the rate of muscle adaptation, which occurs more rapidly than bone adaptation (Margulies et al. 1986). The progression from training every second day to more frequent training should proceed systematically. Training every second day should be increased to training for two successive days followed by a recovery day of no training. This should be followed by three successive days, then four successive days, etc., with an appropriate amount of time at each successive "step" before proceeding to the next. On the extreme end of high training load, it is quite common for elite athletes to train every day, with twice daily training sessions 5 or 6 days each week.

Training duration

Initially, it is more useful to prescribe training duration based on the time spent training each week, rather than the distance covered. The concept of time taken to complete a single training session needs to be considered even in the case of someone who has been training for many years. Consider an elite versus a slow "club" runner. The elite runner will cover a distance of approximately 16 km in 60 min in training, whereas the average club runner may cover approximately 12 km in the same time. Alternatively, to complete 16 km would take the same club runner approximately 1 hour 20 min. Yet 1 hour 20 min of running probably imposes more biomechanical stress to the slower runner than that experienced by the fast elite runner whose training session of 16 km is complete after just 60 min in this example. Thus, at least initially, measuring training load based on time rather than distance is preferable.

Regardless of whether the training prescription is time or distance based, as with training frequency, increases should be progressive and systematic. Initially, the beginner would train for only a short time in any given training session. For someone beginning a running program, this may include a period spent walking, developing later into walking alternating with running, and finally only running. Initial progress may appear to be slow. In the case of a non-weight-bearing sport such as cycling, the rate of progression in training duration can be substantially quicker.

Initially, the duration of each training session should be increased every week, while the frequency remains at every second day, as previously described. Once the duration reaches 30–40 min in the case of a running program, or approximately 60 min in the case of cycling or swimming, the switch can be made to increasing the training frequency.

While 30–40 min of training five times weekly is adequate for health benefits, many people will want to train more than this, with a goal of completing a specific running or cycling race. For these individuals, it will be necessary to increase the duration of specific training sessions to prepare for the particular physiologic requirements of the race. To complete a marathon, for example, will require increasing the duration of one training session each week until the duration of that specific session is approximately 75% of the anticipated finishing time for the marathon. Thus, someone training with the anticipation of completing a marathon race in 4 h will systematically increase the time spent on a single run each week until 3 h of running can be completed comfortably in a single training run. These long duration training sessions are at substantially slower speed than "race" speed. The speed, or percentage of $\dot{V}o_{2max}$ at which training sessions are carried out are unimportant when a training program is started.

Initially, a week of training may consist of a training session every second day of 15 min duration each. Subsequently, the time will be increased systematically to 20, 25, 30, 40 min, etc. This will be followed by more frequent training sessions, and finally one of those sessions will become much longer in duration. Ultimately, the duration of a specific training session will be sports-specific. For example, a runner may build up training duration until capable of running for an hour each training session. On the other hand, a cyclist could build up to more than an hour in a single session on a regular basis.

Throughout this period of increasing training duration, it is not too important that much attention is given to the speed at which the training is done. While it is acceptable that the training speed gradually increases naturally during this time, no direct emphasis should be placed on speed or speed work, or trying to make each training session faster than the one before. This approach is not sustainable. Thus, the key to successful training, at least for the first 12 months or so, is the amount of time spent training each week, rather than the distance covered, or the speed at which the training sessions are done. As fitness improves, speed will increase naturally, and therefore more distance will be covered for the same time spent training. After 12 months or more of training in this way, a plateau in performance will be reached. To improve beyond this, some training will have to be carried out at a faster pace, which will require the introduction of faster paced sessions and speed work into the training program. Speed work should always be approached with caution, preferably with the help of a knowledgeable coach, or after reading widely on the topic, as this type of training is high risk for inducing injury or symptoms of overtraining.

To improve further, elite athletes can also train greater distances. However, the risk of injury and overtraining increases precipitously when, specifically with running, training is increased beyond 120–160 km per week for average and elite runners respectively. However, for someone wanting to perform at the elite or optimal individual level it is necessary to identify the maximum volume of training to achieve their best possible performance. This can be by first finding the training volume that produces the best results. This training threshold can really only be identified by a systematic increase in training until more than the optimum amount is shown by a decline in performance. Accordingly, training volume needs to be increased gradually and progressively until the individual failure threshold is identified. This corresponds to the training volume that produces a deteriorating, not an improved, racing performance. For the elite performer, identification of this training threshold is a crucial exercise in determining optimal training volume. Training beyond this threshold will result in poor performances and training less rather than more will lead to success. Gradually increasing the intensity of some of that training (speed work) will then optimize the entire training program. Thus, a scientific measure of training load that incorporates both duration of training, as well as the quality of the training, is a useful adjunct to monitoring training.

Foster *et al.* (1996) have proposed a method in which training load is calculated as the duration of the session (in minutes) multiplied by the average rating of perceived exertion during the session (a score between 0 and 10, where 0 is perceived as no effort at all and 10 is a very, very strong, almost maximal perception of effort). The total training load for the week is then plotted on a graph depicting the calculated training load against a measure of performance, such as a time trial. Such a graph will show how performance improves as training load per week is increased, until a point is reached in training load where further increases results in no further performance increase, or even a decline in performance. This type of monitoring soon shows that there is a logarithmic relationship between training load and performance. Thus, a given training increase (e.g., 1000 units per week) produces progressively smaller improvements in performance.

An important point to emphasize is that the individual who wishes to be consistently successful, at whatever level, must learn early on in his or her training career to treat everything performed in training as part of an experiment. The athlete who understands the specific effects that each manipulation of training has on his or her body and performance will be the most successful on a regular basis and have a better chance of reaching his or her full potential.

High intensity training

All the training that has been discussed to this point has been considered to be training performed at a relatively low intensity. As the athlete progresses, additional training at a higher intensity must be included at the appropriate phase of development. These training sessions are performed at 80–100% of $\dot{V}o_{2max}$, and are commonly referred to as speed work or interval sessions.

Speed work or high intensity training is not without risk. The common errors are performing the sessions too often and too fast, using an inappropriate distance, inappropriate progression, or recovery between the fast components that is insufficient for the level of fitness of the athlete. Another error is to have the mind-set that each fast training session must be performed at a faster speed than the previous one. This is neither desirable nor possible. For example, an improvement in time trial performance may only be possible every few weeks. The most positive sign that improvement is occurring is if it is possible to perform the same or better times in successive sessions, but with less effort. Conversely, if the sessions become increasingly difficult and time trial or interval times start to become slower rather than faster, then this is a clear indicator that the athlete is trying to progress too rapidly and a period of recovery is required instead of more and harder training. Typically, however, someone in the position of finding that their speed work appears to be getting slower, suspects that they are not training hard enough and compounds their error by trying to train even harder. This will likely lead to development of symptoms of overreaching (Meeusen *et al.* 2006).

Initially one but later two high intensity (speed work) sessions should be introduced into the training regimen once the total weekly training distance has been reached. One of these sessions should be of short duration but of high intensity, corresponding to approximately 60–90 s performed at a fast speed with an equal rest interval before starting the next 60–90 s rest. "Rest" refers to running at a markedly reduced speed. A second high intensity session each week should be of longer duration, of around 3–5 min but somewhat slower. Again, the rest interval will initially be of equal duration. Both types of high intensity sessions must be introduced gradually into the program, progressively building on the number included in each session until 10–12 repeats of the shorter duration speed work can be completed and around 20 min of the longer speed workout. When this is achieved, the next step is a systematic reduction in the rest period. When the athlete has achieved this level a race can be entered. Low profile races can also serve as a type of speed session.

A series of studies in the UCT/MRC Research Unit for Exercise Science and Sports Medicine at the University of Cape Town and the Sports Science Institute of South Africa have attempted to evaluate the effects of specific speed work sessions on performance. One such study showed that replacing 15% of a group of cyclists' usual training with two speed sessions per week for 3 weeks improved cycling time trial performance by 3.6% (Lindsay *et al.* 1996). Doubling the total number of training sessions by increasing the high intensity training program from 3 to 6 weeks produced no additional benefit (Westgarth-Taylor *et al.* 1997). In another study, different groups of subjects performed high intensity training from 30 s duration to longer (8 min) duration from 175% to 80% of $\dot{V}o_{2max}$ (Stepto *et al.* 1999). Interestingly, only speed work at race pace (4 min at

85% of $\dot{V}o_{2max}$) or very high intensity (30 s at 175% of $\dot{V}o_{2max}$) improved cycling performance in a 40 km cycling time trial. These findings demonstrate two important points: (i) certain types of speed work may be more effective than others; and (ii) large changes in performance can be achieved in a relatively short period of time.

The finding of measurable changes in performance was found also by Smith *et al.* (1999) who measured the effects of high intensity training using two interval sessions per week for 4 weeks. Subjects trained at the maximal treadmill speed achieved during a $\dot{V}o_{2max}$ test, with the duration of each interval being 60–75% of the maximum time that each subject could run at their individual peak speed. Each training session involved the repetition of either five or six of these intervals. In this way subjects maintained heart rates of approximately 90–95% of maximum heart rate during the fast repetitions. However, if exercise duration was extended to more than 70–75% of maximum time capable of running at the velocity of $\dot{V}o_{2max}$, then the heart rate would rise to 100% of maximum after the second or third repetition, suggesting that the intervals were too long and too stressful. Second, if the heart rate did not decrease below 125 beats·min^{-1} by the end of the recovery intervals, the next interval would always elicit a maximum heart rate. This supports the principle that more is not necessarily always better. However, the main finding was that this period of high intensity training significantly increased peak treadmill running speed, the time for which this speed could be maintained, and 3000 m time trial performance, the latter by 2.8%. The authors suggested that using the peak speed obtained in the $\dot{V}o_{2max}$ test and 60–75% of the time for which the peak speed could be maintained, might be particularly useful in exercise prescription. This suggestion is appealing for a number of reasons. First, the variables are easily measurable for a number of sports and do not require any sophisticated equipment. Second, this method does not require the measurement of blood lactate concentrations and the use of the so-called "anaerobic" or "lactate threshold," the physiologic basis of which is in doubt (Swart & Jennings 2004). Third, the incorporation of heart rate monitoring provides a tool to determine when the fast component has been too long, or the number too many (Achten & Jeukendrup 2003).

Experience has shown that high intensity speed training cannot be continued indefinitely without risk of injury, overreaching, or overtraining. It is therefore important that after 4–6 weeks of progressive increase in speed work, there is a recovery period of a week of reduced training before the next period of speed work commences.

Additional training sessions that could be added later include resistance training (use of hills for runners and cyclists) and training sessions of 90–120 min at close to race speed (often called "tempo" training). Like the speed work already discussed, these specialized training sessions also require the input of a sports scientist or experienced coach to reduce the risk of injury or overtraining. It should be stressed that these sessions, as with the other high intensity sessions, need to be introduced into the training schedule progressively, but only much later in the development of the training regimen.

Short races are an excellent form of speed training. These sessions can be carried out as hard efforts with the intensity controlled by perceived effort or heart rate. Provided that these sessions are not at all-out racing intensity, it is a perfectly acceptable addition to a structured training program and should not necessarily be viewed as a training error.

In essence, the introduction of speed work into the training regimen should not be a random event. Rather, the introduction of speed work must be carefully planned, particularly with regard to the distance of the speed work sessions, intensity of the sessions, number of sessions per week, recovery between hard intervals, and overall progression of the speed work component of the training regimen. Failure to pay attention to these factors can lead to an increased risk of injury or the manifestation of the symptoms of overtraining. Therefore, the sports medical practitioner should carefully analyze the nature of any speed work carried out by anyone presenting with injury or symptoms of chronic fatigue.

Hard day, easy day principle

Bill Bowermann and Bill Dellinger, coaches who have trained a dynasty of great runners from the University of Eugene, Oregon, were the first coaches to teach that training should not always be at the same intensity and duration every day. They observed that progression was best when the athlete was allowed a suitable recovery period after each hard training session. This period of recovery ranged from as little as 24 h for some athletes to 48 h for others. This became known as the "hard day/easy day" training principle and incorporates the physiologic principle that a recovery period is needed for physiologic adaptation to take place after a training load that has caused a significant physiologic stress (Busso et al. 2002).

For experienced competitors training to improve performance, all training should follow a "hard day/easy day" principle. The training session on one day should be "hard" in intensity rating, followed the next day by a session that is "easy." For those athletes training twice daily, only one session would be a "hard" session on a "hard" training day. Some athletes find it difficult to train easily when they should be on the "easy day," and for these athletes the use of a heart rate monitor to prevent training too hard is a useful tool. All athletes must establish for themselves how frequently they can train hard. Success will, to a large extent, depend on whether or not they achieve this balance.

Tapering

To achieve a best possible performance, at some point every athlete should reduce their overall training load. Typically, this is primarily a reduction in training volume, with a smaller reduction in the high intensity sessions. Many athletes fear that they will lose their fitness by reducing their training load. Contrary to this opinion, however, an appropriate reduction in training load at the right time before a major competition will enhance performance (Bosch et al. 1999). In the third week before competition, training load can be reduced to approximately 80% of the normal training load in terms of weekly duration or distance; 2 weeks before competition the training load can be further reduced to 60–70% of the normal training load. In the final week training should be maintained, but at the reduced, or even more reduced, level. By maintaining the high intensity workouts (at the same speed, but reduced in overall volume) performance will be improved. It is important to note that the high intensity workouts must not be removed from the training regimen.

Many athletes who are training to improve their performances, rather than for health benefits, fail to either engage in speed training or in tapering and get locked into a regimen in which all attention is focused on weekly training distance. These athletes will only perform their best when they understand the importance of speed work in improving performance and the beneficial effects of tapering before important competition. Scientific evidence has confirmed that tapering produces a dramatic improvement in performance (Mujika *et al.* 2004). The effect is greatest if there is a rapid reduction in training volume in the first few days of the taper, but maintenance of the high intensity workouts, although somewhat reduced in total volume. It has not been clearly established how long the optimal tapering period before a competition should be. The shortest period is probably 10 days, to the 3-week period already discussed. It is quite likely that this may be an individual response, also influenced by the preceding training load. The heavier the preceding training, the more likely it is that a longer tapering period will be required for the body to recover fully in order to achieve optimal performance. As with the optimum volume of training that needs to be determined for each individual, so each individual must experiment with different tapering programs to determine which program produces the best results.

Peaking and subsequent decline in competitive performance

After reaching a peak in competitive performance, many athletes do not accept the fact that it is impossible to perform well for more than 3–6 weeks before their performances start to decline. Performance may improve steadily for as long as 10 weeks, but beyond this period the athletes will often become easily tired, sleep badly, become prone to injury, illness and symptoms of overtraining (Meeusen *et al.* 2006). The decline in performance can occur very rapidly. It may take only 3 weeks to go from a best performance to the point at which the athlete is physically incapacitated. These athletes often present to the medical practitioner for help because they are convinced that there is something medically wrong with them. While this may well be the case in some instances, it is important for the sports medicine practitioner to realize that it is quite normal for performances to decline after a period of peaking, tapering, and racing. A period of reduced training should be planned at this phase of training before the next build-up to another peak begins, otherwise overtraining can result. Once in the overtrained state it may take the athlete many weeks to recover and be able to resume normal training (Noakes 2001).

Recovery

Whether the training regimen is one that requires two training sessions each day (e.g., the elite athlete aiming to win races and championship medals), or four training sessions per week (e.g., the person training for health and fitness reasons), the rule discussed previously in this chapter pertaining to regularity of training applies. However, even though regularity is an important principle of training, there should also be periods of rest built into the training program. Indeed, no matter what the level of training, there should be periods during which the training load is strategically reduced. Thus, in a given year, even the elite endurance athlete will have a number of periods during which little training is carried out. Typically, this will be after an important race or after a continuous build-up in the training load. Similarly, the non-elite participant will benefit from the occasional rest period consisting of a significant reduction in the normal training load. These recovery periods, usually consisting of a training week of reduced distance and intensity, can themselves be considered to be a part of the "consistency" rule by virtue of the fact that they appear regularly, about every 6–8 weeks, in the training schedule.

Heart rate monitoring

A popular trend in recent times has been to use heart rate and a heart rate monitor to control training intensity. While scientific in many respects, training entirely on heart rate has many drawbacks, as the so-called heart rate training zone often fails to predict adequately the correct intensity for training (Lambert *et al.* 1998). Reasons for this include the fact that heart rate while exercising is very dependent on factors other than just the work rate. These include temperature, diurnal variation, and prior sleep. Heart rate also does not adequately account for muscular fatigue which may occur from a prior training session incurred on the previous day. Thus, heart rate may indicate that the training intensity is too low, whereas a low intensity may be appropriate for tired muscles resulting from a previous speed workout for example. Therefore it may be better to use a perception rating of intensity to control training speed. Specifically, does the session feel easy, somewhat hard, hard, or very hard? Where heart rate monitoring may be used to advantage is to monitor trends of either an increase or decrease in heart rate for a given controlled training session.

Often, those who wish to use heart rate during exercise as a monitor of training effort will use an equation based on a predicted maximum heart rate using a simple formula of 220 minus age in years. Therefore, the predicted maximum heart rate of a 40-year-old is $(220 - 40)$ beats·min^{-1}, which equals 180 beats·min^{-1}. However, there is little or no scientific basis for this calculation (Edwards 1997). Therefore, should someone wish to use this method to determine the appropriate exercise intensity, true maximum heart rate should first be established, because all younger, highly trained athletes have maximum heart rates that are lower than expected for their ages. In contrast, highly trained athletes older than 50 years have higher maximal heart rates than predicted by this equation.

Maximum heart rate can be established accurately in one of two ways: an exercise scientist can perform a maximum exercise test or an individual can perform their own test while wearing a heart rate monitor while exercising as hard as possible for 4–10 min. This test should not be undertaken in an unsupervised setting by people whose heart conditions are not known. The popular training dogma is that maximum benefit from training is achieved by training at 60–90% of maximum heart rate. Various exercise training prescriptions can be found that are based on different training heart rate zones. However, for the reasons already described, it is not the best method of monitoring training. For certain people, it may be better than no monitoring whatsoever. This may be particularly true for those individuals who tend to train too hard, too often. For these people, a coach could prescribe a training session (particularly the "easy" day) in which a particular heart rate should not be exceeded. More useful in general terms, however, is that as fitness increases, at any particular exercise intensity or speed, the heart rate will be less. Another benefit from heart rate monitoring is that, performed regularly, the heart rate after exercise will return more quickly towards resting values. Conversely, an increased heart rate at a given speed may indicate the onset of overreaching or overtraining. When this is observed, the individual needs to rest from training, or train less, until recovery has occurred.

Weight training

Weight training performed two or three times weekly has a positive effect on endurance performance if it does not replace training sessions in the endurance training program. In contrast, adding endurance training to a strength training program in which the main expected outcome is a gain in muscle strength and power causes reduced adaptation with a resultant compromised gain in strength (Fleck & Kraemer 1997). There are some specific advantages of strength training for "downhill" races because of the damaging effect of eccentric muscle contraction that occurs when running downhill, which can be reduced by the increased strength from a carefully planned weight-training program. Typically, for those athletes who wish to include weight training into their program, there should be no more than two to three sessions per week. When the training load is increased, the supplementary weight training sessions should be reduced to two sessions per week. Weight training is best performed on the "easy" training days of the sports specific training schedule.

Stretching

Training strengthens the active muscles and reduces their flexibility. To maintain flexibility of the muscles, specific stretching exercises can be performed. However, the exact benefit of stretching, particularly to prevent injuries, has not been proven conclusively (Shrier & Gossel 2000). This has not prevented the popular belief that stretching helps in this regard. There is also no published evidence to suggest that regular stretching improves endurance performance. The one condition that may well be prevented by regular stretching is exercise-associated muscle cramping (Schwellnus 1999). When all the evidence is considered, the pragmatic recommendations are that a stretching program should be carried out in moderation and that the stretching exercises should be performed correctly. Importantly, the stretch must always be applied gradually. Ballistic stretching, which involves bouncing up and down, is considered to be an ineffective method as it simply activates the stretch reflex, causing the stretched muscle to contract rapidly. The tension inside the muscle during this type of stretching is much higher than in a static stretch. Although it is often said that this form of stretching increases the risk of injury, there is no convincing published evidence to confirm this.

Static stretching is a specific type of stretching exercise. During static stretching, the stretch position is assumed slowly and held for 30–60 s. The build-up of tension in the muscle is slow, and so the stretch reflex which causes the muscle to contract is not activated. This type of stretching invokes the inverse stretch reflex which causes muscle tension to fall, enabling the muscle to be stretched a little further. More sophisticated techniques include the contract–relax and contract–relax–antagonist contract techniques. The static stretch technique has been shown to be highly effective for increasing the range of motion while being relatively low risk for inducing injury (Hughes 1996).

Overtraining

Overtraining is discussed in detail in Chapter 3. From a practical perspective relating to endurance training, one way to help prevent overtraining is to ensure application of the "hard day, easy day" training principle. A heart rate monitor can be useful to prevent hard training on a day when only light training should be carried out, by prescribing a heart rate that must not be exceeded during training. However, if one day of easy training is insufficient for the athlete to feel adequately recovered, then an extra day of "easy" training should be carried out before the next strenuous workout. Applying this diligently will reduce the risk of developing symptoms of overtraining.

Symptoms of overtraining include one or more of the following: painful muscles, muscle fatigue, general feeling of fatigue, depression, irritability, disturbed sleep patterns, and increased POMS score, weight loss, raised resting pulse rate, an increased susceptibility to upper respiratory tract infections, gastrointestinal disturbances, and a decrease in running performance (Lehmann *et al.* 1993; Meeusen *et al.* 2006).

There is no magical cure for overtraining other than a reduction in training load until the symptoms have passed. Complete rest from training may be necessary. Reducing training or resting is not something that a sportsperson training seriously wants to do, and it is often difficult to convince someone that these are the only options to recover from the overtraining syndrome. The training at which the onset of symptoms commenced should be noted (Foster 1998). This represents somewhat more than the maximum training load that can be tolerated. Subsequently, as that particular training load is reached, the volume and speed should be increased only very gradually as the physiologic adaptations are given every chance to occur. However, it should be recognized that everyone has a genetically determined ceiling in training load above which adaptation will not occur.

TRAINING FOR SKILL ACQUISITION

To be successful in sport athletes must possess great physical attributes such as strength, power, stamina, and flexibility, as well as demonstrate expert motor skill abilities. Indeed, at the elite level the difference between athletes often relates more to the ability to perform skills with high levels of consistency, precision, and smoothness than it does to issues of speed, power, and strength. However, despite the importance of effective skill execution in determining sporting performance, research into the areas of motor learning and skills training have often brought conflicting results, leaving coaches confused about the best training methods to use.

One of the difficulties facing researchers concerns the definitions of skill and skill acquisition. For example, the concept of skill itself is much more difficult to define than the physical capacities such as strength or stamina, as it is more a construct than a physical capacity. Leonard (1998) summarized this issue when he indicated that skill is not a term than represents a singular entity, but rather involves sensory processing, motor learning and control, coordination of muscles, adaptability of control during various conditions, and retention of the acquired skills. Importantly, skill acquisition is also multidisciplinary and involves areas such as neuromuscular physiology, biomechanics, and psychology.

Despite the complexities in defining and categorizing skill acquisition, the goal in training for skill acquisition is to allow the athlete to perform skills with quality, certainty, and with economy of movement, thereby conserving energy and reducing potential injury. In order to do this, the coach must be aware of how the neuromuscular system works, the mechanical principles underpinning movement, and the environments that may facilitate or inhibit skill acquisition. This part of this chapter is divided into two sections: the underpinning physiology that contributes to skill acquisition and theories of skill acquisition, followed by evidence-based concepts influencing motor skill acquisition.

Physiologic basis of motor skill acquisition

Skilled performance is purposeful movement and is reliant on the coordination of agonist, synergist, and antagonist skeletal muscles. Motorneurons innervating skeletal muscles are found in both the central nervous system (CNS) and peripheral nervous system (PNS) and excite or inhibit muscles to produce coordinated movements. The synchronized

and coordinated means by which the nervous system varies the amount of force required to produce meaningful movement is one of the fundamental aspects of motor skill acquisition. Performance with too little or too much muscular force can mean the difference between success and failure. To produce skilful movement, there must be an interaction between the number of motor units recruited, the muscular fibre types involved, and the synchronization and firing rate of motorneurons. For reviews on motor unit recruitment the reader is referred to Binder and Mendell (1990), Enoka and Stuart (1984), and Noth (1992). In addition to the amount of motor unit recruitment, the nervous system must also control agonist–antagonist muscle activity. When an individual performs a goal-directed motor skill of moderate to fast speed, a three burst pattern of agonist–antagonist–agonist muscle is observed allowing for smooth controlled movement from initiation to completion (Enoka 1994).

Skilled movement also requires sensory feedback to the nervous system, particularly from the internal environment. There are two receptors that provide sensory feedback to the CNS: muscle spindles and Golgi tendon organs (GTOs). Muscle spindles, found within each muscle fiber, provide information about the length of a muscle and the rate in change of the length during movement. If a muscle is stretched, these receptors will send impulses to the CNS, which in turn sends a motor command to the muscle to contract, thereby stopping the muscle from overstretching. GTOs, found in the musculotendinous junction, responds to muscle tension either from the muscle being stretched or generated by muscular contraction. Unlike spindles that monitor individual muscle fiber length, GTOs receives information from 10–15 motor units, thereby monitoring whole muscle tension rather than individual muscle fiber tension (Hullinger et al. 1995). For more extensive discussion on sensory feedback the reader is referred to Rothwell (1994).

Central nervous system and motor control systems

The coordination and management of muscle groups during skilled movement is the responsibility of

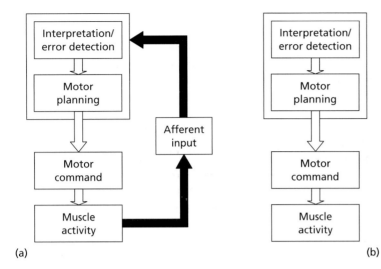

Fig. 1.1 (a) Closed-loop control system. (b) Open-loop control system (Schmidt & Lee 1999, after Hodges, 2003).

higher CNS brain centers, such as the cerebellum, basal ganglia, and cerebral cortex. Unlike reflexes, which are stereotypical responses to a stimulus and controlled primarily at the spinal level, higher brain centers have the ability for modification with voluntary movements. Schmidt and Lee (1999) have suggested two basic systems of motor control. One is via the closed-loop system where movement is continually updated and modified on the basis of feedback through muscle spindles, GTOs, joint, skin vestibular and visual receptors (Fig. 1.1a). The alternative is through open-loop control systems where movement is controlled by means of higher CNS centers independent of sensory feedback (Fig. 1.1b). Movements are preplanned and performed without deliberation of sensory feedback, which may be too slow to make adjustments to the movement, or are just not needed. Despite continuing debate regarding these two theories, Hodges (2003) has suggested that motor control maybe a hybrid of these two theories.

Physiologic mechanisms underpinning motor skill acquisition: Cortical plasticity

The acquisition of skills is associated with changes in the brain's neural networks, otherwise known as plasticity, or functional reorganization (Donoghue 1995; Kaas 1991). Cowan *et al.* (1985) have suggested

that in early life, plasticity occurs through regression of neuronal networks, with up to 50% loss in neurons in brain structure studies. By approximately 3 years, this regression is almost complete with children having a basic ability to modify or control grips and load forces, which by 6–8 years becomes much more adult-like (Forssberg *et al.* 1995). Importantly, neurophysiologic research has demonstrated CNS plasticity in healthy (Pascual-Leone *et al.* 1994, 1995) and diseased adults (Byrnes *et al.* 1999), showing that acquisition or reacquisition of motor skills is possible throughout the life cycle. These findings are contrary to the earlier neuropsychologic learning theories of Freud and Piaget, which viewed neural growth and development as virtually complete by mid to end of adolescence. CNS plasticity is achieved through the process of long-term potentiation (LTP) where changes are activity dependent; synapses will strengthen (or weaken in the case of long-term depression) depending on the strength of the stimuli from practice. For more information on LTP the reader is directed to Leonard (1998) and Perkins and Teyler (1988).

Mechanisms to suggest plastic changes from skill acquisition include the establishment of new connections and/or alterations of the effectiveness of previously existing connections (Donoghue 1995; Kaas 1991; Pascual-Leone & Torres 1993). However, cortical plasticity seen with older children and adults suggests that it is likely changes occur in pre-existing connections that are normally present but physiologically silent (Leonard 1998). Neuro-imaging studies have demonstrated plasticity in the motor cortex in highly skilled adult athletes and musicians who have undertaken structured motor skill acquisition and reinforcement (Elbert *et al.* 1995; Pearce *et al.* 2000). Elbert *et al.* (1995) demonstrated changes in the motor cortex representation in the fingering hand but not the bow hand of skilled violin players. Similar findings have also been identified by Pearce *et al.* (2000) who found differences in the motor cortex (plasticity) and increased neural excitability to the playing hand in elite, but not recreational badminton players. These researchers suggested that the presence of structured practice was the stimulus for the observed changes in both the elite athlete group and in highly skilled musicians.

Physiology of motor learning

A number of sequential models, such as Gentile's (1972, 1987, 2000) two-phase model and the popular Fitts and Posner (1967) three-phase model, are outlined below describing the stages of an individual learning a motor task. More recently, these stages of learning have been used to demonstrate changes in the individual's neural strategy (muscle activation patterns and motor commands) reflecting cortical plasticity. For example, changes in whole muscle activation patterns (reflecting motor learning) using electromyography (EMG) have been demonstrated in a number of sports and activities (Kamon & Gormley 1968; Vorro *et al.* 1978; Jaegers *et al.* 1989; Williams & Walmsley 2000). These studies have shown that during initial stages of skill acquisition (*cognitive* stage) the individual uses muscles inappropriately by both activating excessive or redundant muscle groups, and activating muscle groups with incorrect timing. However, as practice continued (*associative* to *autonomous* stages) the number of muscles activated decreases to a minimal (or optimal) number required to perform the skill effectively, and the timing of muscle activation became appropriate (Magill 2003).

Similar findings have been demonstrated in motor unit recruitment where variability in motor unit recruitment decreases with the acquisition and improvement of a motor skill (Moritani 1993). These authors have also shown changes in motor unit firing frequency following specific practice of skills requiring fast movements.

TIME COURSE OF MOTOR LEARNING

From a practical point of view an area of great interest for coaches concerns the time it takes to learn skills (Baker *et al.* 2003). Ericsson *et al.* (1993) have suggested that it takes approximately 10,000 h (or 10 years) of deliberate practice for a high performance athlete to be developed. However, this view has been questioned recently, with researchers suggesting that approximately 69% of all senior national level athletes had 4 years of experience or less in that sport (Oldenziel *et al.* 2003, 2004). However, these authors noted that these *"quick learners"* had played at least three sports (3.3 ± 1.6) before settling on their main sport, a fact in stark contrast to the limited prior sporting experiences (0.9 ± 1.3) of those athletes who had taken 10 or more years to achieve a similar level of performance.

Theories of motor skill acquisition

Plasticity of the neuromuscular system allows for the acquisition of skills throughout the life cycle. Plasticity is dependent on activity, providing stimulation to strengthen neural pathways to facilitate LTP. Although the old saying "practice makes perfect" holds true to a certain extent, when training for skill acquisition, practice and repetition are not the only variables to consider. To optimize training for skill acquisition, a number of authors have suggested that it is important to understand the conditions that athletes practice under. For example, the type and amount of feedback presented, the grouping and sequencing of practice, and the type of sensory feedback provided all influence the acquisition and retention of motor skills (Leonard 1998; Magill 2003; Schmidt & Lee 1999).

Grouping of practice sessions

BLOCK VERSUS RANDOM PRACTICE

A common question among the coaching fraternity is whether it is better to practice a skill repetitively within a practice session, or whether it is preferential to mix up skills during the session. The former is often referred to as blocked (or massed) practice, while the latter is described as random practice. A typical blocked practice session involves athletes practicing one skill (more skills may be involved but they are practiced independently of each other) in a session with relatively low contextual interference (Battig 1979). Conversely, random practice sessions involve a multiple number of skills practiced simultaneously (or under tactical conditions) and present athletes with higher contextual interference (Battig 1979). Table 1.2 provides an example of the differ-

ences between these two types of practices for a racquet sport.

Research has shown that blocked practice sessions result in faster skill acquisition of complex motor skills (Shea *et al.* 1990), most likely as a result of strengthening of the effectiveness of an existing (but singular) neural pathway (Leonard 1998). However, a large number of studies have shown that random practice results in greater skill retention and adaptation to the sporting environment than blocked practice (Shea & Morgan 1979; Goode & Magill 1986; Hall *et al.* 1994; Landin & Herbert 1997). Leonard (1998) has suggested that this is due to LTP of the skill among a number of neural pathways rather than a singular circuit. In recognizing the value of random practice studies, Rose and Christina (2006) noted that practice sessions should be sport-specific and practice conditions should reflect *real-world* sports

Table 1.2 Example differences between blocked and random practice styles in tennis. The emphasis is on technical development; however, the practice environment differs greatly between the two practice styles. Under random practice, the coach will facilitate skill learning with questions and addressing technical problems within a tactical framework.

Blocked practice	Random practice
Forehand crosscourt	*Zone rally*
Ball racquet feed* from coach to player's forehand side	Rally started with courtesy feed (underarm) from player (or coach) to opponent
Player to return ball to predesignated area (marked by cones)	Rally progresses with a point awarded to the player who can hit a winning or unreturnable forehand. No points given for errors
Service practice	*Service rally* (3 shot rally)
Classic service practice into open service box	Player practices service but under realistic conditions (i.e. with return of serve)
No return from an opponent or coach	Three shot rally includes service (shot #1), return (shot #2), and first shot after return (shot #3)
	Player is instructed to create serves to force weak return from opponent (from good placement of serve) and to set up aggressive third shot after return (ground stroke or volley)
Closed rally drill	*Open rally game*
Players will hit only one shot (e.g., backhand cross-court) and instructed to keep the cross-court rally going for as long as possible	Player gives courtesy feed (underarm) with both players rallying full court to create winning situations. Points awarded for tactical awareness
	One point: Winning point when opponent makes unforced error
	Two points: Forcing opponent into error
	Three points: Hitting outright winning shot

* Also known as "*dead-ball*" drill training.

settings in order to reinforce the skill in a relevant context.

PRACTICE VARIABILITY

Closely linked with random practice is the issue of practice *variability*. Practice variability refers to providing and structuring a practice environment for the learner to apply different parameters, or variations of a motor skill (e.g., in tennis, adapting different swing patterns for low or high bouncing on-coming balls). A number of studies conducted in the 1970s and 1980s (Catalano & Kleiner 1984; Margolis & Christina 1981; McCracken & Stelmach 1977) have demonstrated that variability in the acquisition of a new motor task facilitates transfer of that learning to a similar but novel task. Sports-specific training is important in this regard as studies have shown that practicing variable movement patterns must relate to the performance of that skill (Leonard 1998).

From a practical point of view, the issue of whether to *block* a practice session or to use a *random* style creates a considerable problem for coaches. For example, blocked practice sessions are themed, sequenced smoothly, and athletes tend to improve skill execution during the course of training. Many coaches prefer these sessions because training *looks good*, and sessions are *easier* to plan. In addition, coaches can provide repetitious models, based on their own experiences from which their athletes copy, despite the limited skill retention that tends to occur (Roetert *et al.* 2003). Similarly, some players have been so conditioned by the blocked practice approach that they almost require drills to be performed in a routine order before they can produce a certain skill. This is an obvious problem for performance situations. Typically, excessive use of blocked style training results in the *"We can do it at training, so why can't we do it in the game"* syndrome, which is frustrating for both coaches and athletes alike.

Random style training sessions provide a different set of problems for coaches. While there is little question that random style training results in better skill retention, some coaches, especially those conditioned to using blocked training, are still reluctant to implement it. Even coaches who profess to using both forms of practices generally demonstrate a reliance on repeated closed environments and progress to open environments slowly. Clearly, some coaches need to have the courage to forgo the *perfect looking* training session, in favor of training that may not look as good, but results in genuine skill acquisition.

PART VERSUS WHOLE PRACTICE

Whole practice describes situations where the learner practices the entire skill (movement pattern) from the outset, while *part* practice occurs when the various components of the skill are learned thoroughly first. Considerable debate continues regarding the effectiveness of one over the other. A complicating factor in much of this research has been the choice of skills examined, as it is generally agreed that the type of skill required will dictate whether it is learned best using part or whole methods (Naylor & Briggs 1961; Wightman & Lintern 1985). Rose and Christina (2006) have recommended that complex movement patterns, involving the combination of many individual skills (e.g., gymnastics floor routine), should be taught using the *part* method. Conversely, less complex but highly organized skills (e.g., hitting a baseball) are better suited to the *whole* method.

The *whole–part–whole* practice model is an extension from both the *whole* and *part* practice methods (Swanson & Law 1993). In the *whole–part–whole* model, the subject is provided with the skill in its entirety before having it broken down into parts and taught using the segmentation, simplification, or fractionization methods (Wightman & Lintern 1985). The skill is then taught as a whole a second time to complete the understanding process (Swanson & Law 1993).

Many successful skills coaches prefer to use *whole* or *whole–part–whole* style training, with very few selecting *part* style training during complex technique or skills sessions. One of the key advantages of *whole* and *whole–part–whole* style training over *part* training is the fact that it enables skills to be expressed in the context in which they are to be performed. Whether from an individual or team skill perspective, focusing on just one of the components of a skill ignores the important interaction effects. A traditional approach in some sports has been to focus excessively on the movements of each of the individual segments before *"putting the skill together"* (*part* training). That is, many skills (e.g., kicks, hits, or throws) involve movement of multiple body segments where the coordination, sequencing, timing, and forces produced at each segment must all be optimized for the skill to be executed successfully. For example, the knee extension velocities achieved at ball contact in kicking (approximately 25 rad · s⁻¹) occur primarily through the actions of the preceding segments (e.g., pelvic tilt and rotation, hip flexion) and not through a forceful knee extension via the quadriceps (Davids *et al.* 2000; Lees & Nolan 2002; Lees *et al.* 2005; Robertson & Mosher 1985). Therefore, training drills that isolate the knee extension action and focus on the use of a forceful contraction of the quadriceps actually bear little resemblance to the kicking action. Several coaches still persist with the latter, but their athletes often have problems such as *"My athlete has performed this kicking drill well, but how come he can kick only 30 m?"* A similar argument can be developed for the use of *whole* or *whole–part–whole* style training for game moves practice

sessions (i.e., moves from set pieces in football, rugby, basketball, etc.). That is, while each move involves several players all executing individual tasks, it is the coordination of these actions into the whole that determines the game move's overall effectiveness.

Role of feedback

While practice and repetition are integral components of the skill acquisition process (Newell & Rosenbloom 1981), it is important to realize that practice itself does not guarantee that learning will be either maximized, or occur at all. For example, in a classic study by Bilodeau *et al.* (1959) it was shown that the absence, or removal of feedback during a simple movement task had a direct effect on the execution of that task with practice (Fig. 1.2). While providing somewhat of a simplistic view, this study highlights the important role that feedback has in the skill acquisition process. However, this research did not address other key issues such as *"What sort of feedback should be provided?"* and *"What is the optimal time to provide feedback?"*

There are two basic types of feedback: knowledge of performance, where feedback provides information

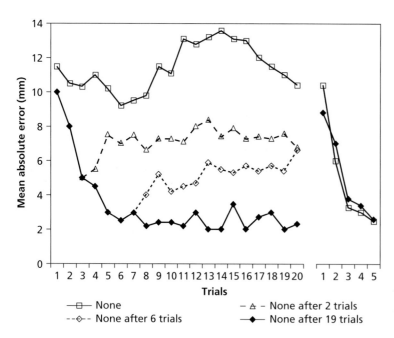

Fig. 1.2 Error in reproducing a simple movement as a function of the amount and type of feedback provided. Following a pause, subjects from the *None* and *None after 19 trials* groups were retested over five trials, but with both groups being given feedback after each trial. (After Bilodeau *et al.* 1959.)

regarding the ongoing sensory or perceptual information provided during the movement, and knowledge of results, providing feedback on the outcome of the movement. Feedback is also obtained *intrinsically* through visual, auditory, or kinaesthetic processes and/or *extrinsically* from the coach or an observer. However, these two processes are not interdependent.

Coaches may often provide excessive feedback or feedback that lacks specificity. The level of feedback needs to be congruent with the skill level of the performer, as less skilled performers are likely to experience overload if too much, or too precise levels of feedback are provided (Magill & Wood 1986; Smoll 1972). It is important here to note that simple praise (e.g. "good shot") is not a true form of feedback, and has been shown to be largely ineffective (Kulhavy & Wager 1993). Research findings have demonstrated that feedback was more effective when provided from the learner's perspective (Magill 1993; Schmidt 1991) because the acquisition of motor skills relies on both internal and external sensory feedback. The *amount* and *timing* of extrinsic feedback is also important (Ho & Shea 1978; Reeve & Magill 1981). Williams and Hodges (2005) have

suggested that disproportionate amounts of extrinsic feedback, stemming from the timing of the feedback (almost immediately after the skill has been executed), may incur an overreliance by the player on the coach and impair the learner's problem-solving processes. Table 1.3 illustrates some feedback examples that coaches can use to facilitate independent thinking.

Instruction versus demonstration

A fundamental issue in coaching is to provide verbal instruction or visual demonstrations (or a combination of both). There is considerable inconsistency regarding the effectiveness of verbal feedback versus visual demonstration. For example, Magill and Schoenfelder-Zohdi (1996) have suggested that visual information is superior to verbal instruction, while other researchers have indicated that the combination of verbal instruction and visual demonstration is far superior to the use of verbal feedback alone (McCullagh *et al*. 1990; Weiss & Klint 1987). Moreover, other researchers have suggested that verbal instructions do not have a positive influence on the learning process (Hodges

Table 1.3 The use of questioning as a form of feedback in comparison to traditional instructions. In order to reduce the potential for overreliance, coaches can pose questions rather than prescriptive feedback to assist learning from the player's perspective. The examples below pertain to racquet sports such as tennis and badminton, but can be adapted for other sports.

Coach's questions	Traditional instructions
When is the best time to go for a winning shot?	When the opponent is out of position I want you to go for it, and put the ball away
In this game, were more points won on outright winners or opponent's errors?	In that game most of your points were won due to your opponent's errors
On a scale of 1–5 (5 being great and 1 being poor), how would you rate your balance during those last couple of forehands?	Your balance was a little off in that last rally, next time keep your weight on the balls of your feet, widen your stance slightly, and stay low
On a scale of 1–5 (5 being great and 1 being poor), how would you rate your weight transfer in those last serves	You are transferring your weight really well. However, make sure that you keep finishing here though (coach points to a position on court)
What are some ways to make it easier for you to play angled cross-court shots?	For all your cross-court shots make sure that you take the ball early and hit it out in front of the body
If your opponent hits short cross-court and is out of position, what would be the best choice of shot?	Hit the ball down the line when your opponent hits his or her cross-court shot short

& Lee 1999; Masters 1992; Wulf & Weigelt 1997). Williams and Hodges (2005) noted that for precise replication of a technique, demonstrations were preferred, as these played a significant part in aiding motor learning (Haguenauer *et al.* 2005; Magill & Schoenfelder-Zohdi 1996). Hodges and Franks (2002) also indicated that demonstrations were effective particularly when the activity being taught was based on combining movements for which the athlete had a prior degree of proficiency. However, in situations involving novice learners it was important to provide some verbal instruction to avoid either overload, or the learner may attend to inappropriate cues during the demonstration (McCullagh *et al.* 1990; Weiss & Klint 1987). Further, demonstrations may be less effective when used to try and refine an existing movement pattern (Horn & Williams 2004). From a coaching perspective, the combination of verbal instruction and demonstration is desirable for most sports, but it does depend on the type of skills being taught, and the level and motivation of the athletes being trained.

Implicit versus explicit perceptual learning

Perceptual skill learning is a relatively new area in the motor skill acquisition literature and has become fashionable in many coaching circles. Underpinning the issue of perceptual learning is the concept that expert performers have an enhanced cognitive knowledge of their sport. This is based on their ability to recognize cues of relevance and patterns of play, superiority in anticipating opponent's actions, and greater accuracy in expectations of what is likely to happen given a particular set of circumstances (Williams & Grant 1999). This expertise is developed primarily as a result of long-term sport-specific experience. However, Abernethy (1993) explored the concepts of whether there were any potential training methods that could be employed to enhance the development of perceptual skill in sport as an alternative to years of task-specific practice.

A key issue within the perceptual skill acquisition domain is the importance of implicit versus explicit learning processes (Magill 1998; Williams & Grant 1999). The arguments surrounding this issue center on whether skill learning is superior when training is based on the learner's internal *feel* and experience (implicit), rather than sessions based on instruction and external feedback (explicit; Gentile 1998; Jackson 2003). The relative merits of each of these training methods have been the subject of considerable debate, with some researchers heavily in favor of implicit training (Masters 1992, 2000), while others emphasize that explicit knowledge has an important role in the learning process (Beek 2000).

The issues surrounding the implicit versus explicit debate have resulted in a great deal of confusion. Apart from the difficulty in conducting interference-free research in this area (Jackson 2003), there is also conflict regarding study design and the applicability of these findings to the training environment (Farrow & Abernethy 2002, 2003; Jackson 2003). From a practical point of view, a major failing of this research is that it tends to promote a bias towards either the implicit or explicit concepts, with many researchers even suggesting the explicit instruction is counterproductive to the skill learning process (Horn & Williams 2005). Such a bias can lead to confusion in skills coaches who must operate in an environment more flexible than that used to meet research methodologic constraints (e.g., coaches must deal with athletes at vary stages of skill development, and over a wide range of contexts).

Regardless of the arguments for and against implicit versus explicit practice, many successful skills coaches lean towards an implicit model in their coaching, while selectively using explicit methods to great success. One important constraint of research in this area relates to the fact that few implicit training studies have been conducted on highly experienced or elite level athletes (i.e., groups with high explicit knowledge of their sport). In particular, an interesting problem arises when coaching a high level athlete who develops a technical problem that interferes with performance (e.g., a golfer who develops the "*yips*" when putting, a rugby goal kicker who starts to push the ball to the right of the posts). It is not uncommon for these athletes to have a great deal of difficulty "feeling" this technical flaw (especially if they have had the error for a long time), negating the effectiveness of using a purely implicit approach during technique correction. In this case, some explicit instruction can often result in very rapid improvements. It appears that both methods sit along a continuum that although favoring the use of implicit practices, must also acknowledge the role of explicit instruction in skill development.

Mental imagery

The bridge between neuropsychology and neurophysiology is demonstrated through the relationship of mental rehearsal, or imagery, and their affect on motor skill acquisition. For example, a number of studies have shown that similar neural circuits and cerebral cortex activation patterns are involved during both mental rehearsal and the performance of the motor skill (Decety 1996; Grafton *et al.* 1996; Jeannerod 1995; Sirigu *et al.* 1996). This provides a possible explanation as to why mental practice using imagery can result in athletic motor performance improvements (Feltz & Landers 1983). However, some differences exist between mental imagery and actual performance, in particular when an individual is performing simple or complex motor skills. Bennet (1997), in research using non-invasive neuroimaging techniques, suggested that during the performance of a simple motor skill an area within the sensorimotor cortex becomes active. However, when a more complex motor skill was required, a secondary motor area (the supplementary motor area [SMA]) becomes active at the same time. During mental imagery performance of the same complex motor skill (without muscular activity) only the SMA is active. This may have implications for coaches to reinforce the value of mental imagery to their athletes in training complex skills pertinent to their sport, as well as to injured athletes who maybe unable to perform the skills physically. For more information regarding the link between mental imagery and the neuromuscular system the reader is referred to Lotze and Halsband (2006).

Physical fatigue and muscle damage

Despite studies dating back to the 1970s suggesting otherwise (Carron 1972; Thomas *et al.* 1975) it is relatively common to observe athletes practicing motor skills while in a state of physical fatigue, or for coaches to follow up heavy or intense training sessions by programing "light" training based around skill acquisition. Research has demonstrated that motor skill acquisition and performance is affected following fatiguing exercise. Arnett *et al.* (2000) showed that anaerobically induced fatigue had a detrimental effect on gross motor skill acquisition. Similarly, although Lyons *et al.* (2006) demonstrated significant detriments in passing performance following fatiguing exercise in both novice and elite basketball players, the decrements in the elite players were not as great as those of the novices. Other studies measuring motor skill decrements have used fatiguing exercise involving eccentric exercise, which produces muscle damage (Pearce *et al.* 1998; Saxton *et al.* 1995), and concentric exercise that fatigues muscle but does not cause as much damage (Bottas *et al.* 2005; Walsh *et al.* 2004). Saxton *et al.* (1995) and Walsh *et al.* (2004) showed position errors in a subject's arm when matched to their non-exercised arm. Despite different time course measures, similar results were found in both eccentric exercise and concentric exercise. Pearce *et al.* (1998) demonstrated that following eccentric exercise subjects exhibited both greater error in a subsequent visuo-motor tracking task and reduced motor skill proficiency than control subjects (Fig. 1.3). Further studies correlated these errors with a drop in muscular force (Pearce *et al.* 1998; Walsh *et al.*

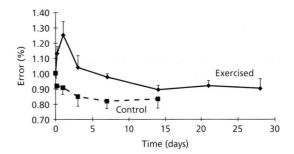

Fig. 1.3 Comparison of change in tracking error in exercised (solid line) and control subjects (dashed line) normalized to initial values. A score lower than 1 shows improvement, whereas values greater than 1 shows greater error (Pearce *et al.* 1998).

2004). Using EMG, Bottas *et al.* (2005) found that reduced force from fatigued muscles impaired activation patterns of agonist and antagonist muscle groups, as well as reduced position sense from muscle damage, contributing to decline in the motor skill task.

Although further research needs to be conducted in the area of fatigue and motor skill training, the coaching implications of this research indicate that undertaking developmental skill-based training sessions with fatigued athletes is contraindicated. Therefore, developmental skills training should precede voluminous or intense training sessions. Contrary to this view, many high performance coaches use light skills-based sessions as a means of active recovery (e.g., the day after an international football match). While this practice should probably be avoided in novice athletes it does not appear to interfere with the skill levels of high performance athletes.

Conclusions

This section has provided a brief overview of the physiologic, biomechanical, and psychologic components underpinning motor skill acquisition. Recent advances in neurophysiology have shown that skill acquisition can occur at any stage of the life cycle, rather than occurring only when athletes are young. For the coach, the main issue is to understand the processes underpinning motor learning and motor control, as well as creating the optimal environment to improve and maintain the athlete's technical skill base. The areas of motor learning, skill acquisition, and motor control are complex and challenging areas which are continually expanding. Results from future studies will provide coaches with more information enabling them to program training practices more effectively and enhance the skill level of their athletes, regardless of chronologic or training age.

References

Abernethy, B. (1993) The nature of expertise in sport. In: *Proceedings of the VIIIth World Congress of Sport Psychology* (Serpa, S., Alves, J., Ferreira, V. & Paula-Brito, A., eds.) International Society of Sport Psychology, Lisbon: 18–22.

Achten, J. & Jeukendrup, A.E. (2003) Heart rate monitoring: applications and limitations. *Sports Medicine* **33**, 517–538.

Allerheiligen, B. (2003) In-season strength training for power athletes. *Strength and Conditioning Journal* **25**, 23–28.

American College of Sports Medicine (1998) ACSM Position Stand. The recommended quantity and quality of exercise for developing and maintaining cardiorespiratory and muscular fitness, and flexibility in healthy adults. *Medicine and Science in Sports and Exercise* **30**, 975–991.

American College of Sports Medicine (2002) Progression models in resistance training for healthy adults. *Medicine and Science in Sports and Exercise* **34**, 364–380.

Arnett, M.G., DeLuccia, D. & Gilmartin, K. (2000) Male and female differences and the specificity of fatigue on skill acquisition and transfer performance. *Research Quarterly for Exercise and Sport* **71**, 201–205.

Baechle, T.R., Earle, R.W. & Wathen, D. (2000) Resistance training. In: *NSCA: Essentials of Strength Training and Conditioning*, 2nd edn. (Baechle, T.R. & Earle, R.W., eds.) Human Kinetics, Champaign, IL: 395–425.

Baker, D. (2001a) A series of studies on the training of high-intensity muscle power in rugby league football players. *Journal of Strength and Conditioning Research* **15**, 198–209.

Baker, D. (2001b) Acute and long-term power responses to power training: observations on the training of an elite power athlete. *Strength and Conditioning Journal* **23**, 47–56.

Baker, D. (2001c) Comparison of upper-body strength and power between professional and college-aged rugby league players. *Journal of Strength and Conditioning Research* **15**, 30–35.

Baker, D., Nance, S. & Moore, M. (2001a) The load that maximizes the average mechanical power output during explosive bench press throws in highly trained athletes. *Journal of Strength and Conditioning Research* **15**, 20–24.

Baker, D., Nance, S. & Moore, M. (2001b) The load that maximizes the average mechanical power output during jump squats in power-trained athletes. *Journal of Strength and Conditioning Research* **15**, 92–97.

Baker, J., Cote, J. & Abernethy, B. (2003) Sport specific training, deliberate practice and the development of expertise in team ball sports. *Journal of Applied Sport Psychology* **15**, 12–25.

Bam, J., Noakes, T.D., Juritz, J. & Dennis, S.C. (1997) Could women outrun men in ultramarathon races? *Medicine and Science in Sports and Exercise* **29**, 244–247.

Battig, W.F. (1979) The flexibility of human memory. In: *Levels of Processing in Human Memory* (Cermak, L.S. & Craik, F.I.M., eds.) Lawrence Erlbaum, Hillsdale, NJ: 23–44.

Beek, P.J. (2000) Toward a theory of implicit learning in the perceptual-motor domain. *International Journal of Sport Psychology* **31**, 547–554.

Bennet, M.R. (1997) *The Idea of Consciousness*. Harwood Academic, Amsterdam.

Bilodeau, E.A., Bilodeau, I.M. & Schumsky, D.A. (1959) Some effects of introducing and withdrawing knowledge of results early and late in practice. *Journal of Experimental Psychology* **58**, 142–144.

Binder, M.D. & Mendell, L.M. (1990) *The Segmental Motor System*. Oxford University Press, New York.

Bird, S.P., Tarpenning, K.M. & Marino, F.E. (2005) Designing resistance training programmes to enhance muscular fitness: a review of the acute programme variables. *Sports Medicine* **35**, 841–851.

Bompa, T.O. (1999) *Periodization: Theory and Methodology of Training*, 4th edn. Human Kinetics, Champaign, IL.

Booth, D., Magdalinski, T., Miah, A. & Phillips, M. (2000) Coaching, science and the professionalism of sport since 1950. Brisbane, Australia, 7–13 September. National Sport Information Centre, Australian Sports Commission and Sports Medicine Australia: 328.

Bosch, A.N., Thomas, A. & Noakes, T.D. (1999) Improved time-trial performance after tapering in well-trained cyclists. *South African Journal of Sports Medicine* **7**, 11–15.

Bottas, R., Linnamo, V., Nicol, C. & Komi, P.V. (2005) Repeated maximal eccentric actions causes long-lasting disturbances in movement control. *European Journal of Applied Physiology* **94**, 62–69.

Brooks, G.A., Fahey, T.D. & Baldwin, K.M. (2005) *Exercise Physiology: Human Bioenergetics and its Applications*, 4th edn. McGraw-Hill, New York.

Budgett, R. (1990) Overtraining syndrome. *British Journal of Sports Medicine* **24**, 231–236.

Busso, T., Benoit, H., Bonnefoy, R., Feasson, L. & Lacour, J.R. (2002) Effects of training frequency on the dynamics of performance response to a single training bout. *Journal of Applied Physiology* **92**, 572–580.

Byrnes, M.L., Thickbroom, G.W., Phillips, B.A., Wilson, S.A. & Mastaglia, F.L. (1999) Physiological studies of the corticomotor projection to the hand after subcortical stroke. *Clinical Neurophysiology* **110**, 487–498.

Campos, G.E.R., Luecke, T.J., Wendeln, H.K., Toma, K., Hagerman, F.C., Murray, T.F., *et al.* (2002) Muscular adaptations in response to three different resistance-training regimens: specificity of repetition maximum training zones. *European Journal of Applied Physiology* **88**, 50–60.

Carpinelli, R.N. & Otto, R.M. (1998) Strength training: single versus multiple sets. *Sports Medicine* **26**, 73–84.

Carroll, T.J., Riek, S. & Carson, R.G. (2001) Neural adaptations to resistance training: implications for movement control. *Sports Medicine* **31**, 829–840.

Carron, A.V. (1972) Motor performance and learning under physical fatigue. *Medicine and Science in Sports and Exercise* **4**, 101–106.

Catalano, J.F. & Kleiner, B.M. (1984) Distant transfer in coincident trimming as a function of practice variability. *Perceptual and Motor Skills* **58**, 851–856.

Chilibeck, P.D., Sale, D.G. & Webber, C.E. (1995) Exercise and bone mineral density. *Sports Medicine* **19**, 103–122.

Coetzer, P., Noakes, T.D., Sanders, B., Lambert, M.I., Bosch, A.N., Wiggins, T., *et al.* (1993) Superior fatigue resistance of elite black South African distance runners. *Journal of Applied Physiology* **75**, 1822–1827.

Cowan, W.M., Fawcett, J.W., O'Leary, D.D.M. & Standfield, B.B. (1985) Regressive events in neurogenesis. In: *Neuroscience* (Abelson, P., ed.) American Association for the Advancement of Science, Washington: 13–29.

Coyle, E.F. (2000) Physical activity as a metabolic stressor. *American Journal of Clinical Nutrition* **72**, 512S–520S.

Cronin, J. & Slievert, G. (2005) Challenges in understanding the influence of maximal power training on improving athletic performance. *Sports Medicine* **35**, 213–234.

Cronin, J.B. & Hansen, K.T. (2005) Strength and power predictors of sports speed. *Journal of Strength and Conditioning Research* **19**, 349–357.

Cronin, J.B. & Henderson, M.E. (2004) Maximal strength and power assessment in novice weight trainers. *Journal of Strength and Conditioning Research* **18**, 48–52.

Cronin, J.B., McNair, P.J. & Marshall, R.N. (2003) Force–velocity analysis of strength-training techniques and load: implications for training strategy and research. *Journal of Strength and Conditioning Research* **17**, 148–155.

Daniels, J. (1998) *Daniels' Running Formula*. Human Kinetics, Champaign, IL.

Daniels, J.T. (1985) A physiologist's view of running economy. *Medicine and Science in Sports and Exercise* **17**, 332–338.

Davids, K., Lees, A. & Burwitz, L. (2000) Understanding and measuring coordination and control in kicking skills in soccer: implications for talent identification and skill acquisition. *Journal of Sports Sciences* **18**, 703–714.

Decety, J. (1996) Do imagined and executed actions share the same neural substrate? *Brain Research Cognitive Brain Research* **3**, 87–93.

Delecluse, C., Van Coppenolle, H., Willems, E., Van Leemputte, M., Diels, R., & Goris, M. (1995) Influence of high-resistance and high-velocity training on sprint performance. *Medicine and Science in Sports and Exercise* **27**, 1203–1209.

Derman, W., Schwellnus, M.P., Lambert, M.I., Emms, M., Sinclair-Smith, C., Kirby, P., *et al.* (1997) The "worn-out athlete": a clinical approach to chronic fatigue in athletes. *Journal of Sports Sciences* **15**, 341–351.

Dollman, J., Norton, K. & Norton, L. (2005) Evidence for secular trends in children's physical activity behaviour. *British Journal of Sports Medicine* **39**, 892–897.

Donoghue, J.P. (1995) Plasticity of adult sensorimotor representation. *Current Opinion in Neurobiology* **5**, 749–754.

Dugan, E.L., Doyle, T.L.A., Humphries, B.J., Hasson, C.J. & Newton, R.U. (2004) Determining the optimal load for jump squats: a review of methods and calculations. *Journal of Strength and Conditioning Research* **18**, 668–674.

Durandt, J., Tee, J.C., Prim, S.K. & Lambert, M.I. (2006) Physical fitness components associated with performance in a multiple sprint test. *International Journal of Sports Physiology and Performance* **1**, 78–88.

Duthie, G.M., Pyne, D. & Hooper, S. (2003) Applied physiology and game analysis of rugby union. *Sports Medicine* **33**, 973–991.

Edwards, S. (1997) *Smart Heart: High Performance Heart Zone Training*. Heart Zones Company, Sacramento, USA.

Elbert, T., Pantev, C., Wienbruch, C., Rockstroh, B. & Taub, E. (1995) Increased cortical representation of the fingers of the left hand in string players. *Science* **270**, 305–307.

Enoka, R.M. (1988) Muscle strength and its development: new perspectives. *Sports Medicine* **6**, 146–168.

Enoka, R.M. (1994) *Neuromechanical Basis of Kinesiology*. Human Kinetics, Campaign, IL.

Enoka, R.M. & Stuart, D.G. (1984) Henneman's size principle. *Trends in Neurosciences* **7**, 226–228.

Ericsson, K.A., Krampe, R.T. & Tesch-Romer, C. (1993) The role of deliberate practice in the acquisition of expert performance. *Psychological Review* **100**, 363–406.

Evans, W.J. (1999) Exercise training guidelines for the elderly. *Medicine and Science in Sports and Exercise* **31**, 12–17.

Farrow, D. & Abernethy, B. (2002) Can anticipatory skills be learned through implicit video-based perceptual training? *Journal of Sports Sciences* **20**, 471–485.

Farrow, D. & Abernethy, B. (2003) Implicit perceptual learning and the significance of chance comparisons: a response to Jackson. *Journal of Sports Sciences* **23**, 511–513.

Feigenbaum, M.S. & Pollock, M.L. (1997) Strength training: rationale for current guidelines for adult fitness programs. *The Physician and SportsMedicine* **25**, 44–64.

Feigenbaum, M.S. & Pollock, M.L. (1999) Prescription of resistance training for health and disease. *Medicine and Science in Sports and Exercise* **31**, 38–45.

Feltz, D.L. & Landers, D.M. (1983) The effect of mental practice on motor skill learning and performance: a meta-analysis. *Journal of Sports Psychology* **5**, 25–57.

Field, R.W. (1988) Rationale for the use of free weights for periodization. *NSCA Journal* **10**, 38–39.

Fitts, P.M. & Posner, M.I. (1967) *Human Performance*. Brooks/Cole, Belmont.

Fleck, S.J. (1983) Body composition of elite American athletes. *American Journal of Sports Medicine* **11**, 398–403.

Fleck, S.J. (1999) Periodized strength training: a critical review. *Journal of Strength and Conditioning Research* **13**, 82–89.

Fleck, S.J. & Kraemer, W.J. (1997) *Designing Resistance Training Programs*, vol. 2, 2nd edn. Human Kinetics, Champaign, IL.

Forssberg, H., Eliasson, A.C., Kinoshita, H., Westling, G. & Johansson, R.S. (1995) Development of human precision grip. IV. Tactile adaptation of isometric finger forces to the frictional condition. *Experimental Brain Research* **104**, 323–330.

Foster, C. (1998) Monitoring training in athletes with reference to overtraining syndrome. *Medicine and Science in Sports and Exercise* **30**, 1164–1168.

Foster, C., Daines, E., Hector, L., Snyder, A.C. & Welsh, R. (1996) Athletic performance in relation to training load. *Wisconsin Medical Journal* **95**, 370–374.

Foster, C., Florhaug, J.A., Franklin, J., Gottschall, L., Hrovatin, L.A., Parker, S., *et al.* (2001) A new approach to monitoring exercise training. *Journal of Strength and Conditioning Research* **15**, 109–115.

Fry, A.C. (2004) The role of resistance exercise intensity on muscle fibre adaptations. *Sports Medicine* **34**, 663–679.

Gabriel, D.A., Kamen, G. & Frost, G. (2006) Neural adaptations to resistive exercise:

mechanisms and recommendations for training practices. *Sports Medicine* **36**, 133–149.

Gentile, A.M. (1972) A working model of skill acquisition with application to teaching. *Quest* **17**, 3–23.

Gentile, A.M. (1987) Skill acquisition: action, movement, and neuromotor process. In: *Movement Science: Foundations for Physical Therapy in Rehabilitation* (Carr, J.H., Shepard, R.B., Gordon, J., Gentile, A.M. & Hinds, J.M., eds.) Aspen, Rockville, MD: 93–154.

Gentile, A.M. (1998) Implicit and explicit processes during acquisition of functional skills. *Scandinavian Journal of Occupational Therapy* **5**, 7–16.

Gentile, A.M. (2000) Skill acquisition: action, movement and neuromotor process. In: *Movement Science: Foundations for Physical Therapy in Rehabilitation* (Carr, J.H., Shepard, R.B., Gordon, J., Gentile, A.M. & Hinds, J.M., eds.) Aspen, Rockville, MD: 111–187.

Getchell, B. (1985) *Physical Fitness: A Way of Life*. MacMillan Publishing, New York.

Gill, N.D., Beaven, C.M. & Cook, C. (2006) Effectiveness of post-match recovery strategies in rugby players. *British Journal of Sports Medicine* **40**, 260–263.

Gleim, G.W. & McHugh, M.P. (1997) Flexibility and its effects on sports injury and performance. *Sports Medicine* **24**, 289–299.

González-Badillo, J.J., Gorostiaga, E.M., Arellano, R. & Izquierdo, M. (2005) Moderate resistance training volume produces more favorable strength gains than high or low volumes during a short-term training cycle. *Journal of Strength and Conditioning Research* **19**, 689–697.

Goode, S. & Magill, R.A. (1986) Contextual interference effects in learning three badminton serves. *Research Quarterly for Exercise and Sport* **57**, 308–314.

Goto, K., Nagasawa, M., Yanagisawa, O., Kizuka, T., Ishii, N., & Takamatsu, K. (2004) Muscular adaptations to combinations of high- and low-intensity resistance exercises. *Journal of Strength and Conditioning Research* **18**, 730–737.

Grafton, S.T., Arbib, M.A., Fadiga, L. & Rizzolatti, G. (1996) Localization of grasp representation in humans by positron emission tomography. 2. Observation compared with imagination. *Experimental Brain Research* **112**, 103–111.

Green, H.J., Jones, L.L. & Painter, D.C. (1990) Effects of short-term training on

cardiac function during prolonged exercise. *Medicine and Science in Sports and Exercise* **22**, 488–493.

Haff, G.G. (2000) Roundtable discussion: Machine versus free weights. *Strength and Conditioning Journal* **22**, 18–30.

Haff, G.G. (2004a) Roundtable discussion: Periodization of training. Part 1. *Strength and Conditioning Journal* **26**, 50–59.

Haff, G.G. (2004b) Roundtable discussion: Periodization of training. Part 2. *Strength and Conditioning Journal* **26**, 56–70.

Haguenauer, M., Fargier, P., Legreneur, E., Dufour, A.B., Cogerino, G., Begon, M., *et al.* (2005) Short-term effects of using verbal instructions and demonstration at the beginning of learning a complex skill in figure skating. *Perceptual and Motor Skills* **100**, 179–191.

Hakkinen, K., Alen, M., Kraemer, W.J., Gorostiaga, E., Izquierdo, M., Rusko, H., *et al.* (2003) Neuromuscular adaptations during concurrent strength and endurance training versus strength training. *European Journal of Applied Physiology and Occupational Physiology* **89**, 42–52.

Hall, K.G., Domingues, D.A. & Cavazos, R. (1994) Contextual interference effects with skilled baseball players. *Perceptual and Motor Skills* **78**, 835–841.

Halson, S.L., Bridge, M.W., Meeusen, R., Busschaert, B., Gleeson, M., Jones, D.A., *et al.* (2002) Time course of performance changes and fatigue markers during intensified training in trained cyclists. *Journal of Applied Physiology* **93**, 947–956.

Hass, C.J., Feigenbaum, M.S. & Franklin, B.A. (2001) Prescription of resistance training for healthy populations. *Sports Medicine* **31**, 953–964.

Hass, C.J., Garzarella, L., De Hoyos, D.V. & Pollock, M.L. (2000) Single versus multiple sets and long-term recreational weightlifters. *Medicine and Science in Sports and Exercise* **32**, 235–242.

Hedrick, A. (2002) Learning from each other: training to increase power. *Strength and Conditioning Journal* **24**, 25–27.

Hellard, P., Avalos, M., Millet, G., Lacoste, L., Barale, F., & Chatard, J.C. (2005) Modelling the residual effects and threshold saturation of training: a case study of Olympic swimmers. *Journal of Strength and Conditioning Research* **19**, 67–75.

Hellenbrandt, F. & Houtz, S. (1956) Mechanism of muscle training in man: experimental demonstration of the overload principle. *Physical Therapy Reviews* **36**, 371–383.

Henriksson, J. (1992) Effects of physical training on the metabolism of skeletal muscle. *Diabetes Care* **15**, 1701–1711.

Higgins, D. & Kaminski, T.W. (1998) Contrast therapy does not cause fluctuations in human gastrocnemius intramuscular temperature. *Journal of Athletic Training* **33**, 336–340.

Ho, L. & Shea, J.B. (1978) Effects of relative frequency of knowledge of results on retention of a motor skill. *Perceptual Motor Skills* **46**, 859–866.

Hodges, N.J. & Franks, I.M. (2002) Modelling coaching practice: the role of instruction and demonstration. *Journal of Sports Sciences* **20**, 793–811.

Hodges, N.J. & Lee, T.D. (1999) The role of augmented information prior to learning a bimanual visual-motor coordination task: do instructions of the movement pattern facilitate learning relative to discovery learning? *British Journal of Psychology* **90**, 389–403.

Hodges, P.W. (2003) Motor control. In: *Physical Therapies and Sport and Exercise* (Kolt, G.S. & Snyder-Mackler, L., eds.) Churchill Livingstone, Edinburgh: 107–125.

Horn, R.R. & Williams, A.M. (2004) Observational learning: Is it time we took another look? In: *Skill Acquisition in Sport: Research, Theory and Practice* (Williams, A.M. & Hodges, N.J., eds.) Routledge, London: 175–206.

Hughes, H.G. (1996) *The effects of static stretching on the musculo-tendinous unit.* MSc thesis, University of Cape Town, South Africa.

Hullinger, M., Sjolander, P., Windhorst, U.R. & Otten, E. (1995) Force coding by populations of cat Golgi tendon organ efferents: the role of muscle length and motor unit pool activation strategies. In: *Alpha and Gamma Motor Systems* (Taylor, A., Gladden, M.H. & Durrbaba, R., eds.) Plenum Press, New York: 302–308.

Irrcher, I., Adhihetty, P.J., Joseph, A.M., Ljubicic, V. & Hood, D.A. (2003) Regulation of mitochondrial biogenesis in muscle by endurance exercise. *Sports Medicine* **33**, 783–793.

Izquierdo, M., Häkkinen, K., González-Badillo, J.J., Ibánez, J. & Gorostiaga, E.M. (2002) Effects of long-term training specificity on maximal strength and power of the upper and lower extremities in athletes from different sports. *European Journal of Applied Physiology* **87**, 264–271.

Jackson, R.C. (2003) Evaluating the evidence for implicit perceptual learning: a re-analysis of Farrow and Abernethy (2002). *Journal of Sports Sciences* **21**, 503–509.

Jaegers, S.M.H.J., Peterson, R.F., Dantuma, R., Hillen, B., Gueze, R. & Schellekens, J. (1989) Kinesiologic aspects of motor learning in dart throwing. *Journal of Human Movement Studies* **16**, 161–171.

Jeannerod, M. (1995) Mental imagery in the motor context. *Neuropsychologica* **33**, 1419–1432.

Jennings, C.L., Viljoen, W., Durandt, J. & Lambert, M.I. (2005) The reliability of the FitroDyne as a measure of muscle power. *Journal of Strength and Conditioning Research* **19**, 859–863.

Jensen, L., Bangsbo, J. & Hellsten, Y. (2004) Effect of high intensity training on capillarization and presence of angiogenic factors in human skeletal muscle. *Journal of Physiology* **557**, 571–582.

Kaas, J.H. (1991) Plasticity of sensory and motor maps in adult mammals. *Annual Review of Neuroscience* **14**, 137–167.

Kamon, E. & Gormley, J. (1968) Muscular activity patterns for skilled performance and during learning of a horizontal bar exercise. *Ergonomics* **11**, 345–347.

Kawamori, N. & Haff, G.G. (2004) The optimal training load for the development of muscular power. *Journal of Strength and Conditioning Research* **18**, 675–684.

Kawamori, N., Crum, A.J., Blumert, P.A., Kulik, J.R., Childers, J.T., Wood, J.A., *et al.* (2005) Influence of different relative intensities on power output during the hang power clean: identification of the optimal load. *Journal of Strength and Conditioning Research* **19**, 698–708.

Kenttä, G. & Hassmen, P. (1998) Overtraining and recovery: a conceptual model. *Sports Medicine* **26**, 1–16.

Kontor, K. (1988) Historical perspectives and future considerations for strength training in athletics. In: *Muscle Development: Nutritional Alternatives to Anabolic Steroids* (Garrett, W.E. & Malone, T.R., eds.) Ross Laboratories, Columbus, OH: 1–7.

Kraemer, W.J., Bush, J.A., Wickham, R.B., Denegar, C.R., Gomez, A.L., Gotshalk, L.A., *et al.* (2001) Influence of compression therapy on symptoms following soft tissue injury from maximal eccentric exercise. *Journal of Orthopedic Sports Physical Therapy* **31**, 282–290.

Kraemer, W.J. & Ratamess, N.A. (2004) Fundamentals of resistance training: progression and exercise prescription.

Medicine and Science in Sports and Exercise **36**, 674–688.

Kuipers, H. & Keizer, H.A. (1988) Overtraining in elite athletes: review and directions for the future. *Sports Medicine* **6**, 79–92.

Kulhavy, R.W. & Wager, W. (1993) Feedback in programmed instruction: historical context and implications for practice. In: *Interactive Instruction and Feedback* (Dempsey, J.V. & Sales, G.C., eds.) Educational Technology, Englewood Cliffs, NJ: 3–20.

Lambert, M.I. (2006) Physiological testing: help or hype? *International Journal of Sports Science and Coaching* **1**, 199–208.

Lambert, M.I. & Borresen, J. (2006) A theoretical basis of monitoring fatigue: a practical approach for coaches. *International Journal of Sports Science and Coaching* **1**, 371–388.

Lambert, M.I. & Noakes, T.D. (1989) Dissociation of changes in $\dot{V}o_{2max}$, muscle Qo_2, and performance with training in rats. *Journal of Applied Physiology* **66**, 1620–1625.

Lambert, M.I., Mbambo, Z.H. & St Clair Gibson, A. (1998) Heart rate during training and competition for long-distance running. *Journal of Sports Sciences* **16**, S85–S90.

Landin, D.L. & Herbert, E.P. (1997) A comparison of three practice schedules along the contextual interference continuum. *Research Quarterly for Exercise and Sport* **68**, 357–361.

Laursen, P.B. & Jenkins, D.G. (2002) The scientific basis for high-intensity interval training: optimising training programmes and maximising performance in highly trained endurance athletes. *Sports Medicine* **32**, 53–73.

Lees, A. & Nolan, L. (2002) Three dimensional kinematic analysis of the instep kick under speed and accuracy conditions. In: *Science and Football*, Vol. 4 (Spinks, W., Reilly, T. & Murphy, A., eds.) Routledge, London: 16–21.

Lees, A., Kershaw, L. & Moura, F. (2005) The three-dimensional nature of the maximal instep kick in soccer. In: *Science and Football*, Vol. 5 (Reilly, T., Cabri, J. & Araujo D., eds.) Routledge, London: 64–69.

Léger, L.A. & Lambert, J. (1982) A maximal multistage 20-m shuttle run test to predict $\dot{V}o_{2max}$. *European Journal of Applied Physiology and Occupational Physiology* **49**, 1–12.

Lehmann, M., Foster, C. & Keul, J. (1993) Overtraining in endurance athletes: a brief review. *Medicine and Science in Sports and Exercise* **25**, 854–862.

Leighton, J.R. (1966) The Leighton flexometer and flexibility test. *Journal of the Association for Physical and Mental Rehabilitation* **20**, 86–93.

Leonard, C.T. (1998) *The Neuroscience of Human Movement*. Mosby, St Louis, MO.

Lindsay, F.H., Hawley, J.A., Myburgh, K.H., Schomer, H.H., Noakes, T.D., & Dennis, S.C. (1996) Improved athletic performance in highly trained cyclists after interval training. *Medicine and Science in Sports and Exercise* **28**, 1427–1434.

Lotze, M. & Halsband, U. (2006) Motor imagery. *Journal of Physiology (Paris)* **99**, 386–395.

Lyons, M., Al-Nakeeb, Y. & Nevill, A. (2006) The impact of moderate and high intensity total body fatigue on passing accuracy in expert and novice basketball players. *Journal of Sports Science and Medicine* **5**, 215–227.

Mader, A. (1988) A transcription–translation activation feedback circuit as a function of protein degradation, with the quality of protein mass adaptation related to the average functional load. *Journal of Theoretical Biology* **134**, 135–157.

Magill, R.A. (1993) *Motor Learning: Concepts and Applications* (4th edn.). Wm C. Brown, Dubuque, IA.

Magill, R.A. (1998) *Motor Learning: Concepts and Applications* (5th edn.). McGraw-Hill, Boston, MA.

Magill, R.A. (2003) *Motor Learning and Control: Concepts and Applications* (7th edn.). McGraw-Hill, Boston, MA.

Magill, R.A. & Schoenfelder-Zohdi, B. (1996) A visual model and knowledge of performance as sources of information in learning a rhythmic gymnastics rope skill. *International Journal of Sport Psychology* **27**, 7–22.

Magill, R.A. & Wood, C.A. (1986) Knowledge of results precision as a learning variable in motor skill acquisition. *Research Quarterly for Exercise and Sport* **57**, 170–173.

Margolis, J.F. & Christina, R.W. (1981) A test of Schmidt's schema theory of discrete motor skill learning. *Research Quarterly for Exercise and Sport* **52**, 474–483.

Margulies, J.Y., Simkin, A., Leichter, I., Bivas, A., Steinberg, R., Giladi, M., *et al.* (1986) Effect of intense physical activity on the bone-mineral content in the lower limbs of young adults. *Journal of Bone and Joint Surgery* **68**, 1090–1093.

Martin, A.D., Spenst, L.F., Drinkwater, D.T. & Clarys, J.P. (1990) Anthropometric estimation of muscle mass in men. *Medicine and Science in Sports and Exercise* **22**, 729–733.

Masters, R.S.W. (1992) Knowledge, nerves and know-how: the role of explicit versus implicit knowledge in the breakdown of a complex motor skill under pressure. *British Journal of Psychology* **83**, 343–358.

Masters, R.S.W. (2000) Theoretical aspects of implicit learning in sport. *International Journal of Sport Psychology* **31**, 530–541.

McBride, J.M., Triplett-McBride, T., Davie, A. & Newton, R.U. (2002) The effect of heavy- vs. light-load jump squats on the development of strength, speed and power. *Journal of Strength and Conditioning Research* **16**, 75–82.

McCracken, H.D. & Stelmach, G.E. (1977) A test of schema theory of discrete motor learning. *Journal of Motor Behaviour* **9**, 193–201.

McCullagh, P., Stiehl, J. & Weiss, M.R. (1990) Developmental modelling effects on the quantitative and qualitative aspects of motor performance. *Research Quarterly for Exercise and Sport* **61**, 344–350.

McNair, D.M., Lorr, M. & Droppleman, L.F. (1971) *Manual for the Profile of Mood States*. Educational and Industrial Testing Service, San Diego, CA.

Meeusen, R., Duclos, M., Gleeson, M., Rietjens, G.J., Steinacker, J.M. & Urhausen, A. (2006) Prevention, diagnosis and treatment of the overtraining syndrome. *European Journal of Sport Science* **6**, 1–14.

Morgan, W.P., Brown, D.R., Raglin, J.S., O'Connor, P.J. & Ellickson, K.A. (1987) Psychological monitoring of overtraining and staleness. *British Journal of Sports Medicine* **21**, 107–114.

Moritani, T. (1993) Neuromuscular adaptations during the acquisition of muscle strength, power and motor tasks. *Journal of Biomechanics* **26**, 95–107.

Morton, R.H. (1997) Modelling training and overtraining. *Journal of Sports Sciences* **15**, 335–340.

Mujika, I., Padilla, S., Pyne, D. & Busso, T. (2004) Physiological changes associated with the pre-event taper in athletes. *Sports Medicine* **34**, 891–927.

Naylor, J. & Briggs, G. (1961) Effects of task complexity and task organization on the relative efficiency of part and whole training methods. *Journal of Experimental Psychology* **65**, 217–244.

Newell, A. & Rosenbloom, P.S. (1981) Mechanisms of skill acquisition and the law of practice. In: *Cognitive Skills and Their Acquisition* (Anderson, J.R., ed.) Erlbaum, Hillsdale, NJ: 1–56.

Newton, R.U., Murphy, A.J., Humphries, B.J., Wilson, G.J., Kraemer, W.J., & Häkkinen, K. (1997) Influence of load and stretch–shortening cycle on kinematics, kinetics and muscle activation that occurs during explosive upper-body movements. *European Journal of Applied Physiology* **75**, 333–342.

Noakes, T.D. (2001) *Lore of Running*. Oxford University Press, Cape Town, South Africa.

Noth, J. (1992) Motor units. In: *Strength and Power in Sport* (Komi, P.V., ed.) Blackwell Scientific Publications, Oxford: 21–28.

Oldenziel, K.E., Gagne, F. & Gulbin, J.P. (2003) *How do elite athletes develop? A look through the "rear-view" mirror: a preliminary report from the National Athlete Development Survey (NADS)*. Australian Sports Commission, Belconnen, Australia.

Oldenziel, K.E., Gagne, F. & Gulbin, J.P. (2004) Factors affecting the rate of athlete development from novice to senior elite: How applicable is the 10-year rule? In: *Proceedings of the 2004 Pre-Olympic Congress* (Klisouras, V., Kellis, S. & Mouratidis, I., eds.) Aristotle University of Thessaloniki, Thessaloniki, Greece: 174.

Papagelopoulos, P.J., Mavrogenis, A.F. & Soucacos, P.N. (2004) Doping in ancient and modern Olympic Games. *Orthopedics* **27**, 1226–1231.

Pascaul-Leone, A. & Torres, F. (1993) Plasticity of the sensorimotor cortex representation of the reading finger in Braille readers. *Brain* **116**, 39–52.

Pascaul-Leone, A., Dang, N., Cohen, L.G., Brasil-Neto, J.P., Cammarota, A. & Hallett, M. (1995) Modulation of muscle responses evoked by transcranial magnetic stimulation during the acquisition of new fine motor skills. *Journal of Neurophysiology* **74**, 1037–1043.

Pascual-Leone, A., Grafman, J. & Hallett, M. (1994) Modulation of cortical motor output maps during development of implicit and explicit knowledge. *Science* **263**, 1287–1289.

Pearce, A.J., Sacco, P., Byrnes, M.L., Thickbroom, G.W. & Mastaglia, F.L. (1998) The effects of eccentric exercise on neuromuscular function of the biceps brachii. *Journal of Science and Medicine in Sport* **1**, 236–244.

Pearce, A.J., Thickbroom, G.W., Byrnes, M.L. & Mastaglia, F.L. (2000) The corticomotor representation of elite racquet sport athletes. *Experimental Brain Research* **130**, 238–243.

Pearson, D., Faigenbaum, A., Conley, M. & Kraemer, W.J. (2000) The National Strength and Conditioning Association's basic guidelines for resistance training of athletes. *Strength and Conditioning Journal* **22**, 14–27.

Perkins, I.V. & Teyler, T.J. (1988) A critical period for long-term potentiation in the developing rat visual cortex. *Brain Research* **439**, 222–229.

Peterson, M.D., Rhea, M.R. & Alvar, B.A. (2004) Maximizing strength development in athletes: a meta-analysis to determine the dose–response relationship. *Journal of Strength and Conditioning Research* **18**, 377–382.

Pollock, M.L., Franklin, B.A., Balady, G.J., Chaitman, B.L., Fleg, J.L., Fletcher, B., *et al.* (2000) Resistance exercise in individuals with and without cardiovascular disease. *Circulation* **101**, 828–833.

Pollock, M.L. & Graves, J.E. (1994) Exercise training and prescription for the elderly. *Southern Medical Journal* **87**, S88–S95.

Radford, P. (2000) Endurance runners in Britain before the 20th century. In: *Marathon Medicine* (Tunstall Pedoe, D., ed.) Royal Society of Medicine Press, London: 15–27.

Reeve, T.G. & Magill, R.A. (1981) The role of the components of knowledge of results information in error correction. *Research Quarterly for Exercise and Sport* **52**, 80–85.

Rhea, M.R., Alvar, B.A. & Burkett, L.N. (2002a) Single versus multiple sets for strength: a meta-analysis to address the controversy. *Research Quarterly for Exercise and Sport* **73**, 485–488.

Rhea, M.R., Alvar, B.A., Ball, S.D. & Burkett, L.N. (2002b) Three sets of weight training superior to 1 set with equal intensity for eliciting strength. *Journal of Strength and Conditioning Research* **16**, 525–529.

Rhea, M.R., Alvar, B.A., Burkett, L.N. & Ball, S.D. (2003) A meta-analysis to determine the dose response for strength development. *Medicine and Science in Sports and Exercise* **35**, 456–464.

Robertson, D.G.E. & Mosher, R.E. (1985) Work and power of the leg muscles in soccer kicking. In: *Biomechanics*, Vol. IX-B (Winter, D.A., Norman, R.W., Wells, R.P., Hayes, K.C. & Patla, A.E., eds.)

Human Kinetics, Champaign, IL: 533–538.

Robinson, J.M., Stone, M.H., Johnson, R.L., Penland, C.M., Warren, B.J., & Lewis, R.D. (1995) Effects of different weight training exercise/rest intervals on strength, power, and high intensity exercise endurance. *Journal of Strength and Conditioning Research* **9**, 216–221.

Roetert, E.P., Crespo, M. & Reid, M.M. (2003) How to become a model. *ITF Coaching and Sports Science Review* **31**, 12.

Rose, D.J. & Christina, R.W. (2006) *A Multilevel Approach to the Study of Motor Control and Learning.* Pearson Benjamin Cummings, San Francisco, CA.

Rothwell, J.C. (1994) *Control of Human Voluntary Movement.* Chapman and Hall, London.

Rushall, B.S. (1990) A tool for measuring stress tolerance in elite athletes. *Journal of Applied Sport Psychology* **2**, 51–66.

Santana, J.C. (2001) Machines versus free weights. *Strength and Conditioning Journal* **23**, 67–68.

Saxton, J.M., Clarkson, P.M., James, R., Miles, M., Westerfer, M., Clark, S., *et al.* (1995) Neuromuscular function following eccentric exercise. *Medicine and Science in Sports and Exercise* **27**, 1185–1193.

Schmidt, R.A. (1991) *Motor Learning and Performance: From Principles to Practice.* Human Kinetics, Champaign, IL.

Schmidt, R.A. & Lee, T.A. (1999) *Motor Control and Learning: A Behavioral Emphasis.* Human Kinetics, Champaign, IL.

Schwellnus, M.P. (1999) Skeletal muscle cramps during exercise. *The Physician and SportsMedicine* **27**, 109–115.

Scully, T.J. & Besterman, G. (1982) Stress fracture: a preventable training injury. *Military Medicine* **147**, 285–287.

Semenick, D.M. (1994) Testing protocols and procedures. In: *Essentials of Strength Training and Conditioning* (Baechle, T.R., ed.) Human Kinetics, Champaign, IL: 258–273.

Shea, C.H., Kohl, R. & Indermill, C. (1990) Contextual interference: contributions of practice. *Acta Psychologica* **73**, 145–157.

Shea, J.B. & Morgan, R.L. (1979) Contextual interference effects on the acquisition, retention, and transfer of a motor skill. *Journal of Experimental Psychology: Human Learning and Memory* **5**, 179–187.

Shellock, F.G. & Prentice, W.E. (1985) Warming-up and stretching for improved physical performance and prevention of sports-related injuries. *Sports Medicine* **2**, 267–278.

Shrier, I. & Gossel, K. (2000) Myths and truths of stretching. *The Physician and SportsMedicine* **28**, 57–63.

Siegel, J.A., Gilders, R.M., Staron, R.S. & Hagerman, F.C. (2002) Human muscle power output during upper- and lower-body exercises. *Journal of Strength and Conditioning Research* **16**, 173–178.

Sirigu, A., Duhamel, J., Cohen, L., Pillon, B., Dubois, B. & Agid, Y. (1996) The mental representation of hand movements after parietal cortex damage. *Science* **273**, 1564–1568.

Smith, D.J. (2003) A framework for understanding the training process leading to elite performance. *Sports Medicine* **33**, 1103–1126.

Smith, T.P., McNaughton, L.R. & Marshall, K.J. (1999) Effects of 4-wk training using Vmax/Tmax on $\dot{V}o_{2max}$ and performance in athletes. *Medicine and Science in Sports and Exercise* **31**, 892–896.

Smoll, F.L. (1972) Effects of precision of information feedback upon acquisition of a motor skill. *Research Quarterly for Exercise and Sport* **43**, 489–493.

Stepto, N.K., Hawley, J.A., Dennis, S.C. & Hopkins, W.G. (1999) Effects of different interval-training programs on cycling time-trial performance. *Medicine and Science in Sports and Exercise* **31**, 736–741.

Stone, M.H., Collins, D., Plisk, S., Haff, G. & Stone, M.E. (2000a) Training principles: evaluation of modes and methods of resistance training. *Strength and Conditioning Journal* **22**, 65–76.

Stone, M.H., O'Bryant, H.S., McCoy, L., Coglianese, R., Lehmkuhl, M., & Schilling, B. (2003a) Power and maximum strength relationships during performance of dynamic and static weighted jumps. *Journal of Strength and Conditioning Research* **17**, 140–147.

Stone, M.H., O'Bryant, H.S., Schilling, B.K., Johnson, R.L., Pierce, K.C., Haff, G., *et al.* (1999) Periodization: effects of manipulating volume and intensity. Part 1. *Journal of Strength and Conditioning Research* **21**, 56–62.

Stone, M.H., Pierce, K.C., Sands, W.A. & Stone, M.E. (2006) Weightlifting: a brief overview. *Strength and Conditioning Journal* **28**, 50–66.

Stone, M.H., Potteiger, J.A., Pierce, K.C., Proulx, C.M., O'Bryant, H.S., Johnson, R.L., *et al.* (2000b) Comparison of the effects of three different weight-training programs on the one repetition maximum squat. *Journal of Strength and Conditioning Research* **14**, 332–337.

Stone, M.H., Sanborn, K., O'Bryant, H.S., Hartman, M., Stone, M.E., Proulx, C.M., *et al.* (2003b) Maximum strength–power–performance relationships in collegiate throwers. *Journal of Strength and Conditioning Research* **17**, 739–745.

Swanson, R.A. & Law, B. (1993) Whole–part–whole learning model. *Performance Improvement Quarterly* **6**, 43–53.

Swart, J. & Jennings, C. (2004) Use of blood lactate concentration as a marker of training status. *South African Journal of Sports Medicine* **16**, 3–7.

Sweet, T.W., Foster, C., McGuigan, M.R. & Brice, G. (2004) Quantitation of resistance training using the session rating of perceived exertion method. *Journal of Strength and Conditioning Research* **18**, 796–802.

Takarada, Y. (2003) Evaluation of muscle damage after a rugby match with special reference to tackle plays. *British Journal of Sports Medicine* **37**, 416–419.

Thomas, J.R., Cotton, D.J., Spieth, W.R. & Abraham, N.L. (1975) Effects of fatigue on stabilometer performance and learning of males and females. *Medicine and Science in Sports and Exercise* **7**, 203–206.

Tipton, C.M. (1997) Sports medicine: a century of progress. *Journal of Nutrition* **127**, 878S–885S.

Tricoli, V., Lamas, L., Carnevale, R. & Ugrinowitsch, C. (2005) Short-term effects on lower-body functional power development: weightlifting vs. vertical jump training programs. *Journal of Strength and Conditioning Research* **19**, 433–437.

Urhausen, A. & Kindermann, W. (1992) Echocardiographic findings in strength- and endurance-trained athletes. *Sports Medicine* **13**, 270–284.

Vorro, J., Wilson, F.R. & Dainis, A. (1978) Multivariate analysis of biomechanical profiles for the coracobrachialis and biceps brachii (caput breve) muscles in humans. *Ergonomics* **21**, 407–418.

Walsh, L.D., Hesse, C.W., Morgan, D.L. & Proske, U. (2004) Human forearm position sense after fatigue of elbow flexor muscles. *Journal of Physiology (London)* **558**, 705–715.

Wathen, D., Baechle, T.R. & Earle, R.W. (2000) Training variation: Periodization. In: *NSCA: Essentials of strength training and conditioning*, 2nd edn. (Baechle, T.R. & Earle, R.W., eds.) Human Kinetics, Champaign, IL: 513–528.

Weiss, M.R. & Klint, K.A. (1987) Show and tell in the gymnasium: an investigation of developmental differences in modelling and verbal rehearsal for motor skills. *Research Quarterly for Exercise and Sport* **58**, 234–241.

Westgarth-Taylor, C., Hawley, J.A., Rickard, S., Myburgh, K.H., Noakes, T.D. & Dennis, S.C. (1997) Metabolic and performance adaptations to interval training in endurance-trained cyclists. *European Journal of Applied Physiology and Occupational Physiology* **75**, 298–304.

Wightman, D.C. & Lintern, G. (1985) Part-task training strategies for tracking and manual control. *Human Factors* **27**, 267–283.

Willardson, J.M. & Burkett, L.N. (2005) A comparison of 3 different rest intervals on the exercise volume completed during a workout. *Journal of Strength and Conditioning Research* **19**, 23–26.

Williams, A.M. & Grant, A. (1999) Training perceptual skill in sport. *International Journal of Sport Psychology* **30**, 194–220.

Williams, A.M. & Hodges, N. (2005) Practice, instruction and skill acquisition in soccer: challenging tradition. *Journal of Sports Sciences* **23**, 637–650.

Williams, L.R. & Walmsley, A. (2000) Response timing and muscular coordination in fencing: a comparison of elite and novice fencers. *Journal of Science and Medicine in Sport* **3**, 460–475.

Wilson, G.J., Newton, R.U., Murphy, A.J. & Humphries, B.J. (1993) The optimal training load for development of dynamic athletic performance. *Medicine and Science in Sports and Exercise* **25**, 1279–1286.

Winett, R.A. & Carpinelli, R.N. (2001) Potential health-related benefits of resistance training. *Preventative Medicine* **33**, 503–513.

Wolfe, B.L., LeMura, L.M. & Cole, P.J. (2004) Quantitative analysis of single- vs. multiple-set programs in resistance training. *Journal of Strength and Conditioning Research* **18**, 35–47.

Wulf, G. & Weigelt, C. (1997) Instructions about physical principles in learning a complex motor skill: to tell or not to tell. *Research Quarterly for Exercise and Sport* **68**, 362–369.

Young, W.B. (2006) Transfer of strength and power to training to sports performance. *International Journal of Sports Physiology and Performance* **1**, 74–83.

Zavorsky, G.S. (2000) Evidence and possible mechanisms of altered maximum heart rate with endurance training and tapering. *Sports Medicine* **29**, 13–26.

Chapter 2

Adaptations to Training

INTRODUCTION

IÑIGO MUJIKA

Performing repeated and systematic bouts of physical exercise over numerous days, weeks, months, or years (i.e., training) is expected to bring about anatomic and physiologic adaptive responses which eventually lead to improvements in sports performance. For these adaptations to be effective, a structured, well-designed training program that adheres to the basic principles of training overload, specificity, individuality, and reversibility should be implemented. In addition, an effective training program should take the concept of fatigue into consideration and include sufficient time for regenerative recovery to allow morphologic and functional adaptations to occur. The emphasis of this chapter is on the adaptations taking place in the various bodily organs and systems as a result of endurance or strength type training in athletes.

The initial section of this chapter deals with the complex issue of fatigue and its elusive underlying mechanisms. To this aim, fatigue is defined, its different manifestations are described, and the various models explaining peripheral and central fatigue are compiled.

The following sections deal with the specific adaptations observed as a result of physical training in the different body organs and systems. Changes in muscle morphology and function induced by aerobic and strength-oriented training are analyzed

The Olympic Textbook of Medicine in Sport, 1st edition. Edited by M. Schwellnus. Published 2008 by Blackwell Publishing, ISBN: 978-1-4051-5637-0.

in the second section of the chapter. These exercise training modalities also induce a series of metabolic adaptations that have direct implications for athletic performance, which are thoroughly discussed in the third section of the chapter. The next section focuses on the adaptations to regular physical activity in relation to acute hormonal responses to physical activity. In this respect, the section deals not only with classic endocrine organs and hormones, but also with recently identified substances with an autocrine, paracrine, and endocrine action. The fifth section of the chapter highlights the major cardiac and respiratory adaptations resulting from endurance training, which improve oxygen transport and promote performance in endurance sporting events. The sixth and final section is dedicated to the structural and mechanical adaptation of bone and connective tissues to the functional demands imposed by athletic training.

It is hoped that this chapter will achieve the goal of providing the sports physician with the most up-to-date compilation of the available knowledge on the physiologic and anatomic adaptations to training, and facilitate the understanding of the adaptation process in the trained athlete.

MODELS OF FATIGUE

SHONA HALSON AND IÑIGO MUJIKA

Introduction

Fatigue is a complex and multifaceted phenomenon, the underlying mechanisms of which remain somewhat elusive. The lack of clear comprehension regarding the sites and mechanisms of skeletal muscle fatigue is indicative of the complexity of the fatigue process.

The common definition of fatigue proposed by Edwards (1983) states that fatigue is a "failure to maintain the required or expected force (or power output)." Others (Bigland-Ritchie & Woods 1984; Vollestad & Sejersted 1988) have chosen to adopt the concept of fatigue as a loss of force generating capacity because losses in force are gradual, do not occur abruptly, and begin at exercise or contraction initiation as determined from electrically stimulated muscle experiments (Bigland-Ritchie *et al.* 1986; Vollestad *et al.* 1988). The definitions used in this chapter are those presented by Gandevia (2001) as the definition of muscle fatigue reflects both peripheral and central fatigue and focuses on the reduction in force that occurs during fatigue.

Muscle fatigue: Any exercise-induced reduction in the ability of a muscle to generate force or power; it has central and peripheral causes.

Peripheral fatigue: Fatigue produced by changes at or distal to the neuromuscular junction.

Central fatigue: A progressive reduction in voluntary activation of muscle during exercise.

These definitions reflect the alternate interpretation of data depending on the experimental model employed and the conditions under which they occur. Thus, muscle contraction and fatigue can vary depending on the type of stimulus (voluntary or electrical), type of contraction (isometric, isotonic, and intermittent or continual), duration, frequency, intensity, type of muscle, and species (Sahlin 1992). Additionally, the physiologic and training status of the individual, contractile history of the muscle (Maclaren *et al.* 1989), and the environmental conditions are also significant factors influencing fatigue (Brooks *et al.* 1996).

As much of the research investigating sites and mechanisms of fatigue has been performed on isolated muscle preparations, it is assumed that changes in the whole muscle reflect metabolic changes in the individual muscle cell (Edwards 1983). Thus, the relevance of results obtained from *in vitro* preparations and muscle stimulation experiments should be considered when examining models of fatigue. In addition, an interactive effect is likely and whether the changes in an isolated fatigueinducing event can represent the gross changes observed in motor behaviour are questionable (Green 1990). However, the failure at one site of fatigue, such as a specific enzyme or cell, or an accumulation of a particular metabolite, is likely to affect other cells, enzymes, and metabolites and thus the cause(s) of fatigue are interactive (Brooks *et al.* 1996). A further issue confounding the identification of the site of fatigue involves compartmentalization of the body into systems and organs through to cells and organelles (Brook *et al.* 1996). Thus, the site of fatigue may be masked when dysfunction occurs in one particular site within a cell, but not in another (i.e., depletion of ATP may occur at the myosin cross-bridge but may be sufficient at other sites within the cell; Brooks *et al.* 1996).

When examining various models of fatigue a description of the chain of command for muscular contraction aids in identifying possible fatigue mechanisms (Fig. 2.1; Edwards 1983). This scheme

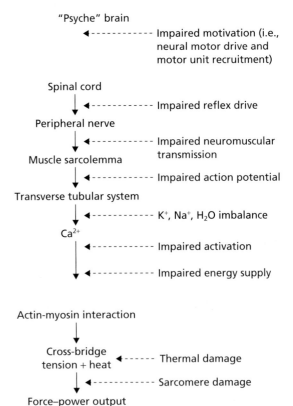

Fig. 2.1 Chain of command for muscular contraction and the possible mechanisms underlying fatigue. (Edwards & Wiles 1981.)

suggests that alterations or impairments at any of these sites may result in fatigue. "Failure" may occur at more than one site and may be interactive among sites.

Central vs. peripheral fatigue

Further division within the scheme highlighted above is often made at the level of the neuromuscular junction, differentiating peripheral from central fatigue (Fig. 2.1). Whether the origin of fatigue resides in the central nervous system or within the muscles is a question that has received much debate. According to Green (1990), altered central motor drive can be the result of changes in the excitability of the motoneuron or an inability of the motor nerve to conduct a repetitive action potential to the presynaptic side of the neuromuscular junction. Altered motoneuron can be the result of intrinsic properties of the motoneurons themselves, higher centers, feedback mechanisms from the muscle, recurrent inhibition, or branch point failure (Fig. 2.2). At the skeletal muscle fiber level, potential sites of fatigue are many and include: failure of the sarcolemma and/or T tubule to conduct a regenerative action potential; failure of the coupling between the T tubule and the sarcoplasmic reticulum; and failure at the level of the sarcoplasmic reticulum itself

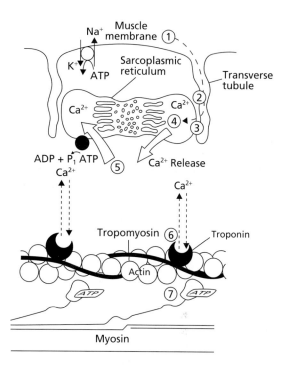

Fig. 2.3 Diagrammatic representation of major components of a muscle cell involved in excitation contraction coupling. Numbers indicate possible sites of muscular fatigue during heavy exercise and include the following: (1) surface membrane; (2) T tubular charge movement; (3) mechanisms coupling T tubular charge movement with sarcoplasmic reticulum (SR) Ca^{2+} release; (4) SR Ca^{2+} release; (5) SR Ca^{2+} reuptake; (6) Ca^{2+} binding to troponin; and (7) myosin binding to actin, ATP hydrolysis and cross-bridge force development and cycle rate. (From Fitts 1994 with permission.)

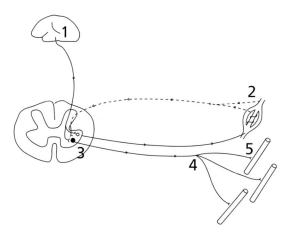

Fig. 2.2 Central fatigue sites: (1) supraspinal failure; (2) segmental afferent inhibition; (3) depression of motoneuron excitability; (4) loss of excitation at branch points; and (5) presynaptic failure. (From Green 1990 with permission.)

(Green 1990). These failure sites are related to alterations in excitation and result in a reduction in calcium in the cytosol. Other peripheral sites of fatigue are related to contraction and can range from disturbances at the level of troponin and tropomyosin to failure at the level of actin and myosin (Fig. 2.3) (Fitts 1994). The models of fatigue outlined below demonstrate the differing opinions on the origins of fatigue.

High and low frequency fatigue

Using electrophysiologic examinations of fatigue, two types of peripheral fatigue have been identified:

high and low frequency fatigue (Maclaren *et al.* 1989). High frequency fatigue is characterized by a selective loss of force at high stimulation frequencies (80–100 Hz) and is thought to be the result of impaired neuromuscular transmission and/or propagation of muscle action potential (Gibson & Edwards 1985). Conversely, low frequency fatigue is believed to be caused by impairments in excitation–contraction coupling and is characterized by selective loss of force at low stimulation frequencies (10–20 Hz; Gibson & Edwards 1985). It is important to note that these two types of fatigue relate only to the method of determination and not the type of activity or impulse pattern (Green 1990).

Jones *et al.* (1979) and Jones (1981) suggest that the loss of force observed during high frequency fatigue is a consequence of accumulation of potassium in the T tubules and muscle interfiber spaces. However, the physiologic relevance of high frequency fatigue is questionable as firing frequencies in voluntary contractions are in the range of 5–30 Hz (Bigland-Ritchie *et al.* 1983; Gibson & Edwards 1985). High tetanic rates of motoneuron discharge may only be evident during the initial phase of muscular contraction (Maclaren *et al.* 1989) and the fall in firing frequency during a sustained voluntary contraction may be a protective mechanism to ensure that high frequency fatigue does not occur (Bigland-Ritchie *et al.* 1983).

Low frequency fatigue is evident following multiple contractions under anaerobic conditions (Edwards *et al.* 1977) and also following dynamic voluntary contractions (Davies & White 1981, 1982; Edwards *et al.* 1977). As low frequency fatigue is believed to represent failure of the muscle despite adequate excitation (Edwards *et al.* 1977), fatigue may result unless a compensatory increase in firing rate occurs (Maclaren *et al.* 1989). Low frequency fatigue is also more pronounced following eccentric than concentric contractions (Newham *et al.* 1983), suggesting that mechanical damage to the muscle may contribute to this form of fatigue.

Models of peripheral fatigue

The decline in skeletal muscle force production that occurs during prolonged activity is often associated with changes occurring at the cellular level (Allen *et al.* 1992). This impairment within the active muscles themselves has been suggested to be the consequence of metabolite depletion or accumulation, alterations in the sodium potassium pump, changes in the ATPase microenvironment, or a combination of these processes. Figure 2.3 outlines the major components of a muscle cell involved in excitation–contraction coupling. Sites 1–4 represent changes associated with excitation–contraction coupling (sarcolemma and transverse tubular action potentials, transverse tubular charge sensor and sarcoplasmic reticulum calcium (Ca^{2+}) release channel), while sites 5–7 are related to metabolic changes that may influence the sarcoplasmic reticulum, the thin filament regulatory proteins, and the cross-bridge (Fitts 1994).

METABOLITE DEPLETION

Phosphagens (ATP and PC)

Adenosine triphosphate (ATP) is the major energy source for cross-bridge cycling and the ionic pumps such as sarcoplasmic reticulum (SR) Ca^{2+} pump and the surface membrane sodium pump (Allen *et al.* 1992). The breakdown of ATP to adenosine diphosphate (ADP) and the rephosphorylation of ADP back to ATP form the ATP–ADP cycle. Phosphocreatine (PCr) is the immediate source of ATP rephosphorylation (Brooks *et al.* 1996). The available quantities of both ATP and PCr are relatively small (27 and 90 mmol·kg^{-1} dry weight ATP and PCr for fast-twitch muscles, respectively, and 19 and 58 mmol·kg^{-1} dry weight ATP and PCr, respectively, for slow-twitch fibers (Fitts 1994)). Thus, one of the classic theories of peripheral fatigue suggests that depletion of ATP and PCr contributes to fatigue during exercise. While a number of studies have found strong correlations between ATP and PCr concentrations at fatigue, debate exists as to whether this is causative or simply a consequence of muscle contraction (Roberts & Smith 1989). The majority of evidence suggests that cell ATP concentrations do not decline to a critical level that would impair contraction, with numerous studies reporting levels rarely declining more than 60–70% of pre-exercise

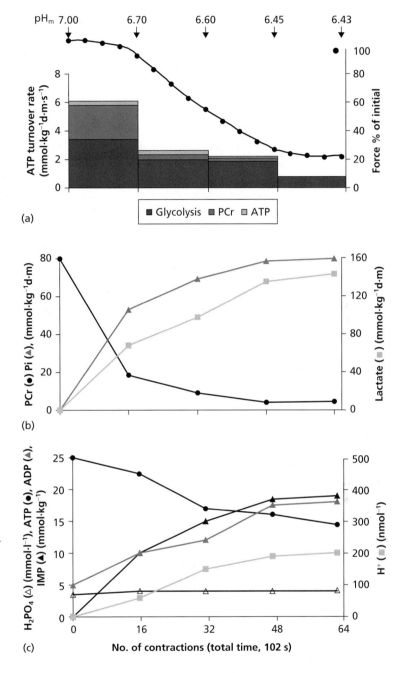

Fig. 2.4 Force generation and energy metabolism in human quadriceps femoris muscle stimulated intermittently at 20 Hz, with 1.6 s tetanus and 1.6 s rest periods. (a) ATP turnover rate, and pH; (b) the concentrations of PCr, P_i, and lactate; (c) ATP, ADP, AMP, H^+, and calculated $H_2PO_4^{-}$ (Hultman *et al*. 1990).

concentrations (Fig. 2.4; Hultman *et al*. 1990). Therefore, it appears that fatigue is produced by other factors, which decrease the rate of ATP utilization before ATP becomes limited (Fitts 1994). This is supported by findings that resting muscle tension and hence rigor does not develop even in the presence of relatively low muscle ATP concentrations (Spriet *et al*. 1987a).

Evidence is also available to suggest that depletion of PCr stores may contribute to fatigue, with low levels of PCr evident at fatigue (Fig. 2.4; Katz *et al.* 1986). Additionally, the ratio of ATP turnover rate to force produced is reduced during ischemia and it may be possible that ATP turnover rate is decreased when PCr is depleted (Vollestad & Sejersted 1988). However, other evidence suggests that the recovery of PCr and the recovery of force do not coincide (McCartney *et al.* 1986). As ATP levels remain relatively high at exhaustion (Fitts 1994), it does not appear that PCr limits performance by limiting ATP resynthesis. Therefore, the role of ATP and PCr depletion in peripheral fatigue is debatable.

Blood glucose and glycogen

Researchers as early as the 1920s recognized that carbohydrate supplementation delayed the development of fatigue during prolonged exercise (Christensen & Hansen 1939a; Dill *et al.* 1932; Levine *et al.* 1924). While research in this area has continued, the exact mechanism by which carbohydrate delays fatigue is unclear, with the exception that carbohydrate ingestion maintains blood glucose concentrations and fatigue coincides with muscle glycogen depletion (Fitts 1994).

During prolonged exercise the contribution of blood glucose to the total energy output increases as the duration of exercise increases and muscle glycogen concentrations decrease (Fitts 1994). According to the findings of Coyle (1991), decreases in blood glucose may lead to fatigue as glucose uptake by the muscle cannot increase sufficiently to offset reduced muscle glycogen availability.

There is a large degree of evidence to support a role for decreased muscle glycogen concentrations in the development of fatigue. Saltin and Karlsson (1971) reported largely depleted glycogen stores following exercise at 50–90% $\dot{V}o_{2max}$. Further, low resting glycogen concentrations have been associated with early onset fatigue (Hargreaves *et al.* 1984; Karlsson & Saltin 1971a) and high resting glycogen concentrations have been associated with a delay in fatigue development (Bergstrom *et al.* 1967; Karlsson & Saltin 1971). Evidence also exists that suggests the consumption of exogenous carbohydrate will spare endogenous sources and delay fatigue (Jeukendrup 2004).

The exact mechanism by which muscle glycogen influences fatigue is unclear and such a mechanism would appear to exist only during prolonged exercise or during repeated high intensity bouts (Fitts 1994). The influence of glycogen depletion on peripheral fatigue may again be questioned by the relatively well-maintained intramuscular ATP concentrations at fatigue. However, recent research suggests a possible role of glycogen in excitation–contraction coupling, in particular at the site of the SR (Marchand *et al.* 2002). Furthermore, a reduced rate of Ca^{2+} release from the SR has been reported in the presence of low muscle glycogen (Chin & Allen 1997). Regardless of the mechanism by which decreased blood glucose and muscle glycogen depletion may influence fatigue, it is clear that supplementation with and an increased availability of carbohydrate delays fatigue. It has recently been suggested that carbohydrate may have a role in central fatigue, and this possibility will be discussed in a later section.

METABOLITE ACCUMULATION

Lactic acid/H^+

The production of lactic acid is a consequence of anaerobic glycolysis, with the highest muscle and blood lactate concentrations observed following maximal intermittent exercise involving a large muscle mass (Fitts 1994). This accumulation of lactate has been implicated in declining maximal force generating capacity during exercise (Fig. 2.4). Studies by Karlsson in the 1970s (Karlsson & Saltin 1970, 1971b; Karlsson *et al.* 1975) reported consistent associations between high muscle lactate concentrations and exhaustion. Associations between increasing lactate concentrations and declining force output during isokinetic exercise have also been reported (Tesch *et al.* 1978). Further, the decrease in lactate accumulation (Holloszy 1973) and the increase in muscle buffering capacity (Sahlin & Henriksson 1984) with training, suggest a relationship between lactate accumulation and fatigue during exercise.

However, there is no conclusive evidence for a direct causal relationship, perhaps with the exception of the development of exhaustion during exercise of 10 s to 15 min in duration (Roberts & Smith 1989).

At a pH of 6.5, 99.8% of lactic acid exists in its ionized form (Sahlin & Henriksson 1984). The dissociation of lactic acid into lactate and H^+ causes marked increases in H^+ concentrations. It is thought that the effects of lactate accumulation on decreases in force production are mediated primarily through this increase in H^+ and subsequent decrease in pH (Roberts & Smith 1989). An increase in the H^+ concentration resulting in direct inhibition of force generating capacity has been reported by numerous studies (Hultman *et al.* 1990). Similar effects on muscle force were observed when pH declines between 7.0 and 6.5 (Hultman *et al.* 1990) as commonly and consistently occurs during exercise (Fig. 2.4; Fitts 1994).

Hydrogen ion accumulation has been reported to have numerous negative effects on force generating capacity (Fig. 2.4). These include: inhibition of phosphofructokinase (PFK) which may slow glycolysis (Brooks *et al.* 1996; Fitts 1994; Maclaren *et al.* 1989; Sahlin 1992); displacement of calcium from troponin thereby interfering with muscle contraction (Brooks *et al.* 1996; Maclaren *et al.* 1989); stimulation of pain receptors; side effects such as nausea and disorientation and limiting the release of free fatty acids into the circulation (Brooks *et al.* 1996); reduction in the number of cross-bridge attachments; reduction in the force per cross-bridge; prolonged muscle relaxation time; inhibition of ATPase (Fitts 1994); and inhibition of the generation of action potentials (Maclaren *et al.* 1989).

Again, it has been reported that factors other than pH may be related to fatigue, evidenced by an inconsistent time course of recovery between force and pH (Fitts & Holloszy 1978; Metzger & Fitts 1987). Further, patients with McArdle's syndrome (a congenital lack of myophosphorylase) who cannot produce lactic acid, demonstrate muscle fatigue at a greater rate than normal (Edwards & Wiles 1981; Wiles *et al.* 1981) and PFK-deficient patients show almost no change in pH during exercise (Edwards *et al.* 1982).

Adenosine diphosphate and inorganic phosphate

ATP is initially degraded to ADP and inorganic phosphate (P_i). The cellular concentration of ADP is approximately 10 times lower than that of ATP. Further, as the major part of ADP is bound, the free and active form is minimal. As was highlighted above (ATP depletion), the small reductions in ATP that occur with exercise may not directly result in significant force loss, but will result in high levels of ADP and P_i. Thus, a small change in ATP may result in relatively large changes in ADP and P_i, which have the potential to cause a decline in force production (Fig. 2.4; Sahlin 1992). It has been suggested that even low concentrations of ADP could interfere with the contraction process as the rate of cross-bridge detachment is dictated by ADP release (McLester 1997). However, several researchers have been unable to demonstrate a relationship between ADP and peak tetanic tension (Cooke & Pate 1985; Kawai & Halvorson 1989), while another group reported *increased* peak tension (Godt & Nosek 1989).

A direct influence of increased P_i on force reduction has been reported using skinned muscle fibers (Brandt *et al.* 1982; Hultman *et al.* 1985) and it has been suggested that an accumulation of P_i is the major limitation in exercise performance (Fig. 2.4; McLester 1997). This suggestion occurs following evidence that P_i increases significantly during exercise (Grimby *et al.* 1981; Harris *et al.* 1976) in hypoxic and ischemic cardiac muscle (Kammermeier *et al.* 1982) and increases in P_i are greater in patients with McArdle's syndrome when compared with controls (Lewis *et al.* 1985). P_i appears to act in a similar manner to that of H^+ in interfering with PFK and hence glycolysis and reducing calcium binding to troponin and therefore altering excitation–contraction coupling (Brooks *et al.* 1996).

CALCIUM FLUX

Altered Ca^{2+} flux has been implicated in the development of skeletal muscle fatigue. Ca^{2+} is stored in high concentrations in the SR and upon initiation of an action potential Ca^{2+} is released from the SR into the myoplasm. This increase in Ca^{2+} results in maximal binding of Ca^{2+} to troponin and maximal interaction between actin and myosin. Relaxation occurs when calcium is pumped out of the myoplasm back into the SR.

According to Allen *et al.* (1992), there are three possible means by which altered Ca^{2+} flux may influence a decline in force during exercise:

1 Reduced intracellular calcium release during activity;

2 Reduced sensitivity of the myofilaments to Ca^{2+}; and

3 Reduced maximal force development (reduced tension achieved at saturated Ca^{2+} concentrations).

Moderate increases in tetanic Ca^{2+} have been observed when tension declined to 80–90% of control levels (Westerblad *et al.* 1991). However, when fatigue has increased and tension declines to a greater extent (30% of control) a substantial decrease in tetanic Ca^{2+} occurs. This Ca^{2+}-dependent change in tension is confirmed through the findings that caffeine increases tetanic Ca^{2+}, which also increases tension when tension declines to relatively low levels (Westerblad *et al.* 1991). Caffeine acts directly on SR Ca^{2+} channels and facilitates Ca^{2+} release during a tetanus (Allen *et al.* 1992). As the effect of caffeine occurred only at the latter stages of fatigue, this suggests that the initiation of fatigue involves Ca^{2+}-independent mechanisms acting on the cross-bridge (Fitts 1994). The finding that caffeine reverses tension loss in fatigued fibers has been observed by other researchers (Garcia *et al.* 1991; Grabowski *et al.* 1972; Lannergren & Westerblad 1989; Nassar-Gentina *et al.* 1981; Vergara *et al.* 1977; Westerblad & Allen 1991).

It appears that fatigue is not the result of Ca^{2+} depletion in the SR as fatigued muscle responds to caffeine through the increased release of Ca^{2+} (Allen *et al.* 1989; Grabowski *et al.* 1972). As the Ca^{2+} transient decreases as fatigue develops (Allen *et al.* 1989; Blinks *et al.* 1978; Gyorke 1993; Westerblas & Allen 1991; Westerblad *et al.* 1990) and depletion of SR Ca^{2+} does not appear to occur, other mechanisms must be responsible. The rate of release of Ca^{2+} from the SR could be decreased during fatigue in the absence of either altered action potential or intramembranous T tubular charge movement (Fitts 1994). Large increases in twitch contraction and relaxation

times are thought to be caused by a prolonged Ca^{2+} transient (Fitts 1994). A redistribution of Ca^{2+} from the SR release site may occur which would result in a decrease in the rate of release of Ca^{2+}. The SR Ca^{2+} pump rate has also been shown to be decreased in the presence of high H^+ (Bezanilla *et al.* 1972; Byrd *et al.* 1989). The slowing of Ca^{2+} transport and progressively decreasing Ca^{2+} transients may be due to reduced Ca^{2+} reuptake by the SR, increased Ca^{2+} binding to Ca^{2+}-binding proteins or depletion of inositol triphosphate (second messenger for Ca^{2+} release; Fitts 1994).

SODIUM POTASSIUM PUMP

A redistribution of sodium (Na^+) and potassium (K^+) during exercise is commonly suggested to be associated with skeletal muscle fatigue. A steep chemical gradient for Na^+/K^+ is necessary for membrane potential and the excitability of the muscle fiber (Nielsen & Clausen 2000). A reduction in this gradient will lower excitability through depolarization and a reduction in the amplitude of action potentials and decrease force production (Nielsen & Clausen 2000). High frequency skeletal muscle stimulation has been shown to result in a shift in Na^+ and K^+ between intra- and extracellular spaces (Sejersted *et al.* 1986; Sjogaard 1983, 1986; Sjogaard *et al.* 1985).

A decrease in M-wave area and a decrease in force occurred when the chemical Na^+/K^+ gradient was decreased through exposure of isolated rat muscle to high K^+ concentrations and low Na^+ concentrations (Overgaard *et al.* 1999). A recovery of force and M-wave occurs when a stimulant (salbutamol) is provided which acts on the Na^+/K^+ pump (Overgaard *et al.* 1999). Other findings to support the role of the Na^+/K^+ pump in skeletal muscle fatigue include: inhibition of this pump results in an inability to maintain Na^+/K^+ homeostasis and a subsequent decrease in force occurs; inhibiting the Na^+/K^+ pump interferes with force recovery in fatigued muscles; and training and detraining results in up- and downregulation respectively of the Na^+/K^+ pump (Nielsen & Clausen 2000).

Medbo and Sejerstad (1990) reported an increase in K^+ concentration during exercise, and exercise at

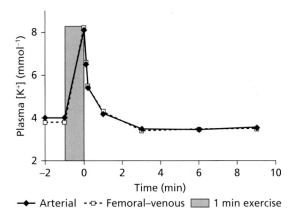

Fig. 2.5 Arterial and femoral–venous plasma potassium concentration before and after 1 min exhausting exercise. (Medbo & Sejersted 1990.)

a reduced intensity resulted in peak post-exercise K^+ concentrations that were linearly related to exercise intensity (Fig. 2.5). Further, the post-exercise plasma K^+ concentrations were lower than baseline, indicating an exercise-induced increased sensitivity of the pump. Therefore, fatigue caused by alterations in the Na^+/K^+ pump should be easily reversed and thus cannot explain the slower recovering phase of muscular fatigue (i.e., the recovery of force that occurs 30–60 min post-exercise; Fitts 1994).

ATPase microenvironment hypothesis

According to the ATPase microenvironment hypothesis (outlined in Fig. 2.6), Korge and Campbell (1995) suggest that alterations in ATP generating enzymes, existing in the vicinity of ATPase, may be involved in fatigue during high intensity exercise. Important to this hypothesis is the limited capacity for local ATP regeneration. During the initial phase of high intensity exercise the creatine kinase–creatine phosphate system is primarily involved in ATP regeneration, followed by glycolysis during prolonged or repeated exercise. A decrease in the efficiency of ATPase function can occur if the rate of ATP regeneration is not sufficient to match ATP consumption. When regeneration of ATP is unable to keep the ADP : ATP ratio low, the rate of ATP hydrolysis is decreased to avoid changes in tissue

adenine nucleotide concentrations. Korge and Campbell (1995) document evidence to suggest that changes in the ATPase microenvironment can result in a depression in Ca^{2+} pump function, resulting in fatigue.

Catastrophe theory of muscular fatigue

The highly integrated and complex nature of fatigue is highlighted in the catastrophe theory of muscular fatigue first proposed by Edwards (1983). In this model, a mathematical/engineering theory of catastrophe is applied to muscle fatigue and infers that failure of one system places stress on other related systems and thus several systems may fail simultaneously. As can be seen in Fig. 2.7, four hypothetical pathways are outlined. While these pathways represent separate mechanisms by which fatigue may occur, they are integrated to reflect the way in which these mechanisms may interact to protect the muscle during exercise (Gibson & Edwards 1985).

Edwards described Pathway 1 as linearly representing pure energy loss without impairment of excitation and if exercise continues may result in muscle ATP concentrations falling to zero and rigor occurring. Edwards states that while it is impossible for rigor to occur in healthy muscle, it may occur in patients with glycolytic disorders. Pathway 4 demonstrates a curvilinear relationship between excitation frequency and force, thus pure excitation or activation occurs without a loss of energy. Fatigue caused by energy loss and excitation failure, but without catastrophe, is highlighted in Pathway 3. Pathway 2 indicates sudden force loss with failure of excitation/activation resulting in catastrophe.

Edwards describes this theory as speculative yet emphasizes the complex interrelation between energy supply required for contraction and energy supply required for excitation/activation processes (Edwards 1983). Protective mechanisms at the cellular level and at the level of the central nervous system are recognised as "fail-safe" mechanisms, of which fatigue is the manifestation. According to Edwards, an important prediction of the catastrophe theory is that it may be difficult if not impossible to determine *the* limiting factor to exercise performance (Edwards 1983).

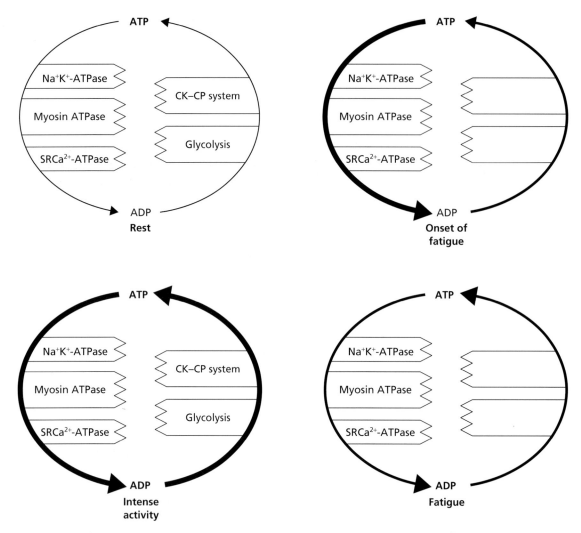

Fig. 2.6 Changes of adenine nucleotide concentration in ATPase microenvironment are regulating the activity of ATP regenerating mechanisms and possibly also that of ATPase during muscular activity and fatigue. The relative width of the arrows indicate qualitatively the rate of a reaction. It is expected that rapid increase in the ATPase activity will increase ADP concentrations in the vicinity of ATPase. At the start of intense activity the significant part of this ADP is not diffusing away, but phosphorylated locally by ATP regenerating system present in this microcompartment. This local ATP regenerating capacity is expected to decrease during intense exercise. As a result ADP : ATP ratio in the vicinity of ATPase will increase. However, this change is not reflected in the tissue adenine nucleotide concentration or ADP : ATP ratio, because the rate of ATP hydrolysis is downregulated, possibly because local change at the "onset" of fatigue. Relatively stable cellular adenine nucleotide concentration in fatigued muscle clearly indicates the existence of sensitive mechanism(s) of downregulation of ATP utilization and ATPase reaction products are expected to be good candidates for accomplishing this downregulation. (Korge & Campbell 1995.)

This theory has recently received criticism (Noakes & St. Clair Gibson 2004; Noakes *et al.* 2004, 2005), with the authors suggesting that absolute system failure does not occur (i.e., skeletal muscle rigor) and there is no single metabolite that has been identified as the cause of fatigue. Further, it is claimed that the catastrophe theory cannot explain the phenomenon of pacing by athletes, whereby

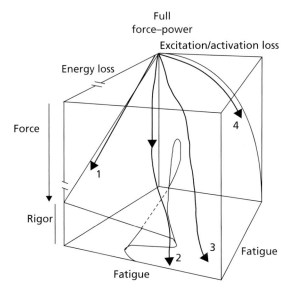

Fig. 2.7 Muscle fatigue: catastrophe theory model. Theoretical pathways for different forms of muscular fatigue: (1) pure energy loss in absence of excitation failure, which if continued would lead to rigor; (2) mixed fatigue with catastrophe–sudden force loss with failure of excitation/activation as (but not only) on steep part of curve 4; (3) mixed energy loss and excitation failure but without "catastrophe"; (4) pure excitation/activation failure thus preventing energy loss. (Gibson & Edwards 1985.)

athletes adopt a strategy at the onset of exercise in the absence of metabolic events in the muscle (Noakes *et al.* 2005). Additionally, Noakes *et al.* (2005) pose the question as to why athletes can increase their pace at the end of an event when inhibitory metabolites at are the highest level, suggesting that peripheral metabolite concentration cannot regulate pacing strategies.

EXERCISE-INDUCED MUSCLE DAMAGE

The development of fatigue in the periphery may also be of non-metabolic origin and is predominantly a consequence of high repetition, high force skeletal muscle contraction which results in damage to the muscle fibers (Green 1997), and delayed onset muscle soreness (DOMS) (Morgan & Proske 2004). Eccentric muscle contractions are known to produce greater muscle damage than either concentric or

isometric muscle contractions (Clarkson & Hubal 2002). Maximal eccentric muscle contractions generate 1.5–1.9 times greater force than isometric contractions (Byrne *et al.* 2004). Further, motor unit activation is less in eccentric contractions than concentric and isometric contractions, and therefore less motor unit activation is required for a given force output (Byrne *et al.* 2004). This is generally considered to be caused by an increased ability to generate tension and a greater distribution of load across the same number of fibers as the muscle lengthens (Clarkson & Hubal 2002). The mechanism by which force is generated during eccentric contractions does not involve ATP breakdown, rather the cross-bridges are mechanically detached (Byrne *et al.* 2004). However, during repeated low intensity eccentric activity (distance running), other factors such as metabolic depletion, calcium influx, and the generation of reactive oxygen species may also contribute to the exercise-induced muscle damage (Byrne *et al.* 2004).

While it is well accepted that prolonged or unaccustomed (unaccustomed muscle length or number of repetitions) eccentric muscle contractions result in DOMS, the initial event that leads to muscle fiber injury remains unclear (Proske & Allen 2005). A number of hypotheses have been proposed to identify and explain the initial event: mechanically induced mechanisms, temperature-induced mechanisms, insufficient mitochondrial respiration; and free radical production (Armstrong *et al.* 1991).

The suggestion that mechanical factors have an integral role in the exercise-induced muscle fiber injury is based on the unique characteristics of eccentric muscle contractions (greater force production and longer muscle lengths). Eccentric muscle contractions have also been shown to result in higher intramuscular temperatures than concentric contractions (Nadel *et al.* 1972), which may have been a consequence of the reported higher metabolic rate in this study. This increased muscle temperature may result in enhanced membrane degradation and is thought to be the result of a reduced rate of heat removal as opposed to higher heat production (Armstrong *et al.* 1991).

Insufficient mitochondrial respiration, which may result in reduced removal of Ca^{2+} from the cytoplasm, is not regarded as one of the more promising explanations to explain the initial event leading to muscle fiber damage. This is primarily because of the reduced metabolic cost of eccentric contractions when compared with concentric contractions (Bonde-Petersen *et al.* 1972), yet increased injury to muscle fibers. Similar concerns are evident with the free radical theory of exercise-induced muscle damage in relation to the question of whether increased free radical production could occur in the presence of a reduced metabolic cost of activity in comparison to concentric contractions. This theory proposes that the high tensions generated during eccentric contractions could disrupt the cytoskeletal framework, impair the electron transport system, increase free radical formation, and oxidize membranous structures and enzymes (Armstrong *et al.* 1991). Empirical support for this theory is minimal, with one investigation reporting protection against a loss of force by antioxidant supplementation in aged, but not young or adult mice (Zerba *et al.* 1990), and another finding no effect of the antioxidant α-tocopherol (Warren *et al.* 1992). Maughan *et al.* (1989) have reported an accumulation of lipid peroxidation products in the plasma after downhill running resulting in muscle soreness, suggesting that muscle damage may cause oxidative damage by enhanced production of free radicals. Further research in this area reported increased nitric oxide content in the muscle of females after 200 eccentric contractions at 60% of maximum isometric contractions (Radak *et al.* 1999). Increased muscular nitric oxide content was associated with a decrease in maximal force generating capacity and increased 8-hydroxydeoxyguanosine, a product of DNA oxidation (Radak *et al.* 1999).

Hellsten *et al.* (1997) reported an increased expression of xanthine oxidase over 4 days following one-legged eccentric exercise. This was attributed to a secondary inflammatory process (Hellsten *et al.* 1997) and would possibly account for the increase in ultrastructural damage evident in the days following eccentric activity (Clarkson & Hubal 2002). Thus, it is possible that free radical production exacerbates the damage that has already occurred and may not be the direct cause or initial event.

The recent popping sarcomere hypothesis (Proske & Morgan 2001) suggests that during stretch of myofibrils while contracting, some sarcomeres resist stretch more than others and thus weaker sarcomeres take up the majority of the stretch. If this occurs during the descending limb of the length–tension curve (i.e., sarcomeres are beyond optimal length), the weakness of the sarcomeres persists until the overlap between the myofilaments no longer exists. As the weakest sarcomeres are not at the same point along each myofibril, this non-uniform lengthening can result in damage to the myofibril (Morgan & Proske 2004). The overstretched sarcomeres lead to membrane damage and is accompanied by an increase in Ca^{2+} into the sarcoplasm (Proske & Morgan 2001). A loss of calcium ion homeostasis may result in further damage through the tearing of membranes or opening of stretch-activated channels (Morgan & Proske 2004).

Evidence exists to support the existence of overstretched sarcomeres in humans (Brockett *et al.* 2001; Jones *et al.* 1987). A change in the length–tension relationship, specifically a shift in the optimal length for peak active tension in the direction of longer muscle lengths, correlates with the amount of damage following eccentric activity (Jones *et al.* 1997). Further, a shift in torque–angle curve has been observed following eccentric activity (Whitehead *et al.* 1998). This shift was characterized by a large shift in torque (lowering of the curve) and a shift of the curve to the right, indicating a shift in the optimal angle for torque generation towards longer muscle lengths (Whitehead *et al.* 1998). Further evidence for this theory has also been provided by Brockett *et al.* (2001), who reported a sustained shift in the skeletal muscle torque–angle curves after a single bout of eccentric activity. This is consistent with the repeated bout effect (Brockett *et al.* 2001), where a single bout of eccentric activity results in an adaptive effect so that there is less evidence of damage up to 6 months post activity (Clarkson & Hubal 2002).

While the initiating event of delayed onset muscle soreness remains speculative, the resultant reduction in force, and increase in pain, is well accepted and documented (Cheung *et al.* 2003). Again, however, the underlying mechanism for this pain stimulus in unclear. Possible theories include: lactic acid, muscle spasm, connective tissue damage, muscle damage, and enzyme efflux theories (Cheung *et al.* 2003). Both the lactic acid and muscle spasm theories have been readily dismissed because of the high clearance rates of lactic acid (does not persist to the time point of maximal pain after eccentric exercise) and inconclusive electromyography results after eccentric exercise, respectively. Increased amino acid components of collagen have been shown to be increased in the urine of subjects following eccentric activity. However, the mechanism behind this is unknown and support for the connective tissue theory is also minimal (Cheung *et al.* 2003). The muscle damage theory is generally well accepted and proposes that the disruption of the contractile components of muscle results in stimulation of nociceptors in muscle connective tissue (Cheung *et al.* 2003). Creatine kinase (CK) is generally considered an indicator of muscle membrane permeability and hence damage. The fact that peak CK levels in serum do not correspond to peak muscle soreness suggests that factors other than damage to the muscle fibers themselves contribute to the pain associated with eccentric exercise (Cheung *et al.* 2003).

The inflammatory response to eccentric exercise occurs to remove debris from the injured area in preparation for regeneration (Clarkson & Hubal 2002). This response involves infiltration of fluid and proteins, increases in cell populations (monocytes and neutrophils), release of reactive oxygen species, and activation of phospholipases and proteases (Clarkson & Hubal 2002). The resultant increase in protein-rich fluid into the muscle exerts an osmotic pressure and pain may occur if group IV sensory neurons are activated (Cheung *et al.* 2003). Finally, the efflux theory of pain states that calcium release into the SR activates phospholipases and proteases, which further injures the cell membrane and produces leukotrienes and prostaglandins. This muscle protein degradation may chemically stimulate pain nerve endings (Cheung *et al.* 2003).

Decreases in force production as a result of exercise are often, correctly, considered the result of metabolic alterations. However, this decrease in force may also be attributable to muscle injury, which can occur independently or concurrently with metabolic alterations.

Models of central fatigue

CENTRAL FATIGUE–SEROTONERGIC SYSTEM

The central fatigue hypothesis (CFH) was first proposed by Newsholme *et al.* (1987) (Fig. 2.8). In

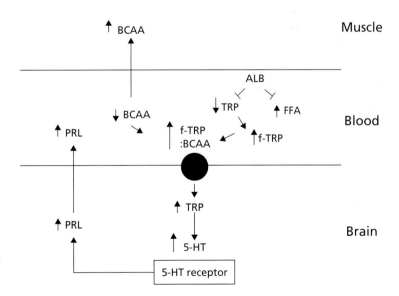

Fig. 2.8 Central fatigue hypothesis. ALB, albumin; BCAA, branched chain amino acids; FFA, free fatty acids; f-TRP, free tryptophan; 5-HT, 5-hydroxytrypamine; PRL, prolactin; TRP, tryptophan. (After Davis & Bailey 1997.)

essence, the CFH suggests that an increase in the activity of the serotonergic system via an increased rate of 5-hydroxytryptamine (5-HT) formation from tryptophan (TRP) can lead to an increased perception of fatigue. The rate of conversion of plasma free-TRP (f-TRP) to brain 5-HT is controlled by the ratio of f-TRP to branched chain amino acids (BCAAs). Thus, either an increase in f-TRP or a decrease in plasma BCAA concentration can lead to an increase in TRP transport across the blood–brain barrier. Once f-TRP has entered the brain it is synthesized to 5-hydroxytryptophan (5-HTP) by the enzyme tryptophan hydroxylase. 5-HTP is then converted to 5-HT by the enzyme aromatic L-amino decarboxylase. Stimulation of 5-HT receptors results in the release of the single polypeptide chain stress hormone prolactin from the anterior pituitary gland (Pan 1991).

The theoretical possibility of altering the influx of TRP into the brain, and hence delaying fatigue, has gained research interest. Investigations have focused on nutritional strategies involving supplementation of BCAAs, carbohydrate, and f-TRP (Blomstrand & Newsholme 1992; Blomstrand et al. 1991, 1995; Struder et al. 1995, 1998; van Hall et al. 1995). BCAA supplementation has been shown to increase endurance performance during a 42.2-km marathon (Blomstrand et al. 1991), and during submaximal cycling (Blomstrand et al. 1995). However, supplementation with BCAAs did not improve performance during a graded incremental exercise to exhaustion (Varnier et al. 1994) and submaximal cycling (Struder et al. 1998; van Hall et al. 1995).

Further efforts to provide scientific validation of the CFH has resulted in a series of investigations into the effects of TRP supplementation on exercise performance (Segura & Ventura 1988; Struder et al. 1996, van Hall et al. 1995). L-tryptophan (L-TRP) supplementation was shown to improve submaximal treadmill running (Segura & Ventura 1988); however, further research could not replicate these findings (Stensrud et al. 1992; Struder et al. 1996; van Hall et al. 1995).

The lack of consistent support for altered exercise performance after nutritional supplementation led researchers to examine the effects of specific drugs that either increase (agonists) or decrease (antagonists) 5-HT activity on fatigue during exercise. Run time to exhaustion is reported to be decreased in a dose–response manner after administration of a 5-HT agonist in rats (Bailey et al. 1992, 1993). In an attempt to replicate the findings of the rat models, Wilson and Maughan (1992) examined the effect of a 5-HT agonist on fatigue in human subjects. Subjects were either administered a placebo or 20 mg paroxetine (5-HT reuptake inhibitor). Subjects who received the placebo exercised for significantly longer than the paroxetine group; however, there were no significant differences in peripheral measures of fatigue. The authors conclude that the difference between the fatigue experienced by the two groups was primarily caused by altered 5-HT activity. Davis et al. (1995) conducted a methodologically comparable study to that of Wilson and Maughan and reported similar results.

Marvin et al. (1997) administered buspirone, a partial 5-HT$_{1A}$ agonist at postsynaptic 5-HT$_{1A}$ receptors, prior to exercise. Time to volitional fatigue was significantly shorter following buspirone ingestion. Rating of perceived exertion (RPE) scores were significantly higher after buspirone during early stages of exercise and prolactin levels were increased throughout exercise and at fatigue despite the fact that subjects receiving buspirone exercised for only two-thirds of the time of the placebo group. The higher RPE scores and thus heightened perception of fatigue as a result of buspirone, in conjunction with a reduced exercise time, supports the theory that 5-HT activity affects endurance performance. Similar results were found by Struder et al. (1998), who showed a significant reduction in exercise time after administration of paroxetine. The subsequent opposing research approach has been used to investigate the effects of a 5-HT receptor *antagonist* on exercise performance and fatigability in human subjects. However, Pannier et al. (1995) and Meeusen et al. (1997) found no differences in exercise time to fatigue after ingestion of a 5-HT antagonist.

Jakeman (1998) suggested that trained individuals should demonstrate a lower f-TRP : BCAA ratio because of a decrease in non-esterified fatty acids resulting from the increase in fat oxidization that occurs following endurance training. Thus, there would be expected to be a reduction in the unbinding of TRP from albumin and hence decrease f-TRP levels and its conversion to 5-HT. However, Jakeman (1998) has reported no differences in the f-TRP : BCAA both at rest and post exercise in trained and non-trained subjects. Thus, an altered ratio cannot explain the lower perception of effort commonly reported by endurance athletes.

Further work by Jakeman *et al.* (1994) involved administration of a serotonergic challenge test to endurance trained and non-endurance trained subjects. This test involves subjects ingesting a 5-HT receptor agonist at rest, in this particular study buspirone, and the amount of prolactin secreted into the blood from the anterior pituitary gland is measured. Prolactin secretion following stimulation of the 5-HT receptor with a standardized dose of a serotonergic agent is considered an indicator of the sensitivity of the 5-HT receptor. Jakeman *et al.* (1994) performed this test on five endurance trained and five untrained matched controls and found that the total prolactin release was significantly lower in trained subjects ($P = 0.042$) and peak prolactin production occurred later in trained individuals (60 vs. 120 min). Further, 16 weeks of endurance training in previously untrained subjects resulted in a reduced response of approximately 30% to a serotonergic agonist (Jakeman 1998). Combined, these data suggest that serotonergic pathways are involved in fatigue mechanisms during exercise and that these pathways may be adaptable following endurance training (Jakeman 1998).

CENTRAL FATIGUE–SUPRASPINAL FACTORS

Muscle behaviour during activity is dependent on drive to the muscles and the manner in which this drive is maintained through feedback mechanisms (Gandevia 2001). Gandevia and colleagues have provided evidence that fatigue may occur at the level of the spinal motoneuron and/or at the supraspinal level (for review see Gandevia 2001). Supraspinal fatigue is defined as fatigue produced by a failure to generate output from the motor cortex and is considered a subset of central fatigue (Gandevia 2001).

The superimposed tetanic twitch technique has been employed to demonstrate a failure in voluntary neural drive. This technique involves superimposing brief tetani on an isometric contraction and examining the possible increase in force produced (i.e., the increase above maximal voluntary force production). This provides an indication of voluntary drive and results from studies employing this technique have demonstrated a decline in motor unit discharge during sustained or intermittent maximal voluntary contractions (MVCs; Lloyd *et al.* 1991; Thomas *et al.* 1989) and hence the development of central fatigue. Transcranial stimulation of the motor cortex during isometric MVCs may also result in the addition of progressively more force above that generated voluntarily, again demonstrating central fatigue during isometric activity (Gandevia 2001).

Gandevia (2001) suggests that the decline in motor unit discharge during fatigue is accompanied by changes in muscle spindles, Golgi tendon organs, small diameter muscle afferents, motoneurons, and Renshaw cells. This may result in reduced spinal reflex facilitation and increase inhibition to corticospinal cells (Fig. 2.9a,b). Changes in intramuscular receptors produce competing excitatory and inhibitory influences on the motoneuron pool that may influence this declining discharge rate. Group III and IV muscle afferents may also reduce voluntary drive through a supraspinal action. Drive to the corticospinal cells is increased during fatigue, which results in the recruitment of additional muscles. The failure of supraspinal drive to the motoneurons may act to protect the muscle and neuromuscular junction against continued fatigue (Gandevia 2001).

Recent research involving motor cortical stimulation has examined the degree of central nervous system activation on muscles at differing levels of fatigue (Todd *et al.* 2003). Using a novel technique involving stimulation of the brachial plexus, stimulation of the biceps brachii/brachialis intramuscular nerve fibers, and transcranial magnetic stimulation of the motor cortex, the authors were able to demonstrate both peripheral and central fatigue. When maximal voluntary force produced by the elbow flexors dropped to 40% of prefatigued values, resting twitch evoked by motor nerve stimulation

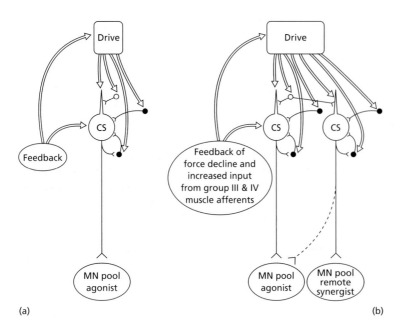

Fig. 2.9 Diagram of possible changes at the motor cortex level with muscle fatigue. Simplified schema for reflex input and "supra" motor cortical input to a corticospinal cell (CS) under control conditions (a) and during fatigue (b). Solid cells are inhibitory and open ones are excitatory. Although shown diagrammatically, the types and locations of connections depicted occur in the motor cortex. During fatigue there is an increased drive to corticospinal cells and more are "recruited." With this scheme local excitation and inhibition would be increased when tested with transcranial magnetic stimulation. (From Gandevia 2001 with permission.)

declined, indicating peripheral fatigue. Additionally, central fatigue was evidenced by an increased superimposed twitch at fatigue than at rest using both motor nerve and transcranial stimulation. By calculating the post-fatigue force that could have been produced if voluntary activation had not fallen, the difference between the calculated and measured force was 10% of MVC. Thus, central fatigue accounted for approximately one-quarter of the 40% decreased in maximal voluntary force (Todd *et al.* 2003). Unique studies such as this will aid in the understanding of fatigue from both a peripheral and central perspective.

CARBOHYDRATE AND CENTRAL FATIGUE

It is possible that carbohydrate has a direct effect on the central nervous system through various mechanisms. First, the role of carbohydrate in the CFH has been suggested through a blunting of exercise-induced increases in free tryptophan (Davis *et al.* 1992). Exogenous carbohydrate inhibits lipolysis during prolonged exercise and thus decreases the unbinding of tryptophan from albumin. This is thought to decrease tryptophan transport across the brain and reduce the formation of serotonin.

Second, carbohydrate may also directly act on the central nervous system through stimulation of receptors in the oral cavity (Jeukendrup 2004). This possibility has arisen through observations that carbohydrate ingestion improves performance during high intensity exercise of around 60 min in duration (Jeukendrup 2004). This improvement appears spurious because muscle glycogen is not depleted, muscle glycogen contributes significantly more to energy expenditure than blood glucose, the amount of carbohydrate that can be absorbed in that time is minimal (approximately 15 g; Jeukendrup *et al.* 1997), and blood glucose concentrations have been shown to increase at these high intensities (80–85% $\dot{V}o_{2max}$) even when no carbohydrate was ingested (Below *et al.* 1995).

Two recent studies by Carter *et al.* (2004a,b) support the suggestion for a role of carbohydrate in central fatigue. In the first study, performance in a approximately 60-min time trial was not different when subjects were infused with either saline or 1 g·min^{-1} glucose (Carter *et al.* 2004b). This suggests that the performance benefits observed with the provision of exogenous carbohydrate in exercise of this duration are not brought about by increased availability of carbohydrate. This was further investigated in a second study where subjects were given either a glucose solution or a placebo and simply asked to rinse their mouth with the solution but not swallow (Carter *et al.* 2004a). The carbohydrate solution in this study resulted in a 2.6% improvement in an approximately 60-min time trial performance when compared with placebo. The authors suggested that receptors may exist in the oral cavity that directly communicate with the brain, potentially the reward/pleasure centers in the brain.

Some of the earliest work in the area of carbohydrate and fatigue examined hypoglycemia and subsequent neuroglucopenia during prolonged exercise (Levine *et al.* 1924). Recently, Nybo (2003) reports evidence that carbohydrate supplementation counteracts central fatigue during prolonged exercise through a maintenance of blood glucose homeostasis. Central fatigue was suggested to be evident when subjects were not provided with carbohydrate during exercise, through lower force production during sustained contractions. This lower force production was associated with a decreased activation from the central nervous system. The author also suggests that the hypoglycemia-induced central fatigue may be the direct effect of a lack of glucose to the brain and hence central fatigue could be the result of depletion of blood glucose in the brain.

A recent hypothesis has also been proposed in which muscle glycogen may have an important signaling role as evidenced by altered pacing strategies in subjects with high and low resting muscle glycogen concentrations (Rauch *et al.* 2005). In this study, seven of eight subjects finished an exercise bout with similar levels of muscle glycogen. This was despite subjects starting the bout with significantly different resting muscle glycogen concentrations on the two occasions. Further, subjects paced themselves at significantly lower workloads when they began with low muscle glycogen concentrations, although subjects had no visual feedback. The authors suggest that there may be a critical level of muscle glycogen at the cessation of exercise, and that athletes may pace themselves to ensure this is reached. Additionally, chemoreceptors were suggested to provide information to the central nervous

system, to allow humans to pace themselves to ensure the exercise task is completed with a specific muscle glycogen concentration. This intramuscular monitor has been termed the "glycostat" and is one element of the central governor theory outlined below.

CENTRAL GOVERNOR THEORY

The central governor or central integrative model proposes that skeletal muscle power output during exercise is regulated in the brain by a governor as part of a complex integrative system (St. Clair Gibson & Noakes 2004). This model predicts that during prolonged exercise the brain does not recruit additional motor units to protect against both premature cessation of exercise and catastrophic organ failure (Noakes *et al.* 2005). An increasing perception of discomfort during exercise is suggested to ensure this safety mechanism remains and thus homeostasis is protected (Noakes *et al.* 2005).

The central control of exercise intensity is suggested to occur through neural integration of peripheral, afferent information and includes both feed forward and feed back mechanisms (Lambert *et al.* 2005). Thus, metabolic variables in the periphery are considered "sensors" and initiate afferent feedback to the brain. The brain then resets metabolic and motor activity through oscillations in power output and physiologic responses in a feed forward manner (Lambert *et al.* 2005).

Scientific support for the central governor model has involved identifying weaknesses or inconsistencies in commonly researched and accepted physiologic and biochemical determinants of fatigue, primarily in the periphery. One of the concepts challenged is the notion that the development of fatigue at moderate to high intensity is the result of an inability to supply oxygen to the active muscle at a sufficient rate. Noakes (2000) suggests that this model is not appropriate for the following reasons:

1 The heart, and not skeletal muscles, is the organ most likely to be affected initially during maximal exercise.

2 There is currently no evidence to suggest that anaerobiosis, hypoxia, or ischemia occurs in skeletal muscle during exercise.

3 The model does not explain the cessation of exercise when skeletal muscle anaerobiosis, hypoxia, ischemia, and full activation of skeletal muscle mass does not occur.

4 The model also does not explain why maximum oxygen consumption and "anaerobic threshold" does not predict exercise capacity in athletes of similar abilities.

Further support for the central governor model is proposed by the fact that ATP concentrations do not fall below 60% of resting values, even during ischemia (Fitts 1994; Spriet *et al.* 1987a). Therefore, it is suggested that one of the commonly accepted causes of fatigue in the periphery, ATP depletion, does not occur as a result of protection by the central governor. Noakes *et al.* (2005) also derive support for their model from the fact that skeletal muscle motor unit recruitment reserve exists when exercising to volitional exhaustion. Thus, it is suggested that fatigue cannot be caused through peripheral-based control, but through regulation of skeletal muscle activation by the central nervous system.

The teleoanticipation model for exercise suggests that efferent information on motion, time, force output, and metabolism and afferent signals then feedback information from mechanoreceptors and chemoreceptors which may change power output to optimize performance (Fig. 2.10; Ulmer 1996). Further, afferent feedback from muscles and/or organs may be altered by prior experience, training, and muscle metabolism to form an integrative control mechanism (Ulmer 1996). This concept of teleoanticipation has been scientifically investigated by providing incorrect information to exercising subjects on exercise intensity (Hampson *et al.* 2001). In this study, subjects who expected an increase in exercise intensity, yet intensity was unchanged, reported increasing perceptions of effort. Thus, anticipation based on expectation occurred and this was suggested to be the result of subconscious setting of exercise intensity based on previous experience. Noakes *et al.* (2005) also suggest that pacing strategies evident during competition cannot be explained by peripheral models of fatigue. It is suggested that athletes pace themselves based on the expected duration of the activity and are supported by increases in power output at the end of events when peripheral fatigue should be at its greatest. Therefore, according to the central governor model all alterations in pace, and including the cessation of exercise, is regulated to protect the body against severe damage (Noakes *et al.* 2005). In this model, fatigue is a sensation based on the conscious perception of exercise and is not a physical event. Therefore, differentiation is made between the sensation/emotion of fatigue and the physical expression of that sensation (Noakes *et al.* 2005).

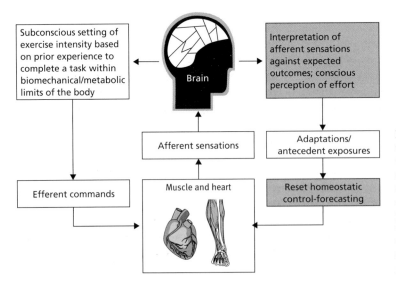

Fig. 2.10 Relation between the teleoanticipatory governor center in the brain and perceived exertion during exercise. Exercise intensity is set at a subconscious level by the central nervous system and the perceived effort is the interpretation of afferent sensations against expected outcomes set by the subconscious teleoanticipatory governor center. (Lambert *et al.* 2005.)

Practical considerations

While the focus of this section has been to highlight possible mechanisms of fatigue during exercise, athletes engaged in intense training often view fatigue from a different perspective. For the elite athlete, the manifestations of fatigue are likely more important than the underlying mechanisms. For these athletes, fatigue may be categorized as perceptual or functional and either short or long term. Further, for athletes, fatigue is considered a typical response both during and after training and is generally considered integral to the adaptive response. Thus, the differentiation between normal fatigue (results in adaptation) and fatigue that is prolonged and severe (results in reduced performance capability and failing adaptation) is of immense practical importance to elite athletes.

The future of fatigue

The future of fatigue research will most likely involve the use of novel and innovative technology. Such techniques may include: near infrared spectroscopy (NIRS), nuclear magnetic resonance (NMR), transcranial magnetic stimulation (TMS), and position emission tomography (PET).

An integrative approach will be required to aid in the determination and differentiation of peripheral and central aspects of fatigue. Intervention, training studies, and studies involving patients with metabolic or neural disturbances may also help provide further insight into the sites and mechanisms of fatigue.

Unfortunately, many of the more sophisticated tools for identifying fatigue are somewhat contrived and are used to investigate obscure or functionally irrelevant forms of fatigue (e.g., fatigue that rarely occurs in healthy, intact humans during intense or prolonged exercise). Further, many approaches to studying fatigue have required a reductionist approach because of difficulties in investigating the numerous integrating elements of fatigue in exercising humans. It is possible that identification of specific genes that may be associated with a genetic predisposition to fatigue, in combination with examining the effects of training, may elucidate fatigue mechanisms in trained individuals. Finally, prolonged training monitoring may provide valuable information on the demarcation between fatigue that results in enhanced adaptation to exercise and fatigue that becomes excessive and results in failed adaptation or overtraining.

NEUROMUSCULAR ADAPTATIONS TO TRAINING

NICHOLAS A. RATAMESS AND MIKEL IZQUIERDO

Introduction

The performance and physiologic adaptations to training are specific to the stimuli applied. *Aerobic training* consisting of continuous exercise of low, moderate, and moderately high intensity produces mostly endurance-related adaptations of the neuromuscular system, whereas *anaerobic training* (i.e., high intensity intermittent bouts of exercises such as weight training, plyometrics, ballistic (power) training, speed, and agility training) produces different types of adaptations. Depending on the specific training program, increases in maximal voluntary strength and muscle power, as well as in maximal rate of force development, will take place. These improvements in performance are directly attributed to either muscle morphology or architecture and/or to neural factors. This section discusses the adaptations that take place within the nervous and muscular systems to both training modalities. Adaptations may take place anywhere along the neuromuscular chain from the higher brain centers (i.e., motor cortex) to ultrastructural changes within muscle fibers (Fig. 2.11). These adaptations ultimately lead to changes in muscle strength and power, hypertrophy, endurance, speed, balance, and agility sought during training.

Muscle perfomance adaptations to training

Heavy resistance and endurance training specificity in the long term, as well as genetic influences, have been shown to induce distinct changes in maximal strength, muscle power, and endurance performance, as a consequence of different neuromuscular, cardiovascular, and hormonal adaptations. Several

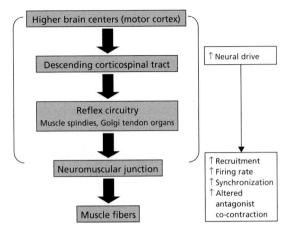

Fig. 2.11 Potential sites of adaptation to training along the neuromuscular chain.

researchers have thus reported sport-related differences in strength/muscle power and endurance performances (Fig. 2.12; Izquierdo *et al.* 2002, 2004; Jürimäe *et al.* 1997; Kanehisa *et al.* 1997). Sport-related differences in strength and/or power may depend on the sport-specific time for force application and to some extent on the sport-specific levels of resistances to be overcome. As expected, high absolute and relative maximal strength and muscle power output has been observed in weightlifters, compared to those of the road cyclists and controls, whereas maximal workload was 44% higher and submaximal blood lactate accumulation was 50–55% lower with increasing workload in road cyclists than in control subjects and weightlifters (Fig. 2.12).

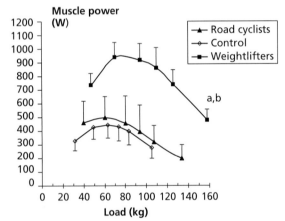

(a)

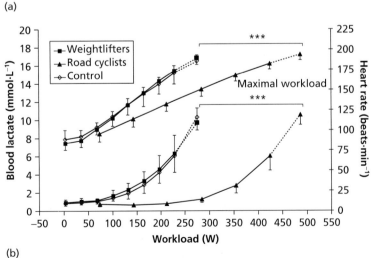

(b)

Fig. 2.12 Mean (±SD) muscle power output of the lower extremity muscles during a half-squat execution at different absolute loads corresponding to the 15%, 30%, 45%, 60%, 70%, and 100% of one repetition maximum from a half-squat position in absolute load values (a) and mean (±SD) heart rate and blood lactate concentrations during a maximal multistage discontinuous incremental cycling test at submaximal and maximal workloads in absolute values (b). [a] Significant difference ($P < 0.05$) between weightlifters and road cyclists. [b] Significant difference ($P < 0.05$) between weightlifters and controls. [c] Significant difference ($P < 0.05$) between road cyclists and controls. *** Significant difference ($P < 0.001$) compared to weightlifters and controls. (After Izquierdo *et al.* 2002, 2004.)

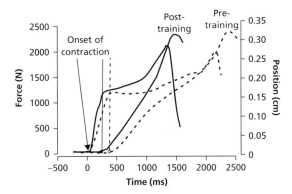

Fig. 2.13 Force–time and position–time curves obtained before and after 10 weeks of heavy resistance training. Onset of movement is denoted by solid circle and vertical line (pre-training) and clear circle and dotted vertical line (post-training). Note that isometric force–time curve during dynamic action is denoted from onset of contraction to onset of movement. Resistance training with heavy loads (i.e., at intensity of 10 repetitions maximum) has been shown to increase during dynamic type of actions the slope of the isometric force–time curve, as well as increases in average velocity of movement, average force and average muscle power (unpublished results).

Systematic strength training can lead to considerable improvements in strength of all muscle groups examined independent of age and gender, when both the loading intensity of training and duration of the resistance training period are sufficient. Depending on the initial physical conditioning level of the subjects, the initial increases in strength can be as large as 10–30% (or even more) during the first weeks or 1–2 months of strength training. Thereafter, strength development takes usually place at a diminished rate during prolonged training periods depending on the intensity, frequency, and type of training. An increase in maximal strength, muscle power, and rate of force development is the most important functional benefit induced by resistance training (Fig. 2.13; Aagard 2003; Kraemer & Ratamess 2004).

Endurance training may complement the adaptation to strength training, especially during the initial phase of training, in previously untrained middle-aged men or subjects with limited training background performing a low frequency training program. Thus, it has been previously suggested that cycling endurance training may also improve the strength of the knee and hip extensor muscles (Izquierdo *et al.* 2002).

Neural adaptations to training

An increase in neural drive has been shown during anaerobic training. Endurance training also imposes specific demands on the nervous system, although the pattern of neural activation appears less complex than that observed with high intensity, intermittent training where high levels of muscle strength, power, and speed are required in a short period of time. The most common method of evaluation has been the use of electromyography (EMG) measurements before and following several weeks of training. The increase in neural drive is thought to occur via increases in agonist motor unit recruitment, firing rate, and synchronization (i.e., timing and pattern of discharge). A reduction in inhibiting stimuli (i.e., Golgi tendon organ reflex, Renshaw cell recurrent inhibition, antagonist muscle activity) or change in sensitivity/threshold is thought to occur (Aagaard 2003; Aagaard *et al.* 2000). It is not exactly clear how these mechanisms coexist. However, it is clear that the adaptations in neuromuscular function are complex. Greater neural drive may precede ultrastructural changes in skeletal muscle, but muscular changes feedback to the central nervous system and affect task-specific neural activation. The next several sections discuss the current thoughts on different potential sites of neuromuscular adaptations to training.

Higher brain centers

The ability to increase motor unit activity begins in the higher brain centers (i.e., motor cortex) with the volitional intent to produce high levels of force or power. This has been shown as neural activity increases in the primary motor cortex as isometric tension increases (Dettmers *et al.* 1996). Motor learning results in functional organization of the cerebral cortex. It has been suggested that most neural adaptations during training (with learned movements) take place within the spinal cord (Carroll *et al.* 2002).

"Imagined" strength training (i.e., performing mental contractions) of the abductor digiti minimi muscle resulted in a 22% increase in strength versus a 30% increase brought about by physical training (Yue & Cole 1992). Similarly, imagined strength training produced a 35% increase in finger abduction strength versus a 13.5% increase in elbow flexion strength with a corresponding increase in electroencephalogram (EEG) derived cortical potentials (Ranganathan *et al.* 2004). These data suggest adaptations in higher brain centers during volitional maximal activation may result in strength gain.

Descending corticospinal tracts

Using twitch-interpolation techniques, it was shown that individuals do not produce as much voluntary force as they do when stimulation is performed simultaneously to maximal contraction (Enoka 1997). This effect is muscle dependent (Belanger & McComas 1981); more evident in fast-twitch (FT) motor units, and demonstrates a limited ability for untrained individuals to maximally recruit motor units. Further evidence has been provided with magnetic resonance imaging (MRI) by Adams *et al.* (1993), who showed that at maximal voluntary contraction only 71% of muscle cross-sectional area (CSA) was activated. A limitation in central drive reduces force production and much of the limitation may originate from descending corticospinal tracts, as evidenced by recent studies using transcranial stimulation before and following strength training (Carroll *et al.* 2002). Training has been shown to reduce this deficit. Pensini *et al.* (2002) examined 4 weeks of eccentric (ECC) plantar flexion training and reported that voluntary activation level increased from 80% pre-study to 91%.

Motor units

The functional unit of the nervous system is the *motor unit* (MU). Motoneurons are multipolar cells that may innervate 5–10 muscle fibers for small muscles and >100 for large trunk and limb muscles. Force modulation is controlled through excitatory and inhibitory synapses which may act on a homonymous motor unit pool or individual motor units. Greater force is produced when excitatory impulses increase, inhibitory impulses decrease, or a combination of both. Agonist force modulation and subsequent training adaptations result from increases in recruitment, firing rate, or synchronization.

RECRUITMENT

Motor units are recruited and decruited in an orderly progression based on the *size principle* which states that MU recruitment order progresses from smaller (slow-twitch [ST]) to larger (FT) units (Henneman *et al.* 1965), although exceptions have been shown. Small units are recruited first for more intricate control and larger units are recruited later to supply substantial force for high intensity contractions. Interestingly, MU threshold depends on previous activation history. Once a MU is recruited, less activation is needed for it to be re-recruited (Gorassini *et al.* 2002). These data have ramifications for acute strength–power performance as higher threshold MUs are more readily recruited over time and in response to fatigue. Variations in recruitment order do exist. Under normal conditions, 84–90% of MUs recruit in accordance with the size principle (Somjen *et al.* 1965). Recruitment order may vary (e.g., *selective recruitment*) during electrical stimulation (Trimble & Enoka 1991), change in direction of exerted forces or task-specific performance (Ter Haar Romeny *et al.* 1982), and ballistic contractions (Nardone *et al.* 1989). It has been suggested that recurrent inhibition of ST alpha motoneurons (via the Renshaw system) may lead to selective activation of FT MUs (Hutton & Enoka 1986), and recruitment of FT units recurrently inhibit smaller ST units (Earles *et al.* 2002). These variations in recruitment order may benefit high velocity, power training where activation of FT MUs can provide the power necessary for contractions of short duration.

TISSUE ACTIVATION

A reduction in EMG with greater muscle strength reflects less neural input is needed to create a specific level of force mostly brought about by muscle hypertrophy (Moritani & deVries 1979). Recently, MRI has enabled the visualization of activated muscle tissue during training. Ploutz *et al.* (1994) examined muscle activation during a resistance exercise protocol before and after 9 weeks of quadriceps femoris strength training (3–6 sets × 12 repetitions) and found strength in the trained leg increased 14% and muscle CSA increased 5%. The amount of activated muscle tissue during the post-study protocol revealed it was less than pre-study. Thus, less muscle mass was activated to lift a standard workload with training and subsequent muscle hypertrophy.

FIRING RATE

An increase in force and contraction velocity necessitates an increase in the rate of MU discharge. Smaller muscles (with low thresholds) tend to have higher firing rates (FR) than larger (high threshold) muscles. Studies have shown a positive sigmoidal relationship between increases in FR and force production (Monster & Chan 1977). In small muscles, recruitment occurs up to low levels of tension (i.e., 50–60% of MVC) and increases in FR are responsible for greater force beyond this point. Large muscles (i.e., deltoid) rely on recruitment to a higher percent of MVC (>80%; DeLuca *et al.* 1982). A disproportionately large increase in EMG relative to strength or rate of force development gains may indicate a greater increase in FR than recruitment (Aagaard *et al.* 2002a). Examining single MUs, Van Custem *et al.* (1998) showed that rate of force development increased following 12 weeks of ballistic training of the ankle dorsiflexors. Accommodating this change was an earlier onset of MU firing, the appearance of "doublets" (i.e., two consecutive discharges within 5 ms), and a higher FR.

CONDUCTION VELOCITY

Conduction velocity is the rate at which action potentials are transmitted along the motoneuron and it has been proposed as an index of MU recruitment according to the size principle. Shifts in the mean or median frequencies should reflect the recruitment of progressively larger and faster MUs. Conduction velocity is higher in type II fibers, is positively related to recruitment threshold (Kernell & Monster 1981), and may increase by >20% as contraction strength increases (Knaflitz *et al.* 1990). Conduction velocity decreases with fatigue, subsequently increases as higher threshold motor units are recruited during sustained contractions, and decreases again as these units fatigue (Houtman *et al.* 2003). Compared to endurance athletes, power athletes demonstrate greater conduction velocity in the tibial nerve (Kamen *et al.* 1981) possibly because of a greater percentage of FT fibers. A longitudinal study has shown no change in conduction velocity in thenar muscles following 18 weeks of strength training (Sale *et al.* 1982). However, highly trained strength athletes (weightlifters, bodybuilders) had 8% greater conduction velocity in thenar muscles than controls (Sale *et al.* 1983a).

MOTOR UNIT SYNCHRONIZATION

Synchronization is when two or more MUs discharge at fixed, grouped time intervals. Isometric contractions >75% MVC have shown synchronization (Stulen & DeLuca 1978). It was shown that synchronization results in higher EMG (65–130%) but not greater force production (Yao *et al.* 2000), and may be more prevalent during high intensity contractions (Kamen & Roy 2000). Greater MU synchronization has been observed after strength training (Felici *et al.* 2001; Milner-Brown 1975; Semmler *et al.* 2004). It is unclear the exact role synchronization has during training. It may be that bursts of grouped MU discharges may be advantageous for the timing of force production, and maybe not the overall level of force produced.

Antagonist co-contraction

Co-contraction of antagonist muscles during movement is a mechanism to increase joint stability, movement coordination, and reduce the risk of injury. However, there are occasions when co-contraction can be counterproductive (e.g., high force production) as it may counteract the kinetic effects of agonist muscle contraction. Several factors including the muscle group, velocity and type of muscle action, intensity, joint position, and injury status affect the magnitude of co-contraction (Sale

2003). Neural adaptations of antagonist musculature show varied responses to training. For sprint or plyometric training, the timing of co-activation may change (i.e., is higher during the pre-contact phase but less during propulsion and braking during drop jumping; Kellis *et al.* 2003). In rapid, ballistic movements requiring agility, co-contraction is triphasic with agonist contraction based on velocity, change of direction, and movement distance (Marsden *et al.* 1983). Cross-sectional studies have shown sprinters possess a greater hamstring co-contraction response to high velocity knee extensions than distance runners (Osternig *et al.* 1986). Antagonist co-contraction may be unchanged after 10–14 weeks of strength training (Aagaard *et al.* 2002a; Seger & Thorstensson 2005) or reduced following 4 weeks to 6 months of strength training (Häkkinen *et al.* 1998a; Pensini *et al.* 2002). Carolan and Cafarelli (1992) showed the degree of hamstring co-activation during extension MVC decreased by approximately 20% (and by 13% in the untrained leg), most of which occurred during the first week. Pearson *et al.* (2002) reported no difference between untrained men and master Olympic weightlifters in hamstring co-activation during isometric knee extension. Thus, co-activation appears to be a mechanism in place when there is a lack of familiarity with the task and the magnitude of reduction is minor compared with the improvements in strength (Enoka 1997; Häkkinen *et al.* 1998a).

Neuromuscular junction

The neuromuscular junction represents the interface between the alpha motoneuron and the muscle fiber. The neuromuscular junction in ST fibers tends to be less complex than FT (Sieck & Prakash 1997), which parallels the type and pattern of stimulation that occurs with each type. Animal studies have shown aerobic training results in greater presynaptic nerve terminal area, increased number of nerve terminal branches, increased perimeter of entire nerve terminal, and increased average length of individual nerve terminals (Deschenes *et al.* 1993). Deschenes *et al.* (1993) compared high to low intensity treadmill training and showed the synapses following high intensity training were more dispersed, asymmetrical, and irregularly shaped

compared to low intensity. Total length of nerve terminal branches, average length/branch, and average number of branches were higher in the high intensity group. Seven weeks of resistance training resulted in increased endplate perimeter length (15%) and area (16%), and greater dispersion of acetylcholine receptors within the endplate region (Deschenes *et al.* 2000).

Reflex potentiation

The effects of training on reflex responses have been studied. Many studies examined stretch reflex potentiation by measuring the Hoffmann reflex (*H reflex*). The H reflex involves simultaneous stimulation (via electrostimulation or voluntary activation) of the afferent and efferent nerves. Stimulation of the alpha motoneuron results in a motor response (M-wave) and the subsequent Ia afferent stimulation results in a detectable muscle response following the M-wave (the H reflex and voluntary [V] waves) which can be detected using surface EMG. The evoked H reflex tends to rely on ST MUs whereas the V waves rely on ST and FT units. The response increases linearly as stimulus intensity increases until maximum values are attained (i.e., $H_{max} : M_{max}$), and is dependent upon feedback from muscle spindles, Golgi tendon organs, and other proprioceptors (Zehr 2002). Larger amplitudes signify greater excitability or potentiation. Following strength training, reflex potentiation average increases of approximately 39–50% have been shown in the soleus, brachioradialis, extensor digitorum brevis, and hypothenar muscles (Sale *et al.* 1983b) but not in the thenar muscles in one study (Sale *et al.* 1982). Fourteen weeks of lower body strength training resulted in a 55% increase in V wave amplitude and 19% increase in H reflex amplitude (Aagaard *et al.* 2002b). Strength trained athletes (weightlifters, bodybuilders) were shown to have greater reflex potentiation in the soleus but not in the thenar muscles than controls (Sale *et al.* 1983a).

The $H_{max} : M_{max}$ ratio has been used to describe the level of reflex excitability. Because H_{max} is highly reliant on ST fiber activation, a higher ratio tends to portray activities/training that rely predominantly on type I MU activation. This ratio has been shown

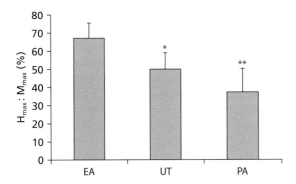

Fig. 2.14 The H_{max} : M_{max} ratio in endurance athletes (EA), untrained controls (UT), and power athletes (PA). Endurance athletes has the highest ratio compared to UT and PA. Power athletes ratio was lower than UT. (Data adapted from Maffiuletti *et al.* 2001.)

to be higher in aerobic athletes than anaerobic athletes, as endurance athletes display much larger H reflex whereas power athletes display higher M-waves. The soleus (predominantly ST) produces a larger H_{max} and the gastrocnemius (predominantly FT) produces a larger M_{max} (Maffiuletti *et al.* 2003). It increases after endurance training (Perot *et al.* 1991) but decreases after power training (i.e., is lower in sprinters and volleyball players than controls; Casabona *et al.* 1990). Endurance athletes have shown ratios of approximately 67% compared to that of approximately 37% in power athletes (Fig. 2.14; Maffiuletti *et al.* 2001).

POST-ACTIVATION POTENTIATION

Activated MUs stay facilitated for a period of time following use. Maximal or near-maximal contractions elicit a *post-activation potentiation* (PAP) for subsequent muscle contractions occurring within several seconds to a few minutes (Baudry & Duchateau 2004). Hamada *et al.* (2000a; 2003) found this to be approximately 71% on average immediately following a 10-s MVC (and elevated by 12% 5 min following the MVC protocol) and 126% in subjects with large amount of FT fibers. However, this same protocol failed to enhance performance of subsequent (i.e., 15 s) maximal isometric knee extensions (Gossen & Sale 2000). PAP is more prominent in FT muscle fibers and in explosive

power athletes (Chiu *et al.* 2003), although endurance athletes demonstrate PAP (Hamada *et al.* 2000b). The mechanism is believed to be related to phosphorylation of myosin regulatory light chains during maximal contraction which renders actin and myosin more sensitive to calcium (Hamada *et al.* 2000a). Performance enhancement has been reported (French *et al.* 2003) but further research is necessary to determine chronic training effects of protocols maximizing PAP.

EMG studies

Most of the evidence supporting neural adaptations to training was attained via EMG studies. EMG measurements are typically made with surface electrodes or with needle or fine wire electrodes. Most often surface electrodes are used because of their ease of application and comfort to the subjects. The signal quantification typically involves the integrated EMG (IEMG) or the root mean square (RMS). An increase in IEMG or RMS signifies greater motor unit activity, which can stem from greater recruitment or rate (these methods cannot differentiate the roots of the signal). Needle electrodes are less commonly used in exercise or training studies.

Table 2.1 depicts some longitudinal training studies using EMG pre- and post-training to examine changes in neural activation. Studies have shown increases and no change in EMG following strength training despite increases in muscle strength (15–73%). Training status of the subjects is critical. It has been shown that the early stage of strength training is characterized predominantly by enhanced motor learning and coordination (Rutherford & Jones 1986). Neural adaptations predominate early (with minimal hypertrophy) and many short-term studies have shown greater IEMG post-training (Aagaard *et al.* 2002a; Narici *et al.* 1989). However, some long-term studies have shown no change, possibly because of changes in muscle architecture, subcutaneous fat, and hypertrophy (Narici *et al.* 1996; Sale 2003). The onset of hypertrophy is associated with declines in EMG (Moritani & deVries 1979) as muscle fibers are capable of providing more tension. It has been suggested that subsequent training exhibits an interplay between neural and

Table 2.1 EMG and training: comparison of selected studies.

Researchers	Subjects	Protocol	Frequency/Duration	Strength Inc.	Outcome
Aagaard *et al.* (2002a)	UT M	4–5×3–12RM leg exercises	2–3×/14 week	16.5%	EMG ↑
Bandy & Hanten (1993)	UT F	ISOM KE	3×/8 weeks		**EMG ↑
Cannon & Cafarelli (1987)	UT M, F	15×80% MVC: 3–4 s thumb adduction	3×/5 weeks	15%	EMG ↔
Carolan & Cafarelli (1992)	UT M	30×ISOM KE	3×/8 weeks	32.8%	EMG ↔
Colson *et al.* (1999)	UT M	5×6 100–120% 1RM ECC elbow flex	3×/7 weeks	11–46%	RMS ↑
Hakkinen & Komi (1983)	RT M	Strength training (80–120% 1RM)	3×/16 weeks	11–15%	EMG ↑
Häkkinen *et al.* (1985a)	RT M	18–30×70–100% 1RM	3×/24 weeks	26.8%	*EMG ↔
Häkkinen *et al.* (1985b)	RT M	Power/jump training	3×/24 weeks	10.8%	EMG ↑
Häkkinen & Komi (1986)	RT M	(a) 18–30×70–120% 1RM (b) jump training	3×/24 weeks	13.9% ns	EMG ↑ EMG ↔
Häkkinen *et al.* (1987)	EWL M	Advanced weightlifting	5×/12 months	1.2–1.7%	*EMG ↔
Häkkinen *et al.* (1996)	UT M, F	Heavy strength training	12 weeks	10–19%	EMG ↑
Häkkinen *et al.* (1998a)	UT M, F	Heavy strength training	6 months	21–66%	EMG ↑
Häkkinen *et al.* (2001)	UT M, F	Strength/power training	2×/6 months	21–35%	EMG ↑
Häkkinen *et al.* (2003)	UT M	Strength & strength/ Endurance training	21 weeks	21–22%	EMG ↑
McBride *et al.* (2002)	RT M	Power jump squats 4–5×30 vs. 80% 1RM	1–2×/8 weeks	8–11%	EMG ↑
McBride *et al.* (2003)	UT M, F	1 vs. 6 sets of leg press, arm curl	12 weeks	7–53%	***EMG ↑
Moritani & deVries (1979)	UT, M, F	2×10 67% max elbow flexion	3×/8 weeks	36%	EMG ↑
Narici *et al.* (1989)	UT M	6×10 ISOK KE	4×/8.5 weeks	20.8%	EMG ↑
Narici *et al.* (1996)	UT M	6×8 80% 1RM KE	6 months	21–30%	EMG ↔
Pensini *et al.* (2002)	UT M	6×6 ECC 120% 1RM	4×/4 weeks	14–30%	EMG ↑
Thorstensson *et al.* (1976)	UT M	3×6RM squats, jumps, abs	3×/8 weeks	16–73%	EMG ↔
Van Custem *et al.* (1998)	UT M, F	10×10 30–40% 1RM	5×/12 weeks	30.2%	EMG ↑

EWL, elite weightlifters; F, female; ISOK, isokinetic; ISOM, isometric; M, male; MVC, maximal voluntary contraction; RT, resistance trained; UT, untrained.
* EMG fluctuated with overall training intensity (decreased during reduced intensity, returned to normal when intensity increased [>80% of 1 RM]).
** EMG increased at non-trained joint angles.
*** EMG increased following multiple-set training only during elbow flexion.

hypertrophic mechanisms for strength and power improvements (Sale 2003). Advanced weightlifters show limited potential for further neural adaptations over the course of 1 year (Häkkinen *et al.* 1987).

The training program may dictate the pattern of adaptation. In a 24-week strength training study, Häkkinen *et al.* (1985a) reported significant increases in EMG during the high intensity (>80% of 1 RM) period. However, when intensity was reduced EMG also decreased but hypertrophy was greatest. Greater neural activation has been observed during

ballistic, high intensity strength, and power training (Häkkinen *et al.* 1985a,b). In weightlifters, high volume, high intensity training (i.e., overreaching) may reduce IEMG during the first few days but returns to baseline within 1 week (Häkkinen & Kauhanen 1989) and may increase during a taper period (i.e., reduced training volume; Häkkinen *et al.* 1991). Although the majority of research has examined EMG changes during strength and/or power training, there is evidence to indicate endurance athletes (i.e., professional road cyclists) may have a greater ability for MU activation during strenuous endurance training periods (Lucia *et al.* 2000).

UNILATERAL VS. BILATERAL TRAINING

Training with one or two limbs simultaneously affects neuromuscular adaptations to training (i.e., bilateral deficit and cross education). *Cross education* refers to strength and endurance gained in the non-trained limb during unilateral training. Several studies have shown strength increases in the contralateral limb. In a recent meta-analysis, Munn *et al.* (2004) reported that contralateral limb strength increased up to 22% with a mean increase of nearly 8% compared to pre-training values. The strength increase is accompanied by greater IEMG activity in the trained and non-trained limbs (Narici *et al.* 1989; Shima *et al.* 2002; Weir *et al.* 1994), especially when ECC training (Hortobagyi *et al.* 1997) and muscle stimulation (Hortobagyi *et al.* 1999) are performed. Endurance may increase in the untrained limb (Yuza *et al.* 2000). *Bilateral deficit* refers to the maximal force produced by both limbs contracting bilaterally being smaller than the sum of the limbs contracting unilaterally. Unilateral training increases unilateral strength to a greater extent and bilateral training increases bilateral strength to a greater extent with a corresponding greater specific IEMG response (Häkkinen *et al.* 1996; Kuruganti *et al.* 2005; Taniguchi 1997). The bilateral deficit is reduced with bilateral training.

Muscular adaptations to training

Fiber type transitions

The pattern of neuromuscular stimulation dictates fiber type composition. Fast-twitch muscle fibers are activated mostly during activities that are short in duration and high in intensity (e.g., weightlifting, sprinting) and are very fatigable whereas ST fibers are fatigue-resistant and predominate during aerobic activities such as distance running and cycling (Table 2.2). Muscle fibers represent a continuum from the most oxidative to the least oxidative. The continuum is as follows: I, IC, IIC, IIAC, IIA, IIAB

Table 2.2 Slow- and fast-twitch muscle fiber characteristics.

Characteristic	Slow-twitch	Fast-twitch
Motoneuron size	Small	Large
Nerve conduction velocity	Slow	Fast
Nerve recruitment threshold	Low	High
Size	Small	Large
Contractile speed	Slow	Fast
Myosin type	Slow	Fast
Myofibrillar ATPase activity	Low	High
Sarcoplasmic reticulum development	Poor	Great
Troponin affinity for calcium	Poor	Great
Force per cross-sectional area	Low	High
Efficiency of force production	Great	Poor
Fatigability	Low	High
Intramuscular ATP/PC stores	Low	High
Relaxation time	Slow	Fast
Glycolytic enzyme activity	Low	High
Glycogen stores	Moderate	High
Endurance	High	Low
Triglyceride stores	High	Low
Myoglobin content	High	Low
Aerobic enzyme activity	High	Low
Capillary density	High	Low
Mitochondrial density	High	Low

(or IIAX), and IIB (IIX) with a concomitant myosin heavy chain expression (i.e., MHCI, IIA, and IIB or IIX; Staron 1997).

Although the proportions of type I and II fibers appear genetically determined, transitions have been shown within each subpopulation. Changes in myosin heavy chain (MHC) content occur within the first few training sessions. Changes from MHCIIb (expressing the MHC-IIX myosin) to MHCIIa have been observed during resistance (Fry *et al.* 1994; Harber *et al.* 2004; Jurimae *et al.* 1997) and sprint cycle training (Allemeier *et al.* 1994) which precede changes in fiber type composition. Several studies have shown a greater proportion of type IIA fibers with a subsequent decrease in type IIX fiber percent during resistance training (Fry *et al.* 1994; Kraemer *et al.* 1995; Staron *et al.* 1989, 1994; Wang *et al.* 1993). These changes have been observed in as little as 2 weeks (four workouts) in women and 4 weeks (eight workouts) in men (Staron *et al.* 1994). It appears that type IIX fibers are "reservoir" fibers which transform into a more oxidative form upon consistent activation along the continuum (i.e., to an intermediate fiber type IIAX to IIA; Campos *et al.* 2002; Hostler *et al.* 2001; Wang *et al.* 1993), as is the case during progressive resistance and endurance training. However, it also appears that the switch from the fast type II to the slow type I is much more difficult to transform. Interestingly, training cessation results in an increase in type IIX fibers and reduction in type IIA fibers (Pette & Staron 1997), with a possible overshoot of type IIX fibers (Andersen & Aagaard 2000).

Similar findings have been shown following aerobic training. O'Neill *et al.* (1999) reported no changes in MHC mRNA following one workout; however, significant downregulation of MHCIIX was found after only 1 week of endurance training (75% of $\dot{V}o_{2max}$). Sixteen weeks of aerobic training (5 times per week, 70% of peak heart rate) resulted in MHC mRNA increases of 63% (MHCI) and 99% (MHCIIA) whereas a 50% reduction was observed in MHCIIX (Short *et al.* 2005). Eight weeks of endurance training resulted in a reduction in type IIX fibers (19% to 14%) and increase in type IIA fibers (37% to 42%; Andersen & Henriksson 1977). The magnitude of type IIX fiber percent reduction is greater following strength than endurance training (Kraemer *et al.* 1995), thereby demonstrating the greater type II fiber recruitment during strength training. Simultaneous aerobic and strength training results in a reduction in MHCIIX (Putnam *et al.* 2004). Although there is some evidence for conversions between type I and II fibers for sprint and endurance training (Jansson *et al.* 1978), it is unclear at this time if this is a common adaptation to training.

Muscle hypertrophy

Muscle hypertrophy is an increase in cross-sectional fiber and muscle area brought about with repeated bouts of physical training. There is a positive relationship between the CSA of skeletal muscle and the amount of force it is capable of producing. The increase in CSA of muscle fibers is proportional to greater size and number of actin/myosin filaments and the addition of peripheral sarcomeres (although the addition of non-structural/contractile proteins

has been suggested). Maximal force production benefits greatly from an increase in myofibrillar proteins (Phillips 2000). Although neural adaptations predominate initially, hypertrophy becomes a critical adaptation to subsequent strength training. Changes in muscle proteins (e.g., MHCs) take place within a couple of workouts (Staron *et al.* 1994). However, a longer period of time (more than eight workouts) is needed to demonstrate significant muscle hypertrophy.

Hypertrophy results from increased net protein accretion (i.e., an increase in protein synthesis, decrease in protein degradation, or combination of both). Protein synthesis increases following an acute bout of resistance exercise, and may be elevated up to 48 h post-exercise (Chesley *et al.* 1992; MacDougall *et al.* 1992, 1995; Phillips *et al.* 1997). Protein synthesis depends on amino acid availability and transport (Biolo *et al.* 1995), post-translational modifications (Jefferson & Kimball 2001), timing of intake (Tipton *et al.* 2001), insulin concentrations (Biolo *et al.* 1999), and other factors such as anabolic hormonal regulation (e.g., growth hormone(s), testosterone, insulin-like growth factor-1 [IGF-1], mechano-growth factor, androgen receptor content) and mechanical stress (Goldspink & Yang 2001; Kraemer & Ratamess 2003, 2005; Ratamess *et al.* 2005), and cellular hydration (Waldegger *et al.* 1997).

The magnitude of hypertrophy depends on several factors. Greater gains in hypertrophy are seen when ECC muscle actions are used (Dudley *et al.* 1991; Hather *et al.* 1991). The intensity and volume of the training program (mechanical stimulus) has significant roles in hypertrophy (Kraemer & Ratamess 2004). Gains in hypertrophy are most evident in FT fibers compared to ST (McCall *et al.* 1996). There is evidence showing the importance of blood flow and/or metabolite accumulation during strength training (Shinohara *et al.* 1998; Smith & Rutherford 1995). This tissue remodeling process is affected by endocrine factors such as the concentrations of testosterone, growth hormone, cortisol, insulin, and IGF-1 (Kraemer & Ratamess 2003, 2005). Men and women increase muscle size substantially. However, men experience greater absolute gains during resistance training (Alway *et al.* 1992). Some caution must be exercised when interpreting the muscle CSA data obtained only at one particular portion of the thigh, because training-induced muscle hypertrophy can also be a non-uniform process along the belly of the muscle (Hakkinen *et al.* 1998b).

Although resistance training is mostly used to enhance muscle hypertrophy, sprint (Linossier *et al.* 1997; Ross & Leveritt 2001) and power training (Häkkinen *et al.* 1985b) have been shown to increase muscle size to a lesser extent. Aerobic training results in no change (Putnam *et al.* 2004) or a reduction in muscle size (Kraemer *et al.* 1995, 2004). Reductions in muscle size occur mostly in type I and IIC fiber populations (Kraemer *et al.* 1995). Simultaneous strength and aerobic training results in substantial increases in CSA of type IIA muscle fibers but only strength training increased CSA of type I fibers (Kraemer *et al.* 1995; Putnam *et al.* 2004).

Hyperplasia

Although hypertrophy is the major mechanism for muscle growth, another proposed mechanism for growth is hyperplasia. *Hyperplasia* involves longitudinal splitting of existing muscle fibers (or new fiber development via satellite cells), subsequently resulting in an increased number of muscle cells. Hyperplasia was first shown in laboratory animals (Gonyea 1980; Gonyea *et al.* 1977). Although methodology used in these studies was questioned by some scientists, later studies in animals showed hyperplasia occurred (Gonyea *et al.* 1986). Hyperplasia has been controversial in humans. Studies comparing body builders and powerlifters with controls have shown greater number of muscle fibers in the lifters (MacDougall *et al.* 1982; Tesch & Larsson 1982). However, it was not determined if this was a result of training or genetics as other studies have shown similar fiber number between strength athletes and controls (MacDougall *et al.* 1984). In a longitudinal study, McCall *et al.* (1996) showed indirect evidence for hyperplasia (i.e., a subpopulation of subjects showed greater fiber number although there was no change when all subjects were analyzed) in the biceps muscle following strength training. If hyperplasia does occur, it may represent an adaptation to strength training when certain muscle fibers reach a theoretical "upper limit" in cell size. If hyperplasia does occur, it may only account for a small portion of the increase in muscle size.

Structural changes in skeletal muscle

Table 2.3 summarizes several skeletal muscle changes following training. Resistance training leads to greater myofibrillar volume, cytoplasmic density, Na^+/K^+ ATPase activity, pennation angle, and fascicle length. Many of these changes support muscular hypertrophy, and subsequent muscular strength enhancement. Sprint training leads to greater calcium kinetics and fascicle length which enable greater muscle contraction velocities. Endurance training leads to slower calcium kinetics and higher Na^+/K^+ ATPase activity characteristic of slow muscle contractions. In addition, endurance training results in increases in aerobic enzyme activity (Costill *et al.* 1976), capillary density (Saltin & Rowell 1980), and mitochondrial density (Hoppeler *et al.* 1985). Other metabolic changes in skeletal muscle (i.e., anaerobic enzyme activity, glycogen content, buffer capacity; Roberts *et al.* 1982; Sharp *et al.* 1986; Tesch 1988) occur enabling higher anaerobic performance.

Conclusions

Aerobic and anaerobic training lead to specific adaptations that accommodate increases in muscle strength, endurance, size, power, speed, agility, and balance. The nervous system adapts to both training modalities, although anaerobic training has been more extensively studied. Adaptations may take place in higher brain centers, descending corticospinal tracts, reflex circuitry (and reduce inhibitions), and at the neuromuscular junction. Greater agonist muscle activity is the result of greater motor unit recruitment, firing rate, and possible synchronization. In addition, timely coordination of antagonist muscle activity is critical to strength, power, and speed training. Muscle fiber types are plastic and may transform within type I and II domains based on the level of activation as training results in greater proportion of type IIA and a reduction of type IIX fiber percentages. Muscle hypertrophy occurs mostly via resistance training, although sprint and power training can lead to

Table 2.3 Training-induced structural changes in skeletal muscle.

Authors	Training protocol	Change
MacDougall et al. (1979)	6 months RT triceps brachii	$\leftrightarrow$ Myofibrillar density*
		$\uparrow$ Myofibrillar volume
Luthi et al. (1986)	6 weeks RT quadriceps	$\leftrightarrow$ Myofibrillar density*
		$\uparrow$ Myofibrillar volume
Claassen et al. (1989)	6 weeks RT quadriceps	$\leftrightarrow$ Space between myosin filaments
MacDougall et al. (1982)	Cross-sectional	$\uparrow$ Cytoplasmic density in PL, BB > C
Claassen et al. (1989)	6 weeks RT quadriceps	$\leftrightarrow$ Sarcomere length
Claassen et al. (1989)	6 weeks RT quadriceps	$\leftrightarrow$ Actin : myosin ratio
Alway et al. (1989)	16 weeks RT triceps surae	$\uparrow$ SR/T tubule density in proportion to myofibrillar volume
Klitgaard et al. (1990)	Cross-sectional, VL B elderly RT vs. C	$\downarrow$ Expression of slow β-tropomyosin Isoform seen in aging
Hunter et al. (1999)	12 weeks RT quadriceps elderly vs. young women	$\uparrow$ Calcium uptake – elderly $\leftrightarrow$ Calcium uptake – young
Ortenblad et al. (2000)	5 weeks sprint training	$\uparrow$ Calcium release, $\leftrightarrow$ uptake
		$\uparrow$ Ryanodine receptor #/ $\leftrightarrow$ density
		$\leftrightarrow$ Ca^{2+} ATPase, $\uparrow$ SERCA-1, SERCA-2
Green et al. (2003)	10 weeks endurance training	$\downarrow$ Ca^{2+} ATPase, Ca^{2+} uptake, & release
		$\downarrow$ SERCA-1, $\leftrightarrow$ SERCA-2
Madsen et al. (1994)	6 weeks endurance training	$\leftrightarrow$ Ca^{2+} ATPase; $\uparrow$ Na^+/K^+ ATPase
Hunter et al. (1999)	12 weeks RT quadriceps elderly vs. young women	$\uparrow$ Ca^{2+} ATPase – elderly $\leftrightarrow$ Ca^{2+} ATPase – young
Green et al. (1998)	12 weeks RT quadriceps	$\leftrightarrow$ Ca^{2+} ATPase
Green et al. (1999)	12 weeks RT quadriceps	$\uparrow$ Na^+/K^+ ATPase
Klitgaard & Clausen (1989)	Cross-sectional	$\uparrow$ Na^+/K^+ ATPase in ST men vs. C
Green et al. (2004)	6 days endurance training	$\uparrow$ Na^+/K^+ ATPase
Aagaard et al. (2001)	14 weeks RT quadriceps	$\uparrow$ Pennation angle
Kearns et al. (2000)	Cross-sectional	Sumo wrestlers > C fascicle length & pennation angle TB & VL
Abe et al. (2000)	Cross-sectional VL, gastrocnemius	Fascicle length: Sprinters > DR Pennation angle: DR > sprinters

B, biceps brachii; BB, body builders; C, control subjects; DR, distance runners; PL, power lifters, RT, resistance training; TB, triceps brachii; VL, vastus lateralis.
* Myofibrillar density is the cross-bridge spacing.

hypertrophy to a lesser extent. Finally, ultrastructural changes occur within skeletal muscles that enable greater force production and endurance.

METABOLIC ADAPTATIONS TO TRAINING

JOHN A. HAWLEY AND GUSTAVO A. NADER

Objectives of training for enhancing athletic performance

The ability of skeletal muscle to adapt to repeated bouts of physical activity over time so that exercise capacity is improved is termed physical training (Booth & Thomason 1991). For the competitive endurance athlete, the primary objective of such training is to increase the ability to sustain the highest *average* power output or speed of movement to overcome resistance (air or water) or drag (friction) for a predetermined distance or time such that performance will be enhanced (Coyle et al. 1994; Hawley 2002). For the strength-trained athlete, the primary objective of training is to develop muscular strength or power. In addition, strength training is often undertaken to improve other sporting skills such as speed, or to enhance performance through "strength-like" or "overloaded" exercises using sports-specific skills or elements typical of a given sport (Deschenes & Kraemer 2002; Kraemer *et al.* 1996). Strength training can also be utilized to increase muscle strength in the absence of an increase in muscle mass (e.g., for improving endurance performance). Importantly, strength training is a fundamental component of many sport rehabilitation programs in which successful implementation of a therapeutic intervention determines the suitability of an athlete to return to competition. Thus, the specificity of strength training is a crucial factor in program design and will likely affect the outcome of the training program.

All sporting endeavours ultimately depend on the rate and efficiency at which chemical energy can be converted into mechanical energy for skeletal muscle contraction. Accordingly, it has been proposed (Coyle *et al.* 1994; Hawley 2002) that training for enhancement of athletic performance should aim to induce multiple physiologic and metabolic adaptations that enable an athlete to:

1 Increase the rate of energy production and force capability from both aerobic (endurance and ultra-endurance events) and oxygen-independent (power/speed events) ATP generating pathways;
2 Maintain tighter metabolic control (i.e., match ATP production with ATP hydrolysis);
3 Minimize cellular disturbances;
4 Increase economy of motion; and
5 Improve the resistance of the working muscles to fatigue during sports-specific contractions.

This chapter summarizes the current knowledge of the metabolic adaptations to endurance and strength training and the implications of such adaptations for athletic performance.

The training stimulus, response, and adaptation continuum

The acute metabolic responses associated with a single bout of exercise and subsequent training-induced adaptations are highly specific to the mode, intensity, and duration of the stimulus (Hildebrandt *et al.* 2003; Nader & Esser 2001), and the corresponding pattern of muscle fiber recruitment (Gollnick *et al.* 1973). Although training-induced metabolic adaptations in skeletal muscle are likely to be the

result of the cumulative effect of repeated bouts of exercise, the initial responses that lead to these chronic changes occur during and after each training session (Pilegaard *et al.* 2000; Widegren *et al.* 2001; Williams & Neufer 1996). For example, at the onset of exercise there are rapid changes in metabolite concentrations (i.e., decreases in [ATP] and increases in [ADP] and adenosine monophosphate [AMP]). Within minutes, these contraction-induced metabolic disturbances in muscle, along with the accompanying mechanical stress (particularly muscle damage caused by eccentric work) activate several key kinases and phosphatases involved in signal transduction. During exercise, and especially in the post-exercise recovery period, there is increased expression of certain transcription factors that promote protein synthesis; the gene expression that allows for these changes in protein concentration is pivotal to the training adaptation (Hansen *et al.* 2005). Accordingly, the training stimulus, response, and adaptation can be viewed as a continuum of coordinated events that elicit a multitude of time-dependent physiologic, biochemical, and molecular changes within the muscle that, depending on the dominant stimuli, produces either mitochondrial biogenesis (an "endurance-like profile") or muscle hypertrophy (a "strength-like profile") and concomitant alterations in muscle phenotype that serve to improve cellular function and thereby enhance exercise capacity (Glass 2003; Hawley *et al.* 2006; Hood 2001).

Metabolic adaptations to endurance training

It is well accepted that sedentary individuals can dramatically increase their endurance capacity by means of regularly performed training. For many years it was believed that this increase in exercise capacity was predominantly the result of "central" cardiovascular adaptations to training (i.e., increased delivery of O_2 to the working muscles and a concomitant increase in maximal aerobic power [$\dot{V}O_{2max}$]), rather than "local" changes in muscle metabolism. While regularly performed endurance exercise induces profound alterations in many physiologic systems (cardiovascular, endocrine,

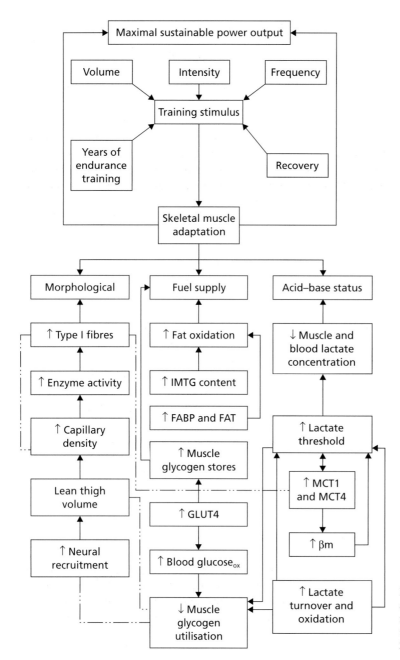

Fig. 2.15 Some of the major adaptations in skeletal muscle that result from regular endurance training. (From Hawley & Stepto 2001.)

hormonal), local muscle adaptations and the accompanying shifts in substrate selection undoubtedly have a key role in the enhanced capacity for prolonged exercise that accrue from such training. Some of the major adaptations in skeletal muscle

resulting from regular endurance exercise are displayed in Fig. 2.15. In this chapter, focus is on the training-induced metabolic perturbations that result in changes in fuel supply and acid–base status. A more detailed discussion of how training affects muscle morphology can be found in several recent reviews (Hawley & Stepto 2001; Zierath & Hawley 2004).

Mitochondrial adaptations to endurance training and their metabolic consequences

Holloszy (1967) was the first to show that endurance exercise training induced an increase in the mitochondrial content of skeletal muscle. This classic study, undertaken in rats, demonstrated that the total protein content of the mitochondria in trained muscle increased by approximately 60%. This increase in mitochondrial content was accompanied by a higher level of respiratory control and tightly coupled oxidative phosphorylation, providing evidence that the increase in electron transport capacity was associated with a concomitant rise in the capacity to generate ATP via oxidative phosphorylation (Holloszy 1967). This finding of increased respiratory capacity and mitochondrial enzyme level in response to training was soon confirmed by other investigators in the muscles of endurance-trained humans (Chi et al. 1983; Costill et al. 1979; Gollnick et al. 1973; Jansson & Kaijser 1977; Orlander et al. 1977). It is now widely recognized that the increase in muscle respiratory capacity is one of the primary mechanisms by which endurance training affects fuel utilization during submaximal exercise.

The effects of endurance training on fuel metabolism have been studied for many decades. Over 60 years ago, Christensen and Hansen (1939a) were the first to demonstrate that endurance training reduced whole-body rates of carbohydrate (CHO) oxidation, as measured by a lower respiratory exchange ratio (RER). Many studies have subsequently confirmed this observation (for review see Coggan & Williams 1995). A similar effect of training is observed when the respiratory exchange quotient (RQ) is measured directly across the exercising limbs (Henriksson 1977). The decreases in whole-body RER and/or muscle RQ with training have been interpreted as a training-induced shift from CHO-based fuels (muscle and liver glycogen, blood glucose, blood, muscle, and liver lactate) towards fat-based fuels (blood-borne free fatty acids [FFA], adipose and intramuscular triglycerides) as a source of energy during exercise. While we know this to be true, measures of RER or RQ alone cannot determine the precise combination of CHO- or fat-based fuels oxidized during exercise. Indeed, it was not until the reintroduction of the needle biopsy technique into exercise physiology in the 1960s, (Bergstrom et al. 1967) in combination with tracer techniques to estimate the fate of endogenous fuel fluxes, that such questions could be addressed.

Utilizing serial muscle biopsies during exercise, Hermanssen et al. (1967) reported that the rate of muscle glycogen disappearance was similar in untrained and trained humans when they exercised at the same *relative* intensity (approximately 75–80% of individual $\dot{V}o_{2max}$). Because the absolute rate of energy expenditure was approximately 20% higher in the trained athletes, these data were the first to demonstrate a marked "glycogen sparing" effect of endurance training. The results from a longitudinal training study in which humans performed exercise at the same *absolute* intensity before and after training confirmed the earlier observations of Hermanssen et al. (Karlsson et al. 1974). Indeed, it is now well accepted that endurance training reduces the rate of muscle glycogen utilization during submaximal exercise. The mechanisms whereby endurance training decreases muscle glycogenolysis include post-transformational regulation of the enzyme controlling glycogen breakdown (glycogen phosphorylase) as well as an attenuated activation of pyruvate dehydrogenase (PDH), the rate-limiting enzyme for entry of CHO-derived acetyl units into oxidative metabolism (LeBlanc et al. 2004).

To investigate the role of endurance training on blood glucose kinetics, Coggan et al. (1990) had seven men perform a standardized bout of cycling before and after 12 weeks of endurance training. Utilizing a continuous infusion of [U-^{13}C] glucose, they observed that the training regimen significantly reduced the production, uptake, and oxidation of plasma glucose during the later stages of prolonged (120 min) submaximal exercise. The finding of a reduced plasma glucose uptake by working muscle seems, at first, paradoxical as endurance training is well known to increase the total concentration of muscle GLUT-4 (Daugaard et al. 2000). The likely mechanism underlying the reduction in blood glucose uptake after training is caused, in part, by a blunted exercise-induced translocation of GLUT-4 protein to the sarcolemma, which in turn, leads to a diminished exercise-induced sarcolemmal glucose transport capacity (Richter *et al*. 1998). From a teleologic viewpoint, the slower rates of muscle glucose uptake and utilization after training makes good sense because the more rapidly glucose (and glycogen) are used during exercise, the sooner the individual is forced to stop exercising, either by the development of hypoglycemia or depletion of endogenous glycogen stores.

Endurance training also reduces the rate of appearance (Ra) of glucose from the liver during exercise (Coggan *et al*. 1995). Reductions in muscle glycogen utilization and liver glycogen utilization seem to contribute equally to the overall CHO-sparing effect of endurance training, at least in moderately trained individuals. As a consequence of these adaptations, trained athletes are better able to maintain plasma glucose concentrations during prolonged exercise compared with their untrained counterparts (Coggan *et al*. 1990, 1992; Mendenhall *et al*. 1994) even when performing exercise at the same relative intensity.

The training-induced reduction in CHO oxidation during submaximal exercise is compensated for by an increase in lipid oxidation. Although the results of tracer infusion studies conducted in the 1960s and early 1970s emphasized the importance of plasma FFA as an energy source during low to moderate intensity exercise (for review see Coggan & Williams 1995), more recent studies have failed to support these findings. Indeed, it is now apparent that intramuscular lipids account for the greater rate of fat oxidation after training (Hurley *et al*. 1986). The precise mechanism(s) responsible for the increased capacity for lipid oxidation after training are not fully understood, but depend, in part, on the ability of the expanded mitochondrial reticulum to suppress glycolysis and increase uptake of fatty acyl-CoA from intracellular triglyceride stores. In addition, Bonen *et al*. (1999) have shown that when the oxidative capacity of muscle is increased, there is a parallel increase in the rate of FA transport and FA transporters at the sarcolemmal membrane, which is associated with the enhanced expression of the membrane transporter FAT/CD36.

ACID–BASE STATUS

Exercise performed at the same relative intensity results in a smaller increase in blood–plasma lactate concentration after endurance training. Furthermore, a considerably higher work rate is required to attain a given lactate level (i.e., 4 mmol·L^{-1}) in the well-trained vs. the untrained state (Hurley *et al*. 1984). To determine whether the reduced blood lactate concentrations during submaximal exercise in humans after endurance training result from a decreased lactate Ra or an increased rate of lactate metabolic clearance (MCR), interrelationships among blood lactate Ra, and lactate MCR were investigated in eight (untrained) men during progressive exercise before and after a 9-week endurance training program. Radioisotope dilution measurements of [U-^{14}C] lactate revealed that the slower rise in blood lactate after training was brought about by a reduced lactate Ra at low work rates (<60% of $\dot{V}o_{2max}$), but a combination of an increased MCR and a lower Ra at higher power outputs (MacRae *et al*. 1992).

There is good evidence that an individual's "lactate threshold" is related to the absolute speed and/or power they can generate during activities lasting longer than about 10 min (Coyle *et al*. 1988; Padilla *et al*. 2000). Indeed, a major attribute of endurance-trained individuals is their ability to sustain high rates of energy production for prolonged periods in the face of (low) steady state lactate levels (Padilla *et al*. 2000). Accordingly, the transport of lactate in and out of the muscle (by the monocarboxylate [MCT] transporters) is important if such conditions are to be maintained. Not surprisingly, individuals with a high proportion of ST fibers in their active musculature have a higher proportion of MCT transporters compared with those individuals who possess fewer ST fibers (Pilegaard *et al*. 1999b). Interestingly, individuals who include a portion of their training as intense interval workouts have the highest MCT transport capacity (Pilegaard *et al*. 1999a), indicating that a large volume of endurance training alone may not be sufficient to induce the necessary muscle adaptations that are responsible for improving the ability to transport lactate. Such an observation may explain why a short-term supramaximal training program (six sessions of 12×30 s all-out sprints) was just as effective in enhancing 40 km cycling performance (lasting approximately 55 min) as longer "aerobic" interval sets (six sessions of 8×4 min at close to race pace; Stepto *et al.* 1999).

Time-course of adaptive changes in skeletal muscle

The time-course of several of the adaptive responses to regular endurance training are known. For example, $\dot{V}o_{2max}$ typically increases 15–25% during the first 2–3 months of endurance training with a further (smaller) improvement occurring over the next 6–24 months (Saltin *et al.* 1977). There are more robust changes in some of the muscle enzymes involved in the citric acid cycle and respiratory chain; most of these enzymes have rather short turnover times, with half-lives in the order of 1–3 weeks (Henrikksson & Reitman 1977). Less precise is the information on the time-course of changes for muscle fiber conversion and capillary density. Transition of fiber types may be quite labile in a similar manner to many of the oxidative enzymes (Saltin *et al.* 1977), whereas capillarization probably occurs at a slower rate. After 1 year or longer of endurance training, the metabolic capacity of muscle is enhanced to a far greater extent than the circulatory capacity of the body to utilize oxygen. The training-induced shift in patterns of muscle substrate utilization (i.e., the "glycogen-sparing" effect) is more pronounced with prolonged training history. Indeed, during the time of peak endurance performance, muscle metabolic adaptations have likely reached their maximal attainable level (Saltin *et al.* 1977).

Goals of a strength training program

Over the years, much attention has been dedicated to the neuromuscular aspects of strength performance. However, much less scientific enquiry has been devoted to understand the metabolic adaptations resulting from strength training. Unfortunately, a coherent interpretation of such adaptations is confounded by the fact that discretely different "populations" can be distinguished as they pertain to the modality of strength training performed (i.e., Olympic lifting induces adaptations that differ from powerlifting and body building despite all three disciplines using "strength training" as the main means to improve performance; Tesch 1987).

Muscle force production is a consequence of both the activation of the nervous system, the intrinsic properties of the muscles, endocrine and metabolic physiology, and a myriad of biomechanical factors that, collectively, directly influence subsequent athletic performance. The force a muscle can produce is directly proportional to the size of the muscle (Close 1972). However, several studies have demonstrated that discrepancies exist between training-induced changes in muscle strength and changes in muscle size (hypertrophy; Howald 1985; Kraemer *et al.* 1996). This anomaly can be explained by the fact that muscle force production is mainly determined by the coordinated action of the neuromuscular system. This force generation paradigm suggests that several components of the adaptive process are likely to ultimately determine strength performance and help explain some of the discrepancies observed in strength gains between athletes undertaking similar training regimens.

Metabolic adaptations to strength training

Although strength training is performed at maximal or near-maximal intensities, such training is sustained for relatively short durations. Accordingly, compared to endurance training, the overall energy requirements are low. Estimates of energy needs during a 30-min workout session involving the lower body musculature suggest that O_2 uptake reaches approximately 50% $\dot{V}o_{2max}$ (Tesch *et al.* 1987). While such estimates are probably conservative and do not take into consideration the rate of ATP turnover, they do suggest that the metabolic demands of strength training are modest.

Despite the apparent low energy requirement of strength training, a single training session taxes all three energy/power systems. Studies examining metabolite changes in response to a strength training session demonstrated significant reductions in the levels of creatine phosphate (CP), ATP, and glycogen, together with increases in blood and intramuscular lactate levels and other glycolytic intermediates (Pascoe *et al.* 1993; Tesch *et al.* 1986). In addition to muscle glycogen utilization, an increase in plasma lipids and glycerol content together with a decrease in muscle triglyceride levels have been observed suggesting that lipids may also be utilized as energy source during recovery both during strength training and the subsequent recovery (Essen-Gustavsson & Tesch 1990).

Because of the nature of the expression of muscle strength, one would expect some adaptive response in enzymes involved in short-term energy generation (i.e., the ATP–CP system). Intriguingly, such enzymatic changes are rather modest in the musculature of individuals who have been participating in long-term strength training. However, the maximal activities of ATPase and creatine kinase (CK) are not increased after short-term training (Thorstensson *et al.* 1976) and in some cases actually decrease in response to long-term (6 month) programs of strength training (Tesch *et al.* 1987). However, myokinase (adenylate kinase), which is responsible for the ATP + AMP $\Leftrightarrow$ ADP + ADP reaction, has been shown to increase after 8 weeks of training in some (Thorstensson *et al.* 1976) but not all studies (Hakkinen *et al.* 1981; Tesch *et al.* 1986). Such differences may be a result of different training modalities and or the initial training state of the subjects. However, taken collectively, these results suggest that some enzymatic adaptations in the anaerobic non-glycolytic system occur after short-term training in previously untrained individuals, although prior training history may attenuate such adaptive metabolic responses.

Similar to the lack of significant adaptations in the immediate energy system are the small changes in enzymes involved in glycolytic energy metabolism. Houston *et al.* (1983) have shown that 10 weeks of strength training did not significantly increase PFK content and the activities/content of other glycolytic enzyme. Furthermore, Tesch *et al.* (1987) reported a decrease in PFK and lactate dehydrogenase among other enzymes following 6 months of training. A potential explanation for the observed decrease in enzyme content resulting from long-term strength training is the dilution effect caused by the increase in skeletal muscle mass as reflected in changes in fiber cross-sectional area. This increased contractile protein content will naturally result in a decrease in enzyme content or activity per unit of muscle mass (milligram of tissue).

Consistent with the observation of a decrease in enzyme content, MacDougall *et al.* (1979) were the first to demonstrate a decrease in mitochondrial volume density following 6 months of strength training. In this study, morphometric analyses of muscle biopsies from the triceps brachii indicated that training resulted in a significant (26%) reduction in mitochondrial volume density and a similar (25%) reduction in the mitochondrial volume to myofibrillar volume ratio. This decrease was accompanied by significant increases in fiber cross-sectional area for both FT (33%) and ST (27%) fibers, which suggests that strength training can result in a dilution of the mitochondrial volume density through the increase in myofibrillar protein content typical of muscle hypertrophy. Similar findings were later confirmed by Luthi *et al.* (1986), who reported a decrease (9.6%) in the volume density of mitochondria only after 6 weeks of training with only a modest increase (8.4%) in both cross-sectional area of the vastus lateralis muscle and myofibrillar volume (10%). Indeed, the decrease in mitochondrial volume density was caused by the dilution effect mentioned above and not by the morphologic or ultrastructural changes intrinsic to the mitochondria as the surface densities of inner and outer mitochondrial membranes remained unchanged.

With mitochondria being the cellular "energy powerhouse" driving oxidative metabolism, it is not surprising that oxidative enzyme content is also reduced (or at least not increased) following strength training. Schantz and Kallman (1989) compared muscles from untrained with strength-trained subjects and found no differences in the levels of enzymes involved in the citric acid cycle, fatty acid oxidation, or glycolysis. No differences were found between the levels of malate-aspartate and alpha-glycerophosphate shuttle enzymes or cytochrome b5 reductase. Similarly, Green *et al.* (1999) reported that 12 weeks of strength training, which resulted in an increase (17%) in fiber cross-section, failed to alter cellular oxidative potential as no changes in succinic dehydrogenase (SDH) activity were induced by training.

In summary, strength training results in substantial increases in muscle mass and strength production capacity. However, it seems that the magnitude of the metabolic adaptations that result from such training are less dramatic and do not accompany the structural and performance changes observed after long-term endurance training. Consequently, and unlike endurance training, enzymatic changes following strength training may not underlie changes in training-induced strength performance.

Performance adaptations to strength and endurance training

Specificity of training and transfer effect during strength performance

Most sports require speed, power, strength, and endurance and hence rely on combinations of several motor abilities in different proportions. Moreover, such combinations are time-dependent and linked to the pattern of fuel utilization (i.e., muscle glycogen and lipid stores, blood-borne substrates). Therefore, the design and structure of a training program for sports performance must take into consideration the specific motor abilities that predominate in that sport and to what extent these components need to be maximized by training in order to optimize the specific metabolic system to elicit the appropriate adaptations. A long-standing issue for coaches in many sports has been the sequence, relative proportion, and amount of training devoted to each of these components. The decision of what type and how much training should be devoted to each component is complicated by the relative amount of time available for training and by evidence suggesting that, in some circumstances, a degree of incompatibility may exist between the different modes of exercise. For example, when endurance training is added to an ongoing strength-training program (i.e., "concurrent training"), a compromise in strength development occurs (Hickson 1980). Such decrements in strength with concurrent training are likely to be underpinned by alterations in the functional properties of individual muscle fibers and the associated biochemical changes (Chilibeck *et al.* 2002; Puttman *et al.* 2004).

Hickson (1980) was the first to determine performance adaptations in response to strength training, endurance training, or a combination of the two training modes. As would be expected, in individuals who undertook only strength-training, leg-strength improved throughout the duration of the training program. Likewise, individuals who performed only endurance training had a progressive increase in $\dot{V}O_{2max}$. Strength training alone did not result in any increase in aerobic capacity, and similarly, endurance training alone did not result in any appreciable gains in strength. The rate of change in strength when undertaking concurrent training was similar to that observed for strength training only for the first 7 weeks, but thereafter strength gains reached a plateau and actually declined during final 2 weeks of training. However, concurrent training did not attenuate the improvement in $\dot{V}O_{2max}$ observed when only endurance training was performed. This study was the first to describe deficits in strength development when endurance training and strength training were undertaken concurrently (Hickson 1980).

From a metabolic standpoint it seems unlikely that skeletal muscle would be able to adapt to two seemingly incompatible training stimuli when they are undertaken simultaneously. One way to circumvent this problem is to take a long-term view of training objectives and plan training to defined goals with appropriate periodization. Such an approach allows more time for the adaptive processes to take place and potentially minimizes any "interference" between the responses to dual-mode training. Evidence to support this model comes from the study of Hakkinen *et al.* (2003) who investigated the effects of 21 weeks of either concurrent strength and endurance training, or strength and endurance training alone. At the completion of the training period similar increases in strength were observed with concurrent and strength training alone (approximately 20%). There were also increases in muscle cross-sectional area in individuals undertaking strength training and concurrent training, indicating that the concurrent training program was successful in inducing both neural and muscular adaptations observed after single-mode (strength) training. Interestingly, rates of force development only increased in individuals who performed only strength training, while $\dot{V}o_{2max}$ improved (18.5%) after concurrent training. These findings demonstrate that when the training stimulus is diluted by a longer period of time with a lower frequency of training, there are gains in strength and muscle hypertrophy. However, the results also suggest that even "low-frequency" concurrent strength and endurance training can interfere with explosive strength development. Such interference may, in part, be mediated by limitations in the adaptive response of the nervous system when endurance and strength training are performed simultaneously. Thus, concurrent training may be successfully employed to improve strength and endurance provided the development of muscle power is not a prerequisite for performance in the athlete's sport.

Strength training has a vital role in general conditioning in a wide range of sporting activities. As such, a common belief among athletic trainers, coaches, and athletes is that there is a transfer effect from strength training to sports performance. Although a structured strength training program may help prevent the occurrence of sporting injuries (Stone 1990), the transfer effect from absolute strength gains to the sporting setting is difficult to determine. This is because strength gains and subsequent performance in a given athlete are dependent on the interaction of many physiologic and biomechanical parameters such as muscle fiber type, working muscle mass, movement pattern, movement velocity, type of contraction (eccentric vs. concentric, isometric vs. isotonic) and force of contractions (Sale & MacDougall 1981). Accordingly, when designing training programs, these factors must be considered in order to obtain maximal gains from strength training.

Can strength training improve endurance performance?

An important aspect of strength training is the potential to improve endurance performance. Hickson et al. (1988) determined whether strength training results in an increase in endurance performance and whether the differences in aerobic power that are normally observed during endurance training can be explained by changes in muscle strength. In that study, endurance-trained men underwent strength training 5 days per week for 10 weeks, during which time they continued with their regular aerobic training. At the completion of the training period, leg muscle strength was increased by approximately 30% without measurable changes in thigh girth or muscle fiber area of the trained musculature. $\dot{V}o_{2max}$ did not change after the training intervention when measured during cycle ergometer or treadmill running. However, short-term (4–8 min) endurance capacity increased 11% and 13% during cycling and running, respectively. Furthermore, submaximal cycling to exhaustion at 80% $\dot{V}o_{2max}$ increased approximately 20% (from 71 to 85 min) when endurance and strength training were combined, whereas 10-km running performance was unaffected (Hickson et al. 1988).

In contrast to these findings, other studies have not been able to detect improvements in endurance performance when such individuals undertake concurrent strength training. Tanaka et al. (1991) studied 24 collegiate swimmers during 14 weeks of their competitive season. Swimmers were divided into two groups and matched for stroke specialties. The two groups performed all swim training sessions together for the season duration, but in addition to pool training, one group performed strength training 3 days per week for 8 weeks. The strength training program was intended to simulate the specific muscles used in front-crawl swimming and utilized weightlifting machines as well as free weights. The most important finding from this study was that resistance training did not improve sprint-swim performance despite the fact that those swimmers who combined strength and swim training increased their strength by 25–35%. Neither did these strength gains result in improved stroke mechanics. These investigators (Tanaka *et al.* 1991) concluded "the lack of positive transfer between dry-land strength gains and swimming propulsive force may be due to the specificity of training." Similar results were obtained by Bell *et al.* (1989) for varsity oarsmen who undertook a variety of strength training programs in the rowers' preseason. These workers suggested that strength training programs might restrict the volume of beneficial, sports-specific training that can be achieved because of the level of fatigue that results from their execution.

Conclusions

Regularly performed endurance and strength training results in a variety of metabolic adaptations in skeletal muscle that function to minimize cellular disturbances during subsequent training sessions. Endurance training leads to a greater utilization of lipid-based fuels and a concomitant "sparing" of CHO-based fuels during exercise performed at the same absolute intensity. The decrease in CHO utilization is caused by both a decrease in muscle glycogenolysis and a decrease in muscle glucose utilization. Although the "sparing" of muscle glycogen accounts for most of the training-induced reduction in whole-body CHO oxidation, this is mostly because glycogen is the major CHO-based fuel for muscle metabolism at the intensities at which most individuals train and compete. The training-induced reduction in CHO oxidation during exercise is compensated for by an increase in the oxidation of fat-based fuels, specifically, intramuscular triglycerides. This shift in the pattern of substrate oxidation during submaximal exercise in trained humans is an important means by which training enhances endurance capacity.

In contrast to endurance training, strength training results in minor metabolic adaptations in skeletal muscle. This is perhaps not surprising given the relatively low energy demands associated with strength performance, which is typically of high intensity (maximal and supra-maximal) and of very low duration (seconds to minutes). Indeed, most data seem to suggest that performance improvements rely on neuromuscular and structural adaptations (i.e., fiber recruitment and muscle

hypertrophy) rather any training-induced alterations in muscle metabolism. Importantly, strength training can improve endurance performance but endurance training compromises strength gains. Athletes engaged in a wide range of sports activities may benefit from concurrent training for both strength and endurance, but individuals who participate in sports in which strength is the main or predominant component may hinder strength gains by engaging in both forms of training.

ENDOCRINE ADAPTATIONS TO TRAINING

MICHAEL KJÆR, SIMON DOESSING AND KATJA PELTOLA MJØSUND

Introduction

Physical activity causes a major response in most endocrine responses that are of importance for the regulation of metabolism whether this is related to carbohydrates, fat, or protein metabolism. In addition to this, several hormones also are involved in blood flow distribution, thermoregulation, immune system regulation, and skeletal muscle contractility. Regular physical activity will – depending on which hormone is studied – in general alter these endocrine responses during exercise either because of an altered magnitude of a given metabolic response required for a specific work task or because of an altered sensitivity towards the hormone in question.

In the following section the focus is on adaptation towards regular physical activity with regards to hormonal responses. In addition to the classic hormones, lately substances such as cytokines have been identified as hormones, and interestingly some of these have been shown not only to be released from the classic endocrine glands, but also to be released from metabolically active tissues themselves. As an example, it has been shown that both adipose tissue and skeletal muscle can release substances that will act as hormones in other parts of the body (e.g., interleukin-6 and adiponectin).

Sympatoadrenergic responses

It is well described that sympathetic activity will rise with increasing activity, whether this is measured directly as electrical activity in superficial sympathetic nerves or determined by the levels of circulating norepinephrine in the blood. In addition to this, release of epinephrine from the adrenal medulla will also rise. The level of norepinephrine and epinephrine in arterial blood will increase with the exercise intensity when this is expressed as a percentage of the maximal individual performance (%$\dot{V}o_{2max}$; Kjaer *et al.* 1985). Based on this it will therefore also be evident that vigorous endurance training will cause a reduction in the catecholamine response to a certain absolute workload. In contrast to this, it has not been possible to show any marked difference in the maximal sympathetic activity that can be found in individuals with different training status. This underlines the view that physical activity in itself does not change the maximal capacity of sympathetic nervous activity, and that sympathetic responses are related to the relative rather than to the absolute workload.

With regards to epinephrine released from the adrenal medulla, it can be shown that increased levels in the blood are not related to changes in clearance but rather directly shows an increased secretion of epinephrine from the adrenal gland. It has also been shown that the epinephrine response in well-trained individuals compared to sedentary individuals is more marked when the adrenal gland is stimulated by a variety of different stimuli such as hypoglycemia, caffeine, glucagon, hypoxia, and hypocapnia. Furthermore, when performing maximal exercise, a release of epinephrine is also larger in well-trained individuals than sedentary counterparts. This indicates that the capacity to secrete epinephrine from the adrenal medulla is improved with training (Kjaer *et al.* 1986). Thus, similar to the adaptation in heart muscle, where one calls it sports heart, it could be argued that the increased capacity to secrete epinephrine from the adrenal medulla develops a so-called sports adrenal medulla. It has been shown in longitudinal studies that animals that undergo prolonged training will actually hypertrophy their adrenal medulla volume and increase the adrenal content of epinephrine (Stallknecht 1990). This increase is specific for physical training rather than for unspecific stress.

Furthermore, it is interesting that physical training in animals causes an increase in the adrenal medulla volume, just closely related to the increase of the entire adrenal gland weight, indicating that the training-induced increase was more pronounced in the adrenal medulla rather than in the cortex of the adrenal gland. Increased size of the adrenal medulla in humans will most likely require several years of training; longitudinal studies have shown that duration has not been able to prove any growth of the adrenal gland. The release of epinephrine from the adrenal gland is regulated by several factors, and both stimulation in parallel with increased motor sensor activity as well as feedback signals from contracting muscle and metabolic changes are important factors. Changes in plasma levels of glucose are an important regulator of epinephrine release, and epinephrine is known to have a role in glycogen depletion in contracting skeletal muscle as well as in release of glucose from the liver, especially at high exercise intensities. It can be shown that epinephrine also plays a part in relation to adipose tissue and that physical activity can increase the sensitivity towards epinephrine. It is thus relevant that the epinephrine response is somewhat reduced during exercise in trained individuals in order to ensure that the metabolic responses are adequate and do not lead to a premature glycogen depletion in either muscle or liver. In general, trained individuals become more sensitive towards adrenergic stimulation in most metabolic tissues such as muscle and fat (Stallknecht 2003).

Growth hormone and insulin-like growth factor-I

Growth hormone (GH) concentrations increase dramatically in relation to exercise and can influence growth, mobilization of FFA from the adipose tissue and stimulate protein synthesis. The release of GH from the pituitary gland is related closely to motor sensor activity and the response is closely related to intensity of the exercise bout. It is clear that a well-trained young person performing high intensity exercise will secrete more GH not only than an untrained person performing exercise at a low intensity, but also compared to an elderly person, because the endocrine response of GH release even in well-trained individuals will decrease with aging.

In studies in which subjects undergo 1 year of systematic training it can be shown that the 24-h GH plasma levels are elevated in persons who have performed regular physical training, and it is also clear that it only is elevated in persons who have performed physical activity of a certain intensity (Weltman *et al.* 1992). GH exists in a variety of molecular isoforms. There is no documentation that training alters the relation between these isoforms. However, it is shown that the most abundant isoform (i.e., the 22-kDa peptide) only represents one-fifth of the total circulating GH, and that during exercise the concentration of non-22-kDa form increases relative to the 22 kDa isoform (Wallace *et al.* 2001). The anabolic influence of GH is predominantly mediated through IGF-1 and GH is a major stimulant of IGF secretion by the liver. IGF-1 binding to IGF-1 cell surface receptors activate intracellular signaling pathway in most human cells. In myofibrils IGF-1 binding initiates at least four different pathways, which ultimately leads to increased protein synthesis, the basis for increased muscle size and strength. Similarly, fibroblast in human tendon increases the synthesis of collagen protein following IGF-1 receptor binding. Hepatic IGF-1 is supplemented by production of IGF-1 by cells in peripheral tissues including skeletal muscle. In myofibers, two different IGF isoforms, with presumed paracrine and autocrine actions, are expressed during exercise. GH probably regulates expression of the IGF-1Ea isoform leading to a stimulation of myoblast differentiation. Somewhat in contrast to this, expression of IGF-1Ec (MGF) appears to be regulated GH independently by exercise per se, and cause myofibrillar proliferation (Hameed *et al.* 2004). It is not clear whether regular physical activity will alter this expression, but it is evident that a more pronounced muscle mass potentially could have a higher possibility for expression of MGF.

In addition to GH and IGF-1, IGF binding proteins and peptides act as carriers prolonging the IGF half-life, and in addition the binding proteins function as modulators of IGF availability and activity. Furthermore, the binding proteins have a biologic IGF-1 independent action in peripheral tissue, but it is not known whether regular physical activity will alter these actions. Whereas lack of GH will have a detrimental effect on myofibrillar protein synthesis, excess amounts of GH is not seen to further stimulate muscle growth. However, increased GH levels are related to markers of formation of connective tissue, and it is likely that the stimulation of collagen production will lead to larger intramuscular connective tissue mass and connective tissue growth (e.g., tendons). These effects are supported by the findings that GH has a positive effect on bone growth and epidermal thickening.

Finally, administration of GH will reduce fat mass during exercise and increase plasma glycerol and fatty acids indicating increased lipolysis but, somewhat surprisingly, trained subjects have shown a substantially decreased exercise performance immediately following GH supplementation despite the fact that GH supplementation and the increased lipolytic activity did not result in any alteration in the combustion pattern during exercise. In some well-trained individuals, GH is used as an ergogenic aid, as it is believed that the GH doping has a beneficial effect of minimizing the fat amount in the individuals and potentially also strengthen the tissue by having a positive effect on the connective tissue. However, there is no evidence that GH will improve the muscle growth as such. Furthermore, side effects of using GH in relation to cardiovascular disease, diabetes, and cancer have not been fully investigated.

Insulin and glucagon

There is no doubt that insulin and glucagon are major hormones regulating to what extent energy fuel should be released from storage sites or should be stored. The relation between insulin and glucagon has a role for glucose release from the liver to the blood, so that simultaneous increase in circulating insulin together with the slight decrease in glucagon concentrations is of importance to direct glucose for storage in skeletal muscle and liver. With exercise, circulating levels of insulin will decrease because of sympathetic inhibition of the beta cell of the pancreas. In contrast, the circulating levels of glucagon with exercise are unchanged or only marginally increased, especially with prolonged exercise. If glucose is taken in during exercise, the decrease in plasma insulin can somewhat be counteracted, but the decrease in circulating insulin is important for mobilization of FFA from adipose tissue, glycogenolysis in skeletal muscle, and release of glucose from the liver (Coker & Kjaer 2005).

Although both exercise and insulin stimulate increases in glucose transport into skeletal muscle, glycogen metabolism, and protein synthesis, these effects are induced through distinctly different signaling pathways, although newer results have shown that they also have some pathways in common. However, it is clear that exercise and insulin have an additive effect upon glucose uptake and metabolism, and physical training will increase the insulin sensitivity of skeletal muscle and thereby increase the insulin-stimulated glucose uptake. During exercise no rise in insulin is needed in order to get glucose transported into the muscle cell, but in the resting state this increased sensitivity will have a major role in decreasing the amount of insulin needed to accomplish the glucose uptake needed (e.g., after a meal). It has been shown that insulin sensitivity valuated as insulin-stimulated glucose uptake in peripheral muscle (and also in fat) will respond to just one single bout of exercise; in contrast, only 5 days of training cessation will reverse insulin sensitivity in previously very well-trained individuals to levels obtained by an untrained individual after just one single bout of exercise (Coker & Kjaer 2005).

In conjunction with these changes in insulin sensitivity level it is important to remember that the beta-cell capacity to secrete insulin will be also altered as a result of more prolonged physical training. Thus, in very well-trained individuals the stimulatable insulin release from the beta cell are reduced. At first sight this seems like the beta-cell function is inhibited and thus potentially simulating a situation that could develop into diabetes. However, it is important to note that this downregulation of the beta-cell function is a physiologic phenomenon, which is caused by the increased insulin sensitivity. Thus, if one decreases the training activity and the insulin sensitivity goes down, the beta-cell secretion

will automatically be upregulated again as individuals detrain. Not only does training in this way provide an intimate interplay between hormonal secretion and hormonal action, in this case for insulin, but it also underlines how important regular physical activity is to the health promoting effect, which is mainly caused through increased insulin sensitivity and decreased circulating levels of insulin.

Reproductive hormones

No distinctively male or female reproductive hormones exist, but there are distinct differences in hormone concentrations between the sexes. Testosterone is secreted from the testes, ovaries, and the adrenal glands. In males, the roles of testosterone can be divided into two major categories: androgenic effects, related to reproductive function and the development of a male's secondary sex characteristics; and anabolic effects, pertaining more generally to stimulation of tissue growth.

Testosterone has direct effects on muscle synthesis, possibly via effects on nuclear receptors, and it also interacts with neural receptors to increase neurotransmitter release, and initiate structural changes that alter the size of neuromuscular junction. These effects lead to enhanced force-generating capacity of the muscle.

The anabolic action of testosterone depends on age, sex, dose, and the basic endocrinologic status of the individual. In hypogonadal or elderly men, testosterone replacement therapy decreases muscle breakdown and increases mucle protein synthesis. On the other hand, supraphysiologic doses are needed to increase muscle protein synthesis in eugonadal young men, and testosterone has severe side effects when used in supraphysiologic doses. Interestingly, several studies have shown disproportionate increases in muscle mass vs. increases in muscle strength with testosterone treatment (Hackney 1998).

The ovaries provide the primary source of estrogens, but estrogens are produced both in gonads and in peripheral tissues. In males, testosterone can be converted into estrogen in peripheral tissues. Estrogens regulate menstruation, ovulation, and the physiologic changes during pregnancy.

Furthermore, estrogen exerts effects on blood vessels, bone, lungs, liver, intestine, prostate, and testes. Estrogen is also a strong antioxidant and a membrane stabilizer, and estrogen receptors have been found in skeletal muscle too. Recently, the expression of estrogen receptor alpha and beta was found to be increased in skeletal muscle of highly endurance trained men, but the significance of this is still unknown (Wiik *et al*. 2005). There is also some recent evidence of estrogen effect on muscle damage and inflammation, mostly from experimental animal studies suggesting a beneficial role of estrogen in muscle repair. However, this must be confirmed in further investigations (Tiidus 2005).

An acute bout of endurance exercise increases plasma testosterone and dehydroepiandrosterone (DHEAS) concentrations in males (Tremblay *et al*. 2005). Also in women, the circulating levels of testosterone, DHEAS, and estradiol as well as progesterone increase in response to an acute bout of endurance exercise (Consitt *et al*. 2002). The hormone response to exercise is dependent on various factors including exercise duration, the training status of the subject, the mode of exercise, and the intensity of exercise. To date, the intensity of exercise is believed to be the most important factor influencing the hormonal response to exercise. Trained endurance athletes display less pronounced increases in testosterone concentrations in response to standardized exercise bouts than untrained subjects, and thus the response is merely related to the relative rather than to the absolute workload (Tremblay *et al*. 2005).

Also resistance exercise has been shown to elicit a significant acute hormonal response with increased testosterone concentration. Anabolic hormones such as testosterone have been shown to be elevated during 15–30 min of recovery from resistance exercise. Resistance training protocols high in volume, moderate to high in intensity, using short rest intervals and stressing a large muscle mass, tend to produce the greatest acute elevation on testosterone (Kraemer & Ratamess 2005).

Regular endurance exercise training can influence the resting hormone profile. Testosterone levels of endurance trained men are found to be 60–85% of the levels of matched, untrained men (Hackney

1998). Endurance trained males may also have other reproductive hormonal abnormalities such as decreased resting levels of prolactin, and more importantly, no significant elevations in resting LH, despite the decreased testosterone concentration. These findings have been labeled by some researchers as a dysfunction of the hypothalamic–pituitary–testicular regulatory axis. However, despite the lower resting levels of testosterone in endurance athletes, there are very few findings to indicate that endurance training disrupts testosterone-dependent anabolic or androgenic processes in the male (Hackney 1998).

Analogous with findings in men, the baseline testosterone levels appear to decline with endurance training in women, and also the concentrations of DHEAS and estradiol decrease (Consitt *et al*. 2002). When energy expenditure exceeds energy intake, female endurance athletes may have disturbances in estrogen production because of GnRH suppression. The hormonal pattern seen in these athletes is a hypothalamic amenorrhea profile. There appears to be a decrease in gonadotropin-releasing hormone (GnRH) pulses from the hypothalamus, which in turn decreases the pulsatile secretion of luteinizing hormone (LH) and follicle-stimulating hormone (FSH) and shuts down stimulation of ovary. Disruption of the hypothalamic–pituitary–ovarian axis appears to be dependent on the body's recognition of an energy imbalance, which may be caused by a lack of compensatory caloric intake in the face of significant energy expenditure, rather than an effect of physical training itself. Athletes with low energy intake are at risk of developing the female athlete triad, which includes amenorrhea, osteoporosis, and disordered eating (Warren & Shantha 2000). Also another type of sports-related amenorrhea characterized by mild hyperandrogenism has been described in swimmers (Constantini & Warren 1995).

Most studies have failed to show any change in plasma hormone concentration during chronic resistance training in males of females, although there is some evidence that resistance-trained males tend to have higher plasma androgen levels compared to sedentary individuals or endurance trained subjects (Consitt *et al*. 2002).

ACTH and cortisol

Physical stress, such as exercise or declining blood glucose, stimulate the release of corticotropin-releasing factor. This stimulates adrenocortico-tropin hormone (ACTH) secretion which, in turn, promotes cortisol secretion from the adrenal cortex, leading to elevation of cortisol concentration in plasma. Endurance exercise-stimulated ACTH and cortisol release are proportional to the relative exercise intensity. In trained subjects, physical conditioning is associated with a reduction of pituitary–adrenal activation in response to exercise. In other words, plasma cortisol tends to rise less in trained subjects compared to untrained when performing the same absolute workload (Luger *et al.* 1987).

Cortisol responds to heavy endurance exercise with significantly higher levels as exercise intensity rises. Even prolonged endurance exercise at moderate intensity increases plasma cortisol levels as the duration increases (Tremblay *et al.* 2005).

Resistance training protocols high in volume, moderate to high in intensity, using short rest intervals, and stressing a large muscle mass tend to produce the greatest acute elevation of cortisol (Kraemer & Ratamess 2005). Following exercise, plasma cortisol levels remain increased for hours and cortisol is believed to affect glucose and glycogen replenishment in the tissues during recovery from prolonged exercise.

Cortisol has a net catabolic effect on muscle by inhibition of muscle protein synthesis, and by inhibitory effects on IGF-1 expression, as well as by increased cytoplasmic protease activity. Cortisol exerts a facilitating effect on substrate use during and after heavy or prolonged exercise; it promotes the breakdown of protein to amino acids for gluconeogenesis in the liver, and also serves as an insulin antagonist by inhibiting cellular glucose uptake and oxidation. Furthermore, cortisol enhances triglyceride breakdown in adipose tissue.

Highly endurance-trained subjects show chronic mild hypercortisolism with increased baseline plasma ACTH and cortisol levels (Luger et al. 1987). The changes in basal hypothalamo–pituitary–adrenal activity during exercise training are believed to be centrally mediated (Park *et al.* 2005).

Cytokines

Cytokines are small secreted proteins that mediate and regulate immunity, inflammation, and hematopoiesis. Traditionally, cytokines have been associated with inflammatory response, for example, but muscle-derived interleukin-6 (IL-6) has additionally been shown to possess several characteristics of an exercise factor, which regulates skeletal muscle substrate metabolism during exercise.

Cytokines typically act on the cells that secrete them (autocrine action) or on nearby cells (paracrine action), but cytokines such as IL-6 may even act on distant cells (endocrine action). They bind to specific membrane receptors, which then signal the cell via second messengers to alter gene expression. The plasma concentrations of several pro- and anti-inflammatory cytokines (tumor necrosis factor α [TNF-α], IL-1β, IL-6, IL-8) and cytokine inhibitors (IL-1 receptor antagonist, TNF-receptors) change during exercise. During endurance exercise, pro-inflammatory cytokine production is downregulated and anti-inflammatory cytokines such as IL-1ra and IL-10 are upregulated, as well as the production of IL-6 (Steinacker *et al.* 2004). Exercise induces IL-6 gene transcription locally in myocytes in contracting skeletal muscle and high amounts of IL-6 are also released to the blood circulation. IL-6 is a myokine: a cytokine produced in skeletal muscle. The plasma concentration of IL-6 increases markedly ($\leq$100-fold) in response to exercise and it appears that IL-6 production in working skeletal muscles is a major source of the exercise-induced increase in arterial IL-6. In the myocytes, the stimuli for IL-6 production are contractions per se, as is a low muscle glycogen content, and the release of IL-6 does not depend on muscle damage or inflammation (Febbraio & Pedersen 2002). Also, the brain has been shown to release some IL-6 during prolonged exercise, but the magnitude of muscle IL-6 release is substantially greater (Nybo *et al.* 2002).

IL-6 exhibits several important biologic roles. IL-6 is proposed to be a strong mediator of anti-inflammatory effects of exercise. It also inhibits the production of the pro-inflammatory cytokine TNF-α and may also inhibit TNF-α-induced insulin resistance. IL-6 may thereby have a role in mediating the beneficial health effects of physical activity (Pedersen *et al.* 2004).

Because IL-6 is activated in exercising skeletal muscle, it is proposed to act as an energy sensor being dependent on the muscle glycogen content and to participate in muscle–adipose tissue cross-talk. IL-6 promotes lipolysis and increases fat oxidation. IL-6 also enhances insulin sensitivity and muscle glucose uptake (Pedersen *et al.* 2004).

Acute exercise also increases the production of the cytokine IL-1, and resting levels of this substance may also be further augmented by exercise training. IL-1 has a direct cytotoxic effect and it also stimulates the T cells to produce increased amounts of IL-1 and IL-2. However, the magnitude of IL-6 change in plasma is manyfold higher than the increase of IL-1, and the appearance of IL-6 precedes that of other cytokines such as IL-1.

In addition to endurance-exercise induced changes in plasma cytokine concentration, there is also a delayed release of cytokines following eccentric exercise that is related to the repair of muscle injury. Because the production of cytokines is greater with endurance than with resistance exercise, it seems unlikely that they have an important role in the hypertrophy of muscle.

Conclusions: Endocrine adaptations to training in athletes

Most classic hormonal changes with exercise result in an increased amount of circulating hormone, and the major exception from this is insulin which will be inhibited during sympathetic activation. Training results in a lower hormonal response because training increases sensitivity towards hormones in the peripheral tissues such as muscle, liver, and fat. Long-term training can result in an increasing capacity from glands such as the adrenal medulla and the pituitary gland. In contrast, training results in a reduced insulin secretion capacity from the pancreas because of elevated peripheral sensitivity of the tissue towards insulin. Finally, cytokines released during exercise, also from the contracting muscle itself, are thought to have a hormonal role in tissues other than muscle.

CARDIORESPIRATORY ADAPTATIONS TO TRAINING

DARREN E.R. WARBURTON, A. WILLIAM SHEEL AND DONALD C. MCKENZIE

Introduction

The physiologic adaptations to endurance exercise training have been evaluated extensively over the last 80 years. In particular, researchers have examined the mechanisms responsible for the enhanced cardiorespiratory fitness of endurance-trained athletes in comparison to untrained individuals (Gledhill *et al.* 1994; Krip *et al.* 1997). Cardiorespiratory fitness refers to the ability to transport and utilize oxygen during sustained strenuous exercise reflecting the combined efficiency of the lungs, heart, vascular system, and exercising muscles. Generally, $\dot{V}o_{2max}$ is considered to be the best indicator of cardiorespiratory fitness and is a key determinant of endurance performance (Bassett & Howley 2000; Warburton *et al.* 1999). Classically defined, $\dot{V}o_{2max}$ refers to the maximum amount of oxygen that can be transported and utilized by the body during strenuous exercise. According to the Fick equation, $\dot{V}o_{2max}$ is the product of cardiac output (Q) and arteriovenous oxygen difference (a-vDo_2). Cardiac output reflects the rate at which the heart transports oxygen to the tissues and is a product of heart rate (HR) and stroke volume (SV; volume of blood ejected with each beat of the heart). The a-vDO_2 refers to difference between the oxygen content of arterial (Cao_2) and venous (Cvo_2) blood reflecting the amount of oxygen extracted at the tissue level.

Owing to the importance of oxygen transport for optimal endurance performance, this chapter highlights the central adaptations resulting from endurance training that improve oxygen transport. In particular, we highlight the major cardiac and respiratory adaptations that promote optimal sport performance. We also review the potential factors that could limit $\dot{V}o_{2max}$ and endurance performance in highly trained endurance athletes.

Endurance performance and its relationship with $\dot{V}O_{2max}$

Endurance performance is affected by numerous factors, in particular $\dot{V}O_{2max}$, the ability to exercise at a high percentage of $\dot{V}O_{2max}$ and metabolic efficiency (Gledhill & Warburton 2000). However, because $\dot{V}O_{2max}$ can vary as much as 300% between healthy individuals (e.g., from <30 to >80 mL·kg^{-1}·min^{-1}; Gledhill & Warburton 2000), many consider $\dot{V}O_{2max}$ to be the major factor explaining the large difference in endurance performances of elite athletes in comparison to normally active or moderately trained individuals (Gledhill *et al.* 1994; Krip *et al.* 1997; Warburton *et al.* 1999).

In highly trained endurance athletes, who have relatively homogeneous $\dot{V}O_{2max}$ values, $\dot{V}O_{2max}$ alone is not the sole predictor of success in endurance events (Bassett & Howley 2000; Joyner 1991). The ability to compete at a high percentage of $\dot{V}O_{2max}$ appears to have a key role in determining success in endurance events (Bassett & Howley 2000). That is, individuals with a similar or lower $\dot{V}O_{2max}$ than their counterpart may compensate for this by performing at a higher percentage of their $\dot{V}O_{2max}$. It is not uncommon for endurance athletes to exercise at levels above 85% of $\dot{V}O_{2max}$ for sustained periods of time.

Some have also argued that metabolic efficiency or economy may explain the enhanced performance of elite athletes, such as the seven-times winner of the Tour de France (Coyle 2005). However, this theory has been recently challenged by several authors (Martin *et al.* 2005; Schumacher *et al.* 2005). In fact, research investigations have reported that metabolic efficiency is not significantly different between novice and elite cyclists (Jeukendrup *et al.* 2003; Moseley *et al.* 2004). It has also been postulated that race tactics, recovery, and training strategies, and a myriad of psychologic and motivational factors may explain why some athletes exhibit superior performance (Myburgh 2003; Schumacher *et al.* 2005).

Although many factors affect elite endurance performance, one should not negate the importance of $\dot{V}O_{2max}$ for success in elite endurance sports. In fact, $\dot{V}O_{2max}$ appears to set the upper limit for elite endurance performance (Bassett & Howley 2000). For instance, Bassett and Howley (2000) calculated

that for an individual to complete a 2:15 marathon they would need to maintain a minimal $\dot{V}O_2$ value of 60 mL·kg^{-1}·min^{-1} throughout the race. As it is not feasible to exercise at 100% of $\dot{V}O_{2max}$ for prolonged periods of time, the authors estimated that a relative intensity of 80–85% of $\dot{V}O_{2max}$ would be possible for a highly trained endurance athlete necessitating a $\dot{V}O_{2max}$ of 70–75 mL·kg^{-1}·min^{-1}. As the current world record for the marathon is 2:04:55, it is clear that elite endurance athletes would require an even higher $\dot{V}O_{2max}$. This is consistent with the reports of elite runners and cyclists possessing $\dot{V}O_{2max}$ values of 80–85 mL·kg^{-1}·min^{-1} (Coyle 2005; Ekblom & Hemnasen 1968). In fact, Lance Armstrong was recently reported to have a $\dot{V}O_{2max}$ of approximately 85 mL·kg^{-1}·min^{-1} (Coyle 2005). Cross-country skiers have also been reported to have $\dot{V}O_{2max}$ of >90 mL·kg^{-1}·min^{-1}. Therefore, it is apparent that a high $\dot{V}O_{2max}$ is a prerequisite for optimal endurance performance (but not the sole determinant) in elite athletes. Furthermore, it explains in large part the enhanced exercise capacity of endurance athletes in comparison to untrained individuals (Gledhill & Warburton 2000). Accordingly, for the purposes of this chapter we restrict our discussion to the physiologic adaptations to chronic endurance training that lead to the enhanced $\dot{V}O_{2max}$ of endurance-trained athletes.

Endurance training and the determinants of $\dot{V}O_{2max}$

Researchers have extensively evaluated the effects of endurance training on $\dot{V}O_{2max}$ and its determinants. This research has identified four major potential limiting factors for $\dot{V}O_{2max}$ including the pulmonary system, maximal Q, the oxygen carrying capacity of arterial blood, and skeletal muscle characteristics responsible for the extraction of oxygen at the tissue level of working muscles (Bassett & Howley 2000). The first three factors are generally considered to be "central factors" related to oxygen transport. The latter factor is referred to as a "peripheral factor" (Bassett & Howley 2000) because it relates to oxygen utilization at the level of the working tissue.

Considerable controversy exists regarding whether central or peripheral factors are more important for

$\dot{V}o_{2max}$ in healthy individuals. Several researchers have shown that the extraction of oxygen by the tissues is more efficient in endurance-trained athletes than in untrained individuals (Blomqvist & Saltin 1983; Scheuer & Tipton 1977). Commonly observed peripheral muscle adaptations that may enhance oxygen extraction include changes in mitochondrial density, capillarization, and increased mitochondrial oxidative enzymes (Bassett & Howley 2000).

An increased a-vDo$_2$ in active tissues may account for 50% of the increased $\dot{V}o_{2max}$ seen after short-term endurance training in previously untrained individuals (Blomqvist & Saltin 1983; Scheuer & Tipton 1977). This has led many researchers to highlight the importance of the periphery for the determination of $\dot{V}o_{2max}$. However, chronic endurance training generally has a greater effect on Q than on a-vDo$_2$ (Blomqvist & Saltin 1983; Hartley et al. 1969; Kilbom & Astrand 1971). Moreover, under conditions of heavy exercise healthy individuals extract near maximal levels of oxygen (irrespective of their training status). The variability in oxygen extraction (in healthy individuals) is markedly lower than that of factors involved in oxygen transport (in particular maximal Q; Bassett & Howley 2000). Furthermore, recent investigators have observed that an enhanced a-vDo$_2$ is not a prerequisite for a high $\dot{V}o_{2max}$ and/ or endurance performance (Gledhill et al. 1994; Krip et al. 1997; Zhou et al. 2001). Therefore, an improvement in the extraction of oxygen after training likely accounts only for a small fraction of the significant differences in $\dot{V}o_{2max}$ between untrained and endurance trained individuals (di Prampero 1985; Gledhill et al. 1994; Saltin 1964; Saltin & Calbet 2006).

The preponderance of available evidence in healthy individuals (in particular, elite athletes) supports the contention that the oxidative capacity of muscles exceeds that of oxygen transport to the working muscles under normoxic, sea level, exercise conditions (involving a large muscle mass such as cycling and running; Gledhill et al. 1994, 1999; Krip et al. 1997; Saltin & Calbet 2006; Warburton & Gledhill 2006). Generally, if oxygen transport is increased the additional oxygen will lead to concomitant changes in $\dot{V}o_{2max}$ and aerobic performance (Gledhill 1992; Gledhill & Warburton 2000; Gledhill et al. 1999; Spriet et al. 1986) irrespective of training status. Thus, factors that affect oxygen transport (i.e., the product of the oxygen content of arterial blood [Cao$_2$] and Q) will have a large effect on $\dot{V}o_{2max}$ and endurance performance (Gledhill 1992; Gledhill & Warburton 2000; Gledhill et al. 1999). As Bassett and Howley (2000) stated: "The evidence that $\dot{V}o_{2max}$ is limited by the cardiac output, the oxygen carrying capacity, and in some cases the pulmonary system, is undeniable." Accordingly, in the remainder of this chapter we focus predominantly on the central adaptations to endurance training including changes in oxygen-carrying capacity, cardiac function, and pulmonary function. We also highlight the potential central limitations to exercise performance in highly trained endurance athletes.

OXYGEN CARRYING CAPACITY

Oxygen is carried within the blood both in combination with hemoglobin and in physical solution (Gledhill & Warburton 2000). The Cao$_2$ is dependent upon the oxygen-carrying capacity of hemoglobin (Hb), the percent oxyhemoglobin saturation (%Sao$_2$), and the partial pressure of oxygen in arterial blood (Pao$_2$), and can be calculated as: (1.39 mL O$_2 \cdot$g^{-1} Hb) $\times$ ([Hb] (g Hb$\cdot$100 mL^{-1} blood)) $\times$ %Sao$_2$ + 0.003 Pao$_2$. Therefore, at sea level, Cao$_2$ is almost entirely determined by the [Hb] of blood (Gledhill 1992; Gledhill & Warburton 2000, Gledhill et al. 1999).

Endurance training has been shown to result in increases in red blood cell production and total Hb; however, the oxygen-carrying capacity of blood is generally maintained as a result of sustained (or slightly lower) [Hb] brought about by a disproportionate training-induced increase in plasma volume (Warburton et al. 2004). As such there is generally little difference in Cao$_2$ between endurance-trained athletes and untrained individuals (approximating 20 mL O$_2 \cdot$100 mL^{-1} blood). However, there are cases wherein athletes exhibit marked reductions in [Hb]. Collectively termed "sports anemia," this may reflect:

1 Foot strike destruction of red blood cells (RBC) (hemolytic anemia);

2 An attenuated erythropoietic drive resulting from improved tissue oxygenation;

3 Expanded plasma volume (PV) leading to a dilutional anemia (pseudoanemia); and

4 Low iron storage (iron deficiency anemia; Gledhill & Warburton 2000).

It has been clearly shown that at a constant Q, an increased [Hb] will result in an improved oxygen transport to the working tissues facilitating concomitant increases in $\dot{V}o_{2max}$ and aerobic performance (Buick *et al.* 1980; Gledhill 1992; Gledhill & Warburton 2000; Gledhill *et al.* 1999; Spriet *et al.* 1980). As reviewed by Gledhill and coworkers (Gledhill 1982, 1992; Gledhill & Warburton 2000; Gledhill *et al.* 1999), the original studies involving blood doping and/or whole blood withdrawal (venesection) revealed that $\dot{V}o_{2max}$ changes by approximately 1% for each $3\ g \cdot L^{-1}$ change in [Hb] over the [Hb] range $120–170\ g \cdot L^{-1}$, with similar changes in endurance performance. Blood doping studies, in particular, clearly established the ability of improvements in oxygen transport to enhance aerobic performance (Buick *et al.* 1980; Spriet *et al.* 1986).

As reviewed by Gledhill and Warburton (2000), there are a variety of means that athletes can utilize to increase their oxygen-carrying capacity including the use of autologous blood infusion, homologous blood infusion, recombinant human erythropoietin injection, and exposure to high altitude ("hypobaric hypoxia"). The three former practices are all banned by the International Olympic Committee, whereas the latter is not a banned practice and is routinely used by athletes and coaches in an attempt to gain an edge over the competition.

Athletes, coaches, and researchers have increasingly used altitude training methodologies (see reviews by Wilber 2001; Wolski *et al.* 1996) and several commercial devices have been created to meet these demands. Altitude training techniques include living at moderate altitude (e.g., 2500 m) combined with low-altitude training (e.g., 1250 m) ("live high, train low"; Levine & Stray-Gundersen 1997), living for sustained periods of time in a hypoxic apartment, sleeping in hypoxic tents or rooms, and being exposed to hypoxia on an intermittent basis. Training techniques that make use of the "live high, train low" theory have in particular shown the ability to improve $\dot{V}o_{2max}$ and endurance performance (Chapman *et al.* 1998; Levine & Stray-Gundersen 1997). The ergogenic effects have generally been associated with the potential to stimulate red blood cell production (erythropoiesis) and increase oxygen transport (Chapman *et al.* 1998; Levine & Stray-Gundersen 1997); however, alternative explanations for the improvement in aerobic capacity after training have also been recently provided including changes in exercise economy (Gore & Hopkins 2005). Although athletes and coaches have widely adopted altitude training methodologies, it is still controversial whether altitude training enhances sea level performance in elite athletes (Friedmann & Bartsch 1997; Wolski *et al.* 1996). Nonetheless, the widespread use of these methodologies clearly indicates that athletes and coaches have recognized the importance of changing oxygen-carrying capacity for optimal endurance performance.

CARDIAC FUNCTION

Perhaps the most important of adaptations to endurance training is an improved cardiac function, so that the heart becomes more effective and efficient in its circulation of blood. Cardiac output, through its central role in oxygen delivery, appears to be particularly important for the enhanced exercise capacity of endurance-trained athletes. In fact, the predominance of evidence indicates that the enhanced $\dot{V}o_{2max}$ after endurance training is predominantly caused by changes in maximal Q, brought about by changes in maximal SV (Blomqvist & Saltin 1983; Ekblom *et al.* 1968; Saltin & Calbet 2006; Warburton & Gledhill 2006; Warburton *et al.* 2004; Wolfe & Cunningham 1982; Wolfe *et al.* 1985). Also, maximal Q is significantly greater in endurance-trained athletes than untrained individuals (Gledhill *et al.* 1994; Krip *et al.* 1997). It is not uncommon for highly trained endurance athletes to have maximal Q of $32–40\ L \cdot min^{-1}$ (Ekblom & Hemnasen 1968; Gledhill *et al.* 1994; Krip *et al.* 1997; Warburton *et al.* 1999) in comparison to maximal Q values of approximately $20–25\ L \cdot min^{-1}$ in untrained individuals (Gledhill *et al.* 1994; Krip *et al.* 1997). The difference in Q accounts for the majority of the difference in $\dot{V}o_{2max}$ between untrained individuals and endurance-trained athletes (Gledhill *et al.* 1994; Krip *et al.* 1997). It has also been postulated that maximal Q accounts for 70–85% of the limitation in $\dot{V}o_{2max}$ (Cerretelli & Di Prampero 1987). As

Blomqvist and Saltin (1983) wrote over 20 years ago, "The improved utilization of the systemic capacity for oxygen transport only accounts for a small fraction of the large difference in maximal oxygen uptake between athletes and sedentary subjects. A superior systemic aerobic capacity clearly requires a superior cardiac pump performance with an increased stroke volume during exercise."

Stroke volume

Endurance training-induced increases in Q come about through changes in HR and/or SV (Q = SV × HR). Bradycardia (a decreased HR) occurs at rest, and during submaximal and maximal exercise in healthy individuals who engage in a physical training program (Convertino 1983; Ekblom et al. 1968; Fortney et al. 1981; Frick et al. 1967; Green et al. 1990; Ritzer et al. 1980). Likewise, the HR of endurance-trained individuals is often reduced slightly during resting and exercise conditions (Blomqvist & Saltin 1983; Gledhill et al. 1994). Therefore, for maximal Q to increase, maximal SV must be increased, by short- and long-term endurance training.

Numerous investigations have revealed an increased SV as the result of endurance training in healthy individuals (Blomqvist & Saltin 1983; Mier et al. 1997; Spina et al. 1992; Warburton et al. 2004). Moreover, the SV of endurance-trained athletes is significantly larger than their non-trained counterparts at rest and throughout incremental exercise (Crawford et al. 1985; Gledhill et al. 1994; Krip et al. 1997). It is not uncommon for highly trained endurance athletes to have maximal SV above 170 mL·beat^{-1} (Krip et al. 1997; Warburton et al. 1999), with reports of elite athletes having maximal SV of 200–210 mL·beat^{-1} (Ekblom & Hemnasen 1968). In comparison, untrained individuals commonly exhibit maximal SV from 100–130 mL·beat^{-1} (Ekblom et al. 1968; Krip et al. 1997).

The increases in SV are attributed to a combination of intra myocardial factors (i.e., heart size, ventricular compliance, and myocardial contractility) and extramyocardial factors (e.g., afterload, blood volume, fibrous pericardium, and venous return; Blomqvist & Saltin 1983; Fagard et al. 1987; Hopper et al. 1988). These factors are now briefly discussed.

Myocardial adaptations to endurance training Cardiac enlargement was first observed in athletes using thoracic percussion and in autopsies (Peronnet et al. 1981). Investigators using echocardiography since the 1970s (and more recently magnetic resonance imaging) have also routinely observed that endurance athletes (Ikaheimo et al. 1979; Morganroth et al. 1975; Pelliccia & Maron 1997; Pelliccia et al. 1991, 1999, 2002, 2005; Pluim et al. 2000; Underwood & Schwade 1977; Zandrino et al. 2000) exhibit left ventricular hypertrophy. Untrained individuals who engage in short-term training (DeMaria et al. 1978; Ehsani et al. 1978) may also exhibit increases in heart dimensions after training. The cardiac morphologic adaptations may occur within weeks or months after the initiation of strenuous training and may be reversed in a similar fashion following the cessation of training (Maron 1986). This left ventricular hypertrophy is generally considered to be physiologic and benign (Pelliccia & Maron 1997), and as such should not be confused with pathologic heart conditions.

Endurance athletes often exhibit an enlarged left ventricular cavity dimension, increased heart mass, and a slightly increased left ventricular wall thickness (Hoogsteen et al. 2003; Pelliccia et al. 2005; Pluim et al. 2000; Spirito et al. 1994). Recent evidence also indicates that endurance athletes have increased left atrial dimensions (Hoogsteen et al. 2003; Pelliccia et al. 2005). These adaptations (often termed the "athlete's heart") are thought to be the result of chronic volume expansion (i.e., training-induced hypervolemia) and exercising at high end-diastolic volumes, SV, HR, and blood pressures for prolonged periods of time. Thus, the endurance athlete's heart appears to adapt to both a chronic volume and pressure overload.

The amount of left ventricular hypertrophy seemingly varies according to the type of endurance activity. In fact, recent evidence indicates that endurance events that combine dynamic and static exercise of large muscle groups (e.g., rowing, triathlon, and cycling) will lead to the greatest changes in left ventricular cavity size and wall thickness (Hoogsteen et al. 2004; Pluim et al. 2000; Spirito et al. 1994) likely owing to the marked volume and pressure overload (Pluim et al. 2000).

Left ventricular dilatation appears to occur early in an athlete's career and progresses with training (Hoogsteen *et al.* 2003). Although the left ventricular cavity dimension returns towards normal after the long-term cessation of training, many athletes do not experience a complete normalization of their left ventricular cavity (Pelliccia *et al.* 2002). In fact, significant chamber dilatation has been shown to persist in over 20% of former elite athletes (Pelliccia *et al.* 2002). Pelliccia *et al.* (2002) revealed that this incomplete remodeling was likely the result of an increase in body weight and consistent recreational physical activity in the former athletes.

It has been postulated that the improvements in left ventricular dimensions lead to an enhanced capacity for diastolic filling, and thus a larger resultant SV (via the Frank–Starling mechanism; Crawford *et al.* 1979, 1985; George *et al.* 1991; Peronnet *et al.* 1981; Wolfe *et al.* 1979). However, enhanced SV and $\dot{V}O_{2max}$ are not necessarily dependent on an increased heart size. In fact, short-term moderate endurance training does not automatically lead to significant increases in ventricular dimensions of previously sedentary subjects despite significant increases in SV and $\dot{V}O_{2max}$ (Wolfe *et al.* 1985).

Ventricular compliance Endurance training has also been associated with an improvement in the compliance of the left ventricle (Arbab-Zadeh *et al.* 2004). Furthermore, there are marked differences between endurance-trained and untrained individuals in the diastolic pressure–volume relationship over a range of end-diastolic pressures (Levine 1993; Levine *et al.* 1991a). As illustrated in Fig. 2.16, there is a rightward shift in the diastolic pressure–volume relationship in endurance-trained athletes, reflecting greater ventricular compliance (Levine 1993; Levine *et al.* 1991a). Furthermore, endurance training results in left ventricular pressure–volume (Starling) curves that facilitate a large change in SV for a given change in preload (Fig. 2.17; Levine 1993; Levine *et al.* 1991a,b). An improvement in ventricular compliance is thought to promote diastolic filling at low pressures and enhance SV (and thus Q) via the Frank–Starling mechanism during exercise (Arbab-Zadeh *et al.* 2004).

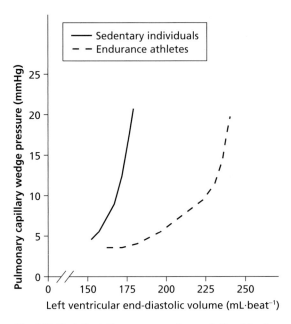

Fig. 2.16 End-diastolic pressure–volume relationships in endurance-trained (dashed line) and sedentary (solid line) humans. (Adapted from information provided by Levine *et al.* 1991.)

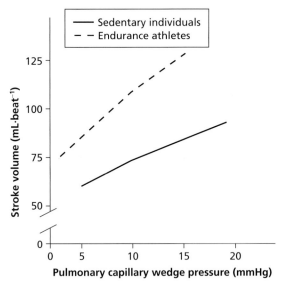

Fig. 2.17 The relationship between stroke volume and pulmonary capillary wedge pressure in sedentary (solid line) and endurance-trained humans (dashed lines). (Adapted from information provided by Levine *et al.* 1991.)

Afterload Afterload, defined as the force required to overcome the impedance or resistance to the ejection of blood (i.e., ventricular emptying), is also affected by endurance training (Blomqvist & Saltin 1983; Clausen 1976, 1977). Afterload varies directly with arterial blood pressure and therefore can be reduced by decreasing total peripheral resistance. Total peripheral resistance is known to decrease as a function of training, which allows for an enhanced ventricular systolic emptying/output and SV (Gledhill *et al.* 1994; Krip *et al.* 1997). An inverse relationship between total peripheral resistance and $\dot{V}o_{2max}$ has also been observed (Clausen 1976, 1977). Therefore, a decreased afterload appears to facilitate an increased SV and $\dot{V}o_{2max}$ after training (Blomqvist & Saltin 1983; Clausen 1976, 1977). Blomqvist and Saltin (1983) postulated that a "marked reduction in peripheral resistance enables the athlete to generate a cardiac output of up to 40 L·min^{-1} compared to 20 L in the sedentary subject at similar arterial pressures during maximal exercise." Without adaptations in total peripheral resistance the arterial blood pressures would have to be twice as high to attain the same Q in endurance athletes (Blomqvist 1991; Blomqvist & Saltin 1983). Several adaptations occur as a result of endurance training that serve to reduce total peripheral resistance (for review see Cornelissen & Fagard 2005). However, it has been shown that short-term training does not necessarily reduce afterload, despite significant increases in SV, Q, and $\dot{V}o_{2max}$ (Wolfe & Cunningham 1982). Therefore, although a reduction in afterload is of clear benefit to cardiac function, caution must be observed when stating that a reduced afterload is a prerequisite for an increased SV, Q, and $\dot{V}o_{2max}$.

Venous return

Venous return, the flow of blood back to the heart, is the major determinant of cardiac preload (i.e., the initial stretch of the myocardium prior to contraction; Rothe 1986) and thus SV. In fact, Q is ultimately limited by the amount of blood returning to the heart. Venous return is determined by venous pressure (P_V) minus right atrial pressure (P_{RA}) and venous resistance (R_V): Venous return = $(P_V - P_{RA})/R_V$.

Several factors favor venous return during exercise conditions: venoconstriction, skeletal muscle contraction (i.e., the muscle pump), and increased inspiratory movements (owing to a decrease in P_{RA} during inspiration).

It appears that endurance training facilitates an improvement in venous return (Gledhill *et al.* 1994, Krip *et al.* 1997; Warburton *et al.* 2002), because end-diastolic volume (an index of cardiac preload) is markedly increased after endurance training (Warburton *et al.* 2002). It is unclear which of the factors that affect venous return explain the enhanced venous return in endurance athletes. It is likely that the increased skeletal and respiratory muscular contractions during high intensity exercise will facilitate venous return in endurance athletes. It is also apparent that the training-induced hypervolemia (as discussed next) will lead to an increase in hemodynamically active blood volume increasing central venous pressure and promoting venous return (Gledhill *et al.* 1994; Krip *et al.* 1997; Warburton *et al.* 2002).

Blood volume expansion

One of the major adaptations to endurance training is an expansion in total blood volume (BV; training-induced hypervolemia; Brotherhood *et al.* 1975; Gillen *et al.* 1991; Gledhill *et al.* 1994; Kjellberg *et al.* 1949; Oscai *et al.* 1968; Warburton *et al.* 1999, 2002, 2004). Total BV is significantly increased within 24 h after exercise (Gillen *et al.* 1991, 1994) and reaches a plateau after 1 week of training (Convertino 1991; Warburton *et al.* 2004). Short-term exercise-induced increases in BV are almost entirely brought about by an increase in plasma volume rather than red blood cell volume (Convertino 1991; Convertino *et al.* 1980a,b; Warburton *et al.* 2004). However, red cell volume does appear to increase after 6 weeks of aerobic training (at sea level in a normoxic environment; Warburton *et al.* 2004).

The average amount of BV expansion resulting from endurance training approximates 6% in previously sedentary males (from 72 to 76 ml·kg^{-1}) and females (67 to 73 ml·kg^{-1}; Warburton *et al.* 2000). In comparison, the BV of endurance-trained athletes is approximately 20–30% larger than that seen in non-trained counterparts (Convertino 1991). Thus, there is a marked difference between the hypervolemia seen in untrained individuals who engage in short-term training versus individuals who are chronically endurance trained. Thus, the duration of intense training for competition likely has an important role in the magnitude of training-induced hypervolemia. However, it is also possible that endurance-trained athletes may naturally have a high BV (Krip *et al.* 1997), which provides them with an augmented SV and Q and hence a high $\dot{V}o_{2max}$. In fact, Gledhill *et al.* (1999) stated that "a high BV results in an enhanced diastolic function, maximal SV, Q_{max}, and $\dot{V}o_{2max}$, which allows these individuals to succeed in endurance events, and success in these events provides the impetus for further endurance training. Endurance training in athletes with a genetically endowed high BV will allow for the development of the high maximal SV, Q_{max}, and $\dot{V}o_{2max}$ commonly observed in endurance athletes." Thus, endurance training simply tops up this high BV. A recent study (Martino *et al.* 2002) supported this postulation. These investigators examined individuals who had high maximal SV and $\dot{V}o_{2max}$ with no history of physical training. The authors revealed that the elevated SV and $\dot{V}o_{2max}$ in the untrained individuals were largely the result of a high BV.

Several reports have indicated that BV may account for a large portion of the difference in maximal SV between trained and untrained individuals (Gledhill *et al.* 1994; Hagberg *et al.* 1998; Krip *et al.* 1997). Warburton *et al.* (2004) revealed that changes in plasma volume explained approximately 30% of the variance in changes in left ventricular function (i.e., end-diastolic volume, SV, and Q) after 12 weeks of endurance training.

The increased SV is thought to be the result of an increased central venous pressure (Convertino *et al.* 1991) and venous return (Gledhill *et al.* 1994; Krip *et al.* 1997; Warburton *et al.* 1999). According to the Frank–Starling law, this increased preload and resultant stretching will lead to a greater end-diastolic volume and thus a larger SV (Gledhill *et al.* 1994; Hagberg *et al.* 1998; Hopper *et al.* 1988; Krip *et al.* 1997; Levine 1993; Warburton *et al.* 1999).

The maintenance of a chronically expanded BV provides a series of cardiovascular and thermoregu-latory benefits (Convertino 1991). Thermoregulatory advantages include an increased sweat rate and evaporative cooling during exercise, which assists in minimizing the increases in core body temperature during exercise (Convertino 1991). Cardiovascular advantages include a reduced HR at rest and during exercise (Convertino 1991; Convertino *et al.* 1980a,b, 1983; Wyndham *et al.* 1976), an increased SV (Coyle *et al.* 1986; Gledhill *et al.* 1994; Krip *et al.* 1997; Warburton *et al.* 1999), and an increased maximal Q (Gledhill *et al.* 1994; Krip *et al.* 1997; Warburton *et al.* 1999).

Recent research has also revealed that an increased BV may account for a significant proportion of the difference in $\dot{V}o_{2max}$ between untrained and trained individuals (Gledhill *et al.* 1994; Krip *et al.* 1997; Warburton *et al.* 2004). Warburton *et al.* (2000, 2004) have revealed that differences in BV explain 53–56% of the variance in $\dot{V}o_{2max}$ between untrained and endurance-trained individuals. Moreover, changes in BV after short-term endurance training (both continuous and interval) explained 47% of the improvements in $\dot{V}o_{2max}$ with training (Warburton *et al.* 2004).

Myocardial contractility

Some authors contend that the enhanced cardiovascular function of endurance athletes suggests that endurance training results in improved myocardial contractility (i.e., the ability of the heart to change contraction vigour without altering end-diastolic fiber length – a positive inotropic effect; Ehsani *et al.* 1991; Ginzton *et al.* 1989; Jensen-Urstad *et al.* 1998; Plotnick *et al.* 1986; Seals *et al.* 1994). An enhanced myocardial contractility may be the result of augmented intrinsic contractile properties of the heart and/or an enhanced response to inotropic stimulation.

Endurance training-mediated improvements in contractility are thought to be of benefit for increasing SV during incremental exercise. However, it is debatable whether changes in myocardial contractility are required for an improvement in SV following endurance training. For instance, when a more sensitive index of contractility (i.e., the ratio of systolic blood pressure to end-systolic volume) has been assessed, many investigations do not support a marked improvement in myocardial contractility with endurance training despite large improvements in SV (Goodman *et al.* 2005; Warburton *et al.* 2004). Also, studies that have shown improvements in indices of myocardial contractility have revealed markedly greater changes in indices of diastolic function (Gledhill *et al.* 1994; Krip *et al.* 1997) providing evidence that supports the contention that improvements in diastolic function are more important for the observed increase in SV after endurance training.

Diastolic function and the Frank–Starling effect

Diastolic function appears to be markedly improved in endurance athletes (Gledhill *et al.* 1994; Krip *et al.* 1997). Also, an enhancement in left ventricular diastolic function after endurance training in previously sedentary individuals is a common finding in the literature (Goodman *et al.* 2005; Warburton *et al.* 2004).

For the purposes of this chapter, we consider diastolic function to reflect the capacity for diastolic filling leading to an enhanced end-diastolic volume. According to the Frank–Starling law of the heart, an increased preload, ventricular filling, and end-diastolic volume will lead to greater stretch on the myocardial fibers resulting in a greater ejection of blood, and thus a larger SV (Gledhill *et al.* 1994; Krip *et al.* 1997; Levine 1993; Warburton *et al.* 1999). An enhanced capacity for diastolic filling is thought to directly explain why endurance-trained athletes are able to achieve such markedly higher maximal SV than untrained individuals (Gledhill *et al.* 1994). Furthermore, endurance training in previously sedentary individuals results in an increased capacity to utilize the Frank–Starling mechanism during exercise allowing for the large increases in SV (Goodman *et al.* 2005; Warburton *et al.* 2004). An enhanced diastolic function is also thought to explain (in large part) why endurance-trained athletes are able to increase their SV throughout incremental exercise.

There are numerous adaptations that serve to promote optimal diastolic filling and allow endurance athletes to utilize more fully the Frank–Starling mechanism to achieve superior SV and Q

during exercise conditions. Key adaptations that serve to augment diastolic filling include increased ventricular compliance, increased left ventricular internal cavity dimensions, increased transmitral pressure gradient (e.g., enhanced diastolic suction), training-induced hypervolemia, increased early filling (i.e., E : A ratio), increased rate of left ventricular pressure decline ($-dP/dt$), and/or increased rate of calcium uptake within the SR (Gledhill *et al.* 1999). A more compliant pericardium may also explain the enhanced diastolic function of endurance-trained athletes (Esch *et al.* 2007).

Stroke volume response to exercise: Mechanisms of primary importance

There is considerable debate as to which factor, myocardial contractility or the diastolic function (via the Frank–Starling effect), has the most influence on cardiovascular function during strenuous exercise in endurance athletes. Several researchers have postulated that at low and moderate exercise intensities, the Frank–Starling mechanism is mainly responsible for increasing SV and thus Q in endurance-trained and untrained individuals (Ginzton *et al.* 1989; Higginbotham *et al.* 1986; Plotnick *et al.* 1986). This occurs because of increased end-diastolic volume, and therefore an increased SV (brought about by the Frank–Starling effect). It is thought that the differences in end-diastolic volume and SV between endurance-trained athletes and untrained individuals remain during moderate and maximal exercise, but do not increase (Ginzton *et al.* 1989; Plotnick *et al.* 1986). That is, both endurance-trained and untrained individuals reach their maximum SV during low intensity exercise.

It is commonly accepted that SV reaches a plateau at a submaximal workload at approximately 40% $\dot{V}o_{2max}$ and HR of 110–130 beats·min^{-1} irrespective of training status (Adams *et al.* 1992; Ginzton *et al.* 1989; Higginbotham *et al.* 1986; McLaren *et al.* 1997; Plotnick *et al.* 1986). Many believe that this plateau occurs because tachycardia limits the time available for diastolic filling, thereby limiting the end-diastolic volume in both trained and untrained individuals (Ginzton *et al.* 1989; Higginbotham *et al.*

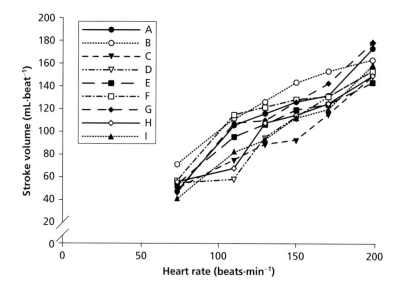

Fig. 2.18 Individual stroke volume responses to incremental cycle ergometer exercise in elite endurance-trained athletes. (Data from Warburton *et al.* 1999.)

1986; Plotnick *et al.* 1986). Concurrently, an increased myocardial contractility is thought to lead to an increased ejection of blood leading to a decreased end-systolic volume that allows SV to be maintained or slightly reduced despite a potential reduction in end-diastolic volume. It is therefore inferred that increased myocardial contractility and tachycardia have more effect on increasing Q than the Frank–Starling mechanism in the later stages of vigorous exercise (Ginzton *et al.* 1989; Higginbotham *et al.* 1986; Plotnick *et al.* 1986).

However, these results were derived from studies using primarily untrained individuals or individuals who were not endurance trained for years. Recent evidence (Gledhill *et al.* 1994; Krip *et al.* 1997; Warburton *et al.* 1999, 2002) and previously overlooked findings (Crawford *et al.* 1985; Spriet *et al.* 1986) indicate that highly trained endurance athletes (unlike untrained individuals) progressively increase their SV throughout incremental to maximal exercise (Fig. 2.18).

The ability to increase SV during strenuous exercise is largely the result of increases in diastolic filling and end-diastolic volume (Warburton *et al.* 2002). This is a result of the series of endurance training-mediated adaptations that optimize diastolic function. Therefore, the enhanced diastolic function of endurance-trained athletes allows them to increasingly use the Frank–Starling mechanism

throughout incremental to maximal exercise (Gledhill *et al.* 1994; Warburton *et al.* 2002; Wiebe *et al.* 1998). The use of the Frank–Starling mechanism is an energy conserving mechanism. The fact that endurance athletes are able to take advantage of the Frank–Starling mechanism during strenuous exercise is likely of great benefit from both cardiac and aerobic performance perspectives.

The pericardium: Has it been overlooked?

Since 1898 (Barnard 1898) the role of the parietal pericardium in restricting cardiac filling and preventing overdistension of the myocardium has been well established; however, the role of the pericardium for the enhanced cardiac performance of endurance athletes has been largely ignored (Esch *et al.* 2007). Recent evidence suggests that the pericardium of endurance athletes adapts to facilitate optimal ventricular filling especially during strenuous exercise conditions (Esch *et al.* 2007).

As a background, the stress–strain relationship of the pericardium is J-shaped, such that it is relatively compliant at low levels of stretch, but shows a sharp decrease in compliance at high levels of stretch (Morris-Thurgood & Frenneaux 2000). With acute changes in myocardial volume and size, the pericardium restricts further cardiac dilatation, limiting the ability of the ventricles to further increase end-diastolic volume and SV (Janicki 1990). The pericardium also enhances the effects of changes in right ventricular volume on left ventricular compliance (Janicki 1990). When the right ventricle is distended, the pericardium that is attached to its free wall is stretched outwards, whereas the pericardium attached to the left ventricular free wall is pulled inward serving to reduce the left ventricular size and compliance (Janicki 1990). Therefore, an increase in right ventricular volume will cause an immediate increase in pericardial pressure and a decrease in the transmural pressure (i.e., pulmonary capillary wedge pressure – pericardial pressure) and area of the left ventricle, reducing left ventricular SV via the Frank–Starling mechanism (Kroeker et al. 2003). This effect (termed diastolic ventricular interaction) only occurs when the increase in right ventricular volume is large enough to shift the pericardium into the stiff portion of its stress–strain relationship resulting in a marked increase in pericardial pressure (Janicki 1990). Thus, the pericardium is thought to have its greatest effects on left ventricular compliance and filling during conditions of heightened heart volumes (as seen during moderate to heavy exercise; Janicki 1990).

With high intercavitary and ventricular filling pressures pericardial restraint to left ventricular filling is significant. Animal studies have shown that pericardial constraint limits left ventricular SV during moderate to high intensity exercise (Hammond et al. 1992; Stray-Gundersen et al. 1986). In fact, the removal of the pericardium in dogs and pigs resulted in an increased left ventricular SV with concomitant improvements in peak Q and $\dot{V}o_{2max}$. The improvements in left ventricular SV were the result of increases in left ventricular end-diastolic volume. Thus, it appears that the pericardium in the normal heart limits left ventricular diastolic filling, making it unable to fully utilize the Frank–Starling mechanism (Kroeker et al. 2003). This is supported by limited human evidence. For instance, one study (Higginbotham et al. 1986) revealed that pulmonary capillary wedge pressure increased throughout incremental upright exercise while SV reached its peak at a submaximal level in healthy untrained individuals. It was postulated that this was the result of a reduced time for diastolic filling during

exercise. The belief that SV plateaus at a submaximal exercise level owing to a limited time for diastolic filling has dominated cardiovascular physiology literature. However, most authors have failed to consider the effects of the pericardium on left ventricular filling during exercise conditions. It is unlikely that a limited time for diastolic filling could explain these findings, because the left ventricular diastolic pressure–volume relation is only affected at HR greater than 170 beats·min^{-1} (Morris-Thurgood & Frenneaux 2000), a HR that is well above where the plateau in SV generally occurs. The invariant filling and SV at much lower HR is supportive of the conclusion that the pericardium limits left ventricular filling during moderate to strenuous exercise in healthy untrained humans (Janicki 1990; Morris-Thurgood & Frenneaux 2000). Additional support for this theory comes from research (including our own) that revealed that acute alterations in venous return via volume expansion or a change in postural position results in minimal changes in exercise SV, despite significantly larger elevations in resting SV (Robinson et al. 1966; Warburton et al. 1999).

Perhaps the most compelling research supporting the significant role of pericardial constraint in limiting left ventricular SV during exercise comes from work with patients with chronic heart failure (Janicki 1990). The landmark work of Janicki (1990) revealed that there are three distinct SV responses to incremental exercise:

1 SV continues to increase throughout incremental exercise. In this group the increase in pulmonary capillary wedge pressure is approximately two- to threefold higher than the increase in right atrial pressure (i.e., minimal pericardial constraint).
2 SV increases at lower exercise intensities, but reaches a plateau at submaximal exercise intensities. This response is associated with equal changes in pulmonary capillary wedge pressure and right atrial pressure (i.e., pericardial constraint is present).
3 SV does not increase at any stage of exercise and is associated with equal changes in pulmonary capillary wedge pressure and right atrial pressure (i.e., pericardial constraint).
In healthy humans, we also commonly observe three SV patterns to exercise (Fig. 2.19). Endurance-trained

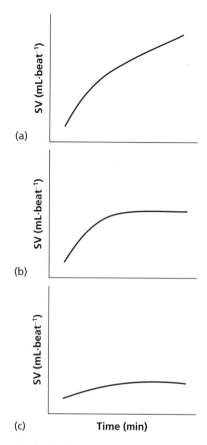

(a)

(b)

(c)   **Time (min)**

Fig. 2.19 Typical stroke volume responses observed during exercise conditions. (a) Reflects minimal pericardial constraint (Janicki 1990). This is the most common pattern observed in highly trained endurance athletes (Warburton *et al.* 2002). (b) Reflects pericardial constraint (Janicki 1990). This is the most common pattern observed in untrained individuals (Warburton *et al.* 2004). (c) Reflects marked pericardial constraint (Janicki 1990). In our practice, we observe this pattern in the least fit sedentary individuals (Warburton *et al.* 2004).

athletes generally exhibit a continual increase in SV during incremental exercise (Figs 2.18 and 2.19a) indicative of less pericardial constraint (Esch *et al.* 2007). Whereas untrained individuals often display the latter SV responses (Fig. 2.19b,c), with the least fit exhibiting the pattern consistent with marked pericardial constraint (Fig. 2.19c).

Warburton *et al.* (1999, 2002) and Kroeker *et al.* (2003) have recently postulated that the pericardium of endurance-trained athletes may remodel in

response to the physiologic stressors placed upon it. This premise is supported by animal research that revealed that the pericardium is capable of growth (i.e., dilatation) in response to chronic volume loading leading to cardiac enlargement (Freeman & LeWinter 1984; Lee *et al.* 1985; Morris-Thurgood & Frenneaux 2000). In fact, it is plausible that endurance-trained athletes undergo pericardial remodeling in response to a chronic volume overload (via training-induced hypervolemia and/or prolonged exercise at high SV). This pericardial remodeling would reduce pericardial constraint during exercise and may explain (in part) why endurance-trained athletes have a more compliant ventricle (Fig. 2.16) and are able to increase their SV throughout incremental exercise (using the Frank–Starling mechanism; Warburton *et al.* 2002), whereas the majority of untrained individuals cannot (Gledhill *et al.* 1994; Krip *et al.* 1997; Warburton *et al.* 1999, 2002). We have recently shown that endurance-trained athletes have less diastolic ventricular interaction during orthostatic stress indicating a more compliant pericardium (Esch *et al.* 2007).

CARDIAC FATIGUE AFTER PROLONGED STRENUOUS EXERCISE

It is well established that cardiovascular drift may occur after approximately 10–20 min of moderate intensity aerobic exercise. Cardiovascular drift is characterized by a reduction in SV and a proportionate increase in HR that allows Q to be maintained (Coyle 1998; Coyle & Gonzalez-Alonso 2001). The mechanisms responsible for this phenomenon are debatable (Coyle 1998; Coyle & Gonzalez-Alonso 2001) but the reduction in SV appears to be the result (in part) of a reduction in preload reserve (i.e., blood volume) from dehydration (Coyle 1998). However, several investigators have also shown a reduction in left ventricular systolic and diastolic function after prolonged strenuous exercise without concomitant changes in preload (Haykowsky *et al.* 2001) or afterload (Douglas *et al.* 1987; Vanoverschelde *et al.* 1991). This phenomenon is distinct from that of cardiovascular drift and indicates that the heart can fatigue (which is contrary to a previously held axiom). Several investigators have revealed that prolonged endurance events can lead to marked reductions in systolic and/or diastolic function (Dawson *et al.* 2003, 2005; Haykowsky *et al.* 2001; Welsh *et al.* 2005; Whyte *et al.* 2000). The impairment in left ventricular function is transient (lasting for less than 24 h; McGavock *et al.* 2002). The reduced left ventricular function has been seen after 60 min of exercise, but appears to be particularly evident and pronounced during competitive endurance events lasting longer than 4 h (McGavock *et al.* 2002). The mechanisms responsible for the left ventricular impairment after prolonged strenuous exercise remain unclear. We have recently shown that the blunted contractile response after prolonged strenuous exercise is caused (in part) by β-adrenoreceptor desensitization (Welsh *et al.* 2005).

Respiratory adaptations to endurance training

During sea level exercise the healthy respiratory system is generally able to maintain the arterial partial pressures of oxygen (Pao_2) carbon dioxide ($Paco_2$) and arterial pH (pHa) at close to resting levels across a wide range of work rates. This is impressive as it occurs despite significant potential impediments to the maintenance of blood-gases at resting levels. For example, there are large decreases in the partial pressure of mixed venous oxygen (Pvo_2) and increases in mixed venous carbon dioxide ($Pvco_2$). The rise in Q that accompanies increasing exercise intensity reduces time for gas exchange equilibrium in the pulmonary capillaries, which could negatively impact on blood gas homeostasis. Regulation of alveolar ventilation is required to be precise in order to maintain the alveolar partial pressures of oxygen and carbon dioxide (PAo_2 and $PAco_2$) within narrow limits. The neural and sensory control of alveolar ventilation (V_A) must therefore be highly coordinated with the muscles of respiration.

It is well known that the regular application of a specific exercise overload enhances physiologic function to bring about a training response. Exercise training induces a variety of highly specific adaptations that enable the body to function more efficiently during exercise and are typically associated with improvements in $\dot{V}o_{2max}$ and athletic performance. The adaptations of the respiratory system to exercise training are considerably less than those observed in other body systems. Other systems (i.e., cardiac, substrate metabolism, skeletal muscle) show significant improvements with long-term training while the respiratory system responses are, for the most part, similar between those who are trained and untrained. This should not be so surprising given that respiratory system can expand its response to exercise to a wider range than other bodily systems. Ventilation can increase 20–40 times that of resting values, implying that the respiratory system is "designed" for maximal function and that any additional adaptations acquired via training are not necessary. However, there are important changes that occur via training to optimize the respiratory response to exercise. In this section, the effects of whole-body endurance training on the respiratory system are reviewed in addition to specific training of the respiratory muscles. While the adaptability of respiratory regulation and respiratory system structures to habitual physical training is less than other links in the oxygen transport system, there are instances where the respiratory system becomes the weak "link" and impairs $\dot{V}o_{2max}$ and exercise performance. Two respiratory limitations with specific reference to exercise performance are presented.

EFFECTS OF PHYSICAL TRAINING ON VENTILATORY RESPONSES TO EXERCISE

Regular aerobic training elicits adaptations in pulmonary ventilation during submaximal and maximal exercise. During maximal exercise, minute ventilation (V_E) increases as $\dot{V}o_{2max}$ increases (Fig. 2.20). The increase in maximal V_E is brought about by increases in both tidal volume (Vt) and breathing frequency (fb). The mechanisms of the increase in V_E are not precisely known but are related to the complex regulatory factors including neural and chemical along with sensory inputs from the lungs and respiratory musculature (Dempsey *et al.* 1995). During submaximal exercise the trained individual has increased ventilatory efficiency as reflected by a lower ventilatory equivalent for

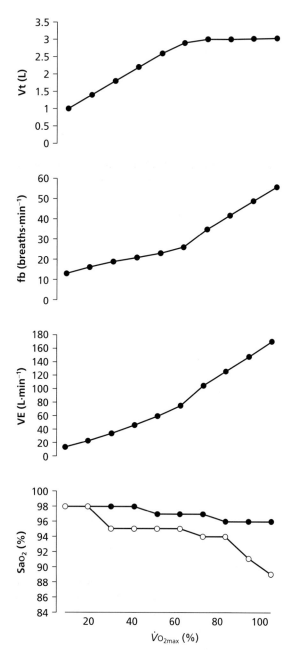

oxygen (V_E/Vo_2; Casaburi *et al.* 1987a,b). It is often viewed that such adaptations indicate a breathing "strategy" that minimizes the cost of respiratory work. Presumably, this allows for greater oxygen utilization by non-respiratory muscles. It should be noted that significant specificity exists for ventilatory responses, where the type of exercise (i.e., arm vs. leg) can dictate the training adaptations (Rasmussen *et al.* 1975). This implies that the ventilatory adjustment to training can partially be explained by local adaptations within the specifically trained muscles rather than strictly within the respiratory regulatory centers within the central nervous system. A consistent adaptation with training is an increase in Vt at rest and during submaximal and maximal exercise (Wilmore *et al.* 1970). This end-result is presumably of benefit because a greater depth of breathing during exercise would ensure appropriate alveolar ventilation.

EFFECTS OF PHYSICAL TRAINING ON RESPIRATORY MUSCLES

Physical training produces a lower V_E/Vo_2 for a given level of exercise intensity. This adaptation implies improvement in respiratory muscle function in terms of strength and endurance. Studies examining the effects of whole-body training on the respiratory muscles (RM) are relatively few and to answer this question, the animal literature must be reviewed. Endurance training elicits small (20–30%) but significant increases in rat diaphragm mitochondrial enzyme activity and antioxidant enzyme activity, resting glycogen levels (Metzger & Fitts 1986; Powers *et al.* 1992, 1994), which is consistent with that seen in locomotor muscle. A consistent finding is that endurance training of sufficient intensity and duration can increase the oxidative capacity of the rat diaphragm. An upregulation of antioxidant enzyme activity in the diaphragm points to an increased ability of the diaphragm to eliminate free radicals during exercise (Vrabas *et al.* 1999). There are also reports of significant decreases in type IIb and an increase in type I myosin heavy chains in trained diaphragms (Vrabas *et al.* 1999). It is presumed that this results in a functional improvement in the endurance properties of the muscle.

Fig. 2.20 Schematic representation of ventilation and oxyhemoglobin saturation during incremental exercise to exhaustion. Note that Sao_2 is maintained throughout exercise in most individuals (solid symbols) whereas some highly trained endurance athletes experience significant decreases in Sao_2 (open symbols) or exercise-induced arterial hypoxemia.

Direct studies examining the effects of RM training on critical bioenergetic enzymes and fatigue resistance in humans are lacking. However, from a functional point of view, studies of human RM adaptation to exercise training have shown improvements in ventilatory performance as evidenced by increases in maximal sustainable ventilatory capacity and maximal voluntary ventilation (MVV; Clanton et al. 1987; O'Kroy & Coast 1993). Comparisons of athletes and non-athletes have shown differences in ventilatory performance (Coast et al. 1990; Martin & Stager 1981). Martin and Stager (1981) showed that athletes could sustain 80% of their 12-s MVV for 11 min; whereas age, gender, vital capacity, and body size matched non-athletes could sustain this ventilatory load for only 3 min. Exercise training is known to increases maximal inspiratory pressure (MIP) or the ability to generate force. Training-induced adaptations to the RM may be of importance to exercise performance for four reasons:

1 There would be a reduction in overall energy demands because of a reduction in the work of breathing;

2 There would be a lowering of lactate production by the RM during high intensity exercise;

3 Training would improve how the RM metabolize circulating lactate as a metabolic fuel; and

4 A reduction in dyspnea or breathlessness is accompanied by training.

Additional well-controlled training studies are necessary to determine the relative importance of each of these possibilities.

SPECIFIC TRAINING OF THE RESPIRATORY MUSCLES

There is evidence to suggest that the RM, as with limb skeletal muscle, respond adaptively to exercise training. In this section the effects of specific RM training with respect to changes in strength and endurance and the consequences for exercise performance and potential physiologic markers of performance are discussed. Different modes of training have been utilized but most RM training studies have employed two modes of training: (i) voluntary isocapnic hyperpnea, or (ii) inspiratory resistive loading. During isocapnic hyperpnea training, subjects maintain a given level of ventilation for up to 30 min. This regime is carried out typically for 3–5 times per week for 4–5 weeks. Using this type of training, several investigators have shown improvements in RM endurance. Inspiratory resistive loading training is consistent of loads (approximately 15–50% MIP) applied to the inspiratory circuit 3–5 times per week for a duration of 5–20 min while at rest (Sheel 2002). This is typically accomplished by using a custom-built apparatus or more recently with a commercially available device. Studies using resistive loading have reported increases in MIP in the range of 8–45% (Sonetti et al. 2001; Volianitis et al. 2001). It is interesting to note that those studies that have utilized the highest percentage MIP and longest duration of training also report the highest change with training in MIP, whereas studies that utilize a lower percentage MIP or training for a shorter duration show less of an improvement in MIP. It is tempting to speculate that, as with other skeletal muscle, the RM respond in a dose–response fashion to a given training stimulus.

On balance it is reasonable to conclude that inspiratory muscle loading can improve the strength of the RM as reflected by MIP. The salient question remains; does RM training result in an improvement in exercise performance? A critical review of the literature reveals that the effects of RM training on exercise performance are controversial. The reason for much of the controversy surrounds the fact that studies have used different RM training regimes, different laboratory tests of exercise "performance," and differences in the training status of subjects. Furthermore, most studies have utilized relatively small sample sizes (typically less than 8–10 and as low as 4), although more recent studies have employed larger samples. From the available studies it appears that RM training can improve time to volitional exhaustion at fixed rate submaximal workloads (Boutellier & Piwko 1992; Boutellier et al. 1992; Morgan et al. 1987b) (although this is not a completely consistent finding) and not at near-maximal exercise intensities. Indeed, the most commonly used laboratory protocols have employed exercise time to exhaustion as a measure of performance. Controversy surrounds the value of fixed work rate laboratory tests for two reasons. First, these tests are not true measures of athletic performance as they do not mimic competitive situations. Athletes often change velocity for strategic or environmental reasons (e.g., hill, wind). Second, those studies that evaluate performance using fixed work rate type performance tests are reported to have poor reliability. Most data suggest that laboratory tests that require subjects to complete a fixed amount of work or to cover a set distance in the shortest possible time are much more reliable than constant load tests. Coefficient of variations (CV) range 1.0–3.1% for cyclists performing time trials (Hickey *et al.* 1992; Palmer *et al.* 1996), and 2.7–3.4% when cyclists perform as much work as possible in 1 h (Jeukendrup *et al.* 1996). This contrasts sharply with fixed work rate tests with CV values of 17–40% (Jeukendrup *et al.* 1996) and 25% (Billat *et al.* 1994). During an 8-km laboratory time trial, cycling performance was increased significantly (+1.8 ± 1.2%) in well-trained athletes who performed 5 weeks of RM training (Sonetti *et al.* 2001). In this study, subjects who performed placebo RM training did not show an improvement in performance; however, the improvement in the RM training group was not significantly different than the placebo group. Improved performance was seen in eight of nine RM training subjects and five of eight placebo subjects. The lack of a consistent effect of RM on exercise performance can be interpreted in two ways:

1 Improvements in 8 km time trial were brought about by a familiarization effect; or

2 The changes can be explained by the placebo effect.

If we operate on the premise that RM training can increase exercise performance (as some have shown), what physiologic mechanisms might be responsible? Usually, increased performance is attributed to improvements of the cardiocirculatory system or to improvements to skeletal muscles. From the available data, it does not appear that RM training has any systematic effect on maximal V_E, Vo_2, HR, SV, blood gas concentrations, or oxyhemoglobin saturation during incremental exercise to exhaustion (Fairbarn *et al.* 1991; Hanel & Secher 1991; Inbar *et al.* 2000; Markov *et al.* 2001; Morgan *et al.* 1987a; Sonetti *et al.* 2001; Spengler *et al.* 1999; Stuessi *et al.*

2001). However, some studies report modest reductions in blood lactate concentrations of approximately 2 mmol·L^{-1} (Spengler *et al.* 1999) while others report no change as a result of RM training (Sonetti *et al.* 2001).

The respiratory system can become fatigued with exercise (see p. 109). Could RM training delay fatigue of the respiratory musculature? This is an attractive possibility, but objective measures of diaphragm fatigue following exhaustive exercise pre- and post-RM training have not been performed. The regulation and distribution of cardiac output during exercise is a highly complex process. It has been hypothesized that during exercise the RM "compete" with limb locomotor muscles for their "share" of Q (Harms *et al.* 1998b; Sheel *et al.* 2001). It remains unknown if RM training can "free" Q from the RM to the locomotor muscles as these measures have not been performed. Dyspneic sensations are commonly cited as factors limiting exercise during exercise. It has been hypothesized that RM training may decrease perception of respiratory exertion and contribute to the observed increase in constant load exercise performance; however, supporting data have been few. Another possibility to explain the effects of RM training is altered ventilatory efficiency. Possibly, V_E is reduced following RM training during submaximal exercise and could contribute to the observed improvements in fixed work rate exercise tests. Reduced V_E for a given workload would reduce the metabolic requirements of the respiratory muscles and result in a diminished competition for blood flow requirements between the RM and locomotor muscles. This remains an interesting possibility that awaits experimental evidence.

In summary, specific respiratory muscle training has been shown to improve the endurance and strength of the respiratory muscles in healthy humans. The effects of respiratory muscle training on exercise performance remain controversial. Mechanisms to explain the purported improvements in exercise performance remain largely unknown. However, candidates include improved ratings of breathing perception, delay of respiratory muscle fatigue, ventilatory efficiency, or blood flow competition between respiratory and locomotor muscle. Future well-controlled studies with larger sample sizes are warranted to ascertain whether delaying or attenuating respiratory muscle fatigue does indeed improve athletic performance and what physiologic mechanisms might be responsible.

RESPIRATORY SYSTEM LIMITATIONS TO EXERCISE PERFORMANCE

The healthy lung and chest wall are remarkably well designed in terms of homeostasis of systemic arterial oxygenation and carbon dioxide elimination. However, the pulmonary system is far from perfect and there are exceptions to its anatomic and regulatory capacities. Here we discuss two specific respiratory system limitations with respect to exercise performance: (i) exercise-induced arterial hypoxemia; and (ii) diaphragm fatigue.

Exercise-induced arterial hypoxemia

Arterial oxygen desaturation of 3–15% below resting levels have been observed to occur at or near maximum exercise intensities (Fig. 2.20; Dempsey *et al.* 1984) (and during submaximal exercise (Rice *et al.* 1999). This phenomenon has been termed exercise-induced arterial hypoxemia (EIAH) which is reported to occur in approximately 50% of highly trained male endurance athletes but not sedentary males (Powers *et al.* 1988). Most recently, studies of smaller numbers of fit females claim higher prevalence of EIAH and that EIAH occurs at lower levels of $\dot{V}o_{2max}$ than in the young adult males (Harms *et al.* 1998a; Richards *et al.* 2004). However, this remains controversial and the true prevalence of EIAH and susceptibility of various subpopulations (females, older athletes) remains unresolved. Why EIAH occurs has been the subject of much speculation, which is based primarily on indirect measures, and explanatory mechanisms remain controversial. Potential mechanisms include:

1 Right-to-left shunt;
2 Ventilation–perfusion (V_A/Q) inequality; and
3 Failure of alveolar–end-capillary diffusion equilibration (for review see Dempsey & Wagner 1999).

Does EIAH negatively influence exercise performance and $\dot{V}o_{2max}$? The factors that provide a limit to $\dot{V}o_{2max}$ have been a source of debate for many years. It has been postulated that in some elite aerobic athletes the limit to $\dot{V}o_{2max}$, and possibly performance, is the respiratory system (Dempsey 1986). Accordingly, the first step in the supply of oxygen to working muscle becomes the "weak link." Elite athletes undergo training adaptations in skeletal muscle and the cardiovascular system, which eventually surpasses the capability of the pulmonary system. Dempsey (1986) speculates further that this occurs because of the inability of the pulmonary system to adapt despite many years of aerobic training. If this supposition holds true then the pulmonary system does in fact pose a constraint to maximal exercise performance because of the inability to match the metabolic requirements of the athlete. To address this issue, experiments have been conducted by providing supplemental inspired oxygen to prevent EIAH (Harms *et al.* 2000). By increasing the FIO_2 from 0.21 to 0.26 there is an improvement in $\dot{V}o_{2max}$ in those athletes with EIAH. Those who demonstrated the most desaturation under normoxic conditions showed the greatest improvement in $\dot{V}o_{2max}$ if desaturation was prevented. The improvement in $\dot{V}o_{2max}$ appears to be 2% increase for each 1% decrease in Sao_2, beginning with >3% desaturation from rest.

The effects of preventing EIAH on exercise performance as opposed to the effects on $\dot{V}o_{2max}$ have not been adequately studied. However, it does appear that reductions in Sao_2 from control values have negative effects on exercise performance (Koskolou & McKenzie 1994). Highly trained cyclists without EIAH performed three 5-min cycle performance tests under normoxia, mild hypoxemia, or moderate hypoxemia. Mean Sao_2 values were 96, 90, and 87%, respectively (Fig. 2.21). As was correctly pointed out by the authors, a linear trend was observed between decreasing levels of Sao_2 and diminished work.

Respiratory muscle fatigue The diaphragm is a highly oxidative, densely capillarized muscle sheet which, in resting subjects, must sustain very high levels of force output to show fatigue. During exercise to exhaustion at intensities ≤80% of $\dot{V}o_{2max}$ the diaphragm does not fatigue, but at higher intensities

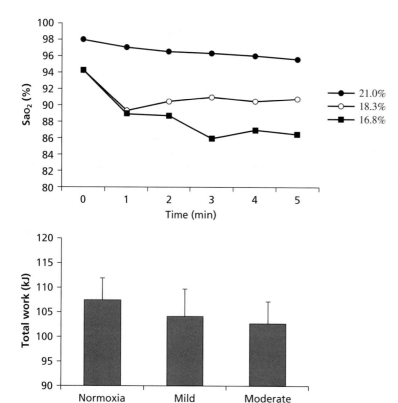

Fig. 2.21 Effects of lowering oxyhemoglobin saturation on cycle exercise performance. Mild refers to mild hypoxemia and moderate refers to moderate hypoxemia. (After Koskolou & McKenzie 1994.)

of sustained exercise the diaphragm shows fatigue at end-exercise, as demonstrated using bilateral phrenic nerve stimulation (Johnson *et al.* 1993). This fatigue occurred even though the force output of the diaphragm during exercise was well below the fatigue threshold of this muscle determined during voluntary hyperpnea at rest (Babcock *et al.* 1995). Does respiratory muscle fatigue impact exercise performance? This was recently addressed by subjecting highly trained cyclists to 9–12 randomly assigned exercise performance trials, consisting of cycling to exhaustion, beginning at 90% $\dot{V}o_{2max}$, under control conditions and during respiratory muscle resistive loading and respiratory muscle unloading (Babcock *et al.* 2002). Unloading increased endurance time in 76% of performance trials by a mean of $14 \pm 5\%$ and respiratory muscle loading reduced performance time in 83% of trials by $15 \pm 3\%$. The rate of rise of $\dot{V}o_2$ over exercise time was reduced with unloading and increased with loading, most likely in response to the accompanying

changes in the work of breathing. Similarly, the rate of rise of the subject's perception of both respiratory and limb discomfort were markedly reduced with unloading and increased with respiratory muscle loading. These significant effects of respiratory muscle unloading on exercise performance are consistent with the deleterious effects of fatiguing the respiratory muscles on subsequent exercise performance.

Conclusions

Endurance training produces a number of central and peripheral adaptations that allow an athlete to have an increased $\dot{V}o_{2max}$ and sustain higher aerobic workloads. Oxygen transport appears to be the ratelimiting factor for elite aerobic performance. Coaches and athletes alike are aware of the importance of oxygen transport for optimal aerobic performance and as such have used a variety of ethical and unethical means to enhance their performance.

The key adaptation to endurance training appears to be an enhancement in cardiac function, specifically SV and Q. A variety of adaptations account for the improved SV in highly trained endurance athletes. Endurance athletes show superior systolic and diastolic function. However, improvements in the capacity for diastolic filling appear to explain a large portion of the enhanced cardiac function of elite endurance-trained athletes.

The adaptability of the respiratory system to endurance training appears to be less than other links in the oxygen transport chain. However, there are several instances wherein the respiratory system becomes the weak link in oxygen transport directly affecting aerobic performance. This is particularly evident in highly trained endurance athletes.

Contrary to widely held axioms, both the heart and respiratory muscles may fatigue after prolonged strenuous exercise. This muscle fatigue limits the ability of the cardiorespiratory system to supply oxygen to the working tissues and as such has a significant effect upon aerobic capacity and performance.

ADAPTATIONS OF BONE AND CONNECTIVE TISSUE TO TRAINING

PEKKA KANNUS, RIKU NIKANDER, HARRI SIEVÄNEN AND IÑIGO MUJIKA

Introduction

Because bone and connective tissues are living tissues, it is not surprising that they show the capacity to adapt their structure and mechanical properties to the functional demands of the entire body. Understanding the adaptation of bone and connective tissue to various levels of loading is important not only for better understanding the basic physiology of these tissues but also for a deeper understanding of their pathologic processes. The old axiom applied to musculoskeletal tissues that "hyperfunction leads to tissue hypertrophy and hypofunction to tissue atrophy" also seems to apply to bone and connective tissue, provided that the activity increase is gradual and within the limits that the tissues can withstand without breakdown and injuries.

Adaptation of bone to training

Phylogeny and associated locomotive and loading issues basically define the specific functional organization and features of the skeleton and musculature. Appendicular and axial skeleton made of rigid bones, shaped for the specific locomotive or functional purpose and interconnected by joints, substantiate the framework for a complex mechanical system comprising skeletal muscles and attached tendons, joints and ligaments, and the underlying neural control system. During locomotion and other movements, body weight induced reaction forces, in most cases substantially magnified by moment arms of the musculoskeleton, cause the net muscle forces to be relatively high – multiples of body weight (Biewener 1991). All body movements are produced by coordinated contractions of skeletal muscles, and the associated concentric or eccentric muscle work comprises the fundamental source of mechanical loading to the skeleton – the resultant loading pattern within the affected bones can naturally vary substantially in terms of magnitude, rate, frequency, direction, and distribution. In order to survive, the musculoskeleton must be able to adapt to altered loading environment by increasing the size and characteristics of its functional units – in concordance with each other.

Mechanical competence of the skeleton per se is principally maintained by a mechanosensory feedback system that senses loading-induced deformations within the bone structures (Frost 2003; Turner 1991). Bone cells located within the mineralized bone matrix (evidently through the interconnected osteocyte network; Martin 2000) sense the strains arising from the muscle work of locomotion and convert a part of this mechanical energy (a part of this energy is dissipated into heat) into chemical energy which eventually results in synthesis of new bone tissue. Details of the microscopic mechanosensory system and associated pathways from mechanical stimulus to formation or resorption of bone tissue are complex and not yet fully established (Karsenty 2003). The macroscopic principle of skeletal adaptation, in turn, is shortly the following: new bone tissue is laid on skeletal regions that are subject to loading that exceeds clearly the customary loading range (deformations are

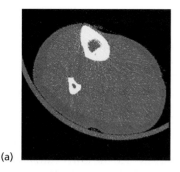 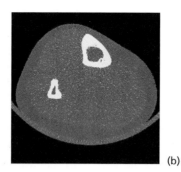

(a)

(b)

Fig. 2.22 The influence of extreme loading (impacts up to 20 times of body weight onto a single leg) on the size and shape of the tibial midshaft. Tibial shaft of the triple jumper (a) and of an age, height, and weight matched non-athletic counterpart (b). Note the substantial difference in the cortical bone. (Adapted from the study by Heinonen *et al.* 2001.)

somehow too large for the given bone region), while bone tissue is removed from regions that experience declined loading well below the customary loading range (deformations are marginal). As deformations can vary substantially from site to site, the bone response to loading is primarily site-specific and can be accomplished through different structural modifications of size, shape, or architecture in bone (Fig. 2.22a,b). The goal of the mechanosensory control system is simply to maintain the mechanical competence of the loaded bone reasonable in terms of the predominant loading environment while keeping the loading-induced deformations well within a specified safety range.

While the clinical studies assessing the skeletal adaptation to training have quite consistently been based on measurements of bone mineral density (BMD) or content (BMC), the bone structure is considered the most relevant factor underlying bone fragility (Currey 2003; Järvinen *et al.* 2005). The amount of bone tissue (~BMC) volume represents only the rudimentary bulk of which the complete bone structure and organ is made but, as such, the bulk is not, and cannot be, fully indicative of the actual bone structure or strength. It is obvious that the strength and rigidity of the whole bone are attributable to interaction of material properties, amount (mass) of material, morphologic, organizational, and (somewhat confusing) quality issues of bone tissue and whole organ. It is ultimately the whole bone structure, not its mass, mineral content or density, that determines the bone's mechanical competence (Järvinen *et al.* 2005).

The exercise intervention trial among postmenopausal women by Adami *et al.* (1999) is a classic example underlining the importance of structural evaluation of bones with appropriate methods (Järvinen *et al.* 1999): no significant training effects were seen using the conventional BMD measurement, while the cortical area increased as a response to loading. In the present paper, we mainly focus on clinical evidence about changes in the bone structure as a response to increased mechanical loading.

Principles of skeletal adaptation to training

The type of mechanical loading (loading modality) is apparently the major modulator of the bone structure (Haapasalo *et al.* 2000; Heinonen *et al.* 2001, 2002; Kaptoge *et al.* 2003; Liu *et al.* 2003; Nikander *et al.* 2005). Skeletal adaptation to mechanical loading is a very slow process taking several months or years to result in measurable effects; degradation of originally competent bone structure is much faster than its improvement (Sievänen *et al.* 1996).

Skeletal adaptation to loading is affected by the magnitude of the strains within the bones, the strain rate, the strain distribution, and the number and frequency of repetitions (Borer 2005; Duncan & Turner 1995; Gross *et al.* 2004; Umemura *et al.* 2002). Turner (1998) has summarized the principles of bone adaptation to mechanical stimuli:

1 Bone adaptation is driven by dynamic, rather than static, loading;

2 Only a short duration of mechanical loading is necessary to initiate adaptive response, while extending the loading has a diminishing effect on further adaptation; and

3 Bone cells accommodate to customary loading environment, making them less responsive to routine loading stimuli.

Thus, to be effective, the duration of a single training session needs not be long. Rubin and Lanyon (1984) stated that only a few jumps or leaps per session, repeated more than once a day, would be an effective way for improving bone strength (Rubin & Lanyon 1984). Bone adaptation is indeed load- and time-dependent and the rest period between the loading sessions can modulate the osteogenic response (Turner *et al.* 2003; Umemura *et al.* 1997, 2002). The mechanosensivity of the loaded bone becomes virtually saturated after only 20 loading cycles, while a 4-h rest period between consecutive loading sessions can double the loading-induced bone formation; the initial mechanosensitivity returns after a 24-h non-loading period (Turner *et al.* 2003). Also, a great number of low magnitude strains at low rate, not believed to be osteogenic as such, may diminish the effect of a

single daily exposure to a highly osteogenic, high magnitude strain stimulus (Mosley 2000). It also seems obvious that dynamic loading is necessary for any skeletal adaptation, and particularly the unusual loading from exceptional directions seems to be more osteogenic than common loading from typical directions (Frost 2003; Turner 1991).

Intense exercise that includes impacts (i.e., jumps and leaps) has been shown to be effective for building a strong bone structure in the lower extremities (Haapasalo *et al.* 2000; Heinonen *et al.* 2001, 2002; Kaptoge *et al.* 2003; Liu *et al.* 2003; Nikander *et al.* 2005). Recently, the intense sports not involving very high impacts in vertical direction but rather the intense sports with small leaps and highly diverging accelerations or decelerations (odd-impact type of loading), especially from unusual directions, have been beneficially associated with mechanically

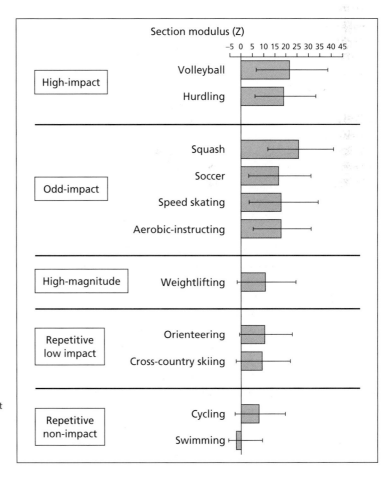

Fig. 2.23 The specific loading modality of sports is associated with the estimated bone strength or section modulus (Z) of the femoral neck. The bars represent the percentage benefits in bone strength among athletes representing different sports relative to non-athletic, but otherwise physically active persons. (Data adapted from the study of Nikander *et al.* 2005.)

competent bone structure (Faulkner *et al.* 2003; Liu *et al.* 2003; Nikander *et al.* 2005) – quite equally to the effects of high impact loading (Fig. 2.23). The apparent reason behind these observations pertains to the fact that the joint moments mediate the effect of sport-specific loading into the bone structure (Moisio *et al.* 2004). The joint moment represents the incident load (body weight together with loading-related reaction and muscle peak forces) multiplied by the lever arms of the skeleton. Because the muscle attachments are often close to the joints, the lever arms are bad in mechanical terms and very high muscle forces are thus needed for locomotion and other movements (Currey 2002). In other words, a similar jump from the same height causes a higher load for a heavier but equally tall person's hip, or conversely, a taller but lighter person can experience high loads at the hip.

At the upper extremities, the association between loading and strong bone structure has been best demonstrated in tennis studies (Haapasalo *et al.* 2000; Kontulainen *et al.* 2002). As the constant weight-bearing component is absent from the upper extremities, the muscle activity, in conjunction with the loading modality, becomes an important determinant of strong bone structure. For example, notwithstanding the fact that swimmers and tennis players load their bones in a very different fashion during the sports activity, these athletes can have almost equally strong bones in the region of humerus where strong shoulder muscles are attached (Nikander *et al.*, unpublished data, 2005). During the hit of the ball, the upper extremities of a tennis player must be able to cope with the very high momentary load (eccentric muscle work) because of the extended lever arm (the extremity and the racket together) and the heavy impact of the high velocity ball. A swimmer should only resist the drag of the water through coordinated and repeated, mostly concentric, muscle activity. Despite the virtually complete lack of eccentric muscle work, which is typical for bones in the lower extremities (e.g., during jumping), the strong humerus in swimmers pinpoints the significance of dynamic muscle activity as an important determinant of skeletal adaptation to training. In this context, it is also important to note that hip abductor muscle activity

is central in stabilizing postural balance and resisting compressive and bending forces, which affect the hip joint during exercise (Biewener 1989, 1991; Hawkins *et al.* 1999; Lovejoy 1988).

Recommendations for improving bone strength through exercise

In principle, the capacity of human skeleton to adapt to mechanical loading (i.e., physical training) is substantially different between childhood (the period of axial growth) and adulthood (Fig. 2.24). Training, already started before or at puberty, seems to be most effective for high accrual of bone mass and consequent strengthening of bone (Kannus *et al.* 1995). During young adulthood, training could continually be effective for bone structure, while during middle age, maintenance of mechanically competent bone structure would remain the main goal. The safety of training comes first at old age and therefore training that improves or maintains balance and coordination, as well as muscle force and power, is of primary importance. In old age, the direct training effect on bone structure may be limited (Karinkanta *et al.* 2005; Uusi-Rasi *et al.* 2002, 2003).

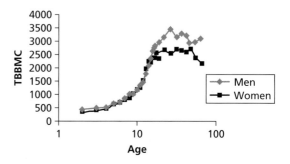

Fig. 2.24 Total body bone mineral content (TBBMC) accumulation from childhood to old age (in logaritmic scale). Data for children and adolescents are adapted from the study by Zanchetta *et al.* (1995) and the adult data from the study by Rico *et al.* (1994). Given the substantial accrual of bone mass, the childhood and young adulthood provide the most opportune time to build a mechanically competent bone structure, while middle age is mainly the time for maintaining the competence of bone structure. Old age represents chiefly the time for specific balance and strength training, while the direct effect of exercise on bone structure may be limited.

Childhood and particularly the growth spurt at puberty seem to be the right time for enhancing bone strength and laying the foundation for mechanically competent bones in later life. Adequate intake of calcium and vitamin D are the prerequisites for building strong bones. In childhood, the most effective training modes for strong bones seem to be sports that involve jumps, leaps, high accelerations, or decelerations through intense exercises. These activities not only benefit bones, but also improve a person's muscle performance and skills for various activities. Parents and professionals should encourage children and adolescents in intense exercise and sports, while keeping in mind the risk for injury. In this group, physical activity sessions should be carried out on a daily basis, according to general health recommendations.

The period of young adulthood, until 30–40 years of age, is good for further strengthening bones and muscles. As athletes have stronger bones than their non-athletic but otherwise physically active counterparts, the following sports can be recommended during young adulthood: soccer, tennis, squash, floorball, basketball, gymnastics, weight training, badminton, step aerobics, and other intense activities such as dancing (line dance, disco dance). However, the risk for injury can be relatively high in some of these sports, and this should be considered in exercise recommendations.

During middle age it is still possible to slightly improve or at least maintain bone mineral and competent bone structure (Uusi-Rasi et al. 1999). The above intense sports could be suitable for people over 50 years of age at somewhat reduced intensity, but previous inexperience of the specific sports and health-related factors such as previous joint injuries and problems should be taken into account in exercise prescription. The main goal of exercise, in addition to producing enjoyment, is to improve health without excess risks. As the risk for sports injury during intense exercise is usually higher than during moderately intense exercise, moderate intensity sports can be more appropriate for many middle-aged people. For example, many dancing activities can be beneficial to balance, coordination, and muscular performance, which all are important factors in preventing falls and related injuries (Kannus et al. 2005a).

At 65 years and over, many of the abovementioned sports such as modified tennis, gymnastics and dancing are still beneficial to many. Lightweight resistance training, walking, and water gymnastics may, in turn, be more suitable and enjoyable for people over 75 years. In old age, the main goal of exercise should concentrate on improving functional ability and quality of life – in addition to many other exercise-induced health benefits. For elderly and frail elderly people, safety should be a major issue when planning exercise sessions: regular health examinations, adequate lightning during exercise sessions, and proper clothing and footwear (hip protectors, slip protectors) can help in avoiding fall-related fractures and other injuries during indoor activities and slippery outdoor conditions (Kannus 1999; Kannus et al. 2000, 2005a,b; McKiernan 2005).

Adaptation of connective tissue to training

Research on the adaptive responses of connective tissue to training has been usually carried out with tendons and ligaments. Tendons and ligaments consist of collagen (mostly type I collagen) and elastin embedded in a proteoglycan–water matrix, with collagen accounting for 65–80% and elastin approximately 1–2% of the dry mass of the structure (Hess et al. 1989; Hooley et al. 1980; Jozsa et al. 1989; Kannus 2000; Tipton et al. 1967, 1970, 1975). These elements are produced by fibroblasts and fibrocytes that lie between the collagen fibers and are organized in a complex hierarchical scheme to form the tendon or ligament proper (Hess et al. 1989; Kannus 2000).

In tendons and ligaments, soluble tropocollagen molecules form cross-links to create insoluble collagen molecules, which then aggregate progressively in electronmicroscopically well-definable units: collagen fibrils. A bunch of fibrils forms a collagen fiber, which is the basic unit of a tendon and ligament. A fiber represents the smallest collagenous structure that can be seen by a light microscope, tested mechanically, and is aligned from end to end in these structures. A bunch of collagen fibers then forms a primary fiber bundle, followed by a

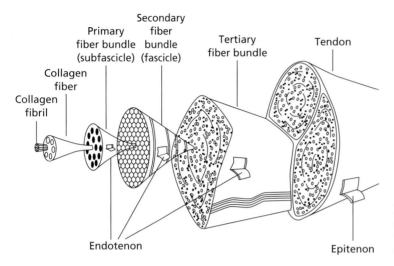

Fig. 2.25 The hierarchical organization of the structure of a tendon from collagen fibrils to the entire tendon.

secondary bundle, tertiary bundle, and finally the entire structure (Fig. 2.25).

Adaptation of a tendon to training

Compared with muscle tissue, the metabolic turnover of tendons is many times slower because of poorer vascularity and circulation (Barfred 1971; Kannus & Jozsa 1991). The adaptive responses to training are therefore also slower but may have great potential if the time-frame is long enough (Barfred 1971; Stanish *et al.* 1985). The same applies for ligamentous tissue (Kannus *et al.* 1992a).

Animal experiments

Inglemark (1945, 1948a,b) was one of the first researchers to study the effects of exercise on animal tendons. He observed that the cross-sectional area of the Achilles tendon grew up to 25% more in rabbits that ran up to 700 m daily on a fast-moving endless band between the ages of 6 and 37 weeks than in unexercised controls. Also, the wet weight and collagen fibril thickness of the tendons of the trained animals were higher. A more detailed study with mice confirmed this, and also revealed an increase in the concentration of nuclei in these hypertrophied tendons. Similar but smaller effects were seen in the tendons of mice trained when

adult. Inglemark (1948b) repeated the experiment with rats and found that training did not affect the water and nitrogen content, or the length of the tendon, and that whereas the increase in weight of the muscle was relatively greater than that of the tendon during normal growth, they remained proportional during exercise-induced hypertrophy.

Rollhäuser (1954) removed one Achilles tendon as a control from each of a number of adult guinea-pigs that were trained for 2–42 days. Although he observed no increase in the thickness of the remaining tendon and no histologic changes, its tensile strength increased up to 12% and the molecular organization of the collagen also improved. Rollhäuser concluded that tendons of growing animals may hypertrophy, whereas the only way for mature tendons to show a positive response is to improve the internal structure. Tittel and Otto (1970) made similar observations when training rats. Viidik (1967) exercised rabbits for 40 weeks and observed that the energy absorbed before failure and the ultimate load of the posterior tibial tendons were higher for trained than for untrained animals but the mass as well as water and collagen content of these tendons were not different. In other words, training was likely to improve the quality of the tendon tissue so that the stress–strain curve had moved upwards as a result of the training stimulus (Fig. 2.26).

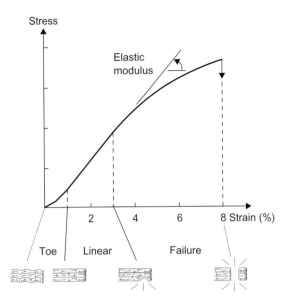

Fig. 2.26 The classic stress–strain curve of a tendon and ligament.

In later animal experiments, controlled, gradually increasing exercise has been shown to result in many positive structural and functional changes in tendons (Archambault *et al.* 1995; Buchanan & Marsh 2001; Curwin *et al.* 1988; Kiiskinen & Heikkinen 1973; Maffulli & King 1992; Michna 1984; See *et al.* 2004; Sommer 1987; Tipton *et al.* 1986; Vilarta & de Campos Vidal 1989; Woo *et al.* 1982; Zamora & Marini 1988). The changes can be explained by exercise-induced acceleration in the synthesis of collagen and proteoglycan matrix as a result of increased fibroblast–fibrocyte activity (Heikkinen & Vuori 1972; See *et al.* 2004; Tipton *et al.* 1970; Vailas *et al.* 1985; Zamora & Marini 1988). Microscopically, in loaded tendons the collagen fibrils and fibers seem to become thicker and their tropocollagen cross-links increase in number, although these observations are not entirely unequivocal (Magnusson *et al.* 2003). With loading, the three-dimensional orientation of tendon fibers becomes more parallel with the stress lines of the tendon (Jozsa 1984; Michna 1984, 1987; Michna & Hartmann 1989).

However, care must be taken in interpreting much of the animal exercise data on connective tissue strength (Stone 1991). Young trained animals are typically compared with untrained caged animals of the same age. Confinement-induced disuse and inactivity are likely to reduce connective tissue size and tensile strength, and therefore training may only return the tissue properties to unconfined values (Butler *et al.* 1978). Also, the strain rates used in many of these exercise studies have been below normal physiologic rates, making generalizations difficult. In addition, because age may be a confounding factor in evaluating the adaptation of the tendon to exercise, results on mature animals might be more applicable to humans (Archambault *et al.* 1995). In older individuals, the effects of long-term training on connective tissue may be related more to retardation of inactivity and aging-induced tissue atrophy and stiffening rather than actual improvements in tissue quality and quantity (Magnusson *et al.* 2003; Simonsen *et al.* 1995; Tuite *et al.* 1997).

Despite these limitations, animal experiments give reason to believe that the tensile strength, load to failure, elastic stiffness, total weight, cross-sectional area, and collagen content of tendons increase by gradually increasing physical exercise (Stone 1991; Tipton *et al.* 1975; Woo *et al.* 1982). In other words, physical training may alter the properties of tendons such that they are larger, stronger, and more resistant to injury. In growing animals, the response seems to be better than in their adult counterparts, although exercise appears to have a beneficial effect on the aging tendon too. However, if training is too strenuous, the sum effect may be harmful; that is, exercise-induced tendon cell apoptosis; inflammation and fiber damage; delayed and reduced collagen maturation; inhibition in collagen fibril cross-linking; and chronic overuse injury (Curwin *et al.* 1988; Kannus 1997; Kannus *et al.* 1992a; Scott *et al.* 2005).

Human studies

The effects of long-term exercise on human tendons have not been studied prospectively and systematically, as far as we know. The Achilles tendons of intensively trained athletes seem to be thicker (larger cross-sectional area) than those of controls, and this suggests that localized physiologic adaptation on loading and mechanical stresses may also occur in human tendons (Maffulli & King 1992; Magnusson *et al.* 2003). This tendon hypertrophy is likely to represent a biologic mechanism to diminish the mean stress imposed on the tendon. However, selection bias and suboptimal control of the potential confounding factors limit the conclusions of the cross-sectional human studies.

Although tendon tissue has been traditionally considered metabolically rather inactive, recent microdialysis studies have shown that human peritendinous tissue is actually metabolically active in response to physical activity (Kjaer *et al.* 2005; Langberg *et al.* 2001; Magnusson *et al.* 2003). An acute bout of exercise immediately reduces collagen synthesis followed by a dramatic rise in subsequent days. Also, chronic loading appears to increase the collagen synthesis (Kjaer *et al.* 2005; Langberg *et al.* 2001; Magnusson *et al.* 2003). An interstitial increase in the collagen synthesis-related growth factors has also been observed (Kjaer *et al.* 2005). All these findings are in line with the concept that human tendons can adapt reasonably to exercise.

Adaptation of a ligament to training

The internal structure of ligaments is very much the same as previously described in tendons, and therefore it is not surprising that the effects of training on ligamentous tissue are similar to those described for tendon tissue. In animal experiments, physical training has been shown to increase the tensile strength, elastic stiffness, and total weight of ligamentous tissue (Cabaud *et al.* 1980; Cornwall & LeVeau 1984; Gomez *et al.* 1991; Tipton *et al.* 1967, 1970, 1975, 1986; Viidik 1968; Zuckermann & Stull 1969) and improve the biomechanical properties of the osseous component of the ligament–bone junction (Laros *et al.* 1971; Tipton *et al.* 1975). However, we must keep in mind that, despite the strengthening effects of exercise on ligamentous tissue, the stability of the joint may not change because the length of the ligament may remain essentially the same

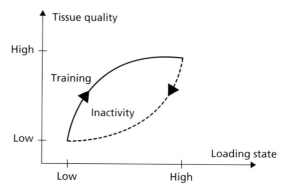

Fig. 2.27 The effects of training and inactivity on the quality of the tendon and ligament tissue.

(Cabaud *et al.* 1980; Kannus *et al.* 1992a). Also, after a ligament rupture and subsequent rehabilitation, the properties of ligament collagen fibers may be still deficient in content, quality, or orientation, and it is unknown if this matter is clinically important concerning the risk of rerupture during later activity (Frank *et al.* 1983; Kannus *et al.* 1992b).

Conclusions

Bones adapt well to mechanical loading. Versatile and relatively intense physical activity maximizes skeletal size, strength, and integrity during childhood and young adulthood, maintains these properties during adulthood, and can prevent aging-related bone fragility. Healthy adults can perform relatively vigorous weight-bearing physical activities until old age, but with increasing age the safety issues of exercise become important. Among elderly people, regular exercise is especially beneficial in preventing falling and consequent injuries (fractures).

Tendons and ligaments also show good ability to adapt to different states of loading and movement, provided that the time-frame for adaptation is sufficient and long enough – weeks, months, and years instead of days. Concerning training and physical activity, the lower the initial loading state, the faster and better the adaptation, and vice versa. For disuse and inactivity, the higher the initial loading state, the faster and more severe the tissue atrophy, and vice versa (Fig. 2.27).

References

Aagaard, P. (2003) Training-induced changes in neural function. *Exercise and Sports Science Reviews* **31**, 61–67.

Aagaard, P., Andersen, J.L., Dyhre-Poulsen, P., *et al.* (2001) A mechanism for increased contractile strength of human pennate muscle in response to strength training: changes in muscle architecture. *Journal of Physiology* **534**, 613–623.

Aagaard, P., Simonsen, E.B., Andersen, J.L., Magnusson, P. & Dyhre-Poulsen, P. (2002a) Increased rate of force development and neural drive of human skeletal muscle following resistance training. *Journal of Applied Physiology* **93**, 1318–1326.

Aagaard, P., Simonsen, E.B., Andersen, J.L., Magnusson, P. & Dyhre-Poulsen, P. (2002b) Neural adaptation to resistance training: changes in evoked V-wave and H-reflex responses. *Journal of Applied Physiology* **92**, 2309–2318.

Aagaard, P., Simonsen, E.B., Andersen, J.L., Magnusson, P., Halkjaer-Kristensen, J. & Dyhre-Poulsen, P. (2000) Neural inhibition during maximal eccentric and concentric quadriceps contraction: effects of resistance training. *Journal of Applied Physiology* **89**, 2249–2257.

Abe, T., Kumagai, K. & Brechue, W.F. (2000) Fascicle length of leg muscles is greater in sprinters than distance runners. *Medicine & Science in Sports and Exercise* **32**, 1125–1129.

Adami S., Gatti, D., Braga, V., Bianchini, D. & Rossini, M. (1999) Site-specific effects of strength training on bone structure and geometry of ultradistal radius in postmenopausal women. *Journal of Bone and Mineral Research* **14**, 120–124.

Adams, G.R., Harris, R.T., Woodard, D. & Dudley, G. (1993) Mapping of electrical muscle stimulation using MRI. *Journal of Applied Physiology* **74**, 532–537.

Adams, K.F. Jr, McAllister, S.M., El-Ashmawy, H., Atkinson, S., Koch, G. & Sheps, D.S. (1992) Interrelationships between left ventricular volume and output during exercise in healthy subjects. *Journal of Applied Physiology* **73**, 2097–2104.

Allemeier, C.A., Fry, A.C., Johnson, P., Hikida, R.S., Hagerman, F.C. & Staron, R.S. (1994) Effects of sprint cycle training on human skeletal muscle. *European Journal of Applied Physiology* **77**, 2385–2390.

Allen, D.G., Lee, J.A. & Westerblad, H. (1989) Intracellular calcium and tension during fatigue in isolated single muscle fibres from *Xenopus laevis*. *Journal of Physiology* **415**, 433–458.

Allen, D.G., Westerblad, H., Lee, J.A. & Lannergren, J. (1992) Role of excitation–contraction coupling in muscle fatigue. *Sports Medicine* **13**, 116–126.

Alway, S.E., Grumbt, W.H., Stray-Gundersen, J. & Gonyea, W.J. (1992) Effects of resistance training on elbow flexors of highly competitive bodybuilders. *Journal of Applied Physiology* **72**, 1512–1521.

Alway, S.E., MacDougall, J.D. & Sale, D.G. (1989) Contractile adaptations in the human triceps surae after isometric exercise. *Journal of Applied Physiology* **66**, 2725–2732.

Andersen, J.L. & Aagaard, P. (2000) Myosin heavy chain IIX overshoot in human skeletal muscle. *Muscle and Nerve* **23**: 1095–1104.

Andersen, P. & Henriksson, J. (1977) Training induced changes in the subgroups of human type II skeletal muscle fibres. *Acta Physiologica Scandinavica* **99**, 123–125.

Arbab-Zadeh, A., Dijk, E., Prasad, A., Fu, Q.T.P., Zhang, R., Thomas, J.D., *et al.* (2004) Effect of aging and physical activity on left ventricular compliance. *Circulation* **110**, 1799–1805.

Archambault, J.M., Wiley, J.P. & Bray, R.C. (1995) Exercise loading of tendons and the development of overuse injuries. *Sports Medicine* **20**, 77–89.

Armstrong, R.B., Warren, G.L. & Warren, J.A. (1991) Mechanisms of exercise-induced muscle fibre injury. *Sports Medicine* **12**, 184–207.

Babcock, M.A., Pegelow, D.F., Harms, C.A. & Dempsey, J.A. (2002) Effects of respiratory muscle unloading on exercise-induced diaphragm fatigue. *Journal of Applied Physiology* **93**, 201–206.

Babcock, M.A., Pegelow, D.F., McLaran, S.R., Suman, O.E. & Dempsey, J.A. (1995) Contribution of diaphragmatic power output to exercise-induced diaphragm fatigue. *Journal of Applied Physiology* **78**, 1710–1719.

Bailey, S.P., Davis, J.M. & Ahlborn, E.N. (1992) Effect of increased brain serotonergic activity on endurance performance in the rat. *Acta Physiologica Scandinavica* **145**, 75–76.

Bailey, S.P., Davis, J.M. & Ahlborn, E.N. (1993) Serotonergic agonists and antagonists affect endurance performance in the rat. *International Journal of Sports Medicine* **14**, 330–333.

Bandy, W.D. & Hanten, W.P. (1993) Changes in torque and electromyographic activity of the quadriceps femoris muscles following isometric training. *Physical Therapy* **73**, 455–467.

Barfred, T. (1971) Experimental rupture of the Achilles tendon.: comparison of various types of experimental rupture in rats. *Acta Orthopaedica Scandinavica* **42**, 528–543.

Barnard, H. (1898) The functions of the pericardium. Proceedings of the Physiological Society. *Journal of Physiology* **22**, 43–48.

Bassett, D.R. Jr. & Howley, E.T. (2000) Limiting factors for maximum oxygen uptake and determinants of endurance performance. *Medicine and Science in Sports and Exercise* **32**, 70–84.

Baudry, S. & Duchateau, J. (2004) Postactivation potentiation in human muscle is not related to the type of maximal conditioning contraction. *Muscle and Nerve* **30**, 328–336.

Belanger, A.Y. & McComas, A.J. (1981) Extent of motor unit activation during effort. *Journal of Applied Physiology* **51**, 381–393.

Bell, G.J., Petersen, S.R., Quinney, H.A. & Wenger, H.A. (1989) The effect of velocity-specific strength training on peak torque and anaerobic rowing power. *Journal of Sports Sciences* **7**, 205–214.

Below, P.R., Mora-Rodriguez, R., Gonzalez-Alonso, J. & Coyle, E.F. (1995) Fluid and carbohydrate ingestion independently improve performance during 1 h of intense exercise. *Medicine and Science in Sports and Exercise* **27**, 200–210.

Bergstrom, J., Hermansen, L., Hultman, E. & Saltin, B. (1967) Diet, muscle glycogen and physical performance. *Acta Physiologica Scandinavica* **71**, 140–150.

Bezanilla, F., Caputo, C., Gonzalez-Serratos, H. & Venosa, R.A. (1972) Sodium dependence of the inward spread of activation in isolated twitch muscle fibres of the frog. *Journal of Physiology* **223**, 507–523.

Biewener, A.A. (1989) Scaling body support in mammals: limb posture and muscle mechanics. *Science* **245**, 45–48.

Biewener, A.A. (1991) Musculoskeletal design in relation to body size. *Journal of Biomechanics* **24** (Supplement 1), 19–29.

Bigland-Ritchie, B., Furbush, F. & Woods, J.J. (1986) Fatigue of intermittent submaximal voluntary contractions: central and peripheral factors. *Journal of Applied Physiology* **61**, 421–429.

Bigland-Ritchie, B., Johansson, R., Lippold, O.C., Smith, S. & Woods, J.J. (1983) Changes in motoneurone firing rates during sustained maximal voluntary contractions. *Journal of Physiology* **340**, 335–346.

Bigland-Ritchie, B. & Woods, J.J. (1984) Changes in muscle contractile properties and neural control during human muscular fatigue. *Muscle & Nerve* **7**, 691–699.

Billat, V., Bernard, O., Pinoteau, J., Petit, B. & Koralsztein, J.P. (1994) Time to exhaustion at $\dot{V}o_{2max}$ and lactate steady state velocity in sub elite long-distance runners. *Archives Internationales de Physiologie, de Biochimie et de Biophysique* **102**, 215–219.

Biolo, G., Maggi S.P., Williams B.D., Tipton K.D. & Wolfe R.R. (1995) Increased rates of muscle protein turnover and amino acid transport after resistance exercise in humans. *American Journal of Physiology* **268**, E514–E520.

Biolo, G., Williams B.D., Fleming R.Y. & Wolfe R.R. (1999) Insulin action on muscle protein kinetics and amino acid transport during recovery after resistance exercise. *Diabetes* **48**, 949–957.

Blinks, J.R., Rudel, R. & Taylor, S.R. (1978) Calcium transients in isolated amphibian skeletal muscle fibres: detection with aequorin. *Journal of Physiology* **277**, 291–323.

Blomqvist, C.G. & Saltin, B. (1983) Cardiovascular adaptations to physical training. *Annual Reviews of Physiology* **45**, 169–189.

Blomqvist, G. (1991) Physiology and pathophysiology of exercise. In: *Cardiology: Physiology, Pharmacology, Diagnosis* (Parmeley, W.W. & Chatterjee, K., eds.) J.B. Lippincott, New York.

Blomstrand, E., Andersson, S., Hassmen, P., Ekblom, B. & Newsholme, E.A. (1995) Effect of branched-chain amino acid and carbohydrate supplementation on the exercise-induced change in plasma and muscle concentration of amino acids in human subjects. *Acta Physiologica Scandinavica* **153**, 87–96.

Blomstrand, E., Hassmen, P., Ekblom, B. & Newsholme, E.A. (1991) Administration of branched-chain amino acids during sustained exercise: effects on performance and on plasma concentration of some amino acids. *European Journal of Applied Physiology and Occupational Physiology* **63**, 83–88.

Blomstrand, E. & Newsholme, E.A. (1992) Effect of branched-chain amino acid supplementation on the exercise-induced change in aromatic amino acid concentration in human muscle. *Acta Physiologica Scandinavica* **146**, 293–298.

Bonde-Petersen, F., Knuttgen, H.G. & Henriksson, J. (1972) Muscle metabolism during exercise with concentric and eccentric contractions. *Journal of Applied Physiology* **33**, 792–795.

Borer, K.T. (2005) Physical activity in the prevention and amelioration of osteoporosis in women: interaction of mechanical, hormonal and dietary factors. *Sports Medicine* **35**, 779–830.

Boutellier, U., Buchel, R., Kundert, A. & Spengler, C. (1992) The respiratory system as an exercise limiting factor in normal trained subjects. *European Journal of Applied Physiology* **65**, 347–353.

Boutellier, U. & Piwko, P. (1992) The respiratory system as an exercise limiting factor in normal sedentary subjects. *European Journal of Applied Physiology* **64**, 145–152.

Brandt, P.W., Cox, R.N., Kawai, M. & Robinson, T. (1982) Regulation of tension in skinned muscle fibres. *Journal of General Physiology* **79**, 997–1016.

Brockett, C.L., Morgan, D.L. & Proske, U. (2001) Human hamstring muscles adapt to eccentric exercise by changing optimum length. *Medicine and Science in Sports and Exercise* **33**, 783–790.

Brooks, G.A., Fahey, T.D. & White, T.P. (1996) Fatigue during muscular exercise. In: *Exercise Physiology: Human Bioenergetics and Its Applications.* Mayfield Publishing, CA: 701–717.

Brotherhood, J., Brozovic, B. & Pugh, L.G. (1975) Haematological status of middle- and long-distance runners. *Clinical Science and Molecular Medicine* **48**, 139–145.

Buchanan, C.I. & Marsh, L. (2001) Effects of long-term exercise on the biomechanical properties of the Achilles tendon of guinea fowl. *Journal of Applied Physiology* **90**, 164–171.

Buick, F., Gledhill, N., Froese, A.B., Spriet, L. & Meyers, E.C. (1980) Effect of induced erythrocythemia on aerobic work capacity. *Journal of Applied Physiology* **48**, 636–642.

Butler, D.L., Grood, E.S., Noyes, F.R. & Zernicke, R.F. (1978) Biomechanics of ligaments and tendons. *Exercise and Sport Sciences Reviews* **6**, 125–181.

Byrd, S.K., McCutcheon, L.J., Hodgson, D.R. & Gollnick, P.D. (1989) Altered sarcoplasmic reticulum function after high-intensity exercise. *Journal of Applied Physiology* **67**, 2072–2077.

Byrne, C., Twist, C. & Eston, R. (2004) Neuromuscular function after exercise-induced muscle damage: theoretical and applied implications. *Sports Medicine* **34**, 49–69.

Bonen, A., Dyck, D.J., Ibrahimi, A. & Abumrad, N.A. (1999) Muscle contractile activity increases fatty acid metabolism and transport and FAT/CD36. *American Journal of Physiology, Endocrinology and Metabolism* **276**, E642–E649.

Booth, F.W. & Thomason, D.R. (1991) Molecular and cellular adaptation of muscle in response to exercise: perspectives of various models. *Physiological Reviews* **71**, 541–585.

Cabaud, H.E., Chatty, A., Gildengorin, V. & Feltman, R.J. (1980) Exercise effects on the strength of the rat anterior cruciate ligament. *American Journal of Sports Medicine* **8**, 79–86.

Campos, G.E., Luecke, T.J., Wendeln, H.K., et al. (2002) Muscular adaptations in response to three different resistance-training regimens: specificity of repetition maximum training zones. *European Journal of Applied Physiology* **88**, 50–60.

Cannon, R.J. & Cafarelli, E. (1987) Neuromuscular adaptations to training. *Journal of Applied Physiology* **63**, 2396–2402.

Carolan, B. & Cafarelli, E. (1992) Adaptations in coactivation after isometric resistance training. *Journal of Applied Physiology* **73**, 911–917.

Carroll, T.J., Riek, S. & Carson, R.G. (2002) The sites of neural adaptation induced by resistance training in humans. *Journal of Physiology* **544**, 641–652.

Carter, J.M., Jeukendrup, A.E. & Jones, D.A. (2004a) The effect of carbohydrate mouth rinse on 1-h cycle time trial performance. *Medicine and Science in Sports and Exercise* **36**, 2107–2111.

Carter, J.M., Jeukendrup, A.E., Mann, C.H. & Jones, D.A. (2004b) The effect of glucose infusion on glucose kinetics during a 1-h time trial: carbohydrate mouth rinse on 1-h cycle time trial performance. *Medicine and Science in Sports and Exercise* **36**, 1543–1550.

Casabona, A., Polizzi, M.C. & Perciavalle, V. (1990) Differences in H-reflex between athletes trained for explosive contractions and non-trained subjects.

European Journal of Applied Physiology **61**, 26–32.

Casaburi, R., Storer, T.W., Ben-Dov, I. & Wasserman, K. (1987a) Effect of endurance training on possible determinants of VO2 during heavy exercise. *Journal of Applied Physiology* **62**, 199–207.

Casaburi, R., Storer, T.W. & Wasserman, K. (1987b) Mediation of reduced ventilatory response to exercise after endurance training. *Journal of Applied Physiology* **63**, 1533–1538.

Cerretelli, P. & di Prampero, P.E. (1987) Gas exchange in exercise. In: *The Respiratory System IV. Handbook of Physiology*, Section 3. (Farhi, L.E. & Tenney, S.M., eds.) American Physiological Society, Bethesda, MD.

Chapman, R.F., Stray-Gundersen, J. & Levine, B.D. (1998) Individual variation in response to altitude training. *Journal of Applied Physiology* **85**, 1448–1456.

Chesley, A., MacDougall J.D., Tarnopolsky M.A., Atkinson S.A. & Smith K. (1992) Changes in human muscle protein synthesis after resistance exercise. *Journal of Applied Physiology* **73**, 1383–1388.

Cheung, K., Hume, P. & Maxwell, L. (2003) Delayed onset muscle soreness: treatment strategies and performance factors. *Sports Medicine* **33**, 145–164.

Chi, M.M., Hintz, C.S., Coyle, E.F., Martin, W.H. 3rd, Ivy, J.L., Nemeth, P.M., *et al.* (1983) Effects of detraining on enzymes of energy metabolism in individual human muscle fibres. *American Journal of Physiology* **244**, C276–C287.

Chilibeck, P.D., Syrotuik, D.G. & Bell, G.J. (2002) The effect of concurrent endurance and strength training on quantitative estimates of subsarcolemmal and intermyofibrillar mitochondria. *International Journal of Sports Medicine* **23**, 33–39.

Chin, E.R. & Allen, D.G. (1997) Effects of reduced muscle glycogen concentration on force, Ca^{2+} release and contractile protein function in intact mouse skeletal muscle. *Journal of Physiology* **498**, 17–29.

Christensen, E.H. & Hansen, O. (1939a) Hypoglykamie, arbeitsfahigkeit and Ermudung. *Skandinavische Archiv fur Physiologie* **81**, 172–179.

Christensen, E.H. & Hansen O (1939b) Respiratorscher quotient und O_2-aufnahme. *Scandinavian Archives of Physiology* **81**, 180–189.

Chiu, L.Z., Fry, A.C., Weiss, L.W., Schilling, B.K., Brown, L.E. & Smith S.L. (2003) Postactivation potentiation response in athletic and recreationally trained individuals. *Journal of Strength and Conditioning Research* **17**, 671–677.

Claassen, H., Gerber, C., Hoppeler, H., Luthi, J.M. & Vock, P. (1989) Muscle filament spacing and short-term heavy-resistance exercise in humans. *Journal of Physiology* **409**, 491–495.

Clanton, T.L., Dixon, G.F., Drake, J. & Gadek, J.E. (1987) Effects of swim training on lung volumes and inspiratory muscle conditioning. *Journal of Applied Physiology* **62**, 39–46.

Clarkson, P.M. & Hubal, M.J. (2002) Exercise-induced muscle damage in humans. *American Journal of Physical Medicine and Rehabilitation* **81**, S52–S69.

Clausen, J.P. (1976) Circulatory adjustments to dynamic exercise and effects of physical training in normal subjects and in patients with coronary artery disease. *Progress in Cardiovascular Disease* **18**, 480–481.

Clausen, J.P. (1977) Effect of physical training on cardiovascular adjustments to exercise in men. *Physiological Reviews* **57**, 779–810.

Close, R.I. (1972) Dynamic properties of mammalian skeletal muscles. *Physiological Reviews* **52**, 129–197.

Coast, J.R., Clifford, P.S., Henrich, T.W., Stray-Gundersen, J. & Johnson, R.L. Jr. (1990) Maximal inspiratory pressure following maximal exercise in trained and untrained subjects. *Medicine and Science in Sports and Exercise* **22**, 811–815.

Coggan, A.R., Kohrt, W.M., Spina, R.J., Bier, D.M. & Holloszy, J.O. (1990). Endurance training decreases plasma glucose turnover and oxidation during moderate-intensity exercise in men. *Journal of Applied Physiology* **68**, 990–996.

Coggan, A.R., Kohrt, W.M., Spina, R.J., Kirwan, J.P., Bier, D.M. & Holloszy, J.O. (1992). Plasma glucose kinetics during exercise in subjects with high and low lactate thresholds. *Journal of Applied Physiology* **73**, 1873–1880.

Coggan, A.R., Swanson, S.C., Mendenhall, L.A., Habash, D.L. & Kien, C.L. (1995) Effect of endurance training on hepatic glycogenolysis and gluconeogenesis during prolonged exercise in men. *American Journal of Physiology* **268**, E375–E383.

Coggan, A.R. & Williams, B.D. (1995) Metabolic adaptations to endurance training: substrate metabolism during exercise. In: *Exercise Metabolism* (Hargreaves, M., ed.) Human Kinetics, Champaign, IL: 177–210.

Coker, R.H. & Kjaer, M. (2005) Glucoregulation during exercise: the role of the neuroendocrine system. *Sports Medicine* **35**, 575–583.

Colson, S., Pousson, M., Martin, A. & Van Hoecke, J. (1999) Isokinetic elbow flexion and coactivation following eccentric training. *Journal of Electromyography and Kinesiology* **9**, 13–20.

Consitt, L.A., Copeland, J.L. & Tremblay, M.S. (2002) Endogenous anabolic hormone responses to endurance versus resistance exercise and training in women. *Sports Medicine* **32**, 1–22.

Constantini, N.W. & Warren, M.P. (1995) Menstrual dysfunction in swimmers: a distinct entity. *Journal of Clinical Endocrinology and Metabolism* **80**, 2740–2744.

Convertino, V.A. (1983) Heart rate and sweat rate response associated with exercise-induced hypervolemia. *Medicine and Science in Sports and Exercise* **15**, 77–82.

Convertino, V.A. (1991) Blood volume: its adaptation to endurance training. *Medicine and Science in Sports and Exercise* **23**, 1338–1348.

Convertino, V.A., Brock, P.J., Keil, L.C., Bernauer, E.M. & Greenleaf, J.E. (1980a) Exercise training-induced hypervolemia: role of plasma albumin, renin, and vasopressin. *Journal of Applied Physiology* **48**, 665–669.

Convertino, V.A., Greenleaf, J.E. & Bernauer, E.M. (1980b) Role of thermal and exercise factors in the mechanism of hypervolemia. *Journal of Applied Physiology* **48**, 657–664.

Convertino, V.A., Keil, L.C. & Greenleaf, J.E. (1983) Plasma volume, renin, and vasopressin responses to graded exercise after training. *Journal of Applied Physiology* **54**, 508–514.

Convertino, V.A., Mack, G.W. & Nadel, E.R. (1991) Elevated central venous pressure: a consequence of exercise training-induced hypervolemia. *American Journal of Physiology* **29**, R273–R277.

Cooke, R. & Pate, E. (1985) The effects of ADP and phosphate on the contraction of muscle fibers. *Biophysical Journal* **48**, 789–798.

Cornwall, M.W. & LeVeau, B.F. (1984) The effects of physical activity on ligamentous strength: an overview. *Journal of Sports Medicine* **5**, 275–277.

Costill, D.L., Fink, W.J., Getchell, L.H., Ivy, J.L. & Witzmann, F.A. (1979) Lipid metabolism in skeletal muscle of endurance-trained males and females.

Journal of Applied Physiology **47**, 787–791.

Costill, D.L., Fink, W.J. & Pollock, M.L. (1976) Muscle fiber composition and enzyme activities of elite distance runners. *Medicine and Science in Sports* **8**, 96–100.

Cornelissen, V.A. & Fagard, R.H. (2005) Effects of endurance training on blood pressure, blood pressure-regulating mechanisms, and cardiovascular risk factors. *Hypertension* **46**, 667–675.

Coyle, E.F. (1991) Carbohydrate metabolism and fatigue. In: *Muscle Fatigue: Biochemical and Physiological Aspects* (Atlan, G., Beliveua, L. & Bouissou, P., eds.) Masson, Paris: 153–164.

Coyle, E.F. (1998) Cardiovascular drift during prolonged exercise and the effects of dehydration. *International Journal of Sports Medicine* **19** (Supplement 2), S121–S124.

Coyle, E.F. (2005) Improved muscular efficiency displayed as Tour de France champion matures. *Journal of Applied Physiology* **98**, 2191–2196.

Coyle, E.F., Coggan, A.R., Hopper, M.K. & Walters, T.J. (1988) Determinants of endurance in well-trained cyclists. *Journal of Applied Physiology* **64**, 2622–2630.

Coyle, E.F. & Gonzalez-Alonso, J. (2001) Cardiovascular drift during prolonged exercise: new perspectives. *Exercise and Sport Sciences Reviews* **29**, 88–92.

Coyle, E.F., Hemmert, M.K. & Coggan, A.R. (1986) Effect of detraining on cardiovascular responses to exercise: role of blood volume. *Journal of Applied Physiology* **60**, 95–99.

Coyle, E.F., Spriet, L., Gregg, S. & Clarkson, P. (1994) Introduction to physiology and nutrition for competitive sport. In: *Perspectives in Exercise Science and Sports Medicine. Volume 7. Physiology and Nutrition for Competitive Sport* (Lamb, D.R., Knuttgen, H.G. & Murray, R., eds.) Cooper Publishing Group, Carmel, Indianapolis: xv–xxix.

Crawford, M.H., Petru, M.A. & Rabinowitz, C. (1985) Effect of isotonic exercise training on left ventricular volume during upright exercise. *Circulation* **72**, 1237–1243.

Crawford, M.H., White, D.H. & Amon, K.W. (1979) Echocardiographic evaluation of left ventricular size and performance during handgrip and supine and upright bicycle exercise. *Circulation* **59**, 1188–1196.

Currey, J.D. (2002) *Bones: Structure and Mechanics*. Princeton University Press.

Currey, J.D. (2003) How well are bones designed to resist fracture? *Journal of Bone and Mineral Research* **18**, 591–598.

Curwin, S., Vailas, A.C. & Wood, J. (1988) Immature tendon adaptation to strenuous exercise. *Journal of Applied Physiology* **65**, 2297–2301.

Daugaard, J.R., Nielsen, J.N., Kristiansen, S., Andersen, J.L., Hargreaves, M. & Richter, E.A. (2000) Fiber type-specific expression of GLUT4 in human skeletal muscle: influence of exercise training. *Diabetes* **49**, 1092–1095.

Davies, C.T. & White, M.J. (1982) Muscle weakness following dynamic exercise in humans. *Journal of Applied Physiology* **53**, 236–241.

Davies, C.T. & White, M.J. (1981) Muscle weakness following eccentric work in man. *Pflugers Archiv* **392**, 168–171.

Davis, J.M. & Bailey, S.P. (1997) Possible mechanisms of central nervous system fatigue during exercise. *Medicine and Science in Sports and Exercise* **29**, 45–57.

Davis, J.M., Bailey, S.P., Jackson, D.A., Strasner, A.B. & Morehouse, S.L. (1995) Effects of a serotonin (5-HT) agonist during prolonged exercise to fatigue in humans. *Medicine and Science in Sports and Exercise* **25**, S78.

Davis, J.M., Bailey, S.P., Woods, J.A., Galiano, F.J., Hamilton, M.T. & Bartoli, W.P. (1992) Effects of carbohydrate feedings on plasma free tryptophan and branched-chain amino acids during prolonged cycling. *European Journal of Applied Physiology* **65**, 513–519.

Dawson, E., George, K., Shave, R., Whyte, G. & Ball, D. (2003) Does the human heart fatigue subsequent to prolonged exercise? *Sports Medicine* **33**, 365–380.

Dawson, E.A., Shave, R., George, K., Whyte, G., Ball, D., Gaze, D, et al. (2005) Cardiac drift during prolonged exercise with echocardiographic evidence of reduced diastolic function of the heart. *European Journal of Applied Physiology* **94**, 305–309.

DeLuca, C.J., LeFever, R.S., McCue, M.P. & Xenakis, A.P. (1982) Behaviour of human motor units in different muscles during linearly varying contractions. *Journal of Physiology* **329**, 113–128.

Demaria, A.N., Neumann, A., Lee, G., Fowler, W. & Mason, D.T. (1978) Alterations in ventricular mass and performance induced by exercise training in man evaluated by echocardiography. *Circulation* **57**, 237–244.

Dempsey, J.A. (1986) J.B. Wolffe memorial lecture. Is the lung built for exercise? *Medicine and Science in Sports and Exercise* **18**, 143–155.

Dempsey, J.A., Forster, H.V. & Ainsworth, D.M. (1995) Regulation of hyperpnea, hyperventilation, and respiratory muscle recruitment during exercise. In: *Regulation of Breathing* (Dempsey, J.A. & Pack, A.I., eds.) Marcel Dekker, New York, pp. 1065–134.

Dempsey, J.A., Hanson, P.G. & Henderson, K.S. (1984) Exercise-induced arterial hypoxaemia in healthy human subjects at sea level. *Journal of Physiology (London)* **355**, 161–175.

Dempsey, J.A. & Wagner, P.D. (1999) Exercise-induced arterial hypoxemia. *Journal of Applied Physiology* **87**, 1997–2006.

Deschenes, M.R., Judelson, D.A., Kraemer, W.J., Meskaitis, V.J., Volek, J.S., Nindl, B.C., et al. (2000) Effects of resistance training on neuromuscular junction morphology. *Muscle and Nerve* **23**, 1576–1581.

Deschenes, M.R. & Kraemer, W.J. (2002) Performance and physiologic adaptations to resistance training. *American Journal of Physical Medicine and Rehabilitation* **81**, S3–16.

Deschenes, M.R., Maresh, C.M., Crivello, J.F., Armstrong, L.E., Kraemer, W.J. & Covault, J. (1993) The effects of exercise training of different intensities on neuromuscular junction morphology. *Journal of Neurocytology* **22**, 603–615.

Dettmers, C., Ridding, M.C., Stephan, K.M., et al. (1996) Comparison of regional cerebral blood flow with transcranial magnetic stimulation at different forces. *Journal of Applied Physiology* **81**, 596–603.

Dill, D.B., Edwards, R.G. & Talbott, J.H. (1932) Factors limiting the capacity for work. *Journal of Physiology (London)* **77**, 49–62.

di Prampero, P.E. (1985) Metabolic and circulatory limitations to VO_{2max} at the whole animal level. *Journal of Experimental Biology* **115**, 319–331.

Douglas, P.S., O'Toole, M.L., Hiller, W.D., Hackney, K. & Reichek, N. (1987) Cardiac fatigue after prolonged exercise. *Circulation* **76**, 1206–1213.

Dudley, G.A., Tesch, P.A., Miller, B.J. & Buchanan, M.D. (1991) Importance of eccentric actions in performance adaptations to resistance training. *Aviation and Space Environmental Medicine* **62**, 543–550.

Duncan, R.L. & Turner, C.H. (1995) Mechanotransduction and the functional response of bone to mechanical strain. *Calcified Tissue International* **57**, 344–358.

Earles, D.R., Dierking, J.T., Robertson, C.T. & Koceja, D.M. (2002) Pre- and post-synaptic control of motoneuron excitability in athletes. *Medicine and Science in Sports and Exercise* **34**, 1766–1772.

Edwards, R.H., Dawson, M.J., Wilkie, D.R., Gordon, R.E. & Shaw, D. (1982) Clinical use of nuclear magnetic resonance in the investigation of myopathy. *Lancet* **1**, 725–731.

Edwards, R.H., Hill, D.K., Jones, D.A. & Merton, P.A. (1977) Fatigue of long duration in human skeletal muscle after exercise. *Journal of Physiology* **272**, 769–778.

Edwards, R.H. & Wiles, C.M. (1981) Energy exchange in human skeletal muscle during isometric contraction. *Circulation Research* **48**, I11–17.

Edwards, R.H.T. (1983) *Biochemical Basis of Fatigue in Exercise Performance*. Human Kinetics, Champaign, IL: 3–28.

Ehsani, A.A., Hagberg, J.M. & Hickson, R.C. (1978) Rapid changes in left ventricular dimensions and mass in response to physical conditioning and deconditioning. *American Journal of Cardiology* **42**, 52–56.

Ehsani, A.A., Ogawa, T., Miller, T.R., Spina, R.J. & Jilka, S.M. (1991) Exercise training improves left ventricular systolic function in older men. *Circulation* **83**, 96–103.

Ekblom, B. & Hemnasen, L. (1968) Cardiac output in athletes. *Journal of Applied Physiology* **25**, 615–625.

Ekblom, B., Astrand, P.O., Saltin, B., Stenberg, T. & Wallstrom, B. (1968) Effect of training on circulatory response to exercise. *Journal of Applied Physiology* **24**, 518–528.

Enoka, R.M. (1997) Neural adaptations with chronic physical activity. *Journal of Biomechanics* **30**, 447–455.

Esch, B.T.A., Bredin, S.S.D., Haykowsky, M.J., Scott, J.M. & Warburton, D.E.R. (2007) The effects of the pericardium on the cardiac function of endurance-trained athletes under conditions of physiological stress. *Applied Physiology, Nutrition and Metabolism*.

Essen-Gustavsson, B. & Tesch, P.A. (1990) Glycogen and triglyceride utilization in relation to muscle metabolic characteristics in men performing heavy-resistance exercise. *European Journal of Applied Physiology, Occupational Physiology* **61**, 5–10.

Fagard, R.H., Van Den Broeke, C., VanHees, L., Staessen, J. & Amery, A. (1987) Noninvasive assessment of systolic and diastolic left ventricular function in female runners. *European Heart Journal* **8**, 1305–1311.

Fairbarn, M.S., Coutts, K.C., Pardy, R.L. & McKenzie, D.C. (1991) Improved respiratory muscle endurance of highly trained cyclists and the effects on maximal exercise performance. *International Journal of Sports Medicine* **12**, 66–70.

Faulkner, R.A., Forwood, M.R., Beck, T.J., Mafukidze, J.C., Russell, K. & Wallace, W. (2003) Strength indices of the proximal femur and shaft in prepubertal female gymnasts. *Medicine and Science in Sports and Exercise* **35**, 513–518.

Febbraio, M.A. & Pedersen, B.K. (2002) Muscle-derived interleukin-6: mechanisms for activation and possible biological roles. *FASEB J* **16**(11), 1335–47.

Felici, F., Rosponi, A., Sbriccoli, P., Filligoi, C., Fattorini, L. & Marchetti, M. (2001) Linear and non-linear analysis of surface electromyograms in weightlifters. *European Journal of Applied Physiology* **84**, 337–342.

Fitts, R.H. (1994) Cellular mechanisms of muscle fatigue. *Physiological Reviews* **74**, 49–94.

Fitts, R.H. & Holloszy, J.O. (1978) Effects of fatigue and recovery on contractile properties of frog muscle. *Journal of Applied Physiology* **45**, 899–902.

Fortney, S.M., Nadel, E.R., Wenger, C.B. & Bove, J.R. (1981) Effect of acute alterations of blood volume on circulatory performance in humans. *Journal of Applied Physiology: Respiratory, Environmental Exercise Physiology* **50**, 292–298.

Freeman, G.L. & Lewinter, M.M. (1984) Pericardial adaptations during chronic cardiac dilation in dogs. *Circulation Research* **54**, 294–300.

French, D.N., Kraemer, W.J. & Cooke, C.B. (2003) Changes in dynamic exercise performance following a sequence of preconditioning isometric muscle actions. *Journal of Strength and Conditioning Research* **17**, 678–685.

Frick, M., Elovinic, R. & Somer, T. (1967) The mechanism of bradycardia evoked by physical training. *Cardiologia* **51**, 46–54.

Friedmann, B. & Bartsch, P. (1997) High altitude training: sense, nonsense, trends. *Orthopade* **26**, 987–992.

Fry, A.C., Allemeier, C.A. & Staron, R.S. (1994) Correlation between percentage fiber type area and myosin heavy chain content in human skeletal muscle. *European Journal of Applied Physiology* **68**, 246–251.

Frank, C., Woo, S.L., Amiel, D., Harwood, F., Gomez, M. & Akeson, W. (1983) Medial collateral ligament healing. A multidisciplinary assessment in rabbits. *American Journal of Sports Medicine* **11**, 379–389.

Frost, H.M. (2003) Bone's mechanostat: a 2003 update. *Anatomical Record* **275A**, 1081–1101.

Gandevia, S.C. (2001) Spinal and supraspinal factors in human muscle fatigue. *Physiological Reviews* **81**, 1725–1789.

Garcia, M.C., Gonzalez-Serratos, H., Morgan, J.P., Perreault, C.L. & Rozycka, M. (1991) Differential activation of myofibrils during fatigue in phasic skeletal muscle cells. *Journal of Muscle Research and Cell Motility* **12**, 412–424.

George, K.P., Wolfe, L.A. & Burggraf, G.W. (1991) The athletic heart syndrome: a critical review. *Sports Medicine* **11**, 300–331.

Gibson, H. & Edwards, R.H. (1985) Muscular exercise and fatigue. *Sports Medicine* **2**, 120–132.

Gillen, C.M., Lee, R., Mack, G.W., Tomarelli, C.M., Nishiyasu, T. & Nadel, E.R. (1991) Plasma volume expansion in humans after a single intense exercise protocol. *Journal of Applied Physiology* **71**, 1914–1920.

Gillen, C.M., Nishiyasu, T., Langhans, G., Weseman, C., Mack, G.W. & Nadel, E.R. (1994) Cardiovascular and renal function during exercise-induced blood volume expansion in men. *Journal of Applied Physiology* **76**, 2602–2610.

Ginzton, L.E., Conant, R., Brizendine, M. & Laks, M.M. (1989) Effect of long term high intensity aerobic training on left ventricular volume during maximal upright exercise. *Journal of the American College of Cardiology* **14**, 364–371.

Glass, D.J. (2003) Signaling pathways that mediate skeletal muscle hypertrophy and atrophy. *Nature Cell Biology* **5**, 87–90.

Gledhill, N. (1982) Blood doping and related issues: a brief review. *Medicine and Science in Sports and Exercise* **14**, 183–189.

Gledhill, N. (1992) Hemoglobin, blood volume and endurance. In: *Endurance in Sport* (Shephard, R. & Astrand, P.O., eds.) Blackwell Scientific Publications, Oxford.

Gledhill, N., Cox, D. & Jamnik, R. (1994) Endurance athletes' stroke volume does not plateau: major advantage is diastolic function. *Medicine and Science in Sports and Exercise* **26**, 1116–1121.

Gledhill, N. & Warburton, D.E.R. (2000) Hemoglobin, blood volume and endurance. In: *Endurance in Sport* (Shephard, R.J. & Astrand, P.O., eds.) Blackwell Scientific Publications, Oxford.

Gledhill, N., Warburton, D. & Jamnik, V. (1999) Haemoglobin, blood volume, cardiac function, and aerobic power. *Canadian Journal of Applied Physiology* **24**, 54–65.

Godt, R.E. & Nosek, T.M. (1989) Changes of intracellular milieu with fatigue or hypoxia depress contraction of skinned rabbit skeletal and cardiac muscle. *Journal of Physiology* **412**, 155–180.

Goldspink, G. & Yang, S.Y. (2001) Effects of activity on growth factor expression. *International Journal of Sports Nutrition and Exercise Metabolism* **11**, S21–S27.

Gollnick, P.D., Armstrong, R.B., Saltin, B., Saubert, C.W., Sembrowich, W.L. & Shepherd, R.E. (1973). Effect of training on enzyme activity and fiber composition of human skeletal muscle. *Journal of Applied Physiology* **34**, 107–111.

Gomez, M.A., Woo, S.Y., Amiel, D., Harwood, F., Kitabayashi, L. & Matys, J.R. (1991) The effects of increased tension on healing medial collateral ligaments. *American Journal of Sports Medicine* **19**, 347–354.

Goodman, J.M., Liu, P.P. & Green, H.J. (2005) Left ventricular adaptations following short-term endurance training. *Journal of Applied Physiology* **98**, 454–460.

Gonyea, W.J. (1980) Role of exercise in inducing increases in skeletal muscle fiber number. *Journal of Applied Physiology* **48**, 421–426.

Gonyea, W., Ericson, G.C. & Bonde-Peterson, F. (1977) Skeletal muscle fiber splitting induced by weight lifting exercise in cats. *Acta Physiologica Scandinavica* **99**, 105–109.

Gonyea, W.J., Sale, D., Gonyea, Y. & Mikesky, A. (1986) Exercise induced increases in muscle fiber number. *European Journal of Applied Physiology* **55**, 137–141.

Gorassini, M., Yang, J.F., Siu, M. & Bennett, D.J. (2002) Intrinsic activation of human motor units: reduction of motor unit recruitment thresholds by repeated contractions. *Journal of Neurophysiology* **87**, 1859–1866.

Gore, C.J. & Hopkins, W.G. (2005) Counterpoint: positive effects of intermittent hypoxia (live high:train low) on exercise performance are not mediated primarily by augmented red cell volume. *Journal of Applied Physiology* **99**, 2055–2057; discussion 2057–2058.

Gossen, E.R. & Sale, D.G. (2000) Effect of postactivation potentiation on dynamic knee extension performance. *European Journal of Applied Physiology* **83**, 524–530.

Grabowski, W., Lobsiger, E.A. & Luttgau, H.C. (1972) The effect of repetitive stimulation at low frequencies upon the electrical and mechanical activity of single muscle fibres. *Pflugers Archiv* **334**, 222–239.

Green, H., Dahly, A., Shoemaker, K., Goreham, C., Bombardier, E. & Ball-Burnett, M. (1999) Serial effects of high-resistance and prolonged endurance training on Na+–K+ pump concentration and enzymatic activities in human vastus lateralis. *Acta Physiologica Scandinavica* **165**, 177–184.

Green, H., Goreham, C., Ouyang, J., Ball-Burnett, M. & Ranney, D. (1999) Regulation of fiber size, oxidative potential, and capillarization in human muscle by resistance exercise. *American Journal of Physiology* **276**, R591–R596.

Green, H.J. (1990) Manifestations and sites of neuromuscular fatigue. In: *Biochemistry of Exercise VII*. Taylor, A.W., Green, H.J., Ianuzzo, D. & Sutton J.R. (eds.) Human Kinetics, Champaign, IL, pp. 13–25.

Green, H.J. (1997) Mechanisms of muscle fatigue in intense exercise. *Journal of Sports Sciences* **15**, 247–256.

Green, H.J., Ballantyne, C.S., MacDougall, J.D., Tarnopolsky, M.A. & Schertzer, J.D. (2003) Adaptations in human muscle sarcoplasmic reticulum to prolonged submaximal training. *Journal of Applied Physiology* **94**, 2034–2042.

Green, H.J., Barr, D.J., Fowles, J.R., Sandiford, S.D., & Ouyang, J. (2004) Malleability of human skeletal muscle Na+-K+-ATPase pump with short-term training. *Journal of Applied Physiology* **97**, 143–148.

Green, H.J., Grange, F., Chin, C., Goreham, C. & Ranney, D. (1998) Exercise-induced decreases in sarcoplasmic reticulum Ca^{2+}-ATPase activity attenuated by high-resistance training. *Acta Physiologica Scandinavica* **164**, 141–146.

Green, H.J., Jones, L.L. & Painter, D.C. (1990) Effects of short-term training on cardiac function during prolonged exercise. *Medicine and Science in Sports and Exercise* **22**, 488–493.

Grimby, L., Hannerz, J. & Hedman, B. (1981) The fatigue and voluntary discharge properties of single motor units in man. *Journal of Physiology* **316**, 545–554.

Gross, T.S., Poliachik, S.L., Ausk, B.J., Sanford, D.A., Becker, B.A. & Srinivasan, S. (2004) Why rest stimulates bone formation: a hypothesis based on complex adaptive phenomenon. *Exercise and Sport Sciences Reviews* **32**, 9–13.

Gyorke, S. (1993) Effects of repeated tetanic stimulation on excitation–contraction coupling in cut muscle fibres of the frog. *Journal of Physiology* **464**, 699–710.

Haapasalo, H., Kontulainen, S., Sievänen, H., Kannus, P., Järvinen, M. & Vuori, I. (2000) Exercise-induced bone gain is due to enlargement in bone size without a change in volumetric bone density: a peripheral quantitative computed tomography study of the upper arms of male tennis players. *Bone* **27**, 351–357.

Hackney, A.C. (1998) Testosterone and reproductive dysfunction in endurance-trained men. In: *Encyclopedia of Sports Medicine and Science* (Fahey, T.D., ed.) Internet Society for Sport Science: http://sportsci.org. 20 Sept 1998.

Hagberg, J.M., Goldberg, A.P., Lakatta, L., O'Connor, F.C., Becker, L.C., Lakatta, E.G., *et al.* (1998) Expanded blood volumes contribute to the increased cardiovascular performance of endurance-trained older men. *Journal of Applied Physiology* **85**, 484–9.

Häkkinen, K., Alen, M. & Komi, P.V. (1985a) Changes in isometric force- and relaxation–time, electromyographic and muscle fibre characteristics of human skeletal muscle during strength training and detraining. *Acta Physiologica Scandinavica* **125**, 573–585.

Hakkinen, K., Alen, M., Kraemer, W.J., Gorostiaga, E., Izquierdo, M., Rusko, H., *et al.* (2003) Neuromuscular adaptations during concurrent strength and endurance training versus strength training. *European Journal of Applied Physiology* **89**, 42–52.

Häkkinen, K., Kallinen, M., Izquierdo, M., Jokelainen, K., Lassila, H., Malkia, E., *et al.* (1998a) Changes in agonist–antagonist EMG, muscle CSA, and force during strength training in middle-aged and older people. *Journal of Applied Physiology* **84**, 1341–1349.

Häkkinen, K., Kallinen, M., Komi, P.V. & Kauhanen, H. (1991) Neuromuscular adaptations during short-term "normal" and reduced training periods in strength athletes. *Electromyography and Clinical Neurophysiology* **31**, 35–42.

Häkkinen, K., Kallinen, M., Linnamo, V., Pastinen, U.M., Newton, R.U. & Kraemer, W.J. (1996) Neuromuscular adaptations during bilateral versus unilateral strength training in middle-aged and elderly men and women. *Acta Physiologica Scandinavica* **158**, 77–88.

Häkkinen, K. & Kauhanen, H. (1989) Daily changes in neural activation, force–time and relaxation–time characteristics in athletes during very intense training for one week. *Electromyography and Clinical Neurophysiology* **29**, 243–249.

Häkkinen, K. & Komi, P.V. (1983) Electromyographic changes during strength training and detraining. *Medicine and Science in Sports and Exercise* **15**, 455–460.

Häkkinen, K. & Komi, P.V. (1986) Training-induced changes in neuromuscular performance under voluntary and reflex conditions. *European Journal of Applied Physiology* **55**, 147–155.

Häkkinen, K., Komi, P.V. & Alen, M. (1985b) Effect of explosive type strength training on isometric force- and relaxation-time, electromyographic and muscle fibre characteristics of leg extensor muscles. *Acta Physiologica Scandinavica* **125**, 587–600.

Häkkinen, K., Komi, P.V., Alen, M. & Kauhanen, H. (1987) EMG, muscle fibre and force production characteristics during a 1 year training period in elite weight-lifters. *European Journal of Applied Physiology* **56**, 419–427.

Häkkinen, K., Komi, P.V. & Tesch, P.A. (1981) Effect of combined concentric and eccentric strength training and detraining on force-time, muscle fiber and metabolic characteristics of leg extensor muscles. *Scandinavian Journal of Sports Science* **3**, 50–58.

Häkkinen, K., Kraemer, W.J., Newton, R.U. & Alen, M. (2001) Changes in electromyographic activity, muscle fibre and force production characteristics during heavy resistance/power strength training in middle-aged and older men and women. *Acta Physiologica Scandinavica* **171**, 51–62.

Häkkinen, K., Newton, R.U., Gordon, S., McCormick, M., Volek, J., Nindl, B., *et al.* (1998b) Changes in muscle morphology, electromyographic activity, and force production characteristics during progressive strength training in young and older men. *Journal of Gerontology: Biological Sciences* **53A**, B415–B423.

Hamada, T., Sale, D.G. & MacDougall, J.D. (2000b) Postactivation potentiation in endurance-trained male athletes. *Medicine and Science in Sports and Exercise* **32**, 403–411.

Hamada, T., Sale, D.G., MacDougall, J.D. & Tarnopolsky, M.A. (2000a) Postactivation potentiation, fiber type, and twitch contraction time in human knee extensor muscles. *Journal of Applied Physiology* **88**, 2131–2137.

Hamada, T., Sale, D.G., MacDougall, J.D. & Tarnopolsky, M.A. (2003) Interaction of fibre type, potentiation and fatigue in human knee extensor muscles. *Acta Physiologica Scandinavica* **178**, 165–173.

Hameed, M., Lange, K.H., Andersen, J.L., Schjerling, P., Kjaer, M., Harridge, S.D., *et al.* (2004) The effect of recombinant human growth hormone and resistance training on IGF-I mRNA expression in the muscles of elderly men. *Journal of Physiology* **555**, 231–240.

Hammond, H.K., White, F.C., Bharga V.V. & Shabetai, R. (1992) Heart size and maximal cardiac output are limited by the pericardium. *American Journal of Physiology* **263**, H1675–H1681.

Hampson, D.B., St. Clair Gibson, A., Lambert, M.I. & Noakes, T.D. (2001) The influence of sensory cues on the perception of exertion during exercise and central regulation of exercise performance. *Sports Medicine* **31**, 935–952.

Hanel, B. & Secher, N.H. (1991) Maximal oxygen uptake and work capacity after inspiratory muscle training: a controlled study. *Journal of Sports Sciences* **9**, 43–52.

Hansen, A.K., Fischer, C.P., Plomgaard, P., Andersen, J.L., Saltin, B. & Pedersen, B.K. (2005) Skeletal muscle adaptation: training twice every second day vs. training once daily. *Journal of Applied Physiology* **98**, 93–99.

Harber, M.P., Fry, A.C., Rubin, M.R., Smith, J.C. & Weiss, L.W. (2004) Skeletal muscle and hormonal adaptations to circuit weight training in untrained men. *Scandinavian Journal of Medicine and Science in Sports* **14**, 176–185.

Hargreaves, M., Costill, D.L., Coggan, A., Fink, W.J. & Nishibata, I. (1984) Effect of carbohydrate feedings on muscle glycogen utilization and exercise performance. *Medicine and Science in Sports and Exercise* **16**, 219–222.

Harms, C.A., McClaran, S.R., Nickele, G.A., Pegelow, D.F., Nelson, W.B. & Dempsey, J.A. (1998a) Exercise-induced arterial hypoxaemia in healthy young women. *Journal of Physiology (London)* **507**, 619–628.

Harms, C.A., McClaran, S.R., Nickele, G.A., Pegelow, D.F., Nelson, W.B. & Dempsey, J.A. (2000) Effect of exercise-induced arterial O_2 desaturation on $\dot{V}O_{2max}$ in women. *Medicine and Science in Sports and Exercise* **32**, 1101–1108.

Harms, C.A., Wetter, T.J., McClaran, S.R., Pegelow, D.F., Nickele, G.A., Nelson, W.B., *et al.* (1998b) Effects of respiratory muscle work on cardiac output and its distribution during maximal exercise. *Journal of Applied Physiology* **85**, 609–618.

Harris, R.C., Edwards, R.H., Hultman, E., Nordesjo, L.O., Nylind, B. & Sahlin, K. (1976) The time course of phosphorylcreatine resynthesis during recovery of the quadriceps muscle in man. *Pflugers Archiv* **367**, 137–142.

Hartley, L., Girmsby, G., Kilbom, A., Nilson, N., Astrand, I., Ekblom, B., *et al.* (1969) Physical training in sedentary-middle-aged and older men III:Cardiac output and gas exchange at submaximal and maximal exercise. *Scandinavian Journal of Clinical Laboratory Investigation* **24**, 335–344.

Hather, B.M., Tesch, P.A., Buchanan, P. & Dudley, G.A. (1991) Influence of eccentric actions on skeletal muscle adaptations to resistance training. *Acta Physiologica Scandinavica* **143**, 177–185.

Hawkins, S.A., Schroeder, E.T., Wiswell, R.A., Jaque, S.V., Marcell, T.J. & Costa, K. (1999) Eccentric muscle action increases site-specific osteogenic response. *Medicine and Science in Sports and Exercise* **31**, 1287–1292.

Hawley, J.A. (2002) Adaptations of skeletal muscle to prolonged, intense endurance training. *Clinical Experimental Pharmacology and Physiology* **29**, 218–222.

Hawley, J.A. & Stepto, N.K. (2001) Adaptations to training in endurance cyclists: implications for performance. *Sports Medicine* **31**, 511–520.

Hawley, J.A., Tipton, K.D. & Millard-Stafford, M.L. (2006) Promoting training adaptations through nutritional interventions. *Journal of Sports Sciences* **24**, 1–13.

Haykowsky, M., Welsh, R., Humen, D., Warburton, D. & Taylor, D. (2001) Impaired left ventricular systolic function after a half-ironman race. *Canadian Journal of Cardiology* **17**, 687–690.

Heikkinen, E. & Vuori, I. (1972) Effect of physical activity on the metabolism of collagen in aged mice. *Acta Physiologica Scandinavica* **84**, 543–549.

Heinonen, A., Sievänen, H., Kyröläinen, H., Perttunen, J. & Kannus, P. (2001) Mineral mass, size, and estimated mechanical strength of triple jumpers' lower limb. *Bone* **29**, 279–285.

Heinonen, A., Sievanen, H., Kannus, P., Oja, P. & Vuori, I. (2002) Site-specific skeletal response to long-term weight training seems to be attributable to principal loading modality: a pQCT study of female weightlifters. *Calcified Tissue International* **70**, 469–474.

Hellsten, Y., Frandsen, U., Orthenblad, N., Sjodin, B. & Richter, E.A. (1997) Xanthine oxidase in human skeletal muscle following eccentric exercise: a role in inflammation. *Journal of Physiology* **498**, 239–248.

Henneman, E., Somjen, G. & Carpenter, D.O. (1965) Excitability and inhibitability of motoneurons of different sizes. *Journal of Neurophysiology* **28**, 599–620.

Henriksson, J. (1977) Training induced adaptation of skeletal muscle and metabolism during submaximal exercise. *Journal of Physiology* **270**, 661–675.

Henriksson, J. & Reitman, J.S. (1977) Time course of changes in human skeletal muscle succinate dehydrogenase and cytochrome oxidase activities and maximal oxygen uptake with physical activity and inactivity. *Acta Physiologica Scandanavica* **99**, 91–97.

Hermansen, L., Hultman, E. & Saltin, B. (1967) Muscle glycogen during prolonged severe exercise. *Acta Physiologica Scandanavica* **71**, 129–139.

Hess, G.P., Cappiello, W.L., Poole, R.M. & Hunter, S.C. (1989) Prevention and treatment of overuse tendon injuries. *Sports Medicine* **8**, 371–384.

Hickey, M.S., Costill, D.L., McConnell, G.K., Widrick, J.J. & Tanaka, H. (1992) Day to day variation in time trial cycling performance. *International Journal of Sports Medicine* **13**, 467–470.

Hickson, R.C. (1980) Interference of strength development by simultaneously training for strength and endurance. *European Journal of Applied Physiology* **45**, 255–263.

Hickson, R.C., Dvorak, B.A., Gorostiaga, E.M., Kurowski, T.T. & Foster, C. (1988) Potential for strength and endurance training to amplify endurance performance. *Journal of Applied Physiology* **65**, 2285–2290.

Higginbotham, M.B., Morris, K.G., Williams, R.S., Mchale, P.A., Coleman,

R.E. & Cobb, F.R. (1986) Regulation of stroke volume during submaximal and maximal upright exercise in normal man. *Circulation Research* **58**, 281–291.

Hildebrandt, A.L., Pilegaard, H. & Neufer, P.D. (2003) Differential transcriptional activation of select metabolic genes in response to variations in exercise intensity and duration. *American Journal of Physiology, Endocrinology and Metabolism* **285**, E1021–E1027.

Holloszy, J.O. (1967) Biochemical adaptations in muscle. Effects of exercise on mitochondrial oxygen uptake and respiratory enzyme activity in skeletal muscle. *Journal of Biological Chemistry* **242**, 2278–2282.

Holloszy, J.O. (1973) Biochemical adaptations to exercise: aerobic metabolism. *Exercise and Sport Sciences Reviews* **1**, 45–71.

Hood, D.A. (2001) Invited Review: Contractile activity-induced mitochondrial biogenesis in skeletal muscle. *Journal of Applied Physiology* **90**, 1137–1157.

Hoogsteen, J., Hoogeveen, A., Schaffers, H., Wijn, P.F. & Van der Wall, E.E. (2003) Left atrial and ventricular dimensions in highly trained cyclists. *International Journal of Cardiovascular Imaging* **19**, 211–217.

Hoogsteen, J., Hoogeveen, A., Schaffers, H., Wijn, P.F., Van Hemel, N.M. & Van der Wall, E.E. (2004) Myocardial adaptation in different endurance sports: an echocardiographic study. *International Journal of Cardiovascular Imaging* **20**, 19–26.

Hooley, C.J., McCrum, N. & Cohen, R.E. (1980) The viscoelastic deformation of tendon. *Journal of Biomechanics* **13**, 521–528.

Hoppeler, H., Howald, H., Conley, K., *et al.* (1985) Endurance training in humans: aerobic capacity and structure of skeletal muscle. *Journal of Applied Physiology* **59**, 320–327.

Hopper, M.K., Coggan, A.R. & Coyle, E.F. (1988) Exercise stroke volume relative to plasma–volume expansion. *Journal of Applied Physiology* **64**, 404–408.

Hortobagyi, T., Lambert, N.J. & Hill, J.P. (1997) Greater cross education following training with muscle lengthening than shortening. *Medicine and Science in Sports and Exercise* **29**, 107–112.

Hortobagyi, T., Scott, K., Lambert, J., Hamilton, G. & Tracy, J. (1999) Cross-education of muscle strength is greater with stimulated than voluntary contractions. *Motor Behavior* **3**, 205–219.

Hostler, D., Schwirian, C.J., Campos, G., *et al.* (2001) Skeletal muscle adaptations in elastic resistance-trained young men and women. *European Journal of Applied Physiology* **86**, 112–118.

Houston, M.E., Froese, E.A., Valeriote, S.P., Green, H.J. & Ranney, D.A. (1983) Muscle performance, morphology and metabolic capacity during strength training and detraining: a one leg model. *European Journal of Applied Physiology* **51**, 25–35.

Houtman, C.J., Stegeman, D.F., Van Dijk, J.P. & Zwarts, M.J. (2003) Changes in muscle fiber conduction velocity indicate recruitment of distinct motor unit populations. *Journal of Applied Physiology* **95**, 1045–1054.

Howald, H. (1985) Malleability of the motor system: training for maximizing power output. *Journal of Experimental Biology* **115**, 365–373.

Hultman, E., Bergstrom, M., Spriet, L.L. & Soderlund, K. (1990) Energy metabolism and fatigue. In: *Biochemistry of Exercise* Vol. VII (Taylor, A.W., Gollnick, P.D., Green, H.J., Ianuzzo, D., Noble, E.G., Metivier, G., *et al.*, eds.) Human Kinetics, Champaign, IL: 73–92.

Hultman, E., Del Canale, S. & Sjoholm, H. (1985) Effect of induced metabolic acidosis on intracellular pH, buffer capacity and contraction force of human skeletal muscle. *Clinical Science (London)* **69**, 505–510.

Hunter, S.K., Thompson, M.W., Ruell, P.A., *et al.* (1999) Human skeletal sarcoplasmic reticulum Ca^{2+} uptake and muscle function with aging and strength training. *Journal of Applied Physiology* **86**, 1858–1865.

Hurley, B.F., Nemeth, P.M., Martin, W.H. 3rd, Hagberg, J.M., Dalsky, G.P. & Holloszy, J.O. (1986) Muscle triglyceride utilization during exercise: effect of training. *Journal of Applied Physiology* **60**, 562–567.

Hurley, B.F., Hagberg, J.M., Allen, W.K., Seals, D.R., Young, J.C., Cuddihee, R.W., *et al.* (1984) Effect of training on blood lactate levels during submaximal exercise. *Journal of Applied Physiology* **56**, 1260–1264.

Hutton, R.S. & Enoka, R.M. (1986) Kinematic assessment of a functional role for recurrent inhibition and selective recruitment. *Experimental Neurology* **93**, 369–379.

Ikaheimo, M.J., Palatsi, I.J. & Takkunen, J.T. (1979) Noninvasive evaluation of the athletic heart: sprinters versus endurance runners. *American Journal of Cardiology* **44**, 24–30.

Inbar, O., Weiner, P., Azgad, Y., Rotstein, A. & Weinstein, Y. (2000) Specific inspiratory muscle training in well-trained endurance athletes. *Medicine and Science in Sports and Exercise* **32**, 1233–1237.

Inglemark, B.E. (1945) Uber den Bau der Sehnen während verschiedener Altersperioden un unter wechselden funktionellen Bedingungen. *Acta Socio Medica Uppsala* **50**, 357–396.

Inglemark, B.E. (1948a) Der Bau der Sehnen während verschiedener Altersperioden un unter wechselden funktionellen Bedingungen. I. *Acta Anatomica* **6**, 113–140.

Inglemark, B.E. (1948b) The structure of tendons at various ages and under different functional conditions. II. An electron microscopic investigation from white rat. *Acta Anatomica* **6**, 193–225.

Izquierdo, M., Häkkinen, K., González-Badillo, J.J., Ibañez, J. & Gorostiaga, E.M. (2002) Effects of long-term training specificity on maximal strength and power of the upper and lower extremity muscles in athletes from different sports events. *European Journal of Applied Physiology* **87**, 264–271.

Izquierdo, M., Ibañez, J., Häkkinen, K., Kraemer, W.J. & Gorostiaga, E.M. (2004) Maximal strength and power, muscle mass, endurance and serum hormones in weightlifters and road cyclists. *Journal of Sports Sciences* **22**, 465–478.

Jakeman, P.M. (1998) Amino acid metabolism, branched-chain amino acid feeding and brain monoamine function. *Proceedings of the Nutrition Society* **57**, 35–41.

Jakeman, P.M., Hawthorne, J.E., Maxwell, S.R., Kendall, M.J. & Holder, G. (1994) Evidence for downregulation of hypothalamic 5-hydroxytryptamine receptor function in endurance-trained athletes. *Experimental Physiology* **79**, 461–464.

Janicki, J.S. (1990) Influence of the pericardium and ventricular interdependence on left ventricular diastolic and systolic function in patients with heart failure. *Circulation* **81**, III15–III20.

Jansson, E. & Kaijser, L. (1977) Muscle adaptation to extreme endurance training in man. *Acta Physiologica Scandanavica* **100**, 315–324.

Jansson, E., Sjodin, B. & Tesch, P. (1978) Changes in muscle fibre type distribution in man after physical training: a sign of fibre type transformation? *Acta Physiologica Scandinavica* **104**, 235–237.

Järvinen, T.L.N., Kannus, P. & Sievänen, H. (1999) Have the DXA-based exercise studies seriously underestimated the effects of mechanical loading on bone? *Journal of Bone and Mineral Research* **14**, 1634–1635.

Järvinen, T.L., Sievanen, H., Jokihaara, J. & Einhorn, T.A. (2005) Revival of bone strength: the bottom line. *Journal of Bone and Mineral Research* **20**, 717–720.

Jefferson, L.S. & Kimball, S.R. (2001) Translational control of protein synthesis: implications for understanding changes in skeletal muscle mass. *International Journal of Sport Nutrition and Exercise Metabolism* **11**, S143–S149.

Jensen-Urstad, M., Bouvier, F., Nejat, M., Saltin, B. & Brodin, L.A. (1998) Left ventricular function in endurance runners during exercise. *Acta Physiologica Scandinavica* **164**, 167–172.

Jeukendrup, A., Brouns, F., Wagenmakers, A.J.M. & Saris, W.H.M. (1997) Carbohydrate-electrolyte feedings improve 1 h time trial cycling performance. *International Journal of Sports Medicine* **18**, 125–129.

Jeukendrup, A., Martin, D.T. & Gore, C.J. (2003) Are world-class cyclists really more efficient? *Medicine and Science in Sports and Exercise* **35**, 1238–1239; discussion 1240–1241.

Jeukendrup, A., Saris, W.H., Brouns, F. & Kester, A.D. (1996) A new validated endurance performance test. *Medicine and Science in Sports and Exercise* **28**, 266–270.

Jeukendrup, A.E. (2004) Carbohydrate intake during exercise and performance. *Nutrition* **20**, 669–677.

Johnson, B.D., Babcock, M.A., Suman, O.E. & Dempsey, J.A. (1993) Exercise-induced diaphragmatic fatigue in healthy humans. *Journal of Physiology (London)* **460**, 385–405.

Jones, C., Allen, T., Talbot, J., Morgan, D.L. & Proske, U. (1997) Changes in the mechanical properties of human and amphibian muscle after eccentric exercise. *European Journal of Applied Physiology and Occupational Physiology* **76**, 21–31.

Jones, D.A. (1981) Muscle fatigue due to changes beyond the neuromuscular junction. *Ciba Foundation Symposium* **82**, 178–196.

Jones, D.A., Bigland-Ritchie, B. & Edwards, R.H. (1979) Excitation frequency and muscle fatigue: mechanical responses during voluntary and stimulated contractions. *Experimental Neurology* **64**, 401–413.

Jones, D.A., Newham, D.J. & Clarkson, P.M. (1987) Skeletal muscle stiffness and pain following eccentric exercise of the elbow flexors. *Pain* **30**, 233–242.

Joyner, M.J. (1991) Modeling: optimal marathon performance on the basis of physiological factors. *Journal of Applied Physiology* **70**, 683–687.

Jozsa, L. (1984) Morphological and biochemical alterations in hypokinetic human tendons. *Finn Sports Exercise Medicine* **3**, 111–115.

Jozsa, L., Lehto, M., Kvist, M., Balint, B.J. & Reffy, A. (1989) Alterations in dry mass content of collagen fibers in degenerative tendinopathy and tendon rupture. *Matrix* **9**, 140–149.

Jürimäe, J., Abernethy, P.J., Blake, K. & McEniery, M.T. (1997) Changes in the myosin heavy chain isoform profile of the triceps brachii muscle following 12 weeks of resistance training. *European Journal of Applied Physiology* **74**, 287–292.

Kamen, G. & Roy, A. (2000) Motor unit synchronization in young and elderly adults. *European Journal of Applied Physiology* **81**, 403–410.

Kamen, G., Kroll, W. & Zignon, S.T. (1981) Exercise effects upon reflex time components in weight lifters and distance runners. *Medicine and Science in Sports and Exercise* **13**, 198–204.

Kammermeier, H., Schmidt, P. & Jungling, E. (1982) Free energy change of ATP-hydrolysis: a causal factor of early hypoxic failure of the myocardium? *Journal of Melecualr and Cellular Cardiology* **14**, 267–277.

Kanehisa, H., Ikegawa, S. & Fukunaga, T. (1997) Force–velocity relationships and fatigability of strength and endurance-trained subjects. International *Journal of Sports Medicine* **18**, 106–112.

Kannus, P. (1997) Etiology and pathophysiology of chronic tendon disorders in sports. *Scandinavian Journal of Medicine and Science in Sports* **7**, 78–85.

Kannus, P. (1999) Preventing osteoporosis, falls, and fractures among elderly people. Promotion of lifelong physical activity is essential [Editorial]. *British Medical Journal* **318**, 205–206.

Kannus, P. (2000) Structure of the tendon connective tissue. *Scandinavian Journal of Medicine and Science in Sports* **10**, 312–320.

Kannus, P., Haapasalo, H., Sankelo, M., Sievänen, H., Pasanen, M., Heinonen, A., *et al.* (1995) Effect of starting age of physical activity on bone mass in the dominant arm of tennis and squash players. *Annals of Internal Medicine* **123**, 27–31.

Kannus, P. & Jozsa, L. (1991) Histopathological changes preceding spontaneous rupture of a tendon: a controlled study of 891 patients. *Journal of Bone and Joint Surgery (American)* **73-A**, 1507–1525.

Kannus, P., Jozsa, L., Renström, P., Järvinen, M., Kvist, M., Lehto, M., *et al.* (1992a) The effects of training, immobilization and remobilization on musculoskeletal tissue. 1. Training and immobilization. *Scandinavian Journal of Medicine and Science in Sports* **2**, 100–118.

Kannus, P., Jozsa, L., Renström, P., Järvinen, M., Kvist, M., Lehto, M., *et al.* (1992b) The effects of training, immobilization and remobilization on musculoskeletal tissue. 2. Remobilization and prevention of immobilization atrophy. *Scandinavian Journal of Medicine and Science in Sports* **2**, 164–176.

Kannus, P., Parkkari, J., Niemi, S., Pasanen, M., Palvanen, M., Jarvinen, M., *et al.* (2000) Prevention of hip fracture in elderly people with use of a hip protector. *New England Journal of Medicine* **343**, 1506–1513.

Kannus, P., Sievänen, H., Palvanen, M., Järvinen, T. & Parkkari, J. (2005a) Prevention of falls and consequent injuries in elderly population. *Lancet* **366**, 1885–1893.

Kannus, P., Uusi-Rasi, K., Palvanen, M. & Parkkari, J. (2005b) Non-pharmacological means to prevent fractures among older adults. *Annals of Medicine* **37**, 303–310.

Kaptoge, S., Dalzell, N., Jakes, R.W., Wareham, N., Day, N.E., Khaw, K.T., *et al.* (2003) Hip section modulus, a measure of bending resistance, is more strongly related to reported physical activity than BMD. *Osteoporos International* **14**, 941–949.

Karinkanta, S., Heinonen, A., Sievanen, H., Uusi-Rasi, K. & Kannus, P. (2005) Factors predicting dynamic balance and quality of life in home-dwelling elderly women. *Gerontology* **51**, 116–121.

Karlsson, J., Funderburk, C.F., Essen, B. & Lind, A.R. (1975) Constituents of human muscle in isometric fatigue. *Journal of Applied Physiology* **38**, 208–211.

Karlsson, J., Nordesjo, L.O., Saltin, B. (1974) Muscle glycogen utilization during exercise after physical training.

Acta Physiologica Scandinavica **90**, 210–217.

Karlsson, J. & Saltin, B. (1970) Lactate, ATP, and CP in working muscles during exhaustive exercise in man. *Journal of Applied Physiology* **29**, 596–602.

Karlsson, J. & Saltin, B. (1971a) Diet, muscle glycogen and endurance performance. *Journal of Applied Physiology* **31**, 203–206.

Karlsson, J. & Saltin, B. (1971b) Oxygen deficit and muscle metabolites in intermittent exercise. *Acta Physiologica Scandinavica* **82**, 115–122.

Karsenty, G. (2003) The complexities of skeletal biology. *Nature* **423**, 316–318.

Katz, A., Sahlin, K. & Henriksson, J. (1986) Muscle ATP turnover rate during isometric contraction in humans. *Journal of Applied Physiology* **60**, 1839–1842.

Kawai, M. & Halvorson, H.R. (1989) Role of MgATP and MgADP in the cross-bridge kinetics in chemically skinned rabbit psoas fibers: study of a fast exponential process (C). *Biophysical Journal* **55**, 595–603.

Kearns, C.F., Abe, T. & Brechue, W.F. (2000) Muscle enlargement in sumo wrestlers includes increased muscle fascicle length. *European Journal of Applied Physiology* **83**, 289–296.

Kellis, E., Arabatzi, F. & Papadopoulos, C. (2003) Muscle co-activation around the knee in drop jumping using the co-contraction index. *Journal of Electromyography and Kinesiology* **13**, 229–238.

Kernell, D. & Monster, A.W. (1981) Threshold current for repetitive impulse firing in motoneurons innervating muscle fibres of different fatigue sensitivity in the cat. *Brain Research* **229**, 193–196.

Kiiskinen, A. & Heikkinen, E. (1973) Effect of physical training on development and strength of tendons and bones in growing mice. *Scandinavian Journal of Clinical and Laboratory Investigation* **29**, Supplement 123.

Kilbom, A. & Astrand, I. (1971) Physical training with submaximal intensities in women. II. Effect on cardiac output. *Scandinavian Journal of Clinical Laboratory Investigation* **28**, 163–175.

Kjaer, M., Christensen, N.J., Sonne, B., Richter, E.A. & Galbo, H. (1985) Effect of exercise on epinephrine turnover in trained and untrained male subjects. *Journal of Applied Physiology* **59**, 1061–1067.

Kjaer, M., Farrell, P.A., Christensen, N.J. & Galbo, H. (1986) Increased epinephrine

response and inaccurate glucoregulation in exercising athletes. *Journal of Applied Physiology* **61**, 1693–1700.

Kjaer, M., Langberg, H., Miller, B.F., Boushel, R., Crameri, R., Koskinen, R., *et al.* (2005) Metabolic activity and collagen turnover in human tendons in response to physical activity. *Journal of Musculoskeletal and Neuronal Interactions* **5**, 41–52.

Kjellberg, S., Rudhe, U. & Sjostrand, T. (1949) Increase of the amount of hemoglobin and blood volume in connection with physical training. *Acta Physiologica Scandinavica* **19**, 146–151.

Klitgaard, H. & Clausen, T. (1989) Increased total concentration of Na-K pumps in vastus lateralis muscle of old trained human subjects. *Journal of Applied Physiology* **67**, 2491–2494.

Klitgaard, H., Mantoni, M., Schiaffino, S., *et al.* (1990) Function, morphology and protein expression of ageing skeletal muscle: a cross-sectional study of elderly men with different training backgrounds. *Acta Physiologica Scandinavica* **140**, 41–54.

Knaflitz, M., Merletti, R. & DeLuca, C.J. (1990) Inference of motor unit recruitment order in voluntary and electrically elicited contractions. *Journal of Applied Physiology* **68**, 1657–1667.

Kontulainen, S., Sievänen, H., Kannus, P., Pasanen, M. & Vuori, I. (2002) Effect of long-term impact-loading on mass, size, and estimated strength of humerus and radius of female racquet-sports players: a peripheral quantitative computed tomography study between young and old starters an controls. *Journal of Bone and Mineral Research* **17**, 2281–2289.

Korge, P. & Campbell, K.B. (1995) The importance of ATPase microenvironment in muscle fatigue: a hypothesis. *International Journal of Sports Medicine* **16**, 172–179.

Koskolou, M.D. & McKenzie, D.C. (1994) Arterial hypoxemia and performance during intense exercise. *European Journal of Applied Physiology* **68**, 80–86.

Kraemer, W.J., Fleck, S.J. & Evans, W.J. (1996) Strength and power training: physiological mechanisms of adaptation. *Exercise and Sports Science Reviews* **24**, 363–397.

Kraemer, W.J. & Ratamess, N.A. (2003) Endocrine responses and adaptations to strength and power training. In: *Strength and Power in Sport* (Komi, P.V., ed.). 2nd edn. Blackwell Scientific Publications Malden, MA: 361–386.

Kraemer, W.J. & Ratamess, N.A. (2004) Fundamentals of resistance training: progression and exercise prescription. *Medicine and Science in Sport and Exercise* **36**, 674–678.

Kraemer, W.J. & Ratamess, N.A. (2005) Hormonal responses and adaptations to resistance exercise and training. *Sports Medicine* **35**, 339–361.

Kraemer, W.J., Patton, J.F., Gordon, S.E., *et al.* (1995) Compatibility of high-intensity strength and endurance training on hormonal and skeletal muscle adaptations. *Journal of Applied Physiology* **78**, 976–989.

Kraemer, W.J., Nindl, B.C., Ratamess, N.A., *et al.* (2004) Changes in muscle hypertrophy in women with periodized resistance training. *Medicine and Science in Sports and Exercise* **36**, 697–708.

Krip, B., Gledhill, N., Jamnik, V. & Warburton, D. (1997) Effect of alterations in blood volume on cardiac function during maximal exercise. *Medicine and Science in Sports and Exercise* **29**, 1469–1476.

Kroeker, C.A., Shrive, N.G., Belenkie, I. & Tyberg, J.V. (2003) Pericardium modulates left and right ventricular stroke volumes to compensate for sudden changes in atrial volume. *American Journal of Physiology. Heart and Circulatory Physiology* **284**, H2247–H2254.

Kuruganti, U., Parker, P., Rickards, J., Tingley, M. & Sexsmith, J. (2005) Bilateral isokinetic training reduces the bilateral leg strength deficit for both old and young adults. *European Journal of Applied Physiology* **94**, 175–179.

Lambert, E.V., St. Clair Gibson, A. & Noakes, T.D. (2005) Complex systems model of fatigue: integrative homoeostatic control of peripheral physiological systems during exercise in humans. *British Journal of Sports Medicine* **39**, 52–62.

Langberg, H., Rosendal, L. & Kjaer, M. (2001) Training induced changes in peritendinous type I collagen turnover determined by microdialysis in humans. *Journal of Physiology* **534**, 397–402.

Lannergren, J. & Westerblad, H. (1989) Maximum tension and force–velocity properties of fatigued, single *Xenopus* muscle fibres studied by caffeine and high K+. *Journal of Physiology* **409**, 473–490.

Laros, G.S., Tipton, C.M. & Cooper, R.R. (1971) Influence of physical activity on ligament insertions in the knees of dogs. *Journal of Bone and Joint Surgery* **53-A**, 275–286.

LeBlanc. P.J., Howarth, K.R., Gibala, M.J. & Heigenhauser, G.J. (2004) Effects of 7 wk of endurance training on human skeletal muscle metabolism during submaximal exercise. *Journal of Applied Physiology* **97**, 2148–2153.

Lee, M.C., Lewinter, M.M., Freeman, G., Shabetai, R. & Fung, Y.C. (1985) Biaxial mechanical properties of the pericardium in normal and volume overload dogs. *American Journal of Physiology* **249**, H222–H230.

Levine, B.D. (1993) Regulation of central blood volume and cardiac filling in endurance athletes: the Frank-Starling mechanism as a determinant of orthostatic tolerance. *Medicine and Science in Sports and Exercise* **25**, 727–732.

Levine, B.D., Buckey, J.C., Fritsch, J.M., Yancy, C.W. Jr., Watenpaugh, D.E., Snell, P.G., *et al.* (1991a) Physical fitness and cardiovascular regulation: mechanisms of orthostatic intolerance. *Journal of Applied Physiology* **70**, 112–122.

Levine, B.D., Lane, L.D., Buckey, J.C., Friedman, D.B. & Blomqvist, C.G. (1991b) Left ventricular pressure-volume and Frank–Starling relations in endurance athletes: implications of orthostatic tolerance and exercise performance. *Circulation* **84**, 1016–1023.

Levine, B.D. & Stray-Gundersen, J. (1997) "Living high-training low": effect of moderate-altitude acclimatization with low-altitude training on performance. *Journal of Applied Physiology* **83**, 102–112.

Levine, S.A., Gordon, G. & Derick, C.L. (1924) Some changes in the chemical constituents of the blood following a marathon race. *Journal of the American Medical Association* **82**, 1778–1779.

Lewis, S.F., Haller, R.G., Cook, J.D. & Nunnally, R.L. (1985) Muscle fatigue in McArdle's disease studied by 31P-NMR: effect of glucose infusion. *Journal of Applied Physiology* **59**, 1991–1994.

Linossier, M.T., Dormois, D., Geyssant, A. & Denis, C. (1997) Performance and fibre characteristics of human skeletal muscle during short sprint training and detraining on a cycle ergometer. *European Journal of Applied Physiology* **75**, 491–498.

Liu, L., Maruno, R., Mashimo, T., Sanka, K., Higuchi, T., Hayashi, K., *et al.* (2003) Effects of physical training on cortical bone at midtibia assessed by peripheral QCT. *Journal of Applied Physiology* **95**, 219–224.

Lloyd, A.R., Gandevia, S.C. & Hales, J.P. (1991) Muscle performance, voluntary activation, twitch properties and perceived effort in normal subjects and patients with the chronic fatigue syndrome. *Brain* **114**, 85–98.

Lovejoy, C.O. (1988) Evolution of human walking. *Scientific American* **259**, 118–125.

Lucia, A., Hoyos, J., Pardo, J. & Chicharro, J.L. (2000) Metabolic and neuromuscular adaptations to endurance training in professional cyclists: a longitudinal study. *Japanese Journal of Physiology* **50**, 381–388.

Luger, A., Deuster, P.A., Kyle, S.B., Gallucci, W.T., Montgomery, L.C., Gold, P.W., *et al.* (1987) Acute hypothalamic–pituitary–adrenal responses to the stress of treadmill exercise. Physiologic adaptations to physical training. *New England Journal of Medicine* **316**, 1309–1315.

Luthi, J.M., Howald, H., Claassen, H., Rosler, K., Vock, P. & Hoppeler, H. (1986) Structural changes in skeletal muscle tissue with heavy-resistance exercise. *International Journal of Sports Medicine* **7**, 123–127.

MacDougall, J.D., Gibala M.J., Tarnopolsky M.A., MacDonald J.R., Interisano, S.A. & Yarasheski, K.E. (1995) The time course for elevated muscle protein synthesis following heavy resistance exercise. *Canadian Journal of Applied Physiology* **20**, 480–486.

MacDougall, J.D., Sale, D.G., Alway, S.E. & Sutton, J.R. (1984) Muscle fiber number in biceps brachii in body builders and control subjects. *Journal of Applied Physiology* **57**, 1399–1403.

MacDougall, J.D., Sale, D.G., Elder, G.C. & Sutton, J.R. (1982) Muscle ultrastructural characteristics of elite powerlifters and bodybuilders. *European Journal of Applied Physiology* **48**, 117–126.

MacDougall, J.D., Sale, D.G., Moroz, J.R., Elder, G.C., Sutton, J.R. & Howald, H. (1979) Mitochondrial volume density in human skeletal muscle following heavy resistance training. *Medicine and Science in Sports* **11**, 164–166.

MacDougall, J.D., Tarnopolsky, M.A., Chesley, A. & Atkinson, S.A. (1992) Changes in muscle protein synthesis following heavy resistance exercise in humans: a pilot study. *Acta Physiologica Scandinavica* **146**, 403–404.

Maclaren, D.P., Gibson, H., Parry-Billings, M. & Edwards, R.H. (1989) A review of metabolic and physiological factors in fatigue. *Exercise and Sport Sciences Reviews* **17**, 29–66.

MacRae, H.S., Dennis, S.C., Bosch, A.N. & Noakes, T.D. (1992) Effects of training on lactate production and removal during progressive exercise in humans. *Journal of Applied Physiology* **72**, 1649–1656.

Madsen, K., Franch, J. & Clausen, T. (1994) Effects of intensified endurance training on the concentration of Na,K-ATPase and Ca-ATPase in human skeletal muscle. *Acta Physiologica Scandinavica* **150**, 251–258.

Maffiuletti, N.A., Martin, A., Babault, M., Pensini, M., Lucas, B. & Schieppati, M. (2001) Electrical and mechanical H_{max}-to-M_{max} ratio in power- and endurance-trained athletes. *Journal of Applied Physiology* **90**, 3–9.

Maffiuletti, N.A., Pensini, M., Scaglioni, G., Ferri, A., Ballay, Y. & Martin, A. (2003) Effect of electromyostimulation training on soleus and gastrocnemii H- and T-reflex properties. *European Journal of Applied Physiology* **90**, 601–607.

Maffulli, N. & King, J.B. (1992) Effects of physical activity on some components of the skeletal system. *Sports Medicine* **13**, 393–407.

Magnusson, S.P., Hansen, P. & Kjaer, M. (2003) Tendon properties in relation to muscular activity and physical training. *Scandinavian Journal of Medicine and Science in Sports* **13**, 211–223.

Marchand, I., Chorneyko, K., Tarnopolsky, M., Hamilton, S., Shearer, J., Potvin, J., *et al.* (2002) Quantification of subcellular glycogen in resting human muscle: granule size, number, and location. *Journal of Applied Physiology* **93**, 1598–1607.

Markov, G., Spengler, C.M., Knopfli-Lenzin, C., Stuessi, C. & Boutellier, U. (2001) Respiratory muscle training increases cycling endurance without affecting cardiovascular responses to exercise. *European Journal of Applied Physiology* **85**, 233–239.

Maron, B.J. (1986) Structural features of the athlete heart as defined by echocardiography. *Journal of the American College of Cardiology* **7**, 190–203.

Marsden, C.D., Obeso, J.A. & Rothwell, J.C. (1983) The function of the antagonist muscle during fast limb movements in man. *Journal of Physiology* **335**, 1–13.

Martin, B.J. & Stager, J.M. (1981) Ventilatory endurance in athletes and non-athletes. *Medicine and Science in Sports and Exercise* **13**, 21–26.

Martin, D.T., Quod, M.J., Gore, C.J. & Coyle, E.F. (2005) Has Armstrong's cycle efficiency improved? *Journal of Applied Physiology* **99**, 1628–1629; author reply 1629.

Martin, R.B. (2000) Toward a unifying theory of bone remodeling. *Bone* **26**, 1–6.

Martino, M., Gledhill, N. & Jamnik, V. (2002) High $\dot{V}o_{2max}$ with no history of training is primarily due to high blood volume. *Medicine and Science in Sports and Exercise* **34**, 966–971.

Marvin, G., Sharma, A., Aston, W., Field, C., Kendall, M.J. & Jones, D.A. (1997) The effects of buspirone on perceived exertion and time to fatigue in man. *Experimental Physiology* **82**, 1057–1060.

Maughan, R.J., Donnelly, A.E., Gleeson, M., Whiting, P.H., Walker, K.A. & Clough, P.J. (1989) Delayed-onset muscle damage and lipid peroxidation in man after a downhill run. *Muscle and Nerve* **12**, 332–336.

McBride, J.M., Triplett-McBride, T., Davie, A. & Newton, R.U. (2002) The effect of heavy- vs. light-load jump squats on the development of strength, power, and speed. *Journal of Strength & Conditioning Research* **16**, 75–82.

McBride, J.M., Blaak, J.B. & Triplett-McBride, T. (2003) Effect of resistance exercise volume and complexity on EMG, strength, and regional body composition. *European Journal of Applied Physiology* **90**, 626–632.

McCall, G.E., Byrnes, W.C., Dickinson, A., Pattany, P.M. & Fleck, S.J. (1996) Muscle fiber hypertrophy, hyperplasia, and capillary density in college men after resistance training. *Journal of Applied Physiology* **81**, 2004–2012.

McCartney, N., Spriet, L.L., Heigenhauser, G.J., Kowalchuk, J.M., Sutton, J.R. & Jones, N.L. (1986) Muscle power and metabolism in maximal intermittent exercise. *Journal of Applied Physiology* **60**, 1164–1169.

McGavock, J.M., Warburton, D.E., Taylor, D., Welsh, R.C., Quinney, H.A. & Haykowsky, M.J. (2002) The effects of prolonged strenuous exercise on left ventricular function: a brief review. *Heart Lung* **31**, 279–292.

McKiernan, F.E. (2005) A simple gait-stabilizing device reduces outdoor falls and nonserious injurious falls in fall-prone older people during the winter. *Journal of the American Geriatrics Society* **53**, 943–947.

McLaren, P.F., Nurhayati, Y. & Boutcher, S.H. (1997) Stroke volume response to cycle ergometry in trained and untrained older men. *European Journal of Applied Physiology* **75**, 537–542.

McLester, J.R. Jr. (1997) Muscle contraction and fatigue: the role of adenosine 5′-diphosphate and inorganic phosphate. *Sports Medicine* **23**, 287–305.

Medbo, J.I. & Sejersted, O.M. (1990) Plasma potassium changes with high intensity exercise. *Journal of Physiology* **421**, 105–122.

Meeusen, R., Roeykens, J., Magnus, L., Keizer, H. & De Meirleir, K. (1997) Endurance performance in humans: the effect of a dopamine precursor or a specific serotonin (5-$HT_{2A/2C}$) antagonist. *International Journal of Sports Medicine* **18**, 571–577.

Mendenhall, L.A., Swanson, S.C., Habash, D.L. & Coggan, A.R. (1994) Ten days of exercise training reduces glucose production and utilization during moderate-intensity exercise. *American Journal of Physiology* **266**, E136–E143.

Metzger, J.M. & Fitts, R.H. (1986) Contractile and biochemical properties of diaphragm: effects of exercise training and fatigue. *Journal of Applied Physiology* **60**, 1752–1758.

Metzger, J.M. & Fitts, R.H. (1987) Role of intracellular pH in muscle fatigue. *Journal of Applied Physiology* **62**, 1392–1397.

Michna, H. (1984) Morphometric analysis of loading-induced changes in collagen-fibril populations in young tendons. *Cell and Tissue Research* **236**, 465–470.

Michna, H. (1987) Tendon injuries induced by exercise and anabolic steroids in experimental mice. *International Orthopaedics* **11**, 157–162.

Michna, H. & Hartmann, G. (1989) Adaptation of tendon collagen to exercise. *International Orthopaedics* **13**, 161–165.

Mier, C.M., Turner, M.J., Ehsani, A.A. & Spina, R.J. (1997) Cardiovascular adaptations to 10 days of cycle exercise. *Journal of Applied Physiology* **83**, 1900–1906.

Milner-Brown, H.S., Stein, R.B. & Lee, R.G. (1975) Synchronization of human motor units: possible roles of exercise and supraspinal reflexes. *Electroencephalogy and Clinical Neurophysiology* **38**, 245–254.

Moisio, K.C., Hurwitz, D.E. & Sumner, D.R. (2004) Dynamic loads are determinants of peak bone mass. *Journal of Orthopaedic Research* **22**, 339–345.

Monster, A.W. & Chan, H. (1977) Isometric force production by motor units of extensor digitorum communis muscles in man. *Journal of Neurophysiology* **40**, 1432–1443.

Morgan, D., Kohrt, W., Bates, B. & Skinner, J. (1987a) Effects of respiratory muscle endurance training on ventilatory and endurance performance of moderately trained cyclists. *International Journal of Sports Medicine* **8**, 88–93.

Morgan, D.L. & Proske, U. (2004) Popping sarcomere hypothesis explains stretch-induced muscle damage. *Clinical and Experimental Pharmacology and Physiology* **31**, 541–545.

Morgan, D.W., Kohrt, W.M., Bates, B.J. & Skinner, J.S. (1987b) Effects of respiratory muscle endurance training on ventilatory and endurance performance of moderately trained cyclists. *International Journal of Sports Medicine* **8**, 88–93.

Morganroth, J., Maron, B., Henry, W. & Epstein, S. (1975) Comparative left ventricular dimensions in trained athletes. *Annuals of Internal Medicine* **82**, 521–524.

Moritani, T. & deVries, H.A. (1979) Neural factors versus hypertrophy in the time course of muscle strength gain. *American Journal of Physical Medicine* **58**, 115–130.

Morris-Thurgood, J.A. & Frenneaux, M.P. (2000) Diastolic ventricular interaction and ventricular diastolic filling. *Heart Failure Reviews* **5**, 307–323.

Moseley, L., Achten, J., Martin, J.C. & Jeukendrup, A.E. (2004) No differences in cycling efficiency between world-class and recreational cyclists. *International Journal of Sports Medicine* **25**, 374–379.

Mosley, J.R. (2000) Osteoporosis and bone functional adaptation: mechanobiological regulation of bone architecture in growing and adult bone, a review. *Journal of Rehabilitation Research and Development* **37**, 189–199.

Myburgh, K.H. (2003) What makes an endurance athlete world-class? Not simply a physiological conundrum. *Comparative Biochemistry and Physiology Part A: Molecular & Integrative Physiology* **136**, 171–190.

Munn, J., Herbert, R.D. & Gandevia, S.C. (2004) Contralateral effects of unilateral resistance training: a meta-analysis. *Journal of Applied Physiology* **96**, 1861–1866.

Nadel, E.R., Bergh, U. & Saltin, B. (1972) Body temperatures during negative work exercise. *Journal of Applied Physiology* **33**, 553–558.

Nader, G.A. & Esser, K.A. (2001) Intracellular signaling specificity in skeletal muscle in response to different modes of exercise. *Journal of Applied Physiology* **90**, 1936–1942.

Nardone, A., Romano, C. & Schieppati, M. (1989) Selective recruitment of high-threshold human motor units during voluntary isotonic lengthening of active muscles. *Journal of Physiology* **409**, 451–471.

Narici, M.V., Roi, G.S., Landoni, L., Minetti, A.E. & Cerretelli, E. (1989) Changes in force, cross-sectional area and neural activation during strength training and detraining of the human quadriceps. *European Journal of Applied Physiology* **59**, 310–319.

Narici, M.V., Hoppeler, H., Kayser, B., Landoni, L., Claassen, H., Gavardi, C., et al. (1996) Human quadriceps cross-sectional area, torque and neural activation during 6 months strength training. *Acta Physiologica Scandinavica* **157**, 175–186.

Nassar-Gentina, V., Passonneau, J.V. & Rapoport, S.I. (1981) Fatigue and metabolism of frog muscle fibers during stimulation and in response to caffeine. *American Journal of Physiology* **241**, C160–166.

Newham, D.J., Mills, K.R., Quigley, B.M. & Edwards, R.H. (1983) Pain and fatigue after concentric and eccentric muscle contractions. *Clinical Science (London)* **64**, 55–62.

Newsholme, E.A., Acworth, I.N. & Blomstrand, E. (1987) Amino acids, brain neurotransmitters and a functional link between muscle and brain that is important in sustained exercise. *Advances in Myochemistry* **1**, 127–133.

Nikander, R., Sievanen, H., Heinonen, A. & Kannus, P. (2005) Femoral neck structure in adult female athletes subjected to different loading modalities. *Journal of Bone and Mineral Research* **20**, 520–528.

Nielsen, O.B. & Clausen, T. (2000) The Na^+/K^+-pump protects muscle excitability and contractility during exercise. *Exercise and Sport Sciences Review* **28**, 159–164.

Noakes, T.D. (2000) Physiological models to understand exercise fatigue and the adaptations that predict or enhance athletic performance. *Scandinavian Journal of Medicine and Science in Sports* **10**, 123–145.

Noakes, T.D. & St. Clair Gibson, A. (2004) Logical limitations to the "catastrophe" models of fatigue during exercise in humans. *British Journal of Sports Medicine* **38**, 648–649.

Noakes, T.D., St. Clair Gibson, A. & Lambert, E.V. (2004) From catastrophe to complexity: a novel model of integrative central neural regulation of effort and fatigue during exercise in humans. *British Journal of Sports Medicine* **38**, 511–514.

Noakes, T.D., St. Clair Gibson, A. & Lambert, E.V. (2005) From catastrophe to complexity: a novel model of integrative central neural regulation of effort and fatigue during exercise in humans: summary and conclusions. *British Journal of Sports Medicine* **39**, 120–124.

Nybo, L. (2003) CNS fatigue and prolonged exercise: effect of glucose supplementation. *Medicine and Science in Sports and Exercise* **35**, 589–594.

Nybo, L., Nielsen, B., Pedersen, B.K., Moller, K. & Secher, N.H. (2002) Interleukin-6 release from the human brain during prolonged exercise. *Journal of Physiology* **542**, 991–995.

O'Kroy, J.A. & Coast, J.R. (1993) Effects of flow and resistive training on respiratory endurance and strength. *Journal of Applied Physiology* **41**, 508–516.

O'Neill, D.S., Zheng, D., Anderson, W.K., Dohm, G.L. & Houmard, J.A. (1999) Effect of endurance exercise on myosin heavy chain gene regulation in human skeletal muscle. *American Journal of Physiology* **276**, R414–R419.

Orlander, J., Kiessling, K.H., Karlsson, J. & Ekblom, B. (1977). Low intensity training, inactivity and resumed training in sedentary men. *Acta Physiologica Scandanavica* **101**, 351–362.

Ortenblad, N., Lunde, P.K., Levin, K., Andersen, J.L. & Pedersen, P.K. (2000) Enhanced sarcoplasmic reticulum Ca^{2+} release following intermittent sprint training. *American Journal of Physiology* **279**, R152–R160.

Oscai, L., Williams, R. & Hertig, B. (1968) Effect of exercise on blood volume. *Journal of Applied Physiology* **24**, 622–624.

Osternig, L.R., Hamill, J., Lander, J.E. & Robertson, R. (1986) Co-activation of sprinter and distance runner muscles in isokinetic exercise. *Medicine and Science in Sports and Exercise* **18**, 431–435.

Overgaard, K., Nielsen, O.B., Flatman, J.A. & Clausen, T. (1999) Relations between excitability and contractility in rat soleus muscle: role of the Na^+-K^+ pump and Na^+/K^+ gradients. *Journal of Physiology* **518**, 215–225.

Padilla, S., Mujika, I., Angulo, F. & Goiriena, J.J. (2000) Scientific approach to the 1-h cycling world record: a case study. *Journal of Applied Physiology* **89**, 1522–1527.

Palmer, G.S., Dennis, S.C., Noakes, T.D. & Hawley, J.A. (1996) Assessment of the reproducibility of performance testing on an air-braked cycle ergometer. *International Journal of Sports Medicine* **17**, 293–298.

Pan, J.T. (1991) Neuroendocrine control of prolactin secretion: the role of the serotonergic system. *Chinese Journal of Physiology* **34**, 45–64.

Pannier, J.L., Bouckaert, J.J. & Lefebvre, R.A. (1995) The antiserotonin agent pizotifen does not increase endurance performance in humans. *European Journal of Applied Physiology and Occupational Physiology* **72**, 175–178.

Park, E., Chan, O., Li, Q., Kiraly, M., Matthews, S.G., Vranic, M., *et al.* (2005) Changes in basal hypothalamo–pituitary–adrenal activity during exercise training are centrally mediated. *American Journal of Physiology Regulatory, Integrative and Comparative Physiology* **289**, R1360–R1371.

Pascoe, D.D., Costill, D.L., Fink, W.J., Roberts, R.A. & Zachwieja, J.J. (1993) Glycogen resynthesis in skeletal muscle following resistive exercise. *Medicine and Science in Sports and Exercise* **25**, 349–354.

Pearson, S.J., Young, A., Macaluso, A., Devito, G., Nimmo, M.A., Cobbold, M., *et al.* (2002) Muscle function in elite master weightlifters. *Medicine and Science in Sports and Exercise* **34**, 1199–1206.

Pedersen, B.K., Steensberg, A., Fischer, C., Keller, C., Keller, P., Plomgaard, P., *et al.* (2004) The metabolic role of IL-6 produced during exercise: is IL-6 an exercise factor? *Proceedings of the Nutrition Society* **63**, 263–267.

Pelliccia, A., Culasso, F., Di Paolo, F.M. & Maron, B.J. (1999) Physiologic left ventricular cavity dilatation in elite athletes. *Annals of Internal Medicine* **130**, 23–31.

Pelliccia, A. & Maron, B.J. (1997) Outer limits of the athlete's heart, the effect of gender, and relevance to the differential diagnosis with primary cardiac diseases. *Cardiology Clinics* **15**, 381–396.

Pelliccia, A., Maron, B.J., De Luca, R., Di Paolo, F.M., Spataro, A. & Culasso, F. (2002) Remodeling of left ventricular hypertrophy in elite athletes after long-term deconditioning. *Circulation* **105**, 944–949.

Pelliccia, A., Maron, B.J., Di Paolo, F.M., Biffi, A., Quattrini, F.M., Pisicchio, C., *et al.* (2005) Prevalence and clinical significance of left atrial remodeling in competitive athletes. *Journal of the American College of Cardiology* **46**, 690–696.

Pelliccia, A., Maron, B.J., Spataro, A., Proschan, M.A. & Spirito, P. (1991) The upper limit of physiologic cardiac hypertrophy in highly trained elite athletes. *New England Journal of Medicine* **324**, 295–301.

Pensini, M., Martin, A. & Maffiuletti, M.A. (2002) Central versus peripheral adaptations following eccentric resistance training. *International Journal of Sports Medicine* **23**, 567–574.

Peronnet, F., Ferguson, R.J., Perrault, H., Ricci, G. & Lajoie, D. (1981) Echocardiography and the athlete's heart. *The Physician and Sports Medicine* **9**, 103–112.

Perot, C., Goubel, F. & Mora, I. (1991) Quantification of T and H responses before and after a period of endurance training. *European Journal of Applied Physiology* **63**, 368–375.

Pette, D. & Staron, R.S. (1997) Mammalian skeletal muscle fiber type transitions. *International Review of Cytology* **170**, 143–223.

Phillips, S.M. (2000) Short-term training: when do repeated bouts of resistance exercise become training? *Canadian Journal of Applied Physiology* **25**, 185–193.

Phillips, S., Tipton, K., Aarsland, A., Wolf, S. & Wolfe, R. (1997) Mixed muscle protein synthesis and breakdown after resistance exercise in humans. *American Journal of Physiology* **273**, E99–E107.

Pilegaard, H., Domino, K., Noland, T., Juel, C., Hellsten, Y., Halestrap, A.P., *et al.* (1999a) Effect of high-intensity exercise training on lactate/H^+ transport capacity in human skeletal muscle. *American Journal of Physiology, Endocrinology Metabolism* **276**, E255–E261.

Pilegaard, H., Ordway, G.A., Saltin, B. & Neufer, P.D. (2000) Transcriptional regulation of gene expression in human skeletal muscle during recovery from exercise. *American Journal of Physiology, Endocrinology Metabolism* **279**, E806–E814.

Pilegaard, H., Terzis, G., Halestrap, A. & Juel, C. (1999b) Distribution of the lactate/H^+ transporter isoforms MCT1 and MCT4 in human skeletal muscle. *American Journal of Physiology, Endocrinology Metabolism* **276**, E843–E848.

Plotnick, G.D., Becker, L.C., Fisher, M.L., Gerstenblith, G., Renlund, D.G., Fleg, J.L., *et al.* (1986) Use of the Frank–Starling mechanism during submaximal versus maximal upright exercise. *American Journal of Physiology* **251**, H1101–H1105.

Ploutz, L.L., Tesch, P.A., Biro, R.L. & Dudley, G.A. (1994) Effect of resistance training on muscle use during exercise. *Journal of Applied Physiology* **76**, 1675–1681.

Pluim, B.M., Zwinderman, A.H., Van der Laarse, A. & Van der Wall, E.E. (2000) The athlete's heart: a meta-analysis of cardiac structure and function. *Circulation* **101**, 336–344.

Powers, S.K., Criswell, D., Lawler, J., Martin, D., Ji, L.L., Herb, R.A., *et al.* (1994) Regional training-induced alterations in diaphragmatic oxidative and antioxidant enzymes. *Respiratory Physiology* **95**, 227–237.

Powers, S.K., Criswell, D., Lieu, F.K., Dodd, S. & Silverman, H. (1992) Diaphragmatic fiber type specific adaptation to endurance exercise. *Respiratory Physiology* **89**, 195–207.

Powers, S.K., Dodd, S., Lawler, J., Landry, G., Kirtley, M., McNight, T., *et al.* (1988) Incidence of exercise induced hypoxemia in elite endurance athletes at sea level. *European Journal of Applied Physiology* **58**, 298–302.

Proske, U. & Allen, T.J. (2005) Damage to skeletal muscle from eccentric exercise. *Exercise and Sport Sciences Reviews* **33**, 98–104.

Proske, U. & Morgan, D.L. (2001) Muscle damage from eccentric exercise: mechanism, mechanical signs, adaptation and clinical applications. *Journal of Physiology* **537**, 333–345.

Putnam, C.T., Xu, X., Gillies, E., MacLean, I.M. & Bell, G.J. (2004) Effects of strength, endurance and combined training on myosin heavy chain content and fibre-type distribution in humans. *European Journal of Applied Physiology* **92**, 376–384.

Radak, Z., Pucsok, J., Mecseki, S., Csont, T. & Ferdinandy, P. (1999) Muscle soreness-induced reduction in force generation is accompanied by increased nitric oxide content and DNA damage in human skeletal muscle. *Free Radical Biology and Medicine* **26**, 1059–1063.

Ranganathan, V.K., Siemionow, V., Liu, J.Z., Sahgal, V. & Yue, G.H. (2004) From mental power to muscle power: gaining strength by using the mind. *Neuropsychologia* **42**: 944–956.

Rasmussen, B., Klausen, K., Clausen, J.P. & Trap-Jensen, J. (1975) Pulmonary ventilation, blood gases, and blood pH after training of the arms or the legs. *Journal of Applied Physiology* **38**, 250–256.

Ratamess, N.A., Kraemer, W.J., Volek, J.S., et al. (2005) Effects of heavy resistance exercise volume on post-exercise androgen receptor content in resistance-trained men. *Journal of Steroid Biochemistry and Molecular Biology* **93**, 35–42.

Rauch, H.G., St. Clair Gibson, A., Lambert, E.V. & Noakes, T.D. (2005) A signalling role for muscle glycogen in the regulation of pace during prolonged exercise. *British Journal of Sports Medicine* **39**, 34–38.

Rice, A.J., Scroop, G.C., Gore, C.J., Thornton, A.T., Chapman, M.A.J., Greville, H.W., et al. (1999) Exercise-induced hypoxaemia in highly trained cyclists at 40% peak oxygen uptake. *European Journal of Applied Physiology* **79**, 353–359.

Richards, J.C., McKenzie, D.C., Warburton, D.E., Road, J.D. & Sheel, A.W. (2004) Prevalence of exercise-induced arterial hypoxemia in healthy women. *Medicine and Science in Sports and Exercise* **36**, 1514–1521.

Richter, E.A., Kristiansen, S., Wojtaszewski, J., Daugaard, J.R., Asp, S., Hespel, P., et al. (1998) Training effects on muscle glucose transport during exercise. *Advances in Experimental and Medical Biology* **441**, 107–116.

Rico, H., Revilla, M., Villa, L.F., Ruiz-Contreras, D., Hernandez, E.R. & Alvarez de Buergo, M. (1994) The four-compartment models in body composition: data from a study with dual-energy X-ray absorptiometry and near-infrared interactance on 815 normal subjects. *Metabolism* **43**, 417–422.

Ritzer, T.F., Bove, A.A. & Carey, R.A. (1980) Left ventricular performance characteristics in trained and sedentary dogs. *Journal of Applied Physiology: Respiratory, Environmental Exercise Physiology* **48**, 130–138.

Roberts, A.D., Billeter, R. & Howald, H. (1982) Anaerobic muscle enzyme changes after interval training. *International Journal of Sports Medicine* **3**, 18–21.

Roberts, D. & Smith, D.J. (1989) Biochemical aspects of peripheral muscle fatigue: a review. *Sports Medicine* **7**, 125–138.

Robinson, B.F., Epstein, S.E., Kahler, R.L. & Braunwald, E. (1966) Circulatory effects of acute expansion of blood volume: Studies during maximal exercise and at rest. *Circulation Research* **19**, 26–32.

Rollhäuser, H. (1954) Funktionelle Anpassung der Sehnenfaser im submikroskopischen Bereich. *Anatomischer Anzeiger* **51**, 318–322.

Ross, A. & Leveritt, M. (2001) Long-term metabolic and skeletal muscle adaptations to short-sprint training: implications for sprint training and tapering. *Sports Medicine* **31**, 1063–1082.

Rothe, C.F. (1986) Physiology of venous return: an unappreciated boost to the heart. *Archives of Internal Medicine* **146**, 977–982.

Rubin, C.T. & Lanyon, L.E. (1984) Regulation of bone formation by applied dynamic loads. *Journal of Bone and Joint Surgery American* **66**, 397–402.

Rutherford, O.M. & Jones, D.A. (1986) The role of learning and coordination in strength training. *European Journal of Applied Physiology* **55**, 100–105.

Sahlin, K. (1992) Metabolic factors in fatigue. *Sports Medicine* **13**, 99–107.

Sahlin, K. & Henriksson, J. (1984) Buffer capacity and lactate accumulation in skeletal muscle of trained and untrained men. *Acta Physiologica Scandinavica* **122**, 331–339.

Sale, D.G. (2003) Neural adaptations to strength training. In: *Strength and Power in Sport*, 2nd edn. (Komi, P.V., ed.) Blackwell Science, Malden, MA: 281–314.

Sale, D.G. & MacDougall, D. (1981) Specificity in strength training: a review for the coach and athlete. *Canadian Journal of Applied Sports Sciences* **6**, 87–92.

Sale, D.G., McComas, A.J., MacDougall, J.D. & Upton, A.R.M. (1982) Neuromuscular adaptation in human thenar muscles following strength training and immobilization. *Journal of Applied Physiology* **53**, 419–424.

Sale, D.G., Upton, A.R.M., McComas, A.J. & MacDougall, J.D. (1983a) Neuromuscular functions in weight-trainers. *Experimental Neurology* **82**, 521–531.

Sale, D.G., MacDougall, J.D., Upton, A.R.M. & McComas, A.J. (1983b) Effect of strength training upon motoneuron excitability in man. *Medicine and Science in Sports and Exercise* **15**, 57–62.

Saltin, B. (1964) Circulatory response to submaximal and maximal exercise after thermal dehydration. *Journal of Applied Physiology* **19**, 1125–1132.

Saltin, B. & Calbet, J.A. (2006) Counterpoint: In health and in a normoxic environment, $\dot{V}o_{2max}$ is limited primarily by cardiac output and locomotor muscle blood flow. *Journal of Applied Physiology* **100**, 744–745.

Saltin, B., Henriksson, J., Nygaard, E., Andersen, P. & Jansson, E. (1977) Fiber types and metabolic potentials of skeletal muscles in sedentary man and endurance runners. *Annals of the New York Academy of Sciences* **301**, 3–29.

Saltin, B. & Karlsson, J. (1971) Muscle glycogen utilization during work of different intensities. In: *Muscle Metabolism During Exercise* (Saltin, P., ed.) Plenum Press, New York: 289–299.

Saltin, B. & Rowell, L.B. (1980) Functional adaptations to physical activity and inactivity. *Federal Proceedings* **39**, 1506–1513.

Schantz, P.G. & Kallman, M. (1989) NADH shuttle enzymes and cytochrome b5 reductase in human skeletal muscle: effect of strength training. *Journal of Applied Physiology* **67**, 123–127.

Scheuer, J. & Tipton, C.M. (1977) Cardiovascular adaptations to physical training. *Annual Reviews of Physiology* **39**, 221–251.

Schumacher, Y.O., Vogt, S., Roecker, K., Schmid, A. & Coyle, E.F. (2005) Scientific considerations for physiological evaluations of elite athletes. *Journal of Applied Physiology* **99**, 1630–1631; author reply 1631–1632.

Scott, A., Khan, K.M., Heer, J., Cook, J.L., Lian, O. & Duronio, V. (2005) High strain mechanical loading rapidly induces tendon apoptosis: an *ex vivo* rat tibialis anterior model. *British Journal of Sports Medicine* **39**, e25.

Seals, D.R., Hagberg, J.M., Spina, R.J., Rogers, M.A., Schechtman, K.B. & Ehsani, A.A. (1994) Enhanced left ventricular performance in endurance trained older men. *Circulation* **89**, 198–205.

See, E.K.N., Ng, G.Y.F., Ng, C.O.Y. & Fung, D.T.C. (2004) Running exercise improves the strength of a partially ruptured Achilles tendon. *British Journal of Sports Medicine* **38**, 597–600.

Seger, J.Y. & Thorstensson, A. (2005) Effects of eccentric versus concentric training on thigh muscle strength and EMG. *International Journal of Sports Medicine* **26**, 45–52.

Segura, R. & Ventura, J.L. (1988) Effect of L-tryptophan supplementation on exercise performance. *International Journal of Sports Medicine* **9**, 301–305.

Sejersted, O.M., Vollestad, N.K. & Medbo, J.I. (1986) Muscle fluid and electrolyte balance during and following exercise. *Acta Physiologica Scandinavica Supplement* **556**, 119–127.

Semmler, J.G., Sale, M.V., Meyer, F.G. & Nordstrom, M.A. (2004) Motor-unit coherence and its relation with synchrony are influenced by training. *Journal of Neurophysiology* **92**, 3320–3331.

Sharp, R.L., Costill, D.L., Fink, W.J. & King, D.S. (1986) Effects of eight weeks of bicycle ergometer sprint training on human muscle buffer capacity. *International Journal of Sports Medicine* **7**, 13–17.

Sheel, A.W. (2002) Respiratory muscle training in healthy individuals: physiological rationale and implications for exercise performance. *Sports Medicine* **32**, 567–581.

Sheel, A.W., Derchak, P.A., Morgan, B.J., Pegelow, D.F., Jacques, A.J. & Dempsey, J.A. (2001) Fatiguing inspiratory muscle work causes reflex reduction in resting leg blood flow in humans. *Journal of Physiology (London)* **537**, 277–289.

Shima, S.N., Ishida, K., Katayama, K., Morotome, Y., Sato, Y. & Miyamura, M. (2002) Cross education of muscular strength during unilateral resistance training and detraining. *European Journal of Applied Physiology* **86**, 287–294.

Shinohara, M., Kouzaki, M., Yoshihisa, T. & Fukunaga, T. (1998) Efficacy of tourniquet ischemia for strength training with low resistance. *European Journal of Applied Physiology* **77**, 189–191.

Short, K.R., Vittone, J.L., Bigelow, M.L., *et al.* (2005) Changes in myosin heavy chain mRNA and protein expression in human skeletal muscle with age and endurance exercise training. *Journal of Applied Physiology* **99**, 95–102.

Sieck, G.C. & Prakash, Y.S. (1997) Morphological adaptations of neuromuscular junctions depend on fiber type. *Canadian Journal of Applied Physiology* **22**, 197–230.

Sievänen, H., Heinonen, A. & Kannus, P. (1996) Adaptation of bone to altered loading environment: biomechanical approach using X-ray absorptiometric data from the patella of a young woman. *Bone* **19**, 55–59.

Simonsen, E.B., Klitgaard, H. & Bojsen-Moller, F. (1995) The influence of strength training, swim training and ageing on the Achilles tendon and m. soleus of the rat. *Journal of Sports Sciences* **13**, 291–295.

Sjogaard, G. (1983) Electrolytes in slow and fast muscle fibers of humans at rest and with dynamic exercise. *American Journal of Physiology* **245**, R25–31.

Sjogaard, G. (1986) Water and electrolyte fluxes during exercise and their relation to muscle fatigue. *Acta Physiologica Scandinavica Supplement* **556**, 129–136.

Sjogaard, G., Adams, R.P. & Saltin, B. (1985) Water and ion shifts in skeletal muscle of humans with intense dynamic knee extension. *American Journal of Physiology* **248**, R190–196.

Smith, R.C. & Rutherford, O.M. (1995) The role of metabolites in strength training. I. A comparison of eccentric and concentric contractions. *European Journal of Applied Physiology* **71**, 332–336.

Somjen, G., Carpenter, D.O. & Henneman, E. (1965) Responses of motoneurons of different sizes to graded stimulation of supraspinal centers of the brain. *Journal of Neurophysiology* **28**, 958–965.

Sommer, H-M. (1987) The biomechanical and metabolic effect of a running regiment on the Achilles tendon in the rat. *Orthopaedics* **11**, 71–75.

Sonetti, D.A., Wetter, T.J., Pegelow, D.F. & Dempsey, J.A. (2001) Effects of respiratory muscle training versus placebo on endurance exercise performance. *Respiratory, Physiology and Neurobiology* **127**, 185–199.

Spengler, C.M., Roos, M., Laube, S.M. & Boutellier, U. (1999) Decreased exercise blood lactate concentrations after respiratory endurance training in humans. *European Journal of Applied Physiology and Occupational Physiology* **79**, 299–305.

Spina, R.J., Ogawa, T., Martin, W.H.D., Coggan, A.R., Holloszy, J.O. & Ehsani, A.A. (1992) Exercise training prevents decline in stroke volume during exercise in young healthy subjects. *Journal of Applied Physiology* **72**, 2458–2462.

Spirito, P., Pelliccia, A., Proschan, M.A., Granata, M., Spataro, A., Bellone, P., *et al.* (1994) Morphology of the "athlete's heart" assessed by echocardiography in 947 elite athletes representing 27 sports. *American Journal of Cardiology* **74**, 802–806.

Spriet, L., Gledhill, N., Froese, A.B. & Wilkes, D. L. (1986) Effect of graded erythrocythemia on cardiovascular and metabolic responses to exercise. *Journal of Applied Physiology* **61**, 1942–1948.

Spriet, L.L., Gledhill, N., Froese, A.B., Wilkes, D.L. & Meyers, E.C. (1980) The effect of induced erythrocythemia on central circulation and oxygen transport during maximal exercise. *Medicine and Science in Sports and Exercise* **12**, 122–123.

Spriet, L.L., Soderlund, K., Bergstrom, M. & Hultman, E. (1987a) Anaerobic energy release in skeletal muscle during electrical stimulation in men. *Journal of Applied Physiology* **62**, 611–615.

Spriet, L.L., Soderlund, K., Bergstrom, M. & Hultman, E. (1987b) Skeletal muscle glycogenolysis, glycolysis, and pH during electrical stimulation in men. *Journal of Applied Physiology* **62**, 616–621.

Stallknecht, B. (2003) Influence of physical training on adipose tissue metabolism – with special focus on effects of insulin and epinephrine. PhD thesis, University of Copenhagen, Denmark.

Stallknecht, B., Bulow, J., Frandsen, E. & Galbo, H. (1990) Diminished epinephrine response to hypoglycemia despite enlarged adrenal medulla in trained rats. *American Journal of Physiology* **259**, R998–R1003.

Stanish, W.D., Curwin, S. & Rubinovich, M. (1985) Tendinitis: the analysis and treatment for running. *Clinical Sports Medicine* **4**, 593–609.

Staron, R.S. (1997) The classification of human skeletal muscle fiber types. *Journal of Strength and Conditioning Research* **11**, 67.

Staron, R.S., Malicky, E.S., Leonardi, M.J., Falkel, J.E., Hagerman, F.C. & Dudley, G.A. (1989) Muscle hypertrophy and fast fiber type conversions in heavy resistance-trained women. *European Journal of Applied Physiology* **60**, 71–79.

Staron, R.S., Karapondo, D.L., Kraemer, W.J., *et al.* (1994) Skeletal muscle adaptations during early phase of heavy-resistance training in men and women. *Journal of Applied Physiology* **76**, 1247–1255.

St. Clair Gibson, A. & Noakes, T.D. (2004) Evidence for complex system integration and dynamic neural regulation of skeletal muscle recruitment during exercise in humans. *British Journal of Sports Medicine* **38**, 797–806.

Stensrud, T., Ingjer, F., Holm, H. & Stromme, S.B. (1992) L-tryptophan supplementation does not improve running performance. *International Journal of Sports Medicine* **13**, 481–485.

Stepto, N.K., Hawley, J.A., Dennis, S.C. & Hopkins, W.G. (1999) Effects of different interval-training programs on cycling time-trial performance. *Medicine and Science in Sports and Exercise* **31**, 736–741.

Stone, M.H. (1990) Muscle conditioning and muscle injuries. *Medicine and Science in Sports and Exercise* **22**, 457–462.

Stone, M.H. (1991) Connective tissue and bone response to strength training. In: *Strength and Power in Sport: The Encyclopedia of Sports Medicine* (Komi, P.V., ed.) Blackwell, Oxford: 279–290.

Stray-Gundersen, J., Musch, T.I., Haidet, G.C., Swain, D.P., Ordway, G.A. & Mitchell, J.H. (1986) The effect of pericardiectomy on maximal oxygen consumption and maximal cardiac output in untrained dogs. *Circulation Research* **58**, 523–530.

Struder, H.K., Hollmann, W., Duperly, J. & Weber, K. (1995) Amino acid metabolism in tennis and its possible influence on the neuroendocrine system. *British Journal of Sports Medicine* **29**, 28–30.

Struder, H.K., Hollmann, W., Platen, P., Donike, M., Gotzmann, A. & Weber, K. (1998) Influence of paroxetine, branched-chain amino acids and tyrosine on neuroendocrine system responses and fatigue in humans. *Hormone and Metabolic Research* **30**, 188–194.

Struder, H.K., Hollmann, W., Platen, P., Duperly, J., Fischer, H.G. & Weber, K. (1996) Alterations in plasma free tryptophan and large neutral amino acids do not affect perceived exertion and prolactin during 90 min of treadmill exercise. *International Journal of Sports Medicine* **17**, 73–79.

Stuessi, C., Spengler, C.M., Knopfli-Lenzin, C., Markov, G. & Boutellier, U. (2001) Respiratory muscle endurance training in humans increases cycling endurance without affecting blood gas concentrations. *European Journal of Applied Physiology* **84**, 582–586.

Stulen, F.B. & DeLuca, C.J. (1978) The relation between the myoelectric signal and physiological properties of constant-force isometric contractions. *Electroencephalography and Clinical Neurophysiology* **45**, 681–698.

Steinacker, J.M., Lormes, W., Reissnecker, S. & Liu, Y. (2004) New aspects of the hormone and cytokine response to training. *European Journal of Applied Physiology* **91**, 382–391.

Tiidus, P.M. (2005) Can oestrogen influence skeletal muscle damage, inflammation, and repair? *British Journal of Sports Medicine* **39**, 251–253.

Tremblay, M.S., Copeland, J.L. & Van Helder, W. (2005) Influence of exercise duration on post-exercise steroid hormone responses in trained males. *European Journal of Applied Physiology* **94**, 505–513.

Tanaka, H., Costill, D.L., Thomas, R., Fink, W.J. & Widrick, J.J. (1993) Dry-land resistance training for competitive swimming. *Medicine and Science in Sports and Exercise* **25**, 952–959.

Taniguchi, Y. (1997) Lateral specificity in resistance training: the effect of bilateral and unilateral training. *European Journal of Applied Physiology* **75**, 144–150.

Ter Haar Romeny, B.M., Dernier Van Der Goen, J.J. & Gielen, C.C.A.M. (1982) Changes in recruitment order of motor units in the human biceps muscle. *Experimental Neurology* **78**, 360–368.

Tesch, P.A. (1987) Acute and long term metabolic changes consequent to heavy resistance exercise. In: *Medicine and Sport Science* (Hebbelinck, M. & Shephard, R.J., eds). Karger, Basel: 26, 67–89.

Tesch, P.A., Colliander, E.B. & Kaiser, P. (1986) Muscle metabolism during intense, heavy-resistance exercise. *European Journal of Applied Physiology* **55**, 362–366.

Tesch, P.A., Komi, P.V. & Hakkinen, K. (1987) Enzymatic adaptations consequent to long-term strength training. *International Journal of Sports Medicine* **8** (Supplement 1), 66–69.

Tesch, P., Sjodin, B., Thorstensson, A. & Karlsson, J. (1978) Muscle fatigue and its relation to lactate accumulation and LDH activity in man. *Acta Physiologica Scandinavica* **103**, 413–420.

Tesch, P.A. (1988) Skeletal muscle adaptations consequent to long-term heavy resistance exercise. *Medicine and Science in Sports and Exercise* **20** (Supplement), S132–S134.

Tesch, P.A. & Larsson, L. (1982) Muscle hypertrophy in bodybuilders. *European Journal of Applied Physiology* **49**, 301–306.

Thomas, C.K., Woods, J.J. & Bigland-Ritchie, B. (1989) Impulse propagation and muscle activation in long maximal voluntary contractions. *Journal of Applied Physiology* **67**, 1835–1842.

Thorstensson, A., Hulten, B., von Dobeln, W. & Karlsson, J. (1976) Effect of strength training on enzyme activities and fibre characteristics in human skeletal muscle. *Acta Physiologica Scandinavica* **96**, 392–398.

Thorstensson, A., Karlsson Viitasalo, J.H.T., Luhtanen, P. & Komi, P.V. (1976) Effect of strength training on EMG of human skeletal muscle. *Acta Physiologica Scandinavica* **98**, 232–236.

Tipton, C.M., James, S.L., Merger, W., Tcheng, T.K. (1970) Influence of exercise on the strength of the medial collateral ligaments of dogs. *American Journal of Physiology* **218**, 894–902.

Tipton, C.M., Matthes, R.D., Maynard, J.A. & Carey, R.A. (1975) The influence of physical activity on ligaments and tendons. *Medicine and Science in Sports and Exercise* **7**, 165–175.

Tipton, C.M., Schields, R.J. & Tomanek, R.J. (1967) Influence of physical activity on the strength of knee ligaments in rats. *American Journal of Physiology* **212**, 783–787.

Tipton, C.M., Vailas, A.C. & Matthes, R.D. (1986) Experimental studies on the influences of physical activity on ligaments, tendons and joints: a brief review. *Acta Medica Scandinavica* **71**, 157–168.

Tipton, K.D., Rasmussen, B.B., Miller, S.L., Wolf, S.E., Owens-Stovall, S.K., Petrini, B.E., *et al.* (2001) Timing of amino acid-carbohydrate ingestion alters anabolic response of muscle to resistance exercise. *American Journal of Physiology* **281**, E197–206.

Tittel, K. & Otto, H. (1970) Der Einfluss eines Lauftrainings Unterschiedlichen Dauer und Intensität auf die Hypertrophie, Zugfestigkeit un Dehnungsfähigkeit des straffen Kollagenen Bindegewebes (am Beispiel der Achillessehne). *Medizin Sport* **10**, 308–312.

Trimble, M.H. & Enoka, R. (1991) Mechanisms underlying the training effects associated with neuromuscular electrical stimulation. *Physical Therapy* **71**, 273–282.

Todd, G., Taylor, J.L. & Gandevia, S.C. (2003) Measurement of voluntary activation of fresh and fatigued human muscles using transcranial magnetic stimulation. *Journal of Physiology* **551**, 661–671.

Tuite, D.J., Renström, P.A.F.H. & O'Brien, M. (1997) The aging tendon. *Scandinavian Journal of Medicine and Science in Sports* **7**, 72–77.

Turner, C.H. (1991) Homeostatic control of bone structure: an application of feedback theory. *Bone* **12**, 203–217.

Turner, C.H. (1998) Three rules for bone adaptation to mechanical stimuli. *Bone* **23**, 309–407.

Turner, C.H., Robling, A.G., Turner, C.H. & Robling, A.G. (2003) Designing exercise regimens to increase bone strength. *Exercise and Sport Sciences Reviews* **31**, 45–50.

Ulmer, H.V. (1996) Concept of an extracellular regulation of muscular metabolic rate during heavy exercise in humans by psychophysiological feedback. *Experientia* **52**, 416–420.

Umemura, Y., Ishiko, T., Yamauchi, T., Kurono, M. & Mashiko, S. (1997) Five jumps per day increase bone mass and breaking force in rats. *Journal of Bone and Mineral Research* **12**, 1480–1485.

Umemura, Y., Sogo, N. & Honda, A. (2002) Effects of intervals between jumps or bouts on osteogenic response to loading. *Journal of Applied Physiology* **93**, 1345–1348.

Underwood, R.H. & Schwade, J.L. (1977) Noninvasive analysis of cardiac function of elite distance runners-echocardiography, vectocardiography and cardiac intervals. *Annals of New York Academy of Science* **301**, 297–309.

Uusi-Rasi, K., Kannus, P., Cheng, S., Sievanen, H., Pasanen, M., Heinonen, A., *et al.* (2003) Effect of alendronate and exercise on bone and physical performance of postmenopausal women: a randomized controlled trial. *Bone* **33**, 132–143.

Uusi-Rasi, K., Sievanen, H., Pasanen, M., Oja, P. & Vuori, I. (2002) Associations of calcium intake and physical activity with bone density and size in premenopausal and postmenopausal women: a peripheral quantitative computed tomography study. *Journal of Bone and Mineral Research* **17**, 544–552.

Uusi-Rasi, K., Sievanen, H., Vuori, I., Heinonen, A., Kannus, P., Pasanen, M., *et al.* (1999) Long-term recreational gymnastics, estrogen use, and selected risk factors for osteoporotic fractures. *Journal of Bone and Mineral Research* **14**, 1231–1238.

Vailas, A.C., Pedrini, V.A., Pedrini-Mille, A. & Holloszy, J.O. (1985) Patellar tendon matrix changes associated with aging and voluntary exercise. *Journal of Applied Physiology* **58**, 1572–1576.

Van Custem, M., Duchateau, J. & Hainut, K. (1998) Changes in single motor unit behaviour contribute to the increase in contraction speed after dynamic training in humans. *Journal of Physiology* **513**, 295–305.

van Hall, G., Raaymakers, J.S., Saris, W.H. & Wagenmakers, A.J. (1995) Ingestion of branched-chain amino acids and tryptophan during sustained exercise in man: failure to affect performance. *Journal of Physiology* **486**, 789–794.

Vanoverschelde, J.L., Younis, L.T., Melin, J.A., Vanbutsele, R., Leclercq, B., Robert, A.R., *et al.* (1991) Prolonged exercise induces left ventricular dysfunction in healthy subjects. *Journal of Applied Physiology* **70**, 1356–1363.

Varnier, M., Sarto, P., Martines, D., Lora, L., Carmignoto, F., Leese, G.P., *et al.* (1994) Effect of infusing branched-chain amino acid during incremental exercise

with reduced muscle glycogen content. *European Journal of Applied Physiology and Occupational Physiology* **69**, 26–31.

Vergara, J.L., Rapoprot, S.I. & Nassar-Gentina, V. (1977) Fatigue and posttetanic potentiation in single muscle fibers of the frog. *American Journal of Physiology* **232**, C185–190.

Viidik, A. (1968) Elasticity and tensile strength of the anterior cruciate ligament in rabbits as influenced by training. *Acta Physiologica Scandinavica* **74**, 372–380.

Viidik, A. (1967) The effect of training on the tensile strength of isolated rabbit tendons. *Journal of Plastic and Reconstructive Surgery* **1**, 141–147.

Vilarta, R. & de Campos Vidal, B. (1989) Anisotropic and biomechanical properties of tendons modified by exercise and denervation: aggregation and macromolecular order in collagen bundles. *Matrix* **9**, 55–61.

Volianitis, S., McConnell, A.K., Koutedakis, Y., McNaughton, L., Backx, K. & Jones, D.A. (2001) Inspiratory muscle training improves rowing performance. *Medicine and Science in Sports and Exercise* **33**, 803–809.

Vollestad, N.K. & Sejersted, O.M. (1988) Biochemical correlates of fatigue: a brief review. *European Journal of Applied Physiology amd Occupational Physiology* **57**, 336–347.

Vollestad, N.K., Sejersted, O.M., Bahr, R., Woods, J.J. & Bigland-Ritchie, B. (1988) Motor drive and metabolic responses during repeated submaximal contractions in humans. *Journal of Applied Physiology* **64**, 1421–1427.

Vrabas, I.S., Dodd, S.L., Powers, S.K., Hughes, M., Coombes, J., Fletcher, L., *et al.* (1999) Endurance training reduces the rate of diaphragm fatigue *in vitro*. *Medicine and Science in Sports and Exercise* **31**, 1605–1612.

Waldegger, S., Busch, G.L., Kaba, N.K., *et al.* (1997) Effect of cellular hydration on protein metabolism. *Mineral & Electrolyte Metabolism* **23**, 201–205.

Wallace, J.D., Cuneo, R.C., Bidlingmaier, M., Lundberg, P.A., Carlsson, L., Boguszewski, C.L., *et al.* (2001) The response of molecular isoforms of growth hormone to acute exercise in trained adult males. *Journal of Clinical Endocrinology and Metabolism* **86**, 200–206.

Wang, N., Hikida, R.S., Staron, R.S. & Simoneau, J.A. (1993) Muscle fiber types of women after resistance training: quantitative ultrastructure and enzyme

activity. *Pflugers Archives* **424**, 494–502.

Warburton, D.E., Gledhill, N. & Quinney, H.A. (2000) Blood volume, aerobic power, and endurance performance: potential ergogenic effect of volume loading. *Clinical Journal of Sport Medicine* **10**, 59–66.

Warburton, D.E., Haykowsky, M.J., Quinney, H.A., Blackmore, D., Teo, K.K., Taylor, D.A., *et al.* (2004) Blood volume expansion and cardiorespiratory function: effects of training modality. *Medicine and Science in Sports and Exercise* **36**, 991–1000.

Warburton, D.E.R. & Gledhill, N. (2006) Comment on Point-Counterpoint: In health and in a normoxic environment, $\dot{V}o_{2max}$ is limited primarily by cardiac output and locomotor muscle blood flow. *Journal of Applied Physiology* **100**, 1415.

Warburton, D.E.R., Gledhill, N., Jamnik, V., Krip, B. & Card, N. (1999) Induced hypervolemia, cardiac function, $\dot{V}o_{2max}$ and performance of elite cyclists. *Medicine and Science in Sports and Exercise* **31**, 800–808.

Warburton, D.E.R., Haykowsky, M.J., Quinney, H.A., Blackmore, D., Teo, K.K. & Humen, D.P. (2002) Myocardial response to incremental exercise in endurance-trained athletes: influence of heart rate, contractility and the Frank–Starling effect. *Experimental Physiology* **87**, 613–622.

Warren, M.P. & Shantha, S. (2000) The female athlete. *Baillieres Best Practice and Research Clinical Endocrinology and Metabolism* **14**, 37–53.

Weir, J.P., Housh, T.J. & Weir, L.L. (1994) Electromyographic evaluation of joint angle specificity and cross-training after isometric training. *Journal of Applied Physiology* **77**, 197–201.

Warren, J.A., Jenkins, R.R., Packer, L., Witt, E.H. & Armstrong, R.B. (1992) Elevated muscle vitamin E does not attenuate eccentric exercise-induced muscle injury. *Journal of Applied Physiology* **72**, 2168–2175.

Welsh, R.C., Warburton, D.E., Humen, D.P., Taylor, D.A., McGavock, J. & Haykowsky, M.J. (2005) Prolonged strenuous exercise alters the cardiovascular response to dobutamine stimulation in male athletes. *Journal of Physiology* **569**, 325–330.

Weltman, A., Weltman, J.Y., Schurrer, R., Evans, W.S., Veldhuis, J.D. & Rogol, A.D. (1992) Endurance training amplifies the pulsatile release of growth hormone: effects of training intensity. *Journal of Applied Physiology* **72**, 2188–2196.

Westerblad, H. & Allen, D.G. (1991) Changes of myoplasmic calcium concentration during fatigue in single mouse muscle fibers. *Journal of General Physiology* **98**, 615–635.

Westerblad, H., Lee, J.A., Lamb, A.G., Bolsover, S.R. & Allen, D.G. (1990) Spatial gradients of intracellular calcium in skeletal muscle during fatigue. *Pflugers Archiv* **415**, 734–740.

Westerblad, H., Lee, J.A., Lannergren, J. & Allen, D.G. (1991) Cellular mechanisms of fatigue in skeletal muscle. *American Journal of Physiology* **261**, C195–209.

Whitehead, N.P., Allen, T.J., Morgan, D.L. & Proske, U. (1998) Damage to human muscle from eccentric exercise after training with concentric exercise. *Journal of Physiology* **512**, 615–620.

Whyte, G.P., George, K., Sharma, S., Lumley, S., Gates, P., Prasad, K., *et al.* (2000) Cardiac fatigue following prolonged endurance exercise of differing distances. *Medicine and Science in Sports Exercise* **32**, 1067–1072.

Widegren, U., Ryder, J.W. & Zierath, J.R. (2001). Mitogen-activated protein kinase signal transduction in skeletal muscle: effects of exercise and muscle contraction. *Acta Physiologica Scandanavica* **172**, 227–238.

Wiebe, C.G., Gledhill, N., Warburton, D.E., Jamnik, V.K. & Ferguson, S. (1998) Exercise cardiac function in endurance-trained males versus females. *Clinical Journal of Sport Medicine* **8**, 272–279.

Wiik, A., Gustafsson, T., Esbjornsson, M., Johansson, O., Ekman, M., Sundberg, C.J., *et al.* (2005) Expression of oestrogen receptor alpha and beta is higher in skeletal muscle of highly endurance-trained than of moderately active men. *Acta Physiologica Scandinavica* **184**, 105–112.

Wilber, R.L. (2001) Current trends in altitude training. *Sports Medicine* **31**, 249–265.

Wiles, C.M., Jones, D.A. & Edwards, R.H. (1981) Fatigue in human metabolic myopathy. *Ciba Foundation Symposium* **82**, 264–282.

Williams, R.S. & Neufer, P.D. (1996) Regulation of gene expression in skeletal muscle by contractile activity. In: *Handbook of Physiology. Exercise: regulation and integration of multiple systems.* Section 12. American Physiological Society, Bethesda, MD: 1124–1150.

Wilmore, J.H., Royce, J., Girandola, R.N., Katch, F.I. & Katch, V.L. (1970) Physiological alterations resulting from a 10-week program of jogging. *Medicine and Science in Sports* **2**, 7–14.

Wilson, W.M. & Maughan, R.J. (1992) Evidence for a possible role of 5-hydroxytryptamine in the genesis of fatigue in man: administration of paroxetine, a 5-HT re-uptake inhibitor, reduces the capacity to perform prolonged exercise. *Experimental Physiology* **77**, 921–924.

Wolfe, L.A. & Cunningham, D.A. (1982) Effects of chronic exercise on cardiac output and its determinants. *Canadian Journal of Physiology and Pharmacology* **60**, 1089–1097.

Wolfe, L.A., Cunningham, D.A., Rechnitzer, P.A. & Nichol, P.M. (1979) Effects of endurance training on left ventricular dimensions in healthy men. *Journal of Applied Physiology* **47**, 207–212.

Wolfe, L.A., Martin, R.P., Watson, D.D., Lasley, R.D. & Burns, D.E. (1985) Chronic exercise and left ventricular structure and function in healthy human subjects. *Journal of Applied Physiology* **58**, 409–415.

Wolski, L.A., McKenzie, D.C. & Wenger, H.A. (1996) Altitude training for improvements in sea level performance. Is the scientific evidence of benefit? *Sports Medicine* **22**, 251–263.

Woo, S.Y., Gomez, M.A., Woo, Y.K. & Akeson, W.H. (1982) Mechanical properties of tendons and ligaments. II. The relationship between immobilization and exercise on tissue remodelling. *Biorheology* **19**, 397–408.

Wyndham, C.H., Rogers, G.G., Senay, L.C. & Mitchell, D. (1976) Acclimatization in a hot humid environment: cardiovascular adjustments. *Journal of Applied Physiology* **40**, 779–785.

Yao, W., Fuglevand, R.J. & Enoka, R.M. (2000) Motor-unit synchronization

increases EMG amplitude and decreases force steadiness of simulated contractions. *Journal of Neurophysiology* **83**, 441–452.

Yue, G. & Cole, K.J. (1992) Strength increases from the motor program: comparison of training with maximal voluntary and imagined muscle contractions. *Journal of Neurophysiology* **67**, 1114–1123.

Yuza, N., Ishida, K. & Miyamura, M. (2000) Cross transfer effects of muscular endurance during training and detraking. *Journal of Sports Medicine and Physical Fitness* **40**, 110–117.

Zamora, A.J. & Marini, J.F. (1988) Tendon and myotendinous junction in an overload skeletal muscle of the rat. *Anatomy and Embryology* **179**, 89–96.

Zanchetta, J.R., Plotkin, H. & Alvarez Filgueira, M.L. (1995) Bone mass in children: normative values for the 2–20-year-old population. *Bone* **16**, 393S–399S.

Zandrino, F., Molinari, G., Smeraldi, A., Odaglia, G., Masperone, M.A. & Sardanelli, F. (2000) Magnetic resonance imaging of athlete's heart: myocardial mass, left ventricular function, and cross-sectional area of the coronary arteries. *European Radiology* **10**, 319–325.

Zehr, E.P. (2002) Considerations for use of the Hoffmann reflex in exercise studies. *European Journal of Applied Physiology* **86**, 455–468.

Zerba, E., Komorowski, T.E. & Faulkner, J.A. (1990) Free radical injury to skeletal muscles of young, adult, and old mice. *American Journal of Physiology* **258**, C429–C435.

Zhou, B., Conlee, R.K., Jensen, R., Fellingham, G.W., George, J.D. & Fisher, A.G. (2001) Stroke volume does not plateau during graded exercise in elite male distance runners. *Medicine and Science in Sports and Exercise* **33**, 1849–1854.

Zierath, J.R. & Hawley, J.A. (2004) Skeletal muscle fiber type: influence on contractile and metabolic properties. *PLoS Biology* **2**, 1523–1527.

Zuckermann, J. & Stull, G.A. (1969) Effects of exercise on knee ligament separation force in rats. *Journal of Applied Physiology* **26**, 716–719.

Chapter 3

The Overtraining Syndrome: Diagnosis and Management

ROMAIN MEEUSEN

The goal in training competitive athletes is to provide training loads that are effective in improving performance. During this process athletes may go through several stages within a competitive season of periodized training. These phases of training range from undertraining, during the period between competitive seasons or during active rest and taper, to overreaching (OR) and overtraining (OT) which include maladaptations and diminished competitive performance (Meeusen *et al.* 2006). When prolonged, excessive training happens concurrent with other stressors and insufficient recovery, performance decrements can result in chronic maladaptations that can lead to the overtraining syndrome (OTS).

Literature on OT has increased enormously; however, the major difficulty is the lack of common and consistent terminology as well as a gold standard for the diagnosis of OTS.

In this chapter we present not only the current state of knowledge on OTS, but we also highlight the difficulties that arise from the literature, especially on the definition of OTS, but also in trying to detect the possible underlying mechanisms that make an athlete to evolve from acute fatigue to a state of OR and eventually OTS.

Definition

Successful training must involve overload but also must avoid the combination of excessive training plus inadequate recovery. The process of intensifying training is commonly employed by athletes in an attempt to enhance performance. As a consequence, the athlete may experience acute feelings of fatigue and decreases in performance as a result of a single intense training session, or an intense training period. The resultant acute fatigue, in combination with adequate rest, can be followed by a positive adaptation or improvement in performance (supercompensation) and is the basis of effective training programs. However, when the athlete's capacity for adaptation becomes oversolicited through insufficient recovery a maladaptive training response may occur.

OTS is not only a complex condition, making it very difficult to diagnose, but until now the literature has been very inconsistent in defining the different training status that are recognized as precursors of OTS. This complicates the detection of a reliable marker for the early diagnosis of OTS.

Training, overreaching and overtraining

Several authors consider OT as a status that evolves from normal training, through OR and finally ending in an OTS. Probably these states (OR/OTS) show different defining characteristics and the "overtraining continuum" may be an oversimplification, because this emphasizes training characteristics, while the features of OTS consist of more than training errors, and coincides with other stressors

The Olympic Textbook of Medicine in Sport, 1st edition. Edited by M. Schwellnus. Published 2008 by Blackwell Publishing, ISBN: 978-1-4051-5637-0.

(Meeusen *et al.* 2006). However, as stated in the recent Consensus Statement of the European College of Sport Science (ECSS; Meeusen *et al.* 2006), these definitions indicate that the difference between OT and OR is the amount of time needed for performance restoration and not the type or duration of training stress or degree of impairment. These definitions also imply that there may be an absence of psychologic signs associated with the conditions. As it is possible to recover from a state of OR within a 2-week period (Halson *et al.* 2002; Jeukendrup *et al.* 1992; Kreider *et al.* 1998; Lehmann *et al.* 1999a; Steinacker *et al.* 2000), it may be argued that this condition is a relatively normal and harmless stage of the training process. However, athletes with OTS may take months or possibly years to recover completely.

Although some studies indicate that the purpose is to detect the "training status" or the "state of tiredness" of athletes (individual athletes or team sport players), they use "overtraining" in the title, as a keyword, or in the introduction or discussion of the papers (Maso *et al.* 2003; Nindl *et al.* 2002; O'Connor *et al.* 1991; Passelergue & Lac 1999), feeding the confusion that exists in the definition and usage of the word "overtraining."

Others have tried to discover OT features by following athletes for short time periods (Kellmann & Gunther 2000; Knopfli *et al.* 2001; Maso *et al.* 2003) ranging from 3 days to 10–14 days of longitudinal data collection. Several different possible "markers" ranging from hormonal and psychological measurements (Barron *et al.* 1985; Kellmann & Gunther 2000; Knopfli *et al.* 2001; Maso *et al.* 2003; Morgan *et al.* 1988), were used to indicate "training disturbances." Again, most of these authors used "overtraining" as an indicator of the process of increased training load, but confound this term with possible indicators of OTS. Morgan *et al.* (1988) studied swimmers before and after a 10-day period of increased training. They showed a clear agreement between psychometric and physiologic measures; however, although the authors used key words such as "overtraining" and "staleness," this was again a study where training load was increased and monitored. Maso *et al.* (2003) performed one measuring point in a group of rugby players, and

tried to correlate metabolic, hormonal, and psychologic data as indicators of training status. Similar design was used by Passelergue and Lac (1999), carrying out measurements during a 2-day competition. O'Connor *et al.* (1991) report on psychobiological effects of 3 days of increased training. They concluded that some values, such as negative mood, perception, and biomechanical factors, are sensitive to 3 days of intensified training, and that males and females respond in a similar way. Another study also used 72 h of extreme training (military stress) on performance, physical, and occupational related performance in military training (Nindl *et al.* 2002). Fry *et al.* (1998) studied the effects of 2 weeks of intensified training in resistance exercise. They found significant decrements in performance in strength tests and called this indicative for OT, again adding to the confusion on usage of the terminology.

When looking at recent literature it seems that several papers use "overtraining" as a verb and therefore indicate the *process* that might lead to training (mal)adaptations (Armstrong & VanHeest 2002; Halson & Jeukendrup 2004; Meeusen *et al.* 2006). In many studies "overtraining" is used to describe both the process of training excessively and the fatigue states that may develop as a consequence (Callister *et al.* 1990; Kuipers & Keizer 1988; Meeusen *et al.* 2006; Morgan *et al.* 1987). When reading those papers it is clear that "overtraining" is used to define the process of more intensive or prolonged training. Callister *et al.* (1990) followed 15 judo athletes through a 10-week training period. They gradually increased training volume and intensity and found that some but not all aspects of performance decreased, without seeing athletes who showed signs of OTS. Several studies used a longitudinal design in order to register training stress in different athletic populations (Chatard *et al.* 2002; Manetta *et al.* 2002; Maso *et al.* 2003; Petibois *et al.* 2003a). When following a group of swimmers over a 37-week period, Chatard *et al.* (2002) clearly showed that for the whole group salivary hormonal levels (cortisol and dehydroepiandrosteron-sulfate; DHEA-S) were not correlated with swimming performance. However, this study did not report on athletes showing signs and symptoms of OTS.

Manetta *et al.* (2002) followed cyclists during one season in order to look at the influence of carbohydrate dependence and the relation with performance, again these authors registered differences in training state, but could not identify athletes with OTS. Petibois *et al.* (2003a) carefully followed rowers for 12 months, they did not perform a specific training intervention, but showed that when using blood parameters to indicate possible metabolic changes resulting from changes in training load, it is very important to perform periodical blood measurements. This last study illustrates that longitudinal training monitoring can provide interesting data on the training status of the athlete, but do not necessarily indicate that OTS occurs.

Study designs to explore increased load on athletes

Recently, more studies use a design where an intensified training period is used in order to explore the effects of increase in training load and therefore obtain insight into possible mechanisms responsible for metabolic, hormonal, and psychological disturbances frequently encountered in athletes and which are often used as indicators of OR or OT. These studies have the common feature that they no longer use "overtraining" to indicate the load put on the athletes, but call the studies "overload," "intensified training," "strenuous training" etc. Ventura *et al.* (2003) had cyclists perform three additional trainings per week for 6 weeks and included hypoxic conditions. The major findings of this study were that there was no improvement in endurance or differences in metabolic parameters, indicating a stagnation of performance resulting from the increased training load. Yet these authors used "overtraining – overreaching" as keywords, although no signs or symptoms were reported. Pichot *et al.* (2002) had their subjects perform during 8 weeks of intensive training, followed by 4 weeks of overload training, and 2 weeks of recovery in order to measure heart rate variability. Hall *et al.* (1999) followed eight male runners plus controls over 8 weeks. After 2 weeks of normal training, they increased their training load by 43% for 2 weeks, followed by an increase of 86% the next 2 weeks,

and then included a taper of 2 weeks (50% of normal training). Both studies registered training adaptations; however, no signs or symptoms of performance decrements were observed. Halson *et al.* (2002, 2003) also used 2 weeks of "normal" training followed by 2 weeks of intensified training, and 2 weeks of recovery. During the intensified training, subjects were spending twice the amount of time in the intensive training zones (heart rate monitoring). In the studies of Halson *et al.*, subjects showed sings of OR, manifested by a decrease in performance, and disturbed mood state. Rietjens *et al.* (2005) investigated the central and peripheral physiological, neuroendocrine, and psychological responses to 2 weeks of increased training. Both volume and intensity of the training load were increased, creating a severe state of fatigue. The purpose was to create a state of temporary OR. Although they did not register performance decrements in the athletes, the authors found that reaction time, performance, and mood state were the first indicators of early OR. Uusitalo *et al.* (1998a,b) increased training volume and intensity in nine athletes and compared the results with a control group ($n = 6$). The athletes were tested 2 weeks before the start of the experiment, after 4, 6 and 9 weeks of training, and after 4 and 6 weeks of recovery. The authors found marked individual differences in training and OT-induced hormonal changes.

Functional overreaching

The above studies illustrate that OR is often utilized by athletes during a typical training cycle to enhance performance. Intensified training can result in a decline in performance; however, when appropriate periods of recovery are provided, a "supercompensation" effect may occur with the athlete exhibiting an enhanced performance compared with baseline levels. These studies are typically those where athletes go on a short training camp in order to create a "functional overreaching (FOR)". They typically follow athletes not only during the increased training (volume and/or intensity), but also register recovery from this training status. Usually, athletes will show temporary performance decrements that will disappear after a taper period. In this situation, the physiological responses will compensate the training-related stress (Steinacker et al. 2004).

Steinacker et al. (2000) made a distinction between OR and OTS. While following rowers preparing for the World Championships they found clear signs of OR after 18 days of intense training. These signs were a decrease in performance, gonadal, and hypothalamic hormone disturbances, and deterioration of recovery in the psychologic questionnaire. The reason why these authors called the athletes "overreached" was that after a tapering period the values returned to normal. This study was a typical example of FOR because here OR was used as an integral part of successful training, although during the intensive training period some markers already showed disturbances. Hooper et al. (1999) showed that some physiologic (norepinephrine) and psychometric variables (Profile of Mood State; POMS) could be indicators of recovery following an 18-week training period.

Non-functional overreaching

When this intensified training continues, the athletes can evolve into a state of extreme OR or non-functional overreaching (NFOR) that will lead to a stagnation or decrease in performance which will not resume for several weeks or months. Hooper et al. (1995) followed swimmers during a 6-month period in an attempt to determine markers of OT and recovery. They classified "staleness" based on performance criteria (decrease or stagnation in performance; i.e. poor training responses); 7 days of consecutive high fatigue scores with no specific illness present at the time the before-mentioned criteria were registered. In a group of 14 subjects, three were considered as "stale." Stale swimmers rate fatigue and muscle soreness significantly higher than non-stale swimmers, significantly poorer sleep and significantly higher levels of stress were also reported. Tapering did not appear to provide the stale swimmers with sufficient time for complete recovery prior to competition, which could indicate that these three subjects were suffering from NFOR. Unfortunately, the authors did not report how long it took these athletes to recover fully.

However, these authors themselves confuse "overtraining" and "staleness" because they report on the same group of swimmers in a previous paper (Hooper et al. 1993) and identify (the same?) three swimmers as "overtrained" and call them "stale" one sentence later, adding to the confusion in terminology.

Urhausen et al. (1998a,b) used a longitudinal prospective study design in order to follow athletes over 19 months. They measured hormones on five occasions. At certain time periods the athletes increased their training load, so that their training frequency was at least five times per week, for 2–3 weeks. If a subject was showing signs and symptoms such as a sports-specific decline in performance (e.g., early fatigue, sleep disorders), they were tested by a double protocol. This test-battery consisted of an incremental grade exercise test and a 30-s maximal anaerobic cycle test. The second day of investigation took place 3–7 days after the first test day and consisted of a constant load test until exhaustion at 110% of the individual's anaerobic threshold. Out of 17 athletes OT was diagnosed 15 times; mostly athletes complained of heavy legs, underperformance, and sleep disorders. The authors defined the OT as a short-term OT or OR, needing at least 2 weeks of recovery. The authors did not make a distinction on the timing of full recovery, and it is presumed that most of the athletes were FOR although some of these athletes could be considered as NFOR.

In their study, Uusitalo et al. (1998a,b) used a control group ($n = 6$) and tested the athletes at different time points during the OT process, (baseline, after 4, 6 and 9 weeks of training, and after 4–6 weeks of recovery). The athletes in the experimental group trained 7 days per week and five of the subjects in the experimental group showed signs of OT with decreased performance during an exercise test as well as changes in hormonal output. The authors state that one of the athletes had recovered within the 5-week recovery period, but do not indicate if this means that the others needed more time to recover. However, this is a well-controlled and well-designed study, with subjects pushed into NFOR.

Both FOR and NFOR athletes will be able to fully recover after sufficient rest. It seems from the literature that also in NFOR the evolution on the "overtraining continuum" is not only "quantitatively" determined (i.e., by the increase in training volume) but that also "qualitative" changes occur (e.g., signs and symptoms of psychological and/or endocrine distress). This is in line with recent neuroendocrine findings using a double exercise test (Meeusen *et al.* 2004; Urhausen *et al.* 1998a,b).

Overtraining syndrome

As it is possible to recover from short-term or "functional" overreaching within a period of 2 weeks, the recovery from the NFOR state is less clear. This is probably because not many studies tried to define the subtle difference that exists between extreme OR, which needs several weeks or even months to recover (Meeusen *et al.* 2006), and OTS. Athletes who experience OTS may need months or even years to completely recover, frequently leading to cessation of a (top) sports career.

The difficulty lies in the subtle difference that might exist between extreme OR athletes and those having OTS. In using the expression "syndrome" we emphasize the multifactorial etiology, and acknowledge that exercise (training) is not necessarily the sole causative factor of the syndrome.

Reports on athletes with OTS are mostly case descriptions, because it is not only unethical, but probably also impossible to train an athlete with a high training load while at the same time including other "stressors," especially because the symptoms of OTS differ between individuals. The most cited study reporting on athletes with OTS is the paper by Barron *et al.* (1985). The authors report clear hormonal disturbances in four long-distance runners. An insulin-induced hypoglycemic challenge was administered to assess hypothalamic–pituitary function in the OT athletes and compared with controls. In this study, performance was not measured, and the authors declared that hormonal function recovered after 4 weeks. This might indicate that the athletes were NFOR and did not have OTS. Hedelin *et al.* (2000b) report on a cross-country skier who after several months of intensive training (up to 20 h per week) showed increased fatigue, reduced

performance, and disturbances on psychometric tests. After exclusion of other illnesses, this athlete was diagnosed as having OTS. In order to investigate changes in the autonomic nervous system, heart rate variability was recorded in the athlete. They registered a shift towards increased heart rate variability, particularly in the high-frequency range, together with a reduced resting heart rate. This indicates an autonomic imbalance, with extensive parasympathetic modulation. Although it is not clear how performance decrements were measured, the authors report that the athlete needed 8 weeks to recover. Rowbottom *et al.* (1995) report on differences in glutamine in OT athletes, but again this study gives no clear indication on how performance decrements were registered. Meeusen *et al.* (2004) report on differences in normal training status, FOR (after a training camp), and compare the endocrinological results with a double exercise test with an OTS athlete. Athletes were tested in a double exercise protocol (two exercise tests with 4 h between) in order to register the recovery capacity of the athletes. Performance was measured as the time to voluntary exhaustion. They compared the first and the second exercise tests in order to verify if the athletes were able to maintain the same performance. The training camp reduced exercise capacity in the athletes. There was a 3% decrease between performances in the first versus the second test, while in the FOR condition there was a 6% performance decrease. The OTS subject showed an 11% decrease in time to exhaustion. The OTS athletes also showed clear psychologic and endocrinologic disturbances.

Uusitalo *et al.* (2004) report on an athlete with OTS who showed abnormal serotonin reuptake. This case presentation was well documented; however, the authors give no indication on the time the athlete needed to recover from OTS.

Summary

The definition used in this chapter is based on the consensus recently developed by the ECSS (Meeusen *et al.* 2006). Table 3.1 illustrates the different stages from training to OTS.

Table 3.1 Different stages of training: overreaching (OR) and overtraining syndrome. (After Meeusen *et al.* 2006.)

Process	Training (overload) ————————————➤		Intensified training ————————————➤	
Outcome	Acute fatigue	Functional OR (short-term OR)	Non-functional OR (extreme OR)	Overtraining syndrome (OTS)
Recovery	Day(s)	Days–weeks	Weeks–months	Months+
Performance	Increase	Temporary performance decrement (e.g. training camp)	Stagnation/decrease	Decrease

Training can be defined as a process of overload that is used to disturb homeostasis that results in acute fatigue leading to an improvement in performance. When training continues or when athletes deliberately use a short-term period (e.g., training camp) to increase their training load they can experience short-term performance decrement, without severe psychologic or other lasting negative symptoms. This FOR will eventually lead to an improvement in performance after recovery.

However, when athletes do not sufficiently respect the balance between training and recovery, NFOR can occur. At this stage, the first signs and symptoms of prolonged training distress, such as performance decrements, psychological disturbance (decreased vigour, increased fatigue), and hormonal disturbances will occur and the athletes will need weeks or months to recover. Several confounding factors, such as inadequate nutrition (energy and/or carbohydrate intake), illness (most commonly upper respiratory tract infections; URTI), psychosocial stressors (work, team, coach, or family-related), and sleep disorders may be present. At this stage, the distinction between NFOR and OTS is very difficult, and will depend on the clinical outcome and exclusion diagnosis. The athlete will often show the same clinical, hormonal, and other signs and symptoms. Therefore, the diagnosis of OTS can often only be made retrospectively when the time course can be overseen. A key phrase in the recognition of OTS might be "prolonged maladaptation" not only of the athlete, but also of several biologic, neurochemical, and hormonal regulation mechanisms.

Prevalence

The borderline between optimal performance and performance impairment caused by OTS is subtle. This applies especially to physiologic and biochemical factors. The apparent vagueness surrounding OTS is further complicated by the fact that the clinical features vary from one individual to another, are non-specific, anecdotal, and numerous.

Probably because of the difference in the definition used, prevalence data on OT athletes are dispersed. Studies have reported up to 60% of distance runners during their careers show signs of OT, while data on swimmers vary between 3% and 30% (Hooper *et al.* 1997; Lehmann *et al.* 1993a; Morgan *et al.* 1987; O'Connor *et al.* 1989; Raglin & Morgan 1994). If the definition of OTS as stated above is used, the incidence figures will probably be lower. We therefore suggest that a distinction be made between NFOR and OTS, and to only define athletes as having OTS when a clinical exclusion diagnosis (see Table 3.3, p. 152) establishes the OTS.

Mechanisms

Probably because of the difficulty in detecting straightforward mechanisms responsible for OTS, much speculation has been made as to the "real" reason for the genesis of OTS. This has led to many papers presenting a possible hypothesis for the origin of OTS.

Hypothetical mechanisms

Increased training loads, as well as other persistent stresses, can influence the human body chronically. This disturbance of the homeostasis will be compensated by reregulating mechanisms, but when the stress becomes excessive, a permanent disorder can occur. However, at this time it is not yet clear which mechanism eventually leads to OTS. Probably because of this, and because there are several possible hypotheses, some recent review articles have focused on hypothetical explanations for the mechanism behind OTS. Table 3.2 shows a selection of possible hypotheses found in recent literature. One of the remarkable features of these papers are that they propose hypotheses that might explain the possible mechanisms of the genesis of OTS, but all use circumstantial evidence without any back-up from research data.

Budget *et al.* (2000) redefined persistent unexplained performance deficits (recognized and agreed by coach and athlete) despite 2 weeks of relative rest, as the "unexplained underperformance syndrome." However, it seems that OTS covers the same aspects, and knowing that 2 weeks of recovery places an athlete rather in the OR status, this definition might add to the confusion surrounding OTS. Others have tried to formulate hypotheses approaching OTS from different perspectives, such as biochemical or biological mechanisms.

Petibois *et al.* (2002, 2003b) explained the onset of OTS as a biochemical alteration in carbohydrate metabolism. Also, Snyder (1998) suggests that general fatigue and complaints of "heavy legs" are because of reduced glycogen stores and might lead to underperformance. There are other hypotheses which include the imbalance of the sympathetic and parasympathetic nervous systems (Lehmann *et al.* 1998a), glutamine (Rowbottom *et al.* 1995, 1996) and other amino acid hypotheses (Gastmann & Lehmann 1998). Smith (2000) proposed a hypothesis where excessive muscular stress (Seene *et al.* 1999) will induce a local inflammatory response which may evolve into chronic inflammation and possibly result in systemic inflammation. Inflammatory agents, such as cytokines (Smith 2000, 2003, 2004), IL-6 (Robson 2003), might act on the central nervous system leading to a sickness behaviour, creating physiologic, biochemical, neuroendocrine, and psychologic disturbances. Many studies report changes in endocrine functioning in OT athletes, and this has led to possible hypotheses going from catabolic–anabolic imbalances indicated by a decrease in the testosterone : cortisol ratio (Adlercreutz *et al.* 1986) and subsequent neuroendocrine disturbances (Keizer 1998), to central nervous system imbalances in neurotransmitters creating similarities with depression (Armstrong & VanHeest 2002; Kreider 1998; Meeusen 1999).

Hypothesis	Reference
Metabolism alteration process syndrome	Petibois *et al.* (2002)
Cytokine hypothesis	Smith (2000)
IL-6 hypothesis	Robson (2003)
Exercise myopathy hypothesis	Seene *et al.* (1999)
Glycogen depletion hypothesis	Snyder (1998)
Glutamine hypothesis	Rowbottom *et al.* (1995)
Branched chain amino acid hypothesis	Gastmann & Lehmann (1998a)
Autonomic imbalance hypothesis	Lehmann *et al.* (1998)
Central nervous system hypothesis	Meeusen (1999)
Neuroendocrine hypothesis	Keizer (1998)
Central fatigue hypothesis and overtraining	Kreider (1998)
Athlete depression syndrome	Armstrong & VanHeest (2002)
Unexplained underperformance syndrome	Budgett *et al.* (2000)
Monotony hypothesis	Foster (1998)

Table 3.2 Selected summary of possible hypotheses found in recent literature to explain overtraining syndrome (OTS). (Consensus statement ECSS: Meeusen *et al.* 2006.)

Although these theories have potential, until more prospective studies are carried out where longitudinal follow-up of athletes (who may develop the OTS) is performed, or specific diagnostic tools are developed, these theories remain speculative. In the following sections, we briefly explain some of these proposed hypothetical mechanisms. In the section on 'diagnosis' we extract those measures that might give an indication of the training (or OT) status of the individual athlete.

Biochemistry

During prolonged training, glycogen stores become almost fully depleted, glycogenolysis and glucose transport are downregulated in muscle and liver, as well as the production in the liver of insulin-like growth-factor I, and catabolism is induced. This catabolic state could be a possible trigger for several disturbances of homeostasis of blood parameters, but measurements of selected enzyme activities and blood markers are in line with these hypotheses; however, the validity of these variables is overestimated for being a diagnostic tool for OTS (Meeusen et al. 2006; Urhausen & Kindermann 2002).

Physiology

There have been several proposals as to which physiologic measures might be indicative of OR or OTS. Reduced maximal heart rates after increased training may be the result of reduced sympathetic nervous system activity, decreased tissue responsiveness to catecholamines, changes in adrenergic receptor activity, or may simply be the result of a reduced power output achieved with maximal effort. Several other reductions in maximal physiologic measures (e.g., oxygen uptake, heart rate) might be a consequence of a reduction in exercise time and not related to abnormalities per se, and it should be noted that changes of resting heart rate are not consistently found in athletes with OTS (Meeusen et al. 2006). Highly controlled and monitored studies that examine possible changes in heart rate variability (HRV) following OR are lacking. Therefore, as with so many of the other physiological measures, it cannot be stated for certain that

changes observed during OR are reflected in athletes with OTS (Meeusen et al. 2006).

Immune system

There are many reports of URTI resulting from increased training, and also in OR and OTS athletes. It seems feasible that intensified training (leading to OR or OTS) may increase both the duration of the so-called "open window" and the degree of the resultant immunodepression. However, the amount of scientific information to substantiate these arguments is limited. It might just be that the increased URTI incidence is likely to reflect the increase in training, regardless of the response of the athlete to the increased physical stress (Meeusen et al. 2006). URTI might be one of the "triggering" factors that can lead to the induction of OTS.

With sustained periods of heavy training, several aspects of both innate and adaptive immunity are depressed. Several studies have examined changes in immune function during intensive periods of military training (Carins & Booth 2002; Tiollier et al. 2005). However, this often involves not only strenuous physical activity, but also dietary energy deficiency, sleep deprivation, and psychologic challenges. These multiple stressors are likely to induce a pattern of immunoendocrine responses that amplify the exercise-induced alterations.

Whether immune function is seriously impaired in athletes with OTS is unknown as there is insufficient scientific data available. However, anecdotal reports from athletes and coaches of an increased infection rate with OTS (Smith 2000) have been supported by a few empirical studies (Kingsbury et al. 1998; Reid et al. 2004).

There are only a few reports of differences in immune function status in OT athletes compared with healthy trained athletes (Gabriel et al. 1998; Mackinnon & Hooper 1994) and most studies on OT athletes have failed to find any differences (Mackinnon et al. 1997; Rowbottom et al. 1995), probably because these studies also report on OR athletes.

Infection might be one of the "triggering" factors that can lead to the induction of OTS or in some cases the diagnosis of OTS cannot be differentiated from a state of post-viral fatigue such as that observed with episodes of glandular fever.

The current information regarding the immune system and OR confirms that periods of intensified training result in depressed immune cell functions with little or no alteration in circulating cell numbers. However, although immune parameters change in response to increased training load, these changes do not distinguish between those athletes who successfully adapt to OR and those who do not and develop symptoms of OTS.

Hormones

For several years it has been hypothesized that a hormonal-mediated central disregulation occurs during the pathogenesis of OTS, and that measurements of blood hormones could help to detect OTS (Fry & Kramer 1997; Fry *et al.* 1991, 2006; Keizer 1998; Kuipers & Keizer 1988; Urhausen *et al.* 1995, 1998a). The results of the research devoted to this subject is far from unanimous, mostly because of the difference in measuring methods, and/or detection limits of the analytical equipment used.

For a long time the plasma testosterone : cortisol ratio was considered as a good indicator of the OT state. This ratio decreases in relation to the intensity and duration of training and it is evident that this ratio indicates only the actual physiological strain of training and cannot be used for diagnosis of OR or OTS (Lehmann *et al.* 1998a, 1999b, 2001; Meeusen 1999; Urhausen *et al.* 1995).

Most of the literature agrees that OR and OTS must be viewed on a continuum with a disturbance, an adaptation, and finally a maladaptation of the hypothalamic–pituitary–adrenal axis (HPA) and all other hypothalamic axes (Keizer 1998; Lehmann *et al.* 1993a, 1998a, 1999b, 2001; Meeusen 1998, 1999; Meeusen *et al.* 2004, Urhausen *et al.* 1995, 1998b). However, it should be emphasized that depending on the training status, the moment the hormone measures are taken (diurnal variation), urinary, blood, and salivary measures create a great variation in the interpretation of the results. In OTS, a decreased rise in pituitary hormones (adenocorticotropic hormone [ACTH], growth hormone [GH], luteinizing hormone [LH], and follicle-stimulating

hormone [FSH]) in response to a stressful stimulus is reported (Barron *et al.* 1985; Lehmann *et al.* 1993b, 1998a,b, 1999a,b; Meeusen *et al.* 2004; Urhausen *et al.* 1995, 1998a; Wittert *et al.* 1996).

This indicates that hormonal markers are potent parameters to register disturbances of homeostasis, but until now the literature has been very diffuse because of a lack of standardization in test methods.

Is the brain involved?

Over the last few years, there has been significant interest in determining specific peripheral markers for the metabolic, physiologic, and psychologic responses to exercise that have been suggested to have an association with OTS. To date, relatively little attention has been placed on the role of the central nervous system in OTS (Meeusen 1999). The neuroendocrine and central nervous system hypotheses, as well as the neuroimmunologic and psychometric data, indicate that OTS occurs with a major disturbance of regulative mechanisms including the "brain–periphery" interaction.

The observation that other stressors in addition to exercise (e.g., job, social, travel, inadequate nutrition) seem to predispose an athlete to OTS (Foster & Lehmann 1997) links OT with the psychosocial signs of the maladaptive response to intense training. The works of Morgan and colleagues (Morgan *et al.* 1987, 1988; O'Connor 1997; O'Connor *et al.* 1989, 1991; Raglin & Morgan 1994) clearly indicated that psychological factors and especially mood state disturbances are effective in predicting the onset of OTS. The symptoms associated with OTS, such as changes in emotional behaviour, prolonged feelings of fatigue, sleep disturbances, and hormonal dysfunctions are indicative of changes in the regulation and coordinative function of the hypothalamus (Armstrong & VanHeest 2002; Meeusen 1998).

Most of the literature agrees that OTS and OR must be viewed on a continuum with a disturbance, an adaptation, and finally a maladaptation of the HPA (Keizer 1998; Lehmann *et al.* 1993a, 1998a, 1999a,b; Meeusen 1998, 1999; Urhausen *et al.* 1995, 1998a). Behind the seemingly uniform acute hormonal response to exercise, explaining the disturbance to the neuroendocrine system caused by OTS is not that simple. The trigger that eventually leads to OTS may be any of a number of mediators with separate regulatory mechanisms.

The hypothalamus is under the control of several "higher" brain centers and several neurotransmitters (Meeusen & De Meirleir 1995). Amongst these transmitters, serotonin (5-HT) is known to have a major role in various neuroendocrine and behavioural functions (e.g., activation of the HPA axis, feeding, and locomotion; Wilckens et al. 1992). The possibility that impaired neurotransmission at the various central aminergic synapses is associated with major disturbances of the central nervous system, such as depression (and possibly OTS), has received more attention over the past few years. It has been suggested that exercise exerts its putative psychologic effects via the same neurochemical substrate (the monoamines) as antidepressant drugs, known to increase the synaptic availability of transmitters (Armstrong & VanHeest 2002; Meeusen et al. 1996, 1997; Uusitalo et al. 2004). In pathological situations, such as in major depression (Dishman 1997), post-traumatic stress disorders (PTSD; Liberzon et al. 1999; Porter et al. 2004), and probably also in OTS, the glucocorticoids and the brain monoaminergic systems apparently fail to restrain the HPA response to stress (Meeusen et al. 2004).

As it has been shown that exercise and training influence neurotransmitter release in various brain nuclei (Meeusen et al. 1994, 1995, 1996, 1997), possible disregulation at this level could have a key role in the maladaptation to the "stress" of exercise, training, and OTS. Meeusen et al. (1997) showed that endurance training decreases basal neurotransmitter outflow in the striatum of rats, while maintaining the necessary sensitivity for responses to acute exercise. These observations raise the possibility that an exercise-induced change in receptor sensitivity could exist (Meeusen et al. 1997).

Traditionally, the main criterion for a stress response is an increase in the secretion of stress hormones. On this basis, a decline in hormonal secretion when stress is repeated or prolonged is commonly interpreted as indicating stress adaptation (Stanford 1993). A large body of evidence indicates that stressful experiences also alter neurotransmitter metabolism and release in several brain areas (Abercrombie et al., 1989; Finlay et al. 1995; Gresch et al. 1994; Imperato et al. 1992; Jordan et al. 1994; Keefe et al. 1990; Kirby et al. 1997; Kuipers & Keizer 1988; Niesembaum et al. 1991; Weizman et al. 1989). Chronic stress and the subsequent chronic peripheral glucocorticoid secretion have an important role in the desensitization of higher brain center's responses during acute stressors, because it has been shown that in acute (and also chronic) immobilization the responsiveness of hypothalamic corticotropin-releasing hormone (CRH) neurons rapidly falls (Cizza et al. 1993). These adaptation mechanisms could be the consequence of changes in neurotransmitter release, depletion of CRH and/or desensitization of hypothalamic hormonal releases to afferent neurotransmitter input (Cizza et al. 1993). In OTS it is assumed that a "maladaptation" to chronic exercise (and other) stress occurs. In trying to distinguish the effects of chronic and acute stress on brain neurotransmitter concentrations we showed that in chronic stressed animals, the central response to an acute stressor (restraint) is impaired (Thorré et al. 1997). In comparison with controls, acute stress did not increase extracellular 5-HT levels in the hippocampus of chronically stressed rats, while the same immobilization stress increased 5-HT release 300–400% in the control animals (Thorré et al. 1997). One might speculate that in OTS (the step beyond coping with stress) a comparable mechanism occurs.

From the above it can be concluded that in OTS the neuroendocrine disorder is a hypothalamic disfunction rather than a malfunction of the peripheral hormonal organs (Kuipers & Keizer 1988). The interactive features of the periphery and the brain could be translated into possible immunologic, psychologic, and endocrinologic disturbances. However, because OTS is athlete-specific, generalization of the signs and symptoms is at present not possible.

Diagnosis

Although in recent years the knowledge of central pathomechanisms has significantly increased, there is still a strong demand for relevant tools for the early diagnosis of OTS. OTS is characterized by a "sports-specific" decrease in performance, together with persistent fatigue and disturbances in mood state (Armstrong & Van Heest 2002; Halson & Jeukendrup 2004; Meeusen *et al.* 2006; Urhausen & Kindermann 2002). This underperformance persists, despite a period of recovery lasting several weeks or months. Importantly, as there is no diagnostic tool to identify an athlete with OTS, diagnosis can only be made by excluding all other possible influences on changes in performance and mood state. Therefore, if no explanation for the observed changes can be found, OTS is diagnosed. Early and unequivocal recognition of OTS is virtually impossible because the only certain sign of this condition is a decrease in performance during competition or training. The definitive diagnosis of OTS always requires the exclusion of an organic disease (e.g. endocrinological disorders such as thyroid or adrenal gland, diabetes; iron deficiency with anaemia; or infectious diseases; Meeusen *et al.* 2006). Other major disorders or eating disorders (e.g., anorexia nervosa, bulimia) should also be excluded. However, it should be emphasized that many endocrinological and clinical findings brought about by NFOR and OTS can mimic other diseases. The borderline between under- and overdiagnosis is very difficult to judge (Meeusen *et al.* 2006).

Exclusion diagnosis

In essence, it is generally thought that symptoms of OTS (e.g., fatigue, performance decline, and mood disturbances) are more severe than those of NFOR. However, there is no scientific evidence to either confirm or refute this suggestion (Meeusen *et al.* 2006). Hence, there is no objective evidence that the athlete is indeed experiencing OTS. Additionally, in the studies that induced a state of OR, many of the physiologic and biochemical responses to the increased training were highly variable, with some measures in some studies demonstrating changes and others remaining unaltered, most likely because conditions and the degree of NFOR and OTS differ and were not comparably described. Furthermore, different definitions for a status of FOR, NFOR, or OTS are used.

One approach to understanding the etiology of OTS involves the exclusion of organic diseases or infections and factors such as dietary caloric restriction (negative energy balance) and insufficient carbohydrate and/or protein intake, iron deficiency, magnesium deficiency, allergies, together with identification of initiating events or triggers (Meeusen *et al.* 2006). One of the most certain triggers is a training error resulting in an imbalance between load and recovery. Other possible triggers might be the monotony of training (Foster 1998; Foster *et al.* 1996), too many competitions, personal and emotional (psychologic) problems, and emotional demands of occupation. Less commonly cited possibilities are altitude exposure and exercise-heat stress. Scientific evidence is not strong for most of these potential triggers. Many triggers, such as glycogen deficiency (Snyder *et al.* 1993) or infections (Gabriel & Kindermann 1997; Hooper & McKinnon 1995; Rowbottom *et al.* 1995), may contribute to NFOR or OTS, but might not be present at the time the athlete presents to a physician. Furthermore, identifying these possible initiating events has not revealed the mechanism of OTS.

In the following paragraphs we present some of the frequently used parameters and critically evaluate the value of this measure in order to diagnose OTS.

Training status

A hallmark feature of the OTS is the inability to sustain intense exercise, and a decreased sports-specific performance capacity when the training load is maintained or even increased (Meeusen *et al.* 2004; Urhausen *et al.* 1995). Athletes with OTS are usually able to start a normal training sequence or a race at their normal training pace, but are not able to complete the training load they are given, or race as usual. The key indicator of the OTS can be considered an unexplainable decrease in performance. Therefore, an exercise or performance test is considered to be essential for the diagnosis of OTS (Budgett *et al.* 2000; Lehmann *et al.* 1999a; Urhausen *et al.* 1995).

It appears that both the type of performance test employed and the duration of the test are important in determining the changes in performance associated with the OTS. Debate exists as to which performance test is the most appropriate when attempting to diagnose OR and OTS. In general, time-to-fatigue tests will most likely show greater changes in exercise capacity as a result of OR and OTS than incremental exercise tests (Halson & Jeukendrup 2004). Additionally, they allow the assessment of substrate kinetics, hormonal responses, and sub-maximal measures can be made at a fixed intensity and duration. In order to detect subtle performance decrements it might be better to use sports-specific performance tests.

Urhausen *et al.* (1998a) and Meeusen *et al.* (2004) have shown that multiple tests or carried out on different days (Urhausen *et al.* 1998a), or that use the two maximal incremental exercise tests separated by 4 h, can be valuable tools to assess the perform-ance decrements usually seen in OTS athletes. A decrease in exercise time of at least 10% is necessary to be significant. Furthermore, this decrease in per-formance needs to be confirmed by specific changes in hormone concentrations (Meeusen *et al.* 2004).

Physiology

Heart rate variability analysis has been used as a measure of cardiac autonomic balance, with an increase in HRV indicating an increase in vagal (parasympathetic) tone relative to sympathetic activity (Uusitalo *et al.* 2000). Numerous studies have examined the effects of training on indices of HRV but, to date, few studies have investigated HRV in OR or OTS athletes, with existing studies showing either no change (Achten & Jeukendrup 2003; Hedelin *et al.* 2000a; Uusitalo *et al.* 1998a,b), inconsistent changes (Uusitalo *et al.* 2000), or changes in parasympathetic modulation (Hedelin *et al.* 2000a).

Hedelin *et al.* (2000a) reported increased HRV and decreased resting heart rate in a single OT athlete compared with baseline measures. In comparison with normally responding subjects examined dur-ing the same period, the OT subject exhibited an increase in high frequency and total power in the supine position during intensified training, which decreased after recovery. The increase in high frequency power was suggested to be most likely the result of increased parasympathetic activity (Hedelin *et al.* 2000a).

However, much more research is necessary before HRV can be considered as a diagnostic measurement for OTS. It might be an indication of the actual training status of the individual, and therefore part of the exclusion diagnosis as a "marker" that needs attention when examining an athlete suspicious of having OTS.

Biochemistry

Although disturbance of the glycogen stores and the concomitant catabolic reaction could be one of the likely triggers of OTS, muscle glycogen is typically normal when athletes are examined (Lehmann *et al.* 1999b). Blood glucose is also not typically altered. Resting blood glucose : insulin ratio may indicate mild insulin resistance (Steinacker *et al.* 2004).

The interaction of training status and glycogen stores could explain the diminished maximal lactate concentrations, while submaximal values remain unchanged or slightly reduced as reported in sev-eral studies (Kuipers & Keizer 1988; Urhausen & Kindermann 2002). However, as previously stated, the validity of biochemical parameters, such as crea-tine kinase (CK), urea, and glutamine variables, are overestimated when it comes to being a diagnostic tool for OTS (Meeusen *et al.* 2006; Urhausen & Kindermann 2002). Urea and/or CK may provide information concerning an elevated muscular and/or metabolic strain, but they are not suitable for indicating an OR or OTS state (Urhausen *et al.* 1998a), and altered plasma glutamine concentra-tions are not a causative factor of immunodepres-sion in OTS.

Although most of the blood parameters (e.g., blood count, C-reactive protein [CRP], CK, urea, creatinine, liver enzymes, glucose, ferritin, sodium, potassium) are not capable of detecting OR or OTS, they are helpful in providing information on the actual health status of the athlete, and are therefore useful in the exclusion diagnosis (Meeusen *et al.* 2006).

Immune system

It is clear that the immune system is extremely sens-itive to stress – both physiologic and psychologic

– and thus, potentially, immune variables could be used as an index of stress in relation to exercise training. Unresolved viral infections are not routinely assessed in elite athletes, but it may be worth investigating in individuals experiencing fatigue and underperformance in training and competition.

Furthermore, at present it seems that measures of immune function cannot really distinguish OTS from infection or post-viral fatigue states (Gleeson 2007).

Hormones

OTS can be understood partly within the context of the general adaptation syndrome (GAS) of Seyle (1936). Concomitant to this "stress-disturbance," the endocrine system is called upon to counteract the stress situation. The primary hormone products (epinephrine, norepinephrine and cortisol) all serve to redistribute metabolic fuels, maintain blood glucose, and enhance the responsiveness of the cardiovascular system. Repeated exposure to stress may lead to different responsivenesses to subsequent stressful experiences, depending on the stressor as well as on the stimuli paired with the stressor, either leading to an unchanged, increased, or decreased neurotransmitter and receptor function (Meeusen 1999). Behavioural adaptation (e.g., neurotransmitter release, receptor sensitivity, receptor binding) in higher brain centers will certainly influence hypothalamic output (Lachuer et al. 1994).

Lehmann et al. (1993b, 1999b) introduced the concept that hypothalamic function reflects the state of OR or OTS because the hypothalamus integrates many of the stressors. It has been shown that acute stress not only increases hypothalamic monoamine release, but consequently corticotropic-releasing hormone (CRH) and ACTH secretion (Shintani et al. 1995). Chronic stress and the subsequent chronically elevated adrenal glucocorticoid secretion could have an important role in the desensitization of higher brain center's response to acute stressors (Duclos et al. 1997, 1998, 1999, 2003), because it has been shown that in acute and chronic stress the responsiveness of hypothalamic CRH neurons rapidly falls (Barron et al. 1985; Cizza et al. 1993; Lehmann et al. 1993a; Urhausen et al. 1998a).

However, it is not sufficient to know the effect of a hormone to understand its actual role in metabolic control. Each hormone has a predefined exercise-induced pattern. When investigating hormonal markers of training adaptation, it is therefore important to target specific hormones for their informational potential and synchronize their sampling in accordance with their response patterns. Research findings (Barron et al. 1985; Meeusen et al. 2004; Urhausen et al. 1998a) support that athletes experiencing maladaptive training and performance adaptation problems seem to have a dysfunctional HPA axis response to exercise, resulting in an altered hormonal response to intense training and competition. When investigating elite athletes, the HPA axis is believed to offer valuable information about an athlete's state of adaptation (Steinacker & Lehmann, 2002). Meeusen et al. (2004) recently published a test protocol with two consecutive maximal exercise tests separated by 4 h. With this protocol they found that in order to detect signs of OTS and distinguish them from normal training responses or FOR, this method may be a good indicator not only of the recovery capacity of the athlete, but also of the ability to perform the second bout of exercise normally. The use of two bouts of maximal exercise to study neuroendocrine variations showed an adapted exercise-induced increase of ACTH, prolactin (PRL) and GH to a two-exercise bout (Meeusen et al. 2004). The test could therefore be used as an indirect measure of hypothalamic–pituitary capacity. In a FOR stage, a less pronounced neuroendocrine response to a second bout of exercise on the same day is found (De Schutter et al. 2004, Meeusen 2004), while in a NFOR stage the hormonal response to a two-bout exercise protocol shows an extreme increased release after the second exercise trigger (Meeusen 2004). With the same protocol it has been shown that athletes with OTS have an extremely large increase in hormonal release in the first exercise bout, followed by a complete suppression in the second exercise bout (Meeusen et al. 2004). This could indicate a hypersensitivity of the pituitary followed by an insensitivity or exhaustion afterwards. Previous reports that used a single-exercise protocol found similar effects (Meeusen et al. 2004). It appears that the use of two exercise bouts is more useful in detecting OR for preventing OTS.

Early detection of OR may be very important in the prevention of OTS. However, testing of central hypothalamic–pituitary regulation requires functional tests that are considered invasive and require diagnostic experience, and these the tests are time-consuming and expensive.

Psychometric measures

There is general agreement that OTS is characterized by psychologic disturbances and negative affective states. It has been suggested that although psychologic processes underpinning OTS are important, the phenomenon occurs only when these psychologic processes are combined with a negative training adaptation (Silva 1990). Sustained failure to adapt to training generates excessive fatigue. Training when the body's adaptivity is lost leads to OTS (Silva 1990; Foster & Lehmann 1997; Urhausen et al. 1995). Athletes then have a neuroendocrine imbalance and typically experience a noticeable drop in performance (Lemyre 2005).

When athletes have OTS, they typically experience chronic fatigue, poor sleep patterns, a drop in motivation, episodes of depression and helplessness (Lemyre 2005). Not surprisingly, their performance is considerably impaired. Full recovery from OTS represents a complex process that may necessitate many months, or even years, of rest and removal from sport (Kellmann 2002; Kentta & Hassmen 1998).

Several questionnaires, such as the Profile of Mood State (POMS; Morgan et al. 1988; O'Connor 1997; O'Connor et al. 1989; Raglin et al. 1991, Rietjens et al. 2005); Recovery Stress Questionnaire (RestQ-Sport; Kellmann 2002); Daily Analysis of Life Demands of Athletes (DALDA; Halson et al. 2002), and the "self-condition scale" (Urhausen et al. 1998b), have been used to monitor psychologic parameters in athletes. Other tests, such as attention tests (finger pre-cuing tasks; Rietjens et al. 2005) or neurocognitive tests (Kubesh et al. 2003), also serve as promising tools to detect subtle neurocognitive disturbances registered in OR or OTS athletes. It is important to register the current state of stress and recovery, and to prospectively follow the evolution for each athlete individually (Kellmann 2002; Morgan et al. 1988). The great advantage of psychometric instruments is the rapid availability of information (Kellmann 2002), especially because psychologic disturbances coincide with physiologic and performance changes and they are generally the precursors of neuroendocrine disturbances. In OTS the depressive component is more expressed than in OR (Armstrong & VanHeest 2002). Changes in mood state may be a useful indicator of OR and OTS; however, it is necessary to combine mood disturbances with measures of performance.

Are there definitive diagnostic criteria?

The need for definitive diagnostic criteria for OTS is reflected in much of the OR and OT research by a lack of consistent findings. There are several criteria that a reliable marker for the onset of the OTS must fulfill: the marker should be sensitive to the training load and, ideally, be unaffected by other factors (e.g., diet). Changes in the marker should occur prior to the establishment of OTS and changes in response to acute exercise should be distinguishable from chronic changes. Ideally, the marker should be relatively easy to measure and not too expensive. However, none of the currently available or suggested markers meets all of these criteria (Meeusen et al. 2006). When choosing several markers that might give an indication of the training or OT status of the athlete, one needs to take into account several possible problems that might influence decision-making.

When testing the athlete's *performance*, the intensity and reproducibility of the test should be sufficient to detect differences (max test, time trial, 2 max test). Baseline measures are often not available, and therefore the degree of performance limitation may not be exactly determined. Many of the performance tests are not sports-specific. HRV seems a promising tool in theory, but needs to be standardized when tested, and at present does not provide consistent results. A performance decrease with more than 10% on two tests separated by 4 h can be indicative of OTS, if other signs and symptoms are present. *Biochemical markers*, such as lactate or urea, as well as *immunologic markers*, do not have consistent reports in literature to consider these as absolute indicators for OTS. Many factors affect *blood hormone concentrations*: these include factors linked to sampling conditions and/or conservation of the sampling; stress of the sampling, intra- and inter-assay coefficient of variability. Others, such as food intake (nutrients composition and/or pre- vs post meal sampling), can modify significantly either the basal concentration of some hormones (cortisol, DHEA-S, total testosterone) or their concentration change in response to exercise (cortisol, GH). Diurnal and seasonal variations of the hormones are important factors that need to be considered. In female athletes, the hormonal response will depend on the phase of the menstrual cycle. Hormone concentrations at rest and following stimulation (exercise = acute stimulus) respond differently. Stress-induced measures (e.g., exercise, prohormones) need to be compared with baseline measures from the same individual. Poor reproducibility and feasibility of some techniques used to measure certain hormones can make the comparison of results difficult. Therefore, the use of two maximal performance (or time trial) tests separated by 4 h could help in comparing the individual results.

Psychometric data always need to be compared with the baseline status of the athlete. The lack of success induced by a long-term decrement of performance could be explained by the depression in OTS. The differences between self-assessment and the questionnaires, given by an independent experimenter, and the timing of the mood state assessment are important. Questionnaires should be used in standardized conditions. Other psychologic parameters different from mood state (attention-focussing, anxiety) might also be influenced (Table 3.3).

Athletes and the field of sports medicine in general would benefit greatly if a specific, sensitive, simple, diagnostic test existed for the identification of OTS. At present no such test meets this criterion, but there certainly is a need for a combination of diagnostic aids to pinpoint possible markers for OTS. In particular, there is a need for a detection mechanism for early triggering factors.

Table 3.3 Diagnosis of overtraining syndrome (OTS): checklist. (Consensus statement ECSS: Meeusen *et al.* 2006.)

Performance – fatigue
Does the athlete have:
- Unexplainable underperformance
- Persistant fatigue
- Increased sense of effort in training
- Sleep disorders

Exclusion criteria
Are there confounding diseases?
- Anaemia
- Epstein–Barr virus
- Other infectious diseases
- Muscle damage (high CK)
- Lyme disease
- Endocrinologic diseases (e.g., diabetes, thyroid, adrenal gland)
- Major disorders of feeding behaviour
- Biological abnormalities (e.g., increased CRP, creatinine, ferritin, increased liver enzymes)
- Injury (musculoskeletal system)
- Cardiologic symptoms
- Adult-onset asthma
- Allergies

Are there training errors?
- Training volume increased (>5%) (h/week, km/week)
- Training intensity increased significantly
- Training monotony present
- High number of competitions
- In endurance athletes: decreased performance at "anaerobic" threshold
- Exposure to environmental stressors (e.g., altitude, heat, cold)

Other confounding factors
- Psychologic signs and symptoms (e.g., disturbed POMS, RestQ-Sport, RPE)
- Social factors (e.g., family, relationships, financial, work, coach, team)
- Recent or multiple time zone travel

Exercise test
- Are there baseline values to compare with (e.g., performance, heart rate, hormonal, lactate)?
- Maximal exercise test performance
- Submaximal or sports-specific test performance
- Multiple performance tests

CK, creatine kinase; CRP, C-reactive protein; POMS, Profile of Mood State; RPE, Ratings of Perceived Exertion.

Therefore, a flowchart as presented in the Consensus Statement of the ECSS could help to establish the exclusion diagnosis for the detection of OTS.

Prevention

One general confounding factor when reviewing literature on OTS is that the definition and diagnosis of OR and OTS is not standardized. One can even question in most of the studies whether subjects had OTS. Because it is difficult to diagnose, authors agree that it is important to prevent OTS (Foster *et al.* 1988; Kuipers 1996; Uusitalo 2001). Moreover, because OTS is mainly caused by an imbalance in the training : recovery ratio (too much training and competitions and too little recovery), it is of utmost importance that athletes record their training load daily, using a training diary or log (Foster 1998; Foster *et al.* 1988). The four methods most frequently used to monitor training and prevent OT are: retrospective questionnaires, training diaries, physiologic screening and the direct observational method (Hopkins 1991). Also, the psychologic screening of athletes (Berglund & Safstrom 1994; Hooper & McKinnon 1995; Hooper *et al.* 1995; Kellmann 2002; McKenzie 1999; Morgan *et al.* 1988; Raglin *et al.* 1991; Steinacker & Lehmann 2002; Urhausen *et al.* 1998b) and the Ratings of Perceived Exertion (RPE; Acevedo *et al.* 1994; Callister *et al.* 1990; Foster 1998; Foster *et al.* 1996; Hooper & McKinnon 1995; Hooper *et al.* 1995; Kentta & Hassmen 1998; Snyder *et al.* 1993) are receiving more and more attention nowadays.

Hooper *et al.* (1995) used daily training logs during an entire season in swimmers to detect staleness (OTS). The distances swum, the dry-land work time, and subjective self-assessment of training intensity were recorded. In addition to these training details, the swimmers also recorded subjective ratings of quality of sleep, fatigue, stress and muscle soreness, body mass, early morning heart rate, occurrence of illness, menstruation, and causes of stress. Swimmers were classified as having OTS if their profile met five criteria. Three of these criteria were determined by items of the daily training logs: fatigue ratings in the logs of more than 5 (scale 1–7) lasting longer than 7 days, comments in the page provided in each log that the athlete was feeling that he or she responded poorly to training, and a negative response to a question regarding the presence of illness in the swimmer's log, together with a normal blood leukocyte count.

Foster *et al.* (1996, 1998) have determined training load as the product of the subjective intensity of a training session using session RPE and the total duration of the training session expressed in minutes. If these parameters are summed on a weekly basis, it is termed the total training load of an individual. The session RPE has been shown to be related to the average per cent heart rate reserve during an exercise session, and to the percentage of a training session during which the heart rate is in blood lactate-derived heart rate training zones. With this method of monitoring training they have demonstrated the utility of evaluating experimental alterations in training and have successfully related training load to performance (Foster *et al.* 1996). However, training load is clearly not the only training-related variable contributing to the genesis of OTS. So, in addition to the weekly training load, daily mean training load, as well as the standard deviation of training load, were calculated during each week. The daily mean divided by the standard deviation was defined as the monotony. The product of the weekly training load and monotony was calculated as strain. The incidence of simple illness and injury was noted and plotted together with the indices of training load, monotony, and strain. They noted the correspondence between spikes in the indices of training and subsequent illness or injury, and thresholds that allowed for optimal explanation of illnesses were computed (Foster 1998).

One of the disadvantages of the traditional "paper and pencil" method is that data collection can be complicated, and that immediate feedback is not always possible. Another problem is that when athletes are at an international training camp or competition, immediate "data computing" is not possible. It might therefore be useful to have an "online" training log (Cumps *et al.* 2005; Pockelé *et al.* 2004) which has specific features for detecting not only slight differences in training load, but also the subjective parameters (muscle soreness, mental and physical well-being) that have been proven to be important in the detection of OTS (Table 3.4).

Table 3.4 Considerations for coaches and physicians.

Until a definitive diagnostic tool for OTS is present, coaches and physicians need to rely on performance decrements as verification that OTS exists. However, if sophisticated laboratory techniques are not available, the following considerations may be useful

- Maintain accurate records of performance during training and competition. Be willing to adjust daily training intensity/volume, or allow a day of complete rest, when performance declines or the athlete complains of excessive fatigue
- Avoid excessive monotony of training
- Always individualize the intensity of training
- Encourage and regularly reinforce optimal nutrition, hydration status, and sleep
- Be aware that multiple stressors such as sleep loss or sleep disturbance (e.g., jet lag), exposure to environmental stressors, occupational pressures, change of residence, and interpersonal or family difficulties may add to the stress of physical training
- Treat OTS with rest. Reduced training may be sufficient for recovery in some cases of overreaching
- Resumption of training should be individualized on the basis of the signs and symptoms because there is no definitive indicator of recovery
- Communication with the athletes (maybe through an online training diary) about their physical, mental, and emotional concerns is important
- Include regular psychologic questionnaires to evaluate the emotional and psychologic state of the athlete
- Maintain confidentiality regarding each athlete's condition (physical, clinical, and mental)
- Importance of regular health checks performed by a multidisciplinary team (e.g., physician, nutritionist, psychologist)
- Allow the athlete time to recover after illness or injury
- Note the occurrence of URTI and other infectious episodes; the athlete should be encouraged to suspend training or reduce the training intensity when affected by infection
- Always rule out an organic disease in cases of performance decrement
- Unresolved viral infections are not routinely assessed in elite athletes, but it may be worth investigating this in individuals experiencing fatigue and underperformance in training and competition

OTS, overtraining syndrome; URTI, upper respiratory tract infections.

Conclusions

A difficulty with recognizing and conducting research into athletes with OTS is defining the point at which OTS develops. Many studies claim to have induced OTS, but it is more likely that they have induced a state of OR in their subjects. Consequently, the majority of studies aimed at identifying markers of ensuing OTS are actually reporting markers of excessive exercise stress resulting in the acute condition of OR and not the chronic condition of OTS. The mechanism of OTS could be difficult to examine in detail, possibly because the stress caused by excessive training load, in combination with other stressors, might trigger different "defence mechanisms," such as the immunologic, neuroendocrine, and other physiologic systems that all interact and probably therefore cannot be pinpointed as the "sole" cause of OTS. It might be that, as in other syndromes (e.g., chronic fatigue syndrome, or burnout), the psychoneuroimmunology (study of brain–behavior–immune interrelationships) might shed a light on the possible mechanisms of OTS. But until there is a definite diagnostic tool, it is of utmost importance to standardize measures that are now thought to provide a good inventory of the training status of the athlete. It is very important to emphasize the need to distinguish OTS from OR and other potential causes of temporary underperformance, such as anaemia, acute infection, muscle damage, and insufficient carbohydrate intake.

The physical demands of intensified training are not the only elements in the development of OTS. It seems that a complex set of psychologic factors are important in the development of OTS, including excessive expectations from a coach or family members, competitive stress, personality structure, social environment, relationships with family and friends, monotony in training, personal or emotional problems, and school- or work-related demands. While no single marker can be taken as an indicator of impending OTS, the regular monitoring of a combination of performance, physiologic, biochemical, immunologic, and psychologic variables would seem to be the best strategy to identify athletes who are failing to cope with the stress of training.

Much more research is necessary to obtain a clear-cut answer to the origin and detection of OTS. We therefore encourage researchers and clinicians to report as much as possible on individual cases of athletes who are underperforming and by following the exclusion diagnosis find that they possibly have OTS.

Acknowledgement

This chapter is based on the Consensus Statement of the European College of Sport Science: Meeusen *et al.* (2006).

References

Abercrombie, E., Keefe, K., DiFrischia, D. & Zigmond, M. (1989) Differential effect of stress on *in vivo* dopamine release in striatum, nucleus accumbens, and medial frontal cortex. *Journal of Neurochemistry* **52**, 1655–1658.

Acevedo, E., Rinehardt, K. & Kraemer, R. (1994) Perceived exertion and affect at varying intensities of running. *Research Quarterly in Exercise Sport* **65**, 372–376.

Achten, J. & Jeukendrup, A.E. (2003) Heart rate monitoring: applications and limitations. *Sports Medicine* **33**, 517–538.

Adlercreutz, H., Harkonen, M., Kuoppasalmi, K., Naveri, H., Huhtaniemi, I., Tikkanen, H., *et al.* (1986) Effect of training on plasma anabolic and catabolic steroid hormones and their response during physical exercise. *International Journal of Sports Medicine* **7**, S27–S28.

Armstrong, L. & VanHeest, J. (2002) The unknown mechanisms of the overtraining syndrome: clues from depression and psychoneuroimmunology. *Sports Medicine* **32**, 185–209.

Barron, G., Noakes, T., Levy, W., Smidt, C. & Millar, R. (1985) Hypothalamic dysfunction in overtrained athletes. *Journal of Clinical Endocrinology and Metabolism* **60**, 803–806.

Berglund, B. & Safstrom, H. (1994) Psychological monitoring and modulation of training load of world-class canoeists. *Medicine and Science in Sports and Exercise* **26**, 1036–1040.

Budgett, R., Newsholme, E., Lehmann, M., Sharp, C., Jones, D., Peto, T., *et al.* (2000) Redefining the overtraining syndrome as the unexplained underperformance syndrome. *British Journal of Sports Medicine* **34**, 67–68.

Callister, R., Callister, R., Fleck, S. & Dudley, G. (1990) Physiological and performance responses to overtraining in elite judo athletes. *Medicine and Science in Sports and Exercise* **22**, 816–824.

Carins, J. & Booth, C. (2002) Salivary immunoglobulin-A as a marker of stress during strenuous physical training. *Aviation Space and Environmental Medicine* **3**, 1203–1207.

Chatard, J., Atlaoui, D., Lac, G., Duclos, M., Hooper, S. & MacKinnon, L. (2002) Cortisol, DHEA, performance and training in elite swimmers. *International Journal of Sports Medicine* **23**, 510–515.

Cizza, G., Kvetnansky, R., Tartaglia, M., Blackman, M., Chrousos, G. & Gold, P. (1993) Immobolisation stress rapidly decreases hypothalamic corticotropin-releasing hormone secretion *in vitro* in the male 344/N fischer rat. *Life Sciences* **53**, 233–240.

Cumps, E., Pockelé, J. & Meeusen, R. (2005) Blits® on-line: an uniform injury registration system for acute and overuse injuries. *Proceedings of the International Conference on IT and Sport* (Seifriz *et al.*, eds.): 22–25.

De Schutter, M.F., Buyse, L, Meeusen, R. & Roelands, B. (2004) Hormonal responses to a high-intensity training period in Army recruits. *Medicine and Science in Sports and Exercise* **36**, S295.

Dishman, R. (1997) The norepinephrine hypothesis. In: *Physical Activity and Mental Health* (Morgan, W.P., ed.) Taylor & Francis, Washington, D.C.: 199–212.

Duclos, M., Corcuff, J.-B., Arsac, L., Moreau-Gaudry, F., Rashedi, M., Roger, P., *et al.* (1998) Corticotroph axis sensitivity after exercise in endurance-trained athletes. *Clinical Endocrinology* **8**, 493–501.

Duclos, M., Corcuff, J.-B., Rashedi, M., Fougere, V. & Manier, G. (1997) Trained versus untrained men: different immediate post-exercise responses of pituitary–adrenal axis. *European Journal of Applied Physiology* **75**, 343–350.

Duclos, M., Gouarne, C. & Bonnemaison, D. (2003) Acute and chronic effects of exercise on tissue sensitivity to glucocorticoids. *Journal of Applied Physiology* **94**, 869–875.

Duclos, M., Minkhar, M., Sarrieau, A., Bonnemaison, D., Manier, G. & Mormede, P. (1999) Reversibility of endurance training-induced changes on glucocorticoid sensitivity of monocytes by an acute exercise. *Clinical Endocrinology* **1**, 749–756.

Finlay, J., Zigmond, M. & Abercrombie, E. (1995) Increased dopamine and norepinephrine release in medial prefrontal cortex induced by acute and chronic stress effects of diazepam. *Neuroscience* **64**, 619–628.

Foster, C. (1998) Monitoring training in athletes with reference to overtraining syndrome. *Medicine and Science in Sports and Exercise* **30**, 1164–1168.

Foster, C., Daines, E., Hector, L., Snyder, A. & Welsh, R. (1996) Athletic performance in relation to training load. *Wisconsin Medical Journal* **95**, 370–374.

Foster, C. & Lehmann, M. (1997) Overtraining. In: *Running Injuries* (Guten, G.N., ed.) W.B. Saunders, Philadelphia: 173–187.

Foster, C., Snyder, A., Thompson, N. & Kuettel, K. (1988) Normalization of the blood lactate profile. *International Journal of Sports Medicine* **9**, 198–200.

Fry, A., Kraemer, W. & Ramsey, L. (1998) Pituitary–adrenal–gonadal responses to high-intensity resistance exercise overtraining. *Journal of Applied Physiology* **85**, 2352–2359.

Fry, A. & Kraemer, W. (1997) Resistance exercise overtraining and overreaching. *Sports Medicine* **23**, 106–129.

Fry, A., Steinacker, J. & Meeusen, R. (2006) Endocrinology of overtraining. In: *The Endocrine System in Sports and Exercise.* Vol. XI. *Encyclopaedia of Sports Medicine* (Kraemer, W. & Rogol, A., eds.) Blackwell Publishing USA.

Fry, R., Morton, A. & Keast, D. (1991) Overtraining in athletes. *Sports Medicine* **12**, 32–65.

Gabriel, H. & Kindermann, W. (1997) The acute immune response to exercise: what does it mean? *International Journal of Sports Medicine* **18**, S28–S45.

Gabriel, H.H., Urhausen, A., Valet, G., Heidelbach, U. & Kindermann, W. (1998) Overtraining and immune system: a prospective longitudinal study in endurance athletes. *Medicine and Science in Sports and Exercise* **30**, 1151–1157.

Gastmann, U. & Lehmann, M. (1998) Overtraining and the BCAA hypothesis. *Medicine and Science in Sports and Exercise* **30**, 1173–1178.

Gleeson, M. (2007) Immune function and exercise. *European Journal of Sport Science* **103**, 693–699.

Gresch, P., Sved, A., Zigmond, M. & Finlay, J. (1994) Stress-induced sensitization of dopamine and norepinephrine efflux in medial prefrontal cortex of the rat. *Journal of Neurochemistry* **63**, 575–583.

Hall, H., Flynn, M., Carroll, K., Brolinson, P., Shapiro, S. & Bushman, B. (1999) Effects of intensified training and detraining on testicular function. *Clinical Journal of Sports Medicine* **9**, 203–208.

Halson, S. & Jeukendrup, A. (2004) Does overtraining exist? An analysis of overreaching and overtraining research. *Sports Medicine* **34**, 967–981.

Halson, S., Lancaster, G., Jeukendrup, A. & Gleeson, M. (2003) Immunological responses to overreaching in cyclists. *Medicine and Science in Sports and Exercise* **35**, 854–861.

Halson, S.L., Bridge, M.W., Meeusen, R., Busschaert, B., Gleeson, M., Jones, D.A., et al. (2002) Time course of performance changes and fatigue markers during intensified training in trained cyclists. *Journal of Applied Physiology* **93**, 947–956.

Hedelin, R., Kentta, G., Wiklund, U., Bjerle, P. & Henriksson-Larsen, K. (2000a) Short-term overtraining: effects on performance, circulatory responses, and heart rate variability. *Medicine and Science in Sports and Exercise* **32**, 1480–1484.

Hedelin, R., Wiklund, U., Bjerle, P. & Henriksson-Larsen, K. (2000b) Cardiac autonomic imbalance in an overtrained athlete. *Medicine and Science in Sports and Exercise* **32**, 1531–1533.

Hooper, S. & Mackinnon, L. (1995) Monitoring overtraining in athletes: recommendations. *Sports Medicine* **20**, 321–327.

Hooper, S., Mackinnon, L., Gordon, R. & Bachmann, A. (1993) Hormonal responses of elite swimmers to overtraining. *Medicine and Science in Sports and Exercise* **25**, 741–747.

Hooper, S., MacKinnon, L. & Hanrahan, S. (1997) Mood states as an indication of staleness and recovery. *International Journal of Sport Psychology* **28**, 1–12.

Hooper, S., MacKinnon, L. & Howard, A. (1999) Physiological and psychometric variables for monitoring recovery during tapering for major competition. *Medicine and Science in Sports and Exercise* **31**, 1205–1210.

Hooper, S.L., Mackinnon, L.T., Howard, A., Gordon, R.D. & Bachmann, A.W. (1995) Markers for monitoring overtraining and recovery. *Medicine and Science in Sports and Exercise* **27**, 106–112.

Hopkins, W. (1991) Quantification of training in competitive sports: methods and applications. *Sports Medicine* **12**, 161–183.

Imperato, A., Angelucci, L., Casolini, P., Zocchi, A. & Puglisi-Allegra, S. (1992) Repeated stressful experiences differently affect limbic dopamine release during and following stress. *Brain Research* **577**, 194–199.

Jeukendrup, A.E., Hesselink, M.K., Snyder, A.C., Kuipers, H. & Keizer, H.A. (1992) Physiological changes in male competitive cyclists after two weeks of intensified training. *International Journal of Sports Medicine* **13**, 534–541.

Jordan, S., Kramer, G., Zukas, P. & Petty, F. (1994) Previous stress increases *in vivo* biogenic amine response to swim stress. *Neurochemistry Research* **19**, 1521–1525.

Keefe, K., Stricker, E., Zigmond, M. & Abercrombie, E. (1990) Environmental stress increases extracellular dopamine in striatum of 6-hydroxydopamine-treated rats: *in vivo* microdialysis studies. *Brain Research* **527**, 350–353.

Keizer, H. (1998) Neuroendicrine aspects of overtraining. In: *Overtraining in Sport* (Kreider, R., Fry, A.C. & O'Toole, M., eds.) Human Kinetics, Champaign, IL: 145–168.

Kellmann, M. (ed) (2002) *Enhancing Recovery: Preventing Underperformance in Athletes.* Human Kinetics, Champaign, IL.

Kellmann, M. & Gunther, K-L. (2000) Changes in stress and recovery in elite rowers during preparation for the Olympic Games. *Medicine and Science in Sports and Exercise* **32**, 676–683.

Kentta, G. & Hassmen, P. (1998) Overtraining and recovery. *Sports Medicine* **26**, 1–16.

Kingsbury, K.J., Kay, L. & Hjelm, M. (1998) Contrasting plasma amino acid patterns in elite athletes: association with fatigue and infection. *British Journal of Sports Medicine* **32**, 25–33.

Kirby, L., Chou-Green, J., Davis, K. & Lucki, I. (1997) The effects of different stressors on extracellular 5-hydroxytryptamine and 5-hydroxyindoleacetic acid. *Brain Research* **760**, 218–230.

Knopfli, B., Calvert, R., Bar-Or, O., Villiger, B. & Von Duvillard, S. (2001) Competition performance and basal nocturnal catecholamine excretion in cross-country skiers. *Medicine and Science in Sports and Exercise* **33**, 1228–1232.

Kreider, R. (1998) Central fatigue hypothesis and overtraining. In: *Overtraining in Sport* (Kreider, R., Fry, A.C. & O'Toole, M., eds.) Human Kinetics, Champaign, IL: 309–334.

Kreider, R., Fry, A.C. & O'Toole, M. (1998) Overtraining in sport: terms, definitions, and prevalence. In: *Overtraining in Sport* (Kreider, R., Fry, A.C. & O'Toole, M., eds.) Human Kinetics, Champaign, IL: vii–ix.

Kubesch, S., Bretschneider, V., Freudenmann, R., Weidenhammer, N., Lehmann, M., Spitzer, M., et al. (2003) Aerobic endurance exercise improves executive functions in depressed patients. *Journal of Clinical Psychiatry* **64**, 1005–1012.

Kuipers, H. (1996) How much is too much? Performance aspects of overtraining. *Research Quarterly in Exercise Sport* **67**, 65–69.

Kuipers, H. & Keizer, H. (1988) Overtraining in elite athletes, *Sports Medicine* **6**, 79–92.

Lachuer, J., Delton, I., Buda, M. & Tappaz, M. (1994) The habituation of brainstem catecholaminergic groups to chronic daily restraint stress is stress specific like that of the hypothalamo-pituitary–adrenal axis. *Brain Research* **638**, 196–202.

Lehmann, M., Foster, C., Dickhuth, H.H. & Gastmann, U. (1998a) Autonomic imbalance hypothesis and overtraining syndrome. *Medicine and Science in Sports and Exercise* **30**, 1140–1145.

Lehmann, M., Foster, C., Gastmann, U., Keizer, H. & Steinacker, J. (1999a) Definitions, types, symptoms, findings, underlying mechanisms, and frequency of overtraining and overtraining syndrome. In: *Overload, Performance Incompetence, and Regeneration in Sport* (Lehmann, M., Foster, C., Gastmann, U., Keizer, H. & Steinacker, J., eds.) Kluwer Academic/Plenum Publishers, New York: 1–6.

Lehmann, M., Foster, C. & Keul, J. (1993a) Overtraining in endurance athletes: a brief review. *Medicine and Science in Sports and Exercise* **25**, 854–862.

Lehmann, M., Foster, C., Netzer, N., Lormes, W., Steinacker, J.M., Liu, Y., *et al.* (1998b) Physiological responses to short- and long-term overtraining in endurance athletes. In: *Overtraining in Sport* (Kreider, Fry, O'Toole eds.) Human Kinetics, Champaign, IL: 19–46.

Lehmann, M., Gastmann, U., Baur, S., Liu, Y., Lormes, W., Opitz-Gress, A., *et al.* (1999b) Selected parameters and mechanisms of peripheral and central fatigue and regeneration in overtrained athletes. In: *Overload, Performance Incompetence, and Regeneration in Sport* (Lehmann, M., Foster, C., Gastmann, U., Keizer, H. & Steinacker, J., eds.) Kluwer Academic/Plenum Publishers, New York: 7–25.

Lehmann, M., Knizia, K., Gastmann, U., Petersen, K.G., Khalaf, A.N., Bauer, S., *et al.* (1993b) Influence of 6-week, 6 days per week, training on pituitary function in recreational athletes. *British Journal of Sports Medicine* **27**, 186–192.

Lehmann, M., Petersen, K.G., Liu, Y., Gastmann, U., Lormes, W., Steinacker, J.M. (2001) Chronische und erschöpfende Belastungen im Sport – Einfluss von Leptin und Inhibin. [Chronic and exhausting training in sports – influence of leptin and inhibin.] *Deutsch Zeitschrift für Sportmedicine* **51**, 234–243.

Lemyre, N. (2005) Determinants of burnout in elite athletes. PhD Thesis, Norwegian University of Sport and Physical Education.

Liberzon, I., Taylor, S., Amdur, R., Jung, T., Chamberlain, K., Minoshima, S., *et al.* (1999) Brain activation in PTSD in response to trauma-related stimuli. *Biology and Psychiatry* **45**, 817–826.

Mackinnon, L.T. & Hooper, S. (1994) Mucosal (secretory) immune system responses to exercise of varying intensity and during overtraining. *International Journal of Sports Medicine* **15**, S179–S183.

Mackinnon, L.T., Hooper, S., Jones, S., Gordon, R. & Bachmann, A. (1997) Hormonal, immunological, and haematological responses to intensified training in elite swimmers. *Medicine and Science in Sports and Exercise* **29**, 1637–1645.

McKenzie, D. (1999) Markers of excessive exercise. *Canadian Journal of Applied Physiology* **24**(1), 66–73.

Manetta, J., Brun, J., Maimoun, L., Galy, O., Coste, O., Maso, F., *et al.* (2002) Carbohydrate dependence during hard-intensity exercise in trained cyclists in the competitive season: importance of training status. *International Journal of Sports Medicine* **23**, 516–523.

Maso, F., Lac, G., Michaux, O. & Robert, A. (2003) Corrélations entre scores au questionnaire de la Société française de médecine du sport et concentrations de cortisol et testostérone salivaires lors du suivi d'une équipe de rugby de haut niveau. *Science and Sports* **18**, 299–301.

Meeusen, R. (1998) Overtraining, indoor and outdoor. *Vlaams tijdschrift voor Sportgeneeskunde & Sportwetenschappen* **19**, 8–19.

Meeusen, R. (1999) Overtraining and the central nervous system, the missing link? In: *Overload, Performance Incompetence, and Regeneration in Sport* (Lehmann, M., Foster, C., Gastmann, U., Keizer, H. & Steinacker, J., eds.) Kluwer Academic/Plenum Publishers, New York: 187–202.

Meeusen, R. (2004) Overtraining and the neuroendocrine system. *Medicine and Science in Sports and Exercise* **36**, S45.

Meeusen, R., Chaouloff, F., Thorré, K., Sarre, S., De Meirleir, K., Ebinger, G., *et al.* (1996) Effects of tryptophan and/or acute running on extracellular 5-HT and 5-HIAA levels in the hippocampus of food-deprived rats. *Brain Research* **740**, 245–252.

Meeusen, R. & De Meirleir, K. (1995) Exercise and brain neurotransmission. *Sports Medicine* **20**, 160–188.

Meeusen, R., Duclos, M., Gleeson, M., Rietjens, G., Steinacker, J. & Urhausen, A. (2006) Prevention, diagnosis and the treatment of the Overtraining Syndrome. *European Journal of Sport Science* **6**, 1–14.

Meeusen, R., Piacentini, M.F., Busschaert, B., Buyse, L., De Schutter, G. & Stray-Gundersen, J. (2004) Hormonal responses in athletes: the use of a two bout exercise protocol to detect subtle differences in (over)training status. *European Journal of Applied Physiology* **91**, 140–146.

Meeusen, R., Sarre, S., Michotte, Y., Ebinger, G. & De Meirleir, K. (1994) The effects of exercise on neurotransmission in rat striatum: a microdialysis study. In: *Monitoring Molecules in Neuroscience* (Louilot, A., Durkin, T., Spampinato, U. & Cador, M., eds.) Talence, University of Bordeaux: 181–182.

Meeusen, R., Smolders, I., Sarre, S., De Meirleir, K., Ebinger, G. & Michotte, Y. (1995) The effects of exercise on extracellular glutamate (GLU) and GABA in rat striatum: a microdialysis study. *Medicine and Science in Sports and Exercise* **27**, S215.

Meeusen, R., Smolders, I., Sarre, S., De Meirleir, K., Keizer, H., Serneels, M., *et al.* (1997) Endurance training effects on striatal neurotransmitter release: an '*in vivo*' microdialysis study. *Acta Physiologica Scandinavica* **159**, 335–341.

Morgan, W., Costill, D., Flynn, M., Raglin, J. & O'Connor, P. (1988) Mood disturbance following increased training in swimmers. *Medicine and Science in Sports and Exercise* **20**, 408–414.

Morgan, W.P., Brown, D., Raglin, J., O'Connor, P. & Ellickson, K. (1987) Psychological monitoring of overtraining and staleness. *British Journal of Sports Medicine* **21**, 107–114.

Nindl, B., Leone, C., Tharion, W., Johnson, R., Castellani, J., Patton, J., *et al.* (2002) Physical performance responses during 72 h of military operations. *Medicine and Science in Sports and Exercise* **34**, 1814–1822.

Nisembaum, L., Zigmond, M., Sved, A. & Abercrombie, E. (1991) Prior exposure to chronic stress results in enhanced synthesis and release of hippocampal norepinephrine in response to a novel stressor. *Journal of Neuroscience* **11**, 1478–1484.

O'Connor, P. (1997) Overtraining and staleness. In: *Physical Activity and Mental Health* (Morgan, W.P., ed.) Taylor & Francis, Washington, D.C.: 145–160.

O'Connor, P., Morgan, W. & Raglin, J. (1991) Psychobiologic effect of 3 d of increased training in female and male swimmers. *Medicine and Science in Sports and Exercise* **23**, 1055–1061.

O'Connor, P., Morgan, W., Raglin, J., Barksdale, C. & Kalin, N. (1989) Mood state and salivary cortisol levels following overtraining in female swimmers. *Psychoneuroendocrinology* **14**, 303–310.

Passelergue, P. & Lac, G. (1999) Saliva cortisol, testosterone and T/C ratio variations during a wrestling competition and during the post-competitive recovery period. *International Journal of Sports Medicine* **20**, 109–113.

Petibois, C., Cazorla, G. & Déléris, G. (2003a) The biological and metabolic adaptations to 12 months in elite rowers. *International Journal of Sports Medicine* **24**, 36–42.

Petibois, C., Cazorla, G., Pootmans, J. & Déléris, G. (2002) Biochemical aspects of overtraining in endurance sports. *Sports Medicine* **32**, 867–878.

Petibois, C., Cazorla, G., Pootmans, J. & Déléris, G. (2003b) Biochemical aspects of overtraining in endurance sports: the metabolism alteration process syndrome. *Sports Medicine* **33**, 83–94.

Pichot, V., Busso, T., Roche, F., Garet, M., Costes, F., Duverney, D., *et al.* (2002) Autonomic adaptations to intensive and overload training periods: a laboratory study. *Medicine and Science in Sports and Exercise* **34**, 1660–1666.

Pockelé, J., Cumps, E., Piacentini, F. & Meeusen, R. (2005) Blits® on-line training diary for the early detection of overreaching and overtraining. *Proceedings of the International Conference on IT and Sport* (Seifriz *et al.*, eds.).

Porter, R., Gallagher, P., Watson, S. & Young, A. (2004) Corticosteroid–serotonin interactions in depression: a review of the human evidence. *Psychopharmacology* **173**, 1–17.

Raglin, J. & Morgan, W. (1994) Development of a scale for use in monitoring training-induced distress in athletes. *International Journal of Sports Medicine* **15**, 84–88.

Raglin, J., Morgan, W. & O'Connor, P. (1991) Changes in mood state during training in female and male college swimmers. *International Journal of Sports Medicine* **12**, 585–589.

Reid, V.L., Gleeson, M., Williams, N. & Clancy, R.L. (2004) Clinical investigation of athletes with persistent fatigue and/or recurrent infections. *British Journal of Sports Medicine* **38**, 42–45.

Rietjens, G., Kuipers, H., Adam, J., Saris, W., Van Breda, E., Van Hamont, D., *et al.* (2005) Physiological, biochemical and psychological markers of strenuous training-induced fatigue. *International Journal of Sports Medicine* **26**, 16–26.

Robson, P. (2003) Elucidationg the unexplained underperformance syndrome in endurance athletes: the interleukin-6 hypothesis. *Sports Medicine* **33**, 771–781.

Rowbottom, D., Keast, D., Goodman, C. & Morton, A. (1995) The haematological, biochemical and immunological profile of athletes suffering from the overtraining syndrome. *European Journal of Applied Physiology* **70**, 502–509.

Rowbottom, D., Keast, D. & Morton, A. (1996) The emerging role of glutamine as an indicator of exercise stress and overtraining. *Sports Medicine* **21**, 80–97.

Seene, T., Umnova, M. & Kaasik, P. (1999) The exercise myopathy. In: *Overload, Performance Incompetence, and Regeneration in Sport* (Lehmann, M., Foster, C., Gastmann, U., Keizer, H. & Steinacker, J., eds.) Kluwer Academic/Plenum Publishers, New York: 119–130.

Selye, H. (1936) A syndrome produced by diverse nocuous agents. *Nature* **138**, 32.

Shintani, F., Nakaki, T., Kanba, S., Sato, K., Yagi, G., Shiozawa, M., *et al.* (1995) Involvement of interleukin-1 in immobilization stress-induced increase in plasma adrenocorticotropic hormones and in release of hypothalamic monoamines in rat. *Journal of Neuroscience* **15**, 1961–1970.

Silva, J. (1990) An analysis of the training stress syndrome in competitive athletics. *Journal of Applied Sport Psychology* **2**, 5–20.

Smith, L. (2000) Cytokine hypothesis of overtraining: a physiological adaptation to excessive stress? *Medicine and Science in Sports and Exercise* **32**, 317–331.

Smith, L. (2003) Overtraining, excessive exercise, and altered immunity. Is this a T helper-1 versus T helper-2 lymphocyte response? *Sports Medicine* **33**, 347–364.

Smith, L. (2004) Tissue trauma: the underlying cause of overtraining syndrome? *Journal of Strength and Conditioning Research* **18**, 184–191.

Snyder, A. (1998) Overtraining and glycogen depletion hypothesis. *Medicine and Science in Sports and Exercise* **30**, 1146–1150.

Snyder, A., Jeukendrup, A., Hesselink, M., Kuipers, H. & Foster, C. (1993) A physiological/psychological indicator of overreaching during intensive training. *International Journal of Sports Medicine* **14**, 29–32.

Stanford, C. (1993) Monoamines in response and adaptation to stress. In: *Stress, From Synapse to Syndrome* (Stanford, S. & Salmon, P., eds.) Academic Press, London: 281–331.

Steinacker, J.M., Lormes, W., Liu, Y., Opitz-Gress, A., Baller, B., Günther, K., *et al.* (2000) Training of Junior Rowers before World Championships: effects on performance, mood state and selected hormonal and metabolic responses. *Journal of Physical Fitness and Sports Medicine* **40**, 327–335.

Steinacker, J.M. & Lehmann, M. (2002) Clinical findings and mechanisms of stress and recovery in athletes. In: *Enhancing Recovery: Preventing Underperformance in Athletes* (Kellmann, M., ed.) Human Kinetics, Champaign, IL: 103–118.

Steinacker, J.M., Lormes, W., Reissnecker, S. & Liu, Y. (2004) New aspects of the hormone and cytokine response to training. *European Journal of Applied Physiology* **91**, 382–393.

Thorré, K., Chaouloff, F., Sarre, S., Meeusen, R., Ebinger, G. & Michotte, Y. (1997) Differential effects of restraint stress on hippocampal 5-HT metabolism and extracellular levels of 5-HT in streptozotocin-diabetic rats. *Brain Research* **772**, 209–216.

Tiollier, E., Gomez-Merino, D., Burnat, P., Jouanin, J.C., Bourrilhon, C., Filaire, E., *et al.* (2005) Intense training: mucosal immunity and incidence of respiratory infections. *European Journal of Applied Physiology* **93**, 421–428.

Urhausen, A., Gabriel, H. & Kindermann, W. (1995) Blood hormones as markers of training stress and overtraining. *Sports Medicine* **20**, 251–276.

Urhausen, A., Gabriel, H. & Kindermann, W. (1998a) Impaired pituitary hormonal response to exhaustive exercise in overtrained endurance athletes. *Medicine and Science in Sports and Exercise* **30**, 407–414.

Urhausen, A., Gabriel, H., Weiler, B. & Kindermann, W. (1998b) Ergometric and psychological findings during overtraining: a long-term follow-up study in endurance athletes. *International Journal of Sports Medicine* **19**, 114–120.

Urhausen, A. & Kindermann, W. (2002) Diagnosis of overtraining: what tools do we have? *Sports Medicine* **32**, 95–102.

Uusitalo, A.L.T. (2001) Overtraining: making a difficult diagnosis and implementing targeted treatment. *Physician and Sportsmedicine* **29**, 35–50.

Uusitalo, A.L.T., Huttunen, P., Hanin, Y., Uusitalo, A.J. & Rusko, H. (1998b) Hormonal responses to endurance training and overtraining in female athletes. *Clinical Journal of Sports Medicine* **8**, 178–186.

Uusitalo, A.L.T., Uusitalo, A.J., Rusko, H.K. (1998a) Exhaustive endurance training for 6–9 weeks did not induce changes in intrinsic heart rate and cardiac autonomic modulation in female athletes. *International Journal of Sports Medicine* **19**, 532–540.

Uusitalo, A.L.T., Uusitalo, A.J. & Rusko, H.K. (2000) Heart rate and blood pressure variability during heavy training and overtraining in the female athlete. *International Journal of Sports Medicine* **21**, 45–53.

Uusitalo, A.L.T., Valkonen-Korhonen, M., Helenius, P., Vanninen, E., Bergstrom, K. & Kuikka, J. (2004) Abnormal serotonin reuptake in an overtrained insomnic and depressed team athlete. *International Journal of Sports Medicine* **25**, 150–153.

Ventura, N., Hoppeler, H., Seiler, R., Binggeli, A., Mullis, P. & Vogt, M. (2003) The response of trained athletes to six weeks of endurance training in hypoxia or normoxia. *International Journal of Sports Medicine* **24**, 166–172.

Weizman, R., Weizman, A., Kook, K., Vocci, F., Deitsch, S. & Paul, S. (1989) Repeated swim stress alters brain benzodiazepine receptors measured *in vivo. Journal of Pharmacology and Experimental Therapeutics* **249**, 701–707.

Wilckens, T., Schweiger, U. & Pirke, K. (1992) Activation of 5-HT$_{1C}$-receptors suppresses excessive wheel running induced by semi-starvation in the rat. *Psychopharmacology* **109**, 77–84.

Wittert, G., Livesey, J., Espiner, E. & Donald, R. (1996) Adaptation of the hypothalamopituitary adrenal axis to chronic exercise stress in humans. *Medicine and Science in Sports and Exercise* **28**, 1015–1019.

Chapter 4

Clinical Exercise Testing and Assessment of Athletes

ROBERT U. NEWTON, PAUL B. LAURSEN AND WARREN YOUNG

A program of ongoing testing for the assessment of any athlete is essential to optimize training program design, reduce injury or illness risk, increase career longevity, and maximize sports performance. The adage "you can't manage what you can't measure" applies equally to athletes as it does to business. A second important function of testing is to provide feedback to the athlete, which increases motivation as well as the athlete's understanding of their responses and adaptations to different training manipulations.

Optimizing training program design and the window of adaptation

Almost all sports require a range of physical performance qualities. These include components of strength, power, speed, agility, endurance, cardiovascular fitness, flexibility, and body composition. While there are other qualities such as skill and psychologic state, our discussion in this chapter is confined to these physical capacities.

For any given sport, and in some case particular positions in team sports, the athlete will have an enhanced chance of success if their body composition, neuromuscular and cardiorespiratory systems are specifically tuned for the tasks required. It is when the underlying "machinery" is correctly built and tuned that the skill, strategy, and psychologic

abilities of the athlete can be best brought to bear and the greatest chance of success realized.

This highlights the multifaceted nature of sports performance, with a mixed training methods approach being most effective as it develops more components of performance. A key principle of training methodology is that of "diminishing returns," whereby the more developed a particular component, the smaller the window for adaptation. This relates to the initial level of fitness or development of a given component. Each can be developed only to a maximum level dictated by genetic endowment, and as the athlete's development moves along this continuum, the same training effort produces ever-decreasing percentage improvement. The practical application of this is that when an athlete develops one component to a high level (e.g., strength), the potential for that component to contribute to further increases in sport performance diminish. Thus, each component can be thought of as a "window of adaptation" to the larger window of adaptation in overall performance. This concept is summarized in Fig. 4.1. For example, if an athlete undertakes a program of training to develop cardiorespiratory fitness, they will exhibit a shrinking window of adaptation to this form of stimulus. As this window shrinks, training time will be more efficiently spent on other training methods such as speed development or muscle strengthening. Further, training must be targeted to increase performance in those components in which the athlete is weakest, because here lies the largest window for adaptation and thus the greatest increase in overall sports performance.

The Olympic Textbook of Medicine in Sport, 1st edition. Edited by M. Schwellnus. Published 2008 by Blackwell Publishing, ISBN: 978-1-4051-5637-0.

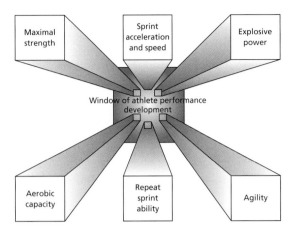

Fig. 4.1 Schematic diagram representing the components contributing to athlete physical performance for a particular sport (e.g., football). Each component can contribute to the overall window for performance adaptation. The greater the development of a single component, the smaller that component's window of adaptation and thus potential to develop overall sporting performance. Thus, it may be more efficient to design the training program to target those components with the greatest windows of adaptation (i.e., the components in which the athlete is weak).

The athlete will be limited in potential by the weakest link.

General principles of testing athletes

Principles of measurement are described in many reference texts (Thomas & Nelson 1990) and the interested reader is advised to make themselves familiar with the key issues prior to developing and implementing a program of athlete assessment. Here we summarize the key aspects.

Validity

To have any meaning the test must: (i) actually measure what it is purported to measure; and (ii) be reliable. An example is the use of bio-impedence to measure body fat mass in the athlete. The technique, described later, actually estimates total body water based on electrical impedance to current flow and then makes inferences about fat content. While a useful technique in some instances,

changes in hydration state for example can impact markedly on the result and yet actual fat content has not changed.

Reliability

For any test result to be meaningful there must be sufficient reliability so that differences between athletes and changes in a given athlete can be effectively detected above the noise of the measurement. How much a given value changes with repeated measurements because of variation in equipment or methods or effects of environment is termed the reliability. The measure is usually expressed as a coefficient of variation or expressed as intra class correlation (ICC) coefficients. An in-depth discussion of the statistics of reliability and methods for determination is beyond the scope of this chapter and the interested reader is referred to the excellent resources provided by Hopkins (http://www.sportsci.org/resource/stats/).

Specificity

Tests should be selected based on their ability to assess key performance components accurately. It is pointless to assess aerobic capacity in sprint runners because the physiologic capacity being measured has no relevance to performance in the target event. Time is valuable to the athlete and coach, and testing can be seen as an imposition if it is not efficient and directly assessing the key aspects that require monitoring and feedback.

Scheduling

Testing must be performed when the athlete is "fresh" and their performance capacity is maximized. Generally, this requires 48 h abstinence from high-intensity training or any competition. This is not always feasible but is desirable to get the best possible scores. In some instances it is the goal of testing to assess levels of fatigue, overtraining, and injury so this principle does not apply. For example, athletes are now routinely tested in the days following a competitive event to assess recovery strategies and readiness to compete in the subsequent competition. Planning of the test schedule must be given careful consideration as test order and rest periods can have large effect on results. For example, a maximum strength test can be performed before an endurance test on the same day but not in the opposite order. Any tests that are fatiguing with persistent effects must be scheduled towards the end of the testing session. In many cases the program will have to be be split over several days to avoid prior tests impacting later ones.

Performance qualities

Certain measures represent specific or independent qualities of neuromuscular performance and these qualities can be assessed and trained independently. Performance diagnosis is the process of determining an athlete's level of development in each of these distinct qualities. By targeting specific performance qualities with prescribed training, greater efficiency of training effort can be achieved resulting in enhanced athlete performance. For most sports and athletic events, there are strength, speed-strength, and strength endurance dimensions. Because elite athletes tend to be genetically predisposed to their sport and train to enhance their abilities, specificity of these qualities is inherent to a particular sport or athletic event. In other words, each sport or event requires a certain level of these performance qualities to underpin a competitive advantage.

Performance diagnosis and prescription

The implementation of performance diagnosis and prescription should flow according to a logical sequence (Fig. 4.2). The initial step requires a determination of the important qualities in the target activity (i.e., a performance needs analysis). A test battery is then established to assess these qualities in an efficient, valid, and reliable manner. A training program is developed based on the performance diagnosis, which will improve performance in the target sport. The final aspect is perhaps the most important as isolated testing has little utility. It is only with frequent, ongoing assessment that a complete profile of the athlete is compiled and

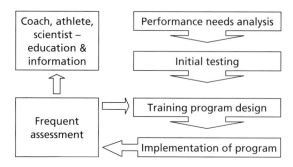

Fig. 4.2 Test–retest cycle for performance diagnosis.

manipulation of training variables can be coordinated to progress the athlete toward performance goals. The test–retest cycle (Fig. 4.2), with frequent adjustments to the training program, is a key feature of the performance diagnosis and prescription process. Various aspects of this process are now addressed.

Determination of key performance characteristics

The first step towards achieving the desired performance goal is to determine the key performance characteristics of the target activity. For example, if the task is to maximize take-off velocity in the high jump, then those strength and power qualities that influence take-off velocity need to be determined. This can be achieved through several processes such as biomechanical evaluation, analysis of high-level athletes, and pre–post testing. The best approach may be to combine all three to gain the greatest understanding of the target performance.

1 Biomechanical evaluation leads to an understanding of the forces exerted by the jump leg, minimum knee angle, and contact times that are observed during the high jump. Speed, range of motion, and contraction type of the other body segments should also be determined.

2 Analysis of high-level athletes in the sport can provide information on strength and power qualities. It can be assumed, although with caution, that if an athlete is performing well in the sport then the athlete possesses the necessary levels of these qualities.

3 A third method is to test athletes before and after phases involving certain training emphases. If they respond with large improvements in the targeted strength and power quality, then it could be that they are deficient in that quality and that this may require further attention. Certainly, if a component is improving rapidly it may be prudent to maintain the emphasis until some plateau occurs. However, there are caveats to this approach. First, it is wasteful to continue to seek improvement if the quality is not of significance to the task, or the athlete has an adequate level such that other qualities may be more limiting. Second, it may be better for the sake of training variety to take note of the large response and return to that quality at a later phase of training.

Assessment of strength and power

An athlete's strength and power profile has many components and the most effective training should involve a "mixed methods" approach (Newton & Kraemer 1994). The degree of adaptation and thus increase in power and strength that can be realized from training is determined to a large extent by how well the particular strength/power quality is already developed in the individual. However, there are biologic limits to how much the body can adapt. Thus, the adaptive capacity can be thought of as being a continuum from novice to elite athlete. For novices, the *window of adaptation* is quite large and starting a training program targeting that quality will elicit large and rapid increases in performance (Newton & Kraemer 1994). However, as the athletes improve and move towards their genetic potential the "window" shrinks and further gains become harder to achieve. Several aspects need to be considered here. First, a beginner will increase in strength and power with even the most basic resistance training program. They will then plateau and gains will become harder to produce. At this point more innovative programming is required. Second, after several years of resistance training the athlete will adapt very quickly and with limited performance gains to a given resistance training program and so variation in programming becomes much more important.

Equipment for measuring power performance qualities

FORCE PLATE

One of the most versatile items for assessing power performance is the force plate (Fig. 4.3). This is a platform containing force transducers which directly measures the force produced by the athlete. Force only needs to be measured in one direction for most tests and so a uniaxial plate will suffice. Triaxial force plates are more versatile as vertical and horizontal components of force output can be measured but they are also much more expensive.

By pushing against a force plate during the leg press or squat, force–time data can be obtained. Alternatively, if the equipment is fixed so that no movement can occur, isometric measures of peak force and rate of force development can also be gathered. During dynamic movements, measures of dynamic strength such as the highest force produced can be measured.

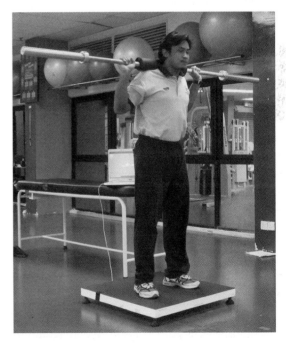

Fig. 4.3 Force platform for measurement of strength and power qualities.

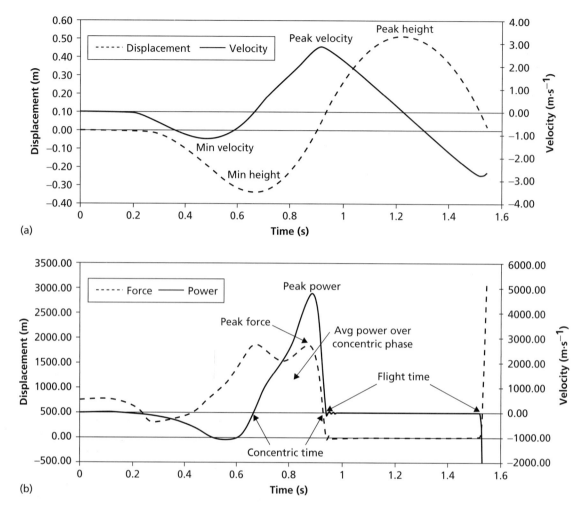

Fig. 4.4 (a) Velocity and displacement, (b) power and force data derived from a vertical jump performed on a force plate. Key summary variables are indicated and demonstrate the utility of this test for detailed performance assessment.

Vertical jumps and similar movements performed on a force plate provide a rich array of performance data. If the athlete is isolated on the plate (i.e., does not touch any other surface) then the impulse–momentum relationship can be used to derive velocity–time and displacement–time data sets from the force–time recording. Combining force and velocity data allows instantaneous power measurements to be derived throughout the jump, and summary variables such as peak and mean power can also be calculated (Fig. 4.4a,b).

LINEAR DISPLACEMENT TRANSDUCER

Transducer systems (Fig. 4.5) can provide very accurate displacement–time data at sampling rates of 500 Hz or more. These data can be used to derive velocity–time, acceleration–time, force–time (if mass is known), and power–time data sets. The transducers have an extendable cable which can be attached to an athlete or implement such as a barbell. As the object moves, the displacement is measured and recorded with a computer system. Such systems are particularly useful for measuring

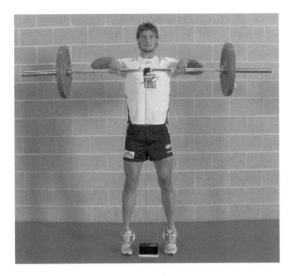

Fig. 4.5 Displacement transducer for measurement of linear movement. Velocity, acceleration, force, and power output can be estimated using the inverse dynamics approach.

performance during jumping with a barbell or during the weightlifting movements. In the latter, attaching the transducer to the barbell provides information on velocity, force, and power applied to the barbell during weightlifting movements (e.g., hang clean, high pull and snatch) which correspond closely to with the athlete's power capacity.

Testing for specific power qualities

Tests (like training) must be specific for the strength/power quality in question. Although opinions within the literature differ, six broad strength/power qualities can be assessed as specific and independent aspects of neuromuscular performance (Newton & Dugan 2002). In sports that involve repeated maximal efforts, such as sprint running or swimming, a seventh quality termed power endurance should be included.

• *Maximum strength* Highest force capability of the neuromuscular system produced during slow eccentric, concentric, or isometric contractions.

• *High load speed-strength* Highest force capability of the neuromuscular system produced during dynamic eccentric and concentric actions under a relatively heavy load (>30% of max) and performed as rapidly as possible.

• *Low load speed-strength* Highest force capability of the neuromuscular system, produced during dynamic eccentric and concentric actions under a relatively light load (<30% of max) and performed as rapidly as possible.

• *Rate of force development* (RFD) The rate at which the neuromuscular system is able to develop force, measured by calculating the slope of the force–time curve on the rise to maximum force of the action.

• *Reactive strength* Ability of the neuromuscular system to tolerate a relatively high stretch load and change movement from rapid eccentric to rapid concentric contraction.

• *Skill performance* Ability of the motor control system to coordinate the muscle contraction sequences to make greatest use of the other five strength/power qualities such that the total movement best achieves the desired outcome.

SELECTION OF MOVEMENT TESTED

The greatest specificity of testing to target performance will be achieved when the movement used as the test closely approximates that of the sport or event being assessed. Often, generic tests of upper and lower body strength are used to achieve a global picture of the athlete's strength which might include bench press, seated row, and a lower body movement such as squat or leg press. For the purposes of informing training program design, more specific testing is required and should be evaluating strength in movements important to the target sport or event. For example, very high leg extensor strength is required in jumping sports so back squat is commonly used as the test movement for these athletes. In rugby and Australian Rules football, the ability to grapple with the opponent and pull them to the ground is critical so upper body pulling tests such as seated row, high pull, and lat pull-down are commonly used. Selection of the appropriate test movement is best achieved through a biomechanical analysis of the movements in the sport or event.

STRETCHING AND OTHER PREPARATION FOR THE TEST

Better performance can be achieved in the strength tests if some prior submaximal efforts are completed in preparation. However, the number of trials must not produce any amount of fatigue that could reduce strength effort. Generally, 3–5 maximal efforts are sufficient. Rest between trials is also important as sufficient recovery requires 3–5 min to avoid fatigue influencing the effort. A final note on preparation is to avoid static stretching because this can reduce force and power output of the muscle (Marek *et al.* 2005).

Maximum strength

Maximum strength can be determined using several methods, each with advantages and disadvantages. The principal modes are isoinertial, isokinetic, and isometric. With all strength testing the force–velocity and length–tension relationships for muscle must be considered, as well as the effect of muscle angle of pull and mechanical advantage influences on the amount of force that can be generated. Briefly, the faster the velocity of muscle shortening the less force can be generated. As the athlete moves through the range of motion for a particular movement, the amount of torque that can be generated about the joints and thus overall force output will change. For example, much less force can be generated from a deep squat position compared to a half squat where the knee angle is 90°. These effects must be considered in the following discussion because they have large influence on the strength measure recorded.

ISOINERTIAL STRENGTH TESTING

Isoinertial refers to constant mass of the resistance. This is perhaps the most simple, inexpensive, and accessible form of strength testing. It involves the use of the gravitational force acting on a mass such as a barbell, dumbbell, or weight resistance machine and the athlete must overcome this force and move the mass through the range of motion. Common examples are the bench press, squat, and deadlift exercises; however, some of the weightlifting movements and derivatives such as hang clean, high pull, and push press are increasingly being used.

Free weight testing as described above has high transference to the sporting environment because almost all sports involve manipulating a freely moving mass against gravity. Also, experienced athletes should have a long training history with the use of free weights and so are very familiar with movements such as bench press, back squat, and hang clean. A disadvantage of free weights is the considerable component of skill that is required, and so to improve test control, possibly reduce injury risk, and limit familiarization required, various forms of resistance machines may be used. The designs of such machines are myriad and many involve cams or levers to alter the resistance force profile. This makes comparison between research studies and athletes groups tested on different equipment difficult whereas free weight testing can be more easily standardized. For example, bench press strength measured with standard Olympic barbell and bench is very repeatable in any weight training facility anywhere in the world.

RATIONALE FOR 1 RM OR REPETITION MAXIMUM TESTING

For isoinertial testing, the maximum weight that can be lifted is determined ideally within 3–5 attempts. The two methods are to determine the maximum weight that can be lifted either once, termed the *one repetition maximum* (1 RM) or, alternatively, lighter weights can be used for a 3–10 RM test. The 1 RM test is a more direct measure of maximal strength as the athlete either has sufficient strength capability to lift the weight or they do not. The principle behind multiple repetition testing is to fatigue the neuromuscular system by prior repetitions to a degree such that the last repetition they can complete is a maximal effort. Multiple repetition testing is preferred by some coaches and scientists because they believe that there is lower risk of injury because a lighter weight is being lifted, although this has not been confirmed or refuted by research. An equally persuasive argument can be made that 1 RM testing involves only a single effort whereas multiple repetition testing involves repeated events for possible injury and thus increases risk. Prefatiguing the athlete in an attempt to elicit a maximal effort may compromise technique resulting in injury and also increases likelihood of muscle damage through the repeated eccentric actions when lowering the

Table 4.1 Protocol for determination of 1 RM: 3–5 min rest between attempts.

Warm-up of 10 repetitions at 50% of 1 RM
5 repetitions at 70% of 1 RM
3 repetitions at 80% of 1 RM
1 repetition at 90% of 1 RM, followed by three attempts to determine their actual 1 RM

weight. Finally, a 6 RM weight for the bench press is approximately 80% of the 1 RM weight, which when lifted six times represents a much higher total work done. Also, because the 6 RM load can be accelerated faster, the peak forces applied to the musculoskeletal system are not appreciably different.

ONE REPETITION MAXIMUM TEST PROTOCOL

A typical protocol for 1 RM testing (McBride *et al.* 1999) is outlined in Table 4.1. Experienced athletes can be asked to estimate their 1 RM and this weight used as a starting point. If the athlete does not know their approximate 1 RM it must be estimated by the personnel performing the test based on the athlete's body weight, age, gender, and lifting experience. This can then be adjusted up or down depending on their performance in the warm-up sets. It should be noted that for 1 RM testing, as any performance test, familiarization can have considerable impact and consideration should be given to employing at least two sessions for accurate determination of 1 RM.

MULTIPLE REPETITION TEST PROTOCOL

There are two approaches to multiple repetition isoinertial strength testing. The first involves selection of a definitive repetition maximum, say 6 RM, and then executing a protocol to determine the maximum weight the athlete can lift six times. The protocol is similar to 1 RM testing with a submaximal warm-up set of 10 repetitions completed first, then an estimated 10 RM load lifted for six repetitions with 1.25–10 kg added until the 6 RM load is obtained. As for the 1 RM protocol, the true 6 RM load should be determined in 3–5 attempts. The other approach is to accurately determine between a 6 RM and 10 RM load and then apply a regression equation to estimate 1 RM strength based on weight lifted and number of repetitions completed. This second method is appealing because an estimate of 1 RM strength is obtained; however, there are limitations in that the regression equations decrease in accuracy of prediction with increasing difference between characteristics of the athlete being tested and the population sample from which the equation was derived. An extensive discussion of protocols and the accuracy of these methods is provided by LeSuer *et al.* (1997).

The range of motion for isoinertial testing must be closely controlled because of the effect on load lifted. For example, the lower the depth in squat testing the less weight the athlete will be able to lift.

ISOMETRIC STRENGTH TESTING

Isometric strength testing involves the athlete performing maximal contractions against an immovable resistance. As no movement occurs this testing is termed *static* or *isometric*. Isometric testing is appealing because the measures are not confounded by issues of movement velocity and changing joint angle already discussed. However, there is also strong argument that isometric testing lacks specificity to the dynamic movements predominant in sports. In fact, research has found isometric measures to be quite poor at predicting dynamic performance (Murphy & Wilson 1996b). Some sports and events involve isometric muscle contractions and such testing may be quite applicable in this instance. One of the advantages of isometric testing is that measures of rate of force development can be obtained which have been suggested (Häkkinen *et al.* 1985) to accurately represent the athlete's ability to rapidly and forcefully contact their muscles, an important aspect of power production to be discussed shortly.

Isometric strength testing can be performed for single (e.g., elbow flexion, knee extension) or multijoint techniques (e.g., squat, bench, mid-thigh pull). Force measuring equipment is required such as a transducer, amplifier, and computer to collect, store, and analyze the force produced. The protocol consists of a warm-up of submaximal efforts followed by a series of maximal efforts. These are continued until no further improvement in maximal force output can be achieved. The instruction to the athlete should be to "push (or pull) against the resistance as hard and fast as possible" for 3–5 s. The force will rise quickly to a peak within this time period and the athlete can then relax once the peak is attained.

ISOKINETIC STRENGTH TESTING

Isokinetic testing involves the use of relatively sophisticated equipment, usually electromechanical, which provides resistance by limiting the speed of movement to a preset linear or angular velocity (Fig. 4.6). The earlier models were limited to concentric only muscle action; however, more contemporary systems incorporate both concentric and eccentric modes, as well as zero velocity (isometric) testing. The advantages of isokinetic strength testing are that the issues of force–velocity effects and changing force capability through the movement are well controlled and quantifiable. Most isokinetic systems are designed primarily for unilateral, single joint movements. For this reason strength measures from isokinetic dynamometers are usually expressed in torque units such as Newton metres. Torque is the angular equivalent of linear force and can be thought of as a "twisting force."

Single joint measurement lacks specificity to most sporting movements which generally involve a

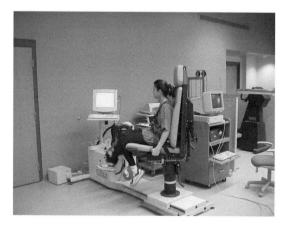

Fig. 4.6 Isokinetic dynamometer set-up for assessment of knee extensor and flexor muscle performance.

coordinated movement of several joints and muscle groups. To address this possible deficiency, manufacturers such as Biodex™ have developed attachments that provide linear as well as rotary isokinetic resistance, thus enabling multi-joint movements such as leg press to be tested.

Perhaps the greatest application of isokinetic testing has been with assessing hamstrings and quadriceps torque production about the knee. Consequently, much research has been directed toward assessing the ratio between these two muscle groups as well as left to right asymmetries in an effort to understand mechanisms, screen and rehabilitate injuries, such as hamstring strain and joint injury of the knee.

By adjusting the resistance (accommodating) continuously to the torque capacity of the musculoskeletal system, a profile throughout the range of movement can be obtained. This is a useful feature of the isokinetic mode as weak portions of the range can be identified as well as shifts in the position at which the peak in torque occurs. Such information has been used to quantify the optimal angle and some researchers have related shifts in this optimal angle to injury events, such as hamstring strains (Brockett *et al.* 2004).

Two issues that clinicians should be aware of when performing isokinetic testing is the torque overshoot phenomenon and gravity correction. At the beginning of each repetition there will be a period when the limb is accelerated from zero to the preset velocity of the dynamometer. This results in an *impact* when the limb attains this velocity and a spike and subsequent damped oscillation occurs in the torque signal. The faster the set speed of the dynamometer for the trial the later into the movement this impact occurs and the larger the spike. Manufacturers have tried to address this problem with electronic and digital filters, as well as ramping the dynamometer speed but, regardless, measurements in the early phase of a movement are problematic. Gravity correction is used to account for the fact that when testing, gravity will assist (increase) torque measured during downward direction movements and impede (decrease) torque measured during upward direction movements. This is easily accounted for by contemporary systems by performing a weighing procedure for the limb and dynamometer arm prior to strength measurement and the torque measurement is then corrected throughout the range of movement.

Ballistic testing

The majority of sports involve striking, kicking, throwing, or projecting the body into free space. The kinetic and kinematic profile of isoinertial, isometric, and isokinetic testing methods are very different to the accelerative, high power output characteristic of sport movements (Newton *et al.*, 1994). As a result, measurement of force, velocity, and power during ballistic movements such as counter-movement jump (CMJ), jump squat (CMJ with additional load to body weight), squat jump (concentric only jump with body weight or load), bench throws, bench pulls, and various weightlifting movements is becoming increasingly used for athlete testing.

The CMJ is a basic test of vertical jump capacity. The athlete dips down and then immediately jumps upward, attempting to maximize the height jumped. With the use of a force plate and position transducer, ground reaction force and displacement can be recorded (McBride *et al.*, 1999). From these data, a number of variables that characterize the performance can be calculated. Jump height is an obvious measure, but the power output during the jump, peak force produced, and time to attain that force can also be calculated.

Sophisticated systems are available to measure force output and displacement as explained earlier in this chapter. From these systems, data such as height (displacement), velocity, force, and power output can be calculated. The loads used depend on the athlete and the task, but a spectrum is useful so that an impression of the athlete's performance under heavy and light loads can be ascertained (i.e., high or low load speed-strength). One scheme is to use loads of 30, 55, and 80% 1 RM (McBride *et al.*, 2001), while another method seeks to determine the *optimal load* for power production (Baker *et al.*, 2001a,b; Wilson *et al.* 1993).

When determining the optimal load for the jump squat, the athlete first performs with a pre-selected load (Fig. 4.7). After each trial the load is

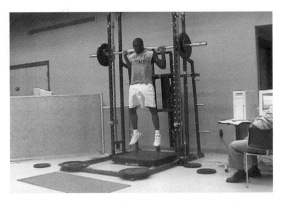

Fig. 4.7 Measurement of power output in a squat jump for determination of optimal load for power production. Ground reaction force measured by force platform is used to calculate velocity and subsequently power output.

adjusted up or down and, because of the relationship between force and velocity, the power output will change. Only one load will produce the highest power output (Wilson *et al.* 1993) and this is termed the optimal load (Fig. 4.8). This may be expressed as an absolute force (or mass), or as a percentage of maximum isometric force or 1 RM. Recent research has suggested that the load at which mechanical power is maximized shifts in response to training demands (Baker, 2001). Although more research is required, this measure may provide a useful tool

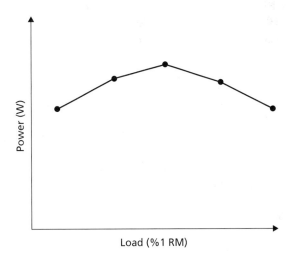

Fig. 4.8 Power output changes with the load that the athlete is working against. One load will produce the highest power output and is termed "optimal."

for monitoring the effects of changing emphasis in program periodization as well as for detecting overtraining, illness, and staleness. For example, Baker (2001) has found that the optimal load increases during phases that emphasize strength and decreases during speed training.

Rate of force development

There are several options to choose from when testing RFD. One common protocol uses isometric squats, but this incorporates many of the same advantages and disadvantages as testing maximal strength with isometrics (Murphy & Wilson 1996b). RFD can also be determined during both concentric and eccentric phases of dynamic tests, which may have greater relevance to task performance (Murphy & Wilson 1996a, 1997; Wilson *et al.* 1995); however, this has not been well researched to date.

Two dynamic tests that are often utilized are the concentric-only jump, often referred to as the squat jump (SJ), and the concentric-only jump squat. For the SJ, the athlete squats down to a self-selected depth and holds that position for 3–4 s, then attempts to jump for maximum height without a preparatory movement. This can be difficult to perform and may require several trials to obtain accurate data. The test is performed with body weight only as the load.

Concentric-only jump squats are SJ but performed with some additional load above body weight. For this variation, mechanical stops are positioned in the squat rack or Smith machine at the appropriate angle for the bottom position of the jump, and this becomes the starting position for the jump. Ground reaction force and bar displacement can be recorded, as well as such derived variables as jump height, power output, and peak force developed. The highest force produced during a concentric-only movement has been termed maximal dynamic strength (MDS; Young 1995) – a strength/power quality with good predictive and discriminatory capability between athletes of different levels. Heavier external loads will result in greater MDS values, and greater test specificity will be obtained if the selected load is similar to the target task. Dynamic concentric-only tests (as with

isometric tests) allow the calculation of several measures of the ability to rapidly develop force (Zatsiorsky 1995), such as maximum RFD or the impulse ($F \times t$) over the initial 100 ms.

Reactive strength

The most common test for assessing an athlete's reactive strength is the depth jump. The athlete drops down from a box, lands, and then jumps upward for maximum height (Fig. 4.9). A contact mat system or force plate can be used to record the characteristics of the performance. Young *et al.* (1995) has shown that the instructions given to the athlete affect the results, and that they should attempt maximum jump height while minimizing ground contact time. Trials completed at increasing drop heights provide insight into how the athlete responds to increasing stretch loads. A common

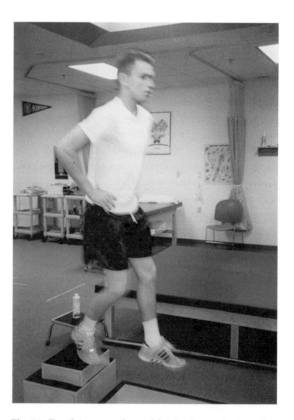

Fig. 4.9 Depth jump performed for the determination of reactive strength index.

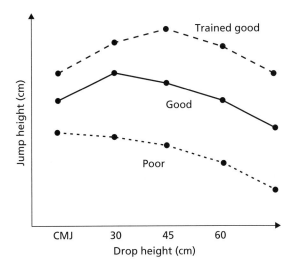

Fig. 4.10 Changes in reactive strength index with increasing drop height. The comparison of novice and athlete subjects and the effect of reactive strength index (RSI) training show a shift in jump height upwards as well as the optimal drop height to the right.

progression is to employ 0.30, 0.45, 0.60, and 0.75 m drop heights. Calculated variables include jump height, flight time, contact time, and flight time to contact time ratio (which is also termed *reactive strength index*; RSI). The "best" drop height can be determined as that which elicits the highest RSI (Fig. 4.10). An athlete with a reasonable level of reactive strength should be able to produce a better jump height following a drop than a CMJ (which effectively has a drop height of zero).

Eccentric strength tests

Many sports involve movements with accentuated eccentric muscle actions. For example, it has been demonstrated that isokinetic eccentric strength of the knee extensors can discriminate elite and sub-elite downhill skiers (Abe *et al.* 1992), which is a reasonable outcome given the repeated eccentric actions experienced by skiers. Therefore, it may be instructive to include tests of eccentric strength and power in the testing program. The most common method of eccentric testing is through the use of isokinetic dynamometers with this capability

(Abe *et al.* 1992) and most commonly applied to hamstrings and quadriceps muscle groups. Eccentric testing of the hamstrings is also performed for the purpose of assessing injury risk and recovery from injury as eccentric strength and endurance have been implicated as possible risk factors. For detailed explanation the reader should consult the many extensive texts on the use of isokinetic dynamometry.

However, for more functional eccentric strength measures the options are much more limited. In one study, an electromechanical device was developed that implemented an isokinetic squat movement (Wilson *et al.* 1997) and it was reported that measures of strength from this device were more highly correlated with cycling performance than single joint tests of the knee. It is possible to use isoinertial loads of greater than 1 RM to assess isokinetic strength by measuring the forces exerted as the subject attempts to slow the rate of decent of the load (Murphy *et al.* 1994). Essentially, a weight such as a barbell is suspended over the subject in the squat or bench press position, and then released using an electromechanical device such as shown in Fig. 4.11. The loads used are between 130% and 150% of maximum isometric strength and so the subject cannot hold the load but attempts to slow the descent. Researchers have recorded measures of eccentric force, power absorption, and rate of force development from such tests and presented evidence that these measures are more informative for sports that rely on high eccentric performance.

"Gold standard" and specific tests/skill performance

It is useful to include a test that is highly task-specific and that incorporates several strength/power qualities. We may refer to this as the "gold standard" for the target task. For example, in volleyball the approach jump and reach is commonly used as a "gold standard" test (Newton *et al.* 1999). In basketball, the athlete could use an approach run on to a contact mat and then jump for maximal height while performing a jump shot action, landing back on the contact mat. In athletics, the actual field event performance (e.g., long jump or shot put distance) can be used.

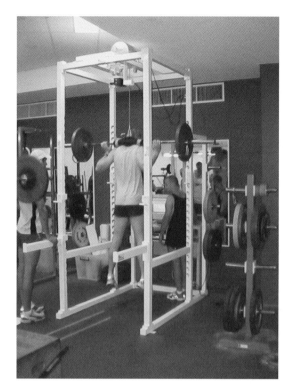

Fig. 4.11 Electromagnetic brake device used to reduce impact forces during ballistic resistance training. The system can also be used to perform eccentric strength testing using loads in excess of the concentric 1 RM.

Sometimes it is necessary to design highly specific tests that assess particular aspects of a sport. For example, power output produced under fatigue and/or following repeated body collisions is important to the sport of rugby. In this instance, an obstacle course could be developed simulating a game, with outcome measures including time to complete certain sections, as well as performance in a power test such as vertical jump.

Relative or absolute measures

Whether the results are expressed as absolute measures or normalized relative to body weight depends on the task and athlete. Both methods have application. When the athlete must move body weight against gravity (e.g., high jump), then relative measures may be more important. However, when momentum or total strength is key (e.g., rugby, American football), then absolute measures may be more instructive. Relative measures allow for better comparison of athletes of different body weights, and most variables can be expressed in relative terms. For example, a 1 RM squat can be expressed as the number of "body weights" (BW) lifted, or power output during jumping expressed as $W \cdot kg^{-1}$ body mass.

Assessing imbalances

In the interests of both injury reduction and performance enhancement it is instructive to investigate imbalances between agonist and antagonist muscle groups, as well as between left and right sides of the body. There is considerable literature (Aagaard *et al.* 1995, 1998) on the former, so we confine our discussion to assessing imbalances between the left and right leg extensors. Most people exhibit some dominance resulting in differences in performance between, for example, hops performed on the left versus right leg. Differences of more than 10–15% may indicate existing pain and injury, inadequate recovery from previous injury, or an undesirable imbalance in muscle strength/power qualities. Such differences are easily assessed by performing unilateral movements such as single leg hops and comparing flight and contact times. Cutting and side-stepping tests using timing lights or contact mats to measure speed in each direction are also useful.

The specific sporting movement should be taken into consideration when assessing left to right side imbalances. In sports that require a one-legged take-off (e.g., high jump or long jump), it may be quite normal for the dominant or take-off leg to be stronger than the contralateral leg. This would be expected because of the nature of the event, so time spent trying to eliminate imbalances in leg power might be counterproductive.

Sophisticated is not necessarily expensive

The number of laboratories and training facilities that have sophisticated equipment for strength/power diagnosis is increasing as the value of this evaluation and training becomes more recognized.

However, one can implement valid and reliable strength/power diagnoses with a minimum of equipment and expense. All of the jump tests can be performed with either jump and reach equipment or a contact mat system, and while not providing the same detailed measures of force and power, they provide adequate information required for basic performance diagnosis. Other tests such as the standing broad jump or medicine ball throw can provide good information and only require a measuring tape.

Speed and agility

Speed and agility are physical qualities required for successful performance in many sports played on a field or court. In science, speed is defined as distance divided by time, and can refer to the movement of part of the body (e.g., the foot in kicking a ball or the whole body such as in running). For the purposes of this section, speed refers to total body running speed. Agility is more difficult to define and this creates difficulties when examining the assessment of this complex quality; however, this is discussed in detail later in the chapter.

Speed

While running speed is normally expressed in $m \cdot s^{-1}$ or $km \cdot h^{-1}$, it is customary to measure and report sprint times at known distances from the commencement of the sprint. Running speed can be classified into three categories:

1 *Acceleration speed* This refers to the speed during relatively short sprints (e.g., 5–20 m), when it is known that running velocity rapidly increases (Bruggemann & Glad 1990).

2 *Maximum speed* This refers to the peak running speed reached by an individual, and typically occurs after 30–60 m of sprinting from a stationary start.

3 *Speed-endurance* This refers to the ability to sustain relatively high running speeds (e.g., 90% of maximum speed). In sport, this quality may be required during long sprints, such as the 200 and 400 m events, or in team sports where sprints may be short (less than 30 m) but are repeated with partial recoveries. This has been termed "repeat sprint ability."

Research has demonstrated that these speed qualities are quite specific (Delecluse *et al.* 1995). Therefore, an athlete who has a high level of one speed quality may be relatively poor at the others, and is likely explained by each quality being influenced by somewhat different physiologic mechanisms. For example, acceleration speed involves relatively more forward lean, shorter steps, longer ground contact times, and greater quadriceps muscle activity than maximum speed sprinting, where hip extensors become relatively more important (Frick *et al.* 1995; Kyrolainen *et al.* 1999; Young *et al.* 2001).

An important implication of the specificity of the speed qualities is that each can be assessed by different tests, and the tester must decide which particular qualities are most important for the sport of interest. A needs analysis should be conducted to assist the tester ascribe an importance to each quality and improve the interpretation of test results.

METHODS OF TESTING SPEED QUALITIES

Running speed can be assessed directly from laser or radar recordings using the Doppler principle. For example, when a radar beam is directed at the back of a runner, the change in frequency between the emitted and reflected signal can be used to measure speed. An advantage of such a system is that it records instantaneous velocity and is therefore useful for measuring peak or maximum speed. A disadvantage is that it can only be used for running in a straight line on an individual athlete.

Another method employed for direct measurement of velocity is the use of a device attached to a light wire attached to the athlete's waist (Volkov & Lapin 1979; Witters *et al.* 1985). With increasing running displacement, the wire is extended which rotates a wheel and this allows displacement and time to be recorded. This kind of device has similar advantages to the radar or laser techniques but a significant disadvantage is that it is obtrusive and cannot be used for testing in competition conditions.

Technologic advances have made global positioning systems (GPS) commercially available, which are able to accurately track the position of the running athlete over time. Although measurement of velocity is accurate, GPS systems with relatively low sampling frequencies (e.g., 1–10 Hz) can introduce significant errors when there is a rapid change in velocity. The latest systems, however, incorporate accelerometers that interpolate acceleration between successive GPS measurements (e.g., www.gpsports.com).

The most common way to assess speed qualities is with time taken to reach known distances or time elapsed between relatively short intervals (e.g., 10 m). Traditionally, stopwatches have been used, but can be expected to result in errors associated with factors such as the variation in the reaction time of the operator. Stopwatches have generally been replaced with electronic timing devices such as "light gates" consisting of an infrared beam that is transmitted and received by a unit mounted on tripods (Fig. 4.12). As the athlete's trunk passes through the beam, the time is recorded and stored.

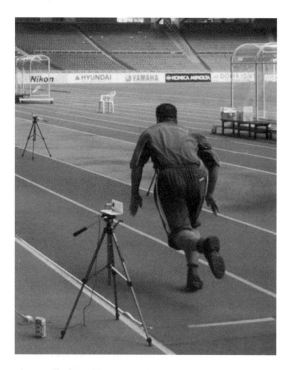

Fig. 4.12 Infrared timing gate systems provide millisecond accuracy in measurement of speed and agility.

This type of system should have a measurement resolution of at least 0.01 s.

Some interest has been generated about whether one beam is adequate for accurate timing of running because of the possibility of time being triggered by a limb rather than the trunk of the body. Because the arms and legs move forward and backward relative to the trunk, limb movement is not a reflection of whole body speed. One solution to this potential problem is the use of multiple beam systems which are programmed to record a time event only when all beams are triggered simultaneously, thereby attempting to capture trunk rather than arm movement. Another solution is the use of real-time computer processing of the light gate pulses with algorithms to predict the time at which the trunk passes through the beam.

An example of a speed test using a timing light gate system would be to use gates at 10 m intervals up to 60 m. Acceleration speed could be represented by time to 10 or 20 m and maximum speed could be estimated by the smallest time elapsed between consecutive gates, expected to be 40–50 m or 50–60 m. Because this procedure requires multiple gates, a more pragmatic approach may be to use four gates placed at the start line, 20 m, 50 m, and the finish line (60 m). The 20 m time is used as a measure of acceleration and the flying 10 m time (50–60 m) is used to represent maximum speed. It should be acknowledged that the latter time indicates an average over the 10 m distance rather than the true peak or maximum running velocity of the individual.

While the above approach to testing is an attempt to separate acceleration and maximum speed qualities, an alternative approach is to simply measure times to distances considered to be critical to a particular sport. For example, the time to sprint to 18 m may be useful for softball because this is the distance between bases. Similarly, a sprint to 10 m rather than 20 m may be more relevant for acceleration speed in tennis.

To assess speed-endurance, times over relatively long sprints (e.g., 300 m) could be used, or to simulate the demands of team sports requiring intermittent sprints, a test involving repeated short sprints would be appropriate. Repeat sprint ability (RSA) can be thought of as a form of speed-endurance and the energy for such activity is derived from a combination of aerobic and anaerobic sources (Glaister 2005). Variables such as the typical length or duration of the sprint, sprint intensity, rest interval between sprints, work to rest ratios, and total number of sprints in a game will influence the precise physiologic demands on the athlete (Spencer *et al.* 2005). Therefore, it is unlikely that one test can suit all needs for assessing RSA in team sports. Further, selection of an appropriate test should be based on a careful evaluation of time–motion data of the sport of interest. An example of a test of RSA is six repetitions of 40 m maximum effort sprints, leaving every 30 s (Dawson *et al.* 1998; Fitzsimons *et al.* 1993). With this protocol, the total time to complete the sprints and the percentage decrement score across the six sprints can be used to monitor training effects (Dawson *et al.* 1998).

STANDARDIZATION OF SPEED TESTING PROCEDURES

Whatever test protocol is selected, there are many variables that must be either controlled or standardized to maximize the reliability and sensitivity of the test.

Environmental conditions

While temperature and humidity cannot always be easily controlled, the influence of wind can have a profound effect on speed and, if possible, should be eliminated by performing the test indoors. A practical consideration of indoor facilities is whether the space is large enough to include a sprint of the required distance, including enough distance for slowing down safely at the end of the sprint. It is important to have enough extra space (at least 20 m) to decelerate while encouraging the athlete to maintain maximum velocity until the finish line is reached.

Floor surface

Assuming an indoor facility can be used, the floor surface can influence the friction between the shoes and surface and therefore the likelihood of slippage. The floor should be clean and free of dust. The footwear used by the athlete must be appropriate for the floor surface and, if possible, the same type of shoes should be worn on repeated tests.

Warm-up

An optimum warm-up is required to maximize test performance and reduce the risk of injury, which may be considered higher than for other physical tests. It is beyond the scope of this section to elaborate on warm-up procedures, but two approaches can been used. The first is to administer a standard warm-up for all athletes to ensure consistency. The problem with this approach is that a single protocol will not be optimum for every individual because of variation in fitness levels. Another preferred approach is to allow each athlete to use their own individualized warm-up as although this will vary, it is more likely to yield an optimum performance, which is a major goal of speed testing. The warm-up should contain some submaximum run-throughs and conclude with some practice of the starting procedure about to be used.

Number of trials

While it is common in research to allow subjects to perform a predetermined number of trials, because the objective is to identify the true best performance of the athlete, the number of trials should not be restricted. If the warm-up is adequate and the test skill has been learned, one or two trials should be enough, but further trials may be needed if test performance is continually improving in successive trials. For relatively short sprint tests, such as 10–20 m, five or six trials could be completed with minimal fatigue effects, but for longer sprints, such as 200 m or longer, a lower number of trials would be necessary, to avoid the influence of fatigue on performance.

Starting procedure

The first consideration is whether reaction time should be included in the test. With track and field sprinters, reacting to the stimulus of the starter's gun is an important component of running speed. In this case, timing should commence from a starting signal and the athlete should use starting blocks. However, with other athletes, it is the running movement time that is of interest, and therefore the timing should commence from the first forward movement. To achieve this, the athlete should adopt a stationary position with the body just behind the beam of the start gate. The usual start position is with one foot forward of the other and the opposing arm forward. The athlete is not permitted to "rock back" prior to forward movement as this would create an advantage. The athlete may start the forward movement when he or she is ready and this should trigger the start of the timing. The position of the front toe relative to the start gate can be controlled, but it is preferable for the athlete to adopt an optimum body position according to his or her unique body dimensions with the trunk just behind the beam.

Recording times from multiple trials

The scores retained as the athlete's test results have been determined as the mean of a number of trials. However, if an unlimited number of trials is used to obtain the best performance, the single best trial should be used. If there are more than one time recorded from a trial (e.g., 20 and 50–60 m), there are two ways the scores can be retained. The first is to use the best 60 m trial (as an example) and then retain the 20 m time from that trial. The second is to retain the best 20 and 50–60 m times regardless of which trial they were obtained. Because arguments can be mounted for both methods, the tester should decide which to use and apply this consistently for the purposes of standardization.

Agility

Agility is a complex quality that is difficult to define. A multitude of definitions refer to elements such as the ability to accelerate, decelerate, and change direction quickly. In most sports, changes in running velocity or direction are usually performed in response to an external stimulus, and therefore agility contains a perceptual and decision-making

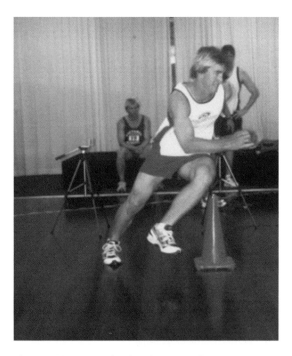

Fig. 4.13 Most tests of agility do not involve a reaction to a stimulus but rather involve preplanned movements around stationary obstacles.

component, as well as change of direction speed (Young *et al.* 2002). An example is a defending soccer player changing direction in response to an attacker's lateral movement. In recognition of this, a new definition of agility in sport is "a rapid whole-body movement with change of velocity or direction in response to a stimulus" (Sheppard & Young, 2006). Most tests of agility do not involve a reaction to a stimulus but rather involve preplanned movements around stationary obstacles (Fig. 4.13). These tests may be described as tests of change of direction (COD) speed as they do not contain the decision-making elements of agility required in most sporting contexts.

Many trainable factors may contribute to agility performance to varying extents (Young *et al.* 2002):
• Anticipation of other players movements;
• Sprinting speed;
• Ability to accelerate and decelerate;
• Body positioning when changing direction;
• Muscle strength, power, and reactive strength;
• Core stability;

- Balance; and
- Reaction time.

Because movement patterns in different sports vary, agility can be considered to be a sport-specific quality. Therefore, a test that may be valid for soccer may not be valid for basketball. Unfortunately, there are no universally accepted tests of agility, and new tests are rapidly emerging.

Evolution of agility testing

GENERIC TESTS

These include movement patterns that may be considered "typical" in many sports. For example, the "505" test involves a 10 m lead-in run followed by a 5 m sprint to a turning line, then a 5 m sprint back. This 5 m up and 5 m back involves a single change of direction and is performed with left leg and right leg trials separately to enable comparison. Although this test has been validated for cricket (Draper & Lancaster 1985), it has been widely used to assess "general" agility for several sports (Ellis *et al*. 2000).

SPORT-SPECIFIC MOVEMENT PATTERNS

Because of the specificity of movement patterns, attempts have been made to analyze the movements of various sports so that these patterns can be incorporated into an agility test. For example, some sports (e.g., basketball, volleyball, and tennis) involve sideways "shuffling" and backwards running, and therefore tests have been devised containing these patterns (e.g., SEMO, "T" test; Buckeridge *et al*. 2000; Semenick 1994).

TESTS INVOLVING A REACTION TO A GENERIC STIMULUS

It has been acknowledged that rapid changes of velocity and direction are often produced in response to an opposition player's movements. In an attempt to include reaction time in agility assessment, tests have been devised that require an athlete to change direction when they see a light, sound, or computer-generated directional stimulus (e.g.,

arrow) appear to indicate the direction of movement (Besier *et al*. 2001; Hertel *et al*. 1999). Although this type of test clearly involves reaction time, the stimulus used to initiate the change of direction is general rather than sport-specific.

Better athletes tend to produce more accurate and faster responses as a result of a superior ability to detect anticipatory information (Abernethy *et al*. 1998). Therefore, a soccer defender may detect the angle of the hips as a cue to anticipate the change of direction of an attacking player. Research suggests that the stimulus must be sport-specific for skilled athletes to use their perceptual skill to advantage (Abernethy *et al*. 1993), and therefore the value of using stimuli such as lights or auditory cues is questionable.

TESTS INVOLVING REACTION TO A SPORT-SPECIFIC STIMULUS

Recently, attempts have been made to assess agility in netball using a videotaped projected image of an attacking player passing the ball (Farrow *et al*. 2005). The athletes were required to step to the left or right and sprint through a timing gate once they detected the direction of the "opposition player's" pass. A unique feature of this test was the use of a video camera to determine the "decision time," defined from ball release to the instant the tested player planted the foot to change direction. The total agility movement time was found to be shorter for highly skilled players than a group of less skilled players. Of importance was the finding that the highly skilled group achieved a negative decision time, whereas the less skilled group had a positive and significantly longer mean decision time. This indicated that the better players anticipated the movement of the netball pass and responded by commencing the change of direction earlier. Recent research on rugby players (Jackson *et al*. 2006) has demonstrated that highly skilled players were better than novices in detecting a deceptive movement ("dummy" side-step) in a change of direction situation.

Another new reactive agility test has been described for use with Australian Rules football (Sheppard *et al*. 2006). In this test, players were

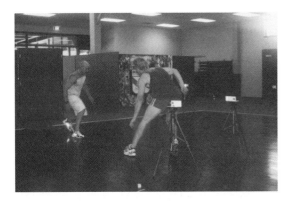

Fig. 4.14 A new reactive agility test has been described for use with Australian Rules football (Sheppard *et al.*, 2006). In this test, players are required to react to the side-stepping movement of a tester running towards them, and sprint to the left or right as soon as they identified the direction.

required to react to the side-stepping movement of a tester running towards them, and sprint to the left or right as soon as they identified the direction (Fig. 4.14). An attempt was made to control for variation in movement time for the tester by using various known foot patterns, but presented in random order to the athlete, and recording a mean of 12 trials. Because of the variability associated with using a real person to present the stimulus to change direction, the protocol was assessed on two occasions for inter-day reliability, and was found to be acceptable (intra-class correlation of 0.88). The validity of the test was evaluated by comparing football players from different levels of competition from the same clubs. The higher and lower performance groups were also compared on a planned change of direction test involving sprinting around an obstacle in a very similar movement pattern to the reactive test. The results indicated that the higher performance group was slightly slower in the planned test (1.9%), but significantly faster in the reactive agility test (5.2%). The common variance between the planned and reactive tests was only 10%, indicating that the reactive test assessed agility that was clearly different and more related to performance than the planned test. Although not discernable from this test, it is

possible that the better players were able to detect cues from the tester's movements about the ensuing change of direction and therefore make a faster response.

Methods of testing agility

The use of radar or laser as described for straight sprint testing is not suitable for assessing agility with changes of direction. While GPS could potentially be used to track an athlete's changes of direction, accurate assessment would require relatively high sampling rates, such as 100 Hz or greater. At this stage it is not possible to recommend this tool for agility assessment. The most common and recommended method for assessing agility is to use timing lights, where a start and stop gate are used to record the total time taken to achieve a given task. The factors relating to standardization of speed protocols also apply to the assessment of agility.

The above examples of agility testing would appear to provide direction for the development of agility assessment in the future. A number of questions still need to be answered:
1 How important is the decision-making speed of the athlete in agility performance?
2 Are the demands different for various playing roles (e.g., attacking and defending?)
3 Is agility completely sport-specific or can an agility test be designed to be valid for multiple sports?

Summary

Before assessing sprinting, the tester must identify which specific speed qualities are of interest and select an appropriate test. If the tester is interested in detecting small changes in speed or times, perhaps as a result of a training intervention, it is crucial that testing procedures are controlled and standardized. Assessment of agility has evolved and many sport-specific tests are now available. Currently, there is a trend to attempt to include decision-making time in agility testing to enhance the specificity and relevance of the test to a particular sport. While this direction seems fruitful, testers must seek evidence for the utility of test protocols.

Testing for endurance activities

The testing of endurance ability is a common practice in the clinical setting, throughout sporting academies, institutes, and universities. It is useful for identifying gifted athletes, for providing coaches with knowledge of an athlete's current performance potential, for determining the effectiveness of a training program or ergogenic aid, and for allowing scientists to understand relationships between testing variables and endurance performance. Before identifying the various methods of endurance testing, the main physiologic factors that make up endurance performance must be understood. Successful endurance performance (i.e., an activity requiring muscle contractions repeated over durations of greater than 1 min) appears to be related to three main physiologic components:

1 The maximal oxygen uptake, or maximal rate of oxygen consumption (also known as $\dot{V}o_{2max}$);
2 The anaerobic threshold, or the exercise intensity that can be completed without the development of high lactic acid levels; and
3 The economy of motion, or the efficient conversion of usable energy into mechanical power (Coyle 1995).

While indices of these three measurements can usually be obtained through the administration of a progressive exercise test ($\dot{V}o_{2max}$ test), not all progressive exercise test protocols will provide an accurate assessment of all three variables. Thus, a more in-depth description of each of these physiologic factors that relate to endurance performance, and a rundown on the various types of progressive exercise test protocols best suited towards accurately measuring each of these distinct variables will be discussed.

While the $\dot{V}o_{2max}$, anaerobic threshold and economy of motion all contribute to and predict endurance performance ability, there is no better measurement of one's endurance performance ability than assessment of performance during an actual endurance performance trial. Endurance performance tests commonly used in assessing endurance capacity include time-to-exhaustion tests (i.e., how long can the athlete exercise for at a given exercise intensity) and time trials (i.e., how fast can the athlete complete a prescribed distance). However, each of these tests has distinctly different characteristics in terms of the reliability, validity, specificity, and practicality, and the practitioner must make careful consideration as to which type of test is most suited to examine the endurance ability pertinent to their situation. Thus, the second half of this section discusses considerations for choosing the most appropriate endurance performance test protocol.

Components of endurance performance

As outlined above, the three main physiologic components that well predict an athlete's actual endurance performance (i.e., performance time achieved over a set distance) include one's maximal oxygen uptake ($\dot{V}o_{2max}$), anaerobic threshold, and economy of motion (Fig. 4.15; Coyle 1999). While each of these variables contribute in some degree to the overall endurance performance, the $\dot{V}o_{2max}$ appears to be a better discriminator of endurance performance within heterogeneous populations (Butts *et al.* 1991), while the anaerobic or lactate threshold and one's economy of motion tends to better predict the endurance performance ability in more homogeneous populations of endurance athletes (Farrell *et al.* 1979; Grant *et al.* 1997; Laursen & Rhodes 2001; Rhodes & McKenzie 1984). Conveniently, all of these variables can be measured using a progressive exercise test protocol, albeit certain progressive exercise test protocols are better suited to measure one variable than others.

MAXIMAL OXYGEN UPTAKE

Maximal oxygen uptake ($\dot{V}o_{2max}$), also referred to as aerobic capacity, is a well-known physiologic factor commonly found to be related not only to endurance performance ability throughout a diverse range of athletes (Butts *et al.* 1991), but also to one's aerobic fitness, functional capacity, and general health (Kohrt *et al.* 1987). As the term implies, $\dot{V}o_{2max}$ reflects the maximal ability of the body to uptake and process oxygen. Broken down, $\dot{V}o_{2max}$ is a product of the capacity of the blood

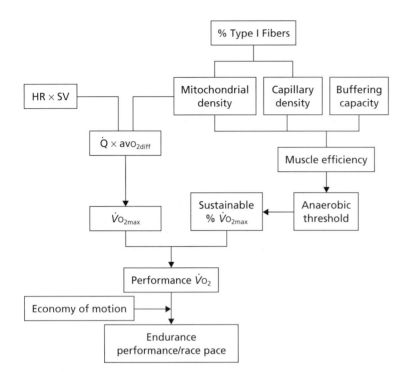

Fig. 4.15 Theoretical model of the main physiologic components contributing to endurance performance. avo_{2diff}, arterial venous oxygen difference; HR, heart rate; $\dot{Q}$, cardiac output; SV, stroke volume; $\dot{V}o_{2max}$, maximal oxygen uptake.

passing through the lungs to take up and load oxygen onto the hemoglobin molecule, the ability of the heart to deliver that oxygenated blood to the working muscles (cardiac output), and the ability of the body's cells to uptake and utilize this oxygen from the blood passing through the capillaries (Fig. 4.15).

$\dot{V}o_{2max}$ is determined directly using a metabolic cart; a machine that measures the volume of air expired and the concentrations of oxygen and carbon dioxide in that expired air (i.e., Fig. 4.16). The difference between the known concentrations of oxygen (20.93%) and carbon dioxide (0.03%) in ambient air and the concentrations of those gases in expired air are used to calculate the oxygen consumed and carbon dioxide produced. While some expert scientists create their own in-house computer-integrated metabolic systems, some of the more commonly used commercial systems include ParvoMedics (Crouter *et al.* 2006), Sensormedics (Webster *et al.* 1998), and Medical Graphics CPX/D (Gore *et al.* 2003). Portable metabolic systems allowing measurement of oxygen uptake ($\dot{V}o_2$) during

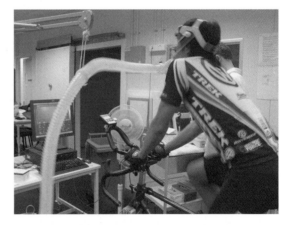

Fig. 4.16 Subject breathing into a metabolic cart while performing a progressive exercise test on a cycle ergometer for the determination of maximal oxygen uptake, anaerobic threshold, and cycling economy.

field-based exercise performance are now available, including the Cosmed K_4 (Nieman *et al.* 2006), Oxycon (Foss & Hallen 2005) and the BodyGem (Nieman *et al.* 2003).

At exercise intensities below the anaerobic threshold, progressive increases in exercise intensity tend to be matched by equivalent increases in $\dot{V}o_2$. At exercise intensities above the anaerobic threshold, further energy requirements (i.e., adenosine triphophate [ATP] levels) can no longer be met with equivalent increases in oxidative phosphorylation, and the energy for these high exercise intensities must be supplemented through anaerobic glycolysis, which temporarily stores electrons and H^+ ions on the pyruvate molecule to form lactate. Thus, $\dot{V}o_2$ tends to plateau, peak, or even decrease during the latter stages of a progressive exercise test. Thus, when a plateau is not evident, the term is no longer referred to as $\dot{V}o_{2max}$, but instead as a $\dot{V}o_{2peak}$, and the highest measurement of $\dot{V}o_2$ that occurs during the exercise test is then used. A $\dot{V}o_2$ plateau appears less frequently in children, possibly because of the unaccustomed high physical and psychologic costs associated with reaching such high exercise intensities (Rowland & Cunningham 1992). The peak in $\dot{V}o_2$ may therefore be caused by early termination of the exercise in this case. Some authors have been of the opinion that a $\dot{V}o_{2max}$ can only truly be obtained during exercise that can stress a very large muscle mass, during exercise modes such as running or cross-country skiing, and that even aerobic capacity values for cycling should be classified as a $\dot{V}o_{2peak}$ (Brooks et al. 1996). Generally, however, "$\dot{V}o_{2max}$" is an accepted term to use when assessing $\dot{V}o_{2max}$ with a cycle ergometer, especially in trained cyclists. Regardless, when a plateau in $\dot{V}o_2$ does not occur during a progressive exercise test, secondary criteria are often used to justify that the capacity of the aerobic system has been reached:

1 A maximum heart rate (HR_{max}) of within ± 10 beats of the age predicted HR_{max} (i.e., 220 − age);
2 A respiratory exchange ratio (RER; $\dot{V}co_2 / \dot{V}o_2$) value greater than 1.10;
3 A blood lactate value of greater than 8 mmol·L^{-1}; and;
4 Volitional fatigue.

When the absolute values of $\dot{V}o_{2max}$ (L·min^{-1}) are compared amongst a normal distribution of individuals there will be large variations in $\dot{V}o_{2max}$ because of body size, muscle mass, age, genetic factors, and body composition, and the ability of this value to consistently predict endurance capacity is not always strong (Laursen & Rhodes 2001). However, when $\dot{V}o_{2max}$ is expressed as a measure relative to an individual's body mass, this tends to improve the relationship between $\dot{V}o_{2max}$ and endurance capacity. This relative measure is expressed in mL·kg^{-1}·min^{-1} by multiplying the $\dot{V}o_{2max}$ in L·min^{-1} by 1000 and then dividing by the body mass in kilograms.

The level of $\dot{V}o_{2max}$ obtained is also highly reliant upon the mode of exercise testing used, with the highest values generally reported during cross-country skiing and treadmill running activities (Droghetti et al. 1985; Kohrt et al. 1987; Schneider et al. 1990). Thus, the higher $\dot{V}o_{2max}$ values generally found with these exercise modes likely relate to the large muscle mass recruited during these activities compared with smaller levels of muscle recruitment in activities such as swimming. Nevertheless, the principle of specificity applies when testing for aerobic capacity. That is, the $\dot{V}o_{2max}$ of a runner should be measured using a running treadmill, the $\dot{V}o_{2max}$ of a cyclist should be measured using a cycle ergometer, the $\dot{V}o_{2max}$ of a rower should be measured on a rowing ergometer, and so on. Indeed, well-trained cyclists measured on a cycle ergometer will regularly record a level of $\dot{V}o_{2max}$ greater than that obtained while treadmill running (Kohrt et al. 1987), and well-trained triathletes can have equivalent measures of $\dot{V}o_{2max}$ measured using both exercise modes (Laursen et al. 2005b).

While obtainment of one's $\dot{V}o_{2max}$ through direct assessment might be ideal, it is often not practical because of the requirements of expensive specialized equipment and the time required to complete such testing. Thus, many non-invasive tests have been developed to predict $\dot{V}o_{2max}$. The Astrand–Rhyming test is a non-invasive submaximal predictor of $\dot{V}o_{2max}$ and conveniently uses the linear relationship between the parallel increases in heart rate with exercise intensity to conveniently predict $\dot{V}o_{2max}$ (Macsween 2001). In this test, subjects cycle, performing progressive increases in exercise intensity until they achieve an age-based submaximal target heart rate; the workload achieved at the desired target heart rate predicts the $\dot{V}o_{2max}$ through a derived formula (Siconolfi et al. 1985). Other commonly used predictive tests of $\dot{V}o_{2max}$ include the Coopers 12-min run test (Grant *et al.* 1995), the 1.5-mile run (Jackson *et al.* 1981), the multistage 20-m shuttle run (i.e., beep test; St Clair Gibson *et al.* 1998) and the Bangsbo Yo-Yo test (Krustrup *et al.* 2003). However, it should be noted that all of these tests require a maximal effort.

For the Coopers 12-min run test and the 1.5-mile run, participants simply run either as far as they can in 12 min or as fast as they can for 1.5 miles, respectively, and equations are used to predict $\dot{V}o_{2max}$ based on their result. The multistage fitness test (the "beep test") consists of multiple levels of running speed over a 20-m distance. The speed needed to run the 20 m distance is dictated by numerous audible "beeps" and subjects need to complete the 20 m distance before the audible "beep" occurs, turn 180° and run the next 20 m in the opposite direction and complete the distance again. The test begins very easy, but slowly progresses until the subject is unable to keep pace with the speed of the repeating beeps. This test, originally developed by the Australian Institute of Sport, is highly correlated to direct measures of aerobic capacity, and is commonly used to assess aerobic fitness by sporting teams throughout the world. The Bangsbo Yo-Yo intermittent endurance test consists of 5–18 s intervals of 20 m running interspersed by regular short rest periods (5 s). The test evaluates an individual's ability to repeatedly perform intervals over a prolonged period of time. The test is particularly useful for an athlete who performs interval sports (e.g., tennis, team handball, basketball, and soccer) and the test usually lasts 5–20 min. For both the multistage fitness test and the Yo-Yo test, equations are used to predict $\dot{V}o_{2max}$, and the longer the athlete lasts, the higher will be the predicted $\dot{V}o_{2max}$.

In summary, the $\dot{V}o_{2max}$, or aerobic capacity, represents the maximal capacity of the cardiovascular system to uptake and deliver oxygenated blood to working musculature, and $\dot{V}o_{2max}$ is an important predictor of endurance performance ability and cardiovascular fitness level.

PEAK AEROBIC POWER

Another factor that is related to the $\dot{V}o_{2max}$ is the highest running speed or peak power output that is attained during a progressive exercise test, and the referred term will be specific to the exercise mode performed (e.g., peak power output for cycle ergometry, maximal aerobic speed for treadmill running). This related variable also does well to predict the endurance performance ability of well-trained endurance athletes (Hawley & Noakes 1992; Noakes *et al.* 1990), but as the level of peak power or speed attained will occur in the latter stages of a progressive exercise test, a partial contribution to this variable will come from anaerobic sources and possibly the anaerobic threshold (Fig. 4.15).

There are a multitude of commercially available treadmills that are applicable for clinical exercise testing. When purchasing a treadmill, however, the reliability and drift of the treadmill speed should be examined, as well as the peak treadmill velocity if the testing of highly trained runners is sought (i.e., >25 km·h^{-1}). There are also a number of commercially available cycle ergometers. The mechanically braked Monark 824E cycle ergometer is probably the most commonly used cycle ergometer found within the teaching and clinical setting, and provides a reliable assessment of power output during cycling (Franklin *et al.* 2005). When assessing the performance of well-trained cyclists, however, the Monark falls somewhat short in terms of its external validity, and adjustable cycle ergometers specific to cyclists include the Lode (Paton & Hopkins 2001), SRM (Smith *et al.* 2001) and Velotron cycle ergometers (McDaniel *et al.* 2005), as well as the Kingcycle ergometer which utilizes the cyclist's own bicycle (Paton & Hopkins 2001).

ANAEROBIC THRESHOLD

Although scientists have in the past debated the existence of an anaerobic threshold (Brooks 1985; Davis 1985), it is generally accepted to be the highest exercise intensity where blood lactate production is equal to the rate of its disappearance (Koike *et al.* 1990), and is therefore considered to be a high exercise intensity that can be maintained for a prolonged period of time (Svedahl & MacIntosh 2003). At high work rates above the anaerobic threshold, the capillary partial pressure of oxygen needed for the muscle cell's oxygen requirements is not met by the cardiovascular oxygen supply (Svedahl &

MacIntosh 2003). This results in the oxygen consumed being less than the oxygen required by the working tissue, with the oxygen equivalent difference necessarily coming from anaerobic metabolism (Koike *et al*. 1990). The consequences are increased lactate formation and metabolic acidosis, and the physiologic and biochemical disturbances that result from the latter; volitional fatigue is the inevitable result.

While $\dot{V}o_{2max}$ is a good predictor of endurance capacity, anaerobic threshold measurements tend to be better predictors of performance ability in homogeneous groups of well-trained endurance athletes (Bentley *et al*., 2001b; Coyle *et al*. 1991; Farrell *et al*. 1979; Rhodes & McKenzie 1984). Indeed, coaches and sports scientists may use measurement of the anaerobic threshold as a tool to forecast and monitor endurance performance ability (Bentley *et al*. 2001b) as the anaerobic threshold varies significantly between individuals and responds favorably to endurance training (Denis *et al*. 1982; Svedahl & MacIntosh 2003). The anaerobic threshold is commonly measured during progressive exercise tests through assessment of changes in blood lactate levels and changes in ventilation, termed the lactate threshold and ventilatory thresholds, respectively.

Lactate threshold

Lactate, or lactic acid when it is dissociated from the H^+ ion, is produced both at rest and during all intensities of exercise from the oxidation of glucose during glycolysis, and is an important source of chemical energy (i.e., fuel substrate) during both exercise and in recovery. During steady state exercise below the lactate threshold, the rate of blood lactate production from glycolysis is matched by the rate of its removal (conversion of lactate to pyruvate via the Cori cycle and lactate shuttle). Lactate produced in working muscle fibers is transported and can flow to adjacent less-recruited muscle fibers to be converted to pyruvate in a process known as the "lactate shuttle" (Brooks 1986). Here pyruvate is converted to acetyl-CoA and oxidized through the central energy pathway. This balanced process is referred to as lactate turnover (Billat *et al*. 2003).

Blood levels of lactic acid are increased at exercise intensities above the anaerobic threshold as a

result of the greater ATP demand and therefore the greater reliance on glycolysis to match the ATP energy requirements. Lactic acid levels begin to accumulate when lactate production rate exceeds its removal rate, and this denotes a high use of the anaerobic glycolytic energy system. Changes in pH and bicarbonate accompany these higher lactic acid levels (Robergs *et al*. 2004). When blood lactate accumulates at a rate in excess of its removal, this causes increases in intracellular acidity, which may cause enzyme disruptions and muscle contraction impairment, and ultimately fatigue (Billat *et al*. 2003). More recent data, however, suggest that a higher level of acidity in the muscle actually assists in the optimization of force production during muscular contraction, making the production of lactic acid during intense exercise beneficial to muscular contraction (Nielsen *et al*. 2001).

Regardless of the possible benefits or encumbrances, lactic acid rises during exercise of increasing intensities, and Coyle *et al*. (1983) define the lactate threshold as a 1 mmol·L^{-1} increase in blood lactic acid levels above steady state levels (Fig. 4.17). Other methods of lactate threshold determination have included the individual lactate threshold, the D-max method, and the log–log lactate threshold method (Bishop *et al*. 1998b). Fixed measurements of the lactate threshold, including the 2.5 mmol·L^{-1} lactate threshold and the 4.0 mmol·L^{-1} onset of

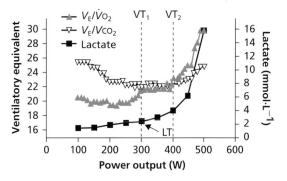

Fig. 4.17 Various anaerobic threshold demarcation points during a progressive exercise test (100 W + 50 W/5 min) in an elite Australian cyclist ($\dot{V}o_{2max} = 78.2 \text{ mL·kg}^{-1}\text{·min}^{-1}$). The first ventilatory threshold (VT_1) and lactate threshold (LT) occurred at 300 W, while the second ventilatory threshold (VT_2) and/or respiratory compensation point occurred at 400 W.

blood accumulation (OBLA), have been used in the past as absolute measures of the lactate threshold (Svedahl & MacIntosh 2003). While these fixed measurements of the lactate threshold have been shown to predict performance ability in earlier studies, it is now established that the lactate threshold occurs at an individualized rate (Myburgh *et al.* 2001). Therefore, a fixed lactate threshold measurement is no longer recommended.

An individual's lactate threshold will be specific to the exercise intensity (power output or running speed) where the imbalance between the muscle cell's lactate formation and clearance occurs. The measurement of one's lactate threshold then provides a means of highlighting an athlete's aerobic ability, and may provide a benchmark for exercise training intensity prescription when incorporated with the associated heart rate, running speed, or power output response. It is important to note that just like the $\dot{V}o_{2max}$ measurement, the lactate threshold is also specific to the mode of exercise because of the neuromuscular blueprint utilized. Recruitment of less trained muscle fibers during unfamiliar exercise modes will alter the lactate threshold. Thus, the lactate threshold needs to be determined using the mode of exercise specific to that athlete's mode of familiarity.

In the clinical setting, lactate levels are commonly measured using benchtop or portable lactate analyzers. A common benchtop analyzer is the YSI Lactate Analyzer (Bishop *et al.* 1992), while the "gold standard" for lactate analysis is thought by many to be the Radiometer (Cobbaert *et al.* 1999). Some of the more common handheld, portable, lactate analyzers are the Accusport (Fell *et al.* 1998), Lactate Pro (van Someren *et al.* 2005), and i-STAT (Dascombe *et al.* 2006).

Ventilatory threshold

The ventilatory threshold is considered to be the point during a progressive exercise test where the minute ventilation ($\dot{V}_E$) rate increases disproportionately to that of the oxygen uptake ($\dot{V}o_2$), and this tends to occur (but not always) at a similar point in time to that of the exponential rise in blood lactate (i.e., the lactate threshold; Brooks 1985; Davis 1985).

As a result of the commonality of these demarcation points, the ventilatory threshold is often used as a tool to predict the lactate threshold (Laursen *et al.* 2005c), particularly in children, as it is seen as being far less invasive. Interestingly, there are generally two distinct points during a progressive exercise test where ventilation increases disproportionately to that of oxygen uptake. These two points are generally referred to as the first and second ventilatory thresholds (Lucia *et al.* 2000) and examples of these are shown in Fig. 4.17.

FIRST VENTILATORY THRESHOLD (VT_1)

The first ventilatory breakpoint is the point during a progressive exercise test where a noticeable increase in the ventilatory equivalent for oxygen uptake ($\dot{V}_E/\dot{V}o_2$) occurs (Lucia *et al.* 2000). Here the volume of air breathed in and out increases at a disproportionate rate to the level of oxygen that is consumed. This point is sometimes referred to as the "aerobic threshold," and is thought to be the exercise intensity where H^+ ions released from lactate are being adequately buffered by the bicarbonate ion to form the weak acid carbonic acid (H_2CO_3), which dissociates into water and carbon dioxide. Increases in carbon dioxide levels and H^+ ion levels trigger an increase rate of breathing through their influence on the central and peripheral chemoreceptors. This increased rate of minute ventilation removes the excess carbon dioxide levels and as a result, pH levels are controlled. While the increase in $\dot{V}_E$ initially falls in line with that of carbon dioxide production ($\dot{V}co_2$), the increase in $\dot{V}_E$ is disproportionate to that of $\dot{V}o_2$. Thus, the ventilatory equivalent for carbon dioxide ($\dot{V}_E/\dot{V}co_2$) does not change at this point (Fig. 4.17; Lucia *et al.* 2000).

SECOND VENTILATORY THRESHOLD (VT_2)

The second ventilatory threshold (VT_2) is associated with very high exercise intensities, where blood lactate accumulates significantly more than it can be cleared (Fig. 4.17). The VT_2 is depicted by another significant increase in the $\dot{V}_E/\dot{V}o_2$, but with a concomitant increase in the $\dot{V}_E/\dot{V}co_2$ (Lucia *et al.* 2000). Here these very high levels of blood lactic acid trigger an exponential increase in the $\dot{V}_E$ to levels much greater than required for oxygen uptake or carbon dioxide removal. While the VT_1 is commonly referred to as the "aerobic threshold," the VT_2 is sometimes referred to as the "anaerobic threshold" or "respiratory compensation point."

The observation of these two distinct ventilatory thresholds (i.e., VT_1 and VT_2) then begs the following two questions. First, how are these points practically related to an athlete's endurance performance? Second, could an athlete use this information in either their training program, or as a pacing tool during an endurance or ultra-endurance event? Few studies to date have examined this. However, a recent study showed in Ironman triathletes that the heart rate associated with VT_1 was related to the heart rate performed at during the running and cycling phases of a 226-km Ironman triathlon (Laursen *et al.* 2005a). Moreover, triathletes who performed above their VT_1 during the cycle phase of the event had slower marathon run performances than those who performed the cycle phase below their VT_1, suggestive to the fact that the heart rate at VT_1 may be a good pacing tool for Ironman triathletes to use to pace their overall triathlon performance. It is possible therefore that the VT_1, or aerobic threshold, may predict an exercise intensity that is maintainable for prolonged endurance and ultra-endurance durations. Conversely, the VT_2 has been shown to be related to endurance performances requiring a very high exercise intensity for durations of around 60 min, such as a 40 km cycling time trial (Laursen *et al.* 2003a).

Economy of motion

The successful endurance athlete is able to maintain a continual high work rate without critically affecting the endogenous energy supplies of their working muscles. Thus, efficient use of accessible energy is an important contributor to the performance ability of the endurance athlete. Economy of motion refers to the relationship between the mechanical work achieved (i.e., running speed or power output) and the total energy expended (i.e., oxygen uptake). For example, running economy is taken by measuring the oxygen uptake at a given submaximal running speed (i.e., $14\ km\cdot h^{-1}$). Imagine two runners, identical in build and stature. The first of those runners is able to run at $14\ km\cdot h^{-1}$ at an oxygen uptake of $2.5\ L\cdot min^{-1}$, while the second runner runs $14\ km\cdot h^{-1}$ at $2.7\ L\cdot min^{-1}$. The first runner is more economical in using a range of physiologic systems (e.g., stretch–shortening cycle, lower respiration rate) to move at the set speed of $14\ km\cdot h^{-1}$. The first runner will also produce less heat than the second runner, as heat is produced relative to the metabolic rate. Thus, it is likely that the first runner will have the capacity to run for longer than the second runner through a sparing of energy reserves (i.e., muscle glycogen), and by a reduction in the amount of heat that is produced from the decreased metabolic rate. Minimizing or eliminating unwanted or counterproductive muscular movements, as well as training adaptations that serve to enhance the stretch–shortening cycle, have the potential to increase one's economy of motion and improve endurance performance (Paavolainen *et al.* 1999).

Similar to the anaerobic threshold measurement, economy of motion has been shown to segregate the performance ability of homogeneous groups of well-trained athletes with comparable levels of $\dot{V}o_{2max}$ (Lucia *et al.* 2002, Weston *et al.* 2000). For example, Weston *et al.* (2000) investigated the $\dot{V}o_{2max}$ and economy of motion in African and Caucasian long-distance runners, and while $\dot{V}o_{2max}$ was 13% higher in the Caucasian group, running economy at $16.1\ km\cdot h^{-1}$ was 5% superior in the faster running African group.

In summary, the $\dot{V}o_{2max}$, peak power output, anaerobic threshold, and economy of motion are the main factors that influence overall endurance performance (Fig. 4.15). While $\dot{V}o_{2max}$ does well to predict performance throughout the general population, peak power output, the anaerobic threshold and the economy of motion may be better discriminators of performance ability in homogeneous groups of well-trained endurance athletes. The extent to which each of these factors has a role in the overall performance outcome depends on the duration and intensity of the endurance performance in question, with a high $\dot{V}o_{2max}$ being more important for shorter duration high-intensity events, and the peak power output, anaerobic threshold, and economy of motion having a higher weighting for longer duration endurance events. Conveniently, all of these factors can be measured using a progressive exercise test.

Progressive exercise tests

A progressive or graded exercise test, sometimes simply referred to as a $\dot{V}o_{2max}$ test (Fig. 4.16), is a common clinical endurance test that can be used to estimate all of the abovementioned variables that well predict endurance performance ability. However, not every type of graded exercise test will measure each of these variables accurately. Thus, it is important for the practitioner to understand how the manipulation of the progressive exercise test protocol can influence the results. Differences in test protocols include aspects such as the stage duration and the rate of increase in exercise intensity (i.e., power or running speed) from one stage to the next. Manipulation of these variables categorizes a progressive exercise test as either a fast or slow ramp protocol (Bentley *et al.* 2001a; Bishop *et al.* 1998a). The suitability of these different types of progressive exercise tests for measuring the main physiologic predictors of performance success will be explained.

TESTING PROTOCOLS

Fast ramp protocols

A progressive exercise test can be classified as having a "fast ramp" protocol when the test is created so that voluntary termination of the exercise from fatigue occurs at 8–15 min (Brooks *et al.* 2000). The reason for the broad range in duration is because if fatigue during a progressive exercise test occurs in less than 8 min, the protocol might have created too great an exercise intensity too soon, and cardiac output might not have been fully challenged. Conversely, for fatigue occurring in a time greater than 15 min, untrained subjects might not be able to push themselves to exercise for such long periods and again cardiovascular capacity might not be fully taxed.

The fast ramp protocol does well to measure $\dot{V}o_{2max}$ and maximum heart rate (HR_{max}) in the broad population (Bishop *et al.* 1998a). A typical fast ramp running protocol used for well-trained runners might begin at 8 $km \cdot h^{-1}$, and increases in speed occur by 1 $km \cdot h^{-1}$ every minute until 18 $km \cdot h^{-1}$. Thereafter, further increases in exercise intensity would be achieved through increases in treadmill incline or grade (i.e., an increase of 1% grade every minute thereafter until volitional fatigue (Laursen *et al.* 2005b). A typical "fast ramp" cycling protocol for well-trained cyclists might have subjects commencing exercise at 100 W for the first minute, with power output increases of 30 W every minute until volitional fatigue (Laursen *et al.* 2002a). However, these fast ramp protocols are not appropriate to measure either economy of motion or the anaerobic threshold, as steady state for each exercise level is not likely to be reached before the next increase in exercise intensity occurs (Bentley *et al.* 2001a). Nevertheless, the "fast ramp" protocol is appropriate for measuring $\dot{V}o_{2max}$ and maximum heart rate, and because of its relatively short time requirement, may be a useful tool for coaches and sports scientists to monitor changes in $\dot{V}o_{2max}$.

Slow ramp protocols

A progressive exercise test is classified as a "slow ramp" protocol when the protocol is designed with prolonged stage durations of 3–8 min. Slow ramp protocols are typically used to assess indices of the anaerobic threshold, peak-sustained power, and in some instances running economy (Noakes *et al.* 1990; Weston *et al.* 2000). Peak-sustained power output has a strong correlation with endurance performance ability, particularly in well-trained athletes (Hawley & Noakes 1992; Noakes *et al.* 1990). The time to fatigue for a slow ramp progressive exercise test will normally be 20–45 min, with 5-min increments generally used as the step duration (Fig. 4.17). These tests may not be suitable for inexperienced or untrained subjects, especially when assessing $\dot{V}o_{2max}$, as fatigue may ensue prior to reaching a level that would challenge cardiovascular capacity. However, in better-trained subjects, slow ramp protocols have been shown to provide equivalent levels of $\dot{V}o_{2max}$ to those of fast ramp protocols (Bentley *et al.* 2001a; Bishop *et al.* 1998a). Therefore, if time permits, the use of a slow ramp protocol would seem to be more valuable to the endurance coach as it provides more useful measures of endurance performance, including the anaerobic threshold and economy of motion, without sacrificing the measurement of $\dot{V}O_{2max}$ (Bentley *et al.* 2001a; Bishop *et al.* 1998a).

Slow ramp protocols implementing 5–6 min progressive stages are typically used for measuring economy to ensure steady state levels of oxygen consumption are attained (Morgan & Daniels 1994). This protocol tends to be more applicable in well-trained athletes, as the longer time frame (20–45 min) fatigues untrained athletes before economy of motion can be properly assessed (Morgan & Daniels 1994). Although not entirely clear as to the exact mechanisms responsible for improving economy of motion, training volume, training intensity, training type (i.e., plyometrics), years of endurance training and genetics all appear to have a role (Franch *et al.* 1998; Paavolainen *et al.* 1999; Sjodin & Svedenhag 1985).

Considerations for endurance performance testing

ERGOMETER SPECIFICITY

A cardinal rule of endurance performance testing is that the ergometer used for the test must be specific to the population being studied. For example, there is no point in measuring the $\dot{V}O_{2max}$ of a cyclist using a running treadmill, as the recruitment patterns used in cycling are different to those used in running, and the resultant $\dot{V}O_{2max}$ score will be significantly lower than that obtained on a cycle ergometer.

Thus, a population of cyclists should be measured using a cycle ergometer in the laboratory or remotely using field power measuring devices, runners must be examined on a running treadmill or on the track, rowers using rowing ergometers. Generally speaking, the more specific the test can be to the actual movements that are performed by the athlete during training and competition the better.

FAMILIARIZATION TRIALS

Familiarity in a performance task is an important variable related closely to variation which is naturally inherent within repeated endurance performance trials. Thus, a familiarization trial of some form should be considered as a requirement for conducting a clinically valid endurance test. The familiarization trial ensures that subjects are comfortable with the equipment and procedures, and this can significantly reduce the within-subject variations that occur from the "learned effect" (Laursen *et al.* 2003a). For example, Laursen *et al.* (2003a) performed a study where cyclists had to perform three indoor 40 km cycle time trials on their own bicycle mounted to a stationary wind-trainer. The coefficient of variation (measure of variability) between the first and second trial, and the first and third trial was 3%. However, when the coefficient of variation was examined between the second and third trials, the variation was markedly reduced to only 1%. Clearly then, a familiarization trial is a vital component of endurance testing research as it significantly reduces the variance between tests.

STANDARDIZED WARM-UP

A standardized warm-up is also an important aspect of an endurance performance test. The warm-up should be specific to the exercise task being performed and will allow for an increase in blood flow into the working muscles that will be recruited for the performance test. The warm-up literally increases the temperature of the muscles and increases the muscles' ability to produce force through an increase in enzyme activity and subsequent increase in energy production, known as the Q-10 effect. A good warm-up for well-trained cyclists could include 3 min of cycling at 25% of peak power output, followed by 5 min of cycling at 60% of peak power output, followed by 2 min of cycling at 80% of peak power output.

TESTS OF ENDURANCE PERFORMANCE

Central to the administration of a meaningful physiologic performance test is the concept of reproducibility or reliability as discussed in the introduction. Reproducibility implies how well a physical performance test is able to give the same result time and time again, which implies a high level of accuracy and precision of the measurement

(Hopkins 2000; Hopkins *et al.* 2001). If a test possesses a high level of reproducibility, it increases the chance of detecting differences in physiologic parameters amongst individuals, or a real change in performance potential, should one exist, following administration of either a training intervention or ergogenic aid.

Current debate exists as to the methodology that should be used to design an endurance performance test. Many endurance performance tests are designed so that the athlete is asked to either "perform for as long as possible at a given exercise intensity," or to "perform a given distance in as fast a time as possible." At first glance these two tasks may seem comparable as both types of tests will challenge one's endurance capacity. Indeed, both types of tests are used extensively within the realm of scientific endurance testing, both in the academic research setting and in national sporting academies and institutes. However, issues surrounding the practicality and reliability of these two types of tests are significant.

Open-loop testing

An exercise performance test that is performed at a constant running speed or power output can be termed an "open-loop" test. This test is deemed "open-looped" because the time to complete the test is determined by the individual; time is therefore unknown, or open-ended. Traditionally, subjects are requested to perform this type of test at set submaximal exercise intensities until they can no longer maintain the required running speed or power output (Jeukendrup *et al.* 1996). These types of tests are better known in the exercise science literature as "time-to-exhaustion" tests and can be run at virtually any set exercise intensity. While time-to-exhaustion tests will be the main focus of the open-loop testing, a progressive exercise test could also be considered to be a type of open-loop test.

PROGRESSIVE EXERCISE TESTS

The progressive exercise test may be considered to be an open-loop test because the subject is asked to perform "to exhaustion." However, this type of test differs from time-to-exhaustion tests in that the exercise intensity is incremental under set time blocks, and the work load is not kept constant. This incremental nature of the progressive exercise tests may assist the subject to allow pacing to occur once a familiarization test has occurred, or if the exercise stages and durations are presented to the subject. In time-to-exhaustion tests, time is typically blinded to the subject. The reliability of progressive tests has been reported to be less than 5% in untrained runners (Kyle *et al.* 1989), with strong reliability coefficients also reported in triathletes performing progressive exercise tests in the modes of running (0.97), cycling (0.93), and swimming (0.97) (Kohrt *et al.* 1987). Thus, progressive exercise tests, which may be considered by some as open-loop tests, appear to be reliable.

TIME-TO-EXHAUSTION TESTS

Time-to-exhaustion tests have been used as an important tool to assess performance changes following a training intervention. During time-to-exhaustion tests, subjects are required to perform at a predetermined exercise intensity that remains constant throughout each trial, until that pace can no longer be maintained and the time-to-exhaustion is recorded (Davis *et al.* 1992; Laursen *et al.* 2002b). The longer an athlete performs, the greater their endurance potential is deemed to be. The submaximal speed or power output is generally established as a percentage of an athlete's $\dot{V}o_{2max}$ or threshold marker (Davis *et al.* 1992; Laursen *et al.* 2002b). During time-to-exhaustion tests, athletes are blinded to feedback on time or distance completed. Billat *et al.* (1994) conducted time-to-exhaustion tests in eight sub-elite runners at the running speed associated with $\dot{V}o_{2max}$ and found no significant differences between the trials repeated within 1 week of each other. Despite this, however, substantial differences existed in the individual subject measurements, and the coefficient of variation was calculated to be high at 25%.

Time-to-exhaustion tests performed at supramaximal exercise intensity (exercise intensity in excess of $\dot{V}o_{2max}$ power output or running speed) also appear to elicit relatively low absolute levels of repeatability. Graham and McLellan (1989) showed that treadmill running tests to exhaustion performed at 120% of the $\dot{V}o_{2max}$ running speed produced a relatively high variation (coefficient of variation [CV] = 10%; r = 0.89), while Laursen *et al.* (2003c) also found that the cycling time-to-exhaustion performed at 150% of the cycling power output associated with $\dot{V}o_{2max}$ was not highly reliable (CV = 11%) in well-trained cyclists and triathletes.

Closed-loop testing

A "closed-loop" exercise test can be defined as an endurance performance test with a known endpoint (i.e., a known amount of work to complete, distance to travel, or time to perform for). Traditionally, subjects are asked to complete the given distance or work as fast as possible, or to complete as much work or distance as they can in a given time period. These types of tests are more commonly referred to as "time-trials."

Closed-loop tests of known distances, work, or time allow the subjects to adjust their exercise intensity according to their perception of fatigue. In these tests, the subject is aware that they have a specific endpoint. In a time-trial of a known distance (most common) the only feedback provided is distance completed or remaining. In these tests, subjects are required to complete every trial in the fastest time possible. The closed-loop protocol shows high absolute levels of reliability, or low coefficient of variation scores (~1%). For example, Palmer *et al.* (1996) showed that the reproducibility of a 20- and 40-km cycling time-trial on a Kingcycle ergometer was highly reproducible (CV = 1.1 and 1.0%, respectively), and similar levels of reliability have been shown by others (Balmer *et al.* 2000; Laursen *et al.* 2003a).

Comparison of open- versus closed-loop tests

In a meta-analysis examining the reliability of cycle performance tests, Hopkins *et al.* (2001) have shown that the test variation of open-loop time-to-exhaustion tests is generally much greater than closed-loop tests which use defined limits (i.e., a known distance). This increased variance for open-loop tests shows the importance placed on "knowing the expected outcome" and the importance of being able to adjust pace in accordance with afferent sensory feedback signals. While some studies have researched each type of test (open- vs. closed-loop test) separately in the same subjects (Laursen *et al.* 2003a–c), there are no known studies that have directly compared the two.

Two recent studies using the same subjects examined the reproducibility of both a closed-loop 40-km cycle time trial (Laursen *et al.* 2003a) and an open-loop time-to-exhaustion test at the power output associated with $\dot{V}o_{2max}$ (Laursen *et al.* 2003b). Both tests were repeated following familiarization tests, at the same time of day, and about 1 week apart. The variation of performance times between the two trials (expressed as the CV) was markedly lower for the time trial ($1 \pm 1\%$; Laursen *et al.* 2003a) compared with the time-to-exhaustion test ($6 \pm 6\%$; Laursen *et al.* 2003b). Thus, "knowing the task at hand" (i.e., test distance) appeared to be responsible for lowering the variation in performance times compared with the open-ended time-to-exhaustion test. In the latter mentioned study, the last of the two time-to-exhaustion tests was found to be significantly longer than the first (Laursen *et al.* 2003b). The authors attributed this finding to the psychologic affect associated with performing "the last test." Physiologic variables in this study were not different between trials, and the performance difference could only be attributed to psychologic factors; the knowledge of the trial being "the last task" somehow influencing performance time (Gleser & Vogel 1971; Hickey *et al.* 1992; Laursen *et al.* 2003b). However, there was no difference found for these same subjects in their 40 km time-trial performances (Laursen *et al.* 2003a).

While all this evidence suggests that closed-loop time-trial tests have a reduced variability compared with those of open-loop time-to-exhaustion tests, no study has directly compared the variation between open- and closed-loop exercise trials of equivalent workloads in the same subjects. In addition, there is some evidence to suggest that prolonged sub-maximal exercise tests have an improved reproducibility when compared with shorter high-intensity exercise trials (Hickey *et al.* 1992; Palmer *et al.* 1996; Stepto *et al.* 1998). For example, in a series of studies by Laursen *et al.* (2003a–c) using trained cyclists, the repeatability of prolonged exercise tests (i.e., 40 km time trials; CV = 1%) was improved compared with higher exercise intensities associated with the time-to-exhaustion tests at $\dot{V}o_{2max}$ (CV = 6%), and at 150% of $\dot{V}o_{2max}$ (CV = 11%). Again, no studies have directly examined the influence of exercise test duration or intensity on the variability between open- and closed-loop exercise tests, and this research is required before clear conclusions on the matter can be made.

Another consideration for sport scientists, when deciding whether to use an open-loop or a closed-loop endurance performance test, comes back to the principle of specificity. That is, is use of an open-loop test a realistic representation of actual athletic performance, as there are very few instances where an endurance athlete must work to exhaustion at set exercise intensity? Thus, time-to-exhaustion tests may be viewed as having less external validity, and have even been labeled as survival tests for athletes who must overcome feelings of boredom and a lack of motivation, rather than an accurate assessment of their endurance performance ability. Termination of the exercise during a time-to-exhaustion test will be dependent upon individual feelings of fatigue, and this will most likely explain the observations of higher levels of variability in these tests (Hopkins *et al.* 2001). Conversely, the closed-loop time-trial protocol has a lower coefficient of variation and is therefore more reproducible, and may be more applicable for the measuring of athletic performance. With this type of test, however, athletes pace themselves and the workload is not even, which can create problems when comparison of physiologic variables throughout the trial is desired.

While the external validity favors selection of the closed-loop test, it has been argued that the signal-to-noise ratio may be greater in the time-to-exhaustion tests than in time-trials. By "noise," this refers to the variability of the measurement (i.e., CV), while by "signal" this refers to the improvement that can be witnessed by the measurement. To illustrate, while the variance in a closed-loop time-trial is generally less than 1%, the change in time-trial performance following a training intervention is also relatively small (usually <5%). Conversely, a time-to-exhaustion test that may have a relatively high variability (35%), may also elicit a very large change following a training intervention (i.e., >20%). Thus, selection of an open-loop time-to-exhaustion test may be appropriate when the goal of the sports scientist is to determine the influence that a particular exercise intervention may have on endurance performance. Research is required to confirm or refute these assumptions.

Summary

To summarize, endurance performance can be broken down into three key physiologic variables: the $\dot{V}o_{2max}$, anaerobic threshold, and economy of motion. Different methods of testing these measures have been used in the past but it would appear prudent that certain protocols be used in accordance with the specific physiologic variable being sought by the clinician. Slow ramp tests or tests with longer incremental progressions (approximately 5 min) enable subjects to attain steady state and are best used to measure running economy and markers of the anaerobic threshold. As a result of the longer increments, the total duration of the test can be more than 25 min. Progressive exercise tests with shorter stages create shorter duration tests (8–15 min), and these fast ramp tests provide a good means of assessing $\dot{V}o_{2max}$ and maximum heart rate and are appropriate for use in untrained subjects.

Matching the testing protocol to that of the athlete's sport, including a familiarization test and a warm-up, were identified as key aspects for the selection of any endurance test and will allow for improved validity, reliability, and therefore greater credibility and acceptance to the findings and conclusions drawn from the results. Laboratory testing is a vital component for establishing and measuring the effectiveness of a training intervention. Although both open- and closed-loop protocols are commonly used throughout the exercise science literature, closed-loop time-trial tests are thought to have a greater reliability and are more like the endurance events commonly performed by endurance athletes. However, some believe that time-to-exhaustion tests have a greater signal: noise ratio and therefore may be a more appropriate test to use when the goal of the researcher is to examine the effectiveness of an intervention on the change in endurance performance.

The future of endurance tests will see improved measures of reliability and validity, and the goal of sports scientists and clinicians will be to design more practical tests based on performances in real competitions so as to reduce the disparity between laboratory results and field performance results.

Body composition

An understanding of the significance of body composition is important for the exercise clinician because of the influence that body composition can have on both exercise performance and general health. For athletes, a reduction in body fat levels means a reduction in the mass that has to be accelerated and thus the force required to change direction, speed, project into the air during jumping, or perform work uphill against gravity. Quite simply, an athlete with more body fat will carry with him or her added non-functional weight that will require more energy to move and produce more heat from the increased metabolic rate. Moreover, additional fat stores provide an added layer of insulation that will shield the body against the dissipation of heat from the central core to the environment. For the general public living in the western world, obesity levels have reached epidemic levels and reducing body fat usually represents a major goal in any exercise training program. High body fat content, and in particular abdominal fat, greatly increases risk of a range of chronic diseases including cardiovascular disease, type II diabetes, hypertension, and some cancers. In light of its obvious importance to the exercise clinician, a general understanding of the science behind body composition and its assessment is a final consideration of this chapter.

Composition of the body

Determination of the body's make-up or composition can be a fairly complex task because of the number of different ways that it can be broken up.

For example, we can separate the composition of our bodies into:
1 Atoms (61% O_2, 23% C, 10% H, 2.6% N, 1.4% Ca, 2% other);
2 Major molecules (carbohydrates, lipids, proteins, mineral compounds, water);
3 Different types of cells and body fluids (fat cells, muscle cells, body fluids);
4 Various tissues (adipose tissue, skeletal muscle, bone, blood); or
5 At a whole body level (using skinfolds, girths, and underwater weighing).

Although the first four methods are considered to be more direct, and have all been completed in prior research, they require expensive analytical equipment or cadaver dissection. However, dual energy X-ray absorptiometry (DEXA) is becoming accepted as the "gold standard" for body composition assessment. This technology is still quite expensive ($100,000–200,000) so more practical alternatives to estimate body composition at the whole body level using indirect methods of assessment are also discussed. Some of the more commonly used indirect assessments include underwater weighing (densitometry), bioelectrical impedence, skinfold thickness, girths, and weight : stature ratios. These indirect anthropometric assessments are attractive because they can easily be conducted in the laboratory or the field.

Dual energy X-ray absorptiometry

Dual energy X-ray absorptiometry involves very low level X-ray radiation to image the body and, based on differential transmission by muscle, fat, and bone tissues, the system is able to separate and provide accurate measures of the quantity of each in grams (Fig. 4.18). This is achieved by simultaneously emitting beams of two different energy levels that are absorbed at different rates by different tissues. DEXA has been used predominantly for determination of bone mineral density but is also finding excellent application for measuring fat and muscle tissue mass (Daly *et al.* 2005).

A further advantage of DEXA is that not only whole body measures can be derived, but also segments including trunk, upper and lower limbs.

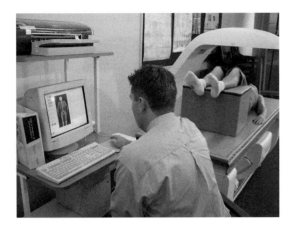

Fig. 4.18 Dual energy X-ray absorptiometry (DEXA) system for assessment of fat, bone, and muscle content of the human body.

For this, DEXA is particularly effective for tracking changes in muscle mass with training interventions (Daly *et al.* 2005).

Underwater weighing (densitometry)

Underwater or hydrostatic weighing (densitometry) can be used to estimate fat mass in relation to fat-free mass in the athlete (literally, the amount of body composition without fat) by calculating the difference between body weights measured in air and in water (Archimedes principle). The proportions of fat and fat-free mass can be calculated from the assumption that the density of fat is 0.9001 g·mL^{-1}, with the remaining tissues (fat-free mass) being approximately 1.100 g·mL^{-1}. Validity of underwater weighing is based on a relatively small number of cadavers that have been analyzed chemically, on animal studies, and on several alternative means used to estimate density and proportions of specific body parts. Thus, it is important to note that underwater weighing, while long felt to be the "gold standard" in body composition assessment, is actually an indirect method of body composition assessment. Indeed, doubt regarding the assumptions relating to the estimation of the density of the fat-free mass used to calculate whole body density has been raised (Martin & Drinkwater 1991). Factors such as the levels of bone mineral density and

muscle mass all serve to influence the 1.100 g·mL^{-1} estimation of the fat-free mass density. For example, underwater weighing often will underestimate levels of body fat in well-trained athletes with high levels of muscle and bone mineral content, and overestimate body fat levels in osteoporotic women with markedly lower levels (Martin & Drinkwater 1991). Another source of error within the estimation of body composition using underwater weighing includes the error associated with the air remaining in the lungs during the measurement (i.e., whether the subject exhaled all of their air, as well as the estimation of the residual volume).

In a more advanced form of this method, residual lung volume can be estimated based on a nitrogen rebreathing technique but it is still an estimate (Wilmore *et al.* 1980). Further, gases in the gastrointestinal tract also can influence the density measure considerably (Martin & Drinkwater 1991). Finally, underwater weighing might not always be a suitable method of body composition assessment with certain populations such as the obese and the elderly because of the difficulty these subjects would have in achieving complete submersion (Martin & Drinkwater 1991). Thus, densitometry is a valid method of body composition assessment that is relatively easily applied with athletic populations, but limitations of the measurement need to be appreciated and caution for appropriateness should be used when assessing other populations.

Bioelectrical impedance

Bioelectrical impedance (Fig. 4.19) is based on the relationship between the volume of the conductor (i.e., the human body), the conductor's length (i.e., height), the components of the conductor (i.e., fat and fat-free mass), and its impedance (Buchholz *et al.* 2004). Estimates of body composition are based on the assumption that the overall conductivity of the human body is closely related to the amount of water it contains. Water is a relatively good conductor of electrical current (i.e., low impedance), particularly when containing electrolytes, which is the case in the body. Fat tissue contains relatively less water and consequently has a much higher impedance. Measurement of this impedance

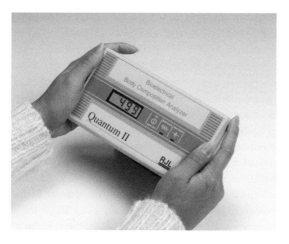

Fig. 4.19 Bioimpedence measurement for the estimation of body composition.

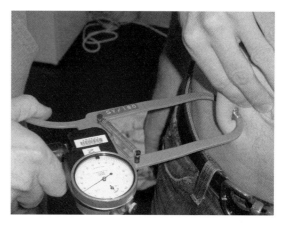

Fig. 4.20 Skinfold calipers are used to measure the thickness of subcutaneous fat and expressed as absolute values, a summed total, or entered into regression formulae for estimation of body composition.

involves placing electrodes to the surface of the lower arms and legs, passing a very low voltage electrical current and measuring the ease of transmission through the body: the impedance. This is combined with anthropometric measures of height, weight, and possibly circumferences to estimate fat and lean body mass. In some machines, the subject stands on a scale with bare feet and the impedance is measured from one foot to the other with weight being recorded simultaneously.

Anthropometric techniques

SKINFOLDS

Largely because of the convenience with which skinfold callipers (Fig. 4.20) can be transported and the comparative ease in measuring subcutaneous fat, skinfold data are now commonly used to estimate total body fat (Clark *et al.* 2002). However, the apparent simplicity in reliable skinfold measures is deceptive. Care in calibration of the callipers, location of sites, and overall consistency in measurement is essential. Indeed, there are a number of possible factors that may reduce the accuracy of a skinfold measurement. The hydration level of the subject or the level of blood flow to the skin caused by showering or sauna can alter skinfold thickness through changes in skin turgidity (Martin &

Drinkwater 1991). As differences in site location will reduce the accuracy of the assessment, the measurement site must be carefully described and accurately located for each measurement made. The type of instrument is also important, where a constant pressure must be applied no matter what the thickness of the skinfold. Standard skinfold callipers are designed to exert a pressure of 10 $g \cdot mm^{-2}$, and commonly used skinfold callipers that do this include Harpenden and Lange.

Skinfold measurement procedures, sites, and body composition prediction equations have been outlined elsewhere (Norton *et al.* 2000). Briefly, when taking the measurement, it should be taken on the right side of the body, with the skinfold being pulled well clear of the underlying muscle using the flat pads of the index finger and thumb. If there is doubt about whether muscle is included, have the subject contract the muscle allowing the subcutaneous fat to be exposed. Callipers should be applied 1 cm from the fingers and placed at a depth of approximately the mid-fingernail. The reading should be taken 2 s after the full pressure of the callipers is applied. Two to three readings should be taken at every site, with the average being taken if two readings are made (first two readings <4 mm difference), and the median used if three readings are made (third reading taken if difference between first and second reading >4 mm).

Once the skinfolds are taken in duplicate and recorded, they are either recorded simply as a sum of skinfolds, or they can be converted to percent body fat using one of many prediction equations (Norton *et al.* 2000).

GIRTH MEASUREMENTS

Girth measurements are simply circumference measurements taken at various sites on the body such as waist, hips, thigh, upper arm, forearm, and calf. Because of muscle mass as well as fat thickness influencing the girth measurements, it is difficult to make meaningful inter-subject comparisons. However, if the limitations are recognized, pre- and post-training measurements may be useful for monitoring the effectiveness of an individual's training program, particularly if a major aim is fat loss and muscle gain. All circumferences are measured with a thin, steel, metric tape measured at right angles to the long axis of a bone or body segment. The perimeter distance with the tape in contact with but not compressing the underlying tissue is recorded in centimeters. This is perhaps the cheapest and easiest measure of body composition. Also, only circumferences are recorded and the measures cannot be converted into estimates of fat and lean mass as is the case in skinfold measurements.

WEIGHT : STATURE RATIOS

The body mass index (BMI) is commonly used to determine body fatness relative to height. The BMI is simply recorded as mass (in kilograms) divided by height (in meters) squared ($kg\cdot m^2$). For the general population, a BMI of 20–25 $kg\cdot m^2$ is desired and is associated with low levels of risk for the development of cardiovascular disease. BMI scores of 26–30 $kg\cdot m^2$ place an individual in the overweight category and at higher risk for cardiovascular disease. A BMI of above 30 $kg\cdot m^2$ places an individual into the obese category, with the greatest risk of developing cardiovascular disease. It is important to note, however, that the BMI scale is most applicable to the general population, and that athletes who have high amounts of muscle (which is much more dense than fat) can have BMI scores above

25 $kg\cdot m^2$. Thus, caution should be used when using the BMI assessment in athletes (Nevill *et al.* 2006).

Summary

In summary, densitometry, bioelectrical impedance, skinfold thickness, girths, and height : stature ratios are commonly used methods of assessing body composition that can be performed both in the laboratory or the field. It is important to note, however, that these methods are all indirect methods of body composition, and that some degree of error in the measurement will always be present. All of these techniques make assumptions about the density of fat and lean tissue in the body and most are based on regression formulae derived from populations that, in all likelihood, will be different to the subject being measured. Validation and regression formula derivation for the skinfold and bioimpedance techniques in most instances has been achieved using underwater weighing as the standard, but as has been observed, there are problems with this technique. Having said this, the routine assessment of body composition during the course of an athlete's season is an important variable to include in the array of physiologic tests that the exercise clinician should apply. However, comparison of one individual with another should be carried out with caution.

Presenting the results

Perhaps the most important aspect of athlete assessment is the provision of simple, concise, informative, and educational reports. Detailed athlete assessment is only of use if the results are used to inform program design for greater effectiveness and efficiency, reduce injury risk, and educate the athlete and coach about responses and adaptations to training and competition. An entire chapter could be devoted to the topic of reporting, particularly when one considers the latest advances on the Internet and database technologies. However, a few key points are pertinent.

Results should be reported graphically whenever possible, and include benchmarks for comparison. Benchmarking might include published results for national or international level athletes in the same or similar sport. If an entire team or squad has been tested, benchmarking to the mean and standard deviation is useful. Z-scores are useful in this regard as they indicate how many standard deviations the athlete's score is from the group mean. The "radar plots" in Microsoft Excel are very effective for presenting this type of data and an example is provided in Fig. 4.21. To produce such a graph, the key components of the athlete assessment battery are listed in the spreadsheet. The mean and standard deviation for each parameter are calculated and then the z-score [(athlete score − mean)/standard deviation] for each athlete's results are determined. These can then be plotted for each athlete and comparisons between athletes or repeated test sessions included.

The future

There are exciting developments occurring, with several sporting bodies making extensive use of Internet technology to provide real-time reports of test results in web-based format that can be accessed from anywhere in the world. This allows the athlete and coach to monitor key variables regardless of where they are traveling for training or competition. The future of athlete testing and assessment is bright, with rapid progress being made in new equipment, which is more portable, less invasive, and can be incorporated with the athlete's training and competition. The result will be improved performance with less injury, greater career longevity, and a more professional management of the careers of athletes and coaches.

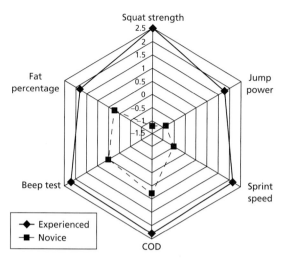

Fig. 4.21 Radar plot for providing benchmarking of performance diagnosis. The athletes' z-scores in selected performance or body composition variables are plotted on a single graph to visually represent their profile relative to the average for the group. Two athletes are presented. One of the most talented in the squad shows a well-rounded profile with consistently strong (well above average – solid line) z-scores while the novice is at or below team average for most scores and particularly weak in strength, power, and speed.

References

Aagaard, P., Simonsen, E.B., Magnusson, S.P., Larsson, B. & Dyhre-Poulsen, P. (1998) A new concept for isokinetic hamstring : quadriceps muscle strength ratio. *American Journal of Sports Medicine* **26**, 231–237.

Aagaard, P., Simonsen, E.B., Trolle, M., Bangsbo, J. & Klausen, K. (1995) Isokinetic hamstring–quadriceps strength ratio: influence from joint angular velocity, gravity correction and contraction mode. *Acta Physiologica Scandinavica* **154**, 421–427.

Abe, T., Kawakami, Y., Ikegawa, S., Kanehisa, H. & Fukunaga, T. (1992) Isometric and isokinetic knee joint performance in Japanese alpine ski racers. *Journal of Sports Medicine and Physical Fitness* **32**, 353–357.

Abernethy, B., Thomas, K.T. & Thomas, J.T. (1993) Strategies for improving understanding of motor expertise (or mistakes we have made and things we have learned!). *Cognitive Issues in Motor Expertise*. Elsevier Science Publishers, B.V.

Abernethy, B., Wann, J. & Parks, S. (1998) Training perceptual motor skills for sport. *Training for Sport: Applying Sport Science*. John Wiley, Chichester.

Baker, D. (2001) Acute and long-term power responses to power training: observations on the training of an elite power athlete. *Strength and Conditioning Journal* **23**, 47–56.

Baker, D., Nance, S. & Moore, M. (2001a) The load that maximizes the average mechanical power output during explosive bench press throws in highly trained athletes. *Journal of Strength and Conditioning Research* **15**, 20–24.

Baker, D., Nance, S. & Moore, M. (2001b) The load that maximizes the average mechanical power output during jump squats in power-trained athletes. *Journal of Strength and Conditioning Research* **15**, 92–97.

Balmer, J., Davison, R.C. & Bird, S.R. (2000) Peak power predicts performance power during an outdoor 16.1-km cycling time trial. *Medicine and Science in Sports and Exercise* **32**, 1485–1490.

Bentley, D.J., McNaughton, L.R. & Batterham, A.M. (2001a) Prolonged stage duration during incremental cycle exercise: effects on the lactate threshold and onset of blood lactate accumulation. *European Journal of Applied Physiology* **85**, 351–357.

Bentley, D.J., McNaughton, L.R., Thompson, D., Vleck, V.E. & Batterham, A.M. (2001b) Peak power output, the lactate threshold, and time trial performance in cyclists. *Medicine and Science in Sports and Exercise* **33**, 2077–2081.

Besier, T.T.F., Lloyd, D.D.G., Cochrane, J.J.L. & Ackland, T.T.R. (2001) External loading of the knee joint during running and cutting maneuvers. *Medicine and Science in Sports and Exercise* **33**, 1168.

Billat, V., Bernard, O., Pinoteau, J., Petit, B. & Koralsztein, J.P. (1994) Time to exhaustion at $\dot{V}o_{2max}$ and lactate steady state velocity in sub elite long-distance runners. *Archives Internationales de Physiologie, de Biochimie et de Biophysique* **102**, 215–219.

Billat, V., Sirvent, P., Py, G., Koralsztein, J.P. & Mercier, J. (2003) The concept of maximal lactate steady state: a bridge between biochemistry, physiology and sport science. *Sports Medicine* **33**, 407–426.

Bishop, D., Jenkins, D.G. & Mackinnon, L.T. (1998a) The effect of stage duration on the calculation of peak $\dot{V}o_2$ during cycle ergometry. *Journal of Science and Medicine in Sport*, **1**, 171–178.

Bishop, D., Jenkins, D.G. & Mackinnon, L.T. (1998b) The relationship between plasma lactate parameters, W_{peak} and 1-h cycling performance in women. *Medicine and Science in Sports and Exercise* **30**, 1270–1275.

Bishop, P.A., Smith, J.F., Kime, J.C., Mayo, J.M. & Tin, Y.H. (1992) Comparison of a manual and an automated enzymatic technique for determining blood lactate concentrations. *International Journal of Sports Medicine* **13**, 36–39.

Brockett, C.L., Morgan, D.L. & Proske, U. (2004) Predicting hamstring strain injury in elite athletes. *Medicine and Science in Sports and Exercise* **36**, 379–387.

Brooks, G.A. (1985) Anaerobic threshold: review of the concept and directions for future research. *Medicine and Science in Sports and Exercise* **17**, 22–34.

Brooks, G.A. (1986) The lactate shuttle during exercise and recovery. *Medicine and Science in Sports and Exercise* **18**, 360–368.

Brooks, G.A., Fahey, T.D. & White, T.P. (1996) *Exercise Physiology. Human Bioenergetics and its Applications.* Mayfield Publishing, CA.

Brooks, G.A., Fahey, T.D., White, T.P. & Baldwin, K.M. (2000) *Exercise Physiology: Human Bioenergetics and its Applications.* McGraw Hill, Sydney.

Bruggemann, G. & Glad, B. (1990) Time analysis of the sprint events. In: *Scientific Research Project at the Games of the XXIVth Olympiad. Seoul, International Athletic Foundation, Monaco* (Bruggemann, G. & Glad, B., eds.)

Buchholz, A.C., Bartok, C. & Schoeller, D.A. (2004) The validity of bioelectrical impedance models in clinical populations. *Nutrition in Clinical Practice* **19**, 433–446.

Buckeridge, A., Farrow, D., Gastin, P., McGrath, M., Morrow, P., Quinn, A. et al. (2000) Protocols for the physiological assessment of high-performance tennis players. *Physiological Tests for Elite Athletes.* Australian Sports Commission, Canberra.

Butts, N.K., Henry, B.A. & McLean, D. (1991) Correlations between $\dot{V}o_{2max}$ and performance times of recreational triathletes. *Journal of Sports Medicine and Physical Fitness* **31**, 339–344.

Clark, R.R., Oppliger, R.A. & Sullivan, J.C. (2002) Cross-validation of the NCAA method to predict body fat for minimum weight in collegiate wrestlers. *Clinical Journal of Sport Medicine* **12**, 285–290.

Cobbaert, C., Morales, C., Van Fessem, M. & Kemperman, H. (1999) Precision, accuracy and linearity of radiometer EML 105 whole blood metabolite biosensors. *Annals of Clinical Biochemistry* **36**, 730–738.

Coyle, E.F. (1995) Integration of the physiological factors determining endurance performance ability. *Exercise and Sport Sciences Reviews* **23**, 25–63.

Coyle, E.F. (1999) Physiological determinants of endurance exercise performance. *Journal of Science and Medicine in Sport* **2**, 181–189.

Coyle, E.F., Feltner, M.E., Kautz, S.A., Hamilton, M.T., Montain, S.J., Baylor, A.M., et al. (1991) Physiological and biomechanical factors associated with elite endurance cycling performance. *Medicine and Science in Sports and Exercise* **23**, 93–107.

Coyle, E.F., Martin, W.H., Ehsani, A.A., Hagberg, J.M., Bloomfield, S.A., Sinacore, D.R., et al. (1983) Blood lactate threshold in some well-trained ischemic heart disease patients. *Journal of Applied Physiology* **54**, 18–23.

Crouter, S.E., Antczak, A., Hudak, J.R., Dellavalle, D.M. & Haas, J. D. (2006) Accuracy and reliability of the ParvoMedics TrueOne 2400 and MedGraphics VO2000 metabolic systems. *European Journal of Applied Physiology* **98**, 139–151.

Daly, R.M., Dunstan, D.W., Owen, N., Jolley, D., Shaw, J.E. & Zimmet, P.Z. (2005) Does high-intensity resistance training maintain bone mass during moderate weight loss in older overweight adults with type 2 diabetes? *Osteoporosis International* **16**, 1703–1712.

Dascombe, B.J., Reaburn, P.R., Sirotic, A.C. & Coutts, A.J. (2007) The reliability of the i-STAT clinical portable analyser. *Journal of Science and Medicine in Sport* **10**, 135–140

Davis, J.A. (1985) Anaerobic threshold: review of the concept and directions for future research. *Medicine and Science in Sports and Exercise* **17**, 6–21.

Davis, J.M., Bailey, S.P., Woods, J.A., Galiano, F.J., Hamilton, M.T. & Bartoli, W.P. (1992) Effects of carbohydrate feedings on plasma free tryptophan and branched-chain amino acids during prolonged cycling. *European Journal of Applied Physiology and Occupational Physiology* **65**, 513–519.

Dawson, B., Fitzsimons, M., Green, S., Goodman, C., Carey, M. & Cole, K. (1998) Changes in performance, muscle metabolites, enzymes and fibre types after short sprint training. *European Journal of Applied Physiology and Occupational Physiology* **78**, 163–169.

Delecluse, C., Van Coppenolle, H., Williams, E. & Goris, M. (1995) Influence of high resistance and high velocity training on sprint performance. *Medicine and Science in Sports and Exercise* **27**, 1203–1209.

Denis, C., Fouquet, R., Poty, P., Geyssant, A. & Lacour, J.R. (1982) Effect of 40 weeks of endurance training on the anaerobic threshold. *International Journal of Sports Medicine* **3**, 208–214.

Draper, J.A. & Lancaster, M.G. (1985) The 505 test: a test for agility in the horizontal plane. *Australian Journal of Science and Medicine in Sport* 15–18.

Droghetti, P., Borsetto, C., Casoni, I., Cellini, M., Ferrari, M., Paolini, A.R., et al. (1985) Noninvasive determination of the anaerobic threshold in canoeing, cross-country skiing, cycling, roller, and ice-skating, rowing, and walking. *European Journal of Applied Physiology and Occupational Physiology* **53**, 299–303.

Ellis, L., Gastin, P., Lawrence, S., Savage, B., Buckeridge, A., Stapff, A., et al. (2000) Protocols for the physiological assessment of team sport players.

Physiological Tests for Elite Athletes. Australian Sports Commission, Canberra.

Farrell, P.A., Wilmore, J.H., Coyle, E.F., Billing, J.E. & Costill, D.L. (1979) Plasma lactate accumulation and distance running performance. *Medicine and Science in Sports* **11**, 338–444.

Farrow, D., Young, W. & Bruce, L. (2005) The development of a test of reactive agility for netball: a new methodology. *Journal of Science and Medicine in Sport* **8**, 52–60.

Fell, J.W., Rayfield, J.M., Gulbin, J.P. & Gaffney, P.T. (1998) Evaluation of the Accusport Lactate Analyser. *International Journal of Sports Medicine* **19**, 199–204.

Fitzsimons, M., Dawson, B., Ward, D. & Wilkinson, A. (1993) Cycling and running tests of repeated sprint ability. *Australian Journal of Science and Medicine in Sport* **25**, 82–87.

Foss, O. & Hallen, J. (2005) Validity and stability of a computerized metabolic system with mixing chamber. *International Journal of Sports Medicine* **26**, 569–575.

Franch, J., Madsen, K., Djurhuus, M.S. & Pedersen, P.K. (1998) Improved running economy following intensified training correlates with reduced ventilatory demands. *Medicine and Science in Sports and Exercise* **30**, 1250–1256.

Franklin, K.L., Gordon, R.S., Baker, J.S. & Davies, B. (2005) Mechanics of a rope-braked cycle ergometer flywheel and its use for physiological measurement. *Research in Sports Medicine* **13**, 331–344.

Frick, U., Schmidtbleicher, D. & Stutz, R. (1995) Muscle activation during acceleration-phase in sprint running with special reference to starting posture. *Xvth Congress of the International Society of Biomechanics, Jyvaskyla*.

Glaister, M. (2005) Multiple sprint work physiological responses, mechanisms of fatigue and the influence of aerobic fitness. *Sports Medicine* **35**, 757–777.

Gleser, M.A. & Vogel, J.A. (1971) Endurance exercise: effect of work-rest schedules and repeated testing. *Journal of Applied Physiology* **31**, 735–739.

Gore, C.J., Clark, R.J., Shipp, N.J., Van der Ploeg, G.E. & Withers, R.T. (2003) CPX/D underestimates Vo_2 in athletes compared with an automated Douglas bag system. *Medicine and Science in Sports and Exercise* **35**, 1341–1347.

Graham, K.S. & McLellan, T.M. (1989) Variability of time to exhaustion and oxygen deficit in supramaximal exercise.

Australian Journal of Science and Medicine in Sport **21**, 11–14.

Grant, S., Corbett, K., Amjad, A.M., Wilson, J. & Aitchison, T. (1995) A comparison of methods of predicting maximum oxygen uptake. *British Journal of Sports Medicine* **29**, 147–152.

Grant, S., Craig, I., Wilson, J. & Aitchison, T. (1997) The relationship between 3 km running performance and selected physiological variables. *Journal of Sports Science* **15**, 403–410.

Häkkinen, K., Alen, M. & Komi, P.V. (1985) Changes in isometric force- and relaxation-time, electromyographic and muscle fibre characteristics of human skeletal muscle during strength training and detraining. *Acta Physiologica Scandinavica* **125**, 573–585.

Hawley, J.A. & Noakes, T.D. (1992) Peak power output predicts maximal oxygen uptake and performance in trained cyclists. *European Journal of Applied Physiology* **65**, 79–83.

Hertel, J., Denegar, C.C.R., Johnson, P.P.D., Hale, S.S.A. & Buckley, W.W.E. (1999) Reliability of the Cybex Reactor in the assessment of an agility task. *Journal of Sport Rehabilitation* **8**, 24–31.

Hickey, M.S., Costill, D.L., McConell, G.K., Widrick, J.J. & Tanaka, H. (1992) Day to day variation in time trial cycling performance. *International Journal of Sports Medicine* **13**, 467–470.

Hopkins, W.G. (2000) Measures of reliability in sports medicine and science. *Sports Medicine* **30**, 1–15.

Hopkins, W.G., Schabort, E.J. & Hawley, J.A. (2001) Reliability of power in physical performance tests. *Sports Medicine* **31**, 211–234.

Jackson, A., Dishman, R.K., La Croix, S., Patton, R. & Weinberg, R. (1981) The heart rate, perceived exertion, and pace of the 1.5 mile run. *Medicine and Science in Sports and Exercise* **13**, 224–228.

Jackson, R., Warren, S. & Abernethy, B. (2006) Anticipation skill and susceptibility to deceptive movement. *Acta Psychologica* **123**, 355–371.

Jeukendrup, A., Saris, W.H., Brouns, F. & Kester, A.D. (1996) A new validated endurance performance test. *Medicine and Science in Sports and Exercise* **28**, 266–270.

Kohrt, W.M., Morgan, D.W., Bates, B. & Skinner, J.S. (1987) Physiological responses of triathletes to maximal swimming, cycling, and running. *Medicine and Science in Sports and Exercise* **19**, 51–55.

Koike, A., Wasserman, K., Beaver, W.L., Weiler-Ravell, D., MCcKenzie, D.K. &

Zanconato, S. (1990) Evidence supporting the existence of an exercise anaerobic threshold. *Advances in Experimental Medicine and Biology* **277**, 835–846.

Krustrup, P., Mohr, M., Amstrup, T., Rysgaard, T., Johansen, J., Steensberg, A., Pedersen, P.K. & Bangsbo, J. (2003) The yo-yo intermittent recovery test: physiological response, reliability, and validity. *Medicine and Science in Sports and Exercise* **35**, 697–705.

Kyle, S.B., Smoak, B.L., Douglass, L.W. & Deuster, P.A. (1989) Variability of responses across training levels to maximal treadmill exercise. *Journal of Applied Physiology* **67**, 160–165.

Kyrolainen, H., Komi, P.P.V. & Belli, A.P.V. (1999) Changes in muscle activity patterns and kinetics with increasing running speed. *Journal of Strength and Conditioning Research* **13**, 400.

Laursen, P.B., Blanchard, M.A. & Jenkins, D.G. (2002a) Acute high-intensity interval training improves Tvent and peak power output in highly trained males. *Canadian Journal of Applied Physiology* **27**, 336–348.

Laursen, P.B., Knez, W.L., Shing, C.M., Langill, R.H., Rhodes, E.C. & Jenkins, D.G. (2005a) Relationship between laboratory measured variables and heart rate during an ultra-endurance triathlon. *Journal of Sports Sciences* **23**, 1111–1120.

Laursen, P.B. & Rhodes, E.C. (2001) Factors affecting performance in an ultraendurance triathlon. *Sports Medicine* **31**, 195–209.

Laursen, P.B., Rhodes, E.C., Langill, R.H., McKenzie, D.C. & Taunton, J.E. (2002b) Relationship of exercise test variables to cycling performance in an Ironman triathlon. *European Journal of Applied Physiology*, **87**, 433–440.

Laursen, P.B., Rhodes, E.C., Langill, R.H., Taunton, J.E. & McKenzie, D.C. (2005b) Exercise-induced arterial hypoxemia is not different during cycling and running in triathletes. *Scandinavian Journal of Medicine and Science in Sports* **15**, 113–117.

Laursen, P.B., Shing, C.M. & Jenkins, D.G. (2003a) Reproducibility of a laboratory-based 40-km cycle time-trial on a stationary wind-trainer in highly trained cyclists. *International Journal of Sports Medicine* **24**, 481–485.

Laursen, P.B., Shing, C.M. & Jenkins, D.G. (2003b) Reproducibility of the cycling time to exhaustion at $\dot{V}o_{2peak}$ in highly trained cyclists. *Canadian Journal of Applied Physiology* **28**, 605–615.

Laursen, P.B., Shing, C.M., Peake, J.M., Coombes, J.S. & Jenkins, D.G. (2005c) Influence of high-intensity interval training on adaptations in well-trained cyclists. *Journal of Strength and Conditioning Research* **19**, 527–533.

Laursen, P.B., Shing, C.M., Tennant, S.C., Prentice, C.M. & Jenkins, D.G. (2003c) A comparison of the cycling performance of cyclists and triathletes. *Journal of Sports Sciences* **21**, 411–418.

LeSuer, D.A., McCormick, J.H., Mayhew, J.L., Wasserstein, R.L. & Arnold, M.D. (1997) The accuracy of prediction equations for estimating 1-RM performance in the bench press, squat, and deadlift. *Journal of Strength and Conditioning Research* **11**, 211–213.

Lucia, A., Hoyos, J., Perez, M. & Chicharro, J.L. (2000) Heart rate and performance parameters in elite cyclists: a longitudinal study. *Medicine and Science in Sports and Exercise* **32**, 1777–1782.

Lucia, A., Hoyos, J., Perez, M., Santalla, A. & Chicharro, J.L. (2002) Inverse relationship between $\dot{V}o_{2max}$ and economy/efficiency in world-class cyclists. *Medicine and Science in Sports and Exercise* **34**, 2079–2084.

Macsween, A. (2001) The reliability and validity of the Astrand nomogram and linear extrapolation for deriving $\dot{V}o_{2max}$ from submaximal exercise data. *Journal of Sports Medicine and Physical Fitness* **41**, 312–317.

Marek, S.M., Cramer, J.T., Fincher, A.L., Massey, L.L., Dangelmaier, S.M., Purkayastha, S., *et al.* (2005) Acute effects of static and proprioceptive neuromuscular facilitation stretching on and muscle strength power output. *Journal of Athletic Training* **40**, 94–103.

Martin, A.D. & Drinkwater, D.T. (1991) Variability in the measures of body fat. Assumptions or technique? *Sports Medicine* **11**, 277–288.

McBride, J.M., Triplett-McBride, N.T., Davie, A. & Newton, R.U. (2001) The effect of heavy versus light load jump squats on the development of strength, power and speed. *Journal of Strength and Conditioning Research* **16**, 75–82.

McBride, J.M., Triplett-McBride, T., Davie, A. & Newton, R.U. (1999) A comparison of strength and power characteristics between power lifters, Olympic lifters, and sprinters. *Journal of Strength and Conditioning Research* **13**, 58–66.

McDaniel, J., Subudhi, A. & Martin, J.C. (2005) Torso stabilization reduces the metabolic cost of producing cycling power. *Canadian Journal of Applied Physiology* **30**, 433–441.

Morgan, D.W. & Daniels, J.T. (1994) Relationship between $\dot{V}o_{2max}$ and the aerobic demand of running in elite distance runners. *International Journal of Sports Medicine* **15**, 426–429. [Published erratum appears in *International Journal of Sports Medicine* **15**, 527.]

Murphy, A.J. & Wilson, G.J. (1996a) The assessment of human dynamic muscular function: a comparison of isoinertial and isokinetic tests. *Journal of Sports Medicine and Physical Fitness* **36**, 169–177.

Murphy, A.J. & Wilson, G.J. (1996b) Poor correlations between isometric tests and dynamic performance: relationship to muscle activation. *European Journal of Applied Physiology and Occupational Physiology* **73**, 353–357.

Murphy, A.J. & Wilson, G.J. (1997) The ability of tests of muscular function to reflect training-induced changes in performance. *Journal of Sports Sciences* **15**, 191–200.

Murphy, A.J., Wilson, G.J. & Pryor, J.F. (1994) Use of the iso-inertial force mass relationship in the prediction of dynamic human performance. *European Journal of Applied Physiology and Occupational Physiology* **69**, 250–257.

Myburgh, K.H., Viljoen, A. & Tereblanche, S. (2001) Plasma lactate concentrations for self-selected effort lasting 1 h. *Medicine and Science in Sports and Exercise* **33**, 152–156.

Nevill, A.M., Stewart, A.D., Olds, T. & Holder, R. (2006) Relationship between adiposity and body size reveals limitations of BMI. *American Journal of Physical Anthropology* **129**, 151–156.

Newton, R.U. & Dugan, E. (2002) Application of strength diagnosis. *Strength and Conditioning Journal* **24**, 50–59.

Newton, R.U., Humphries, B., Murphy, A., Wilson, G.J. & Kraemer., W.J. (1994) Biomechanics and neural activation during fast bench press movements: implications for power training. *National Strength and Conditioning Association Conference*. New Orleans.

Newton, R. U. & Kraemer, W. J. (1994) Developing explosive muscular power: implications for a mixed methods training strategy. *Strength and Conditioning Journal* **16**, 20–31.

Newton, R.U., Kraemer, W.J. & Hakkinen, K. (1999) Effects of ballistic training on preseason preparation of elite volleyball players. *Medicine and Science in Sports and Exercise* **31**, 323–330.

Nielsen, O.B., De Paoli, F. & Overgaard, K. (2001) Protective effects of lactic acid on force production in rat skeletal muscle. *Journal of Physiology* **536**, 161–166.

Nieman, D.C., Austin, M.D., Benezra, L., Pearce, S., McInnis, T., Unick, J. & Gross, S.J. (2006) Validation of Cosmed's FitMate in measuring oxygen consumption and estimating resting metabolic rate. *Research in Sports Medicine* **14**, 89–96.

Nieman, D.C., Trone, G.A. & Austin, M.D. (2003) A new handheld device for measuring resting metabolic rate and oxygen consumption. *Journal of the American Diet Association* **103**, 588–592.

Noakes, T.D., Myburgh, K.H. & Schall, R. (1990) Peak treadmill running velocity during the $\dot{V}o_{2max}$ test predicts running performance. *Journal of Sports Sciences* **8**, 35–45.

Norton, K., Marfell-Jones, M., Whittingham, N., Kerr, D., Carter, L., Saddington, K., *et al.* (2000) Anthropometric assessment protocols. In: *Physiological Tests for Elite Athletes* (Gore, C., ed.) Human Kinetics, Champaign, IL.

Paavolainen, L., Hakkinen, K., Hamalainen, I., Nummela, A. & Rusko, H. (1999) Explosive-strength training improves 5-km running time by improving running economy and muscle power. *Journal of Applied Physiology* **86**, 1527–1533.

Palmer, G.S., Dennis, S.C., Noakes, T.D. & Hawley, J.A. (1996) Assessment of the reproducibility of performance testing on an air-braked cycle ergometer. *International Journal of Sports Medicine* **17**, 293–298.

Paton, C.D. & Hopkins, W.G. (2001) Tests of cycling performance. *Sports Medicine* **31**, 489–496.

Rhodes, E.C. & McKenzie, D.C. (1984) Predicting Marathon time from anaerobic threshold measurements. *The Physician and Sportsmedicine* **12**, 95–99.

Robergs, R.A., Ghiasvand, F. & Parker, D. (2004) Biochemistry of exercise-induced metabolic acidosis. *American Journal of Physiology. Regulatory, Integrative and Comparative Physiology* **287**, R502–516.

Rowland, T.W. & Cunningham, L.N. (1992) Oxygen uptake plateau during maximal treadmill exercise in children. *Chest* **101**, 485–489.

Schneider, D.A., Lacroix, K.A., Atkinson, G.R., Troped, P.J. & Pollack, J. (1990) Ventilatory threshold and maximal oxygen uptake during cycling and running in triathletes. *Medicine and Science in Sports and Exercise* **22**, 257–264.

Semenick, D. (1994) Testing protocols and procedures. *Essentials of Strength and Conditioning*. Human Kinetics, Champaign, IL.

Sheppard, J. & Young, W. (2006) Agility literature review: classifications, training and testing. *Journal of Sports Sciences* **24**, 919–923.

Sheppard, J., Young, W., Doyle, T., Sheppard, T. & Newton, R. (2006) An evaluation of a new test of reactive agility, and its relationship to sprint speed and change of direction speed. *Journal of Science and Medicine in Sport* **9**, 342–349.

Siconolfi, S.F., Garber, C.E., Lasater, T.M. & Carleton, R.A. (1985) A simple, valid step test for estimating maximal oxygen uptake in epidemiologic studies. *American Journal of Epidemiology* **121**, 382–390.

Sjodin, B. & Svedenhag, J. (1985) Applied physiology of marathon running. *Sports Medicine* **2**, 83–99.

Smith, M.F., Davison, R.C., Balmer, J. & Bird, S.R. (2001) Reliability of mean power recorded during indoor and outdoor self-paced 40 km cycling time-trials. *International Journal of Sports Medicine* **22**, 270–274.

Spencer, M., Bishop, D., Dawson, B. & Goodman, C. (2005) Physiological and metabolic responses of repeated-sprint activities specific to field-based team sports. *Sports Medicine* **35**, 1025–1044.

St Clair Gibson, A., Broomhead, S., Lambert, M.I. & Hawley, J.A. (1998) Prediction of maximal oxygen uptake from a 20-m shuttle run as measured directly in runners and squash players. *Journal of Sports Sciences* **16**, 331–335.

Stepto, N.K., Hawley, J.A., Dennis, S.C. & Hopkins, W.G. (1998) Effects of different interval-training programs on cycling time-trial performance. *Medicine and Science in Sports and Exercise* **31**, 736–741.

Svedahl, K. & MacIntosh, B.R. (2003) Anaerobic threshold: the concept and methods of measurement. *Canadian Journal of Applied Physiology* **28**, 299–323.

Thomas, J.R. & Nelson, J.K. (1990) *Research Methods in Physical Activity*. Human Kinetics, Champaign, IL.

Van Someren, K.A., Howatson, G., Nunan, D., Thatcher, R. & Shave, R. (2005) Comparison of the Lactate Pro and Analox GM7 blood lactate analysers. *International Journal of Sports Medicine* **26**, 657–661.

Volkov, N.N.I. & Lapin, V.V.I. (1979) Analysis of the velocity curve in sprint running. *Medicine and Science in Sports and Exercise* **11**, 332–337.

Webster, P.A., King, S.E. & Torres, A. Jr. (1998) An *in vitro* validation of a commercially available metabolic cart using pediatric ventilator volumes. *Pediatric Pulmonology* **26**, 405–411.

Weston, A.R., Ziphelele, M. & Myburgh, K.H. (2000) Running economy of African and Caucasian distance runners. *Medicine and Science in Sports and Exercise* **32**, 1130–1134.

Wilmore, J.H., Vodak, P.A., Parr, R.B., Girandola, R.N. & Billing, J.E. (1980) Further simplification of a method for determination of residual lung volume. *Medicine and Science in Sports and Exercise* **12**, 216–218.

Wilson, G.J., Lyttle, A.D., Ostrowski, K.J. & Murphy, A.J. (1995) Assessing dynamic performance: a comparison of rate of force development tests. *Journal of*

Strength and Conditioning Research **9**, 176–181.

Wilson, G.J., Newton, R.U., Murphy, A.J. & Humphries, B.J. (1993) The optimal training load for the development of dynamic athletic performance. *Medicine and Science in Sports and Exercise* **25**, 1279–1286.

Wilson, G.J., Walshe, A.D. & Fisher, M.R. (1997) The development of an isokinetic squat device: reliability and relationship to functional performance. *European Journal of Applied Physiology and Occupational Physiology* **75**, 455–461.

Witters, J., Heremans, G., Bohets, W., Stijnen, V. & Van Coppenolle, H. (1985) The design and testing of a wire velocimeter. *Journal of Sports Sciences* **3**, 197–206.

Young, W., James, R. & Montgomery, I. (2002) Is muscle power related to running speed with changes in direction? *Journal of Sports Medicine and Physical Fitness* **42**.

Young, W.B. (1995) Laboratory strength assessment of athletes. *New Studies in Athletics* **10**, 89–96.

Young, W.B., Macdonald, C. & Flowers, M.A. (2001) Validity of double- and single-leg vertical jumps as tests of leg extensor muscle function. *Journal of Strength and Conditioning Research* **15**, 6–11.

Young, W.B., Pryor, J.F. & Wilson, G.J. (1995) Effect of instructions on characteristics of countermovement and drop jump performance. *Journal of Strength and Conditioning Research* **9**, 232–236.

Zatsiorsky, V.M. (1995) *Science and Practice of Strength Training*. Human Kinetics, Champaign, IL.

Chapter 5

Clinical Myology in Sports Medicine

WAYNE E. DERMAN, MARTIN P. SCHWELLNUS, DALE E. RAE, YUMNA ALBERTUS-KAJEE AND MICHAEL I. LAMBERT

Although skeletal muscle and its function during exercise is obviously important to the athlete, there is not much information on the disorders of this vital organ in Sports Medicine textbooks. Therefore, the medical professional is often unclear about a systematic diagnostic and therapeutic approach to the athlete who presents with symptoms of muscle disorders that cannot simply be explained by overtraining and overreaching (see Chapter 3).

Symptoms arising from skeletal muscle disorders in the athlete include the following:

- Skeletal muscle pain;
- Skeletal muscle weakness or premature fatigue;
- Skeletal muscle cramps;
- Rhabdomyolysis and red discoloration of the urine; and
- Failure to adapt to training loads.

Of these symptoms, pain, fatigue, cramps and failure to adapt to training are of particular relevance to the athlete.

In this chapter we begin by providing an overview of the function of skeletal muscle and review the concepts of skeletal muscle damage and repair following exercise. Next, we detail two common causative conditions of skeletal muscle pain in athletes: delayed onset muscle soreness (DOMS) and exercise-associated muscle cramps. In the following section we discuss chronic muscle fatigue and underperformance in athletes. Finally, we discuss the clinical approach to the athlete with

symptoms associated with skeletal muscle disorders. Where appropriate, we suggest a clinical diagnostic algorithm to assist in the evaluation of the athlete with these presenting symptoms, as well as suggest the clinical tests of skeletal muscle function that may assist with the diagnosis.

Skeletal muscle physiology with relevance to muscle damage and repair

Skeletal muscle function

Skeletal muscle is a large organ constituting approximately 40% of total body mass in healthy sedentary males, approximately 30% in females (Kim *et al.* 2002), and comprising over 50% of body mass in some athletes. Skeletal muscles are primarily involved in locomotion, posture, and breathing (Chargé & Rudnicki 2004). However, this important metabolic organ also has a role in the energy balance of the human body (Flück & Hoppeler 2003) and is the major organ contributing to thermogenesis (Marino *et al.* 2000).

Skeletal muscle plasticity

Biological stimuli including exercise or denervation cause various adaptations. Such adaptations include modifications of cellular (mitochondria, myofibrils) and extracellular (capillaries, nerves, connective tissue) components. Furthermore, modifications may include altered gene or protein expression and even changes at the levels of transcription, translation, protein translocation, assembly, degradation,

The Olympic Textbook of Medicine in Sport, 1st edition. Edited by M. Schwellnus. Published 2008 by Blackwell Publishing, ISBN: 978-1-4051-5637-0.

and recycling. Collectively, these adaptations contribute to changes in the contractile function of the muscle in response to the initial stimulus and manifest as changes in force production and the ability to resist fatigue (Flück & Hoppeler 2003).

Damage to and repair of skeletal muscle

Skeletal muscle can be injured through a variety of mechanisms including disease, exposure to toxic compounds, direct trauma, ischemia, extreme temperatures, and exercise (Brooks 2003).

EXERCISE-INDUCED MUSCLE DAMAGE

Acute bouts of resistance (Paul *et al.* 1989), sprint (Klapcinska *et al.* 2001), or endurance exercise (Warhol *et al.* 1985) can result in damage to skeletal muscle. The types of injury include sarcolemmal disruption, swelling or disruption of the sarcotubular system, distortion of the myofibrils, contractile components, cytoskeletal damage, and extracellular myofiber matrix abnormalities. In particular, lengthening or eccentric muscle actions elicit greater levels of muscle damage than shortening (concentric) or static (isometric) contractions (Fridén & Lieber 1992). The etiology of muscle damage is discussed in more detail in the section on delayed onset muscle damage.

REPAIR AND REGENERATION OF SKELETAL MUSCLE

Adult skeletal muscle is a post-mitotic stable tissue that easily copes with the wear and tear induced by everyday living. However, this robust organ also has the ability to repair and regenerate very effectively in response to severe injury or damage induced by direct trauma or innate genetic defects. Depending on the severity of the injury, either necrosis occurs or the myofiber is repaired (Chargé & Rudnicki 2004). Minor disruptions to the thick or thin filaments of skeletal muscle only require the resynthesis of the involved molecules. However, more severe damage requires regeneration of the disrupted section of the fiber, or even of the entire myofiber. In cases in which regeneration of a myofiber is required, satellite cells are activated and drawn into the regeneration process (Brooks 2003). Satellite cells are specialized muscle precursor cells that are required for myofiber repair (Renault *et al.* 2000) and for the replacement of any myonuclei lost following damage (Bischoff 1994). These mononucleate cells reside beneath the basal lamina of the myofiber in a state of quiescence (Mauro 1961). During the regeneration phase, quiescent satellite cells along a myofiber are activated which requires the upregulation of muscle transcription factors and muscle specific genes. This is communicated intrinsically through cell–cell and cell–matrix interactions, and extrinsically by extracellular secreted factors. The actual stimulus or stimuli for the activation of satellite cells may be a consequence of the muscle injury itself where growth factors are released from the injured myofiber (Yan 2000). Alternatively, molecules released from inflammatory cells, invading macrophages, soluble factors from connective tissue, and extract from the injured fibers have also been proposed as possible stimuli of satellite cells (Chargé & Rudnicki 2004; Yan 2000).

Skeletal muscle repair is composed of two phases: a degeneration phase followed by a regeneration phase. The degeneration phase is characterized by the activation of inflammatory and myogenic cells. Cytokines from inflammatory cells and growth factors are released from the extracellular matrix or from the injured myofibers (Yan 2000). Within 1–6 h after damage, neutrophils invade the injured site, while macrophages take over as the dominant inflammatory cells about 48 h post injury.

The regeneration phase is characterized by activation and proliferation of satellite cells so that either damaged myofibers can be repaired or new myofibers can be formed. Activated satellite cells can migrate in both directions across the basal lamina and often travel considerable distances to the site of injury (Bischoff 1994). Satellite cells then proliferate to increase the number of myogenic cells available for repair (Chargé & Rudnicki 2004). Following the proliferation phase, some of the satellite cells become terminally differentiated. Differentiation of satellite cells is controlled by a group of myogenic factors such as MyoD and myogenin, which function as transcription factors to activate muscle-specific gene expression. The final decision of whether a myogenic cell will divide or differentiate may be determined by a balance between growth and differentiation signals (Yan 2000). Differentiated satellite cells then fuse either to damaged myofibers for repair, or to each other to form new myofibers. Other satellite cells, however, leave the cell cycle before differentiating, return to the quiescent state, and are restored under the basal lamina (Mauro 1961), presumably to replenish the pool of satellite cells to be used for subsequent rounds of regeneration (Chargé & Rudnicki 2004).

Following fusion of the new myogenic cells, the newly formed myofibers increase in size and the myonuclei move to the periphery of the cell. Signs of regeneration can be visualized using histological staining. Cross-sections of skeletal muscle might show the appearance of smaller fibers and fibers with centrally located nuclei. Splitting or branching fibers, possibly caused by the incomplete fusion of regenerating fibers within the same basal lamina, can also be seen in longitudinal sections (Chargé & Rudnicki 2004).

It is possible that satellite cells are not the only source of myonuclei during muscle repair. Progenitor cells from bone marrow and muscle adult stem cells have been shown to differentiate into muscle cells *in vitro* and to contribute to muscle regeneration *in vivo*. However, this is an unusual occurrence brought on by specific cellular and environmental conditions. Alternatively, regenerating myofibers may gain new myonuclei through the recycling of existing myonuclei from severely injured myofibers (Chargé & Rudnicki 2004).

The potential for repair and regeneration of skeletal muscle is affected by the number of available satellite cells, the proliferative capacity of these satellite cells, and the speed of the response to the injury (Renault *et al.* 2002). Because satellite cells are mortal and have a finite capacity to proliferate, the major determinant of the ability of satellite cells to proliferate appears to be the cell's proliferative history (i.e., the previous number of degeneration and regeneration cycles as determined by growth, disease, or injury; Schultz & McCormick 1994). Extensive proliferation would eventually lead to a reduction in the mitotic reserve of the cells, which

are then said to reach replicative senescence (Campisi 1997). In addition to replicative history, host environment is also responsible for replicative capacity. This has relevance to older athletes, particularly those athletes who have undergone several bouts of damage–regeneration during their training and competition and who have also been exposed to stressors other than the stress of training.

Satellite cells isolated from infants have a greater proliferative capacity than those from older individuals, with little difference existing between young and older adults (Decary *et al.* 1997). However, a gradual decrease in the number of skeletal muscle satellite cells has been observed with increasing age. Furthermore, the satellite cells of older individuals displayed different morphological characteristics such as thinner myotubes and less well-organized desmin filaments than the muscle of the younger individuals.

While everyday wear and tear on adult skeletal muscle does not appear to impact the regenerative capacity of satellite cells, excessive demands may result in premature cell senescence, leading to impaired muscle regeneration. This is illustrated in patients with Duchenne's muscular dystrophy where skeletal muscle undergoes excessive degeneration–regeneration cycles compared to healthy age-matched individuals. The satellite cells of these patients are constantly activated to initiate repair and reach senescence prematurely. Thus, senescent satellite cells are unable to proliferate and therefore cannot aid in regeneration (Decary *et al.* 2000; Renault *et al.* 2000).

Because exercise is often associated with damage to skeletal muscle, it is conceivable that this stressor may increase the demand on the replicative capacity of satellite cells. Both acute and chronic bouts of exercise rapidly activate satellite cells (Schultz & McCormick 1994). Indeed, the pool of satellite cells can be increased within 4 days of a single bout of exercise, presumably reflecting the response to exercise-induced muscle damage. When there is cessation of chronic exercise training, there is a gradual reduction in the number of satellite cells (Kadi *et al.* 2005).

In summary, the potential for skeletal muscle to regenerate depends, in part, on the number of available satellite cells, their remaining proliferative capacity, as well as intrinsic and extrinsic stressors (Mouly *et al.* 2005; Renault *et al.* 2002). The regenerative capacity of skeletal muscle can be determined indirectly through measuring the telomere lengths of the DNA in satellite cells (Renault *et al.* 2002). It is of interest to note that athletes with symptoms of muscle pathology typified by pain, fatigue, and failure to adapt to training also display shortened telomere length (Collins *et al.* 2003).

Delayed onset muscle soreness

One of the consequences of engaging in physical activity is that there is a risk of sustaining a soft tissue injury (Armstrong 1990; Orchard 2001). The severity of this risk varies depending on the type and level of activity and characteristics intrinsic to the individual. One of the most common muscle injuries, experienced by recreational and competitive athletes, is the relatively innocuous muscle damage that is caused by activities that are predominated by eccentric muscle actions. This muscle damage causes delayed onset muscle soreness (DOMS), with the pain becoming noticeable about 12 h after the activity and the intensity of the pain peaking 24–48 h later and disappearing after 5–7 days. The symptoms of DOMS range from being subclinical with mildly tender or stiff muscles with the pain disappearing during daily activities, to severe debilitating pain that restricts movement and alters muscle function (Hume *et al.* 2004). Other symptoms of DOMS include:

- Increase in girth of the affected limb (Clarkson *et al.* 1992; Lambert *et al.* 2002);
- Shortening of muscle (increase in passive tension) (Cleak & Eston 1992; Lambert *et al.* 2002; Proske & Allen 2005);
- Decrease in strength (Byrne & Eston 2002; Clarkson *et al.* 1992; Newham *et al.* 1987);
- Leakage of intramuscular proteins into the circulation (Armstrong 1990; Clarkson & Sayers 1999); and
- Changes in muscle morphology (Friden 1984).

DOMS also has metabolic and physiological consequences which are in accordance with those symptoms that occur after a soft tissue injury. This can be demonstrated as a consequence of the inflammatory response and markers of muscle regeneration (Kuipers 1994; MacIntyre *et al.* 1995; Smith 1991). DOMS has been studied extensively in the laboratory and much of the knowledge from this basic research has resulted in an improved clinical application of the treatment and prevention of more serious soft tissue injuries. For example, the ability of muscle to adapt following damage arising from eccentric exercise allows this form of intervention to be utilized in clinical applications, with the goal of protecting a muscle against further injury (Proske & Morgan 2001).

Initial events causing DOMS

DOMS is caused by the exposure to any exercise that is sufficiently vigorous and to which the subject is not accustomed. DOMS can also be caused by low intensity exercise that consists of predominantly eccentric muscle actions. The term "eccentric" is contentious. However, in the context of this chapter (Faulkner 2003) an eccentric muscle action is one that describes a muscle lengthening under tension, in contrast to a concentric action where the muscle generates force while shortening. Simple examples of activities with predominantly eccentric muscle actions are walking/running downhill, stepping off a bench, or lowering a weight with the elbow flexors. Indeed, these types of activities are often used in experimental laboratory situations to induce DOMS for subsequent study.

There are various explanations for eccentric actions being high risk for causing DOMS. First, eccentric actions require a unique activation strategy by the nervous system and involve preferential recruitment of fast-twitch motor units (Enoka 1996). At any given submaximal workload, the electromyogram (EMG) activity, and by implication muscle fiber recruitment, is less during eccentric vs. concentric muscle action, placing a greater load on each individual muscle fiber (Armstrong 1984). A second explanation is that there is an overstretch of the sarcomeres beyond optimum length during eccentric actions (Morgan & Allen 1999). According to this theory, during an active stretch of a muscle most of the change in length will be accommodated by the weakest sarcomeres. The sarcomeres reach a critical point at which their length changes rapidly and in an uncontrolled way, resulting in no overlap between actin and myosin myofilaments. During the relaxation phase some sarcomeres return to their resting length, allowing the myofilaments to inter-digitate, while other sarcomeres do not and subse-quently become disrupted (Proske & Morgan 2001). This was described as the "popping" sarcomere theory (Morgan 1990). After repeated eccentric actions, with accumulated sarcomere disruption, the sarcolemma becomes damaged. This initiates a self-destructive series of events involving a loss of calcium homeostasis (Armstrong 1990) and an inflammatory response (MacIntyre *et al.* 1995; Smith 1991). Within hours the number of neutrophils increases at the site of the injury. Monocytes and macrophages peak at about 48 h and release prostaglandins which sensitize the nociceptors, innervated by type III and IV afferent fibers, to pres-sure and stretch. This results in a subjective increase in the perception of pain. This phase prepares the muscle cells for subsequent repair and regeneration as discussed previously.

Role of calcium

One of the consequences of exercise-associated injury is that regulation of the sarcoplasmic reticu-lum release and reuptake of calcium (Ca^{2+}) is disturbed (Belcastro *et al.* 1998; Sorichter *et al.* 1999). This results in elevated concentrations of Ca^{2+} in the cytosol which initiates a number of subsequent events. First, elevated Ca^{2+} causes a transient short-ening of the muscle fibers and an increase in their resting tension (Gregory *et al.* 2003). Secondly, elevated Ca^{2+} activates calcium-sensitive phospho-lipase A_2 which changes the permeability of the sarcolemma resulting in the leakage of intramuscu-lar enzymes (e.g., creatine kinase) (Armstrong 1990; Gissel 2005). Thirdly, elevated Ca^{2+} concentrations activate the non-lysosomal cysteine protease, calpain (Belcastro *et al.* 1998). Calpain is assumed to trigger the response of skeletal muscle protein breakdown, inflammatory changes, and regenera-tion processes (Sorichter *et al.* 1999). In particular, calpain splits a variety of protein substrates includ-

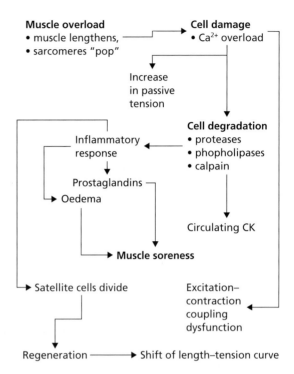

Fig. 5.1 A summary of events that occur after muscle is exposed to eccentric exercises that result in delayed onset muscle soreness. CK, creatine kinase.

ing cytoskeletal and myofibrillar proteins (Belcastro *et al.* 1998). Finally, a calcium overload causes an increased production of reactive oxygen species causing lipid peroxidation. A consequence of this is that the integrity of the muscle cell membrane may be affected. A summary of the events dis-cussed above is shown in Fig. 5.1.

Symptoms

The disruptions to the myofilaments can be seen under light and electron microscopy almost imme-diately after the exercise (Armstrong 1990). Typically, there are also signs of z-line streaming, cytoskeletal disturbances, particularly with respect to the struc-tural protein desmin, and increased lysosomal activity (Friden *et al.* 1984; Yu *et al.* 2003). The urine concentrations of hydroxyproline, an indirect index of collagen breakdown, is increased suggesting an increased breakdown of connective tissue (Brown *et al.* 1997).

PAIN

The time course of the development and disappearance of pain after exposure to the bout of exercise varies depending on the exercise protocol, number of contractions, and muscle group recruited. Peak soreness occurs about 1–3 days after exercise, depending on the type of activity.

The pain is detected by the polymodal nociceptors which can respond to chemical, thermal, and pressure stimuli (Mense 1993). The magnitude of the pain is not closely associated with the extent of the muscle damage (Newham *et al.* 1986). Studies have also shown that other markers (i.e., changes in isometric force, muscle shortening, swelling, and circulating creatine kinase [CK] activity) are not associated with the time course and magnitude of pain (Clarkson *et al.* 1992; Nosaka *et al.* 2002). The reason for this lack of association between pain and markers of muscle damage is not clear.

Pain associated with DOMS is measured either with a visual analog scale (Nosaka *et al.* 2002), a pressure probe (Semark *et al.* 1999), or by means of subjective assessment (Lambert *et al.* 2002).

CIRCULATING CREATINE KINASE ACTIVITY

Creatine kinase is an intramuscular enzyme that catalyzes the conversion of phosphocreatine to creatine, consuming adenosine diphosphate and generating adenosine triphosphate. CK appears in the blood after muscle damage. When the permeability of the cell membrane is altered, as a result of the disturbance in Ca^{2+} homeostasis following exercise-induced muscle damage, CK leaks into the interstitial fluid and enters the lymphatic system. It then filters into the blood and circulates until it is excreted. Circulating CK activities usually peak around 2 days after the exercise and slowly subside by 5–7 days (Ebbeling & Clarkson 1989). Some studies have reported a gender effect, with males having higher levels of CK after exercise than females (Kuipers 1994; Noakes 1987). However, more recent studies have failed to consistently demonstrate a gender effect (Clarkson & Hubal 2001). The theory behind the gender effect was developed based on the premise that estrogen reduced enzyme leakage

out of the cell (Kendall & Eston 2002; Kuipers 1994). It cannot be concluded that reduced leakage of CK reflects reduced muscle damage and therefore more research is required in this area (Kendall & Eston 2002).

Although CK is a general marker for muscle damage it cannot be used to quantify the extent of the damage with any degree of accuracy because of the large intersubject variability (Ebbeling & Clarkson 1989). For example, after an ultra-marathon race there was a 50-fold difference in CK activity (Noakes 1987) despite similar subjective symptoms of pain.

SWELLING

Peak swelling of muscles exposed to eccentric muscle actions occurs about 2–5 days later (Clarkson *et al.* 1992; Lambert *et al.* 2002). Muscle swelling is not associated with the sudden increase in muscle stiffness that occurs immediately after exercise. However, about 48 h thereafter there seems to be an association between swelling and muscle stiffness (Chleboun *et al.* 1998). The swelling is also associated with an increase in intramuscular pressure (Crenshaw *et al.* 1994) and a stimulation of the pressure-sensitive pain receptors.

IMPAIRMENT IN MUSCLE FUNCTION

Muscle function is impaired immediately after the exercise which causes DOMS. This is illustrated by a decrease in maximal torque or maximal voluntary contraction (eccentric, concentric, or isometric) after the exercise-induced damage (Eston *et al.* 1996; Sayers *et al.* 2003). The magnitude of the decrement varies depending on the state of training, the type of activity, muscle group, and speed of movement (Byrne *et al.* 2004). To be able to understand the sites that may be affected and contribute to the muscle dysfunction it is necessary to summarize the events leading to muscle contraction. The signal initiating the recruitment of a muscle originates in the motor center and is promulgated by an action potential which travels along the spinal cord to the peripheral nerve. At the neuromuscular junction the signal passes on to the sarcolemma and then penetrates the muscle via the T tubules to the sarcoplasmic reticulum. Ca^{2+} is released from the sarcoplasmic reticulum and binds to troponin C causing a conformational change which initiates the binding of actin and myosin. Muscle relaxation occurs after Ca^{2+} is pumped back into the sarcoplasmic reticulum (Morgan & Allen 1999). This summary of events illustrates that there are potentially many causes of muscle dysfunction after exercise-induced muscle damage.

During the first 2 days after the exercise the main causes of the muscle dysfunction can be attributed to alteration of the excitation–contraction coupling system (Martin *et al.* 2004), with damage to the force-generating structures accounting for the dysfunction thereafter. There are data to show that the following factors may partially, or in combination, reduce the ability of muscle to function (Morgan & Allen 1999):
• Changes in the central nervous system, motor nerve, or neuromuscular junction;
• Unexcitable muscle cells, presumably resulting from gross cellular damage;
• Failure or reduction of Ca^{2+} release;
• Changes in the Ca^{2+} sensitivity of the contractile machinery; and
• Disorganization of the contractile machinery.
Coupled to the reduced ability of the muscle to produce force is an alteration in proprioception and motor control as a consequence of the altered sensory input to the muscle (Gregory *et al.* 2003).

While most symptoms of muscle damage disappear within about 7 days, there are signs of altered neuromuscular function that last longer, even in the absence of pain (Chambers *et al.* 1998; Deschenes *et al.* 2000).

Metabolic consequences

When a person exercises with DOMS they experience symptoms that are indicative of a higher exercise stress. This can be demonstrated by a significantly higher minute volume, breathing frequency, respiratory exchange ratio, heart rate, rating of perceived exertion, venous blood lactate concentration, and plasma cortisol concentration (Gleeson *et al.* 1995). The higher blood lactate concentration during submaximal exercise may be caused by an increased rate of glycogenolysis (Asp *et al.* 1998; Gleeson *et al.* 1998), possibly arising from an increased recruitment of type II muscle fibers after the damage, or alternatively because of the leaky muscle cell membrane (Gleeson *et al.* 1998). The increased rate of glycogen utilization in the muscle is associated with decreased endurance (Asp *et al.* 1998).

Muscle glycogen concentrations are lower in both type I and II fibers for at least 10 days after the bout of exercise that causes DOMS (O'Reilly *et al.* 1987). A subsequent experiment showed that a diet high in carbohydrate during the recovery phase after exercise-induced muscle damage was not able to replenish glycogen stores more rapidly (Zehnder *et al.* 2004), possibly because of the lower concentration of the protein transporter, GLUT-4, which occurs after muscle damage (Asp *et al.* 1996). The metabolic profile during this phase is similar to that of a mild insulin-resistant condition (Sherman *et al.* 1992).

Prevention of DOMS

Studies have addressed the question of which strategy works best in preventing muscle damage. One study which used a combination of a warm-up, stretching, and massage prior to the exposure to a protocol that induced muscle damage, failed to find a consistent positive effect with any combination of treatments (Rodenburg *et al.* 1994). Another study showed that massage 2 h before a bout of eccentric exercise reduced the symptoms of pain and circulating CK (Smith *et al.* 1994). In this study the infiltration of the neutrophils into the damaged muscle was also reduced in the subjects who received the massage intervention. A recent review paper concludes that while there is general support for massage treatment alleviating the symptoms of pain, there is no convincing evidence to support the use of massage as a preventive strategy (Moraska 2005).

A study has shown that subjects with less passive stiffness (as measured by hamstring flexibility) before a bout of exercise have fewer symptoms of muscle damage after exercise (McHugh *et al.* 1999b). In contrast, the subjects with less flexible muscles experienced more pain after the same bout of exercise. In support of this finding it was shown that yoga training and a single bout of yoga (stretching) reduced the symptoms of soreness after a bout of eccentric exercise (Boyle *et al.* 2004). Based on these studies (Boyle *et al.* 2004; McHugh *et al.* 1999b), there is evidence to support the role of stretching as a prophylactic strategy to prevent the symptoms of DOMS. McHugh *et al.* (1999b) suggested that this finding supports the "popping" sarcomere theory of muscle damage (Morgan 1990) which was described earlier.

EXERCISE TRAINING

There is overwhelming consensus that exercise training is the most effective way to protect against muscle damage (Balnave & Thompson 1993; Brockett *et al.* 2001; Clarkson *et al.* 1992; Ebbeling & Clarkson 1989; McHugh 2003; McHugh *et al.* 1999a; Nosaka *et al.* 2001; Proske & Morgan 2001; Sayers & Dannecker 2004). One of the first studies to highlight this concept exposed eight subjects to exercise that caused muscle damage (Newham *et al.* 1987). After 2 weeks the subjects were re-exposed to the exercise and then they repeated the bout of exercise 2 weeks later. Circulating CK was extremely high after the first bout, less after the second bout, and did not change after the third bout of exercise. Muscle strength decreased after each bout of exercise by 50%, but recovered quicker after each subsequent exercise exposure. Subsequent studies have shown that a single exposure of eccentric exercise stimulates an adaptive response that causes changes in the muscle. These changes provide protection against subsequent exercise-induced damage for at least 6 months (Clarkson *et al.* 1992; Nosaka *et al.* 1991, 2001). This phenomenon is called the "repeat-bout" effect (Clarkson *et al.* 1987). Protection against eccentric damage can occur after as few as six repetitions at low intensity (50% maximum voluntary contraction; Sayers & Dannecker 2004). Many scientists have studied this process in an attempt to explain this adaptation. A summary of the studies are explained in an excellent review paper (McHugh 2003). This paper describes that there is no single explanation for this adaptation but instead the mechanism can be classified as neural, mechanical, or cellular (McHugh 2003).

A summary of studies on the repeat-bout effect suggests that the effectiveness of protection seems to be greater the closer the second bout of exercise was repeated after the initial bout. Furthermore, repeated exercise before the muscle has fully recovered does not worsen the damage or delay the rate of recovery (Hume *et al.* 2004).

Treatment

From a clinical perspective there is obviously an interest in reducing the symptoms of DOMS in athletes. Hundreds of studies have examined the effects of numerous treatments including pharmaceutical agents, herbal remedies, stretching, massage, and nutritional supplements. Many of the studies have yielded different results. This can be attributed to the different research designs, including different exercise protocols, severity of symptoms, and training status of the subjects. Comprehensive reviews have been written on the different treatments in an attempt to summarize these studies and guide clinical management (Cheung *et al.* 2003; Connolly *et al.* 2003; Hume *et al.* 2004).

It is concluded from a comprehensive review of the literature that the following are important practical considerations in reducing the symptoms of DOMS (Hume *et al.* 2004):
• Moderate exercise effectively reduces the symptoms of pain; however, the alleviation is transient;
• Non-steroidal anti-inflammatory drugs (NSAIDs) have a dosage-dependent effect on pain and the effects may be influenced by the timing of administration; and
• Athletes with symptoms of DOMS should be encouraged to reduce both the intensity and duration of exercise for 1–2 days following the initial exercise bout that caused DOMS.

A summary of the various treatments, based on a review of the literature, are shown in the Table 5.1.

Exercise-associated muscle cramping

Skeletal muscle cramping is one of the most common clinical problems encountered by medical staff attending to athletes at endurance events including marathons. The lifetime prevalence of skeletal

Table 5.1 A summary of the treatment methods (*n* = 163 studies) for decreasing the perception of pain associated with delayed onset muscle soreness (DOMS). Hume *et al.* (2004).

Treatment	Limited success*	Moderate success	Some benefits	Little success
Exercise			✓	
NSAIDs	✓			
Compression		✓		
Hot packs		✓		
Ultrasound				✓
Electrical current techniques				✓
Massage	✓			
Stretching				✓
Homeopathy				✓
Cryotherapy				✓
Hyperbaric oxygen therapy				✓
Magnetic exposure		✓†		

NSAIDs, non-steroidal anti-inflammatory drugs.
* Depends on type and timing of treatment.
† Further research is needed.

muscle cramping in marathon runners and triathletes has been reported to be as high as 30–50% and 67%, respectively (Kantorowski *et al.* 1990). The etiology, diagnosis, and management of this condition are not well understood. Muscle cramping can occur in a variety of medical conditions (Miller & Layzer 2005; Parisi *et al.* 2003) but most of these conditions are rare. Most athletes who experience muscle cramps during exercise do not have underlying congenital or acquired medical conditions that cause cramping (Table 5.2).

Definitions and terminology

It is difficult to define muscle "cramping" but it has been suggested that a cramp is a "spasmodic painful involuntary contraction of a muscle" (Layzer 1981). For the purposes of this chapter the definition can be modified to exclude cramps occurring in smooth muscle as well as skeletal muscle cramping that may occur at rest. Exercise-associated muscle cramping (EAMC) is therefore defined as a "painful spasmodic involuntary contraction of skeletal muscle that occurs during or immediately after muscular exercise" (Schwellnus *et al.* 1997).

Pathophysiology and etiology of exercise-associated muscle cramping

The interest in cramps associated with physical exercise was first documented more than 100 years ago by reports of workers who had muscle cramping while performing physical work in hot, humid environments. In these early studies, the proposed pathophysiology for EAMC was a systemic disturbance of fluid and electrolyte balance. These early observations have led to "serum electrolyte" and "dehydration" theories being used to explain EAMC. Although these theories are still accepted by some clinicians (Bergeron 2003), more recent evidence indicates that there is a lack of scientific support for these older theories (Jung *et al.* 2005; Schwellnus *et al.* 2004; Sulzer *et al.* 2005). A critical analysis of: (i) factors associated with EAMC that have been identified from epidemiological studies, (ii) observations from animal experimentation on spinal reflex activity during muscle fatigue, and (iii) recent EMG data obtained during EAMC (Sulzer *et al.* 2005) have led to the development of a novel hypothesis for the etiology of EAMC (Schwellnus *et al.* 1997).

Table 5.2 A novel classification of muscle cramps (Parisi *et al.* 2003).

Paraphysiological cramps
Occasional cramps
Cramps during sporting activity
Cramps during pregnancy

Idiopathic cramps
Familial
Autosomal dominant cramping disease
Familial nocturnal cramps
Continuous muscle fiber activity syndrome

Sporadic
Continuous muscle fiber activity syndrome (Isaacs'
    syndrome, stiff man syndrome, cramp fasciculation
    syndrome, myokymia cramp syndrome)
Syndrome of progressive muscle spasm, alopecia, and
    diarrhea (Satoyoshi's syndrome)
Idiopathic nocturnal cramps
Idiopathic generalized myokymia
Myokymia hyperhidrosis syndrome

Others
Familial insulin resistance with acanthocytosis nigricans
    and acral hypertrophy, muscle cramps in cancer
    patients

Symptomatic cramps
Central and peripheral nervous system diseases
Motoneuron disease
Occupational dystonias
Parkinson's disease
Tetanus
Multiple sclerosis
Radiculopathies
Plexopathies
Peripheral neuropathies (inherited, endocrine–metabolic,
    infectious, toxic, inflammatory demyelinizing)
Others, rare (neurolathyrism, familial paroxysmal
    dystonic choreoathetosis)

Muscular diseases
Metabolic myopathy (deficiency of myophosphorylase,
    phosphofructokinase, phosphoglucomutase,
    phosphoglycerokinase, lactate dehydrogenase,
    adenylate deaminase, glucose-6 phosphate
    dehydrogenase, phosphorylase b-kinase)

Mitochondrial myopathy (carnitine deficiency, carnitine
    palmitoyltransferase 1 and 2 deficiency)
Endocrine myopathy (e.g., Hoffman's syndrome)
Dystrophinopathies (Duchenne, Becker, others)
Myotonia (Thomsen, Becker, rippling syndrome)
Inflammatory myopathies (myositis, myopathy with
    tubular aggregates, rheumatic polymyalgia)
Others, rare (Lambert–Brody disease, Schwartz–Jampel
    syndrome, eosinophilia–myalgia syndrome, type 2
    muscle fiber myopathy)

Cardiovascular diseases
Venous diseases
Arterial diseases
Heart diseases
Hypertension

Endocrine–metabolic disease
Hypo-hyperthyroidism
Hypo-hyperparathyroidism
Cirrhosis
Isolated deficiency of adrenocorticotropic hormone
    accompanied by generalized painful muscle cramp
Bartter's syndrome
Gitelman's syndrome
Conn's disease
Addison's disease
Uremia and dialysis

Hydro-electrolyte disorders
Dehydration with or without electrolytes imbalance
    (e.g., diarrhea, vomiting)
Hypo-hypernatremia
Hypo-hypercalcemia
Hypo-hyperkalemia
Hypomagnesemia
Heat cramps

Toxic and pharmacological causes
Drugs
Pesticides
Black widow bite
Toxic oil syndrome
Malignant hypertermia

Psychiatric disorders

In accordance with this hypothesis, EAMC may result from an abnormality of sustained alpha motor neuron activity, which in turn may be brought about by altered alpha motor neuron control at the spinal level. These alterations of motor neuron control may occur as a result of muscle fatigue. Furthermore, there is evidence to suggest that mus-cle fatigue is also associated with the lack of neural regulation through an imbalance of an excitatory effect on the muscle spindle afferent activity (type Ia and II) and an inhibitory effect on the type Ib Golgi tendon organ afferent activity (Hutton & Nelson 1986; Nelson & Hutton 1985). Thus, muscle fatigue is the central factor in the development of EAMC

(Schwellnus 1999; Schwellnus *et al.* 1997). Contraction of the muscle in its shortest position (inner range) may also be a factor precipitating a muscle cramp. This is probably caused by decreased inhibition of type Ib afferents from the Golgi tendon organ causing impaired muscle relaxation and subsequent cramp (Schwellnus 1999; Schwellnus *et al.* 1997)

Risk factors for EAMC

In an epidemiological study of over 1300 marathon runners, certain risk factors for EAMC were identified (Manjra *et al.* 1996):
- Older age;
- Longer history of running (running years);
- Higher body mass index;
- Shorter daily stretching time;
- Irregular stretching habits; and
- Positive family history of cramping.

In addition, runners identified specific conditions that were associated with EAMC:
- High-intensity running (racing);
- Long duration of running bouts (most cramps occur after 30 km in a standard marathon);
- Subjective muscle fatigue;
- Hill running; and
- Poor race performance.

The two most important observations from these data are first, that EAMC is associated with running conditions that can lead to premature muscle fatigue and, secondly, that poor stretching habits appear to increase the risk for EAMC. In addition, it is well documented that the muscles most prone to cramping are those that span across two joints. These are also the muscles that are often contracted in a shortened position during exercise.

Clinical presentation of EAMC

HISTORY

A typical clinical history of an athlete with EAMC will include the following:
- Pain in the muscle that usually develops gradually over a few minutes during intense or prolonged exercise;
- Cramping is preceded by twitching of the muscle ("cramp prone state") followed by spasmodic spontaneous contractions and frank muscle cramping if activity is continued;
- Onset of EAMC is usually preceded by skeletal muscle fatigue;
- Relief from the "cramp prone state" occurs if the activity is stopped or if the muscle is stretched passively (temporary relief only); and
- Episodes of cramping can be precipitated by contraction of the muscle in a shortened position (inner range).

PHYSICAL SIGNS

The clinical examination of an athlete with localized (confined to one or two muscle groups) acute EAMC reveals the following signs:
- Obvious distress and pain;
- A hard contracted muscle; and
- Visible fasciculation over the muscle belly.

In most instances, the athlete is conscious, responds normally to stimuli, and is able to conduct a conversation. Vital signs and a general examination usually reveal no abnormalities. In particular, most athletes with acute EAMC are not dehydrated or hyperthermic.

The athlete who has generalized severe cramping (i.e., symptoms in non-exercising muscle groups) or is also confused, semi-comatose, or comatose must be treated as a clinical emergency. This patient does have EAMC as a result of fatigued muscle but a systemic disorder may be the cause, and this patient usually requires hospitalization in an intensive care unit for further evaluation.

SPECIAL INVESTIGATIONS IN THE ATHLETE WITH EAMC

In most instances, no special investigations are required. The athlete with severe generalized cramping or associated central nervous system symptoms requires tests to exclude: (i) disturbances of serum electrolyte concentrations; (ii) acute renal failure; (iii) metabolic myopathy; and (iv) intracranial pathology.

Management of acute EAMC

The immediate treatment for acute EAMC is as follows:
• Admission to the medical care facility at the sports event;
• Passive stretching of the affected muscle group(s);
• Maintaining a stretch on the affected muscle until fasciculation ceases;
• General supportive treatment by keeping the patient at a comfortable temperature and providing oral fluids if required; and
• Intravenous diazepam has been used to treat severe forms of cramping, but this is not recommended as it can lead to altered consciousness and respiratory depression.

All patients with acute EAMC should be informed that should they: (i) not pass any urine, or (ii) pass very dark urine in the first 24 h, they should seek medical help immediately. All patients with recurrent acute EAMC should be investigated fully to exclude medical conditions as listed in Table 5.2.

Prevention of EAMC

The key to the prevention of acute EAMC is to protect the muscle from developing premature fatigue during exercise. Athletes should be advised to:
• Be well conditioned for the activity;
• Perform regular stretching of the muscle groups that are prone to cramping;
• Have adequate nutritional intake (carbohydrate and fluid) to prevent premature muscle fatigue during exercise; and
• Perform their activity at a lower intensity and a shorter duration if they are prone to EAMC.

Etiology of chronic exercise-associated fatigue and underperformance

Chronic fatigue and underperformance pose a difficult diagnostic challenge for the sports physician. While a degree of fatigue may be normal for any athlete during periods of intense training, the clinician must be able to differentiate between this appropriate or physiological fatigue, and more prolonged severe fatigue which may be brought about by a pathological condition. Fatigue is a subjective symptom and therefore it is difficult to quantify by means of a good history and physical examination, but with the help of a few well-directed special investigations the practitioner can exclude common underlying reversible causes of persistent fatigue.

Discerning the etiology of fatigue

The causes of fatigue fit into one of two major groups: physiological or pathological.

PHYSIOLOGICAL FATIGUE

Fatigue arising from training may be referred to as physiological fatigue and is described by symptoms of tiredness and underperformance. This is appropriate for the athlete's level of training. Indeed, athletes commonly use the process of overload, or gradually increased workload, as a stimulus for adaptation. During this process, overreaching or an imbalance between exercise and recovery might occur which could lead to symptoms of tiredness and fatigue (Nederhof et al. 2008).

Training overload or overreaching are terms describing the process of undergoing training at loads that are greater than the training load to which the athlete is accustomed (Halson & Jeukendrup 2004; Nederhof et al. 2008). This can be achieved by altering training intensity, frequency and duration, or by reducing the recovery period between training sessions. Physiological fatigue may arise from this form of training. A characteristic of this form of fatigue is that it is reversed by a reduction in training load (Foster 1998).

Monitoring of the athlete's psychological and physiological state during training and competition using subjective and objective tools has proven to be particularly useful (Hooper et al. 1999; Lambert & Borresen 2006). The implementation of a monitoring program can usually alert the clinician prior to the athlete developing serious symptoms of fatigue which may have profound long-term consequences.

Dietary causes of fatigue and underperformance

There are a number of dietary causes of fatigue and tiredness, including undereating, particularly in sports where "making weight" is important. First, it is important that sufficient quantities of carbohydrate are ingested. Skeletal muscle glycogen resynthesis is impaired for up to 10 days following exercise that causes muscle damage (O'Reilly *et al.* 1987). Indeed, it appears that ingestion of carbohydrate, skeletal muscle damage, and symptoms of overtraining are related (Scharf & Barr 1988). Secondly, it is generally accepted that insufficient protein and fluid ingestion has been associated with fatigue in athletes. The role of amino acids, vitamins, micronutrients including magnesium and zinc, and antioxidants in the prevention and treatment of the symptoms of fatigue are currently under study (see Chapter 20).

Endurance athletes are particularly susceptible to depletion of the body iron stores. While the precise mechanism of the reduced iron stores is not known, it is believed that increased iron loss or insufficient dietary intake or absorption can lead to reduced iron stores. This can be diagnosed by measuring blood ferritin concentrations. Reduced ferritin stores can cause the athlete to experience symptoms including fatigue and underperformance without altering the serum iron or hemoglobin concentrations (Garza *et al.* 1997). Thus, ferritin and serum transferrin receptor concentrations should be measured regularly in endurance athletes. While no "normal values" for the athlete population exist, we recommend that symptomatic female athletes embark on iron supplementation programs if their ferritin concentrations are below $40\,\mu g \cdot L^{-1}$. Male athletes should consider iron supplementation if their ferritin concentrations are below $60\,\mu g \cdot L^{-1}$.

Other causes of "physiological fatigue" include inadequate quality and quantity of sleep, international travel across time zones, and pregnancy (Waterhouse *et al.* 2007).

PATHOLOGICAL FATIGUE

Pathological fatigue is defined as fatigue and tiredness that cannot be attributed to physiological causes and is inappropriate for the quantity and intensity of training that the athlete is presently undertaking. Pathological causes of fatigue are outlined in Table 5.3. These causes include unresolved infection, neoplasia, and pathology of the hematological, cardiorespiratory, neuromuscular, or endocrine systems. It is important to note that common allergies including chronic rhinitis, conjunctivitis, or allergy-induced asthma may have a profound effect on the performance of the athlete (Komarow & Postolache 2005). Indeed, the incidence of atopy in the elite athletic populations is far greater than in the general population but prevention and management is relatively simple (Hawarden *et al.* 2002). Psychological or psychiatric disorders including depression, excessive anxiety related to sporting performance or other problems, bulimia, and anorexia nervosa could also present as chronic fatigue in the athlete.

Commonly prescribed medications have the potential to cause chronic fatigue in athletes. These medications include β-adrenergic blockers, other anti-hypertensive agents, drugs acting on the central nervous system, antibiotics, antihistamines, and lipid-lowering agents (Derman *et al.* 1992).

Useful laboratory and other tests to assist in the clinical diagnosis of the athlete with persistent fatigue are presented in the following section of this chapter. Some of the common causes of profound and persistent fatigue warrant further discussion.

Overtraining syndrome

The overtraining syndrome refers to a symptom complex characterized by maladaptation to training, decreased physical performance, and chronic fatigue following high volume and/or high intensity training and inadequate recovery. The overtraining syndrome requires weeks or months of rest or greatly reduced training for complete recovery. Decreased physical performance together with chronic fatigue have been two criteria used most commonly to diagnose the overtraining syndrome. A full discussion of the overtraining syndrome can be found in Chapter 3.

Table 5.3 Common etiology of persistent fatigue in the athlete.

Physiological fatigue (appropriate or training-induced fatigue)
Overreaching
Nutritional
Insufficient sleep
Jet-lag

Pathological fatigue
Medical conditions
Chronic infective conditions: viral, bacterial or paracytic (e.g., hepatitus, infectious mononucleosis, HIV, malaria, tuberculosis, brucellosis)
Hematologic conditions (e.g., iron deficiency anemia)
Neoplastic conditions
Cardiorespiratory conditions (e.g., coronary artery disease, cardiac failure, bacterial endocarditis, asthma, exercise-induced asthma)
Neurogenic–neuromuscular (e.g., post-concussive syndromes, multiple sclerosis, myasthenia, myotonia, paramyotonia)
Endocrine metabolic conditions (e.g., diabetes, hypothyroid, hyperthyroid Addison's disease, Simmond's disease, hyperparathyroid, hypophosphatemia, kalemic periodic paralases, Cushing's syndrome, hypogonadism)
Psychiatric/psychological conditions (e.g., anxiety, depression, psychoneuroses, eating disorders)
Drug-induced (e.g., beta-blockers, other antihypertensive agents, agents acting on the central nervous system, antihistamines, lipid-lowering agents, alcohol, antibiotic agents)
Other (e.g., malabsorption syndromes, allergic conditions, spondyloarthropathies)

Overtraining syndrome
Chronic fatigue syndrome
"Acquired training intolerance"

Chronic fatigue syndrome

The chronic fatigue syndrome is a debilitating illness for both the athlete and the general population. While the etiology, pathophysiology, and management of the condition remain unclear, it is apparent that this disorder is quite different from the usual chronic fatigue and underperformance syndrome and overtraining syndrome experienced by the athletic population (Shephard 2005). In fact, the label of chronic fatigue syndrome is often misused. Criteria for the diagnosis of the chronic fatigue syndrome include (Fukuda *et al.* 1994):

• Clinically evaluated, unexplained persistent or relapsing chronic fatigue that is of new or definite onset (i.e., not lifelong), is not the result of ongoing exertion, is not substantially alleviated by rest, and results in a profound reduction in previous levels of occupational, educational, social, or personal activities.

• The concurrent occurrence of four or more of the following symptoms: substantial impairment in short-term memory or concentration; sore throat; tender lymph nodes; muscle pain; multi-joint pain without swelling or redness; headaches of a new type, pattern, or severity; unrefreshing sleep; and post-exertional malaise lasting more than 24 h. These symptoms must have persisted or recurred during 6 or more consecutive months of illness and must not have predated the fatigue.

Suggested causes of the chronic fatigue syndrome include (Shephard 2005):

• Chronic infection secondary to immunosuppression (seen with overtraining); primary infection;

• Allergic or autoimmune reaction with secondary changes in immune function;

• A reaction to physical or emotional stressors;

• A consequence of nutritional deficits;

• Hormonal disturbance secondary to physical or emotional stress;

• A primary or secondary personality disorder with subsequent anxiety and depression; and

• Autonomic dysfunction secondary to either stressors or physical deconditioning.

Indeed, there are some similarities between the chronic fatigue syndrome and the athletic overtraining syndrome but there are also important differences, in particular the absence of skeletal muscle damage (Urhausen & Kindermann 2002).

Our experience is that while these diagnostic criteria may be appropriate for the general population, very few fatigued athletes fulfill the above criteria. The clinical picture of the chronic fatigue syndrome is also one that can mimic diseases of insidious onset including cancer, tuberculosis, depression, and AIDS. It is always a concern that when making the diagnosis of chronic fatigue syndrome, serious but potentially curable diseases are not overlooked.

Acquired training intolerance

Derman *et al.* (1997) described a group of athletes presenting with exercise-associated fatigue and intolerance to exercise that was accompanied by abnormalities within their skeletal muscles. Historically, this condition has been called fatigued athlete myopathic syndrome (FAMS) and, more recently, acquired training intolerance (ATI) (Grobler *et al.* 2004), because it was agreed that the athletes did not necessarily share a common myopathy or set of myopathies but rather an intolerance to exercise. The athletes with ATI have in common a history of a high training volume and a current inability to tolerate former levels of endurance exercise. They experience a sudden and unexplained decline in performance, often associated with a reduced training volume, both of which are more severe than the decrease that would be expected to accompany the aging process. Medical examination reveals that these athletes are free from physiological fatigue conditions, such as training, diet, travel, or pregnancy-induced fatigue and pathological fatigue conditions, including those listed in Table 5.3. In most cases, the athletes with ATI report general skeletal muscle symptoms including excessive DOMS, muscle stiffness, tenderness, and skeletal muscle cramps. Furthermore, these individuals have usually consulted many physicians, and do not respond to long periods of rest, nutritional or psychological support (Derman *et al.* 1997; Grobler *et al.* 2004).

Biopsies of the vastus lateralis muscles of these athletes showed a greater degree of structural alteration, including fiber size variation, internal nuclei, z-disc streaming, and more lipid and glycogen droplets than healthy, age-matched control athletes (Grobler *et al.* 2004). Endurance training and racing is known to induce such changes in the skeletal muscle of apparently healthy runners and mild levels of structural alteration are thought to be functional adaptations (Sjöström *et al.* 1988), reflective of the continuous state of degeneration and regeneration occurring within the muscle in response to the stimulus of running (Kuipers *et al.* 1989). The greater degree of structural alteration observed in the skeletal muscle of the athletes with ATI, however, may have been an abnormal response. In addition to the structural alterations, these athletes also had significantly shorter skeletal muscle telomeres than asymptomatic athletes (Collins *et al.* 2003). Collins *et al.* (2003) interpreted this as meaning that the muscle of individuals with ATI had undergone more cycles of damage and repair than the age and mileage-matched healthy controls. Alternatively, the shortened telomeres may reflect excessive oxidative damage to the DNA of the skeletal muscle. This too is plausible, as studies have shown that oxidative stress increases as a result of distance running in moderately trained individuals (Dufaux *et al.* 1997). Recent investigation of athletes with ATI has revealed a link with markers of clinical depression in these athletes (St. Clair Gibson *et al.* 2006). The effects of multifactorial interventions including nutritional and psychological intervention (reverse therapy) in these athletes are the topic of ongoing interest and research.

In summary, chronic fatigue and underperformance in the athlete is a complex issue which can involve the muscles, the immune system, the brain, the diet, and the psyche. Occasionally, the management of chronic fatigue and underperformance is easily achieved if an exact diagnosis can be made and the condition appropriately treated. Yet, in most cases, the management of the athlete with chronic fatigue is more complex and involves a sports physician, coach, dietitian, and sports psychologist working together as a coordinated multidisciplinary team. Many of the popular pharmacological treatments for chronic fatigue, including serotonin reuptake inhibitors, tricyclic antidepressants, and high-dose antioxidant supplementation, are still experimental. Only through a comprehensive understanding of the mechanisms underlying this complex topic can appropriate treatments and preventative measures be implemented.

Metabolic myopathies

Metabolic myopathies in the athletic population are uncommon. While most metabolic myopathies would cause profound exercise intolerance that would usually not allow the athlete to perform at the elite level, some partial enzyme defects might indeed still allow some degree of athletic performance (Martin *et al.* 1994). This group of disorders can be differentiated into the disorders of carbohydrate metabolism and disorders of lipid metabolism. The various specific enzyme defects for carbohydrate and lipid metabolism, the age of presentation, clinical features, useful diagnostic tests, as well as management strategies are presented in Tables 5.4 and 5.5. Only the metabolic myopathies that are more common in physically active individuals will be discussed further. These disorders include McArdle's disease, phosphofructokinase (PFK) deficiency, carnitine palmitoyl transferase (CPT) deficiency, myoadenylate deaminase deficiency, and the mitochondrial myopathies (Tarnopolsky 2006; Tarnopolsky & Raha 2005).

Carbohydrate metabolism disorders: McArdle's disease and PFK deficiency

This group of disorders includes the absence or inactivity of enzyme proteins involved in glycolysis and glycogenolysis. While the consequences of glycogen phosphorylase deficiency (McArdle's disease) and PFK deficiency are understood, relatively little is known about the other forms of carbohydrate metabolism enzymatic defects (Martin *et al.* 1994).

CLINICAL PRESENTATION

The clinical features of these conditions include exercise intolerance which usually presents in early adulthood, accompanying skeletal muscle pain, swelling, cramps, fatigue, and rhabdomyolysis during high intensity exercise (Martin *et al.* 1994). These clinical features are caused by the unavailability of muscle glycogen as a fuel and thus energy sources during high intensity exercise are restricted to phosphocreatine and ATP stored within the skeletal muscle. In both PFK deficiency and McArdle's disease there is an inability to use glycogen as a metabolic fuel. Glucose oxidation by muscle is blocked in PFK deficiency but not in McArdle's disease. Individuals with these conditions who attempt to perform high intensity exercise present with muscle cramps that are electrically silent. Failure of blood lactate concentrations to increase following ischemic exercise is a hallmark feature of these conditions (Haller *et al.* 2006; Sahlin *et al.* 1995).

As skeletal muscle glycogen is an important fuel for strenuous submaximal exercise, patients with these disorders also show reduced submaximal exercise capacity. However, after a period of rest or reduced intensity, exercise at the same or higher intensity can sometimes be resumed without incurring premature fatigue or other symptoms. This is known as the "second wind" phenomenon and is attributed to increased delivery of blood-borne free fatty acids to the working muscle (Braakhekke *et al.* 1986).

Cardiac output during exercise in patients with McArdle's disease and PFK deficiency is typically 200–300% greater than controls yet $\dot{V}o_{2peak}$ is 35–50% lower than control values because of low O_2 extraction. Although increases in ammonia production have been associated with the fatigue associated with both McArdle's and PFK deficiency, the exact cause of the fatigue is unclear (Wagenmakers *et al.* 1990). The reduced force production of subjects with these disorders can be attributed to the metabolic factors that result in impaired skeletal muscle activation (Haller *et al.* 1985).

Disorders of fat metabolism: CPT deficiency

The genetic defect in this disorder results in deficient concentrations of the enzyme CPT. This enzyme is normally responsible for the movement

Table 5.4 Clinical features and age of presentation of the disorders of skeletal muscle metabolism.

Disorders of muscle metabolism	Age of presentation	Clinical features
Carbohydrate metabolism disorders		
Non-lysosomal glycogenoses		
Glycogenosis type VIII Phosphorylase *b* kinase deficiency	Young children, infants	Ex intol, cramps, myalgia, muscle weakness, myoglobinuria
Glycogenosis type V (McArdle's) Myophosphorylase deficiency	85% before 15 years	Ex intol (intense isometric or sustained dynamic exercise), cramps, myalgia, muscle weakness, myoglobinuria, muscle swelling
Glycogenosis type VII Phosphofructokinase deficiency	Infants–adults	Ex intol, cramps, myalgia, myoglobinuria, muscle weakness
Gycogenosis type XII Aldolase A deficiency	Children	Myopathic symptoms, anemia, jaundice, rhabdomyolysis
Glycogenosis type III Debrancher deficiency	Children–adults	Child: hepatomegaly and liver dysfunction, FTT, hypoglycemia, Adult: ex intol
Glycogenosis type IV Branching enzyme deficiency	Children	Liver failure and FTT, hepatomegaly, hypotonia, muscle weakness, cardiomyopathy
Glycogenosis type IX Phosphoglycerate kinase deficiency	Children	CNS dysfunction, seizures, mental retardation, myopathy, ex intol, cramps, myoglobinuria
Glycogenosis type XI Lactate dehydrogenase deficiency	Children	Fatigue, ex intol, myoglobinuria
Phosphoglycerate mutase deficiency	Children–adolescents	Ex intol, muscle cramps, myalgia, myoglobinuria after activity
Lysosomal glycogenosis		
Glycogenosis type II Acid maltase deficiency	Infant–adults	Infantile: muscle weakness, cardiomegaly Adult: progressive weakness, respiratory failure
Lipid metabolism disorders		
Carnitine deficiency syndromes		
Primary muscle carnitine deficiency		Progressive proximal muscle weakness, ex intol, myalgia, myoglobinuria
Primary systemic carnitine deficiency with hepatic encephalopathy	Infants	Reye's syndrome encephalopathy, hepatomegaly, hyperketotic hypoglycemia
Primary systemic carnitine deficiency with cardiomyopathy	Infants	Cardiomyopathy
Secondary carnitine deficiency		
Fatty acid transport defects		
Carnitine: acylcarnitine translocase and CPT I defects	Infants	Progressive cardiomyopathy, hypoketotic hypoglycemia, ventricular arrythmia
CPT II deficiency	15–50 years	Myalgia, cramps, muscle stiffness, tenderness, fatigue following prolonged exertion >30 min, weakness, myoglobinuria
Defects of beta oxidation enzymes		Cardiomyopathy

CNS, central nervous system; CPT, carnitine palmitoyl transferase; ex intol, exercise intolerance; FTT, failure to thrive.

Table 5.5 Useful diagnostic tests and management strategies in the disorders of skeletal muscle metabolism.

Disorders of muscle metabolism	Useful diagnostic tests	Management
Carbohydrate metabolism disorders		
Non-lysosomal glycogenoses		
Glycogenosis type VIII Phosphorylase *b* kinase deficiency	s-[CK], FILT, muscle biopsy and immunohistochem, det PBK activity	No specific treatment available
Glycogenosis type V (McArdle's) Myophosphorylase deficiency	s-[CK], FILT, muscle biopsy and immunohistochem staining phosphorylase, P31-NMR spectroscopy, EMG	? High protein diet
Glycogenosis type VII Phosphofructokinase deficiency	s-[CK], FILT, FBC (reticulocytes), [uric-a], muscle biopsy and immunohistochem staining	Nil specific, ketogenic diet
Gycogenosis type XII Aldolase A deficiency	s-[CK], FBC (reticulocytes), hemoglobinuria, myoglobinuria	Nil specific
Glycogenosis type III Debrancher deficiency	s-[CK], FILT, muscle biopsy and immunohistochem, EMG	Infants: glucose infusions, high protein diet
Glycogenosis type IV Branching enzyme deficiency	s-[CK], ECG, muscle biopsy, skin fibroblasts	Liver transplantation
Glycogenosis type IX Phosphoglycerate kinase deficiency	s-[CK], muscle biopsy	Nil specific
Glycogenosis type XI Lactate dehydrogenase deficiency	s-[CK], FILT, [LDH] (reduced in muscle and RBC)	Nil specific
Phosphoglycerate mutase deficiency	s-[CK], muscle biopsy	Nil specific
Lysosomal glycogenosis		
Glycogenosis type II Acid maltase deficiency	s-[CK], FILT (normal), EMG, ECG, muscle biopsy, urine leukocytes	High protein, low CHO diet, ?gene therapy
Lipid metabolism disorders		
Carnitine deficiency syndromes		
Primary muscle carnitine deficiency	[Carnitine] determination in muscle and plasma low, normal liver and cardiac [carnitine], muscle biopsy	Oral: L-carnitine
Primary systemic carnitine deficiency with hepatic encephalopathy	Free [carnitine] reduced in plasma but [esterified carnitine] proportionately reduced as well	Oral: L-carnitine
Primary systemic carnitine deficiency with cardiomyopathy	[Carnitine] in muscle, heart, liver, and plasma is low, lipid storage on muscle biopsy	Oral: L-carnitine
Secondary carnitine deficiency		
Fatty acid transport defects		
Carnitine: acylcarnitine translocase and CPT I defects	Serum [carnitine] is normal or increased, with a high free : total ratio	Nil specific
CPT II deficiency Defects of beta oxidation enzymes	s-[CK] following exercise, [TG] & [Chol], muscle biopsy, FILT, cultured fibroblast and blood assay	High CHO, low fat, low protein diet

CHO, carbohydrate; [Chol], cholesterol concentration; CPT, carnitine palmitoyl transferase; det, determination; ECG, electrocardiography; EMG, electromyography; FBC, full blood count; FILT, forearm ischemic lactate test; [LDH], lactate dehydrogenase concentration; P31-NMR, phosphorus-31 nuclear magnetic resonance spectroscopy; PBK, phosphorylase *b* kinase; RBC, red blood cell; s-[CK], serum creatine kinase concentration; [TG], triglyceride concentration; [uric-a], uric acid concentration.

of long-chain fatty acids, across the inner mitochondrial membrane where they are oxidized to CO_2 and H_2O. Thus, this enzyme defect would result in deficient fatty acid oxidation (Zierz 1994).

Symptoms are usually reported in early adulthood and include skeletal muscle pain, muscle tenderness, muscle swelling, and myoglobinuria. This occurs when exercise is attempted at an intensity that would normally require free fatty acids to be oxidized as a fuel source (Zierz 1994). While muscle strength, $\dot{V}o_{2peak}$, and short duration, high intensity exercise are usually normal (as carbohydrates are mostly used as fuels), longer forms of exercise at lower intensity usually provokes fatigue (Bertocci et al. 1991; Haller 1994). This is exacerbated by an overnight fast or a low carbohydrate diet, because of depletion of muscle glycogen stores. High respiratory exchange ratios at rest and during submaximal exercise are typical (Carroll et al. 1979).

Myoadenlyate deaminase deficiency

Myoadenylate deaminase (AMPD) deficiency is present in 1–2% of the population. AMPD catalyzes the first three reactions of the purine nucleotide cycle resulting in AMP deamination to inosine monophosphate and ammonia. Patients with this condition would possibly have a reduced capacity to buffer ADP accumulation and therefore might be more prone to fatigue. Approximately 50% of patients with AMPD deficiency report exercise intolerance, myalgia, and skeletal muscle cramps. Typically, graded exercise to exhaustion and total work produced during cycling is reduced in these patients; however, high intensity, short duration exercise capacity is unaffected (Fishbein 1985).

Mitochondrial myopathies

Dysfunction of the mitochondria in the body tissues is termed mitochondrial cytopathy, but if the pathology is restricted to muscle the term mitochondrial myopathy is used. There are a number of recognized disorders that bear the acronyms of the condition including MELAS, NARP, LHON, according to which genetic mutations are identified. While the presenting features of these disorders might be a result of consequences of other tissue involvement including heart or brain, exercise intolerance resulting from muscle mitochondrial defects is common (Tarnopolsky & Raha 2005). These defects typically cause profound exercise intolerance; however, milder mutations have been noted in athletes (Taivassalo & Haller 2005). The hallmark clinical features of this group of disorders include very low $\dot{V}o_{2peak}$ because of poor oxygen extraction, a hyperdynamic circulation, and a high respiratory exchange ration (RER) relative to workload (Taivassalo et al. 2003; Tarnopolsky & Raha 2005). Investigation of the athlete would include exercise testing, skeletal muscle biopsy, muscle enzymology, magnetic resonance spectroscopy, and genetic evaluation. Various treatments including coenzyme Q10, creatine monohydrate, uridine prodrugs, dichloroacetate, and various combination cocktails have been attempted with varying success (Tarnopolsky & Raha 2005).

It is important to note that myopathies may also be acquired. Infection and pharmacological agents have been noted to induce myopathy in athletically inclined individuals (Sewright et al. 2007).

Exertional rhabdomyolysis

Extreme levels of exertion that stress muscle causing large increases in serum enzymes, rhabdomyolysis, myoglobinuria, and acute renal failure can be life-threatening (Lott & Landesman 1984). While training provides some degree of resistance to rhabdomyolysis, a mild form of exertional rhabdomyolysis is common. Severe pathological rhabdomyolysis is fortunately uncommon (Knochel 1990).

During rhabdomyolysis, the integrity of the muscle cell membrane is compromised, so that the contents of the cell leak into the plasma within a 24-h period after the event (Warren et al. 2002). Biochemical findings in cases of acute rhabdomyolysis can include the presence of the haem pigment in the urine, elevation of serum CK or aldolase concentrations, hyperkalemia, hypocalcemia, hyperphosphatemia, hyperuricemia, a high creatinine :

BUN ratio, hypoalbuminuria, and even markers of disseminated intravascular coagulation (Knochel 1990). Excessive release of myoglobin from muscle cells is filtered in the kidney and excreted into the urine. This leads to a potentially high risk of acute renal failure because the passage of myoglobin through the kidney may be directly toxic to the renal tubule (Bank 1977).

Clinical causes or precipitators of rhabdomyolysis include infection, metabolic disorders (diabetes, hypokalemia, hyponatremia, hypophosphatemia and hypothyroidism), heat-related syndromes, inflammatory and metabolic myopathies, and medications listed in Table 5.6.

The clinical features of rhabdomyolysis include acute muscle pain, swollen tender muscles, limb weakness, and contractures. This clinical picture may involve specific groups of muscles such as the calves and lower back or may be more generalized. However, a significant proportion of athletes who have rhabdomyolysis may not show any signs of muscle injury. In some instances hemorrhagic discoloration of the overlying skin may be visible. Systemic symptoms might include fever, tachycardia, nausea, vomiting, leukocytosis, myoglobinuria, and clinical features of acute renal failure (Warren *et al.* 2002).

Elevated CK activity is the most sensitive plasma indicator of rhabdomyolysis. Should this enzyme be elevated more than five times above the normal post-exercise concentration (in the absence of cerebral or myocardial infarction), skeletal muscle rhabdomyolysis is likely (Warren *et al.* 2002).

Skeletal muscle is vulnerable to minor levels of damage as induced by acute bouts of exercise through to extreme disruption that can cause potentially life-threatening exertional rhabdomyolysis. Fortunately, this is rare as this organ is well equipped to recover from and adapt to these insults. Typically, the muscle disorder is self-limiting and resolves within days to weeks, because of the good regenerative capacity of muscle.

Clinical investigation of the athlete with muscle symptomatology

Myopathic symptoms in the athlete include skeletal muscle pain, weakness, fatigue, fasiculations, red urine, and skeletal muscle cramps. This section of the chapter focuses specifically on two of these symptoms and provides an approach to investigation of the athlete with chronic fatigue and chronic muscle pain.

Table 5.6 Common medications that can affect skeletal muscle and induce skeletal muscle pain.

Drugs that can cause skeletal muscle pain and weakness
Amphotericin B, chloroquine, clofibrate, ciprofloxacin, colchicine, cyclosporine, certain diuretics, emetine, ε-aminocaproic acid, glucocorticoids, labetalol, niacin, perhexilline, propranolol, statin drugs, antibiotic–statin interactions, vincristine, zidovudine

Drugs that can cause elevated serum creatinine kinase with/without weakness
Clofibrate, statin drugs

Drugs that can cause skeletal muscle inflammation
Cimetidine, penicillamine, procainamide

Drugs that can cause rhabdomyolysis and myoglobinuria
Alcohol, amphetamine, barbiturates, clofibrate, cocaine, ε-aminocaproic acid, gemfibrozil, heroin, lovastatin, phencyclidine

Drugs that can cause myotonia
Propranolol, cyclosporine, iodides, clofibrate, penicillamine

Drugs that can cause focal myopathy
Pentazocine, meperidine, heroin

Evaluation of the athlete with chronic fatigue

All athletes and most exercising individuals have experienced fatigue at some point in their exercise history. Indeed, muscle cramps, pain, and a feeling of fatigue are expected consequences of unaccustomed exercise or activities. With repeated activities, the body usually adapts to the training, and these symptoms abate and performance gains are expected. However, in some athletes the symptoms of fatigue can persist and may lead to training intolerance and chronic underperformance.

Chronic fatigue and underperformance could also potentially be brought about by other pathologies as discussed previously, thus the diagnosis and management of athletes with these symptoms remains difficult. To address this challenge, we have designed a clinical diagnostic evaluation algorithm for athletes presenting with chronic fatigue and underperformance. The outline of the evaluation as used in the Sports Medicine Division of the Sports Science Institute of South Africa is shown in Fig. 5.2. This approach includes a minimum of two visits before the etiology of chronic fatigue and underperformance can be established (Derman *et al*. 1997). However, it is more likely that the athlete with chronic fatigue will have to consult with many members of the multidisciplinary team and visit the clinic and exercise laboratory on a number of occasions before a diagnosis is made.

VISIT 1

The athlete's first visit to our clinic is perhaps the most important. At this consultation, a detailed history is taken and a thorough physical examination is performed by a sports physician. It is preferable that the athlete is accompanied to the consultation by his/her coach and/or exercise physiologist if possible, as this facilitates the collection of accurate training and rest information. It also creates a supportive environment for the athlete.

History

Amongst the standard medical history that is taken, it is noteworthy to determine the following:

- The duration and severity of the fatigue;
- Whether the onset of the fatigue was marked by a particular event (infection or overseas travel);
- If the fatigue is constant or intermittent;
- The extent of impairment of exercise performance or activities of daily living; and
- If the fatigue is associated with particular environmental conditions (venue or climate).

Furthermore, it is important to assess the athlete's quantity and quality of sleep and determine if the athlete is presently ingesting any medications or nutritional supplements. Further enquiry is directed to determine if the athlete has any of the classic symptoms of the overtraining syndrome or if the athlete has any systemic symptoms indicative of abnormalities of the cardiorespiratory, gastrointestinal, neuromuscular, endocrine, ear nose and throat (ENT), or urogenital systems. In the female athlete, a menstrual history should be taken to exclude either pregnancy or possible anemia from excessive blood loss resulting from heavy menstrual bleeding.

With the help of the coach and/or exercise physiologist, it is important to determine the current stage of the athlete's training cycle and what the athlete's intended future training program entails. The volume, intensity, frequency of training, as well as the quantity and quality of rest between training sessions and competitions should be established. If the athlete keeps a log book, the weekly training volumes over the previous few months should be determined and any large changes to the athlete's program should be noted.

The athlete is asked to recall all food eaten during a typical 24-h period and the athlete's attitudes and practices with respect to nutrition and fluid intake before, during, and after competition are determined. This brief screening procedure is performed only to alert the clinician to possible eating disorders and insufficient or incorrect nutritional practices. If these are suspected, the athlete is referred to a dietitian for a more detailed dietary analysis.

Psychological causes possibly contributing to the athlete's fatigue should be determined. Administration of the Profile of Mood States (POMS) Questionnaire might prove to be useful. In young athletes, the "HEADS" questions, which are designed to

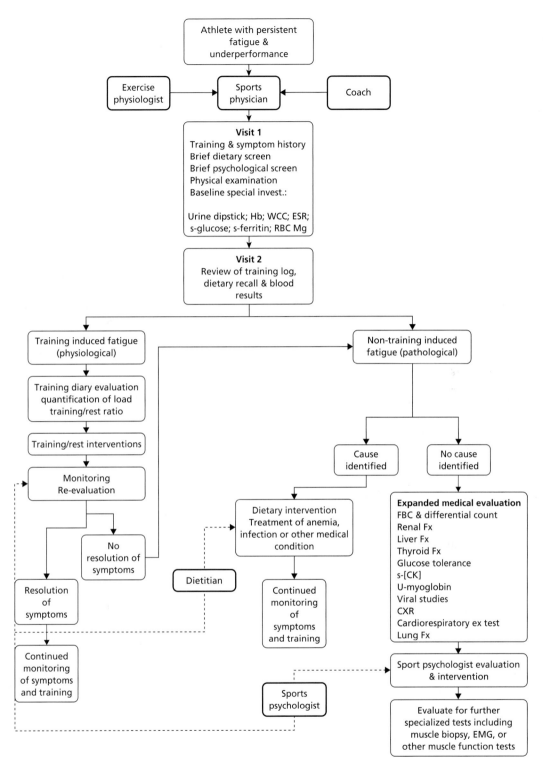

Fig. 5.2 Clinical diagnostic evaluation algorithm for the athlete presenting with persistent fatigue and underperformance as used at the Sports Science Institute of South Africa. CXR, chest X-ray; EMG, electromyogram; ESR, erythrocyte sedimentation rate; ex, exercise; FBC, full blood count; Fx, functions; Hb, hemoglobin; Invest, investigations; s-[CK], serum creatine kinase concentration; s-ferritin, serum ferritin concentration; s-glucose, serum glucose concentration; RBC Mg, red blood cell magnesium concentration; U, urine; WCC, white cell count.

determine stress from Home, Education, Activities, Alcohol, Drugs, Depression, Sex and Sport may be particularly useful to indicate problem areas that would necessitate referral to a sport psychologist (Dyment 1993).

Physical examination

A general medical examination to exclude signs of jaundice, anemia, edema, and lymphadenopathy should be performed, followed by a detailed medical examination of the cardiorespiratory, gastrointestinal, neuromuscular, and ENT systems. The athlete's temperature, resting heart rate, and blood pressure are measured and noted.

Special investigations

While the history and physical examination are the most important components of the first visit to enable the clinician to establish a diagnosis, it is helpful to conduct a number of baseline special investigations, the results of which could indicate specific pathology. At the first visit, we suggest that the athlete's hemoglobin concentration, white cell count, erythrocyte sedimentation rate, red blood cell magnesium, and random blood glucose concentrations are measured. Serum ferritin concentrations are measured particularly in female athletes. A urine dipstick test is performed to exclude renal abnormalities and determine hydration status by measurement of urine osmolality.

The athlete is then provided with a training diary and asked to complete this daily for the following 2–3 week period. During this time, the baseline blood test results are reviewed. It is essential that the athlete continues with his/her normal pattern of training during this time so that the symptomatology can be reviewed.

VISIT 2

At this visit, the completed training diary and results of the baseline tests are reviewed with the athlete and support team. The clinician should, at this stage, be able to distinguish between physiological and pathological fatigue.

If the clinician suspects that the fatigue and underperformance is physiological in origin, the appropriate management is employed and may include training/rest interventions, further specialized determination and manipulation of training/rest ratios, and, if indicated, dietary and psychological support. Ongoing reassessment and monitoring of the athlete by the multidisciplinary team is essential.

Further special investigations should be conducted if: (i) the athlete does not respond to rest, dietary or psychological intervention; (ii) the cause of the chronic fatigue is not directly apparent; or (iii) there are abnormalities of the baseline investigations. These expanded investigations could include a full blood and differential count, serum electrolyte determination (including sodium, potassium, magnesium, and chloride), liver function tests, thyroid function tests, viral serology studies, serum creatinine kinase concentration, and a glucose tolerance test. A chest X-ray, lung function tests, and a cardiorespiratory exercise test could also be conducted if the athlete has signs and symptoms of cardiorespiratory disease as indicated by the results of the initial clinical examination.

VISIT 3

The results of these tests are reviewed at visit 3, and the clinician should now be in a position to: (i) exclude medical conditions that could cause fatigue; (ii) review the criteria and possibly exclude the chronic fatigue syndrome; or (iii) make the diagnosis of the overtraining syndrome and institute a monitoring program as discussed previously.

The role of the dietitian in the management of eating disorders, anemia, chronic infection, and other medical conditions is of specific importance, as is the role of the sport psychologist in specialized evaluation and management of anxiety and depressive-related disorders. If metabolic or other myopathies are considered, the clinician could, at this stage of the evaluation, arrange for further specialized tests of skeletal muscle structure and function to be conducted. These tests might include EMG, muscle biopsy, or P31-NMR spectroscopy and will be discussed in more detail in the following section of this chapter.

While evaluation (and management) of the athlete with physiological or pathological fatigue might appear to be relatively simple in terms of this diagnostic algorithm, chronic fatigue and underperformance in the athlete still remain one of the more difficult challenges in clinical sports medicine. It is important that reversible causes of fatigue and underperformance should systematically be excluded. Thus, the investigation and management of these difficult cases hinges on the participation of a multidisciplinary team. The athlete, coach, dietitian, exercise physiologist, and sport psychologist all play an important part in enabling the physician to make the correct diagnosis and institute appropriate management.

Evaluation of the athlete with chronic skeletal muscle pain

Skeletal muscle pain is a troublesome symptom for both athletes and the general population alike. While some transient muscle pain can be expected following unaccustomed exercise, prolonged or excessive muscle pain can indeed indicate underlying pathology. Muscle pain during and after exercise can also be as a result of excessive forces involved in repetitive contraction leading to muscle strains and tears. However, other pathophysiological processes including compartment syndromes, arterial occlusive disease, and disorders of skeletal muscle metabolism might also cause the symptom of skeletal muscle pain.

The diagnostic algorithm detailing the investigation of the athlete presenting with muscle pain as used at the Sports Science Institute of South Africa is shown in Fig. 5.3. The investigation of the athlete begins with a thorough history and physical examination followed by selected initial special investigations.

HISTORY

The location, duration, frequency, and intensity of the muscle pain and its relationship to the physical activity should be ascertained. Muscle pain is most commonly related to overuse, or muscle injury resulting from exercise. In these situations, the pain tends to involve the specific muscles involved and starts during or just after the activity. Aggravating and relieving factors should be determined.

The patient should be carefully questioned regarding other symptoms that could indicate myopathy. These include the presence of muscle weakness, fatigue, exercise-related skeletal muscle cramps, and myoglobinuria. The onset of these symptoms and their relationship to the exercise bout should be determined. If these symptoms occur shortly after the start of exercise, a disorder of carbohydrate metabolism should be considered; if the symptoms occur only during prolonged duration exercise, the abnormalities of lipid metabolism should be considered. The patient should be questioned to determine the presence of a warm-up phenomenon (McArdle's disease).

If skeletal muscle pain occurs at rest and is unrelated to exercise, other causes including thyroid disease, viral or other infection, fibromyalgia, diabetes, rheumatic conditions, dermatomyositis, polymyositis, circulatory disorders, depression, organ failure, acute alcohol, or drug-induced myopathy should be excluded.

The past medical history, family history (particularly as many of the metabolic myopathies are hereditary), and history of medication use is obtained. Some of the more common medications that can cause (and other) effects on skeletal muscle are listed in Table 5.6.

PHYSICAL EXAMINATION

A complete general and specific systemic examination of the patient should be undertaken. The focus is specifically aimed at the neurological and musculoskeletal systems. In particular, the various groups of muscles should be palpated for tenderness to determine which muscle groups are involved. Tests of resisted contraction should be undertaken to determine if muscle weakness is present. Muscle weakness is often in the proximal muscles, and is generally symmetrical in patients with metabolic myopathy. Patients with mitochondrial myopathy can present with mild proximal weakness, but more often present with prominent eye muscle involvement and ptosis.

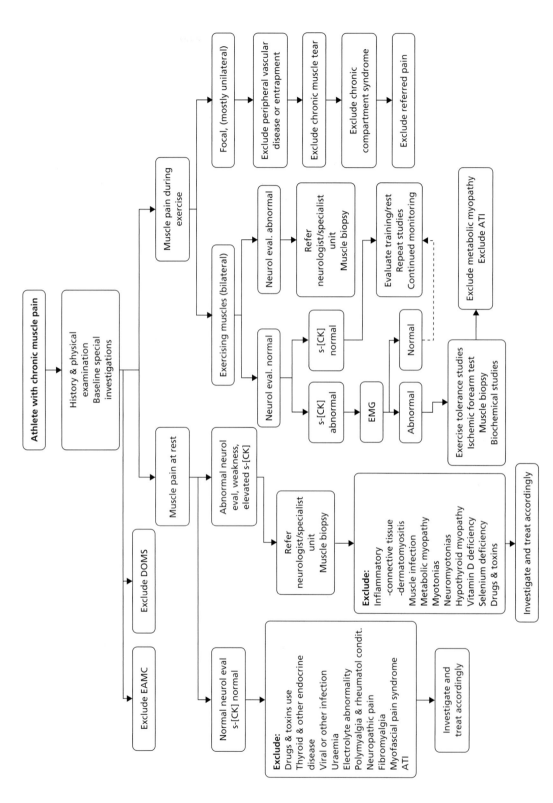

Fig. 5.3 Clinical diagnostic evaluation algorithm for the athlete presenting with chronic muscle pain as used at the Sports Science Institute of South Africa. ATI, acquired training intolerance; DOMS, delayed onset muscle soreness; neurol, neurological; EAMC, exercise-associated muscle cramps; EMG, electromyogram; eval, evaluation rheumatol condit, rheumatological conditions; s-[CK], serum creatine kinase concentration.

Other physical features to note include myotonia, which can be found in patients with hyperkalemic periodic paralysis. Edema is seen in about one-third of patients with hypothyroid myopathy while muscle hypertrophy may be seen in patients with hypothyroid myopathy. Exertional contracture of the skeletal muscle is characteristic of defective carbohydrate metabolism. Delayed reflexes can occur in both hypothyroid myopathy and periodic paralysis.

SPECIAL INVESTIGATIONS

The following baseline special investigations investigations are performed on all patients: full blood count, fasting blood glucose, serum [CK], [urea], creatinine and electrolytes, thyroid function test, and erythrocyte sedimentation rate. A urine dipstick test is also performed on all patients.

Evaluation of the heart (including stress electrocardiogram [ECG] and echocardiogram) and liver functions may be assessed in patients with suspected lipid storage myopathy; and respiratory function tests may be evaluated in patients with suspected maltase deficiency.

Based on the findings from the history and physical examination alone, the clinician can exclude DOMS and EAMC. Should the muscle pain occur at rest, further evaluation of the athlete is based on the findings of the neurological and musculoskeletal assessment as well as the results of the resting CK concentration.

Should the athlete have an abnormal neurological evaluation (including weakness) and have and elevated resting CK concentration, the athlete should be referred to a specialist neurologist or academic neurology unit for further specialized tests to detect myopathy and other conditions listed in Fig. 5.3.

If both the neurological evaluation and resting CK concentration are normal, drugs and toxins (Table 5.6) and other disease entities listed in Fig. 5.3 should be investigated and treated accordingly. The clinician should be aware that acquired training intolerance might present with muscle pain at rest, yet neurological evaluation and CK concentrations are typically within the normal range.

In the athlete who presents with muscle pain during exercise, the clinician should differentiate if this originates from a specific focal area or from the exercising skeletal muscles in general. Should the pain during exercise originate from the bilateral exercising muscles and the neurological evaluation or CK concentrations be abnormal, the athlete should be referred to a specialist neurologist for further tests including a skeletal muscle biopsy. Should the neurological evaluation be unremarkable with either an abnormal or indeed normal CK concentration, further special investigations including exercise tolerance studies, forearm ischemic lactate test, muscle biopsy, and biochemical studies (described below) should be conducted to exclude metabolic myopathy. ATI should be considered in this group of athletes.

Should the skeletal muscle pain during exercise be focal or unilateral in location, a chronic muscle tear, chronic compartment syndrome, and vascular entrapment should be considered. Each of these conditions has a more specific clinical picture.

SKELETAL MUSCLE STRAINS OR TEARS

Skeletal muscle strains or tears occur if excessive loading is placed on the muscle tissue during exercise, resulting in microscopic (strain) or macroscopic tears of the fibers. These injuries usually have an acute onset during an exercise bout which may cause the athlete to stop the exercise activity. Pain on palpation, discoloration of the area, and increased discomfort on resisted contraction of the affected muscle are the clinical hallmark features of the injury. Diagnosis is confirmed by ultrasound evaluation or magnetic resonance imaging (MRI) scan. Management is best achieved by rest, ice, compression, and elevation followed by early physiotherapy intervention and, finally, rehabilitation.

CHRONIC COMPARTMENT SYNDROME

Although the exact etiology of chronic compartment syndrome is unknown, the skeletal muscle becomes too large for its fascial sheath causing muscle pain during and after exercise, tight hard muscles on palpation following exercise, and neuromuscular symptoms including parasthesia distal to the affected compartment. The diagnosis is usually made by monitoring the compartment pressure during provoking exercise and surgical fasciotomy is the most effective form of management. Although the muscle compartments of the lower limb are most commonly affected, this condition may occur in the upper limb, hands, and feet.

ARTERIAL OCCLUSIVE DISEASE

Occlusion of blood flow to the skeletal muscle by atherosclerotic plaque, fibrous bands of connective tissue, or impingement by the muscle bellies themselves might cause pain in the skeletal muscle during exercise. Typically, pain occurs early during exercise and is relieved rapidly following the exercise bout. Peripheral pulses may or may not be palpable during the discomfort. Diagnosis is made using color duplex flow Doppler evaluation and angiography if necessary, and intervention is usually via balloon angioplasty or surgery.

Finally, it is important for the clinician to note that proximal or distal pathology might refer pain to the affected skeletal muscle. Therefore, it would be beneficial to examine the joints both above and below the sight of the muscle pain.

FURTHER USEFUL SPECIAL INVESTIGATIONS

Further invstgations are considered when a secondary metabolic myopathy is suspected. These might include studies for endocrine disorders, periodic paralysis, or drug-induced myopathy.

NERVE CONDUCTION STUDIES AND ELECTROMYOGRAPHY

Nerve conduction studies and nerve stimulation tests might be useful special investigations. Motor and sensory nerve conduction studies are usually normal in the metabolic myopathies, unless there is coexisting neuropathy, as is seen in mitochondrial, drug-induced, and endocrine myopathies. Electromyography can be performed to differentiate between electrically active or electrically silent abnormal motor unit function.

EXERCISE TESTING

Exercise challenge tests are usually performed using a protocol that would challenge the patient with respect to the metabolic pathway where the enzymatic defect would occur. Various parameters, including the cardiorespiratory and metabolic response to the exercise challenge, should be determined. This could include collection of expired gases for determination of $\dot{V}o_{2peak}$ and the RER. The RER provides an indication of fuel use during exercise. Values range from 0.7 at rest to 1.1 at peak exercise, reflecting increased oxidation of carbohydrate relative to lipid during exercise of increasing intensity. Heart rate and blood pressure responses to graded exercise should be measured and cardiac output can also be readily measured by rebreathing techniques.

FOREARM ISCHEMIC EXERCISE TEST

This is a relatively simple screening test to determine the presence of some of the metabolic abnormalities of skeletal muscle (DiMauro & Tsujino 1994). After cannulation of a forearm vein, a blood pressure cuff is pumped up above systolic pressure and the patient performs repetitive handgrip contraction–relaxation cycles for a minimum period of 1–2 min or until contracture occurs. Following release of the circulatory occlusion, blood is collected 1, 3, 5, 10 and 15 min following exercise, the serum is then analyzed to determine lactate and ammonia concentrations. In normal individuals, both lactate and ammonia concentrations increase four- to eightfold and return to baseline 10–15 min following exercise. Increased ammonia without increased lactate concentrations are consistent with glycogen storage disorders including McArdle's syndrome. Myoadenylate deaminase deficiency should be considered if lactate concentrations increase but ammonia concentrations remain the same. If there is no increase in either parameter a poor patient effort must be considered.

NEAR-INFRARED AND PHOSPHORUS MAGNETIC RESONANCE SPECTROSCOPY

These are useful, non-invasive methods of determination of skeletal muscle function and fuel usage during dynamic contraction. Near-infrared spectroscopy uses measurement of oxygenation of blood hemoglobin and skeletal muscle myoglobin to estimate the $a-vO_2$ difference. Phosphorus magnetic resonance spectroscopy measures the concentration of high energy phosphates, inorganic phosphate, and pH in exercising muscle, therefore patterns typical of mitochondrial abnormalities, disorders of glycogenolysis, and muscular dystrophies can be discerned. These techniques are mostly available in specialized units.

SKELETAL MUSCLE BIOPSY

A skeletal muscle biopsy is an important investigation in the patient with suspected myopathy. This can be performed using either an open or needle biopsy technique and the specimen should be flash-frozen immediately after biopsy for best results. The structural and ultrastructural features of the skeletal muscle, as well as enzymatic staining, should be investigated. Skeletal muscle biopsies of patients with metabolic myopathies often show storage of glycogen or triglycerides or excessive accumulation of mitochondria (ragged red fibers) but the muscle can look normal. Changes suggestive of denervation including fiber grouping and angulated atrophic fibers can sometimes be seen in metabolic myopathies. Histochemical evaluation of the skeletal muscle biopsy can allow specific diagnoses or provide evidence of a metabolic myopathy. Myophosphorylase, phosphofructokinase or myoadenylate deaminase deficiency can be diagnosed using specific histochemical techniques.

References

Armstrong, R.B. (1984) Mechanisms of exercise-induced delayed onset muscular soreness: a brief review. *Medicine and Science in Sports and Exercise* **16**, 529–538.

Armstrong, R.B. (1990) Initial events in exercise-induced muscular injury. *Medicine and Science in Sports and Exercise* **22**, 429–435.

Asp, S., Daugaard, J.R., Kristiansen, S., Kiens, B. & Richter, E.A. (1996) Eccentric exercise decreases maximal insulin action in humans: muscle and systemic effects. *Journal of Physiology* **494**, 891–898.

Asp, S., Daugaard, J.R., Kristiansen, S., Kiens, B. & Richter, E.A. (1998) Exercise metabolism in human skeletal muscle exposed to prior eccentric exercise. *Journal of Physiology* **509**, 305–313.

Balnave, C.D. & Thompson, M.W. (1993) Effect of training on eccentric exercise-induced muscle damage. *Journal of Applied Physiology* **75**, 1545–1551.

Bank, W.J. (1977) Myoglobinuria in marathon runners: possible relationship to carbohydrate and lipid metabolism. *Annals of the New York Academy of Sciences* **301**, 942–948.

Belcastro, A.N., Shewchuk, L.D. & Raj, D.A. (1998) Exercise-induced muscle injury: a calpain hypothesis. *Molecular and Cellular Biochemistry* **179**, 135–145.

Bergeron, M.F. (2003) Heat cramps: fluid and electrolyte challenges during tennis in the heat. *Journal of Science and Medicine in Sport* **6**, 19–27.

Bertocci, L.A., Haller, R.G., Lewis, S.F., Fleckenstein, J.L. & Nunnally, R.L. (1991) Abnormal high-energy phosphate metabolism in human muscle phosphofructokinase deficiency. *Journal of Applied Physiology* **70**, 1201–1207.

Bischoff, R. (1994) The satellite cell and muscle regeneration. In: *Myology*, 2nd edn. (Engel, A.G. & Franzini-Armstrong, C., eds.) McGraw-Hill, New York: 97–118.

Boyle, C.A., Sayers, S.P., Jensen, B.E., Headley, S.A. & Manos, T.M. (2004) The effects of yoga training and a single bout of yoga on delayed onset muscle soreness in the lower extremity. *Journal of Strength and Conditioning Research* **18**, 723–729.

Braakhekke, J.P., de Bruin, M.I., Stegeman, D.F., Wevers, R.A., Binkhorst, R.A. & Joosten, E.M. (1986) The second wind phenomenon in McArdle's disease. *Brain* **109**, 1087–1101.

Brockett, C.L., Morgan, D.L. & Proske, U. (2001) Human hamstring muscles adapt to eccentric exercise by changing optimum length. *Medicine and Science in Sports and Exercise* **33**, 783–790.

Brooks, S.V. (2003) Current topics for teaching skeletal muscle physiology. *Advances in Physiology Education* **27**, 171–182.

Brown, S.J., Child, R.B., Day, S.H. & Donnelly, A.E. (1997) Indices of skeletal muscle damage and connective tissue breakdown following eccentric muscle contractions. *European Journal of Applied Physiology and Occupational Physiology* **75**, 369–374.

Byrne, C. & Eston, R. (2002) The effect of exercise-induced muscle damage on isometric and dynamic knee extensor strength and vertical jump performance. *Journal of Sports Sciences* **20**, 417–425.

Byrne, C., Twist, C. & Eston, R. (2004) Neuromuscular function after exercise-induced muscle damage: theoretical and applied implications. *Sports Medicine* **34**, 49–69.

Campisi, J. (1997) The biology of replicative senescence. *European Journal of Cancer* **13**, 703–709.

Carroll, J.E., DeVivo, D.C., Brooke, M.H., Planer, G.J. & Hagberg, J.H. (1979) Fasting as a provocative test in neuromuscular diseases. *Metabolism* **28**, 683–687.

Chambers, C., Noakes, T.D., Lambert, E.V. & Lambert, M.I. (1998) Time course of recovery of vertical jump height and heart rate versus running speed after a 90-km foot race. *Journal of Sports Sciences* **16**, 645–651.

Chargé, S.B. & Rudnicki, M.A. (2004) Cellular and molecular regulation of muscle regeneration. *Physiology Reviews* **84**, 209–238.

Cheung, K., Hume, P. & Maxwell, L. (2003) Delayed onset muscle soreness: treatment strategies and performance factors. *Sports Medicine* **33**, 145–164.

Chleboun, G.S., Howell, J.N., Conatser, R.R. & Giesey, J.J. (1998) Relationship between muscle swelling and stiffness after eccentric exercise. *Medicine and Science in Sports and Exercise* **30**, 529–535.

Clarkson, P.M., Byrnes, W.C., Gillisson, E. & Harper, E. (1987) Adaptation to exercise-induced muscle damage. *Clinical Science* **73**, 383–386.

Clarkson, P.M. & Hubal, M.J. (2001) Are women less susceptible to exercise-induced muscle damage? *Current Opinion in Clinical Nutrition and Metabolic Care* **4**, 527–531.

Clarkson, P.M., Nosaka, K. & Braun, B. (1992) Muscle function after exercise-induced muscle damage and rapid adaptation. *Medicine and Science in Sports* **24**, 512–520.

Clarkson, P.M. & Sayers, S.P. (1999) Etiology of exercise-induced muscle damage. *Canadian Journal of Applied Physiology* **24**, 234–248.

Cleak, M.J. & Eston, R.G. (1992) Delayed onset muscle soreness: mechanisms and management. *Journal of Sports Sciences* **10**, 325–341.

Collins, M., Renault, V., Derman, E.W., Butler-Browne, G.S. & Mouly, V. (2003) Athletes with exercise-associated fatigue have abnormally short muscle DNA telomeres. *Medicine and Science in Sports and Exercise* **35**, 1524–1528.

Connolly, D.A., Sayers, S.P. & McHugh, M.P. (2003) Treatment and prevention of delayed onset muscle soreness. *Journal of Strength and Conditioning Research* **17**, 197–208.

Crenshaw, A.G., Thornell, L.E. & Friden, J. (1994) Intramuscular pressure, torque and swelling for the exercise-induced sore vastus lateralis muscle. *Acta Physiologica Scandinavica* **152**, 265–277.

Decary, S., Ben Hamida, C., Mouly, V., Barbet, J., Hentati, F. & Butler-Browne, G. (2000) Shorter telomeres in dystrophic muscle consistent with extensive regeneration in young children. *Neuromuscular Disorders* **10**, 113–120.

Decary, S., Mouly, V., Ben Hamida, C., Sautet, A., Barbet, J. & Butler-Browne, G. (1997) Replicative potential and telomere length in human skeletal muscle: implications for satellite cell-mediated gene therapy. *Human Gene Therapy* **8**, 1429–1438.

Derman, W., Schwellnus, M., Lambert, M., Emms, M., Sinclair-Smith, C., Kirby, P., *et al.* (1997) The "worn-out athlete": A clinical approach to chronic fatigue in athletes. *Journal of Sports Sciences* **15**, 341–351.

Derman, W.E., Sims, R. & Noakes, T.D. (1992) The effects of antihypertensive medications on the physiological response to maximal exercise testing. *Journal of Cardiovascular Pharmacology* **19** (Suppl. 5), S122–S127.

Deschenes, M.R., Brewer, R.E., Bush, J.A., McCoy, R.W., Volek, J.S. & Kraemer, W.J. (2000) Neuromuscular disturbance outlasts other symptoms of exercise-induced muscle damage. *Journal of the Neurological Sciences* **174**, 92–99.

DiMauro, S. & Tsujino, S. (1994) Nonlysosomal glycogenoses. In: *Myology* (Engel, A. & Banker, B., eds.) McGraw-Hill, New York: 1554–1576.

Dufaux, B., Heine, O., Kothe, A., Prinz, U. & Rost, R. (1997) Blood glutathione status following distance running. *International Journal of Sports Medicine* **18**, 89–93.

Dyment P.G. (1993) Frustrated by chronic fatigue? Try this systematic approach. *Physician and Sportsmedicine* **21**, 47–54.

Ebbeling, C.B. & Clarkson, P.M. (1989) Exercise-induced muscle damage and adaptation. *Sports Medicine* **7**, 207–334.

Enoka, R.M. (1996) Eccentric contractions require unique activation strategies by the nervous system. *Journal of Applied Physiology* **81**, 2339–2346.

Eston, R.G., Finney, S., Baker, S. & Baltzopoulos, V. (1996) Muscle tenderness and peak torque changes after downhill running following a prior bout of isokinetic eccentric exercise. *Journal of Sports Sciences* **14**, 291–299.

Faulkner, J.A. (2003) Terminology for contractions of muscles during shortening, while isometric, and during lengthening. *Journal of Applied Physiology* **95**, 455–459.

Fishbein, W.N. (1985) Myoadenylate deaminase deficiency: inherited and acquired forms. *Biochemical Medicine* **33**, 158–169.

Flück, M. & Hoppeler, H. (2003) Molecular basis of skeletal muscle plasticity: from gene to form and function. *Reviews of Physiology, Biochemistry and Pharmocology* **146**, 159–216.

Foster, C. (1998) Monitoring training in athletes with reference to overtraining sydrome. *Medicine and Science in Sports and Exercise* **30**, 1164–1168.

Friden, J. (1984) Muscle soreness after exercise: implications of morphological changes. *International Journal of Sports Medicine* **5**, 57–66.

Friden, J., Kjorell, U. & Thornell, L.E. (1984) Delayed muscle soreness and cytoskeletal alterations: an immunocytological study in man. *International Journal of Sports Medicine* **5**, 15–18.

Fridén, J. & Lieber, R. (1992) Structural and mechanical basis of exercise-induced muscle injury. *Medicine and Science in Sports and Exercise* **24**, 521–530.

Fukuda, K., Straus, S.E., Hickie, I., Sharpe, M.C., Dobbins, J.G. & Komaroff, A. (1994) The chronic fatigue syndrome: a comprehensive approach to its definition and study. International Chronic Fatigue Syndrome Study Group. *Annals of Internal Medicine* **121**, 953–959.

Garza, D., Shrier, I., Kohl, H.W. III, Ford, P., Brown, M. & Matheson, G.O. (1997) The clinical value of serum ferritin tests in endurance athletes. *Clinical Journal of Sports Medicine* **7**, 46–53.

Gissel, H. (2005) The role of Ca^{2+} in muscle cell damage. *Annals of the New York Academy of Sciences* **1066**, 166–180.

Gleeson, M., Blannin, A.K., Walsh, N.P., Field, C.N. & Pritchard, J.C. (1998) Effect of exercise-induced muscle damage on the blood lactate response to incremental exercise in humans. *European Journal of Applied Physiology and Occupational Physiology* **77**, 292–295.

Gleeson, M., Blannin, A.K., Zhu, B., Brooks, S. & Cave, R. (1995) Cardiorespiratory, hormonal and haematological responses to submaximal cycling performed 2 days after eccentric or concentric exercise bouts. *Journal of Sports Sciences* **13**, 471–479.

Gregory, J.E., Morgan, D.L. & Proske, U. (2003) Tendon organs as monitors of muscle damage from eccentric contractions. *Experimental Brain Research* **151**, 346–355.

Grobler, L.A., Collins, M., Lambert, M.I., Sinclair-Smith, C., Derman, E.W., St. Clair Gibson, A., *et al.* (2004) Skeletal muscle pathology in endurance athletes with acquired training intolerance. *British Journal of Sports Medicine* **38**, 697–703.

Haller, R.G. (1994) Oxygen utilization and delivery in metabolic myopathies. *Annals of Neurology* **36**, 811–813.

Haller, R.G., Lewis, S.F., Cook, J.D. & Blomqvist, C.G. (1985) Myophosphorylase deficiency impairs muscle oxidative metabolism *Annals of Neurology* **17**, 196–199.

Haller, R.G., Wyrick, P., Taivassalo, T. & Vissing, J. (2006) Aerobic conditioning: an effective therapy in McArdle's disease. *Annals of Neurology* **59**, 922–928.

Halson, S.L. & Jeukendrup, A.E. (2004) Does overtraining exist? An analysis of overreaching and overtraining research. *Sports Medicine* **34**, 967–981.

Hawarden D., Baker, S., Toerien, A., Prescott, R., Derman. E.W., Leaver, R., et al. (2002) Atopy in South African Olympic athletes. *South African Medical Journal* **92**, 355–356.

Hooper, S.L., Mackinnon, L.T. & Howard, A. (1999) Physiological and psychometric variables for monitoring recovery during tapering for major competition. *Medicine and Science in Sports and Exercise* **31**, 1205–1210.

Hume, P., Cheung, K., Maxwell, L. & Weerapong, P. (2004) DOMS: An overview of treatment strategies. *International Journal of Sports Medicine* **5**, 98–118.

Hutton, R.S. & Nelson, L.D. (1986) Stretch sensitivity of Golgi tendon organs in fatigued gastrocnemius muscle. *Medicine and Science in Sports and Exercise* **18**, 69–74.

Jung, A.P., Bishop, P.A., Al Nawwas, A. & Dale, R.B. (2005) Influence of hydration and electrolyte supplementation on incidence and time to onset of exercise-associated muscle cramps. *Journal of Athletic Training* **40**, 71–75.

Kadi, F., Charifi, N., Denis, C., Lexell, J., Andersen, J.L., Schjerling, P., et al. (2005) The behaviour of satellite cells in response to exercise: what have we learned from human studies? *Pflugers Archiv: European Journal of Physiology* **451**, 319–327.

Kantorowski, P.G., Hiller, W.D., Garrett, W.E., Douglas, P.S., Smith, R. & O'Toole, M.L. (1990) Cramping studies in 2600 endurance athletes. *Medicine and Science in Sports and Exercise* **22**, S104.

Kendall, B. & Eston, R. (2002) Exercise-induced muscle damage and the potential protective role of estrogen. *Sports Medicine* **32**, 103–123.

Kim, J., Wang, Z., Heymsfield, S.B., Baumgartner, R.N. & Gallagher, D. (2002) Total-body skeletal muscle mass: estimation by a new dual-energy X-ray absorptiometry method. *American Journal of Clinical Nutrition* **76**, 378–383.

Klapcinska, B., Iskra, J., Poprzecki, S. & Grzesiok, K. (2001) The effects of sprint (300 m) running on plasma latctate, uric acid, creatine kinase and lactate dehydrogenase in competitive hurdlers and untrained men. *Journal of Sports Medicine and Physical Fitness* **41**, 306–311.

Knochel, J.P. (1990) Catastrophic medical events with exhaustive exercise: "white collar rhabdomyolysis". *Kidney International* **38**, 709–719.

Komarow, H.D. & Postolache, T.T. (2005) Seasonal allergy and seasonal decrements in athletic performance. *Clinical Sports Medicine* **24**, e35–50, xiii.

Kuipers, H. (1994) Exercise-induced muscle damage [Review]. *International Journal of Sports Medicine* **15**, 132–135.

Kuipers, H., Janssen, G., Bosman, F., Frederik, P. & Geurten, P. (1989) Structural and ultrastructural changes in skeletal muscle associated with long-distance training and running. *International Journal of Sports Medicine* **10**, S156–S159.

Lambert, M.I. & Borresen, J. (2006) A theoretical basis of monitoring fatigue: a practical approach for coaches. *International Journal of Sports Science and Coaching* **1**, 371–388.

Lambert, M.I., Marcus, P., Burgess, T. & Noakes, T.D. (2002) Electro-membrane microcurrent therapy reduces signs and symptoms of muscle damage. *Medicine and Science in Sports and Exercise* **34**, 602–607.

Layzer, R.B. (1981) Leg muscle cramps. *Journal of the American Medical Association* **245**, 2298.

Lott, J.A. & Landesman, P.W. (1984) The enzymology of skeletal muscle disorders. *Critical Reviews in Clinical Laboratory Sciences* **20**, 153–190.

MacIntyre, D.L., Reid, W.D. & McKenzie, D.C. (1995) Delayed muscle soreness: the inflammatory response to muscle injury and its clinical implications. *Sports Medicine* **20**, 4–40.

Manjra, S.I., Schwellnus, M.P. & Noakes, T.D. (1996) Risk factors for exercise associated muscle cramping (EAMC) in marathon runners. *Medicine and Science in Sports and Exercise* **28** (Suppl 5), S167.

Marino, F.E., Mbambo, Z., Kortekaas, E., Wilson, G., Lambert, M.I., Noakes, T.D., et al. (2000) Advantages of smaller body mass during distance running in warm, humid environments. *Pflugers Archiv: European Journal of Physiology* **441**, 359–367.

Martin, A., Haller, R.G. & Barohn, R. (1994) Metabolic myopathies. *Current Opinion in Rheumatology* **6**, 552–558.

Martin, V., Millet, G.Y., Lattier, G. & Perrod, L. (2004) Effects of recovery modes after knee extensor muscles eccentric contractions. *Medicine and Science in Sports and Exercise* **36**, 1907–1915.

Mauro, A. (1961) Satellite cell of skeletal muscle fibers. *Journal of Biophysical and Biochemical Cytology* **9**, 493–495.

McHugh, M.P. (2003) Recent advances in the understanding of the repeated bout effect: the protective effect against muscle damage from a single bout of eccentric exercise. *Scandinavian Journal of Medicine and Science in Sports* **13**, 88–97.

McHugh, M.P., Connolly, D.A., Eston, R.G. & Gleim, G.W. (1999a) Exercise-induced muscle damage and potential mechanisms for the repeated bout effect. *Sports Medicine* **27**, 157–170.

McHugh, M.P., Connolly, D.A., Eston, R.G., Kreminic, I.J., Nicholas, S.J. & Gleim, G.W. (1999b) The role of passive muscle stiffness in symptoms of exercise-induced muscle damage. *American Journal of Sports Medicine* **27**, 594–599.

Mense, S. (1993) Nociception from skeletal muscle in relation to clinical muscle pain. *Pain* **54**, 241–289.

Miller, T.M. & Layzer, R.B. (2005) Muscle cramps. *Muscle Nerve* **32**, 431–442.

Moraska, A. (2005) Sports massage: a comprehensive review. *Journal of Sports Medicine and Physical Fitness* **45**, 370–380.

Morgan, D.L. (1990) New insights into the behavior of muscle during active lengthening. *Biophysics Journal* **57**, 209–221.

Morgan, D.L. & Allen, D.G. (1999) Early events in stretch-induced muscle damage. *Journal of Applied Physiology* **87**, 2007–2015.

Mouly, V., Aamiri, A., Bigot, A., Cooper, R.N., Di Donna, S., Furling, D., et al. (2005) The mitotic clock in skeletal muscle regeneration, disease and cell mediated gene therapy. *Acta Physiologica Scandinavia* **184**, 3–15.

Nederhof, E., Zwerver, J., Brink, M., Meeusen, R. & Lemmink, K. (2008) Different diagnostic tools in nonfunctional overreaching. *International Journal of Sports Medicine*. E-pub ahead of print.

Nelson, L.D. & Hutton, R.S. (1985) Dynamic and static stretch response in muscle spindle receptors in fatigued muscle. *Medicine and Science in Sports and Exercise* **17**, 445–450.

Newham, D.J., Jones, D.A. & Clarkson, P.M. (1987) Repeated high-force eccentric exercise: effects on muscle pain and damage. *Journal of Applied Physiology* **63**, 1381–1386.

Newham, D.J., Jones, D.A., Tolfree, S.E. & Edwards, R.H. (1986) Skeletal muscle damage: a study of isotope uptake, enzyme efflux and pain after stepping. *European Journal of Applied Physiology and Occupational Physiology* **55**, 106–112.

Noakes, T.D. (1987) Effect of exercise on serum enzyme activities in humans. *Sports Medicine* **4**, 245–267.

Nosaka, K., Clarkson, P.M., McGuiggin, M.E. & Byrne, J.M. (1991) Time course of muscle adaptation after high force eccentric exercise. *European Journal of Applied Physiology and Occupational Physiology* **63**, 70–76.

Nosaka, K., Newton, M. & Sacco, P. (2002) Delayed-onset muscle soreness does not reflect the magnitude of eccentric exercise-induced muscle damage. *Scandinavian Journal of Medicine and Science in Sport* **12**, 337–346.

Nosaka, K., Sakamoto, K., Newton, M. & Sacco, P. (2001) How long does the protective effect on eccentric exercise-induced muscle damage last? *Medicine and Science in Sports and Exercise* **33**, 1490–1495.

O'Reilly, K.P., Warhol, M.J., Fielding, R.A., Frontera, W.R., Meredith, C.N. & Evans, W.J. (1987) Eccentric exercise-induced muscle damage impairs muscle glycogen repletion. *Journal of Applied Physiology* **63**, 252–256.

Orchard, J.W. (2001) Intrinsic and extrinsic risk factors for muscle strains in Australian football. *American Journal of Sports Medicine* **29**, 300–303.

Parisi, L., Pierelli, F., Amabile, G., Valente, G., Calandriello, E., Fattapposta, F., *et al.* (2003) Muscular cramps: proposals for a new classification. *Acta Neurologica Scandinavia* **107**, 176–186.

Paul, G., Delany, J., Snook, J., Seifert, J. & Kirby, T. (1989) Serum and urinary markers of skeletal muscle tissue damage after weight lifting exercise. *European Journal of Applied Physiology and Occupational Physiology* **58**, 786–790.

Proske, U. & Allen, T.J. (2005) Damage to skeletal muscle from eccentric exercise. *Exercise and Sport Sciences Reviews* **33**, 98–104.

Proske, U. & Morgan, D.L. (2001) Muscle damage from eccentric exercise: mechanism, mechanical signs, adaptation and clinical applications. *Journal of Physiology* **537**, 333–345.

Renault, V., Piron-Hamelin, G., Forestier, C., DiDonna, S., Decary, S., Hentati, F., *et al.* (2000) Skeletal muscle regeneration and the mitotic clock. *Experimental Gerontology* **35**, 711–719.

Renault, V., Thornell, L.E., Eriksson, P.O., Butler-Browne, G. & Mouly, V. (2002) Regenerative potential of human skeletal muscle during aging. *Aging Cell* **1**, 132–139.

Rodenburg, J.B., Steenbeek, D., Schiereck, P. & Bar, P.R. (1994) Warm-up, stretching and massage diminish harmful effects of eccentric exercise. *International Journal of Sports Medicine* **15**, 414–419.

Sahlin, K., Jorfeldt, L., Henriksson, K.G., Lewis, S.F. & Haller, R.G. (1995) Tricarboxylic acid cycle intermediates during incremental exercise in healthy subjects and in patients with McArdle's disease. *Clinical Science* **88**, 687–693.

Sayers, S.P. & Dannecker, E.A. (2004) How to prevent delayed onset muscle soreness (DOMS) after eccentric exercise. *International Journal of Sports Medicine* **5**, 84–97.

Sayers, S.P., Knight, C.A. & Clarkson, P.M. (2003) Neuromuscular variables affecting the magnitude of force loss after eccentric exercise. *Journal of Sports Sciences* **21**, 403–410.

Scharf, M.B. & Barr, S. (1988) Craving carbohydrates: a possible sign of overtraining. *Annals of Sports Medicine* **4**, 19–20.

Schultz, E. & McCormick, K.M. (1994) Skeletal muscle satellite cells. *Reviews of Physiology, Biochemistry and Pharmacology* **123**, 213–257.

Schwellnus, M.P. (1999) Skeletal muscle cramps during exercise. *The Physician and Sportsmedicine* **27**, 109–115.

Schwellnus, M.P., Derman, E.W. & Noakes, T.D. (1997) Aetiology of skeletal muscle "cramps" during exercise: a novel hypothesis. *Journal of Sports Sciences* **15**, 277–285.

Schwellnus, M.P., Nicol, J., Laubscher, R. & Noakes, T.D. (2004) Serum electrolyte concentrations and hydration status are not associated with exercise associated muscle cramping (EAMC) in distance runners. *British Journal of Sports Medicine* **38**, 488–492.

Semark, A., Noakes, T.D., St. Clair Gibson, A. & Lambert, M.I. (1999) The effect of a prophylactic dose of flurbiprofen on muscle soreness and sprinting performance in trained subjects. *Journal of Sports Sciences* **17**, 197–203.

Sewright, K.A., Clarkson, P.M. & Thompson, P.D. (2007) Statin myopathy: incidence, risk factors, and pathophysiology. *Current Atherosclerosis Reports* **9**, 389–396.

Shephard, R.J. (2005) Chronic fatigue syndrome: a brief review of functional disturbances and potential therapy. *Journal of Sports Medicine and Physical Fitness* **45**, 381–392.

Sherman, W.M., Lash, J.M., Simonsen, J.C. & Bloomfield, S.A. (1992) Effects of downhill running on the responses to an oral glucose challenge. *International Journal of Sports Nutrition* **2**, 251–259.

Sjöström, M., Johansson, C. & Lorentzon, R. (1988) Muscle pathomorphology in m.

quadriceps of marathon runners: early signs of strain disease or functional adaptation? *Acta Physiologica Scandinavia* **132**, 537–542.

Smith, L.L. (1991) Acute inflammation: the underlying mechanism in delayed onset muscle soreness? *Medicine and Science in Sports and Exercise* **23**, 542–551.

Smith, L.L., Keating, M.N., Holbert, D., Spratt, D.J., McCammon, M.R., Smith, S.S., *et al.* (1994) The effects of athletic massage on delayed onset muscle soreness, creatine kinase, and neutrophil count: a preliminary report. *Journal of Orthopaedic and Sports Physical Therapy* **19**, 93–99.

Sorichter, S., Puschendorf, B. & Mair, J. (1999) Skeletal muscle injury induced by eccentric muscle action: muscle proteins as markers of muscle fiber injury. *Exercise Immunology Review* **5**, 5–21.

St. Clair Gibson, A., Grobler, L.A., Collins, M., Lambert, M.I., Sharwood, K., Derman, E.W., *et al.* (2006) Evaluation of maximal exercise performance, fatigue, and depression in athletes with acquired chronic training intolerance. *Clinical Journal of Sports Medicine* **16**, 39–45.

Sulzer, N.U., Schwellnus, M.P. & Noakes, T.D. (2005) Serum electrolytes in Ironman triathletes with exercise-associated muscle cramping. *Medicine and Science in Sports and Exercise* **37**, 1081–1085.

Taivassalo, T. & Haller, R.G. (2005) Exercise and training in mitochondrial myopathies. *Medicine and Science in Sports and Exercise* **37**, 2094–2101.

Taivassalo, T., Jensen, T.D., Kennaway, N., DiMauro, S., Vissing, J. & Haller, R.G. (2003) The spectrum of exercise tolerance in mitochondrial myopathies: a study of 40 patients. *Brain* **126**, 413–423.

Tarnopolsky, M.A. (2006) What can metabolic myopathies teach us about exercise physiology? *Applied Physiology, Nutrition and Metabolism* **31**, 21–30.

Tarnopolsky, M.A. & Raha, S. (2005) Mitochondrial myopathies: diagnosis, exercise intolerance, and treatment options. *Medicine and Science in Sports and Exercise* **37**, 2086–2093.

Urhausen, A. & Kindermann, W. (2002) Diagnosis of overtraining: what tools do we have? *Sports Medicine* **32**, 95–102.

Wagenmakers, A.J., Coakley, J.H. & Edwards, R.H. (1990) Metabolism of branched-chain amino acids and ammonia during exercise: clues from McArdle's disease. *International Journal of Sports Medicine* **11** (Suppl 2), S101–S113.

Warhol, M.J., Siegel, A.J., Evans, W.J. & Silverman, L.M. (1985) Skeletal muscle injury and repair in marathon runners after competition. *American Journal of Pathology* **118**, 331–339.

Warren, J.D., Blumbergs, P.C. & Thompson, P.D. (2002) Rhabdomyolysis: a review. *Muscle Nerve* **25**, 332–347.

Waterhouse, J., Reilly, T., Atkinson, G. & Edwards, B. (2007) Jet lag: trends and coping strategies. *Lancet* **369**, 1117–1129.

Yan, Z. (2000) Skeletal muscle adaptation and cell cycle regulation. *Exercise and Sport Sciences Reviews* **28**, 24–26.

Yu, J.G., Furst, D.O. & Thornell, L.E. (2003) The mode of myofibril remodelling in human skeletal muscle affected by DOMS induced by eccentric contractions. *Histochemistry and Cell Biology* **119**, 383–393.

Zehnder, M., Meulli, M., Buchli, R., Kuehne, G. & Boutellier, U. (2004) Further glycogen decrease during early recovery after eccentric exercise despite a high carbohydrate intake. *European Journal of Nutrition* **43**, 148–159.

Zierz, S. (1994) Limited trypsin proteolysis renders carnitine palmitoyl transferase insensitive to inhibition by malonyl-CoA in patients with muscle carnitine palmitoyltransferase deficiency. *Clinical Investigations* **72**, 957–960.

Chapter 6

Sports Cardiology

CHRISTOS KASAPIS AND PAUL D. THOMPSON

"Walking is a man's best medicine" (Hippocrates (460–357 BC). The concept that physical activity is beneficial for health maintenance is not new. Regular exercise as a way of promoting health can be traced back at least 5000 years to India, where yoga originated. The Ancient Greeks had exercise programs 2500 years ago, which led to the first Olympic Games in 776 BC. Over the past century, the role of habitual exercise in the prevention of coronary heart disease has been documented in numerous epidemiologic and observational studies (Fletcher *et al.* 2001; Thompson *et al.* 2003). Based on this evidence, a consensus has been reached from the Centers for Disease Control and Prevention (CDC) and the American College of Sports Medicine (ACSM) that a minimum of 30 min of moderate intensity physical activity is required on most, preferably all, days of the week to reduce the risk of coronary artery disease (CAD) (Pate *et al.* 1995).

The beneficial effects of exercise "against" CAD are mediated through multiple biologic mechanisms, which may be classified as follows:
• Anti-atherogenic effects resulting from attenuation of traditional risk factors, including reduction of adiposity, blood pressure, and triglycerides as well as increase in high density lipoproteins (HDL) and improvement of insulin sensitivity (Blair 1993; Kraus *et al.* 2002; Mayer-Davis *et al.* 1998; Whelton *et al.* 2002);

• Anti-thrombotic effects secondary to a reduced tendency for platelet aggregation and increased fibrinolytic activity (Lee & Lip 2003);
• Improvement of endothelial function augmenting the release of endothelium-derived nitric oxide (Hambrecht *et al.* 2000);
• Autonomic function changes attributed to enhanced parasympathetic and reduced sympathetic tone in trained individuals (Goldsmith *et al.* 1992);
• Anti-ischemic effects mediated by improving the relative balance between myocardial oxygen supply and demand as reflected in the lowered resting heart rate and blood pressure in athletes as well as by increasing the diameter and dilating capacity of coronary arteries, increasing collateral artery formation and delaying the progression of coronary artery atherosclerosis (Niebauer *et al.* 1997);
• Anti-arrhythmic effects maintained by the reduction in sympathetic tone and the improvement of myocardial oxygen supply–demand balance (Billman 2002); and
• Anti-inflammatory effects, as demonstrated by the reduction of baseline serum C-reactive protein levels and other inflammatory markers in physically active individuals (Kasapis & Thompson 2005).

Despite the overwhelming evidence for the benefits of exercise on the cardiovascular system, occasionally vigorous exercise is associated with sudden cardiac death (Maron 2003; Siscovivk *et al.* 1984; Thompson *et al.* 1982) and myocardial infarction in individuals with both diagnosed and occult heart disease (Giri *et al.* 1999; Mittleman *et al.* 1993). Such cardiac catastrophes in competitive athletes, often in the absence of prior symptoms, have a

The Olympic Textbook of Medicine in Sport, 1st edition. Edited by M. Schwellnus. Published 2008 by Blackwell Publishing, ISBN: 978-1-4051-5637-0.

considerable emotional and social impact on the public and medical communities. Attempts to understand and prevent such events have triggered interest in differentiating physiologic athlete's heart from structural heart disease (Maron *et al.* 1995; Thompson & Estes 2002), as well as in formulating preparticipation screening guidelines and disqualification criteria for athletes (36th Bethesda Conference 2005; Corrado *et al.* 2005; Maron *et al.* 1996b).

This chapter focuses on the cardiovascular evaluation and management of heart disease in athletes. First, the normal physiologic cardiovascular response to exercise and exercise training is discussed briefly to help understand and differentiate the athlete's heart syndrome from cardiovascular disease. Next, the chapter reviews the athlete's heart syndrome and the cardiovascular risks of exercise as well as specific heart disease entities and the preparticipation evaluation of athletes. In addition, because athletes represent a special part of society, because of their unique lifestyle and capability for admirable physical achievements, an overview of special considerations in evaluating this population is included. Finally, future directions and perspectives, especially with the revolution in genetic medicine, is examined.

Cardiovascular response to exercise and exercise training

Types of exercise

There are three types of muscular contraction or exercise: isometric (static); isotonic (dynamic); and resistance (a combination of isometric and isotonic). Isotonic exercise, which is defined as rhythmic physical exertion resulting in movement, such as running, swimming and bicycling, primarily provides a volume load to the left ventricle, and the responses are proportional to the size of the working muscle mass and the intensity of exercise. Isometric exercise is defined as muscular contraction against resistance without movement, such as static handgrip, and imposes a greater pressure than volume load on the left ventricle. Cardiac output is not increased as much as in isotonic exercise because increased resistance in active muscle groups limits blood flow. Resistance exercise combines both isotonic and isometric muscle contraction, such as free weight lifting.

Sports can be classified in terms of their static and dynamic demands and by the level of intensity (low, medium, or high) generally required to perform that sport during competition, as summarized in Fig. 6.1 (36th Bethesda Conference 2005). It should be recognized that this classification is not rigid; athletes in the same sport can be placed in different categories, and many sports involve a mixture of static and dynamic demands. However, this classification is a helpful guide in decision-making regarding eligibility and disqualification for competitive sports.

Endurance athletes, compared to the general population, are characterized by a higher ability to perform maximal dynamic exercise. This ability can be measured as maximal oxygen uptake ($\dot{V}o_{2max}$). $\dot{V}o_{2max}$ is expressed either as liters of oxygen per minute or "normalized" for body weight as milliliters of oxygen per minute per kilogram of body weight. $\dot{V}o_{2max}$ is reflected as the point at which there is no further increase in oxygen uptake despite further increases in workload and is physiologically limited by the ability of the cardiopulmonary system to deliver, and the ability of the exercising muscles to use, oxygen. The determinants of $\dot{V}o_{2max}$ can be demonstrated by the Fick equation for cardiac output (cardiac output = $\dot{V}o_2$/ A–$\dot{V}o_2$ difference) reflecting that $\dot{V}o_{2max}$ is the product of maximal cardiac output and the maximal arteriovenous O_2 difference. Maximal cardiac output is the product of maximal heart rate and stroke volume. Because maximal heart rate among healthy individuals varies primarily by age and because the ability to increase the A–$\dot{V}o_2$ difference is limited, the major factor responsible for the higher $\dot{V}o_{2max}$ among endurance athletes is an increased stroke volume. The major causes of increased stroke volume during exercise are increased myocardial contractility and increased venous return to the heart. The clinical findings typical of the athlete's heart are generally manifestations of this increased stroke volume.

The acute cardiovascular adaptations to exercise in young healthy subjects are mediated by several

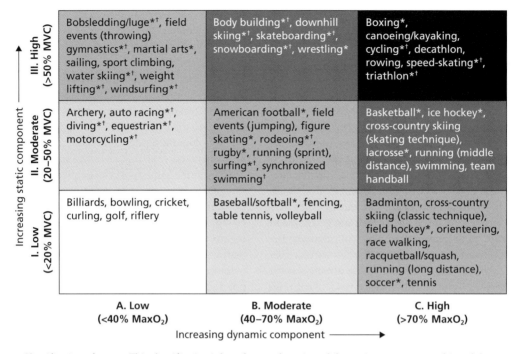

Fig. 6.1 Classification of sports. This classification is based on peak static and dynamic components achieved during competition. It should be noted, however, that higher values may be reached during training. The increasing dynamic component is defined in terms of the estimated percent of maximal oxygen uptake ($MaxO_2$) achieved and results in an increasing cardiac output. The increasing static component is related to the estimated percent of maximal voluntary contraction (MVC) reached and results in an increasing blood pressure load. The lowest total cardiovascular demands (cardiac output and blood pressure) are shown in **white** and the highest in **black**. **Light**, **intermediate**, and **dark gray** depict low moderate, moderate, and high moderate total cardiovascular demands, respectively. Reproduced with permission from 36th Bethesda Conference 2005. * Danger of bodily collision. † Increased risk if syncope occurs.

mechanisms. The increase in heart rate is initially brought about by withdrawal of resting vagal tone. At approximately 50% of maximal heart rate, additional acceleration of heart rate is associated with increased sympathetic nerve activity and norepinephrine spillover into the circulation (Rowell 1986). Peak heart rate is estimated as 220 – age, but the standard deviation of this estimate is ±11–22 beats·min^{-1} (Ferguson et al. 2000). Changes in stroke volume during exertion are influenced by body position, mostly as a result of the effects of the gravity on venous return. During supine exercise, the increase in stroke volume is primarily brought about by increases in end-diastolic volume. During upright exercise, increases in stroke volume are produced by both increases in end-diastolic volume and decreases in end-systolic volume (Rowell 1986).

The increase in A–$\dot{V}o_2$ difference is primarily the result of decreased mixed venous oxygen content, produced by redistribution of blood from non-exercising tissue to the exercising musculature, increased extraction of O_2 over the exercising muscle bed, and hemoconcentration (Rowell 1986). Sweat loss is not required for this hemoconcentration, because plasma fluid moves into exercising muscle to produce the muscle swelling obvious in recently exercised muscle. These changes, and the mediating mechanisms, apply to young, healthy subjects. Altered responses and different mechanisms are observed in elderly subjects and in patients with disease.

It is important for clinicians to recognize that any change in any component of this system can affect maximal exercise capacity. Cardiologists tend to focus on changes in maximum heart rate and stroke volume, but changes in hemoglobin concentration, the ability to oxygenate the red blood cells fully, the capacity to shunt blood to exercising muscle, and the ability of the muscles to extract the available oxygen can affect exercise performance. These factors should be considered in evaluating athletes for problems with exercise performance.

There are differences in mechanical efficiency among different athletes performing identical exercise tasks. Nevertheless, in general, a specific physical task requires approximately the same oxygen uptake when performed by different individuals. Consequently, knowing the work rate of exercise permits a general estimation of the $\dot{V}o_2$ required, even when $\dot{V}o_2$ is not measured. The O_2 consumption required by a physical task is referred to as the external work rate (Amsterdam et $al.$ 1974). The external work rate also determines the cardiac output response to the exercise task. In general, a 1-L increase in O_2 consumption produces a 6-L increase in cardiac output (Wilmore & Gostill 1994). The external work rate is also referred to as the absolute work rate or the absolute $\dot{V}o_2$. The relative work rate refers to the percent of an individual's $\dot{V}o_{2max}$, which is required for that person to perform a certain physical task. In other words, relative work rate is the required $\dot{V}o_2$ relative to the individual's maximum. Individuals differ in their maximal exercise capacity, primarily because maximal stroke volume and maximal cardiac output vary among individuals. Because of differences in individual exercise capacity, the same physical task usually requires approximately the same absolute work rate for different individuals, but often requires markedly different relative work rates.

Identical external work rates can produce markedly different myocardial O_2 demand. Myocardial O_2 demand has been referred to as the internal work rate (Amsterdam et $al.$ 1974). Myocardial oxygen demand increases with increasing heart rate and systolic blood pressure (Gobel et $al.$ 1978). The product of heart rate and systolic blood pressure or the rate–pressure product is used clinically to estimate the myocardial oxygen demand of exertion (Gobel et $al.$ 1978). Both heart rate and systolic blood pressure increase linearly with the relative work rate.

Consequently, identical external work rates can produce markedly different internal work rates or myocardial O_2 demands depending on the individual's $\dot{V}o_{2max}$. The implication of this observation is that the same physical task requires less myocardial oxygen supply for an individual with a high $\dot{V}o_{2max}$ than that task requires for a less fit individual.

Differences in acute cardiovascular responses to dynamic and static exercise

The acute responses of the cardiovascular system to exercise differ according to the type of exercise and are summarized in Table 6.1 (Gallagher et $al.$ 1999; Mitchell & Raven 1994). Dynamic exercise causes a marked increase in oxygen consumption mediated through a substantial increase in cardiac output, heart rate, stroke volume, and systolic blood pressure. There is also a moderate increase in mean arterial pressure and a decrease in diastolic pressure with a marked decrease in systemic vascular resistance. These hemodynamic changes produce a volume load on the left ventricle during dynamic exercise and an increase in myocardial O_2 demand caused by the substantial increase in heart rate and stroke volume. The increase in stroke volume is mediated by both an increase in end-diastolic volume (Frank-Starling mechanism) and a decrease in end-systolic volume (increased contractility). Static exercise produces a small increase in oxygen consumption, cardiac output, and heart rate, and no change in stroke volume. Additionally, there are marked increases in systolic, diastolic, and mean

Table 6.1 Cardiovascular response to dynamic and static exercise (Gallagher et $al.$ 1999; Mitchell & Raven 1994).

	Dynamic exercise	Static exercise
Oxygen consumption $\dot{V}o_2$	↑↑↑	↑
Cardiac output	↑↑↑	↑
Heart rate	↑↑↑	↑
Stroke volume	↑↑↑	—
Mean blood pressure	↑	↑↑↑
Systolic blood pressure	↑↑	↑↑↑
Diastolic blood pressure	↓	↑
Peripheral resistance	↓↓↓	↑

arterial pressure and no significant change in systemic vascular resistance. Thus, static exercise produces primarily a pressure load on the left ventricle and the increase in myocardial O_2 demand is achieved primarily through an increase in arterial pressure and the contractile state of the ventricle and to a lesser extent through a small increase in heart rate.

Effect of exercise training on exercise performance

The chronic adaptation of the cardiovascular system to dynamic exercise training results in an increase in $\dot{V}_{O_{2max}}$ produced by increases in both maximal stroke volume and the maximal A–$\dot{V}_{O_2}$ difference, whereas static exercise training results in little or no increase in $\dot{V}_{O_{2max}}$ (Gallagher et al. 1999). It is generally stated that approximately 50% of the increase in $\dot{V}_{O_{2max}}$ is caused by increases in stroke volume and 50% to changes in A–$\dot{V}_{O_2}$ difference (Mitchell & Blomqvist 1971), but this varies greatly among studies (Sadaniantz et al. 1996). Increases in $\dot{V}_{O_{2max}}$ are greater with increasing duration and intensity of the exercise-training program and with the amount of muscle mass used in training (Rowell 1986). Also, with more prolonged training, more of the increase in exercise capacity is brought about by increased stroke volume. Apparently the increase in A–$\dot{V}_{O_2}$ difference is an early adaptation to habitual exercise, whereas large increases in stroke volume require cardiac adaptations over a longer, albeit undefined, period of time. The average increase in $\dot{V}_{O_{2max}}$ in healthy subjects after jogging or cycling for 3–12 months is approximately 20% (Brooks et al. 1996), but is less in more fit and older individuals. Increments in $\dot{V}_{O_{2max}}$ can be considerably larger if the training is prolonged over years rather than months.

The increase in absolute work capacity produced by exercise training means that the same external workload after training represents less of the individual's relative workload. Because exercise-induced increases in heart rate and systolic blood pressure are related to the relative, as opposed to the absolute, exercise workload, the same external workload after training elicits smaller increments in heart rate, blood pressure, and myocardial oxygen demand.

Athlete's heart

The athlete's heart or athletic heart syndrome was first described by Henschen in 1899, using percussion of the chest to determine the heart size in competitive cross-country skiers (Rost 1997). He concluded that skiing produces a physiologic beneficial cardiac enlargement that enables the heart to perform more work than the heart of sedentary individuals. This finding was later confirmed by a variety of imaging techniques: radiography, echocardiography, computed tomography, and magnetic resonance imaging, as well as by necropsy findings. The athletic heart syndrome is now recognized as a constellation of structural, functional, electrocardiographic, and echocardiographic variants of normal, found in well-trained athletes, who participate in sports requiring prolonged aerobic exercise training. These findings include sinus bradycardia, A-V conduction delay, systolic flow murmurs, and cardiac chamber enlargement with or without thickening of the ventricular wall. The clinical findings of the athletic heart syndrome are limited to athletes involved in aerobic or endurance exercise. It is important to highlight the manifestations of this syndrome. Physicians involved in evaluating athletes prior to participation must differentiate these physiologic changes from pathologic conditions, such as hypertrophic cardiomyopathy, coronary artery anomalies, aortic stenosis and right or left ventricular cardiomyopathy in young athletes as well as coronary artery disease in adults.

Structural and echocardiographic variants of the athlete's heart

Physical exercise is associated with hemodynamic changes that alter the loading conditions of the heart. These changes differ according to the type of exercise. As a result, isotonic (dynamic) exercise causes predominantly a volume load, whereas isometric (static) exercise results in a pressure load on the heart. Long-term, these hemodynamic changes and ventricular loading conditions during exercise can lead to left ventricular hypertrophy (LVH). Volume load would lead to enlargement of the left ventricular internal diameter and proportional increase of wall thickness, termed "eccentric LVH." On the contrary, pressure load would induce thickening of the ventricular wall with unchanged internal dimension, termed "concentric LVH." Thus, the hearts of endurance athletes (dynamic exercise) are characterized primarily by chamber dilatation, whereas strength-trained athletes (static exercise) may show mildly increased wall thickness (Keul et al. 1981; Longhurst et al. 1980). The degree that these changes occur is based on the type of training pursued.

There is ample of evidence that habitual dynamic exercise produces a global cardiac enlargement, which may affect all four chambers, but most consistently the left ventricular chamber. Mild enlargement of the right atrium and right ventricle can occur, but marked enlargement of these chambers is more suggestive of a disease process rather than manifestations of the athlete's heart syndrome. At least 59 studies have used echocardiography to examine cardiac dimensions in athletes compared with sedentary controls and consistently documented increased left ventricular dimensions by an average of 10% in athletes (Thomas & Douglas 2001). Thirteen studies demonstrated increased right ventricular transverse dimension by an average of 24% in athletes (Thomas & Douglas 2001). Fourteen studies demonstrated 16% larger left atrial transverse dimension in athletes and only one study showed larger right atrial size in the athlete group (Thomas & Douglas 2001). The increase in left ventricular end-diastolic dimension (LVEDD) is usually within the normal range (<5.5 cm in males and <4.8 cm in females), but it has been reported to be as high as 6.6 cm for a female and 7 cm for a male athlete (Pelliccia et al. 1999; Thomas & Douglas 2001). Sports that required a large endurance component or a combination of endurance and strength training with increased body size are associated with larger LVEDD. The cardiac enlargement observed in athletes occurs without any evidence of left ventricular systolic or diastolic dysfunction (Pelliccia et al. 1999; Thomas & Douglas 2001).

Left ventricular wall thickness is increased by an average of 15–20% in well-trained athletes compared to sedentary controls and the absolute values are generally within or slightly above the normal range (Thomas & Douglas 2001). LVH is concentric, more pronounced, and occurs secondary to the pressure load in strength-trained athletes, whereas in endurance athletes it is eccentric and occurs as an adaptation to the increased cavity dimensions in order to maintain normal wall stress. Left ventricular wall thickness >12 mm is unusual and rarely exceeds 16 mm even in the most elite athletes (Pelliccia et al. 1991; Thomas & Douglas 2001). Values above this rage should raise the possibility of hypertrophic cardiomyopathy. Noteworthy, LVH above the normal range is generally not observed in female athletes (Pelliccia et al. 1991). The calculated left ventricular mass is also 45–50% greater in well-trained athletes compared to sedentary controls (Thomas & Douglas 2001). Interestingly, the increased left ventricular mass noted in strength-trained athletes is not observed when cardiac size is normalized for skeletal muscle mass; however, the increased left ventricular size of endurance athletes does persist after the adjustment (Keul et al. 1981; Longhurst et al. 1980).

Table 6.2 summarizes the screening echocardiographic limits of normal used in athletes. It should be re-emphasized that only rarely does cardiac hypertrophy and dilation exceed normal values adjusted for body size and there is generally no impact of this structural remodeling on left ventricular systolic or diastolic function. Furthermore, the morphologic changes in the highly trained individuals reverse with detraining and the onset of this regression can become apparent as soon as 1 week after physical deconditioning (Ehsani et al. 1978; Thomas & Douglas 2001).

Nevertheless, these principles are generalizations and exceptions do occur. The largest study to examine cardiac wall thickness in 947 elite athletes observed only 16 athletes (1.7%) with left ventricular wall thickness ≥13 mm (Pelliccia et al. 1991). Fifteen of these athletes were rowers or canoeists and one was a cyclist, sports that require both isotonic and isometric effort and involve large muscle mass. However, only 219 of the 947 athletes examined were rowers, canoeists, or cyclists, so that 16 of 219 (7%) of these athletes had "abnormal" wall thickening. This suggests that such hypertrophy

Table 6.2 Screening echocardiographic morphologic limits in athletes. These limits of "normal" for athletes are based on pooled data from several studies involving large numbers of patients (Thomas & Douglas 2001).

Echocardiographic characteristics	General limits in athletes
Wall thickness (septal and posterior)	<1.3 cm
Septal-to-posterior wall thickness ratio	<1.3
Relative wall thickness*	<0.45
Left ventricular end-diastolic dimension	≤6 cm
Left ventricular mass	≤294 g in men, ≤198 g in women

* Relative wall thickness = mean wall thickness ÷ cavity radius.

may be reasonably common among such endurance athletes. All athletes with wall thickness ≥13 mm had enlarged left ventricular end-diastolic cavities (dimensions 55–63 mm). In another study the same investigators demonstrated that left ventricular dimensions among 1300 elite athletes were related to body size, so physically large, endurance-trained individuals, such as professional basketball players, may demonstrate left ventricular volumes and wall thickness suggesting disease (Pelliccia et al. 1999).

Clinical and electrocardiographic variants of the athlete's heart

RHYTHM CHANGES IN THE ATHLETE'S HEART

Many of the components of the athletic heart syndrome, including resting bradycardia, sinus arrhythmia, and atrioventricular conduction delay, have been attributed to increased parasympathetic tone (Chapman 1982; Kenney 1985). Downregulation of β-adrenergic receptors, a decrease in sympathetic tone and intrinsic mechanisms may also contribute (Furlan et al. 1993). Sinus bradycardia is the most frequent electrocardiographic finding and occurs in more than 50% of endurance athletes, with a recorded resting heart rate as low as 25 beats·min⁻¹ (Chapman 1982). Sinus arrhythmia, defined as respiratory variation in heart rate with an increase in heart rate during inspiration, occurred in 13.5–69% of athletes studied (Huston et al. 1985). In addition to sinus bradycardia and sinus arrhythmia, sinus pauses or sinus "arrest" of more than 2 s have been documented during sleep in endurance athletes (Estes et al. 2001). A wandering atrial pacemaker as well as junctional rhythm is also more common in athletes than in sedentary controls (Huston et al. 1985). Conduction abnormalities are also more frequent in endurance athletes compared to the general population (Estes et al. 2001; Huston et al. 1985). First and second Mobitz type I AV block have been reported in 10–33% and 2.4–10% of endurance athletes, respectively (Huston et al. 1985). However, second-degree Mobitz type II and third-degree AV block are rare in athletes and usually associated with underlying cardiac disease. It is important to emphasize that all of these variants of heart rhythm in the athletic heart syndrome (Table 6.3) resolve during exercise with the subsequent withdrawal of vagal tone and the increased sympathetic drive as well as after detraining (Estes et al. 2001).

OTHER ELECTROCARDIOGRAPHIC CHANGES

Alterations in repolarization are very common in well-trained athletes, with a frequency varying from 10 to 100% in cross-sectional studies (Huston et al. 1985; Serra-Grima et al. 2000). These changes of "early repolarization" are characterized by ST segment elevation ≥0.5 mm in two consecutive leads and by elevated J wave or terminal slurring of the R wave, most frequently in the precordial leads. ST segment depression, in contrast, is found only rarely, if at all, in athletes. Alterations in the T wave, recorded as peaked, biphasic, or inverted T waves, especially in the precordial leads, are also frequently seen in endurance athletes (Serra-Grima et al. 2000). Tall, peaked T waves often occur as part of the early repolarization changes described earlier (Estes et al. 2001; Huston et al. 1985). Frank T wave inversions occurring across the precordium and/or in the limb leads have been documented in a number of cross-sectional studies (Estes et al. 2001;

Table 6.3 Rhythm changes in the athletic heart (Puffer 2001).

Arrhythmia	Frequency in population (%)	Frequency in athletes (%)
Sinus bradycardia	23.7	50–85
Sinus arrhythmia	2.4–20	13.5–69
Wandering atrial pacemaker	–	7.4–19
First-degree AV block	0.65	6–33
Second-degree AV block		
Möbitz I	0.003	0.125–10
Möbitz II	0.003	Not reported
Third-degree AV block	0.0002	0.017
Junctional rhythm	0.06	0.031–7

Huston *et al.* 1985). A variation of T wave inversion is the presence of biphasic T waves, which typically occur in leads V3–V5 (Estes *et al.* 2001). These ST-T wave changes are attributed to training-induced sympathetic nervous system alterations and usually normalize with exertion and possibly with deconditioning (Estes *et al.* 2001). However, not all extreme ST-T wave changes in athletes are brought about by the athletic heart syndrome and underlying pathology must be excluded when ST-T wave changes are accompanied by symmetric deeply inverted T waves, ST depression, prolonged QT interval, or the absence of normal septal Q waves.

In addition to ST-T wave changes, the electrocardiogram (ECG) in well-trained athletes may show mildly increased P wave amplitude suggesting right atrial enlargement, notched P waves consistent with left atrial enlargement, incomplete right bundle branch block (RBBB), as well as voltage criteria for right and left ventricular hypertrophy (Huston *et al.* 1985). Among endurance athletes, 32–76% of subjects meet voltage criteria for LVH, whereas 18–69% of subjects meet criteria for right ventricular hypertrophy (Estes *et al.* 2001). This frequency is brought about by both biventricular enlargement and the thin body habitus of most endurance athletes.

A variety of abnormal ECG patterns occurred in 40% of 1005 competitive athletes, but only 10% of the athletes with striking abnormal ECGs had echocardiographically determined structural cardiac abnormalities (Pelliccia *et al.* 2000). This study indicates that false positive ECGs, representing a component of athletic heart syndrome, may pose a potential limitation to routine ECG testing as part of preparticipation screening.

VASOVAGAL SYNCOPE AND FUNCTIONAL CARDIAC MURMURS IN ATHLETES

Vasovagal syncope appears to occur more frequently in endurance athletes, secondary, in part, to their enhanced parasympathetic tone. Lower body negative pressure is a research technique to examine blood pressure control and an individual's response to orthostatic stress. Endurance athletes have a reduced ability to maintain blood pressure during lower body negative pressure, compared to strength-trained athletes or non-trained individuals (Smith *et al.* 1988). The clinical implication of this is that endurance athletes are more vulnerable to vasovagal syncope and that positive tilt table test responses are almost the norm in well-trained endurance athletes. These athletes have a large venous capacity from exercise training, enhanced vagal tone, and reduced sympathetic tone, all of which contribute to postural hypotension and a positive tilt table response.

Apart from the increased frequency of vasovagal syncope, 30–50% of endurance athletes have functional early systolic "flow murmurs" created by cardiac adaptations to exercise training (Huston *et al.* 1985). Training induces an increase in stroke volume and a decrease in resting heart rate. Consequently, much of the larger stroke volume is delivered more vigorously in early systole by a more dynamic ventricle resulting in an increase in blood velocity and the production of early systolic "flow murmurs." Similarly, the frequency of third and fourth heart sound is 30–100% and 20–60%, respectively, in dynamic athletes (Huston *et al.* 1985).

Clinical implications of the athletic heart syndrome

A thorough understanding of the manifestations of the athletic heart syndrome is essential for the physician in order to differentiate the normal adaptations to exercise training from pathologic conditions that jeopardize the well-being of an athlete.

The majority of ECG changes seen in the athletic heart syndrome results from diminished sympathetic drive and enhanced vagal tone, and therefore any maneuver that increases sympathetic tone may result in disappearance of the "abnormality." More concerning are the echocardiographic findings that fall into the gray zone and can create confusion with respect to distinguishing the heart's remodeling as an adaptation to intense training from hypertrophic cardiomyopathy. This diagnostic ambiguity can often be resolved through the use of non-invasive measurements, such as the response of cardiac mass to a short period (usually 3 months) of discontinuation of training (Ehsani *et al.* 1978; Pelliccia *et al.* 2002; Thomas & Douglas 2001) or assessment of diastolic filling with tissue Doppler echocardiography (Maron *et al.* 1995; Vinereanu *et al.* 2001). Changes reflective of the athletic heart will regress with detraining while those of hypertrophic cardiomyopathy will not, thereby confirming the diagnosis. In the future, DNA-based diagnostic tests may be utilized to help distinguish genetic heart diseases from athlete's heart syndrome (Maron *et al.* 1995).

The extreme alterations in cardiac dimensions evident in some athletes do not fully regress with exercise cessation. A longitundinal echocardiographic study demonstrated incomplete reversal and substantial residual dilatation of the cardiac chambers in 20% of retired, deconditioned, elite athletes (Pelliccia *et al.* 2002). This implies that either the athletes were genetically endowed to have bigger cardiac dimensions or some of the cardiac adaptations to prolonged exercise training are irreversible.

Cardiovascular risks of exercise and sudden cardiac death

Definition and epidemiology of sudden cardiac death

Sudden cardiac death (SCD) is defined as a witnessed or unwitnessed natural death resulting from sudden cardiac arrest occurring unexpectedly within 6 hours of a previously normal state of health.

Vigorous exertion acutely increases the risk of sudden death in individuals with known or occult cardiac disease, but the absolute cardiac risk of exercise is extremely low. The annual incidence of sudden death among high school and college athletes ranges between 1 in 100,000 and 1 in 300,000 (Maron *et al.* 1998a; Van Camp *et al.* 1995). The incidence is significantly higher in males than females (1 in 133,000 in men and 1 in 769,000 in women; Van Camp *et al.* 1995). The risk of exercise-related SCD is considerably higher in adults because of the increased prevalence of CAD and it has been estimated to be one death per year for every 15,000–18,000 asymptomatic middle-aged men (Siscovick *et al.* 1984; Thompson *et al.* 1982). The cardiovascular causes of exercise-related sudden death vary depending on the age of the subject. CAD is by far the most common cause of exercise-related SCD in adults over 35 years old, whereas congenital cardiac abnormalities are the primary cause of SCD in athletes younger than 35 years old (Maron *et al.* 1986a).

Cardiovascular causes of sudden cardiac death in young athletes

A number of largely congenital but clinically unsuspected cardiovascular diseases have been causally linked to sudden death in young trained athletes, often in association with physical exertion (Maron 2003; Maron *et al.* 1986a; Van Camp *et al.* 1995). The frequency of various causes of exercise-related events may vary by geographic distribution. In large autopsy-based surveys of populations of athletes in the USA, hypertrophic cardiomyopathy (HCM) is the most common cardiovascular cause of sudden death (Maron 2003; Maron *et al.* 1986a;

Maron *et al.* 1996a; Van Camp *et al.* 1995), whereas arrhythmogenic right ventricular dysplasia/cardiomyopathy (ARVC) is the primary cause of such events in Italian athletes, especially in the Veneto region of Italy (Thiene *et al.* 1988). Interestingly, a multicenter study in German speaking countries in Europe did not find a predominance of HCM (Raschka *et al.* 1999). CAD and myocarditis were the main reasons of SCD in young athletes less than 35 years old, with a frequency of 36.1% and 30.6% of SCD, respectively (Raschka *et al.* 1999). Possible explanations for these regional differences in the causes of exercise-related SCD might be varying selection of patients, different genetic backgrounds as well as different national screening programs. A report from the National Center for Catastrophic Sports Injury Research analyzing 150 deaths in US athletes occurring during or within 1 h of sports participation attributed 100 deaths to cardiac conditions (Van Camp *et al.* 1995). HCM comprised 56% of the cardiac deaths, which is the highest reported

frequency among different registries, followed by coronary artery anomalies (13%), myocarditis (7%), aortic stenosis (6%), and dilated cardiomyopathy (6%). Less common cardiac causes included CAD (4%), aortic rupture secondary to Marfan syndrome (2%), Kawasaki disease (less than 1%), and non-identified causes (2%). The coronary artery anomalies included anomalous origin, intramyocardial course and an ostial ridge at the coronary origin. In contrast to the Italian results, only one case was attributed to ARVC. Other autopsy-based studies demonstrated similar data for US athletes, but with lower frequencies of HCM (Table 6.4; Maron 2003; Maron *et al.* 1986a; Maron & Shirani *et al.* 1996). It should be noted that about 2% of young athletes who die suddenly have normal cardiac structure at autopsy and no definitive cause of death (Maron *et al.* 1996a; Van Camp *et al.* 1995). Such deaths are probably secondary to conditions that are not associated with gross pathologic cardiac abnormalities, such as ion-channel disorders, including the long

Table 6.4 Causes of sudden cardiac death (SCD) in 387 young athletes. Data are from the registry of the Minneapolis Heart Institute Foundation. Reproduced from Maron (2003) with permission.

Causes of SCD in 387 young athletes	No. of athletes	Percent
Hypertrophic cardiomyopathy	102	26.4
Commotio cordis	77	19.9
Coronary artery anomalies	53	13.7
Left ventricular hypertrophy of indeterminate causation*	29	7.5
Myocarditis	20	5.2
Ruptured aortic aneurysm (Marfan syndrome)	12	3.1
Arrhythmogenic right ventricular cardiomyopathy	11	2.8
Tunneled (bridged) coronary artery[†]	11	2.8
Aortic valve stenosis	10	2.6
Atherosclerotic coronary artery disease	10	2.6
Dilated cardiomyopathy	9	2.3
Myxomatous mitral valve degeneration	9	2.3
Asthma (or other pulmonary condition)	8	2.1
Heat stroke	6	1.6
Drug abuse	4	1.0
Other cardiovascular cause	4	1.0
Long QT syndrome[‡]	3	0.8
Cardiac sarcoidosis	3	0.8
Trauma causing structural cardiac injury	3	0.8
Ruptured cerebral artery	3	0.8

* Findings at autopsy were suggestive of HCM but were insufficient to be diagnostic.

[†] Tunneled coronary artery was deemed the cause of death in the absence of any other cardiac abnormality.

[‡] The long QT syndrome was documented on clinical evaluation.

QT syndromes, the Wolff–Parkinson–White syndrome, structural abnormalities of the conducting system and microvasculature, catecholaminergic polymorphic ventricular tachycardia, right ventricular outflow tract tachycardia, coronary vasospasm, undetected segmental ARVC, or subtle morphologic forms of HCM (Maron 2003).

In athletes with underlying heart disease, the predominant pathophysiologic mechanism of sudden death is the development of ventricular tachyarrhythmias (Maron *et al.* 1996a), with the exception of Marfan's syndrome where death is often a result of aortic rupture.

Sudden cardiac death in athletes in the absence of cardiovascular disease

Although SCD in athletes is usually the consequence of underlying cardiovascular disease, under specific circumstances sudden cardiac death may occur among sports participants in the absence of cardiovascular disease.

COMMOTIO CORDIS

Commotio cordis is an example of SCD in athletes without underlying cardiac disease that occurs as a result of blunt, non-penetrating, and innocent-appearing chest blows triggering ventricular fibrillation unassociated with structural damage to the ribs, sternum, or heart itself (Maron *et al.* 2002). The precise incidence of commotio cordis during athletic events remains unknown, but it may be a more frequent cause of sports-related SCD than previously believed (Maron 2003; Maron *et al.* 1996a). This entity is more common in children and adolescents because of the compliant chest walls in these age groups facilitating the transmission of energy from the impact to the heart (Maron *et al.* 2002). It occurs in a wide variety of sports, but is most commonly caused by projectiles used in such sports as baseball, football, and ice hockey. Deaths from commotio cordis can occur during informal sporting recreational activities.

The uncommon occurrence of commotio cordis is largely explained by its mechanism, which requires the exquisite confluence of several determinants, such as location of the blow directly over the heart and precise timing to the vulnerable phase of repolarization just prior to the T wave peak. This is within a narrow 15–30 ms interval, representing only 1% of the cardiac cycle (Link *et al.* 1998, 2001). Survival after commotio cordis is estimated at 15% and is most likely when there is prompt cardiopulmonary resuscitation and defibrillation (Maron *et al.* 2002).

Strategies to prevent commotio cordis have been suggested (36th Bethesda Conference 2005). These include age-appropriate safety baseballs for children up to 13 years of age as well as automated external defibrillators available within 5 min at sporting events. There is insufficient evidence to recommend chest wall barriers for participants in sports. Survivors of commotio cordis should undergo a thorough cardiac evaluation, including ambulatory Holter monitoring and echocardiogram, whereas standard electrophysiologic testing and implantable cardioverter-defibrillator are not recommended (36th Bethesda Conference 2005). Eligibility for returning to competitive sports in survivors is at present a decision of individual judgment, because there are no data with regard to the susceptibility for recurrent events.

RECREATIONAL DRUGS AND PERFORMANCE-ENHANCING SUBSTANCES

SCD, non-fatal stroke, and acute myocardial infarction (MI) in trained athletes have been associated with the abuse of cocaine, anabolic steroids as well as dietary and nutritional supplements (Lange & Hills 2001; Samenuk *et al.* 2002; Valli & Giardina 2002). Dietary supplements, such as *ma juang*, a herbal source of ephedrine, a potentially arrhythmogenic cardiac stimulant (Samenuk *et al.* 2002, Valli & Giardina 2002), are often taken to enhance athletic performance. Causal linkage of dietary supplements and cardiovascular events is often inferential, based on the close temporal relation of taking the compound and the occurrence of such events in otherwise healthy individuals.

Cardiovascular diseases in athletes and eligibility recommendations

The standard evaluation of potential athletes with known cardiovascular disease includes a medical history emphasizing exercise-related symptoms, a physical examination, echocardiography, and an exercise stress test. The need for additional studies depends on the clinical situation.

Guidelines for determining athletic eligibility among children and adults with diagnosed cardiovascular disease have been expertly presented in the 36th Bethesda Conference (2005). These guidelines are necessarily conservative because they serve as a standard of practice. Physicians can use these guidelines to be more or less restrictive of athletic participation given the individual's disease severity, patient preference, the physician's appreciation of risk, and the patient and family's willingness to tolerate that risk.

Cardiomyopathies, myocarditis, and Marfan syndrome

HYPERTROPHIC CARDIOMYOPATHY

Hypertrophic cardiomyopathy (HCM) is the most common cardiovascular cause of death in young athletes according to autopsy-based surveys in the USA. HCM accounts for 26–56% of exercise-related SCDs (Maron 2003; Maron et al. 1986a; Maron et al. 1996a; Van Camp et al. 1995). HCM is characterized initially by an asymmetrically or symmetrically hypertrophied and non-dilated left ventricle, but in late stages may be indistinguishable from dilated cardiomyopahy. HCM has an incidence of 0.2% in the general population and has heterogeneous clinical, morphologic, and genetic expression (Maron et al. 2003).

While HCM may be suspected during preparticipation sports evaluations by the prior occurrence of exertional syncope, family history of the disease or premature cardiac death, or by a loud systolic heart murmur, these clinical features are relatively uncommon among all individuals with the disease. Detection of HCM by standard screening is unreli-

able because most patients have the non-obstructive form of this disease, characteristically expressed by only a soft heart murmur or none at all (Maron et al. 1996b). One retrospective study showed that potentially lethal cardiovascular abnormalities, including HCM, were suspected by the standard preparticipation history and physical examination in only 3% of young competitive athletes (Maron et al. 1996a). Even when echocardiography is employed in screening athletes for HCM, false negatives may occur when encountering young individuals with incomplete phenotypic expression of the disease (Maron et al. 1986b; Lange & Hills 2001).

Another major challenge in evaluating athletes is the distinction between physiologic LVH caused by athletic heart syndrome from a relatively mild morphologic expression of HCM. This differentiation has significant implications, because proper identification of HCM in an athlete may be the basis for disqualification from competition (36th Bethesda Conference 2005). Criteria that favor the diagnosis of HCM in an athlete with LVH include (Fig. 6.2; Maron et al. 1995):

• Unusual patterns of LVH, including heterogeneous distribution of hypertrophy with prominent asymmetry and adjacent regions of markedly different thicknesses as well as patterns in which the anterior ventricular septum is spared from the hypertrophic process with predominant thickening of the posterior septum or the anterolateral or posterior free wall.
• Non-dilated left ventricle (LV) cavity with end-diastolic dimension less than 45 mm;
• Solitary left atrial enlargement;
• Abnormal Doppler diastolic indexes of left ventricular filling and relaxation;
• Female gender, based on the fact that female athletes rarely show LV wall thickness more than 12 mm (Pelliccia et al. 1991);
• No regression of LVH with deconditioning;
• Family history or gene mutation for HCM.

The latter criterion is the most specific and promising in providing a definite diagnosis of HCM. The most definitive evidence for the presence of HCM in an athlete with LVH comes from demonstration of disease in a relative. Therefore, in those athletes in

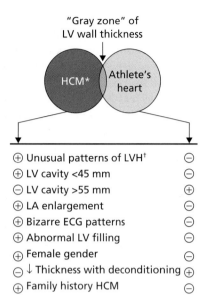

"Gray zone" of
LV wall thickness

HCM*   Athlete's
        heart

⊕ Unusual patterns of LVH†   ⊖
⊕ LV cavity <45 mm   ⊖
⊖ LV cavity >55 mm   ⊕
⊕ LA enlargement   ⊖
⊕ Bizarre ECG patterns   ⊖
⊕ Abnormal LV filling   ⊖
⊕ Female gender   ⊖
⊖ ↓ Thickness with deconditioning ⊕
⊕ Family history HCM   ⊖

Fig. 6.2 Criteria used to distinguish hypertrophic cardiomyopathy (HCM) from athlete's heart when the l eft ventricular (LV) wall thickness is within the shaded gray zone of overlap, consistent with both diagnoses. Reproduced from Maron *et al.* 1995 with permission. ECG, electrocardiogram; LA, left atrium; LVH, left ventricular hypertrophy.

whom the distinction between HCM and athletic heart syndrome cannot be achieved with certainty, one potential approach would be echocardiographic screening of family members. However, absence of HCM in a family does not exclude the diagnosis, because the disease may occur in a "sporadic" pattern (Maron *et al.* 1995). Recent advances in the understanding of the genetic alterations responsible for HCM raise the possibility of DNA diagnosis in athletes suspected of having this disease. The genetic abnormalities that cause HCM, however, are greatly heterogeneous. Mutations of at least 10 different genes can bring about HCM. This substantial genetic heterogeneity of the disease makes it extremely difficult, expensive, and time-consuming at present to use the techniques of molecular biology for the purpose of resolving clinically the differential diagnosis between athlete's heart and HCM (Maron *et al.* 1995).

SCD can occur as the initial disease presentation of HCM, most frequently in asymptomatic or mildly symptomatic young people less than 30–35 years old and often during periods of strenuous exertion. Complex ventricular tachyarrhythmias originating from an electrically unstable myocardial substrate are the most common mechanism by which SCD occurs in HCM. Although there are substantial available data on the stratification of SCD risk, precise identification of all individual high-risk patients by clinical markers is not completely resolved. Nevertheless, it is possible to identify most high-risk patients by the following non-invasive clinical markers (Maron *et al.* 2003):

1 Prior cardiac arrest or spontaneously occurring and sustained VT;

2 Family history of a premature HCM-related SCD;

3 Identification of a high-risk genotype;

4 Exertional or recurrent syncope;

5 Non-sustained VT (of three beats or more and of at least 120 beats·min^{-1}) evident on ambulatory (Holter) ECG;

6 Abnormal (attenuated or hypotensive) blood pressure response during upright exercise; and

7 Extreme LVH ≥30 mm.

These criteria have been used to identify patients with HCM at high risk who would be considered for primary prevention of SCD with prophylactic implantation of cardioverter-defibrillator (Maron *et al.* 2000). However, any extrapolation of risk assessment to highly trained competitive athletes would be very tenuous and this is reflected in the 36th Bethesda Conference (2005) recommendations for athletic eligibility which are necessarily conservative and disqualify athletes with unequivocal or probable diagnosis of HCM from participation in most competitive sports.

With the advances in the availability of preclinical genetic diagnosis of HCM, the clinical significance and natural history of genotype positive–phenotype negative individuals remains unresolved. At present, there are no compelling data available to preclude these patients from competitive sports, particularly in the absence of symptoms or a family history of SCD (36th Bethesda Conference 2005), but each case must be evaluated individually.

ARRHYTMOGENIC RIGHT VENTRICULAR CARDIOMYOPATHY

ARVC is a relatively uncommon cause of SCD in the USA; however, it is the most common cause of SCD in northern Italy (Thiene *et al.* 1988). ARVC is characterized pathologically by fibrofatty replacement primarily of the right ventricle (RV) and clinically by life-threatening ventricular arrhythmias with left bundle branch morphology in apparently healthy young people, elicited by exercise-induced catecholamine discharge (Gemayel *et al.* 2001). The disease has an estimated prevalence of 1 in 5000 individuals and is typically inherited with variable penetrance and incomplete expression (Gemayel *et al.* 2001), whereas an association with myocarditis has also been frequently reported (Bowles *et al.* 2002). Clinical diagnosis is challenging and may be suspected on the basis of familial occurrence, exercise-triggered ventricular tachyarrhythmias and syncope, Twave inversion in right precordial leads (V1–V3), or characteristic epsilon waves on the surface ECG (Fig. 6.3). Echocardiography may demonstrate right ventricular dilatation and dysfunction, and magnetic resonance imaging (MRI)

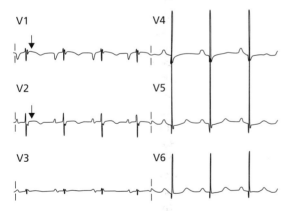

Fig. 6.3 Electrocardiogram (ECG) of an 18-year-old male patient diagnosed with arrhythmogenic right ventricular cardiomyopathy by cardiac angiography and refractory ventricular tachycardia requiring a defibrillator. The ECG is magnified to demonstrate the epsilon waves (arrow). Reproduced from Gemayel *et al.* 2001 with permission.

can sometimes be diagnostic in demonstrating fatty infiltration of the myocardium (Gemayel *et al.* 2001). A definite diagnosis of ARVC requires the histologic finding of transmural fibrofatty replacement of RV myocardium at endomyocardial biopsy. Unfortunately, biopsy is limited by the segmental pattern of the disease and by the fact that the interventricular septum, the area usually biopsied, is rarely involved (McKenna *et al.* 1994).

Treatment is directed to preventing life-threatening cardiac arrhythmias with medications, radiofrequency ablation of the arrhythmogenic focus, and the use of implantable defibrillators. Because of the high risk of exercise-induced SCD in patients with ARVC, athletes with probable or definite diagnosis of the disease should be excluded from vigorous athletic competition, with the possible exception of low intensity sports (36th Bethesda Conference 2005).

MYOCARDITIS

Myocarditis is an inflammatory disease of the myocardium that has been associated with SCD in young athletes (Maron 2003; Maron *et al.* 1996a). The most common cause is acute viral infection by enteroviruses, mainly coxsackie and echoviruses, adenoviruses, or parvoviruses, but myocarditis may also be caused by other infectious agents, such as bacteria, protozoa, and even worms, systemic diseases, drugs, and toxic agents (Feldman & McNamara 2000). The diagnosis may be challenging in the absence of symptoms and may be suggested by ECG abnormalities alone, including heart block, ventricular arrhythmias, or findings mimicking MI or pericarditis (Feldman & McNamara 2000). Using reverse trancriptase polymerase chain reaction assay to amplify the viral genome in endomyocardial biopsy specimens may enhance the diagnostic yield (Pauschinger *et al.* 1999). SCD in myocarditis may be caused by the development of an electrically unstable substrate resulting in ventricular tachyarrhythmias (Vignola *et al.* 1984). Supportive care is the mainstay of therapy of myocarditis.

Athletes with probable or definite evidence of myocarditis should be withdrawn from all competitive sports for 6 months after the onset of clinical manifestations. After this period of time they should be re-evaluated with echocardiographic and/or radionuclide studies at rest and exercise, ambulatory Holter monitoring and repeat 12-lead ECG. If LV function, wall motion, cardiac dimensions, ECG, and serum markers of inflammation return to normal and there are no evident clinical arrhythmias on Holter monitoring, the athlete can resume training and competitive sports (36th Bethesda Conference 2005).

OTHER CARDIOMYOPATHIES

There are a number of other uncommon diseases of the myocardium that may potentially cause SCD in athletes. These include dilated cardiomyopathies, restrictive cardiomyopathies, systemic infiltrative diseases with involvement of the myocardium, such as sarcoidosis, idiopathic left ventricular hypertrophy, and left ventricular non-compaction of the myocardium. Because there are no data regarding the relative risks of athletic activities in patients with these conditions, it is most prudent to exclude athletes with these diseases from highly competitive sports until more information is available (36th Bethesda Conference 2005).

MARFAN SYNDROME

Marfan syndrome is an autosomal dominant disorder caused by mutations in the gene encoding the microfibrillar protein fibrillin-1 (*FBN1*). It has an estimated prevalence of 1 in 5000 in the general population (De Paepe *et al.* 1996). The diagnosis is based largely on clinical criteria as well as on a positive family history for Marfan syndrome, although spontaneous mutations and variable penetrance make the family history somewhat unreliable. Manifestations occur in many systems, involving primarily the ocular, the skeletal, and the cardiovascular system. The ocular abnormalities include ectopia lentis, whereas the skeletal abnormalities include a diverse constellation of findings such as pectus carinatum or excavatum, arm span : height ratio more than 1.05, tall stature, arachnodactyly,

joint hyperextensibility, and scoliosis (De Paepe *et al.* 1996).

The major risks to an athlete with Marfan syndrome are associated with the cardiovascular abnormalities, which are brought about by the two primary defects: aortic root dilatation and mitral valve prolapse (MVP). Progressive dilatation of the aortic root or descending aorta predisposes to dissection and rupture, whereas MVP with associated mitral regurgitation or LV systolic dysfunction may occasionally predispose to ventricular arrhythmias and sudden death (Yetman *et al.* 2003). The risk of aortic dissection is increased considerably when the greatest diameter of the aorta exceeds 5–5.5 cm and these patients should be referred for elective surgical aortic root reconstruction (Kouchoukos & Dougenis 1997). Prophylactic β-adrenergic blockade is effective in slowing the rate of aortic dilatation and reducing the development of aortic complications in some patients with Marfan syndrome (Shores *et al.* 1994). Weightlifting has been specifically associated with aortic dissection in athletes with cystic medial necrosis (de Virgilio *et al.* 1990). Congenital bicuspid aortic valve has also been associated with ascending aortic root dilatation and dissection, independent of Marfan syndrome (Ferencik & Pape 2003).

Athletes with Marfan syndrome can participate in low and moderate static or low dynamic competitive sports if they do not have aortic root dilatation more than 4 cm, moderate to severe mitral regurgitation, or a history of dissection or SCD in a relative with Marfan syndrome (36th Bethesda Conference 2005). However, these athletes should have an echocardiographic measurement of the aortic root dimension every 6 months. If one of the abovementioned conditions is present or there is chronic dissection of the aorta or prior surgical root reconstruction, athletic participation should be limited to low intensity competitive sports. Additionally, athletes with Marfan syndrome, familial aortic aneurysm dilatation, or congenital bicuspid aortic valve with any degree of ascending aortic enlargement should not participate in sports with a potential for bodily collision (36th Bethesda Conference 2005).

Congenital heart diseases

CONGENITAL CORONARY ARTERY ANOMALIES

The second most common cause of SCD in US athletes is congenital coronary artery anomalies in which the artery arises from the wrong sinus of Valsalva, most commonly the left main coronary artery originating from the right sinus (Basso *et al.* 2000; Davis *et al.* 2001). The mechanism of SCD in these circumstances is probably episodic myocardial ischemia.

Several potential mechanisms have been proposed to explain myocardial ischemia and sudden death in patients with wrong sinus coronary anomalies (Basso *et al.* 2000):

1 Reduced coronary flow because of the acute take-off angle of the artery from the aorta. In this instance, the proximal artery segment could be compromised by the increase in stroke volume and aortic dimensions during exercise.
2 Acute angle take-off with "kinking" of the coronary artery as it arises from the aorta.
3 Flap-like closures of the abnormal slit-like coronary orifice.
4 Compression of the anomalous coronary artery between the aorta and pulmonary trunk during exercise as a result of of increased stroke volume.
5 An intramural course of the proximal coronary segment with proximal compression by the exercise-induced increased stroke volume and aortic diameter.
6 Spasm of the anomalous coronary artery, possibly as a result of endothelial injury.

Coronary artery anomalies may be more frequent than previously thought (Davis *et al.* 2001). Their diagnosis requires a high index of suspicion and this possibility should be considered in a young athlete with a history of angina or syncope, especially if these episodes are triggered by exercise (Basso *et al.* 2000). The anatomy of these malformations can occasionally be defined noninvasively by transthoracic or transesophageal echocardiography, ultrafast computed tomography, or MRI, but coronary arteriography is usually required for the definitive diagnosis (Basso *et al.* 2000).

Timely clinical identification of wrong sinus coronary artery anomalies in young trained athletes is crucial for two reasons. First, these coronary anomalies should result in exclusion from participation in intense competitive sports to reduce the risk of a cardiac event or sudden death (36th Bethesda Conference 2005). Second, and more importantly, wrong sinus coronary artery anomalies are surgically correctable with coronary artery bypass grafting (CABG) as the standard procedure (Thomas *et al.* 1991). Participation in all sports 3 months after successful operation would be permitted for an athlete without ischemia, ventricular tachyarrhythmia, or dysfunction during maximal exercise testing (36th Bethesda Conference 2005).

Another uncommon congenital coronary artery anomaly is myocardial bridging (MB) or tunneled coronary artery, which is defined by myocardial muscle overlying and surrounding a segment of a major epicardial coronary artery, most commonly the left anterior descending. It is characterized by systolic compression of the tunneled segment, which remains clinically insignificant in the vast majority of cases, but occasionally can cause angina and SCD in athletes (Mohlenkamp *et al.* 2002).

Treatment options for clinically significant MB include medical management with beta-blockers or calcium-channel antagonists, surgical myotomy and/or CABG, and stenting of the tunneled segment (Mohlenkamp *et al.* 2002). Athletes with MB and no evidence of myocardial ischemia at rest and during exercise can participate in all competitive sports. If there is evidence of myocardial ischemia or prior MI, participation should be restricted to low intensity competitive sports. The same restriction applies for athletes with MB for the first 6 months after surgical correction or stenting of the MB. After this 6-month period, athletes who remain asymptomatic should undergo exercise testing and if there is no evidence of myocardial ischemia, they may resume participation in all competitive sports (36th Bethesda Conference 2005).

Congenital valvular disease

CONGENITAL PULMONARY VALVE STENOSIS

Pulmonary valve stenosis (PS) is diagnosed clinically by the presence of systolic ejection murmur and variable ejection click and is confirmed by echocardiography. Echocardiography is necessary to classify the PS as mild (Doppler peak gradient <40 mmHg), moderate (40–60 mmHg) or severe (>60 mmHg). Asymptomatic athletes with mild PS and normal RV function can participate in all competitive sports with re-evaluation on an annual basis. Athletes with moderate or severe PS can participate in low intensity competitive sports and should be referred for balloon valvuloplasty or surgical valvotomy. Three months after repair, they should be re-evaluated and can resume unrestricted sports participation if they are asymptomatic, with normal RV function and no or mild residual PS (36th Bethesda Conference 2005).

CONGENITAL AORTIC VALVE STENOSIS

Congenital aortic stenosis (AS) is usually caused by a bicuspid aortic valve and can be classified as mild, moderate, or severe based on the measured mean and peak gradient by Doppler echocardiography. Occasionally, the distinction between moderate and severe AS can be more difficult and require cardiac catheterization (Table 6.5). Common presenting symptoms of AS include exertional dyspnea, fatigue, presyncope or syncope, and chest pain. Additional evaluation with cardiac catheterization and exercise testing is necessary in symptomatic patients. SCD can occur in patients with AS with an incidence of 0.3% per year and the risk increases when there is more than 50 mmHg pressure gradient across the aortic valve (severe AS) as well as in patients with symptoms. Children are less likely to have antecedent symptoms (Gersony *et al.* 1993). Between 20% and 80% of sudden deaths in patients with severe AS occur on physical exertion (Doyle *et al.* 1974; Driscoll & Edwards 1985).

Athletes with mild AS can participate in all competitive sports if they are asymptomatic and they have normal ECG and normal exercise tolerance. Athletes with moderate AS can participate in low static/low to moderate dynamic and moderate static/low to moderate dynamic competitive sports, if there is no evidence of LVH by echocardiography or LV strain by ECG, they are asymptomatic, and have a normal exercise test. Athletes with severe AS should be excluded from competitive sports (36th Bethesda Conference 2005).

Other congenital heart diseases

For athletes with other congenital heart diseases, such as congenital heart defects, coarctation of the aorta, cyanotic congenital heart diseases, tetralogy of Fallot, transposition of great arteries, individualized eligibility recommendations have been proposed by the 36th Bethesda Conference (2005).

Patients with congenital heart defects can develop pulmonary hypertension that might persist after the surgical or interventional repair of the defect. Patients with severe pulmonary hypertension are also at risk for SCD during sports activity. In general, if pulmonary artery systolic pressure is less than 30 mmHg, athletes can participate in all sports, whereas for pressures of over 30 mmHg a

Table 6.5 Definitions of mild, moderate, and severe aortic stenosis (AS). Reproduced with permission from 36th Bethesda Conference (2005).

	Peak-to-peak systolic gradient (catheterization) (mmHg)	Mean echo Doppler gradient (CW) (mmHg)	Peak instantaneous echo Doppler gradient (CW) (mmHg)*
Mild AS	<30	<25	<40
Moderate AS	30–50	25–40	40–70
Severe AS	>50	>40	>70

* Gradients obtained from apical window usually most predictive of catheter gradient.

full evaluation and individual exercise prescription are required for athletic participation (36th Bethesda Conference 2005).

Valvular heart disease

The diagnosis of valvular heart disease usually can be made on the basis of the characteristic murmurs and associated findings on clinical examination. However, in athletes the physiologic cardiac adaptations, mentioned in the athletic heart syndrome, can create innocent flow murmurs that are difficult to differentiate from the abnormal (Thompson 2001). Such "flow murmurs" in young athletes are caused by flow across the pulmonary valve and often vary with respiration. Athletes aged over 50 years, however, may have mild sclerosis of the aortic valve and the resultant flow murmur may be secondary to aortic valve turbulence created from both the physiologic changes of exercise training and the aortic valve sclerosis. The latter murmurs are not necessarily "innocent" and may progress to important aortic stenosis (Thompson 2001).

Evaluating the severity of valvular lesions is much more difficult. In general, the presence of symptoms indicates significant valvular disease and, in most cases, represents an indication for valve replacement or repair (Bonow *et al.* 1998). In the absence of symptoms, severity can be determined from the physical examination and Doppler echocardiography. Cardiac catheterization may also be necessary to evaluate the hemodynamic severity of valvular lesions (Bonow *et al.* 1998). In athletes where secondary gain in denying symptoms might be present, the history may be unreliable, thus the evaluation of the severity of valvular disease becomes more complicated.

Aortic stenosis

The most common etiologies of valvular AS are rheumatic, congenital, and calcific or degenerative, whereas the majority of young athletes with AS have congenital lesions (36th Bethesda Conference 2005). The normal aortic valve orifice is approximately 3–4 cm^2 and must be reduced to one-quarter of normal before causing significant hemodynamic obstruction (Bonow *et al.* 1998). The diagnosis of AS is based on the characteristic physical findings and confirmed by two-dimensional and Doppler echocardiography. Symptoms of angina, syncope, or heart failure occur late in the course of AS and their development is a critical point in the natural history of AS, because the likelihood of SCD increases significantly with the onset of symptoms (Carabello 2002). Physicians must be aware that transient symptoms are likely to be unreported in competitive athletes. Although the risk of SCD is higher in symptomatic patients with severe AS, SCD may be the first presentation in asymptomatic patients, especially the younger subjects with congenital AS (Rosenhek *et al.* 2000).

The severity of AS can be measured by Doppler echocardiography and categorized as mild, moderate, or severe according to the calculated valve area and the estimated mean aortic gradient (Table 6.5). Cardiac catheterization may be required to evaluate the severity of AS if the non-invasive testing and the clinical evaluation are non-conclussive or contradictory (Bonow *et al.* 1998). Coronary angiography is also required before valve surgery to detect the presence of CAD and to exclude coronary anomolies that may complicate the surgery.

Because AS has a variable and unpredictable progression, with an estimated rate of valve narrowing of 0.12 cm$^2 \cdot$year^{-1} (Bonow *et al.* 1998), periodic re-evaluation with physical examination and Doppler echocardiography on an annual basis is warranted. Asymptomatic athletes with mild AS can participate in all competitive sports, but should undergo annual evaluations (36th Bethesda Conference 2005). Athletes with moderate AS are restricted to low intensity competitive sports, although selected athletes can particiapte in moderate dynamic or static sports if they have normal exercise tolerance testing without symptoms, ST segment depression, ventricular tachyarrhythmias, or abnormal blood pressure response. Athletes with severe AS or symptomatic patients with moderate AS should be restricted from competitive athletics (36th Bethesda Conference 2005) and should be considered for aortic valve repalcement (Bonow *et al.* 1998). Indeed, if an athlete has "moderate" Doppler measurements, but symptoms, the Doppler results should be re-evaluated with cardiac catheterization.

Chronic aortic regurgitation

Chronic aortic regurgitation (AR) has multiple etiologies, including congenital bicuspid aortic valve, rheumatic heart disease, infective endocarditis, and aortic root diseases, such as Marfan syndrome, ascending aortic aneurysm, and rheumatoid spondylitis (Bonow et al. 1998). Chronic AR represents a condition of combined volume and pressure overload with a gradual progression from normal to abnormal left ventricular function. There is an initial increase in end-diastolic LV volume and stroke volume to maintain normal ejection fraction, which results in increased systolic wall tension and subsequent concentric and eccentric hypertrophy of the LV. Vasodilator therapy may reduce the hemodynamic burden in these patients, especially when there is coexistent hypertension (Bonow et al. 1998). The majority of patients remain asymptomatic during this compensatory phase, which may last for decades, but ultimately progress to asymtopmatic LV systolic dysfunction and then to the development of symtoms such as dyspnea, angina, and overt heart failure. However, some patients may not develop any sentinel symptoms and present with marked LV enlargement and severe systolic LV dysfunction, although this course is unusual in athletes. SCD is rare among asymptomatic patients and occurs at a rate of less than 0.2% per year (Bonow et al. 1998).

Doppler echocardiography is essential in quantifying the severity of the AR, measuring LV end-diastolic and end-systolic dimensions and LV systolic function, whereas serial comparisons of these parameters are important predictors of prognosis and guide management decisions. The upper limits of normal LV end-diastolic size are often increased in highly trained endurance athletes and this may affect the assessment of LV size in the setting of AR. Radionuclide angiography or cardiac MRI may be helpful if echocardiograms are of suboptimal quality. Athletes with AR should be carefully questioned for exercise-induced signs of cardiac decompensation and exercise testing can be useful in assessing exercise capacity, especially in those with equivocal symptoms (Bonow et al. 1998).

The effects of exercise training in athletes with AR have not been examined. However, dynamic exercise acutely increases the heart rate with shortening of diastole and decreases peripheral vascular resistance resulting in a decrease in the regurgitant volume (Dehmer et al. 1981). In contrast, exercise training induces a lower heart rate at rest, which prolongs diastole and the time available for aortic regurgitation. In addition, patients with significant AR are routinely advised to avoid static exercise, which acutely increases aortic regurgitation by increasing afterload (Thompson 2001).

Asymptomatic athletes with mild or moderate AR, with normal LV systolic function, and normal or mildly increased LV end-diastolic size can participate in all competitive sports (36th Bethesda Conference 2005). In selected cases, athletes with AR and moderate LV enlargement (LVEDD = 60–65 mm) can engage in low or moderate static and low, moderate, or high dynamic sports if exercise tolerance testing to the level of activity achieved in competition demonstrates no symptoms or ventricular arrhythmias. Athletes with severe AR and LV systolic dysfunction and/or LVEDD over 65 mm or those with symtoms, regardless of the grade of the AR, should be restricted from all competitive sports and should be considered as candidates for aortic valve replacement (36th Bethesda Conference 2005).

Mitral stenosis

Mitral stenosis (MS) is almost always a consequence of rheumatic fever. The normal mitral valve area is 4–5 cm^2 and a reduction to 2.5 cm^2 is required for the development of symptoms (Bonow et al. 1998). Severe MS is usually symptomatic precluding athletes from competitive activities, but patients with mild to moderate MS may be asymptomatic even with strenuous exercise. Exercise increases the heart rate and decreases the ventricular diastolic filling time with a subsequent increase in left atrial, pulmonary capillary wedge, and pulmonary artery pressures. This produces dyspnea on exertion and, rarely, acute pulmonary edema (Rahimtoola et al.

Table 6.6 Definitions of mild, moderate, and severe mitral stenosis (MS) (36th Bethesda Conference 2005).

	Valve area (cm^2)	Rest pulmonary artery systolic pressure (mmHg)	Exercise pulmonary artery systolic pressure (mmHg)
Mild MS	>1.5	<35	<20
Moderate MS	1.0–1.5	<50	<25
Severe MS	<1.0	>50	>25

2002). A total of 30–40% of patients with MS develop atrial fibrilation which may lead to significant hemodynamic consequences from the loss of atrial contribution to LV filling and the rapid ventricular rate. The presence of atrial fibrillation in MS patients requires anticoagulation therapy to prevent systemic embolization (Bonow *et al.* 1998).

Doppler echocardiography is used to assess the severity of MS, which is classified as mild, moderate, or severe according to the calculated valve area and pulmonary arterial systolic pressure (Table 6.6). When there is a question as to the severity of MS and in athletes with no or equivocal symptoms, exercise stress testing to the level approximating the exercise demands of the specific sport should be performed and pulmonary artery systolic pressure during exercise estimated by Doppler echocardiography (36th Bethesda Conference 2005).

Athletes with mild MS in sinus rhythm with peak pulmonary artery systolic pressure of less than 50 mmHg can participate in all competitive sports. Athletes with moderate MS, either in sinus rhythm or atrial fibrillation, with peak pulmonary artery systolic pressures less than 50 mmHg can participate in low or moderate static or dynamic sports. Athletes with severe MS in either sinus rhythm or atrial fibrillation or those with peak pulmonary artery systolic pressures higher than 50 mmHg should be restricted from all competitive athletics. Patients with MS of any severity in atrial fibrillation or with a history of atrial fibrillation, who require anticoagulation therapy, should not engage in any competitive sports involving the risk of bodily collision or possible trauma (36th Bethesda Conference 2005). Athletes with moderate or severe MS, who are symptomatic on moderate exertion, should be considered for percutaneous valvotomy or open valve repair or replacement if their anatomy

appears unfavorable for the percutaneous approach (Bonow *et al.* 1998).

Chronic mitral regurgitation

In contrast to MS, the etiologies of chronic mitral regurgitation (MR) are various and include mitral valve prolapse, rheumatic heart disease, infective endocarditis, ischemic papillary muscle dysfunction, Marfan syndrome, and dilated cardiomyopathy (Thompson 2001). In chronic severe MR, the increase in LV end-diastolic volume permits an increase in total stroke volume, allowing restoration of forward cardiac output, but sustained volume overload eventually leads to LV systolic dysfunction. Augmented preload and reduced or normal afterload (provided by unloading of the left ventricle into the left atrium) facilitate LV ejection and can mask LV dysfunction. At the same time, the increase in LV and left atrial size allows accommodation of the regurgitant volume at a lower filling pressure. These hemodynamic events result in reduced forward output and pulmonary congestion. However, the still favorable loading conditions often maintain ejection fraction in the low normal range (50–60%) despite the presence of significant muscle dysfunction. Therefore, patients with chronic MR should be followed by serial echocardiograms. A decrease in ejection fraction and/or an increase in end-systolic volume with time are helpful markers of declining LV function. Correction of MR should occur before advanced LV decompensation (Bonow *et al.* 1998).

The severity of chronic MR can be assessed non-invasively by two-dimensional and Doppler echocardiography. Various measures of the severity of MR have been described (Zoghbi *et al.* 2003), but generally the LV end-diastolic volume reflects the severity of chronic MR. However, in endurance athletes the upper limit of normal LV size may be increased as part of the athletic heart syndrome. Nevertheless, an LV end-diastolic dimension of more than 60 mm often represents the effects of volume overload secondary to valvular disease, rather than a physiologic adaptation to exercise training (36th Bethesda Conference 2005). An exercise echocardiographic study may be especially helpful in athletes with possible symptoms and mild to moderate MR at rest. In general, exercise produces no significant change or a mild decrease in the regurgitant jet, because of reduced systemic vascular resistance. However, increases in heart rate and blood pressure, brought about especially with static exercise, can increase the regurgitant volume with a subsequent increase in pulmonary pressures during exercise and the development of symptoms (Thompson 2001).

Athletes with mild to moderate MR, who are in sinus rhythm and have normal LV size and function as well as normal pulmonary artery pressures, can participate in all competitive sports. If there is mild LV enlargement (<60 mm) in a well-trained endurance athlete that may be secondary to athletic training, the athlete can participate in low or moderate static and low, moderate, or high dynamic competitive sports. Athletes with severe MR and definite LV enlargement (>60 mm), pulmonary hypertension, or any degree of LV systolic dysfunction should be excluded from any competitive sports (36th Bethesda Conference 2005).

Mitral valve prolapse

Mitral valve prolapse (MVP) is the most common form of valvular heart disease, with a prevalence of 2–6% in the general population. It is the most common cause of significant MR in the USA (Bonow et al. 1998). The prognosis of MVP is generally benign. Complications, including severe progressive MR, infective endocarditis, embolic events, atrial and ventricular tachyarrhythmias, occur most commonly in patients with a mitral systolic murmur, thickened redundant mitral valve leaflets, and increased LV or left atrial size, especially in men over 45 years of age (Avierinos et al. 2002; Bonow et al. 1998; Marks et al. 1989). Sudden death is a rare complication of MVP,

occurring in less than 2% of known cases during long-term follow-up, with annual mortality rates of less than 1% per year (Bonow et al. 1998).

The diagnosis is based on clinical findings, including the characteristic mid-systolic click and/or murmur, and can be confirmed by echocardiography. Although there is controversy regarding the need for echocardiographic confirmation in asymptomatic patients with classic auscultatory findings for MVP, it is recommended that all patients with a diagnosed MVP have an initial echocardiographic study for risk stratification, because the abovementioned structural abnormalities have been associated with unfavorable clinical sequelae (Bonow et al. 1998). Because MVP is common in Marfan syndrome, the physical examination of patients with MVP should include a search to identify phenotypic stigmata of this condition.

Athletes with MVP and moderate or severe MR should be managed according to the recommendations for chronic MR, including their eligibility for competitive sports. Athletes with uncomplicated MVP can participate in all competitive sports, provided that there is no prior syncope of arrhythmogenic origin, no supraventricular or ventricular tachyarrhythmias on ambulatory Holter monitoring, no LV systolic dysfunction, no prior embolic event, and no family history of MVP-related SCD. Athletes with MVP and any of the abovementioned conditions should engage only in low intensity competitive sports (36th Bethesda Conference 2005).

Tricuspid regurgitation and tricuspid stenosis

Tricuspid regurgitation (TR) is usually secondary to RV dilatation brought about by pulmonary hypertension (Bonow et al. 1998). Other causes of TR include rheumatic heart disease, infective endocarditis especially associated with intravenous drug use, and congenital abnormalities such as Ebstein anomaly (Thompson 2001). Trivial TR may be detected in up to 76% of athletes by Doppler echocardiography and is not associated with any valvular pathology (Thompson 2001). Severity of the TR and estimation of right atrial and RV pressures can be determined by physical examination and echocardiography.

Athletes with primary TR, regardless of severity, and normal RV function in the absence of markedly elevated right atrial pressure (>20 mmHg) or elevated RV systolic pressure, can participate in all competitive athletics (36th Bethesda Conference 2005).

Tricuspid stensois (TS) is generally caused by rheumatic heart disease and is almost always associated with MS. In these cases, recommendations for sports participation are based on the severity of the MS (36th Bethesda Conference 2005).

Pulmonic regurgitation

Pulmonary regurgitation (PR) is usually caused by congenital idiopathic dilatation of the pulmonary artery and is usually asymptomatic (Bonow *et al.* 1998). Mild PR may be a normal finding on Doppler echocardiography, especially in athletes. No exercise limitations are placed for asymptomatic athletes with PR.

Coronary artery disease

Despite the well-documented beneficial effects of physical activity in the primary and secondary prevention of CAD (Thompson *et al.* 2003), vigorous exercise transiently increases the risk of both acute MI (Giri *et al.* 1999; Mittleman *et al.* 1993; Willich *et al.* 1993) and SCD (Albert *et al.* 2000; Maron *et al.* 1986a; Siscovick *et al.* 1984; Thompson *et al.* 1982), especially among the most habitually sedentary individuals older then 35 years of age. Both plaque rupture and possibly plaque erosion have been implicated as the immediate cause of exercise-related events in adults, although plaque rupture is more frequent (Black *et al.* 1975; Burke *et al.* 1999; Giri *et al.* 1999).

The diagnosis of CAD is established by a history of MI confirmed by conventional diagnostic criteria, history of angina pectoris with objective evidence of inducible ischemia and/or evidence of coronary atherosclerosis demonstrated by coronary imaging studies, such as coronary angiography, magnetic resonance angiography, and electron beam or multi-slice gated computerized tomography.

Athletes with CAD diagnosed by any method, including coronary artery calcification score more than 100, coronary angiography, evidence of inducible ischemia, or prior coronary event, and who are undergoing evaluation for competitive sports, should have their LV function assessed. These athletes should also undergo maximal exercise stress testing to the level of exercise approximating the planned competitive sport, in order to assess their exercise capacity and the presence of provocable myocardial ischemia (36th Bethesda Conference 2005). However, it should be noted that, although standard clinical exercise tests are helpful objective measurements in the evaluation of athletes, they cannot accurately simulate the cardiovascular stress produced by sudden bursts of strenuous exercise or the combination of high dynamic and static exercise required by athletic training and competition.

Based on the above tests, athletes with CAD are risk-stratified into two groups: those with mildly increased risk and those with substantially increased risk (Table 6.7; 36th Bethesda Conference 2005). Athletes with mildly increased risk can participate in low dynamic and low to moderate competitive sports but should avoid intensely competitive situations and should undergo re-evaluation of their risk stratification annually. Athletes with substantially increased risk should be restricted to low intensity competitive sports. Those with recent MI or post-revascularization should be evaluated on an individual basis, but generally they should cease their athletic training and competition until recovery is deemed complete (36th Bethesda Conference 2005). All athletes with CAD should be educated regarding the nature of prodromal symptoms such as cardiac chest pain and dyspnea and instructed to cease athletic activities once these symptoms appear. Additionally, all athletes with diagnosed CAD, regardless of the risk stratification, should be informed that exercise transiently poses some increased risk of exercise-related events once CAD is established. It is also important to emphasize that atherosclerotic risk factors should be aggressively treated in all athletes with atherosclerotic CAD, in order to stabilize coronary lesions and potentially reduce the risk of exercise-related events (36th Bethesda Conference 2005).

Table 6.7 Risk stratification of athletes with coronary artery disease (CAD) (36th Bethesda Conference 2005).

Mildly increased risk	Substantially increased risk
Preserved LV systolic function at rest (LVEF>50%)	Impaired LV systolic function at rest (LVEF <50%)
Normal exercise tolerance for age	Abnormal exercise tolerance for age
Absence of exercise-induced ischemia and exercise-induced or post-exercise complex ventricular arrhythmias	Evidence of exercise-induced myocardial ischemia or complex ventricular arrhythmias
Absence of hemodynamically significant stenosis in any major coronary artery	Hemodynamically significant stenosis of a major coronary artery (>50%)
Successful myocardial revascularization by surgical or percutaneous techniques	

LVEF, left ventricular ejection fraction.

Arrhythmias

Evaluating rhythm disturbances in athletes is important, in order to determine whether a particular arrhythmia predisposes an athlete to sudden death or to symptoms, such as syncope or presyncope, that can precipitate severe injury. This evaluation is often challenging for a variety of reasons. First, arrhythmias are commonly intermittent and it is usually unpredictable when they recur. The athlete may not develop the arrhythmia during each athletic event. Second, factors related to the autonomic nervous system probably have an important role in determining whether an arrhythmia occurs, its rate, and its effect on the hemodynamic response. The autonomic nervous system balance varies greatly between different athletes and within different athletic events. Third, there is a broad spectrum of rhythm disturbances, mainly bradyarrhythmias, that are considered normal in the conditioned athlete because of their increased vagal tone.

The search for significant structural heart disease is an important element in evaluating athletes with arrhythmias, because the presence of any structural abnormality or an inherited channelopathy, such as congenital long QT syndrome, greatly increases the risk of an arrhythmia-induced SCD during exercise. An assessment of cardiac function is also essential, because right or left ventricular dysfunction is an additional important predictor of arrhythmic death. Athletes with significant cardiac arrhythmias should

be queried about the presence of exertion-related symptoms, including palpitations, syncope, or presyncope. The evaluation of arrhythmias in athletes should include an echocardiogram, an exercise test, and in some cases event recording or ambulatory Holter ECG recording during the specific type of exercise being considered, if possible. The latter is important because conventional exercise testing cannot replicate the conditions produced by actively participating in the sport. In selected cases, an electrophysiologic study may be necessary to diagnose, manage, and risk stratify arrhythmias in athletes. All athletes with arrhythmias who are permitted to participate in athletics should be re-evaluated at 6–12-month intervals, to determine whether the conditioning process affected the arrhythmia (36th Bethesda Conference 2005).

Syncope

Syncope in athletes is an important symptom that requires a thorough evaluation in order to exclude significant structural heart disease or a primary electrical disorder. Vasovagal syncope is the most common cause of non-exertional and immediately post-exertion syncope in athletes (Colivicchi *et al.* 2004). This is caused by enhanced vagal and reduced sympathetic tone as well as by the large venous capacity secondary to exercise training, all of which contribute to postural hypotension and a positive tilt table response. For this reason, tilt testing in assessing athletes with syncope lacks specificity and requires careful interpretation of the results. Although vasovagal syncope does not restrict an athlete from participation in competitive sports, cardiac pathology must be excluded when syncope occurs during or after exercise.

History and physical examination often determine the etiology of syncope. In inconclusive cases, additional testing in search of arrhythmia or structural heart disease is indicated. Ambulatory ECG recordings, event or loop recorders are used in an attempt to identify any potential arrhythmia and should be performed while recording the ECG during the sport in which the athlete participates, although are often unrevealing. Exercise testing is useful. Echocardiography should be obtained in all patients. Provocative catecholamine testing with epinephrine, procainamide, or isoproterenol may be useful to unmask cases of occult long QT syndrome, Brugada syndrome, or catecholaminergic polymorphic ventricular tachycardia (36th Bethesda Conference 2005). Invasive electrophysiologic testing may be necessary when an arrhythmia is an important consideration in athletes who have underlying cardiac disease, or when no cause for the syncope has been established after other testing has been performed. Athletes with syncope or near-syncope should not participate in sports where the likelihood of even momentary loss of consciousness may be hazardous until the cause has been determined and treated, if necessary (36th Bethesda Conference 2005).

Sinus node rhythm disturbances

Sinus tachycardia and sinus bradycardia appropriate for the clinical situation are considered normal and no further testing or therapy is necessary. As mentioned in the athlete's heart syndrome, sinus bradycardia, sinus arrhythmia, and sinus pauses less than 3 s are frequent in trained athletes mainly as a result of the increased parasympathetic tone at rest (Chapman 1982; Estes *et al.* 2001; Furlan *et al.* 1993; Huston *et al.* 1985; Kenney 1985). Longer symptomatic pauses, sinoatrial exit block, and sick sinus syndrome are considered abnormal (36th

Bethesda Conference 2005). Asymptomatic athletes with no structural heart disease in whom the bradycardic rate is increased appropriately by physical activity can participate in all competitive sports. Symptomatic athletes with tachycardia/bradycardia syndrome or inappropriate sinus tachycardia should be treated and, if there is no structural heart disease and they remain asymptomatic for 2–3 months, can resume participation in all competitive sports (36th Bethesda Conference 2005).

Premature atrial complexes

Premature atrial contractions (PACs) are frequent in endurance athletes. These are usually asymptomatic, but may be symptomatic and present as palpitations or lightheadedness. When symptomatic, beta-blocker therapy could be used as first-line treatment. In the absence of symptoms and without any structural heart disease, no further evaluation other than a 12-lead ECG is required. PACs do not require treatment or restriction from athletic competition (36th Bethesda Conference 2005).

Atrial flutter, atrial fibrillation, and atrial tachycardia (in the absence of Wolff–Parkinson–White syndrome)

In the absence of Wolff–Parkinson–White (WPW) syndrome or an acute illness, sustained atrial flutter is uncommon in athletes without structural heart disease. A full cardiac evaluation, including an echocardiogram, should be performed. Because there is a potential for 1:1 atrioventricular (AV) nodal conduction and very rapid ventricular rates, particularly when there is sympathetic stimulation during exertion, an exercise ECG stress test during treatment is essential. An electrophysiologic study may be necessary for patients with paroxysmal atrial flutter (36th Bethesda Conference 2005).

Atrial fibrillation (AF) is a common arrhythmia in the general population and especially among endurance athletes. Among 1160 individuals with AF, 70 (6%) had no evidence of heart disease, so-called "lone AF," and 32 of these were endurance athletes (Mont *et al.* 2002). The onset of AF in endurance athletes is often during sleep or postprandially, consistent with the concept that increased vagal tone from these activities and exercise training contribute to its onset (Mont *et al.* 2002). AF in young, healthy endurance athletes is often transient and requires no treatment (Furlanello *et al.* 1998). In older athletes, hypertension and CAD are common underlying conditions.

Regardless of the age of the athlete, echocardiography should be performed to exclude structural heart disease. If the rhythm is persistent, an exercise test should be performed to determine the ventricular rate response during physical activity using an exercise stimulus comparable to the intended sport. For some patients with paroxysmal AF, induction of the arrhythmia with electrophysiologic studies may be necessary (36th Bethesda Conference 2005).

The 36th Bethesda Conference eligibility recommendations for competitive athletes are similar for subjects with atrial flutter, atrial fibrillation, or atrial tachycardia (36th Bethesda Conference 2005). Asymptomatic athletes without structural heart disease who maintain a ventricular rate that responds appropriately to the level of activity, while receiving no therapy or on therapy with an AV nodal blocking agent, can participate in all competitive sports. However, in some competitive athletics the use of beta-blockers is prohibited. Athletes with structural heart disease and an appropriate ventricular rate response to exercise can participate in athletics consistent with the limitations of the structural heart disease and the potential need for anticoagulation therapy. If anticoagulation therapy is required, participation in sports with a danger of body collision should be restricted. In addition, athletes without structural heart disease, who have elimination of the atrial fibrillation or flutter by an ablation technique, may participate in all competitive sports after 4 weeks without recurrence or after confirmed non-inducibility by an electrophysiologic study.

Supraventricular tachycardia

Supraventricular tachycardia (SVT) in the athlete is generally caused by AV nodal re-entry tachycardia (AVNRT), occurring with a paroxysmal pattern, and may cause symptoms ranging from mild palpitations to syncope, depending on a number of factors, including the rate of the tachycardia and the blood pressure. Less frequently, SVT may occur as a result of AV re-entry over a concealed accessory pathway. Occasionally, stress testing or ambulatory ECG monitoring may be helpful to identify the rate response of the SVT during exercise. If the exercise does not induce the SVT and the diagnosis cannot be made with certainty, invasive electrophysiologic studies may be warranted to define the mechanism of the tachycardia.

Asymptomatic athletes without structural heart disease who have AVNRT reproducibly provoked by exercise, in whom prevention of the arrhythmia by therapy has been demonstrated by appropriate testing, can participate in all competitive sports. Athletes who do not have exercise-induced AVNRT, but who experience sporadic recurrences, can participate in all sports after an adequate response to therapy has been demonstrated. Asymptomatic patients, who have brief and self-limited episodes of 5–15 s that do not increase in duration during exercise, can participate in all sports (36th Bethesda Conference 2005). Athletes who have syncope, presyncope, palpitations, or other manifestations of hemodynamic impairment secondary to the AVNRT or who have structural heart disease in addition to the arrhythmia should not participate in any competitive sports until they have been adequately treated and have had no recurrence for 2–4 weeks. At that time, participation in low intensity competitive sports is permitted (36th Bethesda Conference 2005). With success rates over 95% and complication rates less than 1%, radiofrequency ablation is the preferred initial curative approach in symptomatic subjects. Athletes can resume high intensity competitive athletics immediately after electrophysiologically proven non-inducibility of the arrhythmia or no recurrence of arrhythmia for 2–4 weeks after the procedure (36th Bethesda Conference 2005).

Wolff–Parkinson–White syndrome

Wolff–Parkinson–White syndrome is a condition found in 3 out of 1000 individuals that manifests on the surface ECG with a short PR interval (<0.12 s) and a delta wave, represented as a slurred upstroke

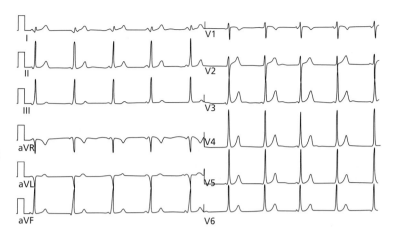

Fig. 6.4 Wolff–Parkinson–White (WPW) pattern. Note the short PR and the subtle "delta" wave at the beginning of the QRS complexes. The delta wave represents early activation of the ventricles in the region where the AV bypass tract inserts. The rest of the QRS is derived from the normal activation sequence using the bundle branches. Reproduced from http://www.ecglibrary.com/wpw.html with permission.

on the QRS complex from early activation of the ventricular myocardium (Fig. 6.4).

This syndrome is clinically associated with tachyarrhythmias, including AV re-entrant tachycardia (AVRT) and less frequently AF or rarely ventricular fibrillation. Sudden cardiac death from ventricular fibrillation in patients with WPW is rare and estimated at 1 in 1000 patients per year (Estes *et al.* 2001). This complication appears to be confined to patients with AF or atrial flutter and rapid conduction to the ventricles over a bypass tract, which has a particularly short functional refractory period (Estes *et al.* 2001).

The evaluation should include an exercise test and an echocardiogram to exclude associated structural heart disease. Occasionally, ambulatory ECG recording during athletic activity may be helpful. Athletes with WPW pattern and symptoms of palpitations, presyncope, or syncope, or with documented arrhythmia should undergo invasive electrophysiologic testing to assess the refractory period of the accessory connection, the minimum RR interval between pre-excited complexes in AF and the number of accessory pathways (36th Bethesda Conference 2005). Individuals with multiple accessory pathways or ventricular rates more than 240 beats·min⁻¹ should be considered for catheter ablation of the accessory pathway, because they are at higher risk for SCD (Pappone *et al.* 2003b).

The evaluation of the athlete with asymptomatic WPW remains controversial and many experts recommend observation without restriction from athletic participation because the risk of SCD is very low (Munger *et al.* 1993). The presence of an accessory AV nodal pathway and the WPW ECG pattern is also likely to be more frequently detected in endurance athletes than in the general population (Huston *et al.* 1985). The enhanced vagal tone in athletes impedes normal AV conduction thereby permitting appearance of the WPW pattern. Exercise testing is useful in such subjects. If the WPW pattern disappears promptly from one beat to the next, without gradual prolongation of the PR interval, and at a heart rate less than 240 beats·min⁻¹, there is very little chance of rapid AV conduction should AF or flutter occur. Nevertheless, some experts suggest that electrophysiologic studies be performed to risk stratify asymptomatic patients with WPW, because inducible AVRT or AF as well as multiple accessory pathways with short refractory period are associated with an increased risk for arrhythmic events (Pappone *et al.* 2003b). Furthermore, the younger the patient, the less time the patient has had to develop symptoms. Because of the cardiovascular demands of high intensity sports, selected asymptomatic athletes, especially those younger than 20–25 years, should be considered for invasive electrophysiologic testing to characterize the bypass tract properties and establish the presence of a tract that has a short refractory period (36th Bethesda Conference 2005). If such a pathway is found to conduct very rapidly antegrade, radiofrequency catheter ablation should be considered, even in asymptomatic athletes (Pappone *et al.* 2003a).

Asymptomatic athletes with WPW pattern without structural heart disease and without tachycardia, particularly those older than 25 years, can participate in all competitive sports. Those with episodes of AVRT should be treated as previously recommended for AVNRT and should undergo electrical induction of AF to determine the shortest RR interval between two complexes during isoproterenol administration or exercise. If this interval is less than 250 ms, ablation of the accessory pathway is recommended (36th Bethesda Conference 2005). Catheter ablation is also recommended for athletes with episodes of atrial flutter/fibrillation or near-syncope whose maximal ventricular rate at rest (without therapy), as a result of conduction over the accessory pathway, exceeds 240 beats·min^{-1}. After successful catheter ablation of the accessory pathway, asymptomatic athletes without structural heart disease, with normal AV conduction, can resume athletic participation in all competitive sports in several days if there is no inducible arrhythmia in follow-up electrophysiologic study, or in 2–4 weeks if there is no spontaneous recurrence of arrhythmia (36th Bethesda Conference 2005).

Premature ventricular complexes

Premature ventricular contractions (PVCs) and occasionally short "runs" of non-sustained ventricular tachycardia are common in trained athletes and are usually unassociated with underlying cardiovascular abnormalities. Such ventricular arrhythmias, if not associated with cardiovascular abnormalities, do not portend adverse clinical events, appear to be an expression of athlete's heart syndrome, and probably do not, per se, justify a disqualification from competitive sports (Biffi *et al.* 2002, 2004).

Evaluation of the athlete with PVCs should include an echocardiogram to exclude structural heart disease. An exercise stress test and a 24-h ECG recording are also helpful to determine if an increase in the number of PVCs or complex ventricular arrhythmias occurs during exercise, which would necessitate further evaluation to rule out otherwise undetected abnormalities, including occult CAD, congenital coronary anomlalies, ARVC, or catecholaminergic polymorphic ventricular tachycardia (CPVT), or cardiomyopathy (36th Bethesda Conference 2005).

Asymptomatic athletes without structural heart disease, who have PVCs at rest and during exercise, can participate in all competitive sports. If the PVCs increase in frequency during exercise and become symptomatic, participation should be restricted to low intenity dynamic/static sports. Similarly, athletes with structural heart disease and PVCs can participate only in low intensity dynamic/static competitive sports (36th Bethesda Conference 2005).

Ventricular tachycardia

Most individuals who present with sustained or non-sustained symptomatic monomorphic or polymorphic ventricular tachycardia (VT) have underlying structural heart disease. Because these arrhythmias are potentially life-threatening, further evaluation is essential and includes 24-h ambulatory monitoring, exercise testing, echocardiography, cardiac catheterization, and electrophysiologic testing to exclude structural heart disease and establish the mechanism and location of the VT.

Athletes without structural heart disease, who have monomorphic non-sustained (defined as less than 30 s in duration) or sustained VT that can be localized to a specific site in the heart, are candidates for catheter ablation (36th Bethesda Conference 2005). Following successful ablation, if electrophysiologic testing with or without isoproterenol does not induce VT, all competitive sports are permitted within 2–4 weeks. For those athletes who choose pharamacologic suppression of the VT, athletic participation should be restricted for at least 2–3 months after the last VT episode. If there are no clinical recurrences, no structural heart disease, and the VT is not inducible by exercise, exercise testing, or electrophysiologic study, all competitive sports should be permitted. Athletes without structural heart disease who have brief episodes of non-sustained monomorphic VT (generally 10 consecutive beats), with rates less than 150 beats·min^{-1}, do not appear to be at increased risk for sudden death. If exercise testing or ambulatory monitoring during the specific competitive sport demonstrates suppression of the VT or no significant worsening compared to baseline, participation in all competitive sports is permitted. Athletes with structural heart disease and sustained or non-sustained VT should not participate in moderate and high intensity competition, regardless of whether or not the VT is suppressed. Only low intensity competitive sports are permitted.

Ventricular flutter and ventricular fibrillation

Athletes who have experienced ventricular flutter or fibrillation or are cardiac arrest survivors, regardless of the presence or absence of structural heart disease, cannot participate in any moderate or high intensity competitive sports and are generally treated with implantable cardioverter defibrillators (ICDs). Athletes with ICDs who have no episodes of ventricular flutter or fibrillation for 6 months with treatment may engage in low intensity competitive sports (36th Bethesda Conference 2005).

Conduction abnormalities

As mentioned in the athlete's heart syndrome, first and type I second degree AV block are common in trained athletes secondary to the increased vagal tone at rest (Estes *et al.* 2001; Huston *et al.* 1985). These conduction abnormalities resolve during exercise with the subsequent withdrawal of vagal tone and the increased sympathetic drive as well as after detraining (Estes *et al.* 2001). Asymptomatic athletes with a structurally normal heart and no worsening of the first or type I second degree AV block with exercise can participate in all competitive sports. If the AV block appears or worsens with exercise or during recovery, further evaluation and possible pacemaker therapy is indicated and restriction to low intensity competitive sports is recommended (36th Bethesda Conference 2005).

In contrast, type II second degree AV block and complete heart block are rare in trained athletes and should be considered a potential marker for underlying cardiovascular disease. Generally, athletes with type II second degree or complete heart block should be treated with permanent pacing before any athletic activity. Athletes with a pacemaker are restricted to those athletic activities in which there is no danger of bodily collision, because trauma may damage the pacemaker system (36th Bethesda Conference 2005).

Intraventricular conduction delays

Incomplete RBBB is the most common form of intraventricular conduction delay and has been noted in up to 51% of athletes in some series (Estes *et al.* 2001). The physiologic basis for incomplete RBBB in the athlete remains unknown, but it may represent right ventricular overload rather than true delayed conduction through the right bundle (Chapman 1982). Asymptomatic athletes with complete or incomplete RBBB, who do not develop AV block or arrhythmias with exercise, can participate in all competitive sports (36th Bethesda Conference 2005).

In contrast, athletes with left bundle branch block (LBBB) should have an evaluation for underlying cardiac disease. Because of the rarity of acquired LBBB in children and its association with syncope from presumed paroxysmal AV block, an invasive electrophysiologic study should be considered in young athletes. Adult athletes with LBBB should follow the same recommendations for participation in sports as for RBBB. Young athletes with normal His-ventricular (HV) interval and normal AV conduction response to pacing can participate in all competitive sports consistent with their cardiac status. Those with abnormal AV conduction, determined by an HV interval greater than 90 ms or a His–Purkinje block, should have pacemaker implantation and avoid sports with danger of bodily collision (36th Bethesda Conference 2005).

Inherited channelopathies and arrhythmia syndromes

LONG QT SYNDROME

Long QT syndrome (LQTS) is a heterogeneous genetic disorder affecting ionic channels of myocardial cells. It is associated with increased risk of ventricular arrhythmias and particularly torsade de pointes, a rapid polymorhic VT that can degenerate into ventricular fibrillation. The diagnosis of congenital LQTS remains complex, because there is debate as to the upper normal limit of corrected QT interval (QTc) and frequent genotype positive–phenotype negative cases with normal QTc intervals. In general, a QTc interval of 470 ms or more in males and 480 ms or more in females requires further investigation as to the presence of congenital or acquired LQTS, and a QTc of 500 ms or more in a patient with LQTS is considered high risk for a significant arrhytmia (Priori *et al.* 2003). A diagnosis of LQTS should be based not only on the QTc interval, but also on history of symptoms, family history, and typical ECG changes (abnormal T waves and T wave alternans). In addition, genetic testing for the five most common forms of congenital LQTS (of the total of seven identified to date) is now available as a commercial diagnostic test (Priori *et al.* 2003).

Physical exertion, particularly swimming, appears to be a common trigger for ventricular arrhythmias in LQTS-1, whereas auditory or emotional triggers are common in LQTS-2. Patients with LQTS-3 may be at increased risk at rest and inactivity (Schwartz *et al.* 2001). Patients with a history of cardiac arrest or suspected LQTS-related syncope, regardless of QTc or underlying genotype, as well as patients with baseline QTc prolongation more than 470 ms in males and more than 480 ms in females, should be restricted to low intensity competitive sports. Asymptomatic athletes with genotype positive–phenotype negative LQTS may be allowed to participate in competitive sports, with the exception of LQTS-1 genotype positive–phenotype negative individuals, who should refrain from competitive swimming (36th Bethesda Conference 2005).

SHORT QT SYNDROME

Short QT syndrome (SQTS) is a novel hereditary channelopathy defined as QTc less than 300 ms, which has been associated with malignant VTs and SCD in young individuals (Brugada *et al.* 2004). Until the phenotype of SQTS is better understood, it is recommended that athletes with SQTS engage only in low intensity athletic activities (36th Bethesda Conference 2005).

CATECHOLAMINERGIC POLYMORPHIC VENTRICULAR TACHYCARDIA

CPVT is characterized by exercise or catecholamine-induced polymorphic ventricular tachyarrhythmias and is associated with an increased risk of SCD (Sumitomo *et al.* 2003). Symptomatic patients diagnosed with CPVT should be treated with an ICD and restricted from all competitive sports with the possible exception of low intensity competitive sports. The same restrictions apply for asymptomatic patients detected as part of familial screening with exercise- or isoproterenol-induced VT (36th Bethesda Conference 2005).

BRUGADA SYNDROME

Brugada syndrome is associated with a specific ECG pattern, including RBBB morphology with an accentuated J wave and ST segment elevation in leads V1–V3, often followed by a negative T wave. The syndrome is related to life-threatening ventricular arrhythmias and SCD, typically during sleep (Brugada & Brugada 1992). Individuals with Brugada syndrome and no previous cardiac arrests may have an increased risk of SCD if they have inducible ventricular arrhythmias and a previous history of syncope (Brugada *et al.* 2003). Hyperthermia can potentially unmask the Brugada ECG pattern and cause fever-induced polymorphic ventricular tachycardia. Athletes with diagnosed Brugada syndrome should be restricted to low intensity competitive sports, although a clear association between exercise and SCD has not been established (36th Bethesda Conference 2005).

Preparticipation screening in young competitive athletes

The ultimate objective of preparticipation screening in athletes is the identification of cardiovascular abnormalities that can progress and impose a risk of SCD. The extent of screening efforts is under ongoing debate because of cost–efficiency considerations, practical limitations and the awareness that zero-risk is not achievable in competitive sports. Furthermore, the prevalence of occult cardiac diseases among athletes is low (Maron *et al.* 1996b).

The American Heart Association (AHA) has issued a medical and scientific statement on the cardiovascular preparticipation screening of competitive athletes (Maron *et al.* 1996b). This document recommends a personal and family history and a physical examination before high school participation, with the examination repeated at least every 4 years (Maron *et al.* 1998c). This statement does not advocate routine echocardiography or ECG because of the high probability of false-positive test results and the cost of this requirement. However, a recent consensus statement from the European Society of Cardiology (ESC) includes 12-lead ECG in the recommended protocol of preparticipation screening (Corrado *et al.* 2005), a recommendation that was adopted by the International Olympic Committee Medical Commission (International Olympic Committee 2004). According to the ESC, the addition of 12-lead ECG has the potential to enhance the sensitivity of the screening process for detection of cardiovascular diseases with risk of sudden death (Corrado *et al.* 2005). For example, the ECG is abnormal in up to 75–95% of patients with HCM, and often before the appearance of hypertrophy (Maron *et al.* 2003). The ECG may also identify many individuals with the LQTS, Brugada syndrome, and other inherited syndromes associated with ventricular arrhythmias and may raise the suspicion of ARVC and myocarditis (Corrado *et al.* 2005). However, the increase in sensitivity by implementing routine 12-lead ECG in the initial preparticipation screening should be balanced against the significant potential socioeconomic impact and the reduction in specificity.

The addition of other non-invasive diagnostic tests to the screening process in young athletes also has the potential to enhance the detection of certain cardiovascular defects. For example, two-dimensional echocardiography is the principal diagnostic tool for the recognition of HCM by demonstrating otherwise unexplained asymmetric LV wall thickening of more than 15 mm. However, any LV wall thickness is theoretically compatible with the presence of a mutant HCM gene (Maron *et al.* 2003). Echocardiography would also be expected to detect congenital structural abnormalities, such as valvular heart disease, aortic root dilatation, and mitral valve prolapse in Marfan syndrome, and LV dysfunction and enlargement. However, even such diagnostic testing cannot itself guarantee identification of all important lesions (i.e., congenital coronary artery anomalies or ARVC; Maron *et al.* 1996b). Thus, cost-efficiency and practical issues are important when assessing the feasibility of screening large athletic populations.

Preparticipation history and cardiac examination of competitive athletes

The AHA consensus recommendations for the preparticipation cardiac examination include a medical history inquiring about:

1 Exertional symptoms including chest discomfort, syncope, dyspnea, and fatigue;

2 Past cardiac murmurs, hypertension, or cardiac diagnoses; and

3 A family history of sudden death or of any of the conditions known to be associated with sudden death.

The physical examination should include:

1 Brachial artery blood pressure measurement;

2 Precordial auscultation with the athlete supine and standing;

3 Simultaneous palpation of the radial and femoral pulses to exclude coarctation; and

4 An assessment for stigmata of Marfan syndrome.

The athletic screening should be performed by a certified health care worker with the requisite training, medical skills, and background to reliably obtain a detailed cardiovascular history, perform a physical examination, and recognize heart disease.

Despite the limitations of the history and physical examination in detecting CAD in older athletes (over 35 years), a personal history of coronary risk factors or a family history of premature ischemic heart disease may be useful for identifying that disease with screening and therefore should be performed before initiating competitive exercise. In addition, it is prudent to selectively perform medically supervised exercise stress testing in men

Table 6.8 American Heart Association (AHA) Consensus Panel Recommendations for Preparticipation Athletic Screening. (Reproduced from Maron *et al.* 1996b with permission.)

Family history
1 Premature sudden cardiac death
2 Heart disease in surviving relatives younger than 50 years old

Personal history
3 Heart murmur
4 Systemic hypertension
5 Fatigue
6 Syncope/near-syncope
7 Excessive/unexplained exertional dyspnea
8 Exertional chest pain

Physical examination
9 Heart murmur (supine/standing*)
10 Femoral arterial pulses (to exclude coarctation of aorta)
11 Stigmata of Marfan syndrome
12 Brachial blood pressure measurement (sitting)

* In particular, to identify heart murmur consistent with dynamic obstruction to left ventricular outflow.

older than 40 years (and women older than 50) who wish to engage in regular physical training and competitive sports, if the examining physician suspects occult CAD on the basis of risk factors, whether multiple (two or more, other than age and gender), or single but markedly abnormal (Maron *et al.* 1996b). Older athletes should also be warned specifically about prodromal cardiovascular symptoms, such as exertional chest pain and their need for prompt medical attention. Specific recommendations for preparticipation screening and evaluation of masters athletes of over 35 years have been published by the AHA (Table 6.8; Maron *et al.* 2001).

When cardiovascular abnormalities are identified or suspected, the athlete should be referred to a cardiovascular specialist for further evaluation and/or confirmation with additional tests. These guidelines should not create a false sense of security on the part of medical practitioners or the general public, because the standard history and physical examination intrinsically lack the capability to reliably identify many potentially lethal cardiovascular abnormalities. Indeed, it is an unrealistic expectation that large-scale standard athletic screening can

reliably exclude most important cardiac lesions (Maron *et al.* 1996b).

Specific considerations in athletes

In evaluating athletes for cardiac abnormalities, a strong distinction should be made between abnormalities discovered during screening examinations and those discovered during the evaluation of symptoms. Frequently, screening examinations do not detect real disease, but detect a high frequency of normal variants, common in young healthy subjects as part of the athletic heart syndrome. Physicians frequently overreact to mild abnormalities detected on screening because of legal concerns and the lack of appreciation for the magnitude of changes that can be produced by extreme endurance exercise. However, symptomatic athletes require a very thorough examination. Excluding important cardiac disease in symptomatic athletes may be the most efficient way to prevent exercise-related complications.

In evaluating symptoms it is extremely important to evaluate any possible cardiovascular disease in the context of the athlete's total physical and psychologic situation. Many young competitive athletes face enormous pressure from coaches, parents, and peers. Failure to achieve the desired level of success is extremely stressful on competitors at any age. Young athletes who present with "fainting", for example, may be simply seeking a medical way out of a difficult, stressful situation. It is easier to claim a medical reason for failure than simply not being good enough. We refer to this condition as the "athletic swoon syndrome." Typically, this is a young athlete in an individual sport who competes well when winning, but collapses dramatically when losing, often within sight of the finish line. We do not mean to minimize the importance of this problem. The athlete often needs reassurance both medically and personally in order to place winning and losing in a more healthy perspective. Also, this athletic swoon syndrome must be differentiated from true exercise-induced syncope and from the LQTS. True exercise-induced syncope is a threatening symptom associated with important cardiac disease, and patients with LQTS are occasionally misdiagnosed as having hysterical syncope (Viskin *et al.* 2000).

It is also strongly recommended that individuals who serve as trainers and coaches or who officiate at sporting events learn and update yearly their cardiopulmonary resuscitation skills, and that when financially feasible automatic defibrillators be available in areas where athletes train and compete. Coaches and officials are often present when athletes collapse. If properly trained in resuscitation and the use of automatic defibrillators, they may be able to resuscitate potential victims of exercise-related sudden death. Competency in these skills should be a prerequisite for physical educators, coaches, and sports officials.

Future directions

Molecular biologic approaches have already led to an understanding of the genetic basis for a number of cardiovascular conditions associated with cardiovascular complications during exercise. This evolution may influence the cardiac care of athletes in multiple ways.

First, the genetic basis for hypertrophic cardiomyopathy, arrhythmogenic right ventricular cadiomyopathy, and the closely related Naxos disease, congenital long QT syndromes, catecholaminergic polymorphic ventricular tachycardia, familial atrial fibrillation, and familial dilated cardiomyopathy have all been partially elucidated. There will be an ongoing evolution of molecular biologic techniques and their application to the diagnosis, prevention, and treatment of cardiovascular disease (Maron *et al.* 1998b).

Second, genetics will likely be used to predict which individuals with a disease phenotype are at risk for an exercise-related complication. A classic example is the evolution of molecular genetics in hypertrophic cardiomyopathy, which represents the leading cause of exercise-related deaths among US athletes. High-risk mutant genes for cardiac troponin T have been identified that are associated with increased risk of SCD (Anan *et al.* 1994; Varnava *et al.* 2001; Watkins *et al.* 1995). Consequently, in the future, genetic analysis may be helpful in the risk stratification of athletes with HCM. Before such techniques can be used clinically, however, there will need to be widespread availability of the testing methods, which are now available only for research, as well as careful clinical studies to determine the ability of genetic analysis to predict prognosis.

Third, genetic analysis may help differentiate the presence of cardiovascular disease from the normal physiologic adaptations to physical training. Some athletes appear to experience especially large changes in cardiac dimensions with endurance training. This response is influenced by genetic variants. The angiotensin-converting enzyme (ACE) gene has two common variants. One, referred to as the D or deletion allele, has a 287 base pair deletion, and is associated with higher ACE blood levels than the I or insertion allele. Among military recruits subjected to 10 weeks of intense physical training, echocardiographic changes in LV mass and ECG evidence of LVH were greatest in individuals with the D allele (Montgomery *et al.* 1997). Additional genetic factors influencing the cardiac response to exercise training will undoubtedly be found. Knowledge of such variants may ultimately help in separating athletes with an excessive physiologic response to training from individuals with HCM.

References

36th Bethesda Conference. (2005) Eligibility recommendations for competitive athletes with cardiovascular abnormalities. *Journal of the American College of Cardiology* **45**, 1313–1375.

Albert, C.M., Mittleman, M.A., Chae, C.U., Lee, I.M., Hennekens, C.H. & Manson, J.E. (2000) Triggering of sudden death from cardiac causes by vigorous exertion. *New England Journal of Medicine* **343**, 1355–1361.

Amsterdam, E.A., Hughes, J.L., DeMaria, A.N., Zelis, R. & Mason, D.T. (1974) Indirect assessment of myocardial oxygen consumption in the evaluation of mechanisms and therapy of angina pectoris. *American Journal of Cardiology* **33**, 737–743.

Anan, R., Greve, G., Thierfelder, L., Watkins, H., McKenna, W.J., Solomon, S., *et al.* (1994) Prognostic implications of novel beta cardiac myosin heavy chain gene mutations that cause familial hypertrophic cardiomyopathy. *Journal of Clinical Investigation* **93**, 280–285.

Avierinos, J.F., Gersh, B.J., Melton, L.J. III, Bailey, K.R., Shub, C., Nishimura, R.A., *et al.* (2002) Natural history of asymptomatic mitral valve prolapse in the community. *Circulation* **106**, 1355–1361.

Basso, C., Maron, B.J., Corrado, D. & Thiene, G. (2000) Clinical profile of congenital coronary artery anomalies with origin from the wrong aortic sinus leading to sudden death in young competitive athletes. *Journal of the American College of Cardiology* **35**, 1493–1501.

Biffi, A., Maron, B.J., Verdile, L., Fernando, F., Spataro, A., Marcello, G., *et al.* (2004) Impact of physical deconditioning on ventricular tachyarrhythmias in trained athletes. *Journal of the American College of Cardiology* **44**, 1053–1058.

Biffi, A., Pelliccia, A., Verdile, L., Fernando, F., Spataro, A., Caselli, S., *et al.* (2002) Long-term clinical significance of frequent and complex ventricular tachyarrhythmias in trained athletes. *Journal of the American College of Cardiology* **40**, 446–452.

Billman, G.E. (2002) Aerobic exercise conditioning: a nonpharmacological antiarrhythmic intervention. *Journal of Applied Physiology* **92**, 446–454.

Black, A., Black, M.M. & Gensini, G. (1975) Exertion and acute coronary artery injury. *Angiology* **26**, 759–783.

Blair, S.N. (1993) Evidence for success of exercise in weight loss and control. *Annals of Internal Medicine* **119**, 702–706.

Bonow, R.O., Carabello, B., de Leon, A.C. Jr., Edmunds, L.H. Jr., Fedderly, B.J., Freed, M.D., *et al.* (1998) Guidelines for the management of patients with valvular heart disease: executive summary. A report of the American College of Cardiology/American Heart Association Task Force on Practice Guidelines (Committee on Management of Patients with Valvular Heart Disease). *Circulation* **98**, 1949–1984.

Bowles, N.E., Ni, J., Marcus, F. & Towbin, J.A. (2002) The detection of cardiotropic viruses in the myocardium of patients with arrhythmogenic right ventricular dysplasia/cardiomyopathy. *Journal of the American College of Cardiology* **39**, 892–895.

Brooks, G., Fahey, T.D. & White, T.P. (1996) *Exercise Physiology: Human Bioenergetics and its Applications.* Mayfield Publishing, Mountain View, CA: 281–299.

Brugada, J., Brugada, R. & Brugada, P. (2003) Determinants of sudden cardiac death in individuals with the electrocardiographic pattern of Brugada

syndrome and no previous cardiac arrest. *Circulation* **108**, 3092–3096.

Brugada, P. & Brugada, J. (1992) Right bundle branch block, persistent ST segment elevation and sudden cardiac death: a distinct clinical and electrocardiographic syndrome. A multicenter report. *Journal of the American College of Cardiology* **20**, 1391–1396.

Brugada, R., Hong, K., Dumaine, R., Cordeiro, J., Gaita, F., Borggrefe, M., *et al.* (2004) Sudden death associated with short-QT syndrome linked to mutations in HERG. *Circulation* **109**, 30–35.

Burke, A.P., Farb, A., Malcom, G.T., Liang, Y., Smialek, J.E. & Virmani, R. (1999) Plaque rupture and sudden death related to exertion in men with coronary artery disease. *Journal of the American Medical Association* **281**, 921–926.

Carabello, B.A. (2002) Evaluation and management of patients with aortic stenosis. *Circulation* **105**, 1746–1750.

Chapman, J.H. (1982) Profound sinus bradycardia in the athletic heart syndrome. *Journal of Sports Medicine and Physical Fitness* **22**, 45–48.

Colivicchi, F., Ammirati, F. & Santini, M. (2004) Epidemiology and prognostic implications of syncope in young competing athletes. *European Heart Journal* **25**, 1749–1753.

Corrado, D., Pelliccia, A., Bjornstad, H.H., Vanhees, L., Biffi, A., Borjesson, M., *et al.* (2005) Cardiovascular pre-participation screening of young competitive athletes for prevention of sudden death: proposal for a common European protocol. Consensus Statement of the Study Group of Sport Cardiology of the Working Group of Cardiac Rehabilitation and Exercise Physiology and the Working Group of Myocardial and Pericardial Diseases of the European Society of Cardiology. *European Heart Journal* **26**, 516–524.

Davis, J.A., Cecchin, F., Jones, T.K. & Portman, M.A. (2001) Major coronary artery anomalies in a pediatric population: incidence and clinical importance. *Journal of the American College of Cardiology* **37**, 593–597.

De Paepe, A., Devereux, R.B., Dietz, H.C., Hennekam, R.C. & Pyeritz, R.E. (1996) Revised diagnostic criteria for the Marfan syndrome. *American Journal of Medical Genetics* **62**, 417–426.

de Virgilio, C., Nelson, R.J., Milliken, J., Snyder, R., Chiang, F., MacDonald, W.D., *et al.* (1990) Ascending aortic dissection in weight lifters with cystic medial

degeneration. *Annals of Thoracic Surgery* **49**, 638–642.

Dehmer, G.J., Firth, B.G., Hillis, L.D., Corbett, J.R., Lewis, S.E., Parkey, R.W., *et al.* (1981) Alterations in left ventricular volumes and ejection fraction at rest and during exercise in patients with aortic regulation. *American Journal of Cardiology* **48**, 17–27.

Doyle, E.F., Arumugham, P., Lara, E., Rutkowski, M.R. & Kiely, B. (1974) Sudden death in young patients with congenital aortic stenosis. *Pediatrics* **53**, 481–489.

Driscoll, D.J. & Edwards, W.D. (1985) Sudden unexpected death in children and adolescents. *Journal of the American College of Cardiology* **5** (Supplement), 118B–121B.

Ehsani, A.A., Hagberg, J.M. & Hickson, R.C. (1978) Rapid changes in left ventricular dimensions and mass in response to physical conditioning and deconditioning. *American Journal of Cardiology* **42**, 52–56.

Estes, N.A. III, Link, M.S., Homoud, M. & Wang, P.J. (2001) Electrocardiographic variants and cardiac rhythm and conduction disturbances in the athlete. In: *Exercise and Sports Cardiology* (Thompson, P.D., ed.) McGraw-Hill, NY: 211–232.

Feldman, A.M. & McNamara, D. (2000) Myocarditis. *New England Journal of Medicine* **343**, 1388–1398.

Ferencik, M. & Pape, L.A. (2003) Changes in size of ascending aorta and aortic valve function with time in patients with congenitally bicuspid aortic valves. *American Journal of Cardiology* **92**, 43–46.

Ferguson, C.M., Myers, J. & Froelicher, V.F. (2000) Overview of exercise testing. In: *Exercise and Sports Cardiology* (Thompson, P.D., ed.) McGraw-Hill, NY: 71–109.

Fletcher, G.F., Balady, G.J., Amsterdam, E.A., Chaitman, B., Eckel, R., Fleg, J., *et al.* (2001) Exercise standards for testing and training: a statement for healthcare professionals from the American Heart Association. *Circulation* **104**, 1694–1740.

Furlan, R., Piazza, S., Dell'Orto, S., Gentile, E., Cerutti, S., Pagani, M., *et al.* (1993) Early and late effects of exercise and athletic training on neural mechanisms controlling heart rate. *Cardiovascular Research* **27**, 482–488.

Furlanello, F., Bertoldi, A., Dallago, M., Galassi, A., Fernando, F., Biffi, A., *et al.* (1998) Atrial fibrillation in elite athletes. *Journal of Cardiovascular Electrophysiology* **9** (Supplement), S63–S68.

Gallagher, K.M., Raven, P.B. & Mitchell, J.H. (1999) Classification of sports and athlete's heart. In: *The Athlete and Heart Disease: Diagnosis, Evaluation and Management* (Williams, P.A., ed.) Lippincott Williams & Wilkins, Philadelphia, PA: 9–21.

Gemayel, C., Pelliccia, A. & Thompson, P.D. (2001) Arrhythmogenic right ventricular cardiomyopathy. *Journal of the American College of Cardiology* 38, 1773–1781.

Gersony, W.M., Hayes, C.J., Driscoll, D.J., Keane, J.F., Kidd, L., O'Fallon, W.M., *et al.* (1993) Second natural history study of congenital heart defects: quality of life of patients with aortic stenosis, pulmonary stenosis, or ventricular septal defect. *Circulation* 87 (Supplement), I52–I65.

Giri, S., Thompson, P.D., Kiernan, F.J., Clive, J., Fram, D.B., Mitchel, J.F., *et al.* (1999) Clinical and angiographic characteristics of exertion-related acute myocardial infarction. *Journal of the American Medical Association* 282, 1731–1736.

Gobel, F.L., Norstrom, L.A., Nelson, R.R., Jorgensen, C.R. & Wang, Y. (1978) The rate–pressure product as an index of myocardial oxygen consumption during exercise in patients with angina pectoris. *Circulation* 57, 549–556.

Goldsmith, R.L., Bigger, J.T. Jr., Steinman, R.C. & Fleiss, J.L. (1992) Comparison of 24-hour parasympathetic activity in endurance-trained and untrained young men. *Journal of the American College of Cardiology* 20, 552–558.

Hambrecht, R., Wolf, A., Gielen, S., Linke, A., Hofer, J., Erbs, S., *et al.* (2000) Effect of exercise on coronary endothelial function in patients with coronary artery disease. *New England Journal of Medicine* 342, 454–460.

Huston, T.P., Puffer, J.C. & Rodney, W.M. (1985) The athletic heart syndrome. *New England Journal of Medicine* 313, 24–32.

International Olympic Committee. (2004) Sudden cardiac death in sport. Lausanne Recommendations adopted 10 December 2004. Lausanne, Switzerland. Accessed from http:// www. olympic.org/uk/news/olympic_news/newsletter_full_story_uk.asp?id=1182, August 25, 2005.

Kasapis, C. & Thompson, P.D. (2005) The effects of physical activity on serum C-reactive protein and inflammatory markers: a systematic review. *Journal of the American College of Cardiology* 45, 1563–1569.

Kenney, W.L. (1985) Parasympathetic control of resting heart rate: relationship to aerobic power. *Medicine and Science in Sports and Exercise* 17, 451–455.

Keul, J., Dickhuth, H.H., Simon, G. & Lehmann, M. (1981) Effect of static and dynamic exercise on heart volume, contractility and left ventricular dimensions. *Circulation Research* 48, 162–170.

Kouchoukos, N.T. & Dougenis, D. (1997) Surgery of the thoracic aorta. *New England Journal of Medicine* 336, 1876–1888.

Kraus, W.E., Houmard, J.A., Duscha, B.D., Knetzger, K.J., Wharton, M.B., McCartney, J.S., *et al.* (2002) Effects of the amount and intensity of exercise on plasma lipoproteins. *New England Journal of Medicine* 347, 1483–1492.

Lange, R.A. & Hillis, L.D. (2001) Cardiovascular complications of cocaine use. *New England Journal of Medicine* 345, 351–358.

Lee, K.W. & Lip, G.Y. (2003) Effects of lifestyle on hemostasis, fibrinolysis, and platelet reactivity: a systematic review. *Archives of Internal Medicine* 163, 2368–2392.

Link, M.S., Maron, B.J., VanderBrink, B.A., Takeuchi, M., Pandian, N.G., Wang, P.J., *et al.* (2001) Impact directly over the cardiac silhouette is necessary to produce ventricular fibrillation in an experimental model of commotio cordis. *Journal of the American College of Cardiology* 37, 649–654.

Link, M.S., Wang, P.J., Pandian, N.G., Bharati, S., Udelson, J.E., Lee, M.Y., *et al.* (1998) An experimental model of sudden death due to low-energy chest-wall impact (commotio cordis). *New England Journal of Medicine* 338, 1805–1811.

Longhurst, J.C., Kelly, A.R., Gonyea, W.J. & Mitchell, J.H. (1980) Echocardiographic left ventricular masses in distance runners and weight lifters. *Journal of Applied Physiology* 48, 154–162.

Marks, A.R., Choong, C.Y., Sanfilippo, A.J., Ferre, M. & Weyman, A.E. (1989) Identification of high-risk and low-risk subgroups of patients with mitral-valve prolapse. *New England Journal of Medicine* 320, 1031–1036.

Maron, B.J. (2003) Sudden death in young athletes. *New England Journal of Medicine* 349, 1064–1075.

Maron, B.J., Araujo, C.G., Thompson, P.D., Flatcher, G.F., de Luna, A.B., Fleg, J.L., *et al.* (2001) Recommendations for preparticipation screening and the assessment of cardiovascular disease in masters athletes: an advisory for healthcare professionals from the working groups of the World Heart Federation, the International Federation of Sports Medicine, and the American Heart Association Committee on Exercise, Cardiac Rehabilitation, and Prevention. *Circulation* 103, 327–334.

Maron, B.J., Epstein, S.E. & Roberts, W.C. (1986a) Causes of sudden death in competitive athletes. *Journal of the American College of Cardiology* 7, 204–214.

Maron, B.J., Gohman, T.E. & Aeppli, D. (1998a) Prevalence of sudden cardiac death during competitive sports activities in Minnesota high school athletes. *Journal of the American College of Cardiology* 32, 1881–1884.

Maron, B.J., Gohman, T.E., Kyle, S.B., Este, N.A. III & Link, M.S. (2002) Clinical profile and spectrum of commotio cordis. *JAMA* 287, 1142–1146.

Maron, B.J., McKenna, W.J., Danielson, G.K., Kappenberger, L.J., Kuhn, H.J., Seidman, C.E., *et al.* (2003) American College of Cardiology/European Society of Cardiology clinical expert consensus document on hypertrophic cardiomyopathy. A report of the American College of Cardiology Foundation Task Force on Clinical Expert Consensus Documents and the European Society of Cardiology Committee for Practice Guidelines. *Journal of the American College of Cardiology* 42, 1687–1713.

Maron, B.J., Moller, J.H., Seidman, C.E., Vincent, G.M., Dietz, H.C., Moss, A.J., *et al.* (1998b) Impact of laboratory molecular diagnosis on contemporary diagnostic criteria for genetically transmitted cardiovascular diseases: hypertrophic cardiomyopathy, long-QT syndrome, and Marfan syndrome. A statement for healthcare professionals from the Councils on Clinical Cardiology, Cardiovascular Disease in the Young, and Basic Science, American Heart Association. *Circulation* 98, 1460–1471.

Maron, B.J., Pelliccia, A. & Spirito, P. (1995) Cardiac disease in young trained athletes: insights into methods for distinguishing athlete's heart from structural heart disease, with particular emphasis on hypertrophic cardiomyopathy. *Circulation* 91, 1596–1601.

Maron, B.J., Shen, W.K., Link, M.S., Epstein, A.E., Almguist, A.K., Daubert, J.P., *et al.* (2000) Efficacy of implantable cardioverter-defibrillators for the prevention of sudden death in patients with hypertrophic cardiomyopathy. *New England Journal of Medicine* **342**, 365–373.

Maron, B.J., Shirani, J., Poliac, L.C., Mathenge, R., Roberts, W.C. & Mueller, F.O. (1996a) Sudden death in young competitive athletes: clinical, demographic, and pathological profiles. *Journal of the American Medical Association* **276**, 199–204.

Maron, B.J., Spirito, P., Wesley, Y. & Arce, J. (1986b) Development and progression of left ventricular hypertrophy in children with hypertrophic cardiomyopathy. *New England Journal of Medicine* **315**, 610–614.

Maron, B.J., Thompson, P.D., Puffer, J.C., McGrew, C.A., Strong, W.B., Douglas, P.S., *et al.* (1996b) Cardiovascular preparticipation screening of competitive athletes. A statement for health professionals from the Sudden Death Committee (clinical cardiology) and Congenital Cardiac Defects Committee (cardiovascular disease in the young), American Heart Association. *Circulation* **94**, 850–856.

Maron, B.J., Thompson, P.D., Puffer, J.C., McGrew, C.A., Strong, W.B., Douglas, P.S., *et al.* (1998c) Cardiovascular preparticipation screening of competitive athletes: an addendum to a statement for health care professionals from the Sudden Death Committee (Council on Clinical Cardiology) and the Congenital Cardiac Defects Committee (Council on Cardiovascular Disease in the Young), American Heart Association. *Circulation* **97**, 2294.

Mayer-Davis, E.J., D'Agostino, R. Jr., Karter, A.J., Haffner, S.M., Rewers, M.J., Saad, M., *et al.* (1998) Intensity and amount of physical activity in relation to insulin sensitivity: the Insulin Resistance Atherosclerosis Study. *JAMA* **279**, 669–674.

McKenna, W.J., Thiene, G., Nava, A., Fontaliran, F., Blomstrom-Lundqvist, C., Fontaine, G., *et al.* (1994) Diagnosis of arrhythmogenic right ventricular dysplasia/cardiomyopathy. Task Force of the Working Group Myocardial and Pericardial Disease of the European Society of Cardiology and of the Scientific Council on Cardiomyopathies of the International Society and Federation of Cardiology. *British Heart Journal* **71**, 215–218.

Mitchell, J.H. & Blomqvist, G. (1971) Maximal oxygen uptake. *New England Journal of Medicine* **284**, 1018–1022.

Mitchell, J.H. & Raven, P.B. (1994) Cardiovascular adaptation to physical activity. In: *Physical Activity, Fitness, Health* (Bouchard, C., Shephard, R. & Stephen, T., eds.) International Proceedings and Consensus Statement. Human Kinetics, Champaign, IL: 286–298.

Mittleman, M.A., Maclure, M., Tofler, G.H., Sherwood, J.B., Goldberg, R.J. & Muller, L.E. (1993) Triggering of acute myocardial infarction by heavy physical exertion: protection against triggering by regular exertion. Determinants of Myocardial Infarction Onset Study Investigators. *New England Journal of Medicine* **329**, 1677–1683.

Mohlenkamp, S., Hort, W., Ge, J. & Erbel, R. (2002) Update on myocardial bridging. *Circulation* **106**, 2616–2622.

Mont, L., Sambola, A., Brugada, J., Vacca, M., Marrugat, J., Elosua, R., *et al.* (2002) Long-lasting sport practice and lone atrial fibrillation. *European Heart Journal* **23**, 477–482.

Montgomery, H.E., Clarkson, P., Dollery, C.M., Prasad, K., Losi, M.A., Hemingway, H., *et al.* (1997) Association of angiotensin-converting enzyme gene I/D polymorphism with change in left ventricular mass in response to physical training. *Circulation* **96**, 74.

Munger, T.M., Packer, D.L., Hammill, S.C., Feldman, B.J., Bailey, K.R., Ballard, D.J., *et al.* (1993) A population study of the natural history of Wolff–Parkinson–White syndrome in Olmsted County, Minnesota, 1953–1989. *Circulation* **87**, 866–873.

Niebauer, J., Hambrecht, R., Velich, T., Hauer, K., Marburger, C., Kalberer, B., *et al.* (1997) Attenuated progression of coronary artery disease after 6 years of multifactorial risk intervention: role of physical exercise. *Circulation* **96**, 2534–2541.

Pappone, C., Santinelli, V., Manguso, F., Augello, G., Santinelli, O., Vicedomini, G., *et al.* (2003a) A randomized study of prophylactic catheter ablation in asymptomatic patients with the Wolff–Parkinson–White syndrome. *New England Journal of Medicine* **349**, 1803–1811.

Pappone, C., Santinelli, V., Rosanio, S., Vicedomini, G., Nardi, S., Pappone, A., *et al.* (2003b) Usefulness of invasive electrophysiologic testing to stratify the risk of arrhythmic events in asymptomatic patients with

Wolff–Parkinson–White pattern: results from a large prospective long-term follow-up study. *Journal of the American College of Cardiology* **41**, 239–244.

Pate, R.R., Pratt, M., Blair, S.N., Haskell, W.L., Macera, C.A., Bouchard, C., *et al.* (1995) Physical activity and public health. A recommendation from the Centers for Disease Control and Prevention and the American College of Sports Medicine. *JAMA* **273**, 402–407.

Pauschinger, M., Bowles, N.E., Fuentes-Garcia, F.J., Pham, V., Kuhl, U., Schwimmbeck, P.L., *et al.* (1999) Detection of adenoviral genome in the myocardium of adult patients with idiopathic left ventricular dysfunction. *Circulation* **99**, 1348–1354.

Pelliccia, A., Culasso, F., Di Paolo, F.M. & Maron, B.J. (1999) Physiologic left ventricular cavity dilatation in elite athletes. *Annals of Internal Medicine* **130**, 23–31.

Pelliccia, A., Maron, B.J., Culasso, F., Di Paolo, F.M., Spataro, A., Biffi, A., *et al.* (2000) Clinical significance of abnormal electrocardiographic patterns in trained athletes. *Circulation* **102**, 278–284.

Pelliccia, A., Maron, B.J., De Luca, R., Di Paolo, F.M., Spataro, A. & Culasso, F. (2002) Remodeling of left ventricular hypertrophy in elite athletes after long-term deconditioning. *Circulation* **105**, 944–949.

Pelliccia, A., Maron, B.J., Spataro, A., Proschan, M.A. & Spirito, P. (1991) The upper limit of physiologic cardiac hypertrophy in highly trained elite athletes. *New England Journal of Medicine* **324**, 295–301.

Priori, S.G., Schwartz, P.J., Napolitano, C., Bloise, R., Ronchetti, E., Grillo, M., *et al.* (2003) Risk stratification in the long-QT syndrome. *New England Journal of Medicine* **348**, 1866–1874.

Puffer, J.C. (2001) Overview of the Athletic Heart Syndrome. In: *Exercise and Sports Cardiology* (Thompson, P.D., ed.) McGraw-Hill, NY: 30–42.

Rahimtoola, S.H., Durairaj, A., Mehra, A. & Nuno, I. (2002) Current evaluation and management of patients with mitral stenosis. *Circulation* **106**, 1183–1188.

Raschka, C., Parzeller, M. & Kind, M. (1999) [Organ pathology causing sudden death in athletes. International study of autopsies (Germany, Austria, Switzerland).] *Medizinisce Klinik (Munich)* **94**, 473–477.

Rosenhek, R., Binder, T., Porenta, G., Lang, I., Christ, G., Scemper, M., *et al.* (2000) Predictors of outcome in severe, asymptomatic aortic stenosis. *New England Journal of Medicine* **343**, 611–617.

Rost, R. (1997) The athlete's heart. Historical perspectives: solved and unsolved problems. *Cardiology Clinics* **15**, 493–512.

Rowell, L.B. (1986) *Human Circulation: Regulation During Physical Stress*. Oxford University Press, NY.

Sadaniantz, A., Yurgalevitch, S., Zmuda, J.M. & Thompson, P.D. (1996) One year of exercise training does not alter resting ventricular systolic or diastolic function. *Medicine and Science in Sports and Exercise* **28**, 1345–1350.

Samenuk, D., Link, M.S., Homoud, M.K., Contreras, R., Theoharides, T.C., Wang, P.J., *et al.* (2002) Adverse cardiovascular events temporally associated with ma huang, an herbal source of ephedrine. *Mayo Clinic Proceedings* **77**, 12–16.

Schwartz, P.J., Priori, S.G., Spazzolini, C., Moss, A.J., Vincent, G.M., Napolitano, C., *et al.* (2001) Genotype–phenotype correlation in the long-QT syndrome: gene-specific triggers for life-threatening arrhythmias. *Circulation* **103**, 89–95.

Serra-Grima, R., Estorch, M., Carrio, I., Subirana, M., Berna, L. & Prat, T. (2000) Marked ventricular repolarization abnormalities in highly trained athletes' electrocardiograms: clinical and prognostic implications. *Journal of the American College of Cardiology* **36**, 1310–1316.

Shores, J., Berger, K.R., Murphy, E.A. & Pyeritz, R.E. (1994) Progression of aortic dilatation and the benefit of long-term beta-adrenergic blockade in Marfan's syndrome. *New England Journal of Medicine* **330**, 1335–1341.

Siscovick, D.S., Weiss, N.S., Fletcher, R.H. & Lasky, T. (1984) The incidence of primary cardiac arrest during vigorous exercise. *New England Journal of Medicine* **311**, 874–877.

Smith, M.L., Graitzer, H.M., Hudson, D.L. & Raven, P.B. (1988) Baroreflex function in endurance- and static exercise-trained men. *Journal of Applied Physiology* **64**, 585–591.

Sumitomo, N., Harada, K., Nagashima, M., Yasuda, T., Nakamura, Y., Aragaki, Y., *et al.* (2003) Catecholaminergic polymorphic ventricular tachycardia: electrocardiographic characteristics and optimal therapeutic strategies to prevent sudden death. *Heart* **89**, 66–70.

Thiene, G., Nava, A., Corrado, D., Rossi, L. & Pennelli, N. (1988) Right ventricular cardiomyopathy and sudden death in young people. *New England Journal of Medicine* **318**, 129–133.

Thomas, D., Salloum, J., Montalescot, G., Drobinski, G., Artigou, J.Y. & Grosgogeat, Y. (1991) Anomalous coronary arteries coursing between the aorta and pulmonary trunk: clinical indications for coronary artery bypass. *European Heart Journal* **12**, 832–834.

Thomas, L.R. & Douglas, P.S. (2001) Echocardiographic findings in athletes. In: *Exercise and Sports Cardiology* (Thompson, P.D., ed.) McGraw-Hill, NY: 43–70.

Thompson, P.D. (2001) Evaluating and managing athletes with valvular heart disease. In: *Exercise and Sports Cardiology* (Thompson, P.D., ed.) McGraw-Hill, NY: 298–314.

Thompson, P.D., Buchner, D., Pina, I.L., Balady, G.J., Williams, M.A., Marcus, B.H., *et al.* (2003) Exercise and physical activity in the prevention and treatment of atherosclerotic cardiovascular disease. A statement from the Council on Clinical Cardiology (Subcommittee on Exercise, Rehabilitation, and Prevention) and the Council on Nutrition, Physical Activity, and Metabolism (Subcommittee on Physical Activity). *Circulation* **107**, 3109–3116.

Thompson, P.D. & Estes, N.A. III. (2002) In: *Textbook of Cardiovascular Medicine* (Topol, E.J., ed.) Lippincot Williams & Wilkins: 889–900.

Thompson, P.D., Funk, E.J., Carleton, R.A. & Sturner, W.O. (1982) Incidence of death during jogging in Rhode Island from 1975 through 1980. *JAMA* **247**, 2535–2538.

Valli, G. & Giardina, E.G. (2002) Benefits, adverse effects and drug interactions of herbal therapies with cardiovascular effects. *Journal of the American College of Cardiology* **39**, 1083–1095.

Van Camp, S.P., Bloor, C.M., Mueller, F.O., Cantu, R.C. & Olson, H.G. (1995) Nontraumatic sports death in high school and college athletes. *Medicine and Science in Sports and Exercise* **27**, 641–647.

Varnava, A.M., Elliott, P.M., Baboonian, C., Davison, F., Davies, M.J. & McKenna, W.J. (2001) Hypertrophic cardiomyopathy: histopathological features of sudden death in cardiac troponin T disease. *Circulation* **104**, 1380–1384.

Vignola, P.A., Aonuma, K., Swaye, P.S., Rozanski, J.J., Blankstein, R.L., Benson, J., *et al.* (1984) Lymphocytic myocarditis presenting as unexplained ventricular arrhythmias: diagnosis with endomyocardial biopsy and response to immunosuppression. *Journal of the American College of Cardiology* **4**, 812–819.

Vinereanu, D., Florescu, N., Sculthorpe, N., Tweddel, A.C., Stephens, M.R. & Fraser, A.G. (2001) Differentiation between pathologic and physiologic left ventricular hypertrophy by tissue Doppler assessment of long-axis function in patients with hypertrophic cardiomyopathy or systemic hypertension and in athletes. *American Journal of Cardiology* **88**, 53–58.

Viskin, S., Fish, R., Roth, A., Schwartz, P.J. & Belhassen, B. (2000) Clinical problem-solving. QT or not QT? *New England Journal of Medicine* **343**, 352–356.

Watkins, H., McKenna, W.J., Thierfelder, L., Suk, H.J., Anan, R., O'Donoghue, A., *et al.* (1995) Mutations in the genes for cardiac troponin T and alpha-tropomyosin in hypertrophic cardiomyopathy. *New England Journal of Medicine* **332**, 1058–1064.

Whelton, S.P., Chin, A., Xin, X. & He, J. (2002) Effect of aerobic exercise on blood pressure: a meta-analysis of randomized, controlled trials. *Annals of Internal Medicine* **136**, 493–503.

Willich, S.N., Lewis, M., Lowel, H., Arntz, H.R., Schubert, F. & Schroder, R. (1993) Physical exertion as a trigger of acute myocardial infarction. Triggers and Mechanisms of Myocardial Infarction Study Group. *New England Journal of Medicine* **329**, 1684–1690.

Wilmore, J.H. & Costill, D.L. (1994) *Physiology of Sport and Exercise*. Human Kinetics, Champaign, IL.

Yetman, A.T., Bornemeier, R.A. & McCrindle, B.W. (2003) Long-term outcome in patients with Marfan syndrome: is aortic dissection the only cause of sudden death? *Journal of the American College of Cardiology* **41**, 329–332.

Zoghbi, W.A., Enriquez-Sarano, M., Foster, E., Grayburn, P.A., Kraft, C.D., Levine, R.A., *et al.* (2003) Recommendations for evaluation of the severity of native valvular regurgitation with two-dimensional and Doppler echocardiography. *Journal of the American Society of Echocardiography* **16**, 777–802.

Chapter 7

Sports Pulmonology

JOSEPH CUMMISKEY, KAI-HÅKON CARLSEN, KEUN-YOUL KIM, CONLETH FEIGHERY, ANDREW GREEN, FABIO PIGOZZI, WALTER CANONICA, VITO BRUSASCO, STEFANO DEL GIACCO, SERGIO BONINI AND MATTEO BONINI

This chapter aims to show the spectrum of pulmonary disease and especially how it may affect the participating sports person. It is not a comprehensive chapter on diagnosis, management, or prognosis of lung disease other than where it might affect the participating athlete. The age group of the participating athlete is childhood to mid thirties. There are older athletes but they are the exception. The pulmonary disorders that affect young athletes differ from the full spectrum of lung disease.

Lung function can be measured by biochemical, physiologic, and anatomic tests. Because airflow obstruction is the most common condition affecting the lung, physiologic studies are most frequently used in lung assessment. Lung flow, as manifested by the forced expiratory volume in 1 s (FEV_1), is the most common and most frequently used test. Other tests include lung volumes and diffusion capacity. Arterial blood gases are a measure of one of the functions of the lung, to move oxygen in and carbon dioxide out of the body.

Lung challenge tests may be pharmacologic and physiologic. Methacholine is the most common pharmacologic challenge test. In a few countries, histamine challenge is used. Physiologic tests include exercise tests as the most commonly available test. Eucapnic voluntary hyperventilation is also available in a small number of laboratories worldwide.

The environment where a sport is practiced is important. Athletes breathe a higher volume of air than the sedentary person so any pollution in the air is more likely to be detrimental. Pollutants in the air that athletes breathe amplify the inflammatory response in the airways.

Measures of the genetic contribution on the incidence of disease are highlighted in relation to asthma. These effects are on the likely incidence of the disease and on inheritance of a specific response to drugs or allergens.

The immune system plays a vital part in the asthmatic process. Atopy has a role in bronchial hyperreactivity. Atopic individuals have an increased eosinophil count in the peripheral blood and in the airways. Levels of total and allergen-specific immunoglobulin E (IgE) are elevated in peripheral blood. The activation of IgE drives the inflammatory response to produce active cytokines.

There is a false differentiation between the lower and the upper respiratory tracts. There is a strong association between diseases of the lower respiratory tract, such as asthma, allergic rhinitis, and conjunctivitis. Other upper respiratory tract diseases, such as aspiration, sleep apnea, and nasal polyps, impact on the lower respiratory tract.

Asthma is the most common respiratory disorder affecting athletes. It is present in as few as 3% and as many as 30%, depending on the environment in which it is measured. We have therefore concentrated on this form of airflow disease in over half of this chapter. Asthma is the most common medical condition for which athletes request Therapeutic Use Exemption (TUE) in the Olympic Games.

The Olympic Textbook of Medicine in Sport, 1st edition. Edited by M. Schwellnus. Published 2008 by Blackwell Publishing, ISBN: 978-1-4051-5637-0.

Because of this, and in order to improve the health of athletes, the criteria for the diagnosis and management of asthma in athletes is important.

Pulmonary physiology, response to exercise, and bronchial hyperresponsiveness

Pulmonary physiology

The fundamental function of the respiratory system is to move air in and out of the lung, thus generating minute ventilation sufficient to assure gas exchange meeting metabolic demands. The ability to accomplish this task is constrained by the static and dynamic properties of all components of the respiratory system (i.e., airways, lung, and chest wall).

Lung volumes

Under static conditions, lung volumes are determined by the balance between forces tending to expand and forces tending to collapse the respiratory system (Fig. 7.1). Total lung capacity (TLC), the volume of gas contained in the lungs at maximal inspiration, is determined by the balance between the maximum force of inspiratory muscles and the elastic recoil of the respiratory system. Thus, TLC is generally increased when lung elastic recoil is reduced (pulmonary emphysema) and reduced when the stiffness of lung (interstitial fibrosis) or chest wall (neuromuscular diseases, ascites, and pregnancy) is increased.

Residual volume (RV) is the volume of gas remaining in the lungs after a maximal expiration. It is determined by the balance between the force of expiratory muscles and the outward recoil of the chest wall.

Vital capacity (VC) is the maximum volume of gas that can be mobilized with a single inspiration or expiration maneuvre, thus representing the difference between TLC and RV. A decrease of VC is generally an index of lung disease, but it does not allow differentiation between restriction and obstruction because it may result from either a decrease in TLC or an increase in RV, which may be increased because of airway closure.

Functional residual capacity (FRC) is the volume of gas remaining in the lungs at end-tidal expiration. At rest, it is determined by the balance between the inward recoil of the lung and the outward recoil of the chest wall, thus corresponding to the relaxation volume of the respiratory system. Decrease in FRC frequently occurs in restrictive respiratory diseases with an increase in lung or chest wall stiffness. Increase in FRC may occur in obstructive disorders because of loss of elastic recoil (emphysema), but also because of expiratory flow limitation (chronic obstructive bronchitis, asthma).

Tidal volume (TV) is the volume of gas inspired and expired during each breath. In healthy subjects its extremes are attained with minimal energy expenditure. At rest, TV is generated by the action of the diaphragm for inspiration and by the inward recoil of the respiratory system for expiration. During exercise, TV increases by increasing end-inspiratory lung volume and decreasing FRC (see below). Expiratory and inspiratory reserve volumes are the volumes below and above TV that are used to increase the TV when required. Although void of importance at rest, they have a critical role during exercise.

Lung flows

Under dynamic conditions, the gas motion in and out of the lung is governed by the pressure losses between alveoli and airway opening (mouth or nose) resulting from convective acceleration, laminar flow, and turbulent flow across the airways. Airway resistance (Raw; i.e., the ratio of alveolar : airway opening pressure to flow) is mostly (40–60%) caused by the nose and larynx, with large variability between and within individuals. Although measurements of Raw may provide direct information on airway caliber, it is not routinely measured because the use of a body plethysmograph is required.

For practical purposes, indirect but useful information about airway caliber is obtainable from the forced expiratory maneuvre. This is because for any lung volume there is a maximum flow that cannot be exceeded by increasing the effort. Thus, plotting forced flow against lung volume gives an estimate of the relationship between size of airways and

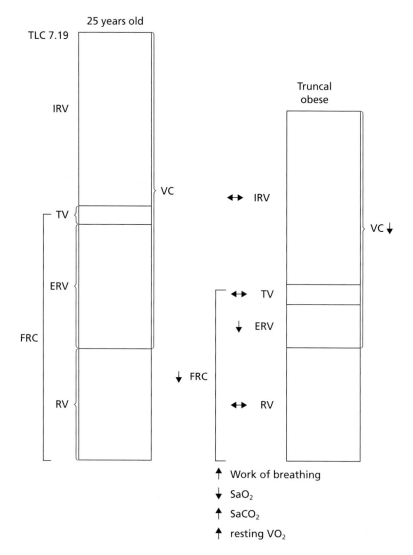

Fig. 7.1 Effects of obesity on exercise testing. ERV, expiratory reserve volume; FRC, functional residual capacity; IRV, inspiratory reserve volume; RV, residual volume; TLC, total lung capacity; TV, tidal volume; VC, vital capacity.

lung. Amongst the parameters derived from forced expiratory maneuvre, the FEV_1 and the forced vital capacity (FVC) are the most important and reproducible. They are generally recommended as a basic assessment of lung function. Because of their dependence on age, height, gender, and race they must be related to the relevant predicted values.

The ratio FEV_1/FVC is widely accepted as an index of airway function, with its decrease being taken as evidence of airway obstruction, although this cannot be excluded if the ratio is within the normal limits. Peak expiratory flow has been proposed as a surrogate of FEV_1 but its variability and dependence on effort make it unreliable for functional diagnosis of respiratory disorders. Reduced expiratory flows at low lung volumes have been proposed as indexes of small airway obstruction, but their wide variability and the dependence on both lung elastic recoil and coexisting large airway narrowing make it unrealistic to assume that they uniquely represent small airway function.

Diffusion

Pulmonary diffusion of oxygen across the blood–gas barrier is a critical link in the oxygen cascade from the atmosphere to the mitochondria. Exercise at high altitude and disease in the interstitium of the lung are the only situations where oxygen transfer is diffusion limited.

Natives of high altitude have a higher diffusion capacity than similar people at sea level. This may be because of an accelerated growth of the lung in a hypoxic environment.

Response to exercise

During exercise, minute ventilation increases to meet the increasing metabolic demands. In normal subjects, this is achieved by increasing tidal volume while breathing frequency increases only at very high exercise levels. With the exception of some highly trained elite athletes, healthy subjects terminate exercise as a result of peripheral muscle exhaustion long before the ventilatory limits are achieved. This is because the maximal flow the normal respiratory system is able to generate in the operational volume range is much higher that the tidal flow usually achieved at maximal exercise. Therefore, the increase in ventilation during exercise is obtained with tidal volume impinging on both inspiratory and expiratory reserve volumes, thus maintaining end-inspiratory lung volume well below TLC. The extent to which airflow can be increased at any given lung volume is critically determined by airway caliber. If this is reduced, minute ventilation can be increased only by breathing at high lung volumes (where greater expiratory flows can be generated), with the consequence that end-inspiratory volume approaches TLC. Because of the elastic characteristics of the respiratory system, breathing at lung volumes close to TLC requires an exaggerated work by inspiratory muscles, eventually resulting in intolerable dyspnea.

In normal subjects, airway caliber may not change or may even increase during exercise as a consequence of a reduction in airway smooth muscle tone. Increased levels of bronchodilator mediators, such as epinephrine, prostaglandin E2, and nitric oxide, or the effect of tidal stretching on airway smooth muscle have been invoked to explain exercise-induced bronchodilatation.

In asthmatic subjects, the effects of exercise hyperpnea on airway caliber may be more variable, with some individuals developing bronchodilatation, as normal subjects do, and some bronchoconstriction. Typically, exercise-induced bronchoconstriction occurs at the end of a submaximal short bout of exercise (e.g., 6 min), but it may also occur during exercise if this is sufficiently prolonged (e.g., 20 min).

The effects of training on pulmonary function are not to increase lung volumes or divisions in lung volumes but to increase $\dot{V}o_{2max}$ by 10–100%, maximum minute ventilation by 20–80%, and to increase the utilization of oxygen by increasing blood volume, and increasing skeletal muscle myoglobin content, number, and size of mitochondria and aerobic enzyme activity. This results in a trained athlete who can recover more quickly from anaerobic exercise.

Bronchial hyperresponsiveness

Airway hyperresponsiveness is defined as an excessive airway narrowing in response to a variety of stimuli that have little or no effects in healthy subjects, and is documented by leftward and upward shifts of the dose–response curve to constrictor agents. There are several mechanisms that may concur to sustain airway hyperresponsiveness, including a dysfunction of the autonomic regulation of airway smooth muscle tone, a release of mediators from immune reactions, changes in airway wall geometry, an increased force generation by airway smooth muscle, and a reduced ability of the lung to maintain the airways open. Although the relative roles of these factors remain unknown, it can be postulated that airway hyperresponsiveness could result from an individual genetic predisposition to develop an abnormal inflammatory response to environmental factors, possibly involving changes in airway smooth muscle characteristics.

Because of its complex nature, challenging the airways using different stimuli can assess airway hyperresponsiveness. Based on their mechanism of action, these stimuli are categorized as direct or indirect, the former causing contraction of airway smooth muscle by activating their specific receptors, the latter through the release of mediators from intermediary cells. The direct stimuli used most commonly are methacholine and histamine, whereas indirect stimuli are exercise, dry air, hypertonic or hypotonic solutions, adenosine, mannitol, and sensitizing agents.

The major difference between the response to direct and indirect stimuli is that the former reflect the behaviour of the target organ, while the latter are critically dependent on the presence of inflammatory cells in the airways. As a consequence, both healthy and asthmatic subjects are expected to respond to direct stimuli, albeit at different doses, while only the latter are expected to respond to indirect stimuli. Therefore, direct stimuli are more sensitive and indirect stimuli more specific for the diagnosis of bronchial asthma.

Diagnosis of asthma in sport

Concerns about asthma and sport are threefold:
1 In diagnosing asthma there should be no distinction between asthma pathogenesis and definition (leading to differences in diagnosis and treatment) as practiced by pulmonary physicians and sports medicine physicians at different sporting events. It is accepted that there is a difference between clinical, research, and sport asthma (e.g., "Cough asthma is not a good reason for allowing stimulants in sport"). This is a measure of severity. It is a potential medicolegal problem if we allow a distinction. Diagnosis must be made by physicians, not by technicians alone.
2 Any test proposed for its diagnosis should be by standard test readily available to the majority of practicing pulmonary physicians throughout the world. The test should be repeated every 4 years to ensure that we are not allowing stimulants in athletes who have "grown out of their childhood asthma."

3 Our eventual diagnosis and management of asthma should not put the health of the athlete or his/her performance at risk. This might arise from provocation testing too close to competition.

Because of the above problems, the academic community in Europe as represented by the European Respiratory Society (ERS) and the European Association of Allergy and Clinical Immunology set up a Task Force to address this problem in 2002. A report was published in the *European Respiratory Monographs* in November 2005 (Carlsen *et al.* 2005) which we believe should be the basis of diagnosing asthma in sport. It now needs to be approved by the European Olympic Committee (EOC), the World Anti-Doping Agency (WADA), other continental Olympic committees, international sporting federations, the International Olympic Committee, Medical Commission (IOC, MC) and eventually the International Olympic Committee (IOC).

Diagnosis and differential diagnosis of asthma in athletes

The diagnosis of asthma is mainly clinical and should be based upon history of symptoms and clinical examination, including signs of bronchial obstruction and variability in lung function spontaneously or from bronchodilators. The main symptoms of asthma are recurring bronchial obstruction, and even in infancy the diagnosis is based upon at least three separate episodes of bronchial obstruction. The competing athlete frequently reports the presence of respiratory symptoms in relationship to exercise, but the diagnosis of asthma or exercise-induced asthma may be difficult because of the variability and non-specificity of symptoms. The diffusion capacity of the lung and pulmonary capillary blood volume remain unaltered in the highly trained athlete, whereas maximum pulmonary blood flow increases with enhanced maximum oxygen uptake. In response to physical training, ventilatory requirement rises with no alteration in the capability of the airways and the lungs to produce higher flow rates or higher tidal volumes, and little or no change in the pressure-generating capability of inspiratory muscles. Furthermore, it has been demonstrated that in healthy, highly trained, elite endurance athletes, exercise-induced hypoxemia occurs in more than 50% of these athletes. Thus, distinguishing exercise-induced asthma (EIA) from physiologic respiratory limitations to physical exercise becomes important.

EIA is the condition with EIA symptoms, whereas exercise-induced bronchoconstriction (EIB) can be understood as the demonstration of EIB by lung function measurements after an exercise test or a naturally occurring exercise (Anderson & Holzer 2000).

A diagnosis of EIA ought to be made before starting treatment. An exact clinical history, examination with lung function measurements before and after inhalation of a β_2-agonist, before and after a standardized exercise test, such as treadmill run and/or a cold air inhalation test, and measurement of bronchial hyperreactivity by methacholine inhalation are parts of the diagnostic process. One important part of the diagnostic process is to follow-up the patient to evaluate the treatment effect.

EIB is rapidly and markedly improved by inhaled steroids, and this puts increased demands upon the standardization of exercise tests with respect to exercise load and environmental factors (ATS 2000).

EIA may be diagnosed in different ways; running provokes EIB more easily than cycling in most athletes except for cyclists. The latest American Thoracic Society (ATS) guidelines recommend that an exercise load of 80–90% of calculated maximum is employed in the testing of EIB with inhalation of air with a relative humidity below 50% and an ambient temperature of 20–25°C while running on a treadmill for 6–8 min. However, it has been shown that the sensitivity of exercise testing increases markedly with an increase in exercise load to 95% of calculated maximum exercise load. Also, the use of inhaled cold air (–20°C) during exercise testing markedly increases the sensitivity, without decreasing specificity. Strict environmental standardization with a sufficiently high exercise load is important in the testing for EIB and using EIB as a monitoring device for asthma. Both the ERS and ATS recommendations set a 10% reduction in FEV_1 as a criterion for EIB.

EIB has been looked as an indirect measure of bronchial responsiveness, causing bronchoconstriction through mediator release. Several other stimuli have also been used as indirect stimuli to assess bronchial responsiveness in athletes: inhalation of cold, dry air; inhalation of dry air; inhalation of hyperosmolar aerosols, such as hypertonic saline and inhaled mannitol; and inhalation of adenosine monophosphate (AMP). Common to all is that a 10% reduction in FEV_1 from the start of the test is taken as the sign of a positive result.

Also, the response to bronchodilators, such as inhaled β_2-agonists, has been used in the diagnosis of asthma. In the guidelines from the IOC, it has been used as a criterion for allowing athletes to use inhaled β_2-agonists in sports. The criterion employed has been that recommended by European Respiratory Society, a 12% increase in FEV_1 expressed as percentage predicted after inhaled bronchodilator or, alternatively, an increase in FEV_1 as a percent of baseline.

Assessment of direct bronchial responsiveness as measured by methacholine bronchial provocation has been recommended as a diagnostic tool by the IOC and its use during the 2002 Winter Olympic Games (Anderson et al. 2003). However, it has been felt among respiratory physicians with sports medicine experience that the levels set were too strict, and a Joint Task Force of ERS and European Academy of Allergy and Clinical Immunology has recently given its recommendations. According to these recommendations (Carlsen et al. 2005), a concentration of methacholine (or histamine) causing a 20% reduction in FEV_1 (PC_{20}) should be less than $4 \ mg \cdot mL^{-1}$ or, alternatively, the total inhaled dose (PD_{20}) less than 4 µmol (compared to 0.8 mg methacholine) in steroid-naïve athletes. In athletes who have been using inhaled steroids for at least 3 months the PC_{20} for methacholine should be less than $16 \ mg \cdot mL^{-1}$ or PD_{20} less than 16 µmol (3.2 mg).

Differential diagnosis of EIA in athletes

As seen from Table 7.1 there are several important differential diagnoses to EIA in athletes. Most of the elite athletes referred for respiratory problems do not have asthma or EIA. Perhaps the most frequent differential diagnosis is exercise-induced inspiratory stridor or vocal cord dysfunction. Dominating

Table 7.1 Differential diagnosis of airflow obstruction.

Localized	Generalized
Vocal cord paresis	Chronic obstructive pulmonary disease
Laryngeal carcinoma	Bronchiectasis
Thyroid enlargement	Cystic fibrosis
Relapsing polychondritis	α_1-Antiprotease deficiency
Tracheal carcinoma	Obstructive sleep apnea
Bronchial carcinoma	Obliterative bronchiolitis
Environmentally induced	Swimming pool pulmonary edema
URT inflammation	Exercise-induced hypoxemia
Post-tracheostomy stenosis	Motile ciliary dysfunction
Foreign body aspiration	Use of bronchoconstrictors prior to PFT
Bronchopulmonary dysplasia	

PFT, pulmonary function test; URT, upper respiratory tract.

symptoms are inspiratory stridor occurring during maximum exercise, and stopping when exercise is terminated unless hyperventilation is maintained. During inspiration there are audible laryngeal sounds with no effect of bronchodilators or other asthma drugs. The condition most often occurs in young, well-trained, 15- to 16-year-old athletic girls. The symptoms are thought to be brought about by the relatively small cross-sectional area of the laryngeal orifice, with the possibility of even further reduction through negative airways pressure created through heavy exercise. One possible differential diagnosis to this syndrome is paradoxical movement of the vocal cords with adduction during inspiration which may also occur without exercise. The diagnoses are made by direct fiberoptic laryngoscopia during exercise.

Swimming-induced pulmonary edema (SIPE) occurs in well-trained swimmers after a forceful swim. This condition was recently reported in 70 previously healthy swimmers, who developed typical symptoms of pulmonary edema, together with a restrictive pattern in pulmonary function, which might remain for up to 1 week after swimming.

Exercise-induced arterial hypoxemia may occur in highly trained athletes, probably because of diffusion limitations and ventilation–perfusion inequality. Physical training will improve muscle strength and endurance, and the ionotropic and chronotropic capacities of the heart increase. No similar training effects occur within the respiratory system. The diffusion capacity of the lung and pulmonary capillary blood volume remain unaltered in the highly trained athlete. Ventilatory requirement rises with no alteration in the capability of the airways and the lungs to produce higher flow rates or higher tidal volumes, and little or no change in the pressure-generating capability of inspiratory muscles. The result is exercise-induced arterial hypoxemia which may occur in up to 50% of highly trained athletes. This reduction in arterial oxygen saturation may be confused with EIA.

Other possible causes of respiratory problems during exercise are listed in Table 7.1. Thus, several differential diagnoses to EIA exist (Table 7.1). It is important to make a thorough examination and rule out possible differential diagnoses as each diagnosis requires a different approach and treatment.

Diagnosis in general

Diagnosis is usually based on etiology. When there is no known etiology, as in asthma, we are left to describe the disease rather than define it. There are many forms of diagnosis:
• Working diagnosis: used until a more definitive diagnosis is made;
• Definite diagnosis: more than 95% certain;
• Probable diagnosis: this can be high or low probability;
• Possible diagnosis: less than 50% certain;
• Clinical diagnosis;

- Physiologic diagnosis;
- Anatomic diagnosis;
- Histologic diagnosis;
- Immunologic diagnosis.

Definition and description

Asthma is defined as a "chronic inflammatory disease of the respiratory tract in which a number of cells have an important pathogenic role, including mast cells, eosinophils, and T lymphocytes. In susceptible individuals this specific inflammation leads to an increase in airway hyperresponsiveness with recurrent episodes of dyspnea, wheezing, coughing, thoracic constriction, and shortness of breath." (www.ginasthma.com, accessed 2007)

SUBJECTIVE AND OBJECTIVE SYMPTOMS

Standardized questionnaires should be used for recording of symptoms suggestive of airways obstruction at rest or in relation to exercise, at night or during the pollen season, as well as previous treatments.

SPIROMETRY

Pulmonary function tests may be normal in athletes whether predicted values are referred to the normal sex- and age-matched population.

According to the current flow-chart, a value of FEV_1 of 75% of predicted is considered as a threshold to suggest differential diagnostic pathways.

EUCAPNIC VOLUNTARY HYPERVENTILATION TEST

A 10% or greater decrease in single stage or multistage eucapnic voluntary hyperventilation (EVH) test has been suggested to document hyperreactive airways in athletes.

REVERSIBILITY AFTER ADMINISTRATION OF A PERMITTED β-AGONIST

A 12% or greater increase of the predicted value of FEV_1 is at present considered by IOC regulations as a sign of reversible airways obstruction. This criterion, adapted by the ERS, differs from the ATS criterion, according to which a positive response is defined as 12% increase from basal value plus 200 mL. For instance, an athlete with a basal FEV_1 of 4.50 L·s^{-1} and a predicted value of 5.00 L·s^{-1}(83% of predicted) with an increase after a permitted inhaled β-agonist of 0.54 L (12% of basal value) would be defined as irreversible by ERS and reversible by ATS.

EXERCISE TESTING

Athletes and amateur exercisers with reactive airways disease may experience bronchoconstriction following or during exercise, thus preventing the successful completion of a given exercise task. EIB has been reported up to 80% of the population with clinically recognized asthma. Therefore, exercise is used as a challenge test to detect EIB in asthmatic patients, with or without respiratory symptoms during or after exertion. EIB cannot be excluded by a negative methacholine test. Moreover, many children and adults with documented EIB have no symptoms of asthma. Recently, a 30% incidence of EIB in a large group of elite athletes has been reported, while respiratory symptoms were only present in 5% of subjects. In a cold environment, the incidence of EIB in subjects without clinical diagnosis of asthma may be even higher. An exercise challenge is therefore often worthwhile for subjects in whom exercise could be limited by EIB.

Respiratory water loss and/or cooling have been invoked as the potential causes of airways narrowing; at present, there is no direct experimental evidence to support either of these hypotheses. However, these proposals led to the conclusion that exercise protocols for the detection of EIB should aim to achieve high levels of ventilation (V_E 15–22 times greater than resting FEV_1) while breathing air containing less than 10 mg·L^{-1} water (20–25°C and less than 50% relative humidity). Breathing compressed air via a Douglas bag, tubing, and valve will ensure the low humidity of inspired air. The required V_E can be achieved by either running on a treadmill or by cycling. Exercise on a cycle ergometer is usually preferred because work rate can be accurately measured. If V_E is not measured, target work rate can be estimated by equations relating V_E to oxygen uptake ($\dot{V}o_2$) and $\dot{V}o_2$ to work rate (e.g., watts = $[53.76 \times$ measured $FEV_1] - 11.07$). Alternatively, 80–90% of predicted maximal heart rate (predicted $HR_{max} = 220 -$ age in years) can be used to monitor exercise intensity.

The exercise protocol recommended comprises a rapid (3–4 min) increase in work rate to the target value which should be maintained for 4–6 min; for the first, second and third minute of cycling work rate may be conveniently set to 60%, 75%, and 90% of the target value. FEV_1 should be measured at rest and in the first 20 min of recovery; a fall of more than 15% (vs. baseline value) is regarded as diagnostic of EIB. In subjects with EIB, FEV_1 generally fails to reach a minimum within the first 10 min after cessation of exercise, with substantial recovery by 30 min post exercise. Airway cooling and drying induced by exercise are also thought to stimulate the release of inflammatory mediators, such as histamine and leukotrienes. Thus, exercise has become an important challenge method for assessing the effects of asthma medications. A drug to be "protective" should reduce the maximal decrease

of FEV_1 after exercise by more than 50%. To maximize the likelihood of a positive response, bronchodilator agents should be withheld prior to exercise for a period commensurate with their duration of action.

Some recommendations should be followed for exercise testing (Table 7.2).

METHACOLINE CHALLENGE

The methacoline challenge, when performed with the available standard procedure, is the most widely used and accurate test to prove airways hyperreactivity.

However, the thresholds indicated by the IOC – a PD_{20} less than 1 μmol (200 μg) or a PD_{20} less than 2 mg·mL^{-1} and a PD_{20} less than 6.6 μmol (1320 μg) or a PC_{20} less than 13.2 mg·mL^{-1} for athletes on topical steroid s – seem to be adequate to identify moderate and severe asthmatic but might fail to identify mild or subclinical asthma or asthma under control with treatment. In fact, the curves of pre-test vs. post-test probability of asthma are largely dependent on the PC_{20} used.

Table 7.2 Prevalence of asthma among winter sports athletes.

Athelete group (n)	Method	Prevalence (%)	Reference
Cross-country skiers (42)	Questionnaire, spirometry, methacholine challenge	54.8	Larsson et al. (1993)
Cross-country skiers (171)	Questionnaire, spirometry, methacholine challenge	12 (Norway) 42 (Sweden)	Sue-Chu et al. (1996)
Figure-skaters	Exercise test	35 (EIB)	Mannix et al. (1996)
Ice-hockey players	Questionnaire, spirometry, methacholine challenge, exercise test	19.2 11.5 (EIB)	Leuppi et al. (1998)
US 1998 Winter Olympic team (196)	Questionnaire	21.9 60.7 (cross-country, etc.) 24 (alpine, etc.) 2.8 (bobsled, etc.)	Weiler et al. (2000)
US 1998 Winter Olympic team	Exercise challenge, spirometry	23 (all, EIB) 50 (cross-country)	Wilber et al. (2000)
Ice-hockey players	Questionnaire, spirometry, histamine challenge	22 (total asthma) 13 (current asthma)	Lumme et al. (2003)

EIB, exercise-induced bronchospasm.

Other special considerations needed in the diagnosis of asthma include:

• Patients with allergic conjunctivitis and rhinitis should be screened for asthma, and vice versa;

• Treatment of mild asthma in athletes should be with anti-inflammatory agents first with due respect to other guidelines;

• Evidence-based studies are needed on all anti-asthma drugs for performance enhancement and safety;

• The use of long-acting β_2-sympathomimetics needs to be clarified in mild asthma in athletes;

• Patients with a history of asthma undocumented for more than 4 years should be considered free of asthma for the purpose of using stimulants in sport;

• Events occurring in special environmental conditions.

Differential diagnoses

There are many differential diagnoses for airflow limitation (Table 7.1). Bronchoscopy and computed tomography (CT) scan of the chest may be useful in better defining the differential diagnosis of airflow limitation. It is seldom indicated in the management of asthma.

Environmental conditions (e.g., swimming halls, ice rinks, pollen)

Several environmental factors are able to influence performances in different sports. Training schedules for top athletes may cause an important stress on the airways. They can increase the respiratory frequency 10- to 15-fold above the normal resting frequency and increase ventilation up to 100 L·min^{-1}. At this high minute ventilation, the lungs are exposed to high ambient levels of pollutants which enhance airways inflammation. This reaction in humans to allergens is measured as decreased pulmonary function. Hyperventilation itself could be a trigger for EIA. The increased uptake of pollutants and their displacement to the smaller airways may worsen respiratory symptoms in professional athletes (Table 7.3). Although the role of substances such as nitrogen dioxide (NO_2), sulfur dioxide (SO_2), particulate matter (PM),

Table 7.3 Air pollutants.

Primary pollutants
CO, CO_2
SO_2, NO_2
Metals
Coal, graphite, lead

Secondary pollutants
Ozone (O_3)
HN_3
H_2SO_4
Nitrate peroxyacetyl
Other inorganics

chlorine derivatives, and smoke has yet to be completely clarified, other factors such as allergens and climatic factors (temperature, humidity, wind speed) have a well-defined influence in inducing respiratory symptoms in the general population as well as in athletes. The proven influence of these factors on the respiratory function of athletes highlights the need for special attention to be paid to the environments in which indoor and outdoor sports are performed.

Relevant pollutants in sport activity

Sports environments may be polluted by exterior pollutants or may be sources themselves of substances able to increase the airways' hyperreactivity (Aekplakorn et al. 2004; D'Amato et al. 2005). There is evidence that urbanization, with its high levels of vehicle emissions and a Westernized lifestyle, is linked directly to the rising frequency of respiratory symptoms in the general population as well as in athletes. An estimated mean increase of 3% in prevalence of lower airways respiratory symptoms and 0.7% increase in upper respiratory tract symptoms every 10 μ·m^3 of airborne particulate matter has been calculated. Furthermore, as concentrations of airborne allergens and air pollutants are frequently increased at the same time, the enhanced airways inflammation, together with an enhanced IgE-mediated response, can worsen respiratory symptoms in allergic subjects.

The pollutants, mainly derived from combustion engines, power generation, and industry, are subdivided into two main categories: primary (those that do not undergo chemical changes after their origin from a certain source) and secondary (those that are produced through a chemical reaction from natural precursors, or emitted from artificial sources; Table 7.3).

NITROGEN DIOXIDE

NO_2 is a combustion-generated oxidant gas (Antò & Sunyer 1995; Bylin et al. 1988). It is widely present in indoor and outdoor environments. Outdoors it is generated mainly by oil combustion and it is a precursor to particles and ozone. Indoors it is generated by kerosene or gas cooking and heating. Its damage on the airways derives from the oxidation of the cell membranes and consequent inflammatory response. It has an important role both in the modulation of the degree and the duration of the inflammatory response itself. Normal subjects have no consistent effects after exposure to NO_2. Subjects with pathologies associated with airway hyperresponsiveness, such as EIB, experience worse symptoms and enhanced airways responsiveness to methacholine. It also enhances the airways response to the hyperventilation of cold air (Poynter et al. 2006).

SULFUR DIOXIDE AND PARTICULATE MATTER

SO_2 and PM are also combustion-generated particles (Dockery & Pope 1994). They can be considered as the most important components of urban smog. Several epidemiologic studies have demonstrated the association of short-term exposure to these components with transient declines in pulmonary function, especially in children.

Particulate matter of less than 10 μm (aerodynamically), PM10, are deposited in the lower respiratory tract. They are associated with both SO_2 and ozone smog. They act as vectors to carry the acidity in the particles to the lower respiratory tract. This gives an increase in respiratory symptom exacerbations and deterioration in lung function.

PM may also act by an oxidative effect. These oxidative effects, such as the catalytic actions of transition metals, may alter viscosity of blood and increase the cardiovascular (CV) risks in patients with previous CV disease.

Symptoms associated with high levels of SO_2 and PM air pollutants are chronic bronchitis, giving rise to wheeze, chest tightness, cough, and sputum. They cause bronchoconstriction in asthmatics and patients with bronchial hyperresponsiveness secondary to methacholine. They can increase morbidity and mortality in patients with underlying chronic bronchitis, asthma, and cardiac disease. Studies from Germany showed it did not increase the prevalence of atopy, hay fever, or asthma in children and adults.

SO_2 is dissolved in the surface fluid layer of the airway epithelium and undergoes a variety of chemical reactions to yield sulfuric acid, sulfites, bisulfites, and sulfates. The final common pathway for damage is the release of inflammatory mediators.

Chlorine

Chlorine is a gas commonly used over the years as a sterilization agent for swimming pools and water supplies in general. It is considered as a strong irritating agent for all human mucous membranes, eyes, and skin, and exposure to this gas may cause pulmonary irritation (Helenius et al. 2002; Proctor et al. 1978).

Ozone

Ozone (O_3) is mainly generated from hydrocarbons and NO_2 in the presence of ultraviolet radiation ("LA smog"). Concentrations of 20–40 p.p.m. may occur in the morning, rising to 100 p.p.m. in the afternoon. Ozone may cause respiratory symptoms and increase the annual rate of decline of FEV_1 at levels as low as 80 p.p.m. when exposure occurs over 6 h per day.

Ozone causes transient increases in airway responsiveness. EIA is not exaggerated by ozone. Allergen responses are exaggerated by ozone. This can occur in 1 h in asthmatics exposed to 120 p.p.m. Nasal allergen responses, in terms of the concentration of eosinophils and eosinophil cationic protein, are increased after exposure to ozone.

The cellular and biochemical effects of O_3 are to increase neutrophils and prostanoids, such as prostaglandins E2 and F2 alpha and thromboxane B2. Treatment or prevention is through the use of bronchodilators, anti-inflammatory agents and, possibly, antioxidants.

Smoke

Smoke is one of the recognized factors influencing both the onset of acute respiratory symptoms and the progression of chronic bronchial inflammation.

Approximately 12,000 compounds have been isolated in the tar, the product of tobacco combustion, and more than 4500 components have been identified. The main compounds are: carbon dioxide, carbon monoxide, cianidric acid, nitrous acid, aldehydes, phenols, alkaloids (such as nicotine), arsenic, radioactive elements, and polycyclic aromatic hydrocarbons. These compounds are also present in the exhaled air and in the surrounding air at the moment in which the smoker is not inhaling from the cigarette, and tar is deposited when smoke is cooled or dissolved, so that their concentration in the environment can be up to four times higher than those present in the inhaled smoke. Therefore, both active and passive smoking are involved in the generation of respiratory diseases.

Active smoking is related to the severity of asthma and to the reduced response to pharmacologic treatment. Also, at least 10% of a smoker's blood is bound to carbon monoxide, which reduces the muscular efficiency and induces a further hyperventilation, thus increasing the possibility of EIA and enhancing the allergens by inhalation.

Smokers were also shown to have increased IgE levels independently from the presence of sensitization to common allergens, which is suggestive of the possibility that smoke promotes a type 2 helper T cell (Th2) response. Moreover, smoke is able to activate the expression of the genes involved in mucus secretion, through activation of the epidermal growth factor receptor (EGFR), this promoting both bronchial obstruction and tissue remodeling.

Epidemiologic studies have suggested that "second-hand smoke", also know as environmental tobacco smoke (ETS) increases the incidence and the severity of allergies and asthma. Recently, it was demonstrated that ETS upregulates the allergic response to inhaled allergens, acting as an adjuvant for Th2 responses, specifically increasing IL-4 and IL-10. Intense exercise can raise the quantity of inhaled air from 5 up to 120 $L \cdot m^{-1}$, thus making the composition of air present in the environment crucial for the induction of respiratory symptoms.

Taken together, these considerations indicate important interactions among allergy, exercise, and smoke and should be seriously considered in organizing physical activity at any level, from elite athletes to amateurs and at any ages, with particular attention to school environment, and student's behaviour, as reported more and more frequently in teenagers' school teams.

However, at present we are missing both epidemiologic data on smoke behaviour in athletes and amateurs, and models for mechanisms study. This gap should be filled starting with epidemiology, and the first possibility is to include, in any survey concerning physical exercise, specific questions about smoking habits and quality of the environment.

Pollens and other allergens

Twenty percent of the general population in industrialized countries experience allergies. This suggests that at least two out of 10 athletes are at high risk of developing allergic symptoms while competing. Indoor and outdoor allergens can influence sport performances in the form of allergic asthma, rhinitis, or conjunctivitis. Epidemiologic data indicate that asthma and allergic rhinitis frequently coexist. At least 80–90% of asthma patients reported rhinitis symptoms, and 19–38% of rhinitic patients reported asthma symptoms. The severity of allergic asthma and rhinitis are correlated.

Pollinosis is frequently used to study the links between air pollution and respiratory allergy. Climatic influences can affect both biologic and chemical components of this interaction. Pollutants, attaching to the surface of pollen grains or of plant-derived particles of paucicromic size, are able to modify the morphology and the allergenic potential of these molecules. Airways inflammation is induced by the pollutants. An increased permeability of the mucosal barrier, at bronchial and nasal level, favors the overcoming of these molecules and a consequent allergic response. Extreme climatic conditions during pollen seasons, such as thunderstorms, can induce severe allergic reactions in pollenosis patients. The rupture of pollen grains induced by a thunderstorm may release their cytoplasmic content, enhancing the number of inhalable, allergen-carrying microparticles.

Positive skin-prick tests were found in 41% of a group of Australian athletes from Olympic sports and in 28% of 118 athletes from the Italian Olympic team. It may therefore be difficult for elite athletes who find themselves participating in competitions which are not determined on the basis of the pollen season.

Therefore, special consideration should be given to aerobiologic and climatic conditions, especially during pollen seasons. The most frequently implicated pollens vary from one country to another. During the 2004 Athens Olympics, an aerobiologic network (www.aeroallergen.gr.) was set up to provide information to athletes, trainers, and medical staff regarding the most frequently implicated pollens. In that region, cypress, hazel, wall pellitory, plane, olive, grasses, goosefoot, mugwort, and fungi spores (*Alternaria spp.*, *Cladosporium spp.*) were most common. This kind of data should be made available at least 1 year before major competitions in order to help allergic athletes to achieve the best performances under the correct prophylactic measures.

In indoor sports, athletes should be aware of other kind of allergens, such as house dust mite (*Dermatophagoides pteronyssinus* and *Dermatophagoides farinae*) and moulds in high-humidity environments (changing rooms of swimming pools and other facilities).

Recently, new potential hazards for allergic subjects have been described. Compressed air diving has been shown to increase airway hyperresponsiveness. This can be enhanced by pollens trapped in the scuba tank, which can also induce very dangerous asthma attacks underwater.

In general, the choice of athletes' accommodation without moquette or carpets can reduce symptoms in sports persons sensitized to house dust mites.

Winter sports

INDOOR ICE-SKATING

Air pollutants, such as CO_2 and NO_2, are present in indoor skating facilities. They may exacerbate a pre-existing pathogenic condition in those people who spend considerable time in these environments, such as professional ice-skaters (ice-hockey, short track, speed-skating, and figure-skating; Table 7.2). The use of propane or gasoline powered ice resurfacers and edgers raised a concern regarding the indoor air quality in these facilities. In studies performed in different ice rinks, the ones with propane fuelled machines had a daily mean indoor concentration of 206 p.p.b., compared to 132 p.p.b. for rinks with gasoline fuelled resurfacers and only 37 p.p.b. for rinks served by an electric powered resurfacer. Other studies (332 rinks studied worldwide) show a mean for NO_2 level of 228 p.p.b. World Health Organization (WHO) recommendations indicate a 1-h guideline value of 213 p.p.b. NO_2 for indoor air. Increased ventilation or resurfacers using reduced NO_2 concentrations reduced pollution. Athletes exposed to this environment show a mixed eosinophilic and neutrophilic infla-mmation, as well as a high prevalence of EIB and a positive methacholine test.

Electric ice resurfacers, increased ventilation, and emission control systems are therefore recommended to avoid the risk of airways hyperresponsiveness-related symptoms in athletes and workers operating in ice rinks.

The presence of CO (also derived from ice resurfacers) in ice rinks is also a problem. It may be adsorbed by athletes, raising their carboxyhemoglobin (COHb) up to 1%. An average environment concentration of 20 p.p.m. for the duration of a hockey game (90 min) should be the warning level for indoor skating rinks to avoid dangerous enhancements of the COHb in athletes' blood.

CROSS-COUNTRY SKIING

It is well-known that dry and cold air exposure, for longer than 5–8 min, is the "perfect" trigger for EIB. These are the typical conditions for cross-country ski sports (cross-country itself and biathlon). The bronchial inflammation shows a different pattern in comparison with the classic asthmatic process. The inflammation shows a prevalence of lymphocytes and mastocytes in bronchoalveoloar lavage of these athletes. A high prevalence of asthma in winter sports athletes is shown also from various studies on different Olympic teams (Karjalainen *et al.* 2000).

Indoor sports

SWIMMING AND INDOOR WATER SPORTS

Swimming is a common sport for both amateurs and competitive athletes with asthma. Clinical evidence suggests that swimming is a low-risk sport for asthmatics. Its protective effect may result, in part, from the high humidity (around 70%) and temperature (24–30°C) of inspired air at water level. This reduces the hyperventilation heat loss and possibly the osmolarity at bronchial level. Increased bronchial hyperresponsiveness in professional swimmers (mainly reversible at the end of career) has been reported in several studies in comparison with controls and other athletes. Chlorine inhalation during the sporting life of the athlete may be the trigger for an increased bronchial inflammation of mixed origin (eosinophilic/neutrophilic). Studies demonstrated that the agitation of water during repeated training sessions may increase the quantity of chlorine inhaled. The high level of eosinophilia in induced sputum (20% of tested athletes) is remarkable. After a 5-year follow-up, eosinophilia was present in 38% of the athletes still practicing their sport and only in 8% of those who quit their activity early. Chlorine may enhance the sensitization of swimmers to aeroallergens.

OTHER INDOOR SPORTS

The risk for people practicing indoor sports is mainly related to the presence of pollutants such as NO_2 and CO from heating systems. It may also come from the presence of house dust mites in communal areas or in devices used to practice special sports (such as *tatami* mats for judo). Athletes should use the correct prophylactic measures in order to avoid airways inflammation.

Outdoor sports

ENDURANCE SPORTS

It is well known that endurance sports (long-distance runners, cyclists) have a higher asthma prevalence than power and speed sports (17% vs. 8%; Helenius & Haahtela 2000; Weiler *et al.* 1998). There is a higher risk of asthma in endurance athletes than power and speed athletes and control subjects (sixfold higher risk vs. 3.5 vs. 1). Endurance sports are usually performed outdoors (Table 7.4).

Treatment of asthma, and the relationship to doping

Rules for the use of inhaled corticosteroids and β-agonists in athletes

In 2005, the following minimal rules applied to the use of inhaled (non-systemic) corticosteroids and β_2-agonists (includes only D and L forms of salbutamol, terbutaline, salmeterol, and formoterol) in sport. When a urinary concentration of salbutamol above 1000 ng·mL^{-1} is found, the athlete has the responsibility to prove that this results from a therapeutic use of inhaled salbutamol.

An athlete who wishes to use inhaled steroids or the above β_2-agonists must submit an abbreviated Therapeutic Use Exemption (aTUE) form to their national anti-doping commission or to their international sports federation. "A medical notification justifying the therapeutic necessity should be included. The diagnosis and when applicable, any tests undertaken in order to establish that diagnosis should be included (without the actual results or details). Such medical notification shall describe the name of the drug, dosage, route of administration, and duration of the treatment" (WADA International Standard for Therapeutic Use Exemptions, version 3.0, 1.1.2004). Approval for the use of prohibited substances, subject to the abbreviated process, is effective on receipt of a completed notification by the anti-doping organization. The anti-doping organization should submit a copy of this TUE to the WADA, international federation, national federation and National Anti-doping Organization (NADO) (as appropriate). The athlete should bring the original TUE to any sporting event where testing is likely to be undertaken and produce it at the time of testing. Most sporting events will ask for or expect a TUE to be declared before the event (Global Strategy for Asthma Management and Prevention 2003).

Table 7.4 Prevalence of asthma among summer sports athletes.

Athlete group (n)	Method	Prevalence (%)	Reference
Australian 1976 Olympic team (185)	Physical examination	9.7	Fitch (1984)
Australian 1980 Olympic team (106)	Physical examination	8.5	Fitch (1984)
US 1984 Olympic team (597)	Questionnaire, treadmill exercise test in selected athletes	4.3	Voy (1984)
1986 football players from University of Iowa (156)	Questionnaire, methacholine challenge	11.5	Weiler et al. (1986)
Swiss athletes from various sport events (2060)	Questionnaire	3.7	Helbling & Muller (1991)
Spanish 1982 Olympic team (495)	Questionnaire	4.4	Drobnic (1994)
Runners from Finnish national team (103)	Questionnaire	15.5	Tikkanen & Helenius (1994)
Swimmers from USA (738)	Questionnaire	13.4	Potts (1996)
US Track and Field Championship Games (73)	Exercise test (competition)	15.1	Schoene et al. (1997)
Track and iield athletes, swimmers (162)	Questionnaire, spirometry, histamine challenge	22.8	Helenius et al. (1998)
US 1996 Olympic team (699)	Questionnaire	15.3	Weiler et al. (1998)
Australian 2000 Olympic team (214)	Questionnaire, skin test	21.9	Katelaris et al. (2000)
Italian 2000 Pre-Olympic team (265)	Questionnaire, skin test, spirometry	10.9	Lapucci et al. (2003)

In winter it reaches prevalence of up to 54.8% (Table 7.2).

ORAL, INTRAVENOUS, OR INTRAMUSCULAR DRUGS

Oral, intravenous, or intramuscular steroids and β-agonists are not permitted in athletes by IOC-WADA regulations.

Allowed and banned asthma drugs in sport

The following respiratory medications are allowed in sport: xanthines, anticholinergics, immunotherapy, antihistamines (with the exception of precision events such as archery and shooting), leukotriene receptor antagonists, anti-tussives, expectorants.

The following stimulants are now on a monitoring list, having been removed from the prohibited list: caffeine, pseudoephidrine, phenylephrine, phenylpropanolamine.

The following respiratory medications are banned in sport: central stimulants of respiration, systemic sympathomimetics, systemic corticosteroids, inhaled clembuterol.

Immunotherapy

Specific immunotherapy is a biologic response modifier. It alters the immune response to allergens at early stages, thus resulting in diminished symptoms and need for drugs. Its efficacy has been proven for both rhinitis and asthma, and the association of the two diseases is the optimal indication. It must be prescribed and administered only by trained physicians, after a careful diagnostic and cost–benefit evaluation. There is no contraindication to immunotherapy in athletes and those practicing sports. The only precaution should be to avoid physical exercise just after receiving the medication. The recent introduction of sublingual immunotherapy has greatly increased the safety of this treatment.

ANTIHISTAMINES

Oral H1 antihistamines are one of the first-line therapeutic options for allergic rhinitis. The new generation molecules have high selectivity, long half-lives and also possess anti-allergic activities. In athletes, the main concern with antihistamines is the possible sedative effect. Although this side-effect is, at least in part, variable from one individual to another, the newest molecules (cetirizine, desloratadine, fexofenadine, levocetirizine, loratadine, mizolastine) proved to be devoid of sedative effect at the usual therapeutic doses. Moreover, those molecules not undergoing liver metabolism (cetirizine, desloratadine, fexofenadine) have the additional advantage of avoiding possible drug–drug interactions and rare but severe cardiotoxic effects.

ANTI-LEUKOTRIENES

The available leukotriene receptor antagonists (zafirlukast and montelukast) are now officially accepted as part of the general therapeutic plan for asthma treatment. In elite and amateur exercisers anti-leukotrienes proved highly effective in protecting against exercise-induced bronchospasm, and can therefore be given in substitution of the β_2-agonists premedication. No particular contraindication for anti-leukotrienes in those practicing sports has so far emerged for anti-leukotrienes, which are included among the drugs for asthmatic athletes permitted by the IOC with no limitations.

TOPICAL STEROIDS

Highly effective as controller drugs for asthma, the use of steroids in athletes has required notification and a physician's certificate from 1993 to 2002. At present, there is no regulation for the use of topical steroids in athletes, although regulations differ among various international sports associations and some of them still follow previous requirements (a TUE is required).

INHALED β-AGONISTS

From the early 1990s there has been a marked concern regarding the use of asthma drugs among elite competitive athletes, especially in endurance sports. In 1993, the IOC, MC decided that only the two short-acting inhaled β_2-agonists, salbutamol and terbutaline, were allowed for use in competitive sports. Use should be declared by the athlete and accompanied by a physician's certificate. The same regulations were made for inhaled steroids. Concern was expressed because of reports that β_2-agonists systemically given in large doses might influence skeletal and heart ventricular muscle fibers in research animals. However, several studies demonstrated that short-acting inhaled β_2-agonists do not improve performance in athletes. New studies confirmed this too for the long-acting β_2-agonists, salmeterol (which was allowed from February 1, 1996) and for inhaled formoterol (allowed from September 1, 2002). At this time WADA had been established, and the doping regulations were the common regulations given by WADA and IOC, MC. From this date, the regulation for asthma drugs only concerned the β_2-agonists, as there were no regulations for the use of inhaled steroids. However, some confusion existed, as regulations differed somewhat between the different international sport associations. FIS (the International Skiing Association) still includes inhaled steroids in their regulations.

Confusion persisted through January 2002. Preliminary regulations for major sporting events were sent out only weeks before the event, including required limits for methacholine provocation (PD_{20}, PC_{20}), levels for responses to bronchodilators and for exercise testing are inadequate. As treatment of asthma has long-term implications, it can be stated that this short-term notice is in conflict with the common guidelines for asthma treatment.

Currently, the latest WADA regulations do not employ predefined limits of bronchial hyper-responsiveness or EIB, but requires extensive documentation.

Because of the extensive use of asthma drugs among top endurance athletes, documentation is clearly required. However, as the current rules and definitions may be confusing, there is clearly a need for defining diagnostic criteria for EIA and bronchial hyperresponsiveness in athletes, guidelines for its treatment, and for refining the present doping regulations. The doping regulations should also be standardized within the different sports associations.

It seems that in some cases an athlete's asthma is difficult to treat. Inhaled corticosteroids are only partly effective, probably because the inflammation has irritant characteristics demonstrated by an increased share of neutrophils, as well as eosinophils, in induced sputum samples. In symptomatic ice-hockey players, even montelukast was ineffective. Bronchodilators offer only limited relief because well-performing athletes do not usually show significant bronchoconstriction even though they may have intensive cough and sputum production.

Limitations for exercise in obstructive airflow disease

The two major physiologic abnormalities in obstructive airflow disease are bronchoconstriction and air trapping. Bronchoconstriction leads to limitation of expiratory flow, which in turn results in air trapping.

The secondary effects of the above two primary abnormalities are limitation in maximum ventilation, hypoxemia of exercise, and disuse atrophy of peripheral muscles, especially in the legs. These are manifested in exercise testing by a reduced $\dot{V}o_{2max}$, low peak ventilation, elevated submaximal ventilation, increased breathing frequency, high dead space, possible hypoxemia, and hypercarbia of exercise. These findings can occur in varying degrees between and within patients at different times. The combination of the above gives rise to dyspnea.

Treatment of these physiologic abnormalities are through the use of bronchodilators to increase airflow, or exercise training to reduce or more efficiently serve demand for oxygen at the mitochondria of skeletal muscles. Pharmacologic and surgical interventions that reduce lung volumes or overexpansion of the lungs during exercise

alleviate exertional dyspnea. Oxygen during exercise (increase in FIo_2) and skeletal muscle conditioning also assists exercise tolerance.

Genetics of asthma

Asthma has been known to have a familial component for many years, and represents the cumulative effects of environmental factors on a predisposed genetic background. Measures of the genetic contribution have been carried out in a wide variety of populations, and have used different definitions of asthma.

However, asthma is not by any means an exclusively genetic disorder. The recent increase in the frequency of asthma cannot be explained by changing genetic background, which only alters over many generations. In addition, the fact that 40% of identical twins are not concordant for asthma indicates that there are many factors unrelated to genetics that influence whether a person develops asthma. The fact that asthma is in a family does not necessarily indicate a major genetic component, as family members share the same environment, including smoking and other environmental exposures.

The genetic component in asthma can be considered polygenic, whereby the predisposition to asthma is contributed to, not by one or two major genes, but a significant number of variants in several lower effect genes. The variants in such genes are likely to be present in the unaffected population as well as people with asthma, but at a higher frequency in those with asthma. Therefore, dissecting out the contribution of such genes becomes a major challenge, requiring large numbers of carefully defined populations, and a great deal of investment in expensive genetic technology and trained staff.

Definitions of asthma

Two main definitions of asthma have been used. The first is the classification of asthma as a manifestation of atopy, thereby including eczema and raised levels of IgE in the definition. The second approach is by defining asthma in the form of induced bronchial hyperreactivity, without reference to atopy.

Defining the genetic contribution

Two main methods of defining the genetic contribution have been used: heritability and twin studies.

HERITABILITY OF ASTHMA

Heritability is the likelihood of a first-degree relative (child or sibling) of a person affected with asthma developing the same condition themselves, when compared with the likelihood in the general population. If the condition has a significant genetic component, then the heritability in families should be increased over the population. The heritability of asthma has been given a wide range of figures, ranging from 30% up to 80% depending on the population and definition used. Nonetheless, all studies have shown a clear familial component.

TWIN STUDIES

Twin studies have compared identical (monozygotic; MZ) with non-identical (dizygotic; DZ) twins, to find out when one twin is affected the likelihood of the other twin also being affected, or concordant. In a genetic condition, the frequency of a condition in MZ twins should be significantly increased compared to DZ twins.

In addition, several twin studies have shown that MZ twins have about 60% concordance for asthma, compared to about 30% concordance for DZ twins.

IDENTIFYING GENES PREDISPOSING TO ASTHMA

The approaches to finding the genes involved in asthma are complex, but all depend on accurate clinical classification of a selected population. Some studies use large numbers of affected sibs with asthma, in a linkage study that does not assume any particular mode of inheritance (non-parametric sib pair study). Other studies use even larger numbers of individuals with asthma, but without any affected family members, and compare with unaffected controls (which also have to be carefully clinically assessed) in an association study.

GENOME SCAN

The form of research genetic testing carried out can also vary. One approach is to study several thousand anonymous gene markers in each patient. These markers are known to vary between individuals, in what is loosely called a genome scan. These markers are either microsatellite markers or, increasingly, single nucleotide polymorphisms (SNPs) which lend themselves to automation and are spread right across all 23 human chromosomes. The aim of such a study is to find chromosome regions where particular variants of a marker are found more frequently than might be expected by chance either in sets of sibs or in individuals with asthma. If such a region is identified, the assumption would be that such a region contains a gene or genes that may contribute to causing asthma.

There have been at least 10 whole genome studies carried out in the last 8 years on populations from France, Germany, USA, UK, and also on the isolated Hutterite community in the USA. However, many of the initial findings have not been reproduced when analyzed in a different population. Such discrepancies may reflect population differences between countries, ascertainment bias, or differences in disease classification. However, there have been consistent findings of linkage to regions on chromosomes 5q, 6p, 12q, and 13q. No specific causative gene has been firmly identified in any of these regions.

CANDIDATE GENE

Another approach on such large populations is to use genetic markers close to a gene that may, based on its known function, have a role in the development of asthma. This is called a candidate gene approach. The aim would be to see whether specific variants of genetic markers in the region of a candidate gene are overrepresented in the asthma population compared with matched controls.

Given that a significant amount is known about the pathobiology of asthma, there are many candidate genes that can be analyzed by linkage or association studies in patients with asthma. The major histocompatibility cluster locus (MHC) encoding the human leukocyte antigen (HLA) genes on 6p21 has been linked in a variety of different asthma phenotypes. This linkage is certainly for class II HLA antigens, but has not been fully elucidated for other MHC loci. The tumour necrosis factor genes in the MHC cluster may also be linked to asthma.

A region on chromosome 5 has been shown to be linked to total serum IgE concentrations in a number of populations, and this linkage is likely to be to a series of interleukin genes, especially IL-13. A polymorphic DNA marker on chromosome 11q13 was reported to be linked to asthma in 1989. This genetic contribution seems to be attributable to the β-chain of the high-affinity receptor for IgE.

PHARMACOGENETICS OF ASTHMA

Pharmacogenetics can be defined as the genetic influence on a person's response to a specific drug, and also whether they might develop side-effects. There are good examples of several genetic influences on a person's response to all three main treatments for asthma: β$_2$-adrenergic agonists, corticosteroids, and leukotriene modifiers. For β-adrenergic agents, the variation can be in the β$_2$ receptor itself, but also in the downstream molecules which transducer the signal generated by the activated β$_2$ receptor, such as several forms of adenyl cyclase. A variant in a T-cell-specific gene transcription factor TBX21 is shown to be associated with better response to inhaled corticosteroids. A variant in the corticotropin-releasing hormone receptor 1 is also associated with response to inhaled steroids. Response to leukotriene modifiers can also be influenced by genetic variants in several genes that are involved in leukotriene metabolism, such as leukotriene C4 synthase. However, none of these gene variants have sufficient predictive power for clinical use currently to predict which form of therapy best suits an individual patient.

There has been a great deal of work on the genetics of asthma over the last 10 years, with a deeper understanding of the biology of the condition. However, as yet none of these genetic advances is clinically applicable. With the pace of both biologic understanding and genetic technology, such genetic findings may well have a place in the management of asthma in years to come.

Effects of exercise on the immune system and respiratory functions

Asthma is a well-recognized clinical syndrome with a complex and hotly debated pathophysiology. Like seasonal rhinitis and atopic eczema, allergic asthma is an atopic disease. Atopic individuals have as yet ill-defined susceptibility genes that combine with environmental influences to predispose the asthmatic state. In the affected airway, cellular infiltration and the release of inflammatory mediators results in the common physiologic denominators of bronchial hyperresponsiveness and transient obstruction, mucous hypersecretion and, ultimately, airway remodeling.

Evidence of substantial inflammation is found in bronchial biopsy specimens of asthmatic patients even in the presence of mild disease. Such biopsies show an increase in the numbers and activation of mast cells, macrophages, eosinophils, and lymphocytes. These cells have been shown in both animal and human studies to be important in the progression of asthmatic inflammation.

TYPE I HYPERSENSITIVITY RESPONSE

Atopic individuals typically have increased levels of total and allergen-specific IgE. IgE is thought to have an important physiologic role in protection against parasitic infections. However, it is a key molecule in the pathologic type I hypersensitivity response, which contributes to inflammation in allergic asthma. In genetically susceptible atopic individuals, ubiquitous environmental proteins act as allergens and drive the onset of IgE-mediated type I hypersensitivity.

In such individuals, inhaled allergens encounter dendritic cells in the airways. These dendritic cells are highly efficient antigen-presenting cells which take up and process the allergen protein. The dendritic cells migrate to regional lymph nodes where they present the offending allergen to helper T cells via interaction with cell surface receptors. Helper T cells communicate with other cells of the immune system by secretion of cytokines and through this mechanism "help" other cells to propagate the immune response. When presented with processed allergen, the helper T cells secrete cytokines, including IL-4, IL-5, and IL-13, which act on antibody secreting B cells. The stimulated B cell, under the influence of these interleukins, then switches to the production of IgE.

After a short period in the circulation, IgE binds to high affinity receptors on the surface of mast cells. In patients with asthma, inhaled allergen interacts with surface bound IgE on mast cells and causes molecular cross-linking. This triggers rapid degranulation of the mast cell with the release of preformed mediators into the surrounding tissue.

The release of histamine, leukotrienes, and interleukins from mast cells causes acute bronchoconstriction and initiates a more prolonged inflammatory reaction which contributes to airway hyperresponsiveness and can continue even in the absence of repeated stimulation with an allergen.

This pathway provides the opportunity to test novel therapeutic agents. A monoclonal antibody that forms complexes with free IgE and blocks its interaction with mast cells is currently being studied in asthmatic patients. Early investigations have shown only a small impact on symptoms but an encouraging reduction in steroid dependence in patients with severe asthma. With use of this agent, IgE levels return to normal but inflammation continues. Clearly, there are other pathways at play.

EOSINOPHILS

Eosinophils are dominant cells in the asthmatic inflammatory infiltrate. These cells were initially associated with asthma in the 1800s when their presence in large numbers was demonstrated in the first pathologic description of fatal status asthmaticus. However, the exact role of this oft forgotten cell remains elusive.

Recent novel animal studies have rejuvenated interest in eosinophils. One study in transgenic mice showed that the absence of eosinophils conferred protection from airway remodeling. Another study, with a different strain of eosinophil-depleted mice, showed reductions in airway hyperresponsiveness

and mucus production. Thus, in mice at least, the eosinophil may have a role in all the key physiologic processes that contribute to the asthma clinical syndrome. The relevance of these animal models to asthma remains to be demonstrated.

In asthma patients, the number of airway eosinophils is directly associated with disease severity and effective corticosteroid therapy reduces the eosinophil count. However, it is not enough to determine the guilt of the eosinophil merely by association. The cytokine IL-5, derived from helper T lymphocytes, is important in the production of eosinophils. A monoclonal antibody that inhibits the action of IL-5 has been studied in patients with mild asthma. These limited studies showed no impact on asthma symptoms despite reducing eosinophil levels in sputum and blood. It remains to be seen if therapies with specific impacts on eosinophil activity will offer symptomatic benefit in asthmatic patients.

Exercise and the immune system

In experimental acute models, intense physical exercise is a stress event inducing several changes of immune functions. Changes of immune parameters during and after exercise include an increase of leukocytes and neutrophils, a reduction of T and B cells with an impaired IgA and IgM production after exercise, a reduction of natural killer (NK) cells and an increase of pro-inflammatory cytokines. In elite athletes, the transient immunodeficiency observed after overtraining is associated with an increased risk of infections, particularly of the upper respiratory tract. The propensity to viral infections as well as to allergic diseases in elite athletes might suggest that strenuous and continuous physical exercise favor a Th1–Th2 imbalance with a prevalent Th2 cytokine profile.

Special attention has also been devoted to the effects of physical exercise on the immune system through its effects on neural and endocrine functions. The mechanisms by which the neuroendocrine system communicates with the immune system and vice versa have been the object of increasing attention from the scientific community over the past 20 years. The set point of these interactions is determined by the central nervous system through the modulation of the hypothalamic–pituitary–adrenal (HPA) axis and the systemic adrenomedullary sympathetic nervous system (SNS), the peripheral limb of the stress system. Exercise and training activate the central components of the system, the corticotropin-releasing hormone (CRH) and locus ceruleus–norepinephrine (LC-NA) autonomic (sympathetic) neurons, which regulate the systemic secretion of glucocorticoids and catecholamines, respectively, mainly epinephrine and norepinephrine and that may in turn influence the immune responses.

The exercise-related stress condition may activate another feedback loop in which cytokines produced by immunocompetent cells act on the hypothalamus to regulate the output of glucocorticoids. In particular, the cytokines tumor necrosis factor α (TNF-α), IL-1, and IL-6, may stimulate CRH secretion and activate both the HPA axis and the SNS. Few data are present in the literature concerning the possibility that strenuous exercise, by these mechanisms, may interfere in the equilibrium between pro-inflammatory (IL-12, TNF-α, γ-interferon) and anti-inflammatory (IL-4, IL-10) cytokine production. Catecholamines released rapidly during exercise, through their specific β_2-adrenergic receptor, might upregulate IL-10 production by monocyte/macrophages without affecting the T helper lymphocyte subclasses Th2 directly even if they may potentiate cytokine production by these cells.

Glucocorticoids, released in the latest response to strenuous exercise, through specific cytoplasmatic/nuclear receptors, might upregulate the zproduction of IL-10 and IL-4 by Th2 cells, then altering the Th1–Th2 balance neuroendocrine immune system. Hormones released after exercise may exert systemic effects on the pro-inflammatory–anti-inflammatory cytokine balance but this evidence may not pertain with local responses in specific compartments of the body. Systemically, exercise-induced release of glucocorticoids and catecholamines seem to be able to stimulate an important immunoendocrine mechanism that protects the athlete from an excess production of pro-inflammatory cytokines and other products of activated macrophages with tissue-damaging

potential. Locally, it may support cytokine production, suppressing or potentiating the regional immune response.

However, hyperventilation associated with exercise is responsible for a limitation in the airflow in a large proportion of subjects as well as with marked nasal pathophysiologic changes, as previously reported.

Functional changes of upper and lower airways induced by exercise are accompanied by an increased number of inflammatory cells in the airways and sputum as well as of circulating CD34+ progenitor cells.

Immunology of asthma in childhood

Epidemiologic studies suggest that exposure to minor respiratory infections and gastrointestinal viruses in early childhood is protective against asthma. Children with older siblings, those who live with pets, and those exposed to daycare facilities at an early stage could be expected to have an increased exposure to minor infections and other potential immunologic stimuli. Such children seem to have a reduced incidence of atopic disease, including asthma.

These findings have resulted in the development of the "hygiene hypothesis." This theory suggests that the epidemic of asthma that is currently gripping the developed world is caused by the lack of immune stimulus in our ultrahygenic Western environment. Efforts to give a scientific explanation for this attractive and media-friendly hypothesis center on the role of the helper T cell.

Helper T lymphocytes have an important role in regulating the immune response and are found in increased numbers in bronchial biopsy specimens of patients with asthma. Current opinion accepts that there are two subtypes of the helper T lymphocyte which are differentiated on the basis of the profile of the cytokine molecules that they secrete and which they use to communicate with and direct other inflammatory cells.

Th1 lymphocytes produce IL-2 and γ-interferon which are important in cell-mediated defense mechanisms. In contrast, Th2 lymphocytes secrete IL-4, IL-5, IL-6, IL-9, and IL-13 which promote allergic inflammation by upregulating mast cells, increasing the production of IgE, and recruiting eosinophils.

It is known that the majority of helper T lymphocytes in the blood of newborn infants are Th2 cells. It is thought that exposure to minor infections upregulates the Th1 cells and leads to a balance between the two subtypes. If exposure to minor infections is limited, then a preponderance of Th2 cells persists predisposing to allergic type inflammation (Bylin *et al.* 1988). This hypothesis implies that a majority of Th1 lymphocyte population should protect against asthma.

However, animal studies tell us that the transfer of allergen-specific Th1 cells to naïve recipients can cause severe airways inflammation. In addition, the cytokine γ-interferon, which is derived from Th1 cells and has been shown to inhibit IgE synthesis and eosinophilia, is present at increased levels in asthma and is thought to be involved in asthma pathogenesis. Thus, the scientific explanation for the hygiene hypothesis is elegant in its simplicity but may not reflect the true complexities of the T-cell involvement in asthma.

Interesting new studies have suggested that exposure to minor infections may allow the development of tolerance to environmental allergens. These studies have suggested a role for a further T cell subtype known as regulatory T cells. Regulatory T cells induce tolerance to antigenic proteins by inhibiting the formation of allergen-specific T cells which contribute to the allergic response. Studies in mice with allergic asthma show that regulatory T cells fail to develop in favor of the Th2 phenotype resulting in a loss of tolerance to a variety of antigens. Production of regulatory T cells is favored by IL-10 secretion by dendritic cells in the respiratory tract that are exposed to antigen and by exposure to viral infections such as hepatitis A. These intriguing regulatory T cells may be another mechanism by which our insulation from environmental antigens may be contributing to the development of asthma.

There is general consensus that asthma is an aberrant immune response to otherwise harmless environmental particles in genetically susceptible individuals. The complexities of this inflammatory response are evident from the often conflicting evidence obtained from experimental models of asthma. It seems that numerous cell types contribute to the inflammatory process and that subtle immunologic differences may differentiate allergic asthma from later onset intrinsic asthma and the exercise-induced asthma variant. Deeper insight into the immunologic mechanisms of asthmatic inflammation should continue to provide new therapeutic targets and may ultimately quiet the asthmatic wheeze.

Upper respiratory tract infection in the athlete: epidemiology and clinical approach to rhinitis and conjunctivitis

Rhinitis in athletes

EPIDEMIOLOGY

Rhinitis occurs frequently in athletes, its prevalence in various studies depending on the criteria used for diagnosis. Helbling and Muller (1991) found that 16.8% of 2060 active Swiss athletes (of 68 different sports) had hay fever, most of them (59%) needing medication during the pollen season.

Athletes with hay fever had significantly more often exercise-related airway symptoms, but received inadequate treatment (Bousquet *et al.* 2001). In a study on 214 athletes, 56% gave a symptom history consistent with allergic rhinoconjunctivitis, 41% also having a positive skin test response to any one allergen, and 29% had seasonal allergic conjunctivitis (a positive seasonal history and at least one positive skin-prick test response to a seasonal allergen). In another series of 265 athletes selected for the Sydney Olympic Games, the prevalence of positive skin tests was 32.6%, and 25.3% of athletes had clinical rhinitis.

As for asthma, the prevalence of allergic rhinitis seems to be on the increase, since the reported prevalence of approximately 8.0% in the 1980s doubled in 1996 (19.6%). Allergic rhinitis was shown to have negative effects on performance scores (ability to train and compete) over the spring. Athletes from aquatic sports were more likely to have symptoms than those from other sports. Athletes who were treated in season with intranasal steroids (once daily for 8 weeks) had statistically significant improvements in symptoms, quality of life, and performance scores.

Epidemiologic data indicate that asthma and allergic rhinitis frequently coexist, even in the absence of atopy, with rhinitis symptoms being reported in 80–90% of asthma patients and asthma symptoms reported in 19–38% of those with allergic rhinitis (Dykewicz *et al*. 1998). A European survey of 1412 subjects with perennial rhinitis and 5198 control subjects found asthma present in 16.2% of subjects with rhinitis and 1% of controls. If epidemiologic studies indicate that up to 40% of patients with allergic rhinitis may have asthma, prospective studies suggest that rhinitis frequently precedes the development of asthma. Moreover, many patients with rhinitis alone demonstrate non-specific bronchial hyperresponsiveness and this may be a risk factor for developing asthma (Bylin *et al*. 1988; Widdicombe 1996).

CLINICAL SYMPTOMS

Reported nasal symptoms in the responses to the United States Olympic Committee (USOC) questionnaire ($n = 67$) were as follows: obstruction 55%, rhinorrea 54%, sneezing 50%, and pruritus 43%. Of athletes with rhinitis, 52% were treated with oral antihistamines and 60% with nasal corticosteroids. However, clinical presentation (and pathophysiologic mechanisms) of rhinitis may vary depending on the type of sports practiced. Accordingly, rhinitis in swimmers, skiers, boxers, and runners are often considered as distinct clinical entities.

Severity of allergic rhinitis and asthma has also been shown to be correlated. Patients with allergic rhinitis exhibit increased eosinophil activity in both upper and lower airways. In these patients, nasal allergen challenge can induce increased bronchial hyperresponsiveness, suggesting that upper and lower airway disorders share common inflammatory features.

TREATMENT

Proper management of allergic rhinitis also improves asthma control, reinforcing the link between both diseases. In fact, intranasal steroids prevent the seasonal increase in non-specific bronchial hyper-reactivity and asthma symptoms associated with pollen exposure. In patients with perennial rhinitis, intranasal corticosteroids were also shown to reduce asthma symptoms, exercise-induced bronchospasm, and bronchial responsiveness to methacholine. In addition to being safe and effective, inhaled corticosteroids are permitted by WADA and IOC, MC following notification by an aTUE form.

The pathophysiologic connections between the upper and lower airways are not completely understood and different mechanisms have been proposed.

EIA occurs in up to 40% of patients with allergic rhinitis. However, EIA frequently goes undiagnosed in children and athletes. Among high school adolescent athletes, 7–12% of subjects not considered to be at risk by baseline spirometry or negative history (asthma, EIA, or rhinitis) tested positive in an exercise challenge.

On the basis of the above reported data, every rhinitic athlete should be screened for asthma and EIA according to Allergic Rhinitis and its Impact on Asthma (ARIA) guidelines. Standard asthma diagnosis procedures for the athlete with rhinitis should include resting spirometry with bronchodilator test, bronchial provocation with methacholine, and field exercise challenge in the usual sport environment or in controlled environment in the laboratory. For the diagnosis of exercise-induced rhinitis, nasal peak inspiratory flow monitoring in the field and/or laboratory exercise challenge with specific nasal evaluation (functional rhinomanometry and morphologic acoustic rhinometry) may be especially useful. Ideally, as in other occupational diseases, these tests should be performed and recorded before therapeutic interventions.

Athletes practicing and competing outdoors should also be screened for the possibility of intermittent rhinitis and/or asthma associated with pollen allergy, which will have a negative impact on their expected peak performances. In major national and international competitions local pollen counts and forecasts (www.polleninfo.org) should be made available in advance to allergic athletes, their coaches, and medical teams.

Conjunctivitis in athletes

The lack of a common nomenclature and of standardized diagnostic procedures and flow charts makes it particularly difficult to determine the prevalence of conjunctivitis in elite athletes. In fact, most of the studies refer to hay fever or allergic rhino-conjunctivitis or seasonal rhino-conjunctivitis, accompanying nasal and eye symptoms and do not give information on different forms and severity of allergic conjunctivitis in individual cases. Data about non-allergic conjunctivitis are even more scarce and anecdotal.

In a study of 214 athletes, 56% gave a symptoms history consistent with allergic rhino-conjunctivitis, 41% had a positive response to any one allergen, and 29% had seasonal allergic rhino-conjunctivitis defined as a positive seasonal history and at least one positive skin-prick test to a three-seasonal allergen.

In another study of 265 Italian Olympic athletes, conjunctivitis was found in 18.8% of athletes. Certainly, from data of epidemiologic studies of allergic diseases in the general population, allergic conjunctivitis seems widely underdiagnosed, because conjunctival symptoms are often considered of less importance than lung and nose symptoms both by the patient and by the doctor. However, allergic conjunctivitis has a significant effect on the athlete's well-being and sports activity. Moreover, oral antihistamines often used to control symptoms may significantly affect vigilance, further influencing the quality of performances.

Atopic conjunctivitis and contact ocular allergy (contact dermatitis of the eyelids) also frequently occur in athletes, in whom increased sweating and use of detergents modify the hydrolipid film of the skin and reduce its defensive capacity. In a study of professional football players, a diagnosis of atopic conjunctivitis or contact dermatitis was made in 5.8% of cases (Ventura *et al.* 2001). Thiourans and mercaptobenzothiazole were the prevalent haptens responsible for positive patch tests in contact dermatitis of the eyelids. The study also showed the increasing relevance of sensitization to latex, favored by the many rubber items in sports equipment (eyeglasses, masks, gloves, clothes, shoes).

Epidemiology of allergic and infectious diseases of the respiratory tract

Exercise increases minute ventilation approximately 20 times (or 20-fold) at rest and changes nasal to mouth breathing. Therefore, athletes are exposed to large amounts of pollutants, including aeroallergens and microbial products. Moreover, intense and prolonged physical activity induces several changes in immune parameters and response to environmental agents, which result in an increased susceptibility to infections and to a preferential Th2 (allergic) phenotype. Accordingly, allergic and infectious diseases of the respiratory tract represent a major concern in sports medicine.

Epidemiology

The prevalence of asthma in elite athletes has been reported to range between 3.7% and 28.8%, depending on the study population and methods used for diagnosis.

Studies performed on comparable population samples indicate that the disease is on the increase, because its prevalence in comparable studies of US Olympic athletes was 9.7% in 1976 and 16.7% in 1996, and values as high as 21.9% have been reported both at the 1998 Nagano Winter Games and at the 2000 Sydney Olympics.

Certainly, the prevalence of bronchial hyperreactivity to methacholine in elite athletes (49%) is higher than that in controls (28%). The highest prevalence of bronchial hyperreactivity has been reported in swimmers and in athletes exercising in humid air.

Accordingly, asthma and asthma-like symptoms are more common in elite athletes than age-matched controls. Asthma is most commonly found in athletes performing endurance events such as cycling, swimming, or long-distance running. Asthma risk is closely associated with atopy and its severity among athletes. When the two risk factors, sporting event and atopy, were combined in a logistic regression model, the increases of relative risk of asthma were surprisingly large: 25-fold in an atopic speed and power athlete; 42-fold in an atopic long-distance runner; and even 97-fold in an atopic swimmer compared with non-atopic controls.

Swimmers and ice-hockey players have shown a mixed type of eosinophilic and neutrophilic inflammation in induced sputum samples. This inflammation correlates with clinical parameters (i.e., exercise-induced bronchial symptoms and bronchial hyperresponsiveness). Karjalainen *et al.* (2000) observed increased T lymphocytes, neutrophils, and eosinophils in the lamina propria of bronchial biopsy samples from highly trained cross-country skiers. It was also shown that mild eosinophilic and lymphocytic airway inflammation was aggravated in swimmers who remained active during a 5-year prospective follow-up study. In contrast, in swimmers who stopped active training, eosinophilic airway inflammation, bronchial responsiveness, and clinical asthma attenuated or even disappeared. This prospective study indicated for the first time that intensive training is associated with long-term airway irritation as well as clinical asthma in susceptible individuals, and these changes are at least partly reversible when training is stopped.

Similar inflammatory changes have also been reported in endurance athletes who show an increase in airway inflammatory cells associated with changes in exhaled NO after exercise.

Because some anti-asthmatic drugs are banned by the current anti-doping regulations, methods for diagnosis of asthma in athletes must be accurate and standardized, but should also ensure that criteria requested should not come in conflict with an optimal treatment of the disease as codified by Global Initiative for Ashthma (GINA) guidelines.

The sensitivity and specificity of parameters used for diagnosis of asthma in athletes largely depends on the thresholds chosen as limits of normality. Accordingly, a distinction should be made between asthmatic athletes or athletes with a history of asthma and apparently healthy athletes or rhinitic athletes (who should always be studied for asthma).

Seventeen per cent of 253 Finnish elite summer sport athletes used anti-asthmatic drugs (most commonly inhaled β_2-agonists) and 17% of the US Winter Olympic team (Nagano) were current users of asthma medication. The figure was twice as high (36%) among Swedish cross-country skiers.

The prevalence of asthma in athletes has significantly increased even in studies with comparable methodology: from 9.7% in 1976 to 21.9% in 1996 in the Australian Olympic delegation and from 4.3% in 1984 to 15.3% in 1996 in the US delegation. In Australian Olympic swimmers the prevalence of asthma was 21.0% in 1976 and 25.9% in 1996.

Asthma is commonly found in swimmers and athletes performing endurance events, such as cross-country skiing or long-distance running. However, speed and power athletes (e.g., ice-hockey players and track and field athletes) also have an increased risk of asthma.

As for rhinitis, atopy is a major risk factor for a higher asthma prevalence and severity. When the two risk factors – type of sport and atopy – were combined in a logistic regression model, the relative risk of asthma was particularly high compared to non-atopic control subjects: 25-fold in atopic speed and power athletes; 42-fold in atopic long-distance runners; and 97-fold in atopic swimmers.

Clinical asthma symptoms are usually related to bronchial hyperreactivity, but the relationship is not straightforward. Bronchial hyperreactivity has been reported to be particularly prevalent in swimmers independently from the presence of clinical asthma. Zwick *et al.* (1990) found competitive swimmers to have significantly more often bronchial hyperreactivity than matched controls (78% vs. 36%). In another study, bronchial hyperreactivity was detected in 60% of swimmers and in 12% of non-swimming athletes.

Asthma symptoms and bronchial hyperreactivity are associated in athletes with a mixed type of eosinophilic and neutrophilic airway inflammation. Sputum eosinophilia (>2% in differential cell count) was found in 20% of highly trained swimmers and in 10% of ice-hockey players. After a 5-year follow-up, sputum eosinophilia was detected in 38% (6% at baseline) of those swimmers who continued their sport activity and in 8% (19% at baseline) of those who had stopped intensive training. Thus, athletes' asthma is at least partly revertible, and intensive training seems to cause airway inflammation and asthmatic symptoms in susceptible individuals.

Rhinitis–asthma link

Epidemiologic data indicate that asthma and allergic rhinitis frequently coexist, even in the absence of atopy, with rhinitis symptoms being reported in 80–90% of asthma patients and asthma symptoms reported in 19–38% of those with allergic rhinitis. A European survey of 1412 subjects with perennial rhinitis and 5198 control subjects found asthma to be present in 40% of patients with allergic rhinitis (Leyneart et al. 1999). Prospective studies suggest that rhinitis frequently precedes the development of asthma. Moreover, many patients with rhinitis alone demonstrate non-specific bronchial hyperresponsiveness and this may be a risk factor for developing asthma.

Severity of allergic rhinitis and asthma has also been shown to be correlated. Patients with allergic rhinitis exhibit increased eosinophil activity in both upper and lower airways. In these patients, nasal allergen challenge can induce increased bronchial hyperresponsiveness, suggesting that upper and lower airway disorders share common inflammatory features. Proper management of allergic rhinitis also improves asthma control, reinforcing the link between both diseases. In fact, intranasal steroids prevent the seasonal increase in non-specific bronchial hyperactivity and asthma symptoms associated with pollen exposure. In patients with perennial rhinitis, intranasal corticosteroids were also shown to reduce asthma symptoms, exercise-induced bronchospasm, and bronchial responsiveness to methacholine.

The pathophysiologic connections between the upper and the lower airways are not completely understood and different mechanisms have been proposed (Table 7.5).

On the basis of the above reported data, every rhinitic athlete should be screened for asthma and EIA according to ARIA guidelines.

Respiratory tract infections

The transient immunodeficiencies observed after overtraining – particularly those involving IgA and the mucosal immune system – are responsible for the reported increased incidence of upper respiratory tract infections (URTI) in athletes.

Endurance athletes appear to be at higher risk of URTI, particularly close to competitions. In runners, not only the number of URTI is increased – in relation to the race time and training – but also the

Table 7.5 Possible mechanisms linking rhinitis and asthma.

Direct effects
Nasal–bronchial reflex (irritant receptors–cholinergic nerves)
Postnasal drip of inflammatory cells/mediators
Mucosal hyperosmolarity (exercise-induced rhinitis and asthma)

Indirect effects
Oral breathing pattern (loss of nasal air conditioning because of obstruction)
Systemic propagation of a localized allergic inflammation

duration of the infectious episodes. However, recurrent episodes of URTI are not confined to runners but have been reported for different sports in national Olympic delegations.

Both viruses (rhinovirus – particularly in spring – influenza and parainfluenza virus, adenovirus and coronavirus) and bacteria (streptococci, staphylococci) are claimed to be involved in causing URTI in athletes, although data from large systematic studies including the isolation and identification of the responsible agents are still very limited.

There is growing evidence that lifestyle factors related to sports activity (stress, traveling and jet-lag, sleep deprivation, community living) contribute to decrease immunity and increased susceptibility to infections.

Several dietary supplements have been reported to restore a normal immune function and reduce the increased risk of URTI in athletes, including vitamin C, glucose, lipids, zinc and other minerals, and echinacea. However, data available are scarce and sometimes conflicting; recent systematic reviews and metanalysis failed to show any effect for most of the remedies suggested. The high prevalence of URTI in athletes has induced some authors to recommend an yearly vaccination against influenza (and hepatitis A and B immunization).

Infections: bacterial, viral, mycobacteriae, fungal, parasitic, SARS, bird flu

Infections of the respiratory tract are a cause of concern in athletes for two reasons: airflow obstruction and systemic manifestations likely to cause myocarditis or other serious conditions. It is a rule of thumb that athletes with upper respiratory manifestations may compete. An athlete with lower respiratory manifestations and a temperature above 38°C should be advised to rest until the findings clear in a matter of days.

The most common lower respiratory infections acquired in the community are viral infections, *Mycoplasma pneumoniae*, *Chlamydia*, Legionnaires' disease, and pneumococcal pneumonia. These four latter conditions respond quickly to macrolides which should be the drug of first choice if an antibiotic is considered necessary. Supportive care with paracetamol is also used. Both these drugs are allowed without notification.

SARS and sporting events

Severe acute respiratory syndrome (SARS) is a viral respiratory condition, less contagious than influenza or viral pneumonia. It has a high mortality and morbidity and can only be treated symptomatically. Diagnosis is best carried out with the aid of a CT scan of the chest. Treatment is by supportive care only, with best outcome after the use of systemic corticosteroids (www.hongkonguniversity.edu).

SARS affected athletes should not be allowed to compete as this is a serious, systemic, lower respiratory tract infection.

WHO countries affected by SARS

WHO recommendations of the countries affected should be taken into consideration when athletes travelling abroad are being prepared for competition (www.who.org). Recommendations for competition in the presence of SARS were outlined in 2003 and are as follows: The EOC, MC, at their meeting in Hasselt, Belgium on May 17, 2003, taking into consideration the recent epidemic of SARS and the need for the continuation of sporting events, recommended the following measures.

Preventive measures for SARS

Training or isolation camps are recommended for athletes from countries on the WHO list affected by the epidemic. Teams or individuals attending from countries with a WHO SARS alert should be invited to attend these camps for at least 10 days after leaving their country. This is being carried out to prevent spread of disease and for the adaptation for circadian rhythm disturbances.

Respiratory isolation (using an N-95 face mask, surgical gloves, gowns, glasses, and head cover) is only indicated for athletes with possible exposure to SARS or symptoms suggestive of lower respiratory tract infection.

These principles can be extrapolated to other infectious lower respiratory tract disorders.

Other pulmonary conditions

Nasal polyps

These are a form of upper airway obstruction. The grape-like polyps block the nasal passage and require the use of mouth breathing. Mouth breathing removes the effects of the nose and sinuses in heating and humidifying the inspired air. Treatment is by surgical removal. Prevention is by the use of steroids by nasal insufflations.

Sleep apnea

Good quality sleep is essential to all athletes' preparation and participation in sporting events. The lack of good quality sleep will lead to underperformance. The modern sleep laboratory has taught us a great deal about event preparation. For example, a normal structured sleep night does not occur on the first night in a strange bed and environment. The value of sleeping in the same bed for three nights before a major event can ensure a normal performance the next day.

Sleep apnea is a severe form of snoring. Snoring is present in up to 40% of the general population. It is upper airway (oropharyngeal soft tissue) obstruction during sleep. It is defined as more than five apneic episodes per hour, each occurring for longer than 10 s each.

The effect of sleep apnea is to interfere with sleep structure thereby causing awakening (often as a result of hypoxemia) during the night. If there are numerous awakenings during the night the athlete will have excessive daytime sleepiness. This will affect competition and can lead to physical underperformance.

Numerous awakenings also lead to less stage 4 sleep. It is in stage 4 sleep that growth hormone and other hormones are released to help the body repair the wear and tear of training and competition.

The treatment of sleep apnea is by means of a physical mask, worn all night, with continuous positive airway pressure (CPAP). This prevents the collapse of the soft tissue in the pharynx and allows normal sleep.

Aspiration

One of the most common causes of palpitations in athletes is reflux esophagitis. Even in a mild form it can give rise to reflex bronchospasm of the lower respiratory tract. If this is of a more severe degree it can cause aspiration, inflammation, and infection with anaerobes in the upper and lower respiratory tract. It must always be included in the differential of upper and lower respiratory tract symptoms.

Diagnosis is carried out through history, barium swallow studies, or 24-h continuous monitoring with a pH meter at the distal esophagus.

The use of antacids or histamine 2 inhibitors is the most common form of therapy. Both these drugs are allowed without notification.

Control of ventilation

HIGH ALTITUDE AND HYPOXEMIA

High altitude training is used by endurance athletes in order to train or sleep at the lower oxygen saturation found at altitude. This causes low oxygen at the kidneys, which releases erythropoietin which goes to the bone marrow where it releases more red cells into the circulation in order to carry more oxygen to all tissues.

HYPOXIA HUTS

These may be seen as a way of delivering nitrogen and oxygen. They should be dealt with as the scientific literature suggests.

The best study to date is a French study which included climbers. It showed the methods were:
• Performance enhancing;
• There was a risk if not properly controlled; and that
• Ethical considerations need further discussion.

A suggestion of an oximeter for safety was considered to be a two-edged sword: it might improve safety but could be seen to assist hypoxia usage.

Due consideration must be given to the effects of hypoxemia on tissues other than the kidney and bone marrow, such as skeletal muscle, cardiac muscle, pulmonary vasculature, and brain. The effects on these tissues are detrimental and are a good reason not to use hypoxemia as a part of training. It is not banned by the IOC, but is not encouraged. The use of hypoxic tents is banned in the Olympic village.

Interstitial lung disease

This is the second most common category of lung disease after obstructive lung disease (Crystal et al. 1981; Hunninghake & Kalica 1995). It accounts for approximately 10% of all lung disease. There are over 200 known causes of interstitial lung disease (ILD). For practical purposes they are divided into ideopathic pulmonary fibrosis, external allergic alveolitis, sarcoidosis, eosinophilic lung disease, and others.

The diseases are manifested by a restrictive pattern on pulmonary function tests. The main physiologic abnormality is a reduced diffusion at the alveolar level. This does not favor endurance sports but would allow a patient to compete in power and precision events.

When the severity of these diseases progresses, a need for systemic corticosteroids may arise thereby precluding athletes competing in high intensity sports where drug testing is mandatory, unless a TUE is obtained.

ILD is a term encompassing diseases that injure the distal airways, producing a disease with similar clinical, radiographic, and physiologic features. However, many ILDs affect not only the alveolar structures (alveolitis) but also the lumen and walls of small airways (alveolar ducts, respiratory bronchioles, terminal bronchioles).

More than 100 agents are known to cause ILD, but in two-thirds of all cases no cause can be identified. Although ILD has diverse forms, one common denominator is the presence of fibrosis of the alveolar interstitium. Thus, the terms "fibrotic lung disease" and "interstitial lung disease" are used interchangeably.

Once considered relatively rare, it is now known that ILD is quite common. The 1972 Task Force Report on Lung Disease estimated that, outside of the infectious disorders, ILD represents 15% of the diseases in all patients seen by pulmonary physicians in the USA. Subsequent statistics of 1977 suggested that in the USA, 89,000 inpatients per year have chronic interstitial fibrosis. It is now considered that ILD is one of the most common diseases worldwide. The clinical difficulties of early detection, because of its diversity and insidious onset of the disease, make it difficult to diagnose.

The typical patient with ILD presents with the insidious onset of dyspnea, occasionally associated with non-productive (dry) cough. Therefore, breathlessness during exercise can be the first symptom of these diseases.

Most patients are detected by simple chest radiograph and routine pulmonary ventilatory function measuring FVC and FEV_1. Although standard chest radiography remains invaluable for verifying and classifying ILD, it is not as sensitive for early detection as the high-resolution CT (HRCT) scan.

The classic findings of ILD on a chest radiograph are those of a "reticular, nodular, or reticulonodular pattern and ground glass appearance." HRCT is necessary to confirm further differentiation, staging the various kinds of ILD, and for prognosis.

The classification of ILD of such diverse causes and clinical entities is not simple nor easy. There is not yet a satisfactory classification system for ILD. For practical purpose, it is useful to categorize the disorders by whether the cause is known or unknown. An alternative criterion is the presence or absence of granuloma as a feature of the inflammatory process.

Known causes of ILD include infection, occupational exposure, neoplasm, congenital and metabolic causes, drug reaction, recurrent aspiration, lipoid pneumonia, amyloidosis, microlithiasis, diseases of heart, liver, kidney, bowel, graft-versus-host disease, acute respiratory distress syndrome (ARDS), and acute eosinophilic pneumonia. Unknown causes of ILD include idiopathic pulmonary fibrosis (IPF), sarcoidosis, vasculitis, collagen vascular diseases, diffuse alveolar hemorhage syndromes, eosinophilic granuloma, chronic eosinophilic pneumonia, bronchiolitis obliterans with organizing pneumonia (BOOP), respiratory bronchiolitis, pulmonary alveolar proteinosis, lymphangioleiomymatosis, tuberous sclerosis, ataxic telangiectasia, lymphoid interstitial pneumonitis, and acute interstitial pneumonitis.

An alternative classification of ILD is the presence or absence of granuloma. Granulomas are present in hypersensitivity pneumonitis, sarcoidosis, eosinophilic granuloma, Wegener's granulomatosis, Churg–Strauss syndrome, and silicosis. IPF, connective tissue disorders, asbestosis, and diseases caused by drugs, radiation, and toxic gas exposure are not associated with granuloma formation.

The course of ILD is unpredictable. It may remain static for a long period of time or it may progress quickly (Hamman–Rich syndrome). If it progresses, the lung tissue thickens and becomes stiff. The work of breathing then becomes more difficult and demanding. Some ILD improve with medication if treated when the inflammatory process is ongoing. Very rarely, ILD may improve spontaneously by protective immunologic processes of the human body's defense mechanism.

It is important for these patients to stay in touch with their team of doctors once these diseases are identified and to report any changes of symptoms. All involved need to work together for effective management of these ILD.

Diagnosis of ILD takes a long period of follow-up (average 3.5 years) before specific diagnostic procedures to differentiate what form of ILD and what medical treatment is indicated and implemented.

1 Careful medical history and meticulous physical examination are important. The history should include environmental and occupational factors, hobbies, legal (prescribed) and illegal drug use, arthritis, and risk factors for diseases that affect the immune system. Environmental monitoring of indoor/outdoor air pollution is needed too.

2 Physical examination, including chest auscultation, chest X-ray, resting and exercise pulmonary function tests, and blood tests (including immunologic parameters) are important. Inspiratory crackles on chest auscultation are a hallmark finding of ILD.

3 Pulmonary function tests will show evidence of a restrictive lung function with decreased VC, TLC, and decreased diffusion capacity ($D_L CO$). Decreased $D_L CO$ can be the most sensitive of pulmonary function test parameter for ILD and may be abnormal even when lung volumes are preserved, and/or in the presence of normal chest radiographic findings. Hypoxia at rest or on exertion, decreased oxygen uptake, and a 6-min walk test are useful. Testing with a finger oximeter is a well-tolerated and simple test that will provide a measure of oxygen requirement, and can be a quantifiable index of disease progression.

4 Bronchoalveolar lavage (BAL) examination during a fiberoptic bronchoscopic procedure may be used to make differential diagnosis and/or to confirm the progressing stages of ILD. However, BAL procedure still needs to be elucidated before it becomes a standard diagnostic measure of ILD.

5 Gallium lung scan using gallium-67 isotope is useful, although not diagnostically specific. It characterizes the severity and anatomic location of alveolitis. It is capable of giving a longitudinal assessment of the degree of inflammation in the parenchyma as a whole.

6 Lung biopsy is a surgical procedure that removes a small sample of lung tissue. It is particularly helpful in establishing the specific diagnosis, treatment, and predicting prognosis. It is usually performed during the flexible fiberoptic bronchoscopic examination. Fiberopic bronchoscopic procedure is simple and easy under local anesthesia and sedation. A lung biopsy is performed by a transbronchial procedure during bronchoscopy. Open lung biopsy is sometimes necessary to make definite diagnosis, depending on how unusual or rare the category of suspected ILD.

Management and therapy of ILD

The most important step of therapy is to remove the causative agent of injury to the lung. This may mean an exhaustive search for a causative agent. If no agent is found, therapy may be directed toward suppression of inflammatory and cellular immune responses.

Effective, specific therapy is not available when the etiology or mechanism of disease is not recognized. The alveolitis may be suppressed with either corticosteroid and/or immunosuppressive or cytotoxic agents (cyclophosphamide and azathioprine). These medications do not cure the disease and should only be used after a definitive diagnosis has been made.

Meticulous supportive care can improve the quality of life of patients with ILD. Supportive therapy includes vaccines, antibiotics for episodes of purulent sputum, bronchodilators for wheezing, supplemental oxygen when partial pressure of arterial oxygen (Pao_2) drops below 55 mmHg, psychosocial therapy, and pulmonary rehabilitation.

The pulmonary physician's world is divided between "lumpers" and "splitters" of ILD diagnosis. The lumpers say ILD is similar in all patients. The splitters recognize a behavior pattern for individually defined conditions, some of which are now described.

Idiopathic pulmonary fibrosis

A large number of ILD patients have ILD of unknown etiology, including idiopathic pulmonary fibrosis (IPF). IPF (also called cryptogenic fibrosing alveolitis) is a common ILD of unknown etiology. It is a well-defined clinical entity with characteristic clinical, radiographic, physiologic, and pathologic manifestations. The characteristics of IPF are summarized as a disease that predominantly affects men in the fifth to seventh decade of life, with a history of exertional dypnea, a chest radiograph that correlates poorly with clinical findings, an HRCT showing the disease's highly distinctive distribution and pattern of lesions. Transbronchial biopsy is not diagnostic, and most patients require an open surgical lung biopsy or a minimally invasive thoracoscopy biopsy. The disease currently is diagnosed by histologic exclusion of other specific entities. The mortality rate is approximately 50% at 5 years. Initial trial of prednisolone (40–60 mg o.d. orally for

3 months) is a reasonable treatment choice. The continuation of therapy depends on an objective response.

Sarcoidosis

Sarcoidosis is the most common ILD of unknown etiology. The characteristics of sarcoidosis are summarized as follows. The disease causes non-caseating granuloma in several organ systems. Most cases are seen in patients 20–45 years old. The disease is common in African-Americans. The lung is the organ most frequently involved. The chest radiograph shows bilateral hilar lymph node enlargement (stage I), pulmonary infiltrates with lymph node enlargement (stage II), and ILD alone (stage III). The adenopathy and ILD frequently regresses spontaneously. Extrapulmonary involvement is common. A transbronchial biopsy demonstrates non-caseating granulomas. Thoracoscopic or open lung biopsy is rarely needed for diagnosis. Corticosteroids are given when functional impairment of one or more organs is present. A TUE is needed for an athlete to compete while using systemic corticosteroids.

Eosinophilic granuloma of the lung

Eosinophilic granuloma was first described as a bone disease but is now recognized as predominantly a pulmonary disorder. The disease is also called Langerhans' cell granuloma. It has the following characteristics. The disease occurs almost exclusively in smokers or former smokers aged 10–40 years. The etiology is unknown. The common presenting symptoms are a non-productive cough, chest pain, and dyspnea on exertion. The extrapulmonary features include diabetes insipidus and lytic bone lesions. An HRCT scan is highly distinctive. A light microscopy examination of tissue shows the cleft nuclei of the Langerhans' cells and stellate pattern of fibrosis in 80% of patients. Spontaneous remissions are the rule. Patients must stop smoking if the disease is to resolve.

Pleural disease

In lung disease, the pleura is most often affected from secondary disease in the lung. There is a major finding of pleural disease of thickening of the pleura secondary to disease which may give rise to an extrapulmonary restriction. This is usually a manifestation of chronic disease and is treated expectantly.

An acute involvement of the pleura usually gives rise to an inflammation (pleurisy), often as a manifestation of an acute pulmonary infection. When that is severe, a pleural effusion may occur, which will need to be sampled for diagnosis or if a large accumulation is to be removed by needle or tube drainage for therapeutic relief of restriction of the lung tissue.

Another acute manifestation of acute pleural disease is barotrauma. This can occur secondary to congenital or acquired bullae of the lung. The acquired bullae usually occur secondary to obstructive airflow disease. These are a relative contraindication to diving to depths as practiced in sport or in industry because of the likelihood of a pneumothorax. The treatment of a pneumothorax is by expectant behaviour or by placing a chest tube in the pleural space and draining the air via an underwater seal.

Pulmonary vascular disease

PULMONARY EMBOLI

Modern airline travel for longer than 4 h causes a threefold risk for pulmonary emboli even in young, otherwise healthy individuals. Therefore, all athletes traveling long distances must be aware of the condition. The best approach to this disease of high morbidity and mortality is prevention.

The predisposing factors to deep venous thrombosis (the forerunner to pulmonary embolism) are stagnation of blood flow in the legs and pelvis, inflammation of vessel walls, and dehydration. These predisposing factors allow thrombi to form on a flight and may only manifest up to 5 days later.

Pulmonary emboli give rise to a lowering of oxygen saturation and possibly to infarction of the lung. This latter effect is manifested by pleuritic chest pain. The diagnosis can be made by non-invasive or invasive radiologic scanning techniques. Treatment is with subcutaneous, low molecular weight heparin for 5 days followed by oral war-farin for at least 6 weeks. A long-term effect of pulmonary emboli is pulmonary hypertension.

Prevention can be achieved by regular movement of the ankles and legs for 5 min in every hour, the wearing of fitted elastic stockings, drinking copious amounts of water or sports drinks, and, if there is a family or patient history of deep venous thrombosis, the use of anti-coagulants. The most common anticoagulants used, from least powerful to most powerful, are salicylic acid, clopidogrel, or warfarin orally. Low molecular weight heparin can be used by subcutaneous injection and is equally as efficacious as warfarin.

Systemic disease causing secondary pulmonary disease

OBESITY

Obesity is an excess of adipose tissue. It is most meaningfully quantified by measures of the mass and distribution of adipose tissue. It is commonly inferred as more than 2 standard deviations above the mean for sex, age, and height, of the body mass index (BMI: weight in kilograms divided by the height in meters squared). Excess fat must be distinguished from lean body mass which may be an increase in muscular hypertrophy.

RESTING PULMONARY FUNCTION TESTS

Excess abdominal fat will decrease the lung volumes to a maximum of 15% in TLC by elevation of the hemidiaphragms. It can also decrease the VC. FRC is reduced earlier than TLC and VC. Residual volume is preserved and therefore the reduction in FRC is the result of a reduction in expiratory reserve volume (ERV).

These reductions in lung volumes are responsible for the hypoxemia that occurs at rest in the supine position which is relieved by the upright position. A parenchymal shunt occurs in the base of the lungs is one cause of hypoxemia.

Another effect of obesity on the work of breathing is when pulmonary system compliance is reduced by the increased mass of the chest wall and the resistance to the decrease of the descent of the diaphragm because of increased abdominal mass. Both of these effects increase the work of breathing. In severe obesity, there may be a resetting of the control of ventilation leading to the onset of hypoxemia and hypercarbia. It is as if the central control of ventilation says to the bellows of the lungs, the extra work of breathing is not worth the effort, so let the carbon dioxide drift upwards from its normal 40 mmHg partial pressure to as high as 48 mmHg partial pressure thereby reducing the oxygen partial pressure a similar amount. The A–a O_2 gradient remains the same because of the normal lung tissue. This is a second cause of the hypoxemia of severe obesity. A third cause of hypoxemia of obesity in the supine position at night-time is the onset of sleep apnea.

There are secondary effects on the lungs from the effects of obesity on the cardiovascular system and the body metabolism. There is a correlation between obesity and hypertensive heart disease. Obesity gives rise to increased blood volume and an eccentric cardiomegaly that leads to increased left ventricular filling pressures and, at its extreme, to heart failure and pulmonary edema. The hypoxemia and sleep apnea of obesity can give rise to right heart failure.

The metabolic effects of obesity are seen secondary to the added metabolic activity of the adipose tissue. This gives rise to an increased metabolic cost, an increased work to support the added body mass, which then increases further on ambulation. This ironically may give rise to a higher $\dot{V}o_{2max}$ secondary to the chronic training effect of obesity on muscle and breathing in obesity. Another major metabolic problem with obesity is insulin resistance. This can impair carbohydrate metabolism, vascular reactivity, and muscle mass.

Sudden death in athletes

It is accepted that cardiac disease is responsible for 90% of sudden death in athletes. It has an incidence of 3 per 100,000 compared to 1 per 100,000 in the non-athletic population of an age and sex-matched group. However, there are other causes and predisposing factors to sudden death in sport.

Non-cardiac sudden death

ASTHMA AND SUDDEN DEATH

An acute exacerbation of asthma during exercise can cause hypoxemia. This, added to the acidosis of exercise, the increased sympathetic outflow of exercise, the steepness of the P-R interval with tachycardia, and possibly the use of excessive β_2-sympathomimetics, can be a cause of cardiac arrhythmia and death in athletes. Although possibly considered a cardiac death, the asthmatic attack is the predisposing factor. The best treatment of EIA is prevention by better control during the non-exercising time of day.

HEAT AND DEHYDRATION

During exercise there is competition between the skeletal muscles and the skin for the increased cardiac output. If the skin does not get enough of the circulation because of dehydration or excessive temperature, the core temperature rises to such a degree (>41°C) that rhabdomyolysis and disseminated coagulopathy occur. Heat stress is more common in unconditioned, unacclimatized, and dehydrated athletes. Some of the banned drugs in sport that contribute to performance enhancement may contribute to sudden death. These include diuretics, amphetamines, and other stimulants.

SICKLE CELL TRAIT

Heterozygotes for the hemoglobin S gene (8% of African-Americans) have an increased risk of sudden death during exercise. This is triggered by hypoxemia and dehydration. This is more likely to occur in unacclimatized athletes at altitude where hypoxemia is more common.

Conclusions

This chapter attempts to show the various pulmonary conditions likely to be seen and how they affect the participating athlete. A short chapter like this cannot hope to be fully comprehensive but aims to highlight the areas of pulmonology that impact most on athletes.

Asthma in athletes has a high prevalence and consequently a major part of this chapter has been devoted to it. It is the one condition that dominates pre-event medical officer discussion. A discrepancy has crept into the sports world whereby some events have different ways of handling the same disease. An attempt is ongoing to correct this discrepancy.

The assessment of the athlete is most often performed with physiologic tests. It is worth mentioning that asthma is the most commonly encountered medical condition at major sporting events when a TUE is requested. The pulmonary physiologic tests are needed to best define the presence and severity of asthma.

We have also tried to show that there are other environmental, systemic (including central), pulmonary vascular, pleural, and interstitial pulmonary diseases that contribute to the limitation of the pulmonary system and hypoxemia. A small section on the major categories of lung disease has been devoted to limitations of exercise in those categories.

References

Aekplakorn, W., Loomis, D., Vichit-Vadakan, N. & Bangdiwala, S. (2004) Heterogeneity of daily pulmonary function in response to air pollution among asthmatic children. *Southeast Asian Journal of Tropical Medicine and Public Health* **35**, 990–998.

American Thoracic Society (ATS). (2000) ATS guidelines for methacoline and exercise challenge testing, 1999. *American Journal of Respiratory and Critical Care Medicine* **161**, 309–329.

Anderson, S.D. & Holzer, K. (2000) Exercise-induced asthma: is it the right diagnosis in elite athletes? *Journal of Allergy and Clinical Immunology* **106**, 419–428.

Anderson, S.D., Fitch, K., Perry, C.P., Sue-Chu, M., Crapo, R., McKenzie, D., *et al.* (2003) Responses to bronchial challenge submitted for approval to use inhaled β_2-agonists before an event at the 2002 Winter Olympics. *Journal of Allergy and Clinical Immunology* **111**, 45–50.

Antò, J.M. & Sunyer, J. (1995) Nitrogen dioxide and allergic asthma: starting to clarify an obscure association. *Lancet* **315**, 402–403.

Bousquet, J, van Cauwenberge, P., Khaltaev, N.; Aria Workshop Group, World Health Organization. (2001) Allergic rhinitis and its impact on asthma. *Journal of Allergy and Clinical Immunology* **108** (5 Suppl), S147–334.

Bylin, G., Hedenstierna, G., Lindvall, T. & Sundin, B. (1988) Ambient nitrogen dioxide concentrations increase bronchial responsiveness in subjects with mild asthma. *European Respiratory Journal* **1**, 606–612.

Carlsen, K-H., Delgado, L. & Del Giacco, S. (2005) Diagnosis, prevention and treatment of exercise-related asthma, respiratory and allergic disorders in sports. *European Respiratory Monographs* **10**, Monograph 33.

Crystal, R.G., Gadek, J.E., Ferrans, V.J., Line, B.R. & Hunninghake, G.W. (1981) Interstitial lung disease: current concepts of pathogenesis, staging and therapy. *American Journal of Medicine* **70**, 542–568.

D'Amato, G., Liccardi, G., D'Amato, M. & Holgate, S. (2005) Environmental risk factors and allergic bronchial asthma. *Clinical and Experimental Allergy* **35**, 1113–1124.

Dockery, D.W. & Pope, C.A. III. (1994) Acute respiratory effects of particulate air pollution. *Annual Review of Public Health* **15**, 107–132.

Dykewicz, M.S., Fineman, S., Skoner, D.P., Nicklas, R., Lee, R., Blessing-Moore, J., et al. (1998) Diagnosis and management of rhinitis: complete guidelines of the Joint Task Force on Practice Parameters in Allergy, Asthma and Immunology. American Academy of Allergy, Asthma, and Immunology. *Annals of Allergy, Asthma and Immunology* **81** (5 Part 2), 478–518.

Global Strategy for Asthma Management and Prevention. Update April 2002. (2003) NIH Publ. No 02-3659 http://www.ginasthma.com Accessed on April 22, 2003.

Helbling, A. & Muller, U. (1991) Bronchial asthma in high performance athletes. *Schweiz Z Sportmed* **39**, 77–81.

Helenius, I.J. & Haahtela, T. (2000) Allergy and asthma in elite summer sport athletes. Rostrum. *Journal of Allergy and Clinical Immunology* **106**, 444–452.

Helenius, I.J., Rytilä, P., Sarna, S., Lumme, A., Helenius, M., Remes, V., et al. (2002) Effect of continuing or finishing high-level sports on airway inflammation, bronchial hyperresponsiveness, and asthma: a 5-year prospective follow-up study of 42 highly trained swimmers. *Journal of Allergy and Clinical Immunology* **109**, 962–968.

Hunninghake, G.W. & Kalica, A.R. (1995) Approaches to the treatmet of pulmonary fibrosis (workshop summary). *American Journal of Respiratory and Critical Care Medicine* **151**, 915–918.

Karjalainen, E.M., Laitinen, A., Sue-Chu, M., Altraja, A. & Bjermer, L. (2000) Evidence of airway inflammation and remodelling in ski athletes with and without bronchial responsiveness to metacholine. *American Journal of Respiratory and Critical Care Medicine* **161**, 2086–2091.

Leynaert, B., Bousquet, J., Neukirch, C. et al. (1999) Perennial rhinitis: An independent risk factor for asthma in non-atopic subjects: Report from the European Community Respiratory Health Survey. *J Allergy & Clin Immunol* **104**, 301–304.

Poynter, M.E., Persinger, R.L., Irvin, C.G., et al. (2006) Nitrogen dioxide enhances allergic airway inflammation and hyperresponsiveness in the mouse. *American Journal of Physiology. Lung Cellular and Molecular Physiology* **290**, L144–152.

Proctor, N.H., Hughes, J.P. & Wesenberg, G.J. (1978) Chlorine. In: *Chemical Hazards of the Workplace.* (Proctor, N.H. & Hughes, J.P., eds.) JB Lippincott, Philadelphia: 157–158.

Ventura, M.T., Dagnello, M., Matino, M.G. et al. (2001) Contact dermatitis in students practicing sports: incidence of rubber sensitization. *Br J Sports Med* **35**, 100–102.

Weiler, J.M., Layton, T. & Hunt, M. (1998) Asthma in United States Olympic athletes who participated in the 1996 Summer Games. *Journal of Allergy and Clinical Immunology* **102**, 722–726.

Widdicombe, J.G. (1996) Neuroregulation in the nose and bronchi. *Clinical and Experimental Allergy* **26** (Suppl 3), 32–35.

Zwick, H., Popp, W., Budik G. et al. (1990) Increased sensitisation to aeroallergens in competitive swimmers. *Lung* **168**, 111–115.

Chapter 8

Endocrinology

JEFFREY M. ANDERSON, THOMAS H. TROJIAN AND WILLIAM J. KRAEMER

The cybernetic control of a variety of different pathologies is mediated by the endocrine system. The endocrine system interfaces with almost every physiologic system in the body and its control and function are tightly regulated under most conditions. In this chapter we examine a few of the major endocrine-related disorders that challenge medical professionals in sport.

Diabetes mellitus

Diabetes mellitus (DM) is a group of metabolic diseases characterized by hyperglycemia resulting from defects in insulin secretion, insulin action, or both (Expert Committee 1997). The chronic hyperglycemia of diabetes is associated with the development of several adverse medical conditions including neuropathy, nephropathy, and retinopathy. Individuals with DM are also at an increased risk for developing cardiovascular disease, which remains a major cause of morbidity and mortality in this population.

There are several types of DM. The vast majority of cases of DM fall into two broad categories. In type 1 DM, the cause is an absolute deficiency of insulin secretion, often related to pancreatic beta-cell destruction. In the absence of exogenous insulin, individuals with type 1 DM are prone to develop ketoacidosis. In the other, much more common, type 2 DM, the cause is a combination of resistance to insulin action and an inadequate compensatory insulin

secretory response (Expert Committee 1997). Other major categories of DM include gestational diabetes and diabetes that develops secondary to other disease states (e.g., Cushing's syndrome, hyperthyroidism, hemochromatosis) or secondary to medication use (e.g., glucocorticoids, pentamidine, α-interferon).

The diagnosis of DM can be made based on one or more of the following criteria:

1 Symptoms of diabetes plus a random plasma glucose concentration ≥ 200 mg·dL^{-1};
2 Fasting plasma glucose ≥ 126 mg·dL^{-1};
3 2-h post-prandial glucose ≥ 200 mg·dL^{-1} following a 75-g glucose load during an oral glucose tolerance test (Expert Committee 1997).

In the USA alone, it is estimated that over 16 million people currently have been diagnosed with DM (Danese *et al.* 1996). By the year 2025, this number will climb to approximately 22 million. The increasing prevalence of DM is not only occurring in the USA but is being witnessed worldwide. By 2025, approximately 300 million people will be diagnosed with DM. As a result, diabetes and its complications will result in an increasing burden on health care costs (Peirce 1999).

Role of exercise in treating diabetes mellitus

For years, the traditional cornerstones of therapy for patients with DM have been dietary modification and medication. Exercise has been encouraged in patients with DM because regular physical

The Olympic Textbook of Medicine in Sport, 1st edition. Edited by M. Schwellnus. Published 2008 by Blackwell Publishing, ISBN: 978-1-4051-5637-0.

Please note to get blood glucose values in mmol·L^{-1} please divide mg·dL^{-1} by 18.

activity may help to control hyperglycemia through improved glucose utilization. However, a variety of factors can influence the effect that exercise can have on blood glucose. Variables that should be considered include the type of DM involved (type 1 vs. type 2), the type of exercise performed (aerobic vs. anaerobic), the duration and intensity of physical activity, concurrent use of medications (e.g., sulfonylureas, insulin), and the patient's baseline cardiorespiratory fitness level (Colberg & Swain 2000).

In order to better understand the effect that exercise can have on glycemic control, it is important to appreciate the relationship between exercise and glucose utilization. In a person without diabetes, during a single episode of exercise, the muscles initially utilize glucose in the muscle and later convert muscle glycogen to glucose to provide energy. Additionally, exercising muscle takes up glucose from the circulation, a process that is dependent on insulin. As the blood glucose concentration drops, insulin secretion decreases and the release of glucagon increases. These hormonal changes result in enhanced hepatic glucose production secondary to increased glycogenolysis and to gluconeogenesis. With further exercise, other counterregulatory hormones (e.g., epinephrine, norepinephrine, growth hormone, and cortisol) begin to have a role in helping to maintain adequate blood glucose levels (McCulloch 2001).

With regular, moderate intensity physical activity, training effects occur that result in more efficient use of energy by muscle. These changes include the development of new muscle capillaries and increases in the quantity of mitochondrial enzymes (McCulloch 2001). Studies have also demonstrated that regular endurance exercise training increases the concentration of GLUT-4 mRNA and protein in skeletal muscle. GLUT-4 is a protein that serves as a glucose transporter. The exercise-related increase in muscle GLUT-4 is physiologically important because elevated GLUT-4 augments muscle glucose transport and enhances whole-body glucose tolerance (MacLean et al. 2000).

GLUT-4 is predominantly found in association with intracellular vesicles which translocate to the cell membrane in order to increase glucose transport.

The maximal rate of muscle glucose transport is determined by both the total number of GLUT-4 molecules and the proportion of the GLUT-4 receptors that are translocated to the cell membrane in response to insulin and/or muscle contraction (MacLean et al. 2000). It has been demonstrated that in type 2 DM, impairment in insulin-stimulated GLUT-4 translocation exists. This defect is felt to be one of the primary contributors to diabetes-related insulin resistance. In contrast, there does not appear to be any decrement in muscle contraction-induced translocation of GLUT-4 during exercise (Goodpaster & Kelley 2001).

In patients with DM, several physiologic responses to exercise are altered based upon the plasma insulin concentration at the time of exercise and the degree of pre-exercise glycemic control. Additionally, the use of exogenous insulin can have a profound effect on glucose concentrations during exercise. Well-controlled diabetics on insulin therapy often will have a much larger drop in blood glucose concentrations than that seen in diabetics not on insulin therapy, or in those individuals without diabetes. Because the effects of exogenous insulin cannot be turned off, muscle glucose uptake and the inhibition of hepatic glucose production may continue to occur despite dropping levels of blood glucose (McCulloch 2001).

In patients with poor glucose control, exercise can actually result in blood glucose elevations. This can occur when inadequate amounts of insulin result in impaired glucose uptake at the muscle and when counterregulatory hormones (e.g., epinephrine, cortisol, and growth hormone), which are released during exercise, increase hepatic glucose production (McCulloch 2001). Plasma glucose remains elevated after exercise because of the absence of elevation in insulin level post exercise. This typically occurs after intense exercise in the poorly controlled diabetic where pre-exercise glucose levels are elevated. In the hypoinsulinemic state, glucose uptake is impaired while hepatic glucose production, lipolysis, and ketogenesis are all elevated (Wasserman & Zinman 1994). This may result not only in hyperglycemia but also hyperlipidemia and, in the more severe cases, ketoacidosis and coma.

Exercise and long-term glycemic control

With regard to the long-term effects of routine exercise on glucose control, the effects differ between patients with type 1 DM and those with type 2 DM. The results of several studies have found that exercise interventions can reduce glycosylated hemoglobin levels (HbA1C) in people with type 2 DM. Many of the studies demonstrating a beneficial effect of regular aerobic exercise on long-term glucose control in type 2 DM utilized physical activity performed for 30–60 min, at 50–80% of maximal oxygen uptake ($\dot{V}o_{2max}$), 3–4 sessions per week. With this type of exercise program, reductions in HbA1C of 10–20% from baseline could be achieved (American Diabetes Association 2001).

Studies utilizing resistance training have also demonstrated a beneficial effect on long-term glucose control in type 2 DM. For example, Eriksson et al. (1997) examined the effects of an individualized, progressive, resistance-training program. Subjects performed circuit-type resistance exercises twice weekly. After 3 months of training, the average HbA1C dropped from 8.8 down to 8.2% ($P < 0.05$). The investigators found that glycemic control correlated strongly with changes in muscle size which were able to be quantified using magnetic resonance imaging.

In 2001, Boule et al. (2001) published a meta-analysis of controlled trials that evaluated the effects of exercise interventions (duration >8 weeks) on glycemic control in patients with type 2 DM. Twelve aerobic training studies and two resistance training studies were included in the analysis. The investigators found that the weighted mean post-intervention HbA1C was lower in the exercise groups than control groups (7.65% vs. 8.31%; $P < 0.001$). It is important to note that the difference in post-intervention body mass between exercise groups and control groups was not statistically significant. The weighted mean difference in HbA1C of −0.66 demonstrated between the exercise and control groups has important clinical implications. This degree of improvement in glycemic control is associated with significant reductions in diabetic complications. Results of the UK Prospective Diabetes Study (Thompson et al. 1997;

UKPDS 1998) demonstrated a continuous relationship between the risks of microvascular and cardiovascular complications and glycemia. For every percentage point decrease in HgA1C (e.g., 9% to 8%) there was a 35% reduction in the risk of microvascular complications, a 25% reduction in diabetes-related deaths, an 18% reduction in combined fatal and non-fatal myocardial infarction, and a 7% reduction in all-cause mortality.

In contrast to the response in type 2 DM, improvement in long-term glucose control through exercise training in type 1 DM has not been demonstrated (Metcalf-McCambridge & Colby 2000; Ramalho et al. 2006). Presumably, the lack of HgA1C lowering in patients with type 1 DM is becase of the difference in etiology of disease. The lack of endogenous insulin in patients with type 1 DM and the importance of insulin resistance in patients with type 2 DM differentiates the response to exercise (McCulloch 2001). Studies have demonstrated, in patients with type 1 DM, a single bout of exercise can have a blood glucose lowering effect (Landt et al. 1985). However, as determined by HgA1C values, these effects of exercise in isolation have not been shown to result in long-term improvement in glucose control (ADA 2001; Landt et al. 1985; Zinker 1999). In order to achieve reductions in HbA1C, intensive insulin therapy and/or dietary restriction needs to be implemented (Perry et al. 1997).

Exercise, diabetes, and mortality

Despite the inadequacy of exercise to improve long-term glycemic control in patients with type 1 DM, physical activity is associated with a decreased risk of overall mortality in this population. The benefits of physical activity on overall mortality were demonstrated in a cohort of 548 type 1 diabetic patients enrolled in the Pittsburgh Insulin-Dependent Diabetes Mellitus Morbidity and Mortality Study (Moy et al. 1993). Physical activity was measured by survey in 1981, and mortality was ascertained through 1988. After controlling for numerous potential confounders (e.g., age, body mass index [BMI], tobacco use), the investigators found that overall activity level was inversely related to mortality risk. Sedentary males (energy expenditure <1000 kcal·week^{-1}) were three times more likely to die than active males (energy expenditure >1000 kcal·week^{-1}).

The beneficial effect of physical activity on overall mortality has also been demonstrated in type 2 diabetics. Wei *et al.* (2000) performed a prospective cohort study of over 1200 men with type 2 DM. The subjects completed a maximal exercise treadmill test to determine cardiopulmonary fitness. Based on performance, subjects were categorized as "low fit, moderately fit, or high fit." Participants also completed an extensive self-report of personal and family history, including physical activity patterns. These individuals were followed for an average of 11.7 years. Adjustments were made for a variety of factors that might affect overall mortality (e.g., age, tobacco use, hypercholesterolemia, hypertension). The investigators found that the low-fitness group had an adjusted risk for all-cause mortality of 2.1 (95% CI, 1.5–2.9) compared with fit men. Additionally, men who reported being physically inactive had an adjusted risk for all-cause mortality of 1.7 (95% CI, 1.2–2.3) compared with men who reported being physically active.

Additional benefits of exercise in diabetes mellitus

Independent of its action of blood glucose control, regular exercise can have several beneficial effects for patients with DM (Table 8.1). One area in which exercise can have a significant impact is in cardiovascular disease risk reduction. In patients with both type 1 and 2 DM, routine exercise can decrease

Table 8.1 Beneficial effects of regular physical activity (primary prevention of chronic disease). (From Kesaniemi *et al.* 2001.)

Coronary heart disease
Cerebrovascular disease
Obesity
Type 2 diabetes mellitus
Colon cancer
Hypertension
Depression
Osteoporosis
Dyslipidemia

risk factors for cardiovascular disease such as dyslipidemia, hypertension, and coagulation abnormalities (Zinker 1999).

Additionally, behavioral characteristics that are considered to be positively related to health and disease prevention, such as stress management and reductions in tobacco use and alcohol consumption, occur with regular physical activity (Zinker 1999).

Regular exercise has also been shown to have mental health benefits for diabetic patients. Although difficult to determine, routine exercise has been associated with an elevated "sense of well-being," increased "self-esteem," and an enhanced "quality of life" (Zinker 1999). Some these psychologic benefits may be derived from the ability of active participation in exercise and organized sports activities to promote socialization and peer acceptance (White & Sherman 1999).

As a result of the many beneficial effects of exercise, the ADA (2001) concludes its position statement on diabetes and exercise by stating, "all patients with diabetes should have the opportunity to benefit from the many valuable effects of exercise."

Exercise risks in diabetes mellitus

Although exercise can be highly beneficial for patients with DM, at the same time it can pose certain risks (Table 8.2). Before initiating an exercise program, individuals with DM should undergo a medical evaluation to screen for microvascular and macrovascular complications that may be exacerbated by exercise (ADA 2001). A complete discussion of all the exercise-associated risks for diabetic patients and the specific recommendations regarding the preparticipation medical evaluation of these individuals is beyond the scope of this chapter. This information can be found in several recent publications (ADA 2001; Peirce 1999; White & Sherman 1999). However, this section reviews two of the major complications, hypoglycemia and myocardial ischemia, that are seen in diabetic patients who exercise.

HYPOGLYCEMIA

Hypoglycemia remains the most common risk encountered for diabetic patients who exercise.

Table 8.2 Risks of exercise for patients with diabetes mellitus. (From ADA 2001; Albright 1997; Peirce 1999; White & Sherman 1999.)

Organ system	Potential adverse event
Metabolic	Hyperglycemia
	Hypoglycemia
Cardiovascular	Coronary artery disease
	Myocardial ischemia
	Cardiac arrest
	Sudden cardiac death
	Arrhythmia
	Abnormal blood response
	Peripheral vascular disease
	(claudication)
Kidneys	Proteinuria
Eyes	Retinal hemorrhage
Musculoskeletal	Ulcerations
	Degenerative joint disease

Although this can occur in patients with type 2 DM, particularly those taking sulfonylureas, it is of greater concern for those patients taking exogenous insulin. Because the effects of exogenous insulin continue despite declining blood glucose levels, muscle glucose uptake, and the inhibition of hepatic glucose production may continue resulting in profound hypoglycemia. Additionally, many diabetics, particularly those who have had the disease for 5 years or more, have impaired counterregulatory mechanisms for combating hypoglycemia (White & Sherman 1999). Exercise can also enhance the absorption of exogenous insulin, particularly if it has been injected into an exercising extremity. This can further increase the risk of exercise-related hypoglycemia (White & Sherman 1999).

Once hypoglycemia has occurred there is an increased risk of further hypoglycemic episodes. The acute counterregulatory failure appears to be a dose-dependent fashion by differing depths of antecedent hypoglycemia (Galassetti et al. 2006). The loss of counterregulatory hormones appears to last 3 days after a hypoglycemic episode (Ertl & Davis 2004). Care to prevent a hypoglycemic episode in an athlete is needed but once it occurs an increase in carbohydrates will be needed during exercise to prevent further episodes.

Even if blood glucose levels remain stable during exercise, patients with diabetes may subsequently develop delayed hypoglycemia. This often occurs at night, 6–15 h after exercise, but may develop as long as 28 h after exercise. This insidious drop in blood glucose results from the residual effect of exercise-enhanced insulin sensitivity. Additionally, hepatic glycogen synthesis to replenish stores depleted by exercise may also contribute to delayed hypoglycemia. Because liver glycogen is replaced more slowly than muscle glycogen, carbohydrate requirements may be increased for up to 24 h after prolonged exercise (White & Sherman 1999). Strategies to help reduce the risk of exercise-related hypoglycemia are outlined in Table 8.3.

MYOCARDIAL ISCHEMIA

Another concern for diabetic patients who exercise is the development of myocardial ischemia or sudden death. These adverse events are related to underlying atherosclerotic coronary artery disease. In many diabetic patients, atherosclerosis is more extensive and develops earlier than in the general non-diabetic population. Although routine exercise can help improve many of the risk factors for coronary artery disease and decrease the long-term risk of developing cardiovascular disease, in fact, during vigorous physical activity, there is an actual transient increased risk for myocardial infarction, cardiac arrest, and sudden death (Thompson 1996).

The ADA has recommended a graded exercise stress test if a patient, about to embark on a moderate- to high-intensity exercise program, is at high risk for underlying cardiovascular disease based on specific criteria (Table 8.4). If the patient will only be participating in low-intensity physical activities (<60% maximal heart rate), then formal exercise stress testing may not be necessary, although appropriate clinical judgment still needs to be executed (ADA 2001).

Additionally, in patients with known coronary artery disease, the ADA recommends that these individuals undergo a supervised evaluation of the ischemic response to exercise, ischemic threshold, and the propensity to arrhythmia during exercise (ADA 2001). It is important to remember that even

Table 8.3 Risk reduction strategies for exercise-related hypoglycemia in patients with diabetes mellitus. (From ADA 2001; Colberg & Swain 2000; White & Sherman 1999.)

Close monitoring of glucose levels before, during, and after activity
Adjust medication dose and/or food intake before exercise
Perform daily, rather than sporadic, exercise performed at the same time in order to facilitate diet and medication adjustments
Morning exercise recommended
Multidose insulin regimens make it easier to adjust dosage when exercise is anticipated
Consider use of lispro (Humalog) insulin (faster onset and shorter half-life)
If pre-exercise blood glucose <100, take a carbohydrate snack (15 g carbohydrate will raise blood glucose approximately 50 mg·dL^{-1})
Avoid exercise when insulin is at its peak activity
Inject insulin in abdomen, not exercising extremities
Eat a well-balanced meal 2–3 h before a planned bout of exercise
Ingest carbohydrate containing foods/beverages during sustained activity (30–60 g·h^{-1} if activity lasts >1 h)
Replete glycogen stores immediately post-exercise
Have easy access to carbohydrate containing foods should hypoglycemia begin to develop
Have easy access to glucagon (1 mg) for s.c./i.m. injection
Train coaches, athletic trainers, fellow athletes to recognize the early warning signs of hypoglycemia

Table 8.4 Criteria that should prompt consideration for exercise stress testing in diabetics before moderate- or high-intensity exercise (From ADA 2001.)

Type 2 DM >10 years' duration
Type 1 DM >15 years' duration
Age >35 years
Presence of any additional risk factors for coronary artery disease
Presence of microvascular disease
Peripheral vascular disease
Autonomic neuropathy

DM, diabetes mellitus.

patients who are identified as low risk for exercise-related complications and are participating in low to moderate intensity activities cannot be completely assured that such activity will not acutely increase the risk of an adverse cardiac event. Nevertheless, it does appear that the long-term health benefits of regular exercise outweigh the acute cardiovascular risks. Therefore, regular exercise should be encouraged in this population of patients with diabetes.

Managing the athlete with type 1 diabetes

It is important in the care of athlete with type 1 DM to prevent hypoglycemia and hyperglycemia. Educating each athlete about the disease and how best to manage glucose levels will aid in avoidance of complications. The diabetic athlete must have good metabolic control prior to undertaking exercise (HgA1C < 9). It is advisable that the athlete begins a consistent daily routine of insulin administration and caloric intake, as well as frequent home blood glucose recordings on a glucometer that stores fingerstick values. Exercising daily will lead to a more reliable understanding of an athlete's insulin and carbohydrate needs. Each athlete is unique and will require individualization of insulin adjustments and carbohydrate intake. In new onset diabetes, the person might be naïve to insulin; this "honeymoon period" of small need for insulin might be prolonged in athletes. Once past, it will necessitate an increase in insulin dosage.

The intensity and duration of exercise will determine specific modifications in the insulin regimen. These include: eat a meal 1–3 h before exercise; exercise after the peak action of subcutaneous insulin injection; delay exercise until glucose and ketones are under control (White & Sherman 1999). Prior to exercise, depending on the predicted intensity, athletes should modify insulin dosage accordingly. Typically, this reduction ranges from 20% to 50%. A recent table was proposed in order to better adjust carbohydrate intake and insulin dosing (Table 8.5; Grimm *et al.* 2004). The dose of insulin that would

Duration →	<20 min	20–60 min	>60 min	>60 min
Intensity ↓				Insulin dosage
<60%	0 g	15 g	30 g	−20%
60–75%	15 g	30 g	75 g	−20%
>75%	30 g	75 g	100 g	−30%

Table 8.5 Extra carbohydrate and insulin adjustment for different physical activity depending on duration and intensity (percentage of maximal heart rate). (After Grimm *et al.* 2004.)

peak during an upcoming sporting event should be decreased. For a morning workout, the morning dose of short-acting insulin (regular insulin – onset, 1–2 h; peak, 2–4 h) should be reduced while an afternoon activity requires reduction of the morning dose of intermediate-acting insulin (NPH or Lente insulin – onset, 1–3 h; peak, 4–10 h). The physician must understand that some trial and error occurs to meet each individual athlete's insulin and carbohydrate modifications. If hyperglycemia (blood glucose >250 mg·dL^{-1}) and ketonuria exists prior to exercise, athletic activity should be postponed until adequate glycemic control is achieved (Boule *et al.* 2001).

During exercise, athletes with type 1 DM do not have the endogenous insulin feedback mechanism that decreases insulin levels in response to exercise. This needs to be accounted for when timing insulin injections. When administering exogenous insulin, the insulin level may remain elevated during exercise leading to inhibition of both glycogenolysis and gluconeogenesis. To avoid the resultant hypoglycemia, adequate calorie intake and vigilant blood glucose monitoring is critical. During prolonged exercise (>1 h duration), blood glucose monitoring should take place every half hour. The athlete needs to replace fluid losses adequately. The contact or collision athlete with diabetes if appropriately managed should initially get a drop in glucose levels. As insulin levels begin to drop off the insulin pump or after subcutaneous injection, frequent monitoring is necessary to assess subsequent glucose elevation to avoid hyperglycemia. Because it is important for the athlete to replenish glycogen stores during and immediately after exercise, they should ingest 30–40 g carbohydrate for every half hour of intensive exercise.

Following exercise, the athlete with diabetes should be aware of the potential of late-onset hypoglycemia and recognize the precursor symptoms in order to prevent it. If the exercise intensity was unusually high, blood glucose monitoring should occur frequently in the hours following activity, even throughout the night. Any sense of exhaustion, weakness, or increase in appetite hours after exercise may warn the athlete of possible hypoglycemia. Prevention requires upward adjustments of caloric intake, lowering of longer acting insulin dosage that typically would peak overnight, and frequent blood glucose checks.

For the athlete with diabetes using multiple injections, the site of injection and rate of absorption is important. Insulin absorption is more rapid and less predictable when injected into the leg prior to exercise (Kovisto & Felig 1978). Care should be taken to avoid accidental intramuscular injection. The most common site used by athletes for injection is the abdomen given its ease of access during meals and more predictable insulin absorption time (White & Sherman 1999).

As the size of insulin pumps have decreased, their popularity has risen. Insulin pumps infuse short-acting insulin via a catheter which is replaced every 3–4 days. The insulin pump (also known as continuous subcutaneous insulin infusion; CSII) is most frequently used in athletes with type 1 DM and has some clear advantage over multiple subcutaneous injections, especially for athletes. The CSII method allows more flexibility for skipped meals, sleeping late, and spontaneous exercise. The subcutaneous insulin delivery with the pump allows for precise dosing – even incremental doses as small as 0.05 units are possible. Appropriate basal rates can be set for each individual, and adjusted according to periods of rest and exercise. The pump can be used to administer boluses of insulin for pre-meal insulin coverage. In order to reduce hypoglycemia, the athlete will precede intense exercise by reducing the action of the pump by 50% about 1 h prior to activity (Sonnenberg *et al.* 1990). For exercise of lower intensity or shorter duration, the standard basal rate can be maintained and a simple reduction in the pre-meal bolus is sufficient.

Insulin pumps can malfunction during exercise. The athlete must be mindful of displacement of the infusion set which can lead to a hypoinsulinemic state and diabetic ketoacidosis (DKA) in a short period of time. Continuing to exercise unaware of a displaced catheter results in lower insulin levels than expected and can easily quicken the progression to DKA.

Sweating can displace the pump and liquid skin preparations can be used to prevent displacement. The use of antiperspirants around the infusion site has helped reduce sweating around the infusion set. The environment can affect the overall effectiveness of an insulin pump. Insulin is heat sensitive and overheating can occur when exercising in the heat with the pump next to the body. If unexplainable hyperglycemia occurs, the infusion catheter and insulin cartridge should be replaced. Proper care and monitoring of the equipment is essential to successful use of the pump during exercise.

If removal of the pump is needed during contact and collision sports, it should be stopped 30 min prior to short duration exercise (<1 h) because of the persistent action of insulin after pump removal. Care should be taken in order to ensure protection of the catheter that will remain in the athlete. Small boluses during exercise may be needed for longer activities (>1 h) in order to prevent hypoinsulinemic states in activities such as marathons and soccer matches. These boluses should be given every hour and the amount of insulin given should represent approximately 50% of the usual hourly basal rate (Danese *et al.* 1996).

The athlete with diabetes should be aware of the warning signs of hypoglycemia which tend to be reproducible for each individual. Symptoms typically involve headache, hunger, and dizziness which indicate mild hypoglycemia (blood glucose levels 50–70 mg·dL^{-1}). Both the practitioner and athlete should be prepared to treat acute hypoglycemia with glucose-containing liquids, hard candy, or oral glucose tablets. More severe hypoglycemia occurs when glucose levels drop below 40 mg·dL^{-1} and athletes with diabetes may be unconscious, combative, or severely obtunded. If the level of consciousness does not allow for protection of the airway, glucose by the oral route should be avoided. In these cases, intravenous glucose administration is indicated. It is always preferable to have confirmation of hypoglycemia by fingerstick; however, this should not delay glucose therapy. In those experiencing severe hypoglycemia, glucagon (1 mg s.c. or i.m.) should be given to produce a rapid release of liver glycogen. This is ineffective if all liver glycogen stores have been depleted after prolonged, intense exercise. Given that glucagon is relatively shortacting, once mental status has improved, oral carbohydrate supplements should be given to avoid rebound hypoglycemia. A glucagon emergency kit is a required addition to every field-side coverage bag.

Thyroid disease

Thyroid disease is common, affecting approximately 5% of the population over their lifetime. Women have a 5–7 times higher incidence of thyroid disease than men. The peak incidence of the disease is over the age of 40 years but is common in the college age population.

Screening for thyroid disease is controversial in the general population, and in the athletic population it is even more controversial. The recommendation for the general population is every 5 years in women over 35 years (Danese *et al.* 1996). Thyroid problems will affect performance and should be considered in athletes with reduced performance. Thyroid screening has been proposed for the elite athlete during the preparticipation physical examination (Mellman & Podesta 1997). This is hardly justifiable in the elite Olympic athlete and should not be recommended in the general asymptomatic athletic population. Screening should start with thyroid-stimulating hormone (TSH) because it is a very sensitive screening test for thyroid disease. Once an abnormal value is obtained further testing should be carried out based on symptoms and clinical suspicion.

Function

Thyroxine (T4) is a tyrosine-based hormone which is iodinated in the thyroid gland. T4 is released from the thyroid upon stimulation from TSH. TSH is released from the anterior pituitary gland by thyroid-releasing factor (TRH), made in the hypothalamus. T4 is then converted to triiodothyronine (T3) at the peripheral tissues by a selenium-dependent enzyme. Thyroid hormone functions by increasing oxidative metabolism in mitochondria and by increasing tissue responsiveness to catecholamines. Problems in the thyroid system stem from interference of proper stimulation of the gland, production of thyroxine, or peripheral conversion. Most frequently, it is a primary thyroid problem. Uncommon are the problems at the hypothalamus or peripheral tissues.

Exercise intolerance

While the scientific literature is sparse on the direct effects of thyroid disease on the competitive athlete, studies on the effects of thyroid dysfunction on cardiac function, pulmonary function, and muscle metabolism have indicated that thyroid disorders are generally deleterious to exercise performance. Kahaly *et al.* (1996, 1998, 1999) have observed the effects of the hyperthyroid state on both cardiac and pulmonary function. This group showed hyperthyroid patients had diminished forced vital capacity, tidal volume, and work load at anaerobic threshold. They also used stress echocardiography to reveal expected elevations in stroke volume index, ejection fraction, and cardiac output at rest, but the responses of these parameters to an exercise load were blunted. These restrictions were normalized, once the hyperthyroid patients were treated and were in the euthyroid state.

Hypothyroidism is not conducive to athletics. There is a decrease in exercise tolerance. A large reduction in $\dot{V}o_{2max}$ and endurance is seen. Specific abnormalities in cardiac function that have been documented in the literature include decreased ejection fraction, decreased stroke volume, decreased cardiac output, and decreased anaerobic threshold, along with an increase in total peripheral resistance (TPR; Biondi *et al.* 2002; Klein & Ojamaa 2001).

At the muscle, there is decreased oxidative capacity. A decrease in perfusion to the muscle has been noted. This is seen in type IIa and I muscle fibers but not in type IIb fibers (McAllister *et al.* 1995). There is also a change in muscle types from fast-twitch to slow-twitch fibers. The normal energy supply is altered and there is a decrease of lipid (free fatty acid; FFA) substrate and an increase dependence on muscle glycogen and this results in early fatigability.

Hyperthyroidism causes an increase in cardiac output and reduction in TPR. Yet, maximum O_2 consumption is decreased by 10% and endurance is also reduced during hyperthyroidism (Martin *et al.* 1991). An increase in blood flow to muscles occurs which might predict an advantage during exercise but there are other mechanisms that decrease total endurance with hyperthyroidism. For example, glycogen is depleted at a much faster rate with elevated lactate levels (Sestoft & Saltin 1985). These metabolic changes and the hyperthermia seen with hyperthyroidism both account for the decreased endurance with this disorder.

Hypothyroidism

There are many different causes of hypothyroidism. Hashimoto's thyroiditis and subclinical hypothyroidism are common problems seen in the athletic population. The prevalence of overt hypothyroid disease is 1.0–1.5% (Tunbridge *et al.* 1977). The athlete with thyroid disease will often present complaining of fatigue (91% of patients with hypothyroidism have fatigue) among other complaints. However, fatigue is a common complaint in athletes and is most often not caused by thyroid disease. Besides fatigue, the female athlete with thyroid dysfunction will frequently present with menstrual dysfunction, either menorrhagia with hypothyroidism or amenorrhea with hyperthyroidism. It is important to consider thyroid disease in female athletes with menstrual irregularities. The main sign and symptoms are slow movement, puffiness, slowed ankle reflex, and dry skin (Table 8.6).

Musculoskeletal problems seen in patients with hypothyroidism are often associated with myopathy (Duyff *et al.* 2000). Carpal tunnel syndrome is found at a higher rate in patients with hypothyroidism,

Table 8.6 Signs and symptoms of hypothyroidism. (After Zulewski *et al*. 1997.)

Symptoms and signs	Positive likelihood ratio	Sensitivity (%)
Slow movement	27.7	36
Puffiness	16.2	60
Ankle reflex	11.8	77
Hearing	8.8	22
Sweating	3.9	54
Constipation	3.2	48
Coarse skin	3.2	60
Paraethesia	3.0	52
Hoarseness	2.7	34
Cold skin	2.5	50
Weight increase	2.4	54
Dry skin	2.1	76

even after they become euthyroid (Cakir *et al.* 2003; Palumbo *et al.* 2000). Cases of rhabdomyopathy have been reported resulting from hypothyroid myopathy (Kisakol *et al.* 2003). Creatine kinase levels should be considered in patients with myalgia and hypothyroidism. Bone mineral density is often higher in hypothyroidism but increased fractures are seen similar to hyperthyroidism. This is because of the poor micro-architecture of the bone secondary to the hypothyroidism.

HASHIMOTO'S THYROIDITIS

Hashimoto's thyroiditis is the most common cause of primary hypothyroidism, with the peak occurrence in middle age. However, it is seen frequently in the college athlete. It is an autoimmune disorder. The two most important autoimmune antibodies are the anti-thyroglobulin antibodies and the anti-thyroid peroxidase. It has a genetic disposition with an increased rate in human leukocyte antigen (HLA) DR3 and DR5. The relative risk is only 4.7 compared to the more common associations of HLA-B27 with ankylosing spondylitis (relative rate [RR] of 150), DQ8 and type 1 DM (RR of 14) and B35 and subacute thyroiditis (RR of 14) (Barbesino & Chiovato 2000).

The usual presentation is with a goiter. The gland is rubbery and both lobes are enlarged but not necessarily symmetrically. The patient is usually euthyroid with an elevated TSH. The presence of autoantibodies is found. The level of T4 will eventually decrease, so monitoring is needed on a bimonthly basis. Occasionally, the patient will present with hyperthyroidism, either from concurrent Graves' disease or anti-TSH receptor antibody.

Treatment is recommended when patients have increased TSH and antibody present. The exogenous thyroxine can reduce the goiter size. Pregnant women with elevated antibody levels have increased miscarriage rates, despite treatment.

SUBCLINICAL HYPOTHYROIDISM

Screening for subclinical hyperthyroidism in women over 35 years, or during first prenatal visit is recommended by some authors (Cooper 2001). The disease is disproportionately seen in women. There is an increase in the incidence of the disorder with age. Reports vary from 1% to 10% of patients depending on age group and location. People with subclinical hypothyroidism describe slightly more thyroid-related symptoms than controls.

Treatment benefit of symptom reduction is seen in one in four patients treated for subclinical hypothyroidism (Cooper *et al.* 1984). Long-term benefits of treatment are postulated because of the changes in cholesterol with treatment and the noted increase in atherosclerosis in patients with untreated subclinical hypothyroidism. Additionally, it has been well-documented that endothelial dysfunction, another risk factor for coronary and vascular disease, is more common in hypothyroid patients, even those with subclinical hypothyroidism. Moreover, endothelial dysfunction can be improved with the administration of thryroxine and restoration of the euthyroid state (Biondi & Klein 2004; Cikim *et al.* 2004; Dagre *et al.* 2005; Papaioannou *et al.* 2004). Prevention of overt hypothyroidism by treatment of subclinical hypothyroidism is postulated as elevated TSH or presence of thyroperoxidase antibodies in population studies correlate with an increased rate of 2.1% and 2.6% per year of developing overt hypothyroidism.

Treatment is recommended in patients with TSH >10 mU·L^{-1} along with either antithyroid antibodies or elevated lipid panel. Treatment with thyroxine should start at 0.05–0.075 mg·day^{-1}. Caution in treatment is needed in patients with coronary artery disease because overtreatment can precipitate angina. Patients should be retested in 4–6 weeks to check that thyroid tests are normalized.

Hyperthyroidism

GRAVES' DISEASE

Graves' disease is the most common cause of hyperthyroidism. It is seen seven times more frequently in females than males. Graves' disease is most common in adults 20–50 years old, with peak incidence in the third and fourth decade of life (McIver & Morris 1998). The exact cause is unknown but it is characterized by the presence of thyrotropin receptor antibodies (TRAb) and familial predisposition. The TRAb are immunoglobulin G (IgG) autoantibodies. There is an increased frequency in haplotypes HLA-B8, HLA-DRw3, and HLA-DRB3 in Caucasians, HLA-DRB3*020 and HLA-DQA1*0501 in African-Americans (Chen et al. 2000), HLA-Bw36 in Japanese, and HLA-Bw46 in Chinese (Gough 2000).

Patients who have hyperthyroidism commonly have nervousness, fatigue, a rapid heartbeat or palpitations, heat intolerance, and weight loss. These symptoms are seen in more than 50% of all patients who have the disease. Ophthalmologic changes, such as proptosis, are probably the most well-known physical characteristic with Graves' disease. They are only seen in 50–75% of patients. The most common eye findings are eyelid retraction or lag, and periorbital edema. Even though exophthalmos (proptosis) is commonly described with Graves' disease, it occurs in only one-third of patients. The ophthalmologic changes seem to be a cross-reactivity with receptor antibodies seen in Graves' disease affecting a pre-adipose subpopulation of the orbital fibroblast.

Some patients who have Graves' disease (1–2%) may develop dermopathy over the shin area. This pretibial myxedema is typified by hyperpigmented patches and plaques that indurate with touch. The dermopathy is seen almost exclusively with severe ophthalmopathy. As with ophthalmopathy, dermopathy may develop the year prior to or into the course of the disease.

Musculoskeletal problems seen with Grave's disease (hyperthyroidism) are well accepted or controversial. The decrease in bone mineral density is seen with hyperthyroid. Even with correction of the hyperthyroid, there is an increase in osteoporosis-associated fractures (Vestergaard & Mosekilde 2003). Adhesive capsulitis is found in patients with hyperthyroidism at a higher rate (Cakir et al. 2003). The association of adhesive capsulitis with hyperthyroidism was attributed to the close resemblance of hyperthyroidism to activation of the sympathetic nervous system (Cakir et al. 2003). Carpal tunnel syndrome is controversial as some studies have found associations (Cakir et al. 2003; Duyff et al. 2000) while other have not (Roquer & Cano 1993). The association of hypothyroidism with carpal tunnel syndrome is more convincing at this time.

Diagnosis of Graves' disease is improved with new second generation assays, with reported sensitivity and specificity of 99.6% and 98.8% (Costagliola et al. 1999). The radioactive iodine uptake (RAIU) scan can help differentiate Graves' disease (diffusely increased uptake) from toxic nodules (with focal uptake) and subacute, chronic, or postpartum thyroiditis (with low uptake).

Treating Graves' disease includes reducing symptoms and controlling the overactive thyroid. Beta-blockers are useful in reducing the symptoms of tremor and tachycardia until the patient is euthyroid. Controlling the overactive thyroid can be accomplished in three ways: antithyroid medications, radioactive iodine ablation, and thyroidectomy.

The medications propylthiouracil and methimazole inhibit thyroid hormone synthesis by inhibition of the thyroid peroxidase enzyme. Rates of remission of 40–65% have been reported with 2-year use of anti-thyroid medication and thyroid replacement (Hashizume et al. 1991). Thyroxine addition prevents TSH production and theoretically reduces anti-receptor antibody production. Side effects of anti-thyroid medications include leukopenia, rash, pruritus, arthralgias, and, rarely (0.3%), agranulocytosis. Complete blood count (CBC) should be monitored appropriately while on this medication. Total

T3 (TT3) and free T4 (FT4) should be monitored every 6 weeks until euthyroid then every 3–4 months for 2 years. Once medication is stopped TSH, TT3, and FT4 should be monitored every 6 weeks for 18 weeks.

Radioactive iodine is the treatment of choice in North America. It is a safe and common treatment (Singer *et al.* 1995). The treatment should not be used in patients who are pregnant or might become pregnant in the next 4 months. The main side effect of radioactive iodine treatment is hypothyroidism post-treatment. It can initiate or exacerbate the oph- thalmologic symptoms of Graves' disease. This can be treated with prednisone. Anti-thyroid medica- tions should not be used immediately before or after radioactive iodine. Medication such as propylth- iouracil can be radioprotective for up to 55 days. Patients' thyroid state usually stabilizes 6–12 months after treatment, and they can be followed every 3–4 months, or as needed, with a T4 index and TSH tests. Once euthyroid, these patients should be followed yearly with a serum TSH test.

Subtotal thyroidectomy is the preferred treatment for certain subgroups of Graves' disease: patients who are pregnant, and in those allergic to anti- thyroid medications. After surgery patients may be hypothyroid and will need supplemental thyroid hormone. It is important to follow patients over the next 6 months as hypothyroidism may develop over that period of time. Yearly thyroid testing is recommended, whether the patient needs thyroid replacement or is euthyroid postoperatively.

Graves' ophthalmopathy may not improve with thyroid treatment, because the antibodies attack the eye as well as the thyroid. Mild to moderate ophthalmopathy may improve without a thyroid treatment and supportive care is all that is needed. Proptosis can produce symptomatic corneal expos- ure, which can be treated by taping the eyelids closed overnight. Other eye symptoms can be usu- ally treated with sunglasses and artificial tears. Ophthalmology should be consulted for any severe symptoms (such as for severe proptosis, orbital inflammation, or optic neuropathy). Approximately two-thirds of patients with severe ophthalmopathy improve with high dose glucocorticoid and/or orbital radiation (Bartalena *et al.* 1997).

SUBACUTE (DE QUERVAIN'S) THYROIDITIS

This is viral in origin. It presents after an upper respiratory infection with prolonged malaise, asthenia, and pain over the thyroid from stretching of the capsule. The symptoms may smolder and be vague in nature. The thyroid is most often tender to palpation.

The diagnosis is made with an elevated erythro- cyte sedimentation rate (ESR) and a depressed RAIU. Other tests (FT4, TT3, and TSH) can vary depending on the stage of the illness. The painless thyroid with hyperthyroidism can mirror Graves' disease and be difficult to separate clinically.

Treatment is mostly supportive because the problem will resolve. Propranolol is used to control the thyrotoxicosis. To decrease the inflammatory response aspirin is used if the case is mild or pred- nisone if more severe. When the RAIU and FT4 return to normal therapy can be stopped.

SUBCLINICAL HYPERTHYROIDISM

Subclinical hyperthyroidism is defined by low TSH but normal T4 and T3. The incidence varies by location, associated thyroid abnormalities, and increasing age. Reported amounts vary from 2% to 16%. The disease may be transient or persistent in nature (Shrier & Burman 2002).

There is a very small likelihood of subclinical hyperthyroidism developing into overt hyperthy- roidism. The main concerns and controversies in treatment are the associated increase risk in cardio- logic and musculoskeletal diseases.

Population studies have shown an increase chance of atrial fibrillation (AF) over 10 year incid- ences of 8%, 12%, and 21% for TSH concentrations of normal, 0.1–0.4 $\mu U \cdot mL^{-1}$, and less than 0.1 $\mu U \cdot mL^{-1}$, respectively (Sawin *et al.* 1994). These increases in AF are correctable with treatment. This is not a reason for immediate therapy as the natural course of the disease is often transient. Monitoring is appropriate.

An increase in bone demineralization is noted in subclinical hyperthyroidism (Faber & Galloe 1994). In premenopausal women the rate was not significant but increased. In postmenopausal women the rate was higher and significant. The athlete with subclinical hyperthyroidism and stress fractures should be considered for earlier treatment.

The female athlete

The problem of amenorrhea in female athletes, and its association with other pathologies specifically disordered eating and loss of bone mineral density, has been discussed at great length in the sports medicine literature. The combination of these three entities has been termed the "female athlete triad" (Otis *et al.* 1997; Yeager *et al.* 1993). Amenorrhea has been recognized as a common issue in physically active women and many of the questions surrounding it have been answered to one degree or another. However, there still remain challenges in understanding the complete etiology of the clinical findings, optimal methods for identifying those at risk, and establishing optimal therapeutic interventions for those affected. As the number of girls and women participating in strenuous physical activity continues to grow, the answers to these questions continue to grow in importance. The understanding of amenorrhea in female athletes incorporates the appreciation of the underlying basic science of the hypothalamic–pituitary–ovarian (HPO) axis, the etiology of menstrual dysfunction in female athletes, the common presenting signs and symptoms of amenorrheic athletes, appropriate evaluation of the amenorrheic athlete, and scientifically based therapeutic intervention.

Endocrinology of the hypothalamic–pituitary–ovarian axis

The HPO axis is governed by both negative and positive feedback loops. It is predominantly controlled by five hormones: gonadotropin-releasing hormone (GnRH) from the hypothalamus, luteinizing hormone (LH), and follicle-stimulating hormone (FSH) from the anterior pituitary, estrogen, and progesterone. GnRH is released in a pulsatile fashion from the hypothalamus. This cyclic release of GnRH, in turn, stimulates the release of LH and FSH from the anterior pituitary. LH, in particular,

stimulates the production of androgens from the ovarian theca cells, which, in turn, migrate to the ovarian granulosa cells and are converted to estradiol via aromatization (Bulun & Adashi 2003).

At low levels of secretion, estrogens exert negative feedback on LH and FSH production. However, as levels of estrogen climb during the follicular phase of the menstrual cycle, the effect of estrogen switches to one of positive feedback on both LH and FSH. This leads to the mid-cycle LH surge, which stimulates ovulation. After ovulation, the remaining components of the follicle that were not ovulated – the granulosa and theca cells – convert to the corpus luteum under the influence of the LH surge. The corpus luteum undertakes the role of secretion of progesterone. The corpus luteum has a limited lifespan, and unless it receives the stimulus of human chorionic gonadotropin, secreted by the fertilized ovum, it undergoes regression and ceases its production of progesterone. It is this drop off in progesterone that stimulates the sloughing of the uterine endometrium and the onset of menstruation.

The uterine endometrium has two functional layers: the basalis layer and the functionalis layer. At the level of the uterine endometrium, the thickness and vascularity of the endometrium are at their lowest levels near the end of the first week of the menstrual cycle, correlating with the end of menstruation. At this point of the cycle, the functionalis layer has been shed, leaving just the basalis layer of the endometrium. During the follicular phase of the menstrual cycle, estrogen levels rise and stimulate the proliferation of the functionalis layer of the uterine endometrium. After ovulation, the functionalis layer is maintained predominantly via the action of progesterone and estrogen from the corpus luteum upon it. Progesterone has a significant role in stimulating the transformation of a proliferative functionalis layer to a secretory functionalis layer that is optimal for providing nutrition and implantation of the fertilized ovum. The drop in progesterone that corresponds with regression of the corpus luteum if fertilization does not occur is a stimulus for the shedding of the functionalis layer, which results in menses.

Alterations in the HPO axis and their relationship to amenorrhea in athletes

It has long been understood that athletic females exhibit a higher rate of amenorrhea than do their non-athletic peers (Otis *et al.* 1997; Warren & Perlroth 2001). For many years, this was felt to be a normal variant, and because of the low numbers of female athletes and the general lack of clinical concern regarding it, there was little scientific investigation into its etiology. The first connection between exercise-associated amenorrhea and compromised bone density was established by Drinkwater *et al.* (1984) and Cann *et al.* (1984). It was then that more focused investigation into this phenomenon was undertaken.

Exercise-associated amenorrhea has been classified as a hypothalamic amenorrhea. In this situation, a stimulus causes a disruption in the normal pulsatile secretion of GnRH from the hypothalamus. Specifically, GnRH pulse frequency diminishes. In response to this diminution in GnRH pulse frequency, the pulse frequency of LH secretion from the anterior pituitary also decreases. This decrease in LH secretion has the effect of decreasing estrogen production from the ovary. As a result, the functionalis layer of the endometrium does not proliferate normally, ovulation does not occur on a predictable basis, the corpus luteum fails to develop normally, progesterone production during the luteal phase of the menstrual cycle suffers, and normal menstruation fails to occur.

Historically, various causes of this abnormal hormonal milieu have been proposed. Frisch and Revelle (1971) noted the difference in body composition between amenorrheic and eumenorrheic females and postulated that the ability to menstruate was tied to having a minimal percentage body fat. This theory was challenged when it was noted that amenorrheic dancers would begin to menstruate after being injured despite experiencing no change in percentage body fat (Warren 1980). Conversely, overweight women who had undergone bariatric surgery and sustained a dramatic weight loss ceased to menstruate despite having body compositions that were still dramatically higher than normal (Di Carlo *et al.* 1999).

Another theory was that the stress of heavy exercise triggered the hormonal abnormalities that translate into the amenorrheic state. This was based on the knowledge that abnormalities in the hypothalamic–pituitary–adrenal (HPA) axis can alter normal menstrual function via corticotropin-releasing hormone (CRH), cortisol, opioids, and pro-opiomelanocortin (POOMC) (Loucks 2005). Subsequent studies demonstrated a correlation between elevated cortisol levels in athletes and the likelihood of amenorrhea in both animals and humans (Bullen *et al.* 1985; Chatterton 1990; Manning & Bronson 1989, 1991). However, the difference between correlation and causation was not clearly delineated and it was unclear whether or not the hormonal abnormalities were simply independent variables caused by another stress. The same authors who produced these studies questioned, at the time, whether exercise stress and its effect on the HPA was actually the causative mechanism of menstrual dysfunction and whether energy imbalance could have a role (Bronson & Manning 1991; Chatterton 1990).

Subsequently, it was demonstrated (Loucks *et al.* 1998) that if sedentary females were started on an exercise protocol, LH pulsatility was unaffected, as long as energy balance was maintained via increasing caloric intake. However, if energy balance was disrupted, either via energy restriction in the form of diminished caloric intake while remaining sedentary or via uncompensated energy expenditure in the form of exercise, LH pulse frequency decreased. This study was able to isolate the effects of energy imbalance from the effects of absolute body composition or "exercise stress." Subsequent investigations have reinforced this finding in both human and non-human primates (Hilton & Loucks 2000; Williams *et al.* 2001a,b). These findings have led to the current belief that energy availability, not body composition or exercise stress, is the driving force behind hypothalamic amenorrhea in athletes (Loucks 2005).

Spectrum of menstrual disorders in female athletes

The menstrual disturbances experienced by female athletes occur along a continuum (De Souza 2003).

These abnormalities range from very subtle changes such as luteal phase deficiency and anovulatory cycles to oligomenorrhea and amenorrhea. These abnormalities are associated with the degree of exercise in which competitive athletes participate. However, the exercise, while it correlates with the menstrual disturbance, is not likely to be causative. Each of these menstrual disturbances are related to the energy-deficient state to which exercise contributes.

LUTEAL PHASE DEFICIENCY

Athletes affected by luteal phase deficiency rarely present for clinical evaluation. Luteal phase deficiency or insufficiency arises because of inadequate progesterone stimulus of the uterine endometrium. After ovulation and the formation of the corpus luteum, glycogen-filled vacuoles begin to form under the influence of progesterone. These vacuoles rise to the surface of the uterine endometrium and empty into the uterine cavity providing a glycogen-rich environment for the fertilized ovum. Without the influence of progesterone, the uterine environment can be inadequate for the appropriate implantation of the developing embryo, resulting in high rates of infertility and spontaneous abortion. Unless the athlete is attempting to become pregnant, the clinical manifestations of this disturbance are minimal. Cycle lengths may be variable with shortened luteal phases, but unless fertility problems are encountered, the athlete will rarely notice problems that would cause them to seek care. Despite the paucity of women seeking care, this disturbance has been found to be extremely common in exercising women. In a group of 24 moderately exercising, regularly menstruating women, De Souza *et al.* (1998) found an incidence of 79% over a 3-month span.

ANOVULATION

Women who experience luteal phase deficiency still have enough estrogen to ovulate appropriately. However, the next step along the exercise-associated menstrual disturbance continuum is the development of anovulation. It is felt that lower levels of estradiol and FSH during the follicular phase of the menstrual cycle fail to stimulate the development and propagation of a dominant follicle for ovulation. The absence of ovulation and the formation of the corpus luteum blunt the progesterone production necessary to transform the uterine endometrium from a proliferative to a secretory endometrium. The progesterone decline that stimulates menstruation is also absent and sloughing of the endometrium fails to occur.

OLIGOMENORRHEA

Oligomenorrhea has been described as menstrual cycles that last 36–90 days (Loucks & Horvath 1985). For the purpose of research that has been carried out previously, it has been described as women having between three and four menstrual periods in a year (Cobb *et al.* 2003). Menstrual cycles are unpredictable and irregular in their occurrence. Serum estradiol levels are very inconsistent, but are generally diminished. It is widely held that oligomenorrhea is more common in athletes that in the general population.

AMENORRHEA

Amenorrhea is the most extreme manifestation of the spectrum of menstrual abnormalities caused by energy imbalance in athletes. Amenorrhea has been defined variably in the literature, and variable groups of athletes have been studied, resulting in a broad range of estimates regarding its prevalence in athletes. A common definition requires the athlete to be without menstrual bleeding for at least 6 months. Therapeutically, it is important to use more liberal criteria for initiating evaluation and treatment. Commonly, the absence of menstrual periods for three consecutive months should stimulate further investigation on the part of the clinician.

Link to bone mineral density

HYPOESTROGENISM

The presence of estrogen is necessary for appropriate osteoblast function and the production of new bone. In low energy states, such as with hypothalamic amenorrhea, estrogen levels fall, and in turn, it has been thought that bone formation suffers. Indeed, the evidence that women with hypothalamic amenorrhea have diminished estrogen levels and bone mineral density. Because of the association between postmenopausal estrogen diminution, its replenishment, and subsequent bone mineral density, it has been widely postulated that the loss of bone mineral density associated with hypothalamic amenorrhea is caused by low estrogen levels in these women.

ENERGY DEFICIENCY

It has been noted that the overall hormonal status of amenorrheic female athletes is very similar to that found in patients with anorexia nervosa. These hormonal abnormalities include elevated cortisol levels, growth hormone resistance, and suppressed serum T3 levels, which are all associated with compromised bone mineral density. Additionally, it has been shown that estrogen replacement alone has not been helpful in restoring bone mineral density in anorectics, and its efficacy in restoring bone mass in athletic amenorrheics have not been consistently documented (Zanker & Cooke 2004). These findings lead to the postulate that the loss of bone mineral density noted in athletes with amenorrhea may have a more complex basis than solely the documented hypoestrogenemic state, and may be secondary to a more complex hormonal influence that is triggered by the athletes' energy deficient state.

CARDIOVASCULAR RISK

To date, the primary complication of hypothalamic amenorrhea to be addressed has been the loss of bone mineral density in these women. However, more recent investigations have raised the concern that these women may also be at increased cardiovascular risk. Endothelial dysfunction can be measured non-invasively by measuring, with ultrasound, the degree of endothelial dilation of the brachial artery in response to the flow through it, known as flow-mediated dilation (FMD) (Anderson et al. 1995; Celermajer 1997; Celermajer et al. 1992). The presence of abnormal FMD is highly correlated with endothelial function in the coronary arteries and has been firmly established as a coronary risk factor. Hoch et al. (2003) and Rickenlund et al. (2005) showed that amenorrheic female athletes display a significantly greater degree of endothelial dysfunction is than do their eumenorrheic peers, as evidenced by impaired FMD. Furthermore, each group demonstrated reversal of these abnormalities with therapeutic intervention (Hoch et al. 2003; Rickenlund et al. 2005). The Hoch group used an educational intervention that resulted in the resumption of normal menstrual function in seven of nine subjects. These seven subjects showed significant improvement in their FMD. The Rickenlund group used oral contraceptives for 9 months, and their amenorrheic athletes also showed significant improvements in their FMD. While research in this area remains young, the initial data indicate that young athletes with hypothalamic amenorrhea may face increased cardiovascular risk, despite their highly active lifestyles, and that this risk is potentially improved with restoration of energy balance or estrogen supplementation.

Clinical evaluation of the female athlete with amenorrhea

The clinical evaluation of a female athlete with amenorrhea begins with an understanding of the differential diagnosis of amenorrhea. Too often, the assumption is made that the woman's amenorrhea is coming from her athletic participation without appropriate investigation into other potential causes. Too often, as well, the patient is told that she is experiencing a benign phenomenon about which she need not worry. The starting point for evaluating a female athlete with amenorrhea is with a differential diagnosis for both primary and secondary amenorrhea that includes the hypothalamic amenorrhea discussed above, but also goes beyond it to other causes. A careful history and physical examination followed by a focused laboratory examination is also essential.

Reindollar et al. (1989) broke down the differential diagnosis of primary amenorrhea into three broad categories: hypergonadotrophic hypogonadism, hypogonadotrophic hypogonadism, and eugonadism.

The hypergonadotrophic hypogonadic group can be further broken down into those individuals with abnormal sex chromosomes, such as Turner's syndrome, and those with normal sex chromosomes, either 46,XX or 46,XY. They hypogonadotrophic hypogonadic group has normally functioning gonads, but impaired stimulation, either resulting from congenital abnormalities (GnRH deficiency, hypopituitarism, or congenital CNS defects), constitutional delay of puberty, acquired lesions of either endocrine (congenital adrenal hyperplasia, Cushing's syndrome, pseudoparathyroidism or hypoparathyroidism, or hyperprolactinemia) or neoplastic origin (pituitary adenoma, craniopharyngioma), systemic illness, or eating disorders. The eugonadic group most commonly had an anatomic abnormality, such as congenital absence of the uterus and vagina, cervical atresia, imperforate hymen, or a transverse vaginal septum. Of these, imperforate hymens and transverse vaginal septae are readily amenable to surgical correction. The eugonadic group less commonly was found to have intersex disorders, such as androgen insensitivity. Of all of the possible causes of primary amenorrhea, the most common were ovarian failure (48.5%), congenital absence of the uterus and vagina (16.2%), GnRH deficiency (8.3%), and constitutional delay of puberty (6.0%) (Reindollar *et al.* 1989).

The differential diagnosis of secondary amenorrhea includes many of the same items as the differential for primary amenorrhea. However, some more common etiologies emerge as potential causes. The most common cause of secondary amenorrhea in young females is pregnancy. To proceed with an evaluation and even treatment of secondary amenorrhea without ruling out pregnancy is, at best, embarrassing and, at worst, potentially harmful to the developing fetus. A test for pregnancy is at the top of all secondary amenorrhea work-ups. Other common causes of secondary amenorrhea can be broken down into disorders of the hypothalamus, the pituitary, the gonads, metabolism, and anatomy. Hypothalamic disorders include those caused by lesions such as craniopharyngiomas or granulomatous disease, drugs such as phenothiazines or birth control pills, and energy imbalances as described above. The pituitary gland can also be affected by neoplastic growth, either prolactin-secreting tumors or tumors secreting chromophobe hormones, such as growth hormone and adenocorticotropic hormone (ACTH). Additionally, cells of the pituitary can be injured or destroyed by anoxia, thrombosis, or hemorrhage. If this occurs in relationship to pregnancy, it is termed Sheehan's syndrome. If unrelated to pregnancy, it is termed Simmonds' disease. It is important to recognize these entities because the production of other pituitary hormones, such as TSH and ACTH can lead to more immediate and dangerous health outcomes than decreases in LH or FSH.

Gonadal sources of secondary amenorrhea predominantly involve premature ovarian failure (POF). POF is defined as the depletion of ovarian follicles prior to the age of 40. The age is set somewhat arbitrarily, and is based upon the fact that only 1% of women cease menstruation before the age of 40 (Bolun & Adashi 2003). Damage to the ovaries from radiation therapy or chemotherapy is one source of POF. Another cause of POF is autoimmune illness, and the diagnosis of such in a woman with no history of radiation or chemotherapy damage to the ovaries necessitates an evaluation for other autoimmune illnesses and endocrinopathies such as hypothyroidism, hypoparathyroidism, or Addison's disease. The diagnosis of POF is established by finding postmenopausal FSH levels ($>30 \ \text{mIU}\cdot\text{mL}^{-1}$) on two separate occasions.

Metabolic diseases are also a relatively common source of secondary amenorrhea. Of these, polycystic ovarian syndrome (PCOS) is the most common. Thyroid disease, both hyperthyroidism and hypothyroidism, is also a relatively common cause. PCOS was initially described by Stein and Leventhal (1935) as a complex of amenorrhea, hyperandrogenism, and polycystic ovaries. Those with this disorder are classically hirsute and obese. For years, this was viewed as a primarily ovarian problem. However, with the further detection of hyperinsulinism and insulin resistance in 1980 (Burghen *et al.* 1980), the realization that the classic "Stein–Leventhal" syndrome was more likely a broader, multifactorial syndrome. While women with PCOS tend to be hirsute and obese, the hyperandrogenism associated with the syndrome may only present as acne and not all women will be obese. PCOS needs to be on the list of differential diagnoses for any woman who presents with either primary or secondary oligomenorrhea or amenorrhea. The diagnosis of PCOS is made by presence of irregular uterine bleeding and androgen excess without other cause of androgen excess (Cushing's syndrome, glucocorticoid resistance, non-traditional congenital adrenal hyperplasia, or ovarian or adrenal tumors; Bolun & Adashi 2003; Lobo & Carmina 2000). The presence of polycystic ovaries on ultrasound (>10 cysts per ovary) helps confirm the diagnosis, but is not a necessary component of the syndrome, despite its name.

Thyroid disease, whether hypothyroidism or hyperthyroidism, can also lead to menstrual dysfunction, including menorrhagia, oligomenorrhea, or amenorrhea. Other signs and symptoms of hypothyroidism include weight gain, fatigue, diminished energy, thinning hair, constipation, and cold intolerance. Hyperthyroidism, on the other hand, can exhibit unintentional weight loss, palpitations, excessive sweating, symptoms of anxiety, and heat intolerance. Often, on careful questioning and examination, women whose menstrual disturbances are caused by thyroid disease will have some of these findings. However, it is possible for the menstrual disturbance to be the presenting symptom of an underlying thyroid disorder.

The most likely anatomic cause of secondary amenorrhea is the presence of intrauterine adhesions (IUAs), also referred to as Asherman's syndrome. IUAs are usually the result of a previous endometrial procedure, especially associated with pregnancy. They are known sequelae of surgical removal of either a dead or live fetus, or either postpartum or post-abortal curettage. Curettage after missed abortion can cause a 30% rate of IUAs (Stenchever et al. 2001). If the patient's amenorrhea began after such a procedure, the diagnosis must be considered. Diagnosis is confirmed with either hysteroscopy or hysterography.

HISTORY

In any patient who presents with oligomenorrhea or amenorrhea, a careful history must be taken. The diagnosis of hypothalamic amenorrhea, although common in the athletic population, is only reached after other etiologies for menstrual disturbances have been ruled out. The history obtained should include the patient's personal menstrual history, including age of menarche, and the timing of the development of secondary sexual characteristics. Sexual activity should be assessed and the date of the last menstrual period should be noted. If possible, maternal age of menarche and any family history of menstrual disorders should also be sought. The patient should also be questioned about symptoms of CNS neoplasms, such as headaches, visual changes, and galactorrhea. All medications should also be known, especially any psychotropic medications or recent use of oral contraceptives. Female athletes should be asked about the use of anabolic steroids and any symptoms that could result from them. A history of male pattern baldness, clitoromegaly, breast shrinkage, extensive acne, male distribution of body hair, or particularly greasy skin can be symptoms of hyperandrogenism associated with anabolic steroid use. PCOS will also cause some symptoms of hyperandrogenism, but will not typically cause high enough androgen levels to effect male pattern baldness, clitoromegaly, or breast shrinkage. Past and current medical problems should be uncovered, including surgical procedures, especially those involving the reproductive system. Symptoms of thyroid disease, noted above, should also be sought.

On initial evaluation, a rough dietary recall on the part of the patient is adequate to begin assessing the adequacy of her caloric intake, but often a more thorough nutritional assessment by a registered dietitian becomes necessary. The volume of exercise being performed is also important to ascertain. Often, competitive athletes keep a training log that can be very beneficial in assessing their energy demands. A few screening questions for eating disorders are also appropriate. If the athlete's dietary history indicates either poor dietary intake or a dietary history that is "too good," further inspection into the possibility of disordered eating is appropriate. Other red flags in the nutritional history may include multiple food allergies, lactose intolerance, vegetarianism, and a strong interest in the nutritional field. While these signs are certainly not all pathologic, the presence of several of them may be an indication that further investigation would be useful. Questions about body image, desired weight, and food attitudes may be helpful, but many athletes are fully versed in the "right" answers, and the diagnosis of disordered eating may take multiple visits with a patient.

PHYSICAL EXAMINATION

The focus of the physical examination should be on evaluating for the above problems. An appropriate examination should be performed with the patient unclothed and involves a pelvic examination. Male physicians who work in the intercollegiate athletics setting, where they have repetitive professional and social contact with the student athletes, are best served to share the evaluation of the patient with a female colleague who can perform the more intimate components of the physical examination.

On general examination, body habitus should be assessed, with hypothalamic amenorrhea being more likely in very thin athletes and PCOS more likely in overweight athletes. Stigmata of growth hormone excess (coarsening of features), Cushing's disease (centripetal obesity and a "buffalo hump"), and Graves' disease (exophthalmos) can be assessed with general inspection. Height and weight are necessary for calculating BMI. Although BMI is not diagnostic in assessing energy balance, it can still be a useful data point. Skin examination is important for assessing the presence and distribution of body hair. Also, the presence of fine lanugo hair may imply disordered eating and acanthosis nigricans is indicative of insulin resistance that accompanies PCOS. In the head region, visual acuity and visual fields should be assessed because the pituitary sits right above the optic chiasm, and a mass in this region can present with visual disturbances. It is very rare for such a mass to cause a rise in intracranial pressure, but funduscopic examination can assess for evidence of papilledema. Intraoral examination assesses dentition. Purging via vomiting can cause erosion of the dental enamel and a surprising amount of tooth decay. In the neck, thyroid size and the presence of nodules should be assessed.

Cervical adenopathy should also be noted. The presence of unsuspected adenopathy should lead to the consideration of systemic illness, such as either a Hodgkin's or non-Hodgkin's lymphoma which is acting as a physiologic stress.

Cardiac examination will likely yield the common findings of the athlete's heart. While bradycardia can be a physical sign of an eating disorder, its presence is common in well-trained athletes and rarely causes concern. However, the presence of mild tachycardia in a conditioned athlete may alert the examiner to underlying hyperthyroidism. Abdominal examination focuses on the presence of organ enlargement.

Neurologic examination is performed both to look for abnormalities that may indicate an intracranial process and to assess reflexes for thyroid disease. Brisk reflexes are characteristic of hyperthyroidism, while more sluggish reflexes with a slow return after contraction are more indicative of hypothyroidism. Any evidence of focal neurologic abnormality or ataxia, while extremely unlikely, should focus attention on the brain.

The pelvic examination is performed to assess for normal reproductive anatomy. Imperforate hymens and transverse vaginal septae are causes of primary amenorrhea. A normal appearing cervix and a normal feeling uterus and ovaries on bimanual examination help to assure normal anatomy. Unfortunately, it will not rule out the possibility of intrauterine adhesions (Asherman's syndrome). In an athlete with a history of endometrial procedures that are temporally related to her menstrual dysfunction, consideration must be given to referral for visualization of the intrauterine cavity, either by hysteroscopy or hysterography. Most female athletes with amenorrhea will be thin enough that adequate evaluation of the ovaries via bimanual examination should be possible. Along with the pelvic examination, a breast examination is performed to assure normal breast development and the absence of galactorrhea.

LABORATORY EVALUATION

In the athlete with no historical or physical examination findings to suggest other causes of menstrual dysfunction, a simple laboratory screen is appropriate. A pregnancy test should not be overlooked and should be performed in athletes of childbearing age. Additionally, a screening TSH, FSH, and prolactin level are recommended. Low TSH levels are almost always indicative of hyperthyroidism, given the suppression of TSH synthesis at the pituitary by T3 and T4. Elevated levels are indicative of hypothyroidism, given the lack of the same feedback inhibition. FSH levels will be elevated in cases of hypergonadotrophic hypogonadism, such as Turner's syndrome or POF. Prolactin levels are elevated with prolactinomas or medications such as phenothiazines, oral contraceptives, cimetidine, and metoclopramide. They will also be normally elevated with lactation and may be elevated by nipple stimulation. Although levels above 20 ng·mL^{-1} are considered abnormal, elevations of more than 200 ng·mL^{-1} are virtually diagnostic of pathologic hyperprolactinemia. In athletes with findings of virilization, a serum testosterone, dehydroepiandrostone (DHEAS), and LH levels are important. In PCOS, serum LH : FSH ratio will typically be greater than 3 : 1, and serum testosterone and DHEAS levels will be elevated. A normally high LH level can be obtained if the sample is drawn during the LH surge of the menstrual cycle. Testosterone and DHEAS levels will be normal. Redrawing the LH levels in 2 weeks should show the expected decrease in LH levels.

In the amenorrheic athlete whose laboratory values are unremarkable, a progestin challenge is recommended. The exogenous administration of an oral progestin will convert the normal proliferative uterine endometrium to a secretory endometrium, and the removal of the progestin should stimulate a withdrawal bleed. If a bleed fails to occur, it is likely the uterine endometrium did not proliferate normally. This can be caused by Asherman's syndrome, but it is more commonly the result of estrogen deficiency failing to stimulate endometrial proliferation. While POF can cause this, the most likely explanation in the amenorrheic athlete is hypoestrogenism secondary to hypothalamic amenorrhea caused by underlying energy deficiency. It is reasonable to make that clinical diagnosis once the evaluation has reached this point.

Management of the athlete with hypothalamic amenorrhea

Once of the diagnosis of hypothalamic amenorrhea has been made with the female athlete, attention turns to appropriate management of the problem. The issue of the amenorrhea is actually not of great clinical concern. The problem lies with the other correlates of hypoestrogenism and energy deficiency in the female athlete, particularly their effect on bone mineral density and potential effect on cardiovascular risk factors. Given that the underlying problem is one of energy deficiency, optimal management is directed at correcting it. The energy equation has two variables: energy intake and energy expenditure. While it is easy to recommend a reduction in energy expenditure via diminished activity, the training volume of an elite athlete is often a fixed variable. It is possible to judiciously work with an athlete and her coach to try to find areas in which her training schedule can be reduced, these energy savings will have relatively little effect on the energy equation. The more fruitful area on which to work is the energy intake component of the equation. In some athletes, education and skilled guidance regarding appropriate volume and composition of nutritional intake can be fruitful. Unfortunately, there is frequently at least a moderate component of psychologically driven disordered eating. For many female athletes, the suggestion of increasing caloric intake to meet energy needs can be a terrifying proposition. It is often necessary to provide coordinated care between the treating physician, a registered dietitian, and either a psychologist or psychiatrist with skill in treating eating disorders.

Concern needs to be relayed to the amenorrheic athlete regarding her risk of bone loss, whether from hypoestrogenemia, energy deficiency, or both. Of concern is that even women who regain their menstrual cycles have not been shown to regain bone at a rate that restores peak bone mass (Drinkwater et al. 1986). The theory that bone mineral density loss is secondary to hypoestrogenemia has led to the hypothesis that estrogen replacement, commonly in the form of oral contraceptive pills, would be beneficial to bone density. The use of estrogen replacement in the form of oral contraceptive pill (OCP) has been investigated. Although not all results are consistent, there appears to be some benefit to bone mineral density with the use of low dose OCPs (Grinspoon *et al.* 2003; Hergenroeder *et al.* 1997; Rickenlund *et al.* 2004). Because of the concern that loss of bone mineral density is caused by a variety of hormonal alterations brought on by a state of energy deficiency, it would seem unlikely that manipulation of only one hormonal parameter would have the optimal effect on bone density, and while prescription of OCPs may be somewhat beneficial, it should not be the only therapeutic intervention undertaken. For optimal results, the energy imbalance faced by the athlete needs to be addressed.

With all of this in mind, our current state of understanding is that it should be emphasized to the athlete with hypothalamic amenorrhea that their body faces a complex constellation of hormonal abnormalities. The complications of their hormonal state include a loss of bone density and potential risk for premature cardiovascular disease. While it is possible that estrogen supplementation may have some beneficial impact on their bone density, it is more important to achieve energy balance, either by increasing caloric intake or decreasing training volume. It is not uncommon that these patients will need continuing support and direction from a variety of health professionals in order to meet these goals.

Conclusions

Many different pathologies have a distinct maladaptation of the endocrine system. Such dysfunction in the cybernetic control of metabolism is but one of the vectors for the pathologies discussed in this chapter. Proper diagnosis, prevention, treatment, and management of the disease are vital for the athlete.

References

American Diabetes Association (ADA). (2001) Diabetes mellitus and exercise. *Diabetes Care* **24**, S51–S55.

Albright, A.L. (1997) Diabetes. In: *American College of Sports Medicine's Exercise Management for Person's with Chronic Disease and Disabilities* (Durstine, J.L., ed.) Human Kinetics, Champaign, IL: 94–100.

Anderson, T.J., Uehata, A., Gerhard, M.D., Meredith, I.T., Knab, S., Delagrange, D., *et al.* (1995) Close relation of endothelial function in the human coronary and peripheral circulations. *Journal of the American College of Cardiology* **26**, 1235–1241.

Barbesino, G. & Chiovato, L. (2000) The genetics of Hashimoto's disease. *Endocrinology and Metabolism Clinics of North America* **29**, 357–374.

Bartalena, L., Marcocci, C. & Pinchera, A. (1997) Treating severe Graves' ophthalmopathy. *Bailliere's Clinical Endocrinology and Metabolism* **11**, 521–536.

Biondi, B. & Klein, I. (2004) Hypothyroidism as a risk factor for cardiovascular disease. *Endocrine* **24**, 1–13.

Biondi, B., Palmieri, E.A., Lombardi, G. & Fazio, S. (2002) Effects of subclinical thyroid dysfunction on the heart. *Annals of Internal Medicine* **137**, 904–914.

Boule, N.G., Haddad, E., Kenny, G.P., Wells, G.A. & Sigal, R.J. (2001) Effects of exercise on glycemic control and body mass in type 2 diabetes mellitus: a meta-analysis of controlled clinical trials. *JAMA* **286**, 1218–1227.

Bronson, F.H. & Manning, J.M. (1991) The energetic regulation of ovulation: a realistic role for body fat. *Biology of Reproduction* **44**, 945–950.

Bullen, B.A., Skrinar, G.S., Beitins, I.Z., von Mering, G., Turnbull, B.A. & McArthur, J.W. (1985) Induction of menstrual disorders by strenuous exercise in untrained women. *New England Journal of Medicine* **312**, 1349–1353.

Bulun, S.E., & Adashi, E.Y. (2003) The physiology and pathology of the female reproductive axis. In: *Williams Textbook of Endocrinology* (Larsen, P.R., Kronenberg, H.M., Melmedm S. & Polonsky, K.S., eds.) W. B. Saunders, Philadelphia, PA.

Burghen, G.A., Givens, J.R. & Kitabchi, A.E. (1980) Correlation of hyperandrogenism with hyperinsulinism in polycystic ovarian disease. *Journal of Clinical Endocrinology and Metabolism* **50**, 113–116.

Cakir, M., Samanci, N., Balci, N. & Balci, M.K. (2003) Musculoskeletal manifestations in patients with thyroid disease. *Clinical Endocrinology (Oxford)* **59**, 162–167.

Cann, C.E., Martin, M.C., Genant, H.K. & Jaffe, R.B. (1984) Decreased spinal mineral content in amenorrheic women. *JAMA* **251**, 626–629.

Celermajer, D.S. (1997) Endothelial dysfunction: does it matter? Is it reversible? *Journal of the American College of Cardiology* **30**, 325–333.

Celermajer, D.S., Sorensen, K.E., Gooch, V.M., Spiegelhalter, D.J., Miller, O.I., Sullivan, I.D., *et al.* (1992) Non-invasive detection of endothelial dysfunction in children and adults at risk of atherosclerosis. *Lancet* **340**, 1111–1115.

Chatterton, R.T. (1990) The role of stress in female reproduction: animal and human considerations. *International Journal of Fertility* **35**, 8–13.

Chen, Q-Y., Nadell, D., Zhang, X-Y., Kukreja, A., Huang, Y-J., Wise, J., *et al.* (2000) The human leukocyte antigen HLA DRB3*0202/DQA1*0501 haplotype is associated with Graves' disease in African Americans. *Journal of Clinical Endocrinology and Metabolism* **85**, 1545–1549.

Cikim, A.S., Oflaz, H., Ozbey, N., Cikim, K., Umman, S., Meric, M., *et al.* (2004) Evaluation of endothelial function in subclinical hypothyroidism and subclinical hyperthyroidism. *Thyroid* **14**, 605–609.

Cobb, K.L., Bachrach, L.K., Greendale, G., Marcus, R., Neer, R.M., Nieves, J., *et al.* (2003) Disordered eating, menstrual irregularity, and bone mineral density in female runners. *Medicine and Science in Sports and Exercise* **35**, 711–719.

Colberg, S.R. & Swain, D.P. (2000) Exercise and diabetes control: a winning combination. *Physician and Sportsmedicine* **28**, 63–81.

Cooper, D.S. (2001) Subclinical hypothyroidism. *New England Journal of Medicine* **345**, 260–265.

Cooper, D.S., Halpern, R., Wood, L.C., Levin, A.A. & Ridgway, E.C. (1984) L-thyroxine therapy in subclinical hypothyroidism: a double-blind, placebo-controlled trial. *Annals of Internal Medicine* **101**, 18–24.

Costagliola, S., Morgenthaler, N.G., Hoermann, R., Badenhoop, K., Struck, J., Freitag, D., *et al.* (1999) Second generation assay for thyrotropin receptor antibodies has superior diagnostic sensitivity for Graves' disease. *Journal of Clinical Endocrinology and Metabolism* **84**, 90–97.

Dagre, A.G., Lekakis, J.P., Papaioannou, T.G., Papamichael, C.M., Koutras, D.A., Stamatelopoulos, S.F., *et al.* (2005) Arterial stiffness is increased in subjects with hypothyroidism. *International Journal of Cardiology* **103**, 1–6.

Danese, M.D., Powe, N.R., Sawin, C.T. & Ladenson, P.W. (1996) Screening for mild thyroid failure at the periodic health examination: a decision and cost-effectiveness analysis. *JAMA* **276**, 285–292.

De Souza, M.J. (2003) Menstrual disturbances in athletes: a focus on luteal phase defects. *Medicine and Science in Sports and Exercise* **35**, 1553–1563.

De Souza, M.J., Miller, B.E., Loucks, A.B., Luciano, A.A., Pescatello, L.S., Campbell, C.G., *et al.* (1998) High frequency of luteal phase deficiency and anovulation in recreational women runners: blunted elevation in follicle-stimulating hormone observed during luteal-follicular transition. *Journal of Clinical Endocrinology and Metabolism* **83**, 4220–4232.

Di Carlo, C., Palomba, S., De Fazio, M., Gianturco, M., Armellino, M. & Nappi, C. (1999) Hypogonadotropic hypogonadism in obese women after biliopancreatic diversion. *Fertility and Sterility* **72**, 905–909.

Drinkwater, B.L., Nilson, K., Chesnut, C.H., Bremner, W.J., Shainholtz, S. & Southworth, M.B. (1984) Bone mineral content of amenorrheic and eumenorrheic athletes. *New England Journal of Medicine* **311**, 277–281.

Drinkwater, B.L., Nilson, K., Ott, S. & Chesnut, C.H. 3rd. (1986) Bone mineral density after resumption of menses in amenorrheic athletes. *JAMA* **256**, 380–382.

Duyff, R.F., Van den Bosch, J., Laman, D.M., van Loon, B-JP. & Linssen, W.H.J.P. (2000) Neuromuscular findings in thyroid dysfunction: a prospective clinical and electrodiagnostic study. *Journal of Neurology, Neurosurgery and Psychiatry* **68**, 750–755.

Eriksson, J., Taimela, S., Eriksson, K., Parviainen, S., Peltonen, J. & Kujala, U. (1997) Resistance training in the treatment of non-insulin-dependent diabetes mellitus. *International Journal of Sports Medicine* **18**, 242–246.

Ertl, A.C. & Davis, S.N. (2004) Evidence for a vicious cycle of exercise and hypoglycemia in type 1 diabetes mellitus. *Diabetes Metabolism Research and Reviews* **20**, 124–130.

Expert Committee on the Diagnosis and Classification of Diabetes Mellitus (1997) Report of the Expert Committee on the Diagnosis and Classification of Diabetes Mellitus. *Diabetes Care* **20**, 1183–1197.

Faber, J. & Galloe, A.M. (1994) Changes in bone mass during prolonged subclinical hyperthyroidism due to L-thyroxine treatment: a meta-analysis. *European Journal of Endocrinology* **130**, 350–356.

Frisch, R.E. & Revelle, R. (1971) Height and weight at menarche and a hypothesis of menarche. *Archives of Disease in Childhood* **46**, 695–701.

Galassetti, P., Tate, D.B., Neill, R.A., Richardson, A., Leu, S.Y. & Davis, S.N. (2006) Effect of differing antecedent hypoglycemia on counterregulatory responses to exercise in type 1 diabetes. *American Journal of Physiology. Endocrinology and Metabolism* **290**, E1109–E1117.

Goodpaster, B.H. & Kelley, D.E. (2001) Exercise and diabetes. In: *Exercise and Sports Cardiology* (Thompson, P.D., ed.) McGraw-Hill, New York: 430–451.

Gough, S.C. (2000) The genetics of Graves' disease. *Endocrinology and Metabolism Clinics of North America* **29**, 255–266.

Grimm, J.J., Ybarra, J., Berne, C., Muchnick, S. & Golay, A. (2004) A new table for prevention of hypoglycaemia during physical activity in type 1 diabetic patients. *Diabetes and Metabolism* **30**, 465–470.

Grinspoon, S.K., Friedman, A.J., Miller, K.K., Lippman, J., Olson, W.H. & Warren, M.P. (2003) Effects of a triphasic combination oral contraceptive containing norgestimate/ethinyl estradiol on biochemical markers of bone metabolism in young women with osteopenia secondary to hypothalamic amenorrhea. *Journal of Clinical Endocrinology and Metabolism* **88**, 3651–3656.

Hashizume, K., Ichikawa, K., Sakurai, A., Suzuki, S., Takeda, T., Kobayashi, M., *et al.* (1991) Administration of thyroxine in treated Graves' disease: effects on the level of antibodies to thyroid-stimulating hormone receptors and on the risk of recurrence of hyperthyroidism. *New England Journal of Medicine* **324**, 947–953.

Hergenroeder, A.C., Smith, E.O., Shypailo, R., Jones, L.A., Klish, W.J. & Ellis, K. (1997) Bone mineral changes in young women with hypothalamic amenorrhea treated with oral contraceptives, medroxyprogesterone, or placebo over 12 months. *American Journal of Obstetrics and Gynecology* **176**, 1017–1025.

Hilton, L.K. & Loucks, A.B. (2000) Low energy availability, not exercise stress, suppresses the diurnal rhythm of leptin in healthy young women. *American Journal of Physiology. Endocrinology and Metabolism* **278**, E43–49.

Hoch, A.Z., Dempsey, R.L., Carrera, G.F., Wilson, C.R., Chen, E.H., Barnabei, V.M., *et al.* (2003) Is there an association between athletic amenorrhea and endothelial cell dysfunction? *Medicine and Science in Sports and Exercise* **35**, 377–383.

Hoch, A.Z., Jurva, J., Staton, M., Vetter, C., Young, C. & Gutterman, D.D. (2003) Is endothelial dysfunction that is associated with athletic amenorrhea reversible? *Medicine and Science in Sports and Exercise* **35**, S12.

Kahaly, G., Hellermann, J., Mohr-Kahaly, S. & Treese, N. (1996) Impaired cardiopulmonary exercise capacity in patients with hyperthyroidism. *Chest* **109**, 57–61.

Kahaly, G.J., Nieswandt, J., Wagner, S., Schlegel, J., Mohr-Kahaly, S. & Hommel, G. (1998) Ineffective cardiorespiratory function in hyperthyroidism. *Journal of Clinical Endocrinology and Metabolism* **83**, 4075–4078.

Kahaly, G.J., Wagner, S., Nieswandt, J., Mohr-Kahaly, S. & Ryan, T.J. (1999) Stress echocardiography in hyperthyroidism. *Journal of Clinical*

Endocrinology and Metabolism **84**, 2308–2313.

Kesaniemi, Y.K., Danforth, E., Jensen, M.D., Kopelman, P.G., Lefebvre, P. & Reeder, BA. (2001) Dose–response issues concerning physical activity and health: an evidence-based symposium. *Medicine and Science in Sports and Exercise* **33**, S351–358.

Kisakol, G., Tunc, R. & Kaya, A. (2003) Rhabdomyolysis in a patient with hypothyroidism. *Endocrine Journal* **50**, 221–223.

Klein I, & Ojamaa K. (2001) Thyroid hormone and the cardiovascular system. *New England Journal of Medicine* **344**, 501–509.

Koivisto, V.A. & Felig, P. (1978) Effects of leg exercise on insulin absorption in diabetic patients. *New England Journal of Medicine* **298**, 79–83.

Landt, K.W., Campaigne, B.N., James, F.W. & Sperling, M.A. (1985) Effects of exercise training on insulin sensitivity in adolescents with type I diabetes. *Diabetes Care* **8**, 461–465.

Lobo, R.A., & Carmina, E. (2000) The importance of diagnosing the polycystic ovary syndrome. *Annals of Internal Medicine* **132**, 989–993.

Loucks, A.B. (2005) Influence of energy availability on luteinizing hormone pulsatility and menstrual cyclicity. In: *The Endocrine System in Sports and Exercise: Encyclopaedia of Sports Medicine*, Vol. XI (Kraemer, W.J. & Rogol, A.D., eds.) Blackwell, Malden: 232–249.

Loucks, A.B. & Horvath, S.M. (1985) Athletic amenorrhea: a review. *Medicine and Science in Sports and Exercise* **17**, 56–72.

Loucks, A.B., Verdun, M. & Heath, E.M. (1998) Low energy availability, not stress of exercise, alters LH pulsatility in exercising women. *Journal of Applied Physiology* **84**, 37–46.

MacLean, P.S., Zheng, D. & Dohm, G.L. (2000) Muscle glucose transporter (GLUT-4) gene expression during exercise. *Exercise and Sport Sciences Reviews* **28**, 148–152.

Manning, J.M. & Bronson, F.H. (1989) Effects of prolonged exercise on puberty and luteinizing hormone secretion in female rats. *American Journal of Physiology. Regulatory, Integrative and Comparative Physiology* **257**, R1359–1364.

Manning, J.M. & Bronson, F.H. (1991) Suppression of puberty in rats by exercise: effects on hormone levels and reversal with GnRH infusion. *American Journal of Physiology* **260**, R717–723.

Martin, W.H., Spina, R.J., Korte, E., Yarasheski, K.E., Angelopoulos, T.J., Nemeth, P.M., *et al.* (1991) Mechanisms of impaired exercise capacity in short duration experimental hyperthyroidism. *Journal of Clinical Investigation* **88**, 2047–2053.

McAllister, R.M., Delp, M.D. & Laughlinm M.H. (1995) Thyroid status and exercise tolerance: cardiovascular and metabolic considerations. *Sports Medicine* **20**, 189–198.

McCulloch, D.K. (2001) Effects of exercise in diabetes mellitus. UpToDate Online 9.3, Available: http://www.uptodate.com.

McIver, B. & Morris, J.C. (1998) The pathogenesis of Graves' disease. *Endocrinology and Metabolism Clinics of North America* **27**, 73–89.

Mellman, M.F. & Podesta, L. (1997) Common medical problems in sports. *Clinics in Sports Medicine* **16**, 635–662.

Metcalf-McCambridge, T. & Colby, R. (2000) Exercising with type 1 diabetes: guidelines for safe and healthy activity. *Your Patient and Fitness* **14**, 22–27.

Moy, C.S., Songer, T.J., LaPorte, R.E., Dorman, J.S., Kriska, A.M., Orchard, T.J., *et al.* (1993) Insulin-dependent diabetes mellitus, physical activity, and death. *American Journal of Epidemiology* **137**, 74–81.

Otis, C.L., Drinkwater, B., Johnson, M., Loucks, A. & Wilmore, J. (1997) American College of Sports Medicine position stand. The Female Athlete Triad. *Medicine and Science in Sports and Exercise* **29**, I–ix.

Palumbo, C.F., Szabo, R.M. & Olmsted, S.L. (2000) The effects of hypothyroidism and thyroid replacement on the development of carpal tunnel syndrome. *Journal of Hand Surgery* **25**, 734–739.

Papaioannou, G.I., Lagasse, M., Mather, J.F. & Thompson, P.D. (2004) Treating hypothyroidism improves endothelial function. *Metabolism* **53**, 278–279.

Peirce, N.S. (1999) Diabetes and exercise. *British Journal of Sports Medicine* **33**, 161–172.

Perry, T.L., Mann, J.I., Lewis-Barned, N.J., Duncan, A.W., Waldron, M.A. & Thompson, C. (1997) Lifestyle intervention in people with insulin-dependent diabetes mellitus (IDDM). *European Journal of Clinical Nutrition* **51**, 757–763.

Ramalho, A.C., de Lourdes Lima, M., Nunes, F., Cambui, Z., Barbosa, C., Andrade, A., *et al.* (2006) The effect of

resistance versus aerobic training on metabolic control in patients with type-1 diabetes mellitus. *Diabetes Research and Clinical Practice* **72**, 271–276.

Reindollar, R.H., Tho, S.P.T. & McDonough, P.G. (1989) Delayed puberty: an updated study of 326 patients. *Transactions of the American Gynecological and Obstetrical Society* **8**, 146–162.

Rickenlund, A., Carlstrom, K., Ekblom, B., Brismar, T.B., von Schoultz, B. & Hirschberg, A.L. (2004) Effects of oral contraceptives on body composition and physical performance in female athletes. *Journal of Clinical Endocrinology and Metabolism* **89**, 4364–4370.

Rickenlund, A., Eriksson, M.J., Schenck-Gustafsson, K. & Hirschberg, A.L. (2005) Amenorrhea in female athletes is associated with endothelial dysfunction and unfavorable lipid profile. *Journal of Clinical Endocrinology and Metabolism* **90**, 1354–1359.

Rickenlund, A., Eriksson, M.J., Schenck-Gustafsson, K. & Hirschberg, A.L. (2005) Oral contraceptives improve endothelial function in amenorrheic athletes. *Journal of Clinical Endocrinology and Metabolism* **90**, 3162–3167.

Roquer, J. & Cano, J.F. (1993) Carpal tunnel syndrome and hyperthyroidism: a prospective study. *Acta Neurologica Scandinavica* **88**, 149–152.

Sawin, C.T., Geller, A., Wolf, P.A., Belanger, A.J., Baker, E., Bacharach, P., *et al.* (1994) Low serum thyrotropin concentrations as a risk factor for atrial fibrillation in older persons. *New England Journal of Medicine* **331**, 1249–1252.

Sestoft, L. & Saltin, B. (1985) Working capacity and mitochondrial enzyme activities in muscle of hyperthyroid patients before and after 3 months of treatment. *Biochemical Society Transactions* **13**, 733–734.

Shrier, D.K. & Burman, K.D. (2002) Subclinical hyperthyroidism: controversies in management. *American Family Physician* **65**, 431–438.

Singer, P.A., Cooper, D.S., Levy, E.G., Ladenson, P.W., Braverman, L.E., Daniels, G., *et al.* (1995) Treatment guidelines for patients with hyperthyroidism and hypothyroidism. Standards of Care Committee, American Thyroid Association. *JAMA* **273**, 808–812.

Sonnenberg, G.E., Kemmer, F.W. & Berger, M. (1990) Exercise in type 1 (insulin-dependent) diabetic patients treated with continuous subcutaneous insulin infusion: prevention of exercise induced hypoglycaemia. *Diabetologia* **33**, 696–703.

Stein, I. & Leventhal, M. (1935) Amenorrhea associated with bilateral polycystic ovaries. *American Journal of Obstetrics and Gynecology* **29**, 181.

Stenchever, M.A., Droegemuller, W., Herbst, A.L. & Mishell, D.R. (2001) *Comprehensive Gynecology*. Mosby, St. Louis.

Thompson, P.D. (1996) The cardiovascular complications of vigorous physical activity. *Archives of Internal Medicine* **156**, 2297–2302.

Thompson, P.D., Yurgalevitch, S.M., Flynn, M.M., Zmuda, J.M., Spannaus-Martin, D., Saritelli, A., *et al.* (1997) Effect of prolonged exercise training without weight loss on high-density lipoprotein metabolism in overweight men. *Metabolism* **46**, 217–223.

Tunbridge, W.M., Evered, D.C., Hall, R., Appleton, D., Brewis, M., Clark, F., *et al.* (1977) The spectrum of thyroid disease in a community: the Whickham survey. *Clinical Endocrinology* **7**, 481–493.

UK Prospective Diabetes Study (UKPDS) Group. (1998) Effect of intensive blood-glucose control with metformin on complications in overweight patients with type 2 diabetes (UKPDS 34). *Lancet* **352**, 854–865.

Vestergaard, P. & Mosekilde, L. (2003) Hyperthyroidism, bone mineral, and fracture risk: a meta-analysis. *Thyroid* **13**, 585–593.

Warren, M.P. (1980) The effects of exercise on pubertal progression and reproductive function in girls. *Journal of Clinical Endocrinology and Metabolism* **51**, 1150–1157.

Warren, M.P. & Perlroth, N.E. (2001) The effects of intense exercise on the female reproductive system. *Journal of Endocrinology* **170**, 3–11.

Wasserman, D.H. & Zinman, B. (1994) Exercise in individuals with IDDM. *Diabetes Care* **17**, 924–937.

Wei, M., Gibbons, L.W., Kampert, J.B., Nichaman, M.Z. & Blair, S.N. (2000) Low cardiorespiratory fitness and physical inactivity as predictors of mortality in men with type 2 diabetes. *Annals of Internal Medicine* **132**, 605–611.

White, R.D. & Sherman, C. (1999) Exercise in diabetes management: maximizing benefits, controlling risks. *Physician and Sportmedicine* **27**, 63–76.

Williams, N.I., Caston-Balderrama, A.L., Helmreich, D.L., Parfitt, D.B., Nosbisch, C. & Cameron, J.L. (2001a) Longitudinal changes in reproductive hormones and menstrual cyclicity in cynomolgus monkeys during strenuous exercise training: abrupt transition to exercise-induced amenorrhea. *Endocrinology* **142**, 2381–2389.

Williams, N.I., Helmreich, D.L., Parfitt, D.B., Caston-Balderrama, A. & Cameron, J.L. (2001b) Evidence for a causal role of low energy availability in the induction of menstrual cycle disturbances during strenuous exercise training. *Journal of Clinical Endocrinology and Metabolism* **86**, 5184–5193.

Yeager, K.K., Agostini, R., Nattiv, A. & Drinkwater, B. (1993) The female athlete triad: disordered eating, amenorrhea, osteoporosis. *Medicine and Science in Sports and Exercise* **25**, 775–777.

Zanker, C.L. & Cooke, C.B. (2004) Energy balance, bone turnover, and skeletal health in physically active individuals. *Medicine and Science in Sports and Exercise* **36**, 1372–1381.

Zinker, B.A. (1999) Nutrition and exercise in individuals with diabetes. *Clinics in Sports Medicine* **18**, 585–606, vii–viii.

Zulewski, H., Muller, B., Exer, P., Miserez, A.R. & Staub, J.J. (1997) Estimation of tissue hypothyroidism by a new clinical score: evaluation of patients with various grades of hypothyroidism and controls. *Journal of Clinical Endocrinology and Metabolism* **82**, 771–776.

Chapter 9

Dermatology

BRIAN B. ADAMS

Skin disorders are the most common ailments of athletes so all sports clinicians should possess a working knowledge of the optimal approach to skin disease. This chapter reviews the diagnosis and management of common dermatoses of the athlete and skin disorders that are specific to participation in sporting activities. While athletes exhibit the common dermatoses present in non-athletic individuals, sports enthusiasts risk other diseases as a result of their intense activity. For instance, the extensive skin-to-skin contact with other competitors experienced by some athletes places the exposed individual at risk to develop myriad cutaneous infections.

Specifically, this chapter examines four main aspects of sports dermatology. First, the diagnosis and management of common cutaneous disorders such as acne and psoriasis are discussed. Second, the chapter discusses the role of exercise in the transmission of skin infections and offers practical care guidelines for these disorders. Third, this chapter reviews an evidence-based approach to therapy and prevention of sun damage and, finally, evaluates the diagnosis and management of exercise-related skin allergies. This chapter strives to present the most up-to-date information regarding sports medicine as it relates to the skin.

The Olympic Textbook of Medicine in Sport, 1st edition. Edited by M. Schwellnus. Published 2008 by Blackwell Publishing, ISBN: 978-1-4051-5637-0.

Diagnosis and management of common disorders in the athlete

Acne vulgaris

Acne vulgaris affects both adolescents and adults. The typical lesions involve the face, neck, back, and chest. Acne is classified by grades: grade 1, comedones; grade 2, erythematous (red) papules; grade 3, pustules; grade 4, erythematous nodules. A variant of acne, termed acne mechanica, occurs in athletes who may or may not have predilection for acne vulgaris. Acne mechanica preferentially occurs beneath protective (often heavy) equipment (Fig. 9.1).

Therapy depends on the specific grade. All forms of acne vulgaris require topical retinoids and specific types relate to the sensitivity of the athlete's skin. Adapalene cream is best suited for athletes with dry skin, especially in the winter. Oily skin can tolerate tazarotene gel and neutral skin tretinoin cream. Athletes should apply these creams very sparingly (a pea-sized dose for the face) at bedtime; physicians should warn about initial redness, scaling, and burning. Unavoidable facial stinging may also occur in athletes while sweating; this side effect most often occurs in individuals with sensitive skin.

Athletes with only a few erythematous papules and pustules may try topical antibiotics (clindamycin and erythromycin) with or without benzoyl peroxide (varying strengths). Combination products with both of these medications exist and increase compliance. Athletes with nodules or many erythematous papules or pustules require chronic oral

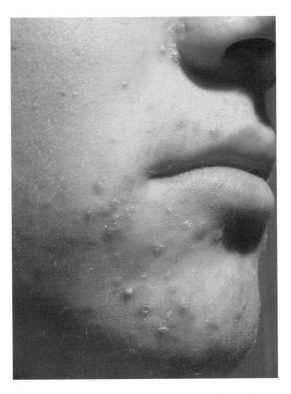

Fig. 9.1 Numerous erythematous papules and pustules with comedones can be seen beneath protective equipment in acne mechanica.

antibiotics (minocycline, doxycycline, tetracycline). Clinicians should warn outdoor athletes that these antibiotics will result in sun sensitivity and the athletes should vigilantly, as always, wear sunscreen on exposed skin and lips. Instead of oral antibiotics, spirolactone at low doses is particularly useful for adult female athletes. Physicians should carefully weigh the risks and benefits of isotretinoin use in highly competitive athletes; arthralgias and myalgias, occasionally severe, are not uncommon.

Acne rosacea

While rosacea shares the term "acne" with its vulgaris counterpart, the disorders differ in their epidemiology, etiology, clinical presentation, treatment, and prevention. Acne rosacea typically affects older athletes (older than 30 years) and its distribution and lack of comedones help to distinguish it from acne vulgaris. Typical acne rosacea presents as discrete, small to medium sized, erythematous papules and microsized pustules on the malar region, over the nose and forehead. While comedones do not appear, telangiectasias do and confer a significant proportion of the "redness" troublesome to the affected athlete. It is important to note that acne rosacea and seborrheic dermatitis can coexist in the same athlete and occasionally can be challenging to distinguish.

Treatment includes not only pharmacologic intervention but also avoidance of triggers, such as spicy food, alcohol (especially red wine), citrus fruits, and caffeine; not all athletes react to each of these stimuli and a careful systematic approach will allow the athlete to identify their specific trigger. Mild disease (with few papules and pustules) warrants chronic daily topical therapy with metronidazole cream or gel (gel for those athletes with oily skin and cream for those with dry skin) or azelaic acid cream (which is limited by increased incidence of redness and irritation). Athletes with many lesions or disease resistant to topical therapy may require brief (a few months) therapy with oral doxycycline (50 or 100 mg) or minocycline (50 or 100 mg) twice daily. Clinicians should warn outdoor athletes that these antibiotics will result in sun sensitivity and the athletes should vigilantly, as always, wear sunscreen on exposed skin and lips.

Seborrheic dermatitis

Seborrheic dermatitis is a fairly common chronic dermatosis characterized by ill-defined greasy scaling, occasionally erythematous plaques distributed on the nasolabial folds, eyebrows, scalp, central chest, and posterior auricular area. Occasionally, seborrheic dermatitis may be confused with psoriasis vulgaris, especially on the scalp. The distinction may be a bit academic as both are steroid responsive, but seborrheic dermatitis will respond to ketoconazole therapy while psoriasis vulgaris will not. For scalp seborrheic dermatitis, athletes should use either ketoconazole or ciclopirox shampoo three times weekly. Non-scalp lesions respond to twice daily ketoconazole cream (for scaling areas) and hydrocortisone cream 2.5% (for red areas). Athletes may enjoy a therapeutic holiday if the lesions are clear.

Atopic dermatitis

Atopic dermatitis is a chronic, pruritic condition typically presenting first in childhood, although adult onset occurs. Affected athletes may also demonstrate seasonal allergies, asthma, and a family history of similar conditions. Typically, atopic dermatitis displays erythematous, scaling, often excoriated plaques in the antecubital and popliteal fossa, and neck; the trunk may also exhibit similar lesions. Follicular papules may occur in dark-skinned athletes.

Therapy first begins with fastidious, regular skin care and moisturization. Affected athletes should use only mild soaps such as Dove, Cetaphil, and Olay. Areas of the body other than the face, axillae, and groin may not require *any* soap at all during dry and cold seasons or in environments with low humidity. Athletes should take brief and lukewarm showers and should lightly pat dry and immediately liberally apply a moisturizer to all areas in an effort to trap the water soaked into the skin during the shower. The choice of moisturizer is athlete-specific and no one moisturizer is universally recommended although Cetaphil, Olay, and Aquaphor are among the favorites. Bedroom humidifiers also provide significant skin moisturization.

During flares, athletes will require topical medications and oral antihistamines. The mainstay of therapy has been triamcinolone 0.1% ointment for mild to moderate flares on the trunk or extremities. Lower potency topical steroids such as hydrocortisone 2.5% ointment or desonide 0.05% ointment should be used in the intertriginous regions and face. For chronic use the clinician should consider pimecrolimus cream or tacrolimus ointment, which do not possess the ability to thin skin as topical steroids do. For intermittent use, during periods of severe flares on the trunk and extremities, super potent topical steroids such as clobetasol ointment are effective. For severe flares on the face and in intertriginous regions, very brief (1 week or less), judicious use of triamcinolone 0.1% ointment may be used.

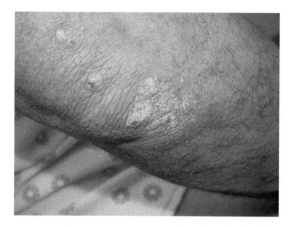

Fig. 9.2 Well-defined, silvery, scaling plaques over the extensor surfaces typify psoriasis.

Psoriasis vulgaris

Typical plaque psoriasis affects 2% of the population and presents as erythematous, silvery scaling plaques on the elbows, knees, scalp, trunk, and buttocks (Fig. 9.2). The soles and the palms may also be affected; nails may become brittle and discolored. The type of therapy primarily relates to the body surface area of involvement. Limited disease (less than 10–15% of involved body surface area) necessitates topical therapy with solo or combination use of topical steroids, calcipotriene, and tazarotene. Potent topical steroids such as clobetasol or diprolene must be used carefully and for only brief periods of time (less than 1 month). Chronic use of these potent steroids can cause tachyphylaxis, wherein the athlete's psoriasis no longer responds to the previously effective, high strength steroid. More severe disease, as represented by surface area greater than 15%, requires systemic therapy. These therapies include oral retinoids, phototherapy, cyclosporine, methotrexate, and the more recent so-called biologics. The risks and benefits as they specifically relate to the athlete must be ascertained; referral to a dermatologist with an appreciation of the level of sporting activity is important. Psoriasis vulgaris is a chronic lifelong disease punctuated by periodic flares; debilitating arthritis can rarely occur.

Actinic keratosis

Outdoor athletes experience an inordinate amount of ultraviolet exposure as they practice and compete during the peak hours of ultraviolet intensity (10AM to 4PM). Furthermore, studies have demonstrated that sweat actually enhances sunburns. Excessive and chronic exposure to ultraviolet irradiation leads to premature aging of the skin (discoloration, wrinkling) and skin cancer.

Skin cancer is the most common cancer and the three main types are basal cell carcinoma, squamous cell carcinoma, and melanoma. The diagnosis and management of these skin cancers is beyond the scope of this chapter and the remainder of this section focuses on the far more prevalent precancers (actinic keratosis). Most actinic keratoses occur on the extremities (especially the arms and hands) and the face and appear as well-defined, erythematous, rough, scaling papules (Fig. 9.3). Not infrequently, the lesions can be more easily felt than seen. Therapy includes both destructive methods such as liquid nitrogen or topical treatments such as imiquimod or 5-fluorouracil. Athletes apply imiquimod three times weekly for up to 12 weeks or 5-fluorouracil twice daily for 4–6 weeks, depending on the response. Athletes must recognize that the medications create extensive erythema, crusting, stinging, and burning.

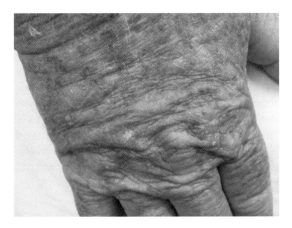

Fig. 9.3 Numerous red, relatively ill-defined, thick scaling papules characterize actinic keratosis; these lesions can be felt often better than they can be seen.

Exercise in the transmission of skin infections (practical clinical guidelines)

Several characteristics of athletes increase the likelihood of developing cutaneous infections. Most micro-organisms enjoy optimal growth in warm, moist, and dark environments. Sweating hyperhydrates the epidermis and occlusive clothing and protective wear further macerates and warms the skin. In addition to offering the optimal microenvironment for infectious agents, athletes' skin is ripe for cutaneous infection because it facilitates the entry of the micro-organism. First, the supersaturation of the epidermis not only provides a hospitable microenvironment, but also allows easier passage for the infectious agent through the epidermis. Second, abrasions and cuts, inherent to all sports, facilitate entrance of the micro-organisms through the epidermis. Finally, many athletes experience close skin-to-skin contact which permits intercompetitor transmission.

Viral infections

HERPES LABIALIS

All outdoor athletes experiencing prolonged exposure to ultraviolet radiation risk reactivating prior herpes simplex virus (HSV) infection (Mills *et al.* 1987). Winter athletes seem particularly prone as ultraviolet irradiation exposure is increased because of snow reflectance and the fact that at high altitudes the atmosphere absorbs less ultraviolet irradiation. A similar level of ultraviolet B radiation is experienced by a winter athlete at 11,000 feet on a snow-covered mountain in Colorado as an aquatic athlete at the beach at Orlando, Florida.

Oral lesions first begin with a tingling sensation without noticeable skin changes. After 1–4 days, a painful, well-defined, erythematous, papulovesicle develops on the lip or perioral area. Treatment includes valacyclovir, two 1-g tablets taken in the morning and two 1-g tablets taken in the evening for just 1 day. Athletes who chronically develop herpes labialis (more than six lesions per year) should take suppressive therapy of valacyclovir 1 g·day^{-1} for 1 year. The incidence of herpes labialis should be reassessed after 1 year and if the frequency remains above six times per year, the athlete should again take daily valacyclovir for 1 year. Sunscreen, applied regularly to the lips, also should protect against herpes labialis reactivation.

HERPES SIMPLEX IN CONTACT SPORTS (HERPES GLADIATORUM – WRESTLING)

All athletes (although rugby players and wrestlers are almost exclusively reported) with close and intense skin-to-skin contact risk acquiring HSV infection. Multiple epidemics in wrestling teams have occurred and the median prevalence of HSV reported in the literature is 20%. HSV-1, which may survive in spas at temperatures above 100°F for 4.5 min, causes this skin infection although typing is not routinely performed (Nerurkar *et al.* 1983).

Before experiencing the skin lesions associated with HSV, the athlete will notice stinging, burning, or pruritus in the area (the prodrome). HSV lesions, in their mature form, demonstrate well-defined, grouped vesicles upon an erythematous base; late lesions become crusted and the grouped nature of the lesion may be obscured (Fig. 9.4). These lesions occur predominately on the head and neck. Systemic signs and symptoms are not uncommon and include fever, sore throat, malaise, myalgias, arthralgias, and swollen lymph glands (Adams 2001b).

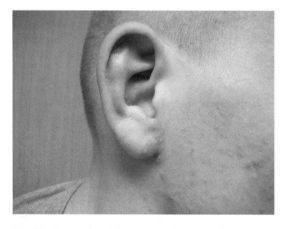

Fig. 9.4 Grouped vesicles on an erythematous base are typical of herpes gladiatorum.

Table 9.1 Dosage regimens for treatment of contact sport-related herpes simplex virus (HSV).

Medication	Dose (mg)	Frequency	Duration
Acyclovir	200	5 times daily	5 days
Famciclovir	500	b.i.d.	5 days
Valacyclovir	2000	b.i.d.	1 day

The constellation of findings, including a prodrome history, suspicious lesions, and associated systemic findings indicates the diagnosis but Tzanck smear, culture, or direct immunoflourescence confirms HSV. Very early lesions are non-specific and can be easily confused with acne vulgaris, atopic dermatitis, molluscum contagiosum, tinea corporis gladiatorum, and impetigo. Complications of contact sport-related HSV include herpes conjunctivitis, blepharitis, and keratitis (Selling & Kibrick 1964), monoarticular arthritis (Shelley 1980), and HSV-related meningitis (White & Grant-Kels 1984).

Therapy for HSV includes oral acyclovir, famciclovir, and valacyclovir (Table 9.1). Athletes with skin-to-skin contact may return to competition and practice 96 h after starting oral therapy as long as all lesions are dried, the athlete has had no new blisters for 3 days, and has no systemic symptoms. Unfortunately, the transmission of HSV among athletes is enhanced by the fact that infected athletes are often contagious before the development of obvious lesions; a 33% probability of HSV transmission in the setting of infected wrestlers has been documented. The distribution of lesions casts doubt on any role the mats have in transmission of HSV, so efforts should rather be directed toward educating coaches, trainers, and athletes to perform daily skin checks to detect lesions as early as possible. Athletes should also avoid sharing equipment and towels. Susceptible athletes or athletes with a history of contact sport-related HSV should take 1 g·day^{-1} oral valacyclovir during the season (Anderson 1999).

MOLLUSCUM

Molluscum contagiosum, caused by a virus, has occurred in multiple contact (rugby players and wrestlers) and non-contact sports (volleyball players,

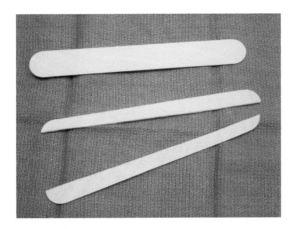

Fig. 9.5 A tongue depressor split longitudinally makes an ideal molluscum scraper.

swimmers, and gymnasts; Cyr 2004). Tight-fitting occlusive shorts facilitate autoinoculation once there is a solitary molluscum. Asymptomatic, small (few millimeters), well-defined, white or skin colored, umbilicated (has a central dell) papules occur over areas of skin-to-skin or skin-to-equipment contact. The differential diagnosis includes acne vulgaris, folliculitis, infected eczema, and verrucae.

Lesions can resolve spontaneously; however, curettage (with a commercially available curette or the end of a tongue depressor broken longitudinally) quickly removes the lesions (Fig. 9.5). Liquid nitrogen for 5 s repeated twice works but can be painful and does not remove the molluscum as rapidly and dramatically as curettage. Clinicians can also apply trichloroacetic acid or cantharidin to the lesion to cause a blister. Other effective athlete applied agents include topical imiquimod, tretinoin, and tazarotene. To prevent team epidemics, athletes should routinely and immediately shower after practice and competition and they should not share equipment. Athletes who are treated and bandaged early will not transmit molluscum to other athletes.

WARTS (VERRUCAE)

Warts appear in any athlete but contact sports with intense skin-to-skin contact transmit the human papillomavirus that causes warts (Adams 2002b); swimming pool decks, weightlifting, rowing, and gymnastic equipment, and locker room and shower floors have also transmitted warts. There are several types of warts that may affect athletes. Periungual warts occur around nails; plantar warts develop on the soles, while verruca plana (flat warts) can appear on many parts of the body. Warts present as well-defined, rough surfaced, papules or plaques and attain large sizes; lesions on the foot grow inward potentially creating intense discomfort for the athlete. Clinicians should pare suspected plantar warts with a #15 blade, not only to facilitate destructive therapies, but also to insure that the lesion is not a callus (skin markings remain intact) or a corn (has a central core upon paring). A wart displays black pinpoint spots upon paring. Verruca plana can be confused with non-pigmented seborrheic keratoses.

Destruction with liquid nitrogen, laser, or curettage may lead to residual pain; if the lesion is large several therapies are necessary. Chemical methods also work and include the application of salicylic acid, cantharidin, and trichloroacetic acid. After paring and soaking, the athlete may apply topical imiquimod under an adhesive bandage such as plastic wrap or duct tape. This method may be less painful and disrupt the athlete's training regimen the least. Oral cimetidine (30–400 mg·kg^{-1}·day^{-1}) can also be employed although the evidence to support its use is controversial. Recalcitrant warts should be referred to a dermatology expert for further advanced therapies. To prevent transmission or contraction of warts, athletes should avoid sharing equipment and should routinely wear sandals in the locker room and showers.

Fungal infections

TINEA PEDIS

Swimmers, runners, and soccer, water polo, and basketball players develop tinea pedis 2–4 times more commonly than non-athletes (Caputo *et al.* 2001; Mailler & Adams 2004). Species of *Trichophyton*, *Epidermophyton*, and *Microsporum* (types of dermatophytes) cause most types of tinea pedis, although *Candida* is occasionally pathogenic. The classic type of tinea pedis, moccasin type, demonstrates fairly

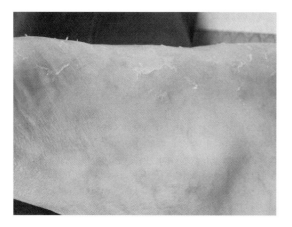

Fig. 9.6 Moccasin type tinea pedis displays scaling plaques on the sole and lateral aspect of the foot.

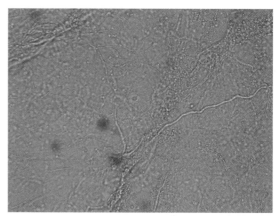

Fig. 9.8 Branching, long, slender hyphae crossing cell borders of keratinocytes characterize a positive potassium hydroxide (KOH) preparation.

ill-defined scaling, minimally to moderately erythematous plaques on the lateral aspects of the soles (Fig. 9.6). The interdigital variety demonstrates macerated, scaling plaques in the web spaces; superinfection with bacteria is not unusual in this type (Fig. 9.7). *Trichophyton rubrum* causes both of these tinea variants. The last type of tinea pedis termed vesicular or inflammatory presents as very pruritic, well-defined, moderately erythematous, scaling papules, plaques, and vesicles in the instep of the sole; *Trichophyton mentagrophytes* induces this tinea pedis. Asymptomatic teammates or competitors may unwittingly transmit these dermatophytes.

The differential diagnosis includes subacute dermatitis, psoriasis, and pitted keratolysis. To confirm the diagnosis, the clinician scrapes scale from the foot onto a glass slide for microscopic evaluation. Another glass slide or a scalpel blade makes an ideal scraper. Under the microscope at low power magnification, long branching hyphae will be seen traversing the cell borders (Fig. 9.8). Cultures confirm the diagnosis and permit species identification; bacterial cultures alert the clinician to superinfection. A Wood's lamp examination yielding a greenish color indicates *Pseudomonas* superinfection.

To clear tinea pedis, topical therapy twice daily for several weeks is necessary. Fungicidal (allylamines) creams such as ciclopirox are effective and also possess antibacterial properties. It appears that the fungistatic azoles are much slower in the onset of action although both topical fungicidal and fungistatic agents have similar cure rates (Millikan *et al.* 1988). Topical aluminum chloride 30% dries the skin and creates an inhospitable microenvironment for dermatophytes (Leyden & Kligman 1975).

Oral antifungal therapy with 200 mg itraconazole once daily or 250 mg terbinafine once daily for 2 weeks clears severe tinea pedis. Several medications adversely interact with oral terbinafine or itraconazole and these agents should be used with care; furthermore, clinicians should obtain baseline liver function tests and complete blood counts.

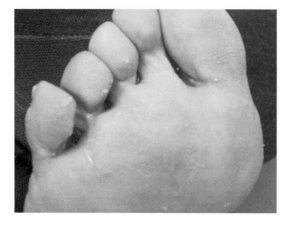

Fig. 9.7 Interdigital tinea pedis demonstrates scaling red plaques in the web spaces.

Concomitant topical therapy is also recommended twice daily.

Occasionally, the scale of tinea becomes hyperkeratotic, preventing the penetration of topical antifungal medications; concomitant application of urea 40% cream enhances therapy. Athletes with blistering lesions may also soak their feet twice daily in a footbath containing warm water and Domeboro crystals or a mixture of vinegar and water. Moderate potency topical corticosteroids, such as triamcinolone 0.1% ointment, combat an athlete's related pruritus. Prevention of tinea pedis is paramount. Athletes can wear synthetic moisture wicking socks that keep sweaty feet dry. Athletes need to wear sandals in the locker room and showers. Particularly susceptible athletes can apply daily ciclopirox.

TINEA CORPORIS GLADIATORUM

Epidemics of tinea corporis have affected up to three-quarters of wrestling teams; however, any athlete with close skin-to-skin contact may develop tinea corporis. *Trichophyton tonsurans* causes most cases of tinea corporis gladiatorum with over 100 reported cases; this dermatophyte may reside asymptomatically in the scalp of carriers who act as reservoirs (Adams 2002a). Lesions demonstrate well-defined, erythematous, scaling, round papules and plaques on the head, neck, and arms; the annular feature of typical ringworm is frequently absent in athletes. The differential diagnosis includes acne vulgaris, atopic dermatitis, early herpes gladiatorum, and early impetigo. The clinician can confirm the diagnosis by scraping scale onto a glass slide for microscopic evaluation. Long branching hyphae will be seen traversing the cell borders. Culture confirms the diagnosis and identifies the organism type.

The only evidence-based recommendation for therapy is once weekly oral fluconazole (200 mg) for 3 weeks which resulted in complete clearance (Kohl *et al.* 1999). Topical clotrimazole twice daily for 3 weeks only cleared 50% of athletes. Other suggested oral therapies that lack evidence-based support include 200 mg·day^{-1} ketoconazole for 2–4 weeks and 200 mg·day^{-1} itraconazole for 1–2 weeks. With oral therapy, clinicians should obtain baseline liver function tests for those athletes on prolonged

daily therapy and should also recall that several medications are contraindicated with oral azole therapy. No studies have examined the newer topical or oral fungicidal agents but athletes should apply topical ciclopirox twice daily. Infected athletes should not compete or practice for 3 days after starting therapy.

Before practicing or competing, infected athletes may, to be conservative, wash with ketoconazole or selenium sulfide shampoo. The athlete then can protect the infected area with gas-permeable dressing such as Op-site or Bioclusive followed by ProWrap and stretch tape. Clinicians should culture competitors' scalps to identify asymptomatic carriers of tinea during epidemics.

Most studies have not cultured any fungus from the wrestling mats and while no study has confirmed that equipment transmits tinea, athletes should avoid sharing equipment. Clinicians, coaches, and athletes need to perform daily skin checks to prevent epidemics. Season long oral prophylaxis with itraconazole (400 mg every other week (Hazen & Weil 1997) or 100 mg fluconazole once weekly (Kohl *et al.* 2000) decreases the incidence of tinea corporis gladiatorum. Clinicians should order liver function tests before starting these medications and at mid-season; review of the athlete's medication list is necessary to avoid adverse cross-reactions.

TINEA VERSICOLOR

Any athlete risks developing tinea versicolor. *Pityrosporum ovale*, the cause of tinea versicolor, flourishes in hot and humid conditions. Tinea versicolor presents as asymptomatic, well-defined, hypo- or hyperpigmented, scaling, discrete, and confluent macules and patches over the upper extremities, neck, and trunk. Occasionally, lesions do not demonstrate scale until they are scraped. Microscopic evaluation of scale from the eruption coupled with a few drops of potassium hydroxide reveals spores and short hyphae (the so-called spaghetti and meatballs). Wood's lamp examination of the affected skin also may reveal a yellow color.

Selenium sulfide 2.5% lotion applied to the affected area and washed off 15 min later clears the eruption. This regimen may be repeated once daily for 1 week. A single dose of two 200-mg tablets keto-conazole also clears tinea versicolor; ketoconazole concentrates in sweat so the athlete should exercise after ingestion to increase efficacy. Repeating this regimen 1 week later further maximize efficacy. Athletes must acknowledge that while the treatment clears the athlete of the dermatophyte's overgrowth, the light or dark areas on the skin may take months to normalize in color. Athletes can prevent tinea versicolor by wearing synthetic moisture wicking clothing and by using selenium sulfide 2.5% once weekly for 10 min before rinsing.

Bacterial infections

IMPETIGO

Multiple sports teams (wrestling, soccer, sea water swimming, rugby and American football) have experienced epidemics of impetigo. Both *Staphylococcus aureus* and *Streptococcus* (including nephrogenic *Streptococcus* [M-type 2]) species can cause impetigo. The clinical presentation depends primarily on the age of the lesion. Very young lesions demonstrate well-defined, erythematous papules and can be confused with acne vulgaris, atopic dermatitis, folliculitis, herpes gladiatorum, and tinea corporis gladiatorum. Mature lesions demonstrate honey-colored, crusted, erythematous plaques with or without obvious pustules; tense, clear, fluid-filled bullae may occur. The lesions occur as a result of skin-to-skin contamination and appear typically on the face and extremities. Lymphadenopathy, pharyngitis, and post-streptococcal glomerulonephritis may also result. Urinalysis and serum complement levels (C3) are indicated if a *Streptococcus* species is cultured; post-streptococcal nephritis may occur up to 3 weeks after skin infection.

The diagnosis of mature lesions is often quite straightforward but in indeterminate lesions and when methicillin-resistant *Staphylococcus aureus* is suspected cultures should be performed. Cultures of the perianal region and nares may identify *Staphylococcus aureus* carriage. Clinicians should consider throat cultures to identify chronic streptococcal carriage. Initial therapy is directed at repairing the perturbed stratum corneum; this therapy includes applying a warm, moist cloth on the lesion for 5–10 min three times daily until the lesion is clear. Athletes should apply mupirocin ointment twice daily and oral antibiotics (500 mg oral dicloxacillin three times daily or 500 mg cephalexin three times daily for 10–14 days). Erythromycin or clindamycin can be substituted in athletes allergic to penicillin. Methicillin-resistant *Staphylococcus aureus* requires trimethoprim-sulfamethoxazole or clindamycin for at least 14 days; depending on culture sensitivities, tetracycline, vancomycin, linezolid, or dactinomycin may be necessary.

Infected athletes who experience skin-to-skin contact with competitors should not compete for 3 days after starting therapy. Athletes may continue to practice if the lesions can be adequately and securely covered. Bleach and water, at least at a temperature of 71°C, is necessary for laundering. Whirlpools need to be regularly drained and cleaned. Athletes should avoid sharing equipment, towels, ointments, and tape. Athletes must shower with antibacterial soap and body shaving should be discouraged in contact sport athletes. Athletes should wear loose fitting, moisture wicking, and synthetic clothing to decrease the exposed skin area. Trainers and other sports clinicians need to conscientiously sanitize their hands between seeing patients.

Athletes who demonstrate positive nasal or crural cultures require topical mupirocin to each nares and the perianal area twice daily for 1 week; to ensure clearance of *S. aureus* carriage, athletes should repeat this procedure every 6 months.

FOLLICULITIS AND FURUNCULOSIS

There have not been any epidemiologic studies of folliculitis but epidemiologic studies have revealed multiple epidemics of furunculosis in fencers, canoeists, swimmers, and American football, rugby, and basketball players (Bartlett *et al.* 1982). *Staphylococcus aureus* causes both folliculitis and furunculosis and the methicillin resistant variant of *Staphylococcus aureus* has produced furunculosis in fencers, American football and rugby players, and weightlifters (Begier *et al.* 2004). Acquiring turf burns, shaving body hair cosmetically, wearing

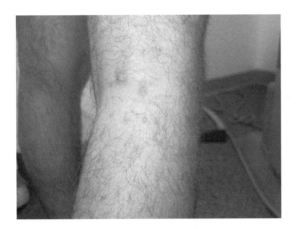

Fig. 9.9 Scattered, red, pustules typify folliculitis.

athletic tape and elbow pads, and not showering before using communal whirlpools increase the risk of transmission of disease.

Folliculitis presents as well-defined, few millimeters, follicular, red papules and pustules scattered on exposed skin in athletes and on areas covered by protective equipment (Fig. 9.9). Furuncles on the other hand tend to be much larger and in their mature stage are erythematous nodules with or without an overlying pustule. The differential diagnosis of *Staphylococcus aureus* folliculitis includes pityrosporum folliculitis, eosinophilic folliculitis, acneiform folliculitis, and hot tub folliculitis. A complete athlete history coupled with cultures and biopsies of the pustules and an evaluation of the response to empiric therapy help differentiate among the various types of folliculitis. Very early furuncles may be confused with acne vulgaris, atopic dermatitis, folliculitis, herpes gladiatorum, and tinea corporis gladiatorum. Repeated infection with either folliculitis or furunculosis should alert the clinician to latent bacterial colonization; cultures of the nares and perianal region will be positive.

All infected athletes first require warm water soaks for 5–10 min three to four times daily. Topical mupirocin, twice daily, for 7–10 days will clear mild disease. Athletes with many lesions or severe lesions require 500 mg oral dicloxacillin three times daily or 500 mg cephalexin three times daily for 10–14 days along with topical antibiotics (erythromycin or clindamycin are alternatives for penicillin-allergic athletes). Methicillin-resistant *Staphylococcus aureus* is sensitive to topical mupirocin but may necessitate oral trimethoprim-sulfamethoxazole or clindamycin for at least 10 days for any disease not amenable to topical treatment alone. During team epidemics, regular use of povidine-iodine liquid soap or 4% chlorhexidine gluconate liquid detergent may be suggested.

Infected athletes who experience skin-to-skin contact with competitors should not compete for 3 days after starting therapy. Athletes may continue to practice if the lesions can be adequately and securely covered. Bleach and water, at least at a temperature of 71°C, is necessary for laundering. Whirlpools need to be regularly drained and cleaned. Athletes should avoid sharing equipment, towels, ointments, and tape. Athletes must shower with antibacterial soap and body shaving should be discouraged in contact sport athletes. Athletes should wear loose fitting, moisture wicking, and synthetic clothing to decrease the exposed skin area. Trainers and other sports clinicians need to sanitize their hands conscientiously between patients.

Athletes who demonstrate positive nasal or crural cultures require topical mupirocin to each nares and the perianal area twice daily for 1 week; to ensure clearance of *S. aureus* carriage, athletes should repeat this procedure every 6 months.

Atypical mycobacterial infections

SWIMMING POOL GRANULOMA

Mycobacterium marinum, an acid-fast atypical mycobacteria, causes swimming pool granuloma in both fresh and sea water. Several epidemics of swimming pool granuloma have occurred and affected athletes include boaters, swimmers, and water polo players (Fisher 1988; Galbraith 1980; Johnston & Izumi 1987). Percutaneous injury from rough pool or sea surfaces allows the organism entry into the dermis. Lesions begin as erythematous papules most commonly on the upper extremities; these lesions progress to verrucous nodules which may ulcerate. Migration along the lymphatics creates multiple linear nodules.

The differential diagnosis includes sporotrichosis, furunculosis, gout, leishmaniasis, sarcoidosis, squamous cell carcinoma, and verruca vulgaris. Correct diagnosis requires biopsy and culture of the lesion. Clinicians should encourage three times daily warm water soaks for 10 min each time. Oral minocycline (100 mg twice daily) or clarithromycin (500 mg twice daily) for at least 6 weeks clears the eruption. Other effective medications include doxycycline, tetracycline, ciprofloxacin, and trimethoprim-sulfamethoxazole; nearly all lesions clear within 2–4 months. Surgical excision has also been suggested (Johnston & Izumi 1987).

Parasitic infections

CUTANEOUS LARVAE MIGRANS

Ancylostoma braziliense, a cutaneous hookworm found in sand, may attach to the lower extremities of athletes who come in contact with the sand (Biolcati & Alabiso 1997). The diagnosis is unmistakable as a brightly erythematous, serpiginous, thin line weaves along the lower extremity. Clinicians should obtain a complete blood count (associated eosinophilia) and a chest radiograph (pulmonary infiltrates can occur). Topical or oral thiabendazole (400 mg twice daily for 5 days) clears the hookworm; oral ivermectin may also work. Athletes should wear protective footwear in infested areas. Officials should ensure any sand area is free from animal feces which may contain the eggs that produce the offending larva.

PEDICULOSIS/SCABIES

Any athlete with close skin-to-skin contact risks development of lice or scabies from other infested athletes. However, wrestling dominates the literature and guideline recommendations.

LICE

The three types of lice include pediculosis corporis (body lice), pediculosis capitis (head lice), and pediculosis pubis (genital lice). Once exposed to any of these parasites, the athlete will develop the condition in up to 14 days and typically will complain of pruritus in the area affected. Direct visualization of the nits or live lice confirms the diagnosis. These lice reside on the hair or on the seams of clothes. Lice-infested athletes require permethrin 5% cream, lindane shampoo, or petrolatum applied to the affected area once daily for 1 week.

SCABIES

The parasite *Sarcoptes scabiei* causes the skin manifestations of scabies. It is critical to note that athletes develop pruritus not limited to the direct area of scabies infestation. Systemic sensitization to the mite, its eggs, and feces occurs and eczematous skin reactions can occur on the trunk, extremities, and the groin. The actual organism (less than 1 mm in size) preferentially locates to the wrists, digital web spaces, and elbows. To confirm the diagnosis, the clinician should gently scrape a #15 surgical blade over linear burrows in these areas (a very small black speck at the end of the burrow represents the tiny parasite). The clinician should first dip the surgical blade in a drop of mineral oil before scraping and then apply to the scrapings to a large drop of mineral oil residing on a glass slide. Direct microscopic examination of the slide will reveal the organism, eggs, and small, brown, oval feces. Scabies-infested athletes require application of permethrin 5% cream applied to every skin surface from the neck down and repeated in 1 week. Oral ivermectin at a dose of 200 $\mu m \cdot kg^{-1}$ with a repeat dose 1–2 weeks later is also an option.

For both lice and scabies infested athletes, athletes' clothes, equipment worn, and bed sheets slept upon within 3–5 days prior to diagnosis should be laundered and dried in a hot cycle. If laundering is not possible, then all clothing and equipment should be placed in an airtight bag for 3–5 days. Upholstered furniture upon which they have sat should be avoided for 3–5 days; intimate contacts need also to be treated.

Athletes with lice or scabies should not participate in sports with skin-to-skin contact. Before the infested athletes returns to practice, they should have been treated and possess no documented organisms.

Prevention and treatment of sun damage

Athletes experience excessive ultraviolet irradiation which acutely can result in painful, debilitating sunburn and sunstroke and chronically, many years later, cause skin cancer such as basal cell carcinoma (Fig. 9.10), squamous cell carcinoma (Fig. 9.11), and melanoma.

Treatment modalities

Neither oral nor topical steroids is effective in the acute management of sunburn based on double-blind, placebo-controlled studies. Evidence does exist that topical non-steroidal agents and oral non-steroidal agents such as aspirin, ibuprofen, and indomethacin taken immediately after sun exposure can decrease the erythema and symptoms associated with ultraviolet irradiation. Studies have noted, however, that this protective effect dissipates after 36 h and erythema related to sun exposure after this time is not affected by the use of non-steroidal agents. One study found no effect with topical aloe vera use on the erythema of sunburned subjects. Emollients may decrease the symptoms related to sunburn but studies investigating this issue are scant. Several studies have also noted a lack of efficacy of antihistamines in the acute management of sunburn. Evidence-based recommendations are scant in the acute management of sunburn but a reasonable approach would include cool water soaks and immediately taking a non-steroidal agent after ultraviolet exposure (Han & Maibach 2004).

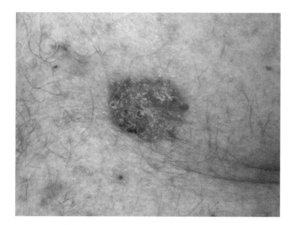

Fig. 9.10 The superficial type of basal cell carcinoma can be confused with psoriasis or dermatitis.

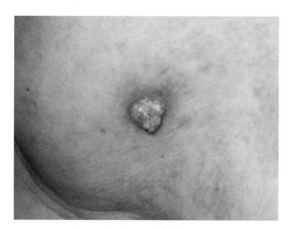

Fig. 9.11 Squamous cell carcinoma typically is a well-defined, thick, scaling nodule, often with erythema.

Preventative techniques

Sunscreen remains the mainstay approach to prevent the untoward side effects of the sun. Unfortunately, recent studies note that most outdoor college athletes do not wear sunscreen during practice and competition (Hamant & Adams 2005). Furthermore, this study documented that over 50% of the reasons for lack of sunscreen use related to lack of availability. As such, having sunscreen readily available at practice sites and competition venues may be a fairly simple method to overcome the main barrier to sunscreen use among athletes.

Athletes should wear a sunscreen with an SPF of 30, broadband (UVA, UVB, UVC) blocking, and be sweatproof and waterproof. Despite the claims of being able to stand up to sweat and water, sunscreen should be reapplied after intense exposure to water or sweat, hourly or at whatever time intervals are allowed with continued athletic performance. The many varied types of vehicles used to dispense sunscreen allow each athlete to tailor their sunscreen use to their unique needs and skin type. In general, athletes prefer sunscreens that are in gel or spray form, although some lotions are quite good (e.g., Blue Lizard and Ocean Potion).

Advanced technologic athletic wear may specifically possess an UPF rating. It is important to note that all colors and knits are not created equally. Dark-colored clothing, dry clothing, and certain types of fabric (nylon, wool, and silk) provide superior ultraviolet irradiation-blocking capabilities. Interestingly, laundering, up to a point, increases the UPF of clothing. Athletes should also wear hats as often as possible in training and, when appropriate, in competition.

Diagnosis and management of exercise-related skin allergies

Irritant contact dermatitis

Unlike allergic contact dermatitis, all athletes are susceptible to irritant contact dermatitis as the only rate-limiting step is the concentration of the irritant. The substances that cause this type of dermatitis exist on the playing "field" and in sporting implements. Specific types of irritant contact dermatitis affect *canoeists and other boaters* whose hands are exposed to rocks and cold water (Descamps & Puechal 2002), or *swimmers* exposed to brominated compound in pools (Rycroft & Penny 1983) or to pulverized seaweed (which produces skin toxins) caught in the bathing suit (Izumi & Moore 1987). *Hockey players* experience fiberglass exposure from their sticks (Levine 1980), *trapshooters* endure friction between their gun and their cheek or neck (Exum & Scott 1992), and *gymnasts* may develop an irritant reaction to chalk (Strauss *et al.* 1988). Finally, male *swimmers* can experience repeated irritation on their shoulder from an unshaven face (Koehn 1991).

Most cases of irritant contact dermatitis have similar clinical presentations. In a distribution related to the athlete's irritant exposure, clearly demarcated, erythematous, occasionally vesicular, mildly scaling plaques develop (Fig. 9.12). In areas of chronic irritant exposure, the skin may acquire lichenification (very thick skin). Athletes develop irritant contact dermatitis rather rapidly after exposure, as its genesis is unrelated to the athlete's immune system. The differential diagnosis mainly consists of subacute to chronic dermatitis of various non-sport-related causes and tinea. Clinicians should

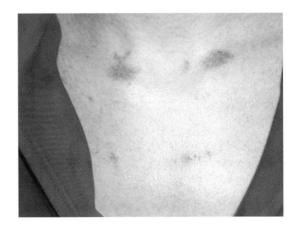

Fig. 9.12 Irritant contact dermatitis displays well-defined, erythematous, scaling, often eroded plaques.

perform a potassium hydroxide examination and patch tests, both of which are negative if the eruption is irritant contact dermatitis. The severe exudates of dermatitis often exhibit yellow-crusted plaques mimicking secondary impetigo; bacterial cultures differentiate the two conditions.

Open wounds should be covered with petroleum jelly and topical antibiotics (e.g., mupirocin or erythromycin ointment) may be necessary. Keeping affected areas moist and covered with bandages decreases pain and healing time. Oral antibiotics are only necessary if the lesions become secondarily infected. Medium potency topical steroids (class II–III) are effective for the pruritic and erythematous components of the eruption. Topical immunomodulators (e.g., pimecrolimus) may be used for mild, facial, or chronic conditions; oral steroids are rarely required. Prevention of irritant contact dermatitis depends primarily on avoiding the primary irritant.

Allergic contact dermatitis

Allergic contact dermatitis is the classic type IV delayed-type hypersensitivity reaction. In a sensitive athlete, exposure to an antigen contained in sports equipment, clothing, topical medications, or objects in the environment of the athletic venue results in allergic contact dermatitis (Table 9.2). Affected athletes will present with pruritic, patterned, very well-defined, erythematous, scaling

Table 9.2 Skin allergens and sport.

Sport	Item	Allergen	Alternative
Equipment			
Swimming	Goggles (Fisher 1987)	Rubber, neoprene	Foamless, air blown neoprene, polyvinyl chloride
	Caps (Cronin 1980)	Mercaptobenzo-thiazole	Silicone swim cap
	Ear plugs	Rubber accelerators	Non-rubber plugs
Landsports	Shoes (Roberts & Hanifin 1979)	Rubber accelerators, dyes	Polyurethane
Racquet sports	Racquet handle	Isophorone diamine or epoxy resin	Handles without resin or add overlying tape
Any	Shin/knee guards (Sommer *et al.* 1999; Vincenzi *et al.* 1992)	Urea-formaldehyde resin, para-tertiary-butylphenol-formaldehyde resin	Barrier beneath guard (coban, liquid adhesive, or petroleum jelly)
Head protection sports	Helmets	Epoxy resin	Silicone
Weightlifting	Metal weights (Guerra *et al.* 1988)	Pallidium	Cloth or petroleum jelly covering contact points
Any	Athletic tape	Para-tertiary-butylphenol-formaldehyde	Acrylate tape
Medications			
Any	Topical analgesics (Camarasa 1990)	Salicylate sprays, methyl salicylate (oil of wintergreen)	Avoidance
Any	Topical anesthetics (Ventura *et al.* 2001)	Benzocaine	Ice
Any	Topical antibiotics	Neosporin	Polysporin, petroleum jelly
Environment			
Outdoor	*Rhus* (plants)	Uroshiol (poison ivy)	Ivyblock

(vesicular, if acute) papules and plaques. The diagnosis is based on the characteristic history and typical clinical morphology and pattern. The differential diagnosis includes psoriasis, atopic dermatitis, eczematous drug eruption, viral exanthems, and tinea. Patch testing suspected chemicals confirms the diagnosis. It is also critical to distinguish the severe exudates of dermatitis from secondary impetigo which can appear very similar.

The treatment of choice includes topical steroids and the choice of steroid potency depends on the severity of the eruption and the anatomic location. Topical immunomodulators (e.g., pimecrolimus) may be used for more mild or chronic conditions. A rapid burst of oral steroids may be necessary for severe outbreaks.

Urticaria (hives)

It is often quite difficult to identify the etiology of urticaria; in the population at large, physical causes represent less than 3% of all causes of urticaria. Conversely, among athletes, at least 15% of all urticaria can be classified as physical urticaria (Mikhaliov *et al.* 1977). The types of physical urticaria include cholinergic, cold, solar, and aquagenic and differ foremost in the inciting factor (Table 9.3).

CHOLINERGIC URTICARIA

Cholinergic urticaria can result from a rapid rise in core body temperature; the exact etiology is unclear.

Table 9.3 Distinguishing tests for physical urticaria.

	Application of room temperature water	Introduction into sauna	Application of ice cube	Application of ultraviolet radiation
Aquagenic	+	−	−	−
Cholinergic	−	+	−	−
Cold	−	−	+	−
Solar	−	−	−	+

Susceptible athletes experience pruritus, burning, warmth, and irritation before the appearance of urticarial lesions. Cholinergic urticaria presents as well-defined, erythematous, edematous, discrete (and frequently confluent when severe), small (1–5 mm) papules anywhere on the body; systemic findings are unusual. Individual lesions lasting longer than 24 h require expert dermatologic evaluation to rule out urticarial vasculitis.

The constellation of clinical signs (especially the distinct, small wheals) and symptoms supports the diagnosis. To confirm the diagnosis, the clinician can reproduce lesions of cholinergic urticaria by having the athlete passively warm while sitting in a sauna. Regular use of antihistamines can treat and prevent recurrent urticaria; protease inhibitors may also work (Adams 2001b; Briner 1993).

COLD URTICARIA

Among athletes, cold urticaria is not uncommon and occurs in swimmers and outdoor winter athletes. Most cases of cold urticaria are idiopathic (essential acquired urticaria) but secondary cold urticaria may result from cryoglobulins and connective tissue disorders. Cold urticaria development results not from cold temperatures necessarily, but rather from a significant drop in temperature. The skin lesions mimic those of cholinergic urticaria and appear on surfaces exposed to the cold environment. Loss of consciousness associated with cold urticaria (e.g., after diving into cold water) is a rare but serious concern (Sarnaik *et al.* 1986).

Clinicians confirm the diagnosis with the "ice cube test." Upon removing an ice cube placed on the athlete's forearm, a hive will develop on the skin (Adams 2001a). The treatment of cold urticaria is

similar to cholinergic urticaria and the clinician should consider secondary causes of cold urticaria. If appropriate, protective equipment can be worn to prevent cold urticaria and athletes may find that the use of cyproheptadine hydrochloride allows continued athletic involvement (Briner 1993).

DERMATOGRAPHISM

Dermatographism is not uncommon in the population at large and can occur beneath rubbing protective athletic equipment or when the athlete scratches (Briner 1993). Sensitive mast cells which degranulate after trauma to the skin likely induce this condition. Distinctive, often linear (corresponding to scratching or rubbing equipment), edematous, erythematous plaques occur (Fig. 9.13). The clinician can confirm the diagnosis by scratching the athlete's back with a pen tip and observing the

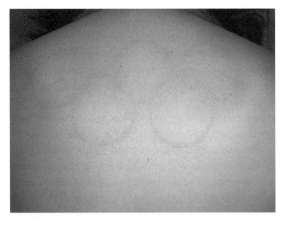

Fig. 9.13 Once scratched, athletes with dermatographism promptly develop edematous, erythematous plaques.

resultant wheal. Routine use of oral antihistamines controls dermatographism (Adams 2001b).

SOLAR URTICARIA

Very rarely, outdoor athletes can develop urticaria induced by UVA, UVB, or visible light. Wheals develop on exposed skin within minutes of exposure to the light source and resolve spontaneously within an hour. Typical wheals are distributed on sun-exposed areas (but not chronically so). Systemic findings such as headache and nausea are rare. Phototesting with UVA, UVB, and visible light will not only reproduce the urticarial lesions but also demonstrate a greater propensity to burn than would be expected.

Treatment of solar urticaria with antihistamines is similar to other physical urticaria. In severe cases, athletes may require antimalarial agents or referral to a dermatologist for ultraviolet desensitization therapy (Adams 2001a). Athletes should focus on prevention with broadband blocking sunscreens and protective clothing; they should also note that typical windows do not shield UVA rays.

AQUAGENIC URTICARIA

While true aquagenic urticaria (urticaria after exposure to ambient temperature water) is exceedingly rare, it is worth noting as it may have serious consequences. The treatment is similar to that for other physical urticaria; affected athletes appear to derive some benefit from applying inert oils to their skin before immersing in water (Panconesi & Lotti 1987).

TRAUMATIC PLANTAR URTICARIA

Traumatic plantar urticaria, an unusual condition previously reported in young basketball players and runners, presents with plantar pain that increases over several days (Metzker & Brodsky 1988). Exquisitely tender, well-defined, small, erythematous to violaceous macules and papules appear on the soles. This condition can be confused with neutrophilic hidradenitis. Only biopsies of the two conditions differentiate them. Both skin disorders resolve spontaneously.

EXERCISE-INDUCED ANGIOEDEMA/ANAPHYLAXIS

Although any athlete may develop exercise-induced angioedema/anaphylaxis (EIA), runners seem particularly prone, with 78% of outbreaks occurring while running (Shadick et al. 1999). Cyclists, downhill skiers, and basketball, handball, racquetball, and tennis players have also all developed EIA (Adams 2004). Females preferentially develop EIA at a ratio of 2:1. Histaminemia, resulting from mast cell degranulation, likely causes EIA (Nichols 1992).

The term EIA is slightly misleading as not all athletes develop anaphylaxis; in fact, there is a range of manifestations that typically begin 5 min after exercise but may still occur even after stopping their activity (Adams 2002c). More than 90% of affected athletes complain of pruritus and urticaria presents in 86% of athletes. Transient facial and palmar angioedema occurs in 70–80%, 50% develop wheezing, and 33% experience syncope. Less common symptoms and signs include nausea, diarrhea, hoarseness, headache, and flushing.

The constellation of clinical findings including angioedema and pruritus, with or without respiratory or vascular collapse, establishes the diagnosis. Clinicians should differentiate cholinergic urticaria from EIA. Both disorders can have dyspnea and skin eruptions, although athletes with EIA demonstrate dyspnea as a result of laryngeal edema and the dyspnea in cholinergic urticaria results from bronchospasm. In terms of the skin eruptions, EIA displays angioedema and those with cholinergic urticaria produce smaller (few millimeters to 1 cm in size), discrete, erythematous papules that may coalesce into larger plaques. Finally, cholinergic urticaria will not present with hypotension, while EIA may. Athletes may require vascular and respiratory support; the subacute treatment of EIA includes antihistamines and epinephrine (Adams 2002c); no evidence exists that β-agonist inhalers or corticosteroids are helpful.

Half of affected athletes can prevent EIA attacks by avoiding extreme temperatures while exercising (Adams 2002c). By avoiding eating before competing, one-third of afflicted athletes may exercise without developing EIA. Specific food triggers include barley, beans, broccoli, cheese, chicken, egg, garlic, grapes, lettuce, peaches, peanuts, rye, shellfish, tomatoes, and wheat (Adams 2004). By avoiding aspirin, beta-lactam antibiotics, and non-steroidal anti-inflammatory products before competing, some athletes can prevent EIA. Affected athletes regularly take antihistamines even though there is no evidence to support this practice. Ketotifen and cromolyn can prevent angioedema and the respiratory symptoms, respectively, in EIA (Adams 2002c). Afflicted athletes should never practice alone and should always carry an epinephrine pen.

Conclusions

Athletes have the same propensity to develop the skin disorders inherent to the normal population; however, their sports participation place them at higher risk to exacerbate those skin problems. Furthermore, athletes develop multiple conditions directly related to their sporting participation. Knowledge of the intimate relationship between an athlete and their skin will enhance the clinician's ability to diagnose and manage adeptly the cutaneous conditions related to sports.

References

Adams, B.B. (2001a) Sports dermatology. *Adolescent Medicine: State of the Art Reviews* **2**, 305–322.

Adams, B.B. (2001b) Sports dermatology. *Dermatology Nursing* **13**, 347–363.

Adams, B.B. (2002a) Tinea corporis gladiatorum. *Journal of the American Academy of Dermatology* **47**, 286–290.

Adams, B.B (2002b) Dermatologic disorders of the athlete. *Sports Medicine* **32**, 309–321.

Adams, B.B. (2002c) Exercise-induced anaphylaxis in a marathon runner. *International Journal of Dermatology* **41**, 394–396.

Adams, E.S. (2004) Identifying and controlling metabolic skin disorders. *The Physician and Sportsmedicine* **32**, 29–40.

Anderson, B.J. (1999) The effectiveness of valacyclovir in preventing reactivation of herpes gladiatorum in wrestlers. *Clinical Journal of Sport Medicine* **9**, 86–90.

Bartlett, P.C., Martin, R.J. & Cahill, B.R. (1982) Furunculosis in a high school football team. *American Journal of Sports Medicine* **10**, 371–374.

Begier, E.M., Frenette, K., Barrett, N.L., Mshar, P., Petit, S., Boxrud, D.J., *et al.* (2004) A high-morbidity outbreak of methicillin-resistant *Staphylococcus aureus* among players on a college football team, facilitated by cosmetic body shaving and turf burns. *Clinical Infectious Diseases* **39**, 1446–1453.

Biolcati, G. & Alabiso, A. (1997) Creeping eruption of larva migrans: a case report in a beach volley athlete. *International Journal of Sports Medicine* **18**, 612–613.

Briner, W.W. (1993) Physical allergies and exercise. *Sports Medicine* **15**, 365–373.

Camarasa, J.G. (1990) Analgesic spray contact dermatitis. *Dermatologic Clinics* **8**, 137–138.

Caputo, R., DeBoulle, K., DelRosso, J. & Nowicki, R. (2001) Prevalence of superficial fungal infections among sports-active individuals: results from the Achilles survey. *Journal of the European Academy of Dermatology and Venereology* **15**, 312–316.

Cronin, E. (1980) Rubber. In: *Contact Dermatitis* (Cronin, E., ed.) Churchill Livingstone, New York: 714.

Cyr. (2004) Viral skin infections. *The Physician and Sportsmedicine* **32**, 33–38.

Descamps, V. & Puechal, X. (2002) 'Canyoning hand': a new recreational hand dermatitis. *Contact Dermatitis* **47**, 363–364.

Exum, W.F. & Scott, M.J. (1992) Trapshooter's stigma. *Cutis* **50**, 110.

Fisher, A.A. (1988) Swimming pool granulomas due to *Mycobacterium marinum*: an occupational hazard of lifeguards. *Cutis* **41**, 397–398.

Fisher, A.A. (1987) Contact dermatitis to diving equipment, swimming pool chemicals, and other aquatic denizens. *Clinical Dermatology* **5**, 36–40.

Galbraith, N.S. (1980) Infections associated with swimming pools. *Environmental Health* **Feb**, 31–33.

Guerra, L., Misciali, C., Borrello, P. & Melino, M. (1988) Sensitization to palladium. *Contact Dermatitis* **19**, 306–307.

Hamant, E.S. & Adams B.B. (2005) Sunscreen use among collegiate athletes. *Journal of the American Academy of Dermatology* **53**, 237–241.

Han, A. & Maibach, H.I. (2004) Management of acute sunburn. *American Journal of Clinical Dermatology* **5**, 39–47.

Hazen, P.G. & Weil, M.L. (1997) Itraconazole in the prevention and management of dermatophytosis in competitive wrestlers. *Journal of the American Academy of Dermatology* **36**, 481–482.

Izumi, A.K. & Moore, R.E. (1987) Seaweed (*Lyngbya majuscula*) dermatitis. *Clinical Dermatology* **5**, 92–100.

Johnston, J.M. & Izumi, A.K. (1987) Cutaneous *Mycobacterium marinum* infection. *Clinical Dermatology* **5**, 68–75.

Koehn, G.G. (1991) Skin injuries in sports medicine. *Journal of the American Academy of Dermatology* **24**, 152.

Kohl, T.D., Martin, D.C. & Berger, M.S. (1999) Comparison of topical and oral treatments for tinea gladiatorum. *Clinical Journal of Sports Medicine* **9**, 161–166.

Kohl, T.D., Martin, D.C., Nemeth, R., Hill, T. & Evans, D. (2000) Fluconazole for the prevention and treatment of tinea gladiatorum. *Pediatric Infectious Disease Journal* **19**, 717–722.

Levine, N. (1980) Dermatologic aspects of sports medicine. *Journal of the American Academy of Dermatology* **3**, 415–424.

Leyden, J.J. & Kligman, A.M. (1975) Aluminum chloride in the treatment of symptomatic athlete's foot. *Archives of Dermatology* **111**, 1004–1010.

Mailler, E.A. & Adams, B.B. (2004) The wear and tear of 26.2: dermatological injuries reported on marathon day. *British Journal of Sports Medicine* **38**, 498–501.

Metzker, A. & Brodsky, F. (1988) Traumatic plantar urticaria: an unrecognized entity? *Journal of the American Academy of Dermatology* **18**, 144–146.

Mikhailov, P., Berova, N. & Andreev, V.C. (1977) Physical urticaria and sport. *Cutis* **20**, 381–390.

Millikan, L.E., Galne, W.K., Gewirtzman, G.B., Horwitz, S.N., Landow, R.K., Nesbitt, L.T., *et al.* (1988) Naftifine cream 1% versus econazole cream 1% in the treatment of tinea cruris and tinea corporis. *Journal of the American Academy of Dermatology* **18**, 52–56.

Mills, J., Hauer, L., Gottlieb, A., Dromgoole, S. & Spruance, S. (1987) Recurrent herpes labialis in skiers. *American Journal of Sports Medicine* **15**, 76–78.

Nerurkar, L.S., West, F., May, M., Madden, DL. & Sever, JL. (1983) Survival of herpes simplex virus in water specimens collected from hot tubs in spa facilities and on plastic surfaces. *JAMA* **250**, 3081–3083.

Nichols, A.W. (1992) Exercise-induced anaphylaxis and urticaria. *Clinics in Sports Medicine* **11**, 303–312.

Panconesi, E. & Lotti, T. (1987) Aquagenic urticaria. *Clinical Dermatology* **5**, 49–51.

Roberts, J.L. & Hanifin, J.M. (1979) Athletic shoe dermatitis: contact allergy to ethyl butyl thiourea. *JAMA* **241**, 275–276.

Rycroft, R.J. & Penny, P.T. (1983) Dermatoses associated with brominated swimming pools. *British Medical Journal (Clinical Research Ed.)* **287**, 462.

Sarnaik, A.P., Vohra, M.P., Sturman, S.W. & Belenky, W.M. (1986) Medical problems of the swimmer. *Clinics in Sports Medicine* **5**, 47–64.

Selling, B. & Kibrick, S. (1964) An outbreak of herpes simplex among wrestlers (herpes gladiatorum). *New England Journal of Medicine* **270**, 979–982.

Shadick, N.A., Liang, M.H., Partridge, A.J., Bingham, C., Wright, E., Fossel, A.H., *et al.* (1999) The natural history of exercise induced anaphylaxis: survey results from a 10-year follow-up study. *Journal of Allergy and Clinical Immunology* **104**, 123–127.

Shelley, W.B. (1980) Herpetic arthritis associated with disseminate herpes simplex in a wrestler. *British Journal of Dermatology* **103**, 209–212.

Sommer, S., Wilkinson, S.M. & Dodman, B. (1999) Contact dermatitis due to urea-formaldehyde resin in shin-pads. *Contact Dermatitis* **40**, 159–160.

Strauss, R.H., Lanese, R.R. & Leizman, D.J. (1988) Illness and absence among wrestlers, swimmers, and gymnasts at a large university. *American Journal of Sports Medicine* **16**, 653–655.

Ventura, M.T., Dagnello, M., Matino, M.G., Di Corato, R., Giuliano, G. & Tursi, A. (2001) Contact dermatitis in students practicing sports: incidence of rubber sensitisation. *British Journal of Sports Medicine* **35**, 100–102.

Vincenzi, C., Guerra, L., Peluso, A.M. & Zucchelli, V. (1992) Allergic contact dermatitis due to phenol-formaldehyde resins in a knee-guard. *Contact Dermatitis* **27**, 54.

White, W.B. & Grant-Kels, J.M. (1984) Transmission of herpes simplex virus type 1 infection in rugby players. *JAMA* **252**, 533–535.

Chapter 10

Exercise and Infections

MARTIN P. SCHWELLNUS, AUSTIN JEANS, SELLO MOTAUNG
AND JEROEN SWART

Athletes are not immune to developing infections. In fact, during intensive training, competition, and international travel, athletes appear to be more prone to developing infections (Gani *et al.* 2003; Nieman 2003). Furthermore, depending on the nature of the sports athletes participate in, they may be exposed to infections transmitted through direct skin contact, contaminated water, blood or tissue products (Kordi & Wallace 2004), or via respiratory droplets (Friman & Wesslen 2000).

An acute bout of exercise, as well as regular exercise training, may alter various components of immune function. The net effect of these changes may result in either protection from or susceptibility to infection. However, there is little direct evidence linking the specific exercise-induced changes to immune function and subsequent rates of infection (Malm 2004). The purpose of this chapter is to review briefly the effects of exercise on systemic and mucosal immunity and then discuss the clinical approach to some of the more common infections that can occur in athletes:

- Upper respiratory tract infections (URTI)
- Systemic viral infections
- Water-borne infections
- Tropical infections
- Blood-borne infections
- Infections of the central nervous system
- Genitourinary infections

The Olympic Textbook of Medicine in Sport, 1st edition. Edited by M. Schwellnus. Published 2008 by Blackwell Publishing, ISBN: 978-1-4051-5637-0.

A brief summary on immunization of athletes is included. Other infections in athletes are also discussed in other chapters of this book.

Exercise and immunology

The effect of exercise training on immune function is a research endeavor in which almost 80% of all the scientific literature has appeared in the past 15 years (Nieman 2000). The effects of exercise on immune function can be categorized into either systemic or local (mucosal) immune effects and the response of these systems to acute or chronic exercise training.

Both self-reported data from athletes and randomized training studies indicate that chronic exercise reduces the incidence of viral illness and URTI (Nieman 2000; Shephard *et al.* 1995). However, the incidence of URTI is increased following heavy training or participation in endurance competition (Malm 2004; Nieman 2000). In addition, training or racing following inoculation with a pathogen may increase the rate of clinical infection as well as associated morbidity and mortality (Chao *et al.* 1992; Malm 2004; Nieman 2000). A single bout of exercise results in changes to various immune parameters that last 3–72 h. These changes may predispose the athlete to viral or bacterial infections. This is known as the "open window" phenomenon (Pedersen & Ullum 1994). Repeated exposure to high intensity exercise or prolonged exercise bouts without sufficient recovery may lead to a cumulative decline in immune function. This may be responsible for the high rates of infection seen in overtrained athletes.

Recent emphasis has been placed on the relative balance between humoral and cell-mediated immunity. The regulation of these two systems appears to be associated with the relative preponderance of two distinct subsets of T helper (Th) lymphocytes. Th1 lymphocytes are associated with cell-mediated immunity, while Th2 lymphocytes are associated with humoral immunity. Downregulation of Th1 cell-mediated immunity results in reduced protection against numerous infectious agents. The cytokine profiles produced by cells of the non-specific immune system in response to infection determines whether the immune response is predominantly cellular or humoral in nature. Interleukin 12 (IL-12) is responsible for the upregulation of Th1 lymphocytes while γ-interferon (IFN-γ) inhibits Th2 proliferation. In contrast IL-4 upregulates Th2 lymphocytes while IL-10 is considered profoundly immunosuppressive in inhibiting Th1 cell-mediated immunity and macrophage function. Excessive exercise, the overtraining syndrome, and trauma can alter the cytokine profile and thereby predispose the athlete to infection (Lakier 2003).

Exercise and systemic immunity

SYSTEMIC IMMUNE RESPONSE TO ACUTE EXERCISE

Acute exercise bouts are associated with changes in the number and function of white blood cells. High intensity endurance exercise is associated with the greatest changes: an increase in circulating granulocytes and monocytes and a reduction in lymphocytes. This leads to an increased neutrophil : lymphocyte ratio (Brenner *et al.* 1998; Nieman 2000). These changes are attributable to elevated concentrations of serum cortisol following intense exercise as well as to several other mechanisms including changes in cytokine concentrations, elevated body temperature, increased blood flow, lymphocyte apoptosis, and dehydration. Natural killer cytotoxic activity (NKCA) is reduced for at least 6 h following intense exercise bouts (Nieman 2000). This reduction in NKCA is linked to decreased numbers of circulating natural killer (NK) cells but the individual NK cell function is maintained. In contrast,

individual granulocytes show reduced oxidative burst activity and mitogen-induced lymphocyte proliferation falls 30–40% following acute exercise bouts (Nieman 2000).

An acute bout of strenuous exercise has been shown to alter the concentration of various cytokines that are responsible for the balance between humoral and cell-mediated immunity. Moderate exercise may promote a Th1-type cytokine response (Malm 2004) while prolonged and strenuous exercise results in elevated concentrations of IL-10 and IL-6. Elevated concentrations of IL-6 stimulate the production of IL-4. In addition, IL-12 and IFN-γ concentrations remain either unchanged or are suppressed following intense exercise. These changes favor a Th2 immune response and suppression of cell-mediated immunity, placing the athlete at risk for viral and bacterial infection (Lakier 2003). This response to intense or prolonged exercise may become more pronounced with increasing age (Malm 2004).

SYSTEMIC IMMUNE RESPONSE TO EXERCISE TRAINING

The adaptive immune response remains relatively unaffected by either intense or prolonged exercise training. Evidence for mitogen-induced lymphocyte proliferation following chronic or strenuous training is inconsistent with some studies showing an increased response in endurance trained athletes vs. controls (Baj *et al.* 1994) while other studies have failed to show any significant change (Nieman 2000). Most comparisons between athletes and controls fail to show any differences in resting serum immunoglobulin G (IgG) concentrations. Particularly intense training may result in reduced serum concentrations of IgA, IgG, and IgM, as seen in swimmers following an intense 7-month training season. Despite low serum IgG concentrations, antibody response to antigenic challenge remained normal (Mackinnon 2000). This indicates that the adaptive immune response (T and B cell function) remains relatively unaffected by either intense or prolonged exercise training.

Various components of the innate immune system are affected by chronic exposure to exercise.

NKCA is enhanced in response to chronic exercise and NK cell numbers are normal or reduced in athletes subjected to prolonged intense training in comparison to sedentary controls (Mackinnon 2000). In comparison to sedentary controls, athletes tend to have enhanced NKCA (Nieman 2000). There is also seasonal variation in NKCA in response to training load, with increased function during high intensity training periods (Nieman 2000). This evidence is not supported by prospective studies using moderate endurance training and suggests that the NKCA response to training may be induced selectively during high intensity or large volumes of training (Nieman 2000). In contrast, overtraining and excessive exercise may suppress NKCA because of the direct suppressive effect of glucocorticoids on NKCA activity (Lakier 2003).

Neutrophils appear to be particularly susceptible to prolonged periods of intense exercise training (Mackinnon 2000). Studies comparing neutrophil activity during low volume training show no difference between athletes and controls (Nieman 2000). During periods of intensive training, neutrophil function is suppressed (Baj *et al.* 1994; Nieman 2000). Neutrophil activation is suppressed in trained cyclists in comparison with non-cyclists, and neutrophil phagocytosis and activation are reduced following intense exercise in runners. Elite swimmers have shown reduced resting neutrophil activity directly related to training intensity (Mackinnon 2000). However, this effect has not been confirmed in a study of elite female rowers 3 months prior to the World Championships (Nieman 2000) while reduced neutrophil activation has not been correlated with rates of URTI in swimmers during intense training (Mackinnon 2000). Despite the effects of chronic exercise on the abovementioned parameters, there is no direct evidence linking these changes with any increased incidence of systemic or URTI (Nieman 2000).

Repeated bouts of prolonged or high intensity exercise may result in a cumulative effect of the cytokine profile on suppression of cell-mediated immunity (Pedersen 2000). In addition, excessive exercise and the overtraining syndrome result in elevated glucocorticoid and catecholamine concentrations as a result of changes in the hypothalamic–pituitary–adrenal axis. Elevated glucocorticoids and catecholamines directly inhibit the production of IL-12 and IFN-ā and stimulate the production of IL-10. This leads to further suppression of the Th1 cell-mediated immune response, possibly increasing susceptibility to infection. Elevated concentrations of Th2 lymphocytes promote atopy and allergies in keeping with increased reports of allergic manifestations in overtrained athletes (Lakier 2003).

Exercise and local immunity

The mucosal immune system and the innate non-specific immune system together form the body's primary first defense mechanism against pathogenic organisms and allergens that present at mucosal surfaces. The common mucosal immune system incorporates the gut-associated lymphoid tissue (GALT), mammary glands, urogenital tracts, lacrimal glands, the bronchus-associated lymphoid tissue (BALT), nasal-associated lymphoid tissue (NALT), and the salivary glands.

At these sites, secretory IgA antibodies have the greatest role in providing specific immunity. The IgA1 subclass predominates in the salivary glands and NALT. To a lesser extent, secretory IgM and serum derived and locally produced IgG also provide immunity, with the latter being important in the protection of the upper respiratory tract and the female urogenital tract (Gleeson & Pyne 2000).

LOCAL IMMUNE RESPONSE TO ACUTE EXERCISE

Numerous studies have documented a reduction in salivary IgA concentrations following an acute exercise bout and these studies have been summarized in an excellent review by Gleeson and Pyne (2000). A number of studies have found a reduction in IgA concentrations following intense endurance exercise or maximal exercise in both elite and recreational athletes. In contrast, a small number of studies have reported increased salivary IgA concentrations following either maximal exercise or prolonged endurance exercise but these studies have been limited to recreational or moderately exercising athletes. In response to moderate exercise intensities, most studies have failed to show any post-exercise change in salivary IgA secretions. Studies of team sports have found either an increase or no change in IgA concentration following competition or training respectively (Gleeson & Pyne 2000). In general, salivary IgM concentrations parallel the changes in IgA concentration in response to exercise while IgG concentrations generally fail to show any response.

In general, the recovery of salivary immunoglobulins to normal concentrations occurs within 1 h after cessation of exercise. However, maximal exercise bouts in elite athletes may prolong the return to normal values, while repetitive bouts of exercise during periods of heavy training may results in a cumulative reduction in IgA concentration from one training day to the next (Gleeson & Pyne 2000).

LOCAL IMMUNE RESPONSE TO EXERCISE TRAINING

Tomasi *et al*. (1982) first reported reduced IgA concentrations in the saliva of cross-country skiers. This finding has subsequently been supported by research showing that concentrations of salivary IgA are reduced in response to extended short periods of training (Gleeson & Pyne 2000; Mackinnon & Hooper 1994; Mackinnon & Jenkins 1993) as well as to prolonged seasonal exposure to training loads (Gleeson & Pyne 2000). The change in salivary immune function parallels the changes in whole body mucosal immunity following high volume or intense training (Gleeson & Pyne 2000).

Specific studies of salivary IgM and IgG concentrations have either been conflicting or have found no changes. In contrast to studies that show a reduction in immunoglobulins in response to training, two studies have found an increase in pre-exercise salivary IgA, IgM, and IgG in well-trained swimmers in comparison to a moderately exercising control group (Gleeson & Pyne 2000) An increase in salivary IgA but not IgM or IgG in well-trained rowers in comparison with non-athletes has also been found (Nehlsen-Cannarella *et al*. 2000). The reduction in secretory immunoglobulins during periods of intense training and competition is associated with an increased susceptibility to URTIs (Gleeson & Pyne 2000).

In summary, moderate or high intensity exercise can result in a temporary decrease in mucosal secretory immunoglobulins which may increase the risk of infection. Repetitive high intensity exercise may cause a cumulative suppression of secretory IgA. High volume training is also associated with a chronic but reversible decline in secretory immunoglobulins which can predispose the athlete to URTI. However, there are limitations in the existing literature that need to be addressed. These include differences in training stimuli, age, gender, and physical activity of subjects, methodologic issues pertaining to assessment of mucosal immunity, and biologic variability in mucosal immunity (Gleeson & Pyne 2004).

Conclusions: Exercise and immunity

The current literature suggests that low or moderate intensity exercise can enhance immune function and thus increase resistance to viral infection. In contrast, high intensity or high volume training suppresses various components of the immune system and increases susceptibility to infection (Shephard 2000). This appears to be related to overall immune system signaling and changed in the cytokine profile which may be related to microtrauma sustained during exercise bouts (Table 10.1; Lakier 2003).

Upper respiratory tract infections in athletes

URTIs can be defined as an acute illness affecting the nasopharynx caused by microbial agents and that results in local and sometimes systemic symptoms. They are not a single illness and are caused by a number of different microbes, mostly viruses. URTIs are the most common infections that affect the adult population including athletes. Adults acquire an average of 2–5 URTIs per year.

Acute exercise and the risk of developing an URTI

There is some scientific evidence to support the hypothesis that an exercise bout that is prolonged

Table 10.1 Summary of exercise-induced immune change.

Acute exercise	Chronic exercise	Overtraining
Systemic immunity		
↑ Granulocyte and monocyte concentration	↔ ↓ Granulocyte activation and phagocyctic activity	
↓ Granulocyte oxidative activity		
↓ Lymphocyte concentration and proliferative response	↔ ↑ Lymphocyte proliferative response	
↓ NKCA	↑ NKCA	↓ NKCA
	↓ ↔ NK cell concentrations	
↓↑ Th1–Th2 balance	↔ ↓ Th1–Th2 balance	↓ Th1–Th2 balance
	↔ ↓ Serum immunoglobulin concentrations	
Local immunity		
↓ IgA concentration (trained athletes)	↑ ↓ IgA concentrations	↓ IgA concentrations
↔ ↑ IgA concentrations (sedentary/moderately trained athletes, moderate intensity and team sports)	↑ ↔ IgM/IgG	

Ig, immunoglobulin; NK, natural killer; NKCA, natural killer cytotoxic activity; Th, T helper.

(>60 min sessions) and performed at high intensity (>80% of maximum ability) is associated with a depression in the immune system. This decrease in immunity can last from a few hours to a few days after an acute exercise bout. During this period, which has been termed the "open window" period, there appears to be an increased risk of developing an URTI.

It has consistently been found that 30–50% of athletes participating in endurance events such as marathon and ultramarathon running will develop symptoms of an URTI. In these studies, the runners at highest risk to developed symptoms were the faster runners (increased running speed), and the runners with an increased training load (>65 km·week^{-1}).

Until recently it has been assumed that these symptoms are caused by an infection resulting from a depressed immune system. However, in two recent scientific studies, viral and bacterial cultures taken from the upper respiratory tracts of symptomatic athletes after an ultramarathon have not shown any growth, indicating that there is no infection. These studies suggest that the symptoms that athletes experience are not caused by an infection; other causes such as allergies or pollution are possibly responsible for these symptoms. The cause of these symptoms therefore requires further investigation.

Regular exercise training and the risk of developing an URTI

Epidemiologic studies have shown that sedentary individuals have a higher incidence of URTI symptoms compared with individuals who regularly perform exercise training at moderate "dose" of exercise (50–70% of maximum ability) and moderate weekly duration (3–5 sessions per week for 30–60 min per session). It has also been shown that athletes who engage in regular intense and prolonged training bouts have a chronic depression of the immune system, and this may result in an increased incidence of URTI symptoms. These findings have therefore shown that the risk of URTI symptoms is:

1 Lowest when individuals are exposed to a moderate "dose" of exercise;

2 Slightly higher in sedentary individuals; and

3 Highest in athletes performing intense and prolonged exercise.

This has resulted in a hypothesis that the relationship between the "dose" of exercise and the risk of URTI symptoms is a "J-shaped" curve (Fig. 10.1).

Advice to athletes to reduce the risk of developing URTI symptoms after an acute exercise bout

Recently, there has been evidence to suggest that adequate nutrition may protect the athlete from the

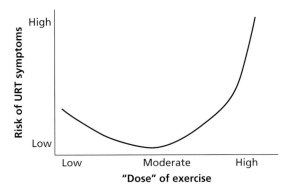

Fig. 10.1 Risk of upper respiratory tract infections (URTI).

Table 10.3 Contraindications to exercise participation in athletes with upper respiratory tract infection (URTI).

Presence of a fever
Presence of myalgia (muscle pains)
Presence of chest pain
Resting tachycardia (increased resting pulse rate)
Excessive shortness of breath
Excessive fatigue
Swollen painful lymphadenopathy

immunosuppressive effects of high intensity or prolonged exercise. Vitamin C (500 mg·day^{-1}), glutamine and, more recently, carbohydrate supplementation may protect against the development of URTI symptoms during sport. However, further scientific study is required to verify these early reports. However, it can be suggested that the following precautions can be taken by athletes to reduce the risk of developing URTI symptoms (Table 10.2).

Advice to athletes on return to play following URTI

One of the most common clinical problems that medical staff attending to athletes face is when a player can return to full activity after injury or illness. URTIs are caused mainly by viral infections. A number of these viruses can affect other organs, including skeletal muscle and cardiac muscle. Viral

Table 10.2 Precautions for athletes to decrease the risk of developing upper respiratory tract infection (URTI).

Space high intensity and prolonged exercise session and race events as far apart as possible
Avoid overtraining and chronic fatigue
Maintain a well-balanced diet
Get adequate sleep
Take 500 mg·day^{-1} vitamin C during periods of heavy training
Ensure adequate carbohydrate intake during intense prolonged exercise

myocarditis following an URTI can occur, and this has been associated with sudden death in athletes. The attending clinician must therefore make sure that an athlete does not return to full activity if there is a risk of myocarditis.

Viral myocarditis should be suspected in any athlete presenting with non-specific symptoms such as fatigue, dyspnea, palpitations, or chest discomfort. In particular, myocardial involvement should be ruled out in athletes who present with viral illness where there are prominent systemic symptoms such as headache, malaise, fever, myalgia, palpitations, and chest discomfort.

In an athlete where viral myocarditis is suspected, the findings on physical examination are usually non-specific. There may be general signs of a systemic viral infection. It is important to note that the presence of a tachycardia, which is out of proportion to the degree of pyrexia, is a useful pointer to myocardial involvement.

On cardiac auscultation the first heart sound may be muffled and there may be a gallop. A transient apical systolic murmur may appear. In severe cases, clinical signs of congestive cardiac failure are present. A pericardial friction rub may be present if there is associated pericarditis.

In an athlete when there is any suspicion that there are systemic symptoms, or signs of viral myocarditis, sports participation must be avoided until symptoms have disappeared (Table 10.3).

If the URTI is not associated with any of the above symptoms, mild exercise may in some cases (to be discussed with a doctor) be permitted during the URTI. If the athlete does not develop any symptoms during this "trial" of exercise, moderate intensity exercise may be resumed.

URTI and the effect on exercise performance after clinical recovery

Athletes who have recovered after URTIs often complain of a residual decrease in performance. Although this may be a result of the effects of a period of detraining during the recovery period, there is a possibility that there may be residual negative effects from the infection. This has never been well investigated in a scientific study. A pilot study has been undertaken during which athletes were followed during recovery from URTI and later during an equivalent period of detraining. The results of this study showed that there was a measurable decrease in exercise performance (treadmill running time) which lasted for 2–4 days after full clinical recovery from an URTI. The practical suggestion resulting from this study is that athletes may experience a decline in performance for a few days following full clinical recovery from a URTI. However, this is an area that requires further scientific study.

Systemic viral infections

Infectious mononucleosis

Epstein–Barr virus (EBV) or infectious mononucleosis (IM) is a DNA herpes virus that is transmitted by oropharyngeal secretions, infecting the squamous epithelial cells of the oropharynx and B cells (Auwaerter 2004). The virus may also be transmitted by parenteral methods (Hosey & Rodenberg 2005). The prevalence of EBV infection varies from 50 to 70% in early adulthood in developed societies to almost 100% by age 4 in less developed countries. The risk of developing clinical symptoms with infection increases with age. Fewer than 10% of children develop clinical signs of infection while adolescents and adults develop symptoms 50–70% of the time. The incidence of clinical infection decreases with age, with the incidence of symptomatic IM in early adulthood being approximately 1–3% and falling to 2–4 per 100,000 by age 35 (Auwaerter 2004).

EBV classically presents as a triad of fever, tonsillar pharyngitis, and lymphadenopathy, which typically begins after an incubation period of 30–50 days. A 3–5 day prodromal period may manifest with headaches, malaise, myalgia, and loss of appetite. This is followed by an acute phase lasting 5–15 days during which exudative pharyngitis, tonsillar enlargement, fever, and posterior cervical lymphadenopathy are the most common symptoms. Symptoms and signs can be variable, with some patients presenting with prolonged fever and flu-like illness which persists for more than 2 weeks and absence of pharyngitis and lymphadenopathy. These patients are often older (>35 years) and may also have prominent gastrointestinal symptoms such as anorexia, nausea, vomiting, and diarrhea.

Lymphocytic infiltration of the spleen results in splenomegaly that is clinically detectable in 40–60% of patients (Hosey & Rodenberg 2005). One study, using ultrasonography, detected splenomegaly in all of the 29 cases who presented with IM (Auwaerter 2004).

Less frequent symptoms and signs include jaundice, hepatomegaly, and rashes (ranging from macular rashes to erythema nodosum). Rare neurologic presentations that occur in less than 0.5% of patients include encephalitis, myelitis, and optic neuritis and are the leading cause of death resulting from IM.

The diagnosis of IM in patients who present with suggestive symptoms and signs is confirmed by several objective tests. White blood cell (WBC) count is typically elevated at 12,000–18,000 cells·mm^{-3} with atypical lymphocytes accounting for up to 30% of the differential. The presence of heterophile antibodies (Monospot test) may confirm the diagnosis in 85–90% of cases who present with clinical findings compatible with IM. EBV antibodies are both specific and sensitive for EBV infection. Viral capsid antigen (VCA) IgM is usually positive by the time of clinical presentation and remains elevated for 1–2 months. VCA IgG antibodies rise concurrently and persist lifelong and are therefore not valuable in making a diagnosis of acute infection. EBV nuclear antigen (EBNA) appears later (6–12 weeks) and the presence of this antibody excludes a primary infection.

Treatment for most cases is essentially supportive as the illness is generally self-limiting. Fatigue and somnolence are best treated by early light activity and avoiding prolonged bed rest. There is no role for pharmacologic management of these symptoms, and this includes antiviral medication or corticosteroids which may increase complications and should be reserved for life-threatening complications such as airway obstruction, profound thrombocytopenia, hemolytic anemia, disseminated intravascular coagulation, and myocarditis (Auwaerter 2004).

Splenic rupture, the most feared and potentially fatal complication of IM, occurs in approximately 0.1–0.5% of cases and is the primary concern in the sports physician assessing the patient's fitness to return to play. The majority of IM patients will have splenomegaly with a resultant increased risk of splenic rupture and should therefore be restricted from participation in sports. This includes non-contact sports as splenic rupture occurs in 50% of cases with no history of antecedent trauma (Auwaerter 2004; Hosey & Rodenberg 2005).

Participants in non-contact sports should be considered fit for return to play after 3 weeks, providing there are no other complications. Activity should be commenced at approximately 50% of the previous training volume with the athlete's subjective response to training tolerance acting as a guide to increasing training intensity and volume. Some athletes may only reach full fitness after approximately 3 months or more. Individuals participating in contact sports should avoid returning to play for at least 4 weeks, at which time most patients will have resolution of splenic enlargement (Auwaerter 2004). If there is a significant risk of abdominal trauma during competition, the patient should undergo ultrasound examination or computed tomography scan at 4 weeks to confirm resolution of splenomegaly. Those patients with persistent splenic enlargement at 4 weeks should be reviewed after a further 1–2 weeks, at which stage persistent splenic enlargement may represent a normal variant and clinical judgment should dictate when to allow resumption of sport (Table 10.4; Auwaerter 2004).

Cytomegalovirus infection

Cytomegalovirus (CMV) infection may be acquired by exposure to infected oropharyngeal secretions, through sexual intercourse, or by parenteral spread. As with other herpes viruses, it lies latent after an

Table 10.4 Return to play (RTP) following Epstein–Barr virus (EBV) infection.

Non-impact sports
Encourage light activity for first 3 weeks
Return to 50% previous training load at 3 weeks
Assess response to training and increase activity as tolerated

Impact sports
Encourage light activity for first 4 weeks
Clinical examination at 4 weeks to rule out splenomegaly prior to RTP
Ultrasound/CT for high risk sports

CT, computed tomography.

initial acute infection. Reactivation may occur as a result of stress or immunocompromise. The prevalence of CMV exposure is approximately 50% in early adulthood but lifetime prevalence is in excess of 80%. The majority of acute infections do not produce clinical symptoms but symptomatic infection resembles acute IM. Acute cytomegalovirus infection can share other characteristics with IM: splenomegaly, hepatomegaly, lymphocytosis, atypical lymphocytosis, and false-positive heterophile antibody tests (Ho-Yen & Martin 1981). The differential diagnosis of IM should therefore always include CMV infection. Confirmation of infection is by serology, with specific IgM antibodies implying acute infection.

In immunocompromised patients, CMV infection can cause serious and potentially life-threatening infections: pneumonia, hepatitis, encephalitis, esophagitis, colitis, and retinitis. Treatment with antiviral agents (ganciclovir) should be reserved for these patients.

Measles

Measles is a highly contagious infectious disease and is transmitted primarily by airborne means. Indoor sporting events therefore present a risk for measles outbreaks. International travel to sporting events places the athlete at risk of infection from indigenous strains of measles. This has occurred at an international gymnastics event, while other measles outbreaks have occurred at a number of indoor athletic competitions held within domed stadiums (Turbeville *et al.* 2006). Despite the American College Health Association (ACHA) recommendations in conjunction with the Centers for Disease Control and Prevention (CDC) recommendation in 1983 that all colleges and universities within the USA provide proof of immunization against measles, mumps, and rubella, a number of outbreaks have occurred during college sporting events as a result of poor compliance with these recommendations. Current recommendations by the ACHA/CDC for collegiate level athletes in the USA are that each incoming student receive two vaccinations with live attenuated measles vaccine. This is because of the 5% failure rate after one vaccination. Adherence to these recommendations would provide adequate protection from measles infection for athletes (Dorman 2000). Susceptible individuals who have been exposed to measles may receive some protection through prophylactic vaccination within 72 h of exposure.

Water-borne infections

A number of other microbial agents may infect athletes who come into contact with contaminated water sources (Beck 2000): leptospirosis, *Aeromonas hydrophilia*, giardiasis, and cryptosporidiosis. In addition, otitis externa is a common localized infection affecting swimmers.

Leptospirosis is a spirochetal infection that present with a flu-like illness 2–20 days following water contact. After a few days this progresses to a syndrome characterized by fever, aseptic meningitis, skin rash, and uveitis. Weil's disease is severe leptospirosis that is characterized by progression to hepatitis, jaundice, renal failure, and coagulopathy. Treatment is by penicillin or doxycycline.

Aeromonas hydrophilia is an infection of the soft tissue following exposure to contaminated water (swimmers, skiers, paddlers). Giardiasis and cryptosporidiosis as well as other gastrointestinal infections may be acquired during swimming and paddling in contaminated water. A wide range of gastrointestinal symptoms can occur, which require specific diagnosis and treatment. Giardiasis requires antibiotic treatment, typically oral metronidazole.

The term "swimmer's ear" has been used to describe any inflammatory condition of the ear that commonly occurs in athletes participating in water sports. This single term describes a variety of conditions that affect the external auditory canal or the middle ear in swimmers. The most common disease of the external auditory canal associated with water sports is otitis externa (Beck 2000; Roland & Marple 1997). Other conditions include bony exostoses of the external auditory canal and infections of the middle ear (otitis media).

Otitis externa is an inflammatory condition of the external auditory canal, which can be caused by chemical irritation, allergies, or infections. Infections can be either bacterial or fungal. The main reason for an increased risk of otitis externa in swimmers is because water that repeatedly enters the canal washes cerumen out. Water that remains in the canal for some time causes maceration of the skin, leaving the damaged epithelium unprotected against invading organisms such as bacteria and fungi (Table 10.5).

The diagnosis of otitis externa is made clinically. The swimmer with otitis externa will initially complain of ear fullness, ear discomfort, and hearing loss. Pain becomes prominent if the condition persists, and discharge from the ear may be observed. An allergic type otitis usually presents with severe pruritus (itch).

On examination of the ear canal there may initially only be erythema and edema observed. Other signs such as a discharge, absence of cerumen, a dull tympanic membrane, and hyperkeratotic epithelium are characteristic of otitis externa at a later and chronic stage. Cultures of otitis externa show that *Pseudomonas aeruginosa* is the most common bacteria and *Aspergillus* is the most common fungus causing the infection. Fungal infections are characterized by a fuzzy lining dotted with black specks and a discharge with a musty odor.

Otitis externa should be managed by a qualified medical practitioner. The first step is to clean out the canal thoroughly by irrigation or the use of instruments (only if experienced). Topical anti-infective agents must be used with caution. In case of bacterial infections, drops containing neomycin or polymyxin B may be used. Acidification of the canal

Table 10.5 Risk factors for developing otitis externa in swimmers.

Spending long period in the water with the ears submerged swimming in unchlorinated, fresh, hot, or contaminated water

Not removing water from the ears after swimming

Introducing bacteria by inserting a dirty finger, contaminated swabs, or other objects into the ear

Contact with water containing sensitizing agents to which the athlete is allergic, or agents that are known irritants such as chemicals

Constant use of over-the-counter ear drops that denude the ear canal further

will discourage bacterial growth; provided there is no perforation of the eardrum, topical acidifiers such as 2% acetic acid may be used. Fungal infections can be treated with a 1% tolnaftate solution. Pain and pruritus must be relieved by analgesics and hydrocortisone, respectively. Hydrocortisone drops must be used with care and only after the infection is controlled. The swimmer should ideally abstain from water sports for 7–10 days. Athletes with less severe infections can return to swimming after 2–3 days, provided the necessary precautions are taken (Table 10.6).

Tropical infections

Bilharzia (schistosomiasis)

Schistosomiasis is a tropical infection caused by a digenetic trematode (Jeans 2003). The two predominant species are *Schistosoma mansoni* and *Schistosoma haematobium*. Less commonly, infection is by *Schistosoma intercalatum*. Human infection in athletes has been documented principally in Africa and involves athletes who participate in water sports where the trematode is prevalent. Human infection occurs on entry into shallow freshwater that contains the schistosome larvae. These larvae penetrate

Table 10.6 Preventing otitis externa in swimmers.

Dry the ear after swimming by tilting the head vigorously, jumping up and down, or drying gently with a towel

Avoid touching or scratching the ear

Use newer silicone-type earplugs for protection

Wear a hood when surfing or sail-boarding

Put a dropper full of drying agent into the ear after each swim

the skin, and the immature parasites migrate via the lungs to the portal circulation. Here they develop into adult worms, who migrate to the veins of the intestines (*S. mansoni*) or bladder (*S. haematobium*). After 7–12 weeks the worms produce eggs which are excreted and can be observed in the feces or urine.

Clinical presentation of bilharzia is as a cercarial dermatitis (swimmer's itch), acute infection (Katayama fever), and later as chronic schistosomiasis (Table 10.7). Laboratory diagnosis is by microscopy (urine or stool) or through a serologic test. Once diagnosed, treatment is by single dose of praziquantel (40 mg·kg^{-1}).

Malaria

Although not strictly speaking a blood-borne infection, malaria is a tropical protozoal vector-borne infection. It is transmitted by the female *Anopheles* mosquito who is a voracious nocturnal blood feeder. It is the most prevalent vector-borne disease and is endemic in 92 countries. In sub-Saharan Africa, 95% of malaria is caused by *Plasmodium falciparum*, the remainder mainly by *Plasmodium vivax*. Malaria is a disease associated with a considerable morbidity and mortality.

Athletes may have to travel frequently to attend events held in endemic malaria areas, and this means that malarial prophylaxis must be taken. A number of specific guidelines for preventing malaria in traveling athletes have been issued (Table 10.8).

It is recommended that athletes who travel to endemic malarial areas take malarial chemoprophylaxis. The effects of common malarial prophylactic agents on exercise performance have not been evaluated in scientific studies, but anecdotal reports

Table 10.7 Prevention of bilharzia in athletes.

Be aware of endemic bilharzia areas
Water sports should avoid areas of shallow or static (non-flowing) water
If water sports are conducted in freshwater in endemic areas, enquire if molluscicide treatment of the water has been undertaken
Athletes should perform vigorous toweling and drying or application of alcohol immediately after water contact
Athletes who have been exposed should be assessed clinically, and tested for the presence of bilharzia (eggs in stool or urine, serologic test)

Table 10.8 Prevention of malaria in traveling athletes.

Be aware of endemic malarial areas
Chemoprophylaxis is recommended (enquire at WHO website or local travel clinic)
Wear clothing with long sleeves and long trousers at dusk and dawn
Use mosquito repellents containing 15–30% DEET on exposed skin and clothing
Use sleeping nets that are treated with insecticide
Spray rooms with insecticide aerosol/surface spray
Use of mosquito vapor mats and/or burning coils at night

DEET, diethylmetatoluamide; WHO, World Health Organization.

indicate that these agents can have negative effects on exercise performance. Current advice to athletes should thus be to:
1 Use the common agents beforehand when in training, to establish whether the agents are tolerated;
2 Use agents that are prescribed only once a week if possible; and
3 Schedule the first dose in such a way that the competition date is on day 6 after administration, rather than on the first day or second day.

Exercise and blood-borne infections

There are a number of important blood-borne infections that team physician must be aware of (Kordi & Wallace 2004): viral hepatitis (B, C, and D; Harrington 2000) and the human immunodeficiency virus (HIV; Beck 2000; Kordi & Wallace 2004).

Viral hepatitis infection

Viruses causing hepatitis include hepatitis A (spread by fecal–oral route), hepatitis B, C, and D (spread by blood, perinatal transmission, and through sexual contact), and hepatitis E (fecal–oral transmission). Infections by hepatitis B, C, and D are associated with a high risk of chronicity (ranging 15–80%) and a higher risk of mortality (1–2%) once infected (Harrington 2000).

Athletes participating in contact sports may be exposed to blood and blood-borne products, and therefore may be at risk for acquiring hepatitis infections. Although the risk of transmission of hepatitis through contact sport is very low, athletes traveling to or living in areas where hepatitis (in particular hepatitis B) is endemic should be vaccinated. Furthermore, the general guidelines for decreasing the risk of blood-borne infections in contact sports should be followed (Table 10.9).

HIV disease and exercise

The acquired immune deficiency syndrome (AIDS) was first described as a clinical entity by the CDC in 1981 with the description of five cases of *Pneumocystis carinii* infection and 26 cases of Kaposi's sarcoma in homosexual males.

The causative agent, HIV, was first discovered in 1983 and isolated in a French laboratory as lymphadenopathy-associated virus (LAV). In 1984 it was designated HTLV-III and later AIDS-associated retrovirus (ARV). The International Committee on

Table 10.9 Guidelines for athletes for return to play following viral hepatitis.

Following acute viral hepatitis, mild to moderate intensity exercise is permitted once clinical condition has normalized
Following acute viral hepatitis, high intensity exercise is permitted once the clinical condition is normalized and liver function test have returned to normal
Athletes with chronic persistent hepatitis should only be allowed to participate in moderate intensity exercise and regular medical follow-up is advised
Athletes with chronic active hepatitis and cirrhosis should not participate in high intensity exercise but low intensity supervised exercise is permitted

the Taxonomy of Viruses chose the designation human immunodeficiency virus (HIV) in 1986. With the discovery in late 1986 of the related HIV-2 virus in West Africa, the original virus became HIV-1. The virus thus currently exits in two forms: commonly HIV-1 and the less common HIV-2.

Regular physical exercise is an essential component of a healthy lifestyle. The health benefits of regular participation in exercise are well established. Public awareness about these benefits and promotion of participation in exercise activities has led to many young people taking part in sports of all types (contact and non-contact).

However, the HIV pandemic has continued to rise in alarming proportions, especially in sub-Saharan Africa. Sub-Saharan Africa has just over 10% of the world's population but has well over 60% of all people living with HIV. The highest prevalence of HIV is in young adults (15–35 years) who form the majority of participants in competitive sports. The association between physical activity and HIV infection can therefore not be ignored. In particular, the following issues need consideration:

• Prevalence of HIV/AIDS in sport;
• Risk of transmission during sports participation;
• Effect of the HIV infection on sports performance; and
• Effect of regular physical activity on the disease process or clinical outcome.

PREVALENCE OF HIV/AIDS IN SPORTS

There are at present no epidemiologic data on the prevalence of HIV/AIDS in athletes. However, the global prevalence rate of HIV is about 1.1%, while the prevalence in selected geographic areas is higher. In sub-Saharan Africa the prevalence of HIV is about 7.4%, while in specific countries in southern Africa the prevalence is estimated to be at least 25%. It is also well established that the majority of those infected are young adults (15–35 years), and that young women are disproportionately at risk of HIV infection compared to young men.

It could therefore be assumed that athletes in sub-Saharan Africa, in particular southern Africa, have a high prevalence of HIV. This statement is based the assumption that:

• Athletes fall into the age category 15–35 years;
• Risk behavior for HIV in athletes is no different from that of their peers in the same age category; and
• Participation in sports does not put athletes at any higher or lower risk of contracting HIV.

In two studies the prevalence of HIV in athletes has been reported. In one study amongst National Football League (NFL) players in the USA, the prevalence of HIV was estimated to be 0.5% which is similar to the estimated prevalence rate for northern America (0.5%). In another study in boxers from South Africa, the prevalence of HIV in over 900 boxers tested in 1995 was determined to be 9%. It is clear that more accurate data on the HIV prevalence amongst sports people is required.

RISK OF TRANSMISSION OF HIV DURING SPORTING ACTIVITY

Prior to 1989, there has been no documentation of HIV infection occurring as a result of participation in sports. However, the theoretical possibility of HIV transmission through open bleeding wounds in contact sports has been recognized by sports physicians. The first case of possible HIV transmission as a result of sports participation was published in 1990. This involved an Italian soccer player in whom HIV seroconversion was documented weeks after a traumatic incident during a soccer match. During the soccer match the player collided with another player who was later documented as being HIV seropositive. Both players sustained open bleeding wounds at the eyebrows resulting in possible mixing of blood. There was no indication that the player may have been infected through any other route of HIV transmission. The authors concluded that this was the first case of HIV transmission that occurred directly as a result of sports participation. Although this case report has been criticized on epidemiologic grounds, it nevertheless has clear implications for the risk of HIV transmission during sports participation. In particular, those sports people who participate in contact sports such as boxing, wrestling, rugby, and soccer are potentially at risk.

It must be emphasized that to date no cases of HIV transmission have been recorded in either the sporting or the non-sporting population through contact with saliva, social contact, or sharing facilities such as living space, toilets, bathrooms, eating and cooking facilities. It must also be borne in mind that the risk of HIV infection in sports people is the same as that in the general population if there is a history of engaging in well-established high risk behaviors for HIV transmission.

Although there is documentation of only a single possible case of HIV disease as a result of sports participation in contact sports, there is a need to establish clear guidelines for the prevention of HIV transmission during sports participation. As early as 1989, the International Sports Medicine Federation (FIMS), together with the World Health Organization (WHO), published guidelines for the prevention of HIV transmission during contact sport (WHO position statement 1989). Subsequently, other organizations such as the Australian Sports Medicine Federation, the American Academy of Pediatrics, and the NFL in the USA have published similar guidelines.

The question that is foremost in the minds of sports administrators and participants is: what is the risk of HIV transmission in sport? In answer to this, there are no epidemiologic data available to date to calculate the risk of HIV transmission during sports participation. At best, a theoretical risk of transmission in a sport can be calculated by considering the following variables:
- Estimated carrier rate of HIV in the sports participants (% participants who are HIV positive);
- Estimated chance of an open bleeding wound in a sports participant (incidence of open bleeding wounds);
- Estimated chance of two players with open bleeding wounds making contact that could result in blood to abrasion or blood to mucous membrane exposure (incidence of physical contact between two participants);
- Estimated chance of transmission of the virus when infected blood makes contact with an open bleeding wound (estimated to be 0.3–0.5% which is similar to that calculated for a needlestick injury).

If all the above data are available for a particular sport, the estimated risk of HIV transmission can be calculated using the following formula:

$$\text{Risk} = \text{Seroprevalence of HIV (\%)} \times \text{Risk of open bleeding wound (\%)} \times \text{Risk of contact with a bleeding player (\%)} \times 0.03^*$$

At present, data are only available for American football and professional boxers in South Africa. In American football, the risk of HIV transmission in a game has been calculated as 0.0000000104. This can be translated to approximately one player becoming infected per 100 million games. Clearly, this is a very low risk and is probably the reason why there is no widespread documentation of HIV infection in American football players. However, it must be pointed out that the seroprevalence in American football players was estimated to be 0.5%, and that both the risk of an open bleeding wound (0.9%) and the risk of contact between players (7.7%) were low. These estimates will differ between different populations (higher seroprevalence) and sports (higher risks of bleeding and player contact). For instance, in a boxing fight of 12 rounds, the risk of an open bleeding wound has been documented as 47%. In 1995, the prevalence of HIV disease in one study of

---

* Estimated to be similar to the risk of seroconversion after a needlestick injury.

952 boxers in South Africa was determined as 9%, and the risk of contact between boxers during a fight is 100%. The risk of seroconversion in professional South African boxers has been calculated as 0.00021 or 1 in 4760 fights. If we were to recalculate the risk using the current prevalence rate of 25%, the risk of seroconversion in professional boxers in South Africa would be 0.000583 or 1 in 1714 fights. This is considerably higher than the previous estimate in 1995 and the calculated risk in American football. The risk of seroconversion after contact between two boxers may also be higher than that of a needlestick injury for at least two reasons:

1 Blood may be forced into the wound by the nature of the blow; and
2 Contact may be repetitive.

PREVENTION OF HIV DISEASE IN ATHLETES

Despite the lack of accurate scientific data in other contact sports, the prevention of HIV disease in sports people has to be addressed by establishing clear guidelines for sports participants, administrators, and medical personnel involved in sport.

Role of the team physician

The preseason or preparticipation examination (PPE) presents the team physician with an excellent opportunity to interact closely with the athlete. Physicians must take advantage of this time to counsel and educate athletes on HIV/AIDS:

• Athletes must be educated on all aspects of HIV, including transmission, consequences of being infected, and, most importantly, prevention.
• It must be made clear to athletes that risk of transmission is greater off the field than on the field. Physicians must therefore educate the athletes on risk behavior off the field.
• All athletes in whom HIV testing is advisable or indicated must be counseled fully.
• All tests must be voluntary and preceded by informed consent. Under no circumstances should the athlete be coerced to submit to testing.
• There should also be post-test counseling of all athletes irrespective of the result.
• All those who test negative must be counseled to remain negative.

Athletes with HIV infection present a slightly different challenge to the team physician. The challenge is to ensure that the disease is closely monitored, contained, and not spread to others who might be in close contact (on or off the field) and to also ensure that continued participation in sports does not worsen the condition. It is also necessary to monitor performance to ensure that it is not negatively affected by the disease state (Table 10.10).

Medical personnel can assist in preventing the transmission of HIV disease in sports people are by treating all open skin lesions sustained during sports participation appropriately before allowing the sports person to return to the playing field (Table 10.11).

The team physician also has a duty to educate sports administrators, including coaches, trainers,

Table 10.10 Guidelines for the team physician in caring for the HIV infected athlete.

Athletes must be adequately counseled on HIV disease
Initially, the severity of the disease must be determined by assessing the clinical state and baseline CD4 count and viral load
Ensure that athletes get adequate nutrition (as with all other athletes)
Assess intake of nutritional supplements and where necessary advice accordingly – ensure safety against inadvertent doping
Avoid overtraining and advice on the safe intensity of exercise. The athlete (and where possible the trainer) should fully understand the effects of, especially, strenuous exercise on the HIV disease state
Ensure confidentiality at all times. While it may be necessary to disclose to the coach or trainer, this should only be at the full consent of the athlete
Continue to closely monitor the disease progression or clinical status of the athlete
Perform serial immune monitoring tests (CD4 count and viral load)
In those athletes on anti-retroviral (ARV) therapy, monitor side effects that may potentially negatively affect performance

Table 10.11 Suggested treatment of open skin lesions to prevent transmission of HIV in sports.

Immediate cleaning of the wound with a suitable antiseptic such as hypochloride (bleach, Milton), 2% gluteraldehyde (Cidex), organic iodines or 70% alcohol (ethyl alcohol, isopropyl alcohol)
The open wound should be covered securely prior to returning to the playing field, so that there is no risk of exposure to blood or blood products
All sports clothing or equipment stained with blood must be cleaned or changed before allowing further participation
It is recommended that all first aiders and medical personnel attending to sports people with open wound lesions wear protective gloves to decrease the risk of HIV transmission to themselves and other sports persons

and managers, on all aspects of HIV disease, especially prevention. When traveling with athletes, always carry enough condoms to be made available to athletes, especially where there is a possibility of social events.

HIV INFECTION AND EXERCISE PERFORMANCE

In analyzing the relationship between HIV infection and exercise or physical performance, studies in medical literature can be categorized as follows:
• Effects of HIV on physical performance;
• Effect of training on physical performance in the HIV infected athlete; and
• Effect of regular exercise on the clinical outcome of HIV.

There are very few studies that address the effect of HIV infection on exercise performance. One study characterized physical performance in ambulatory patients with HIV (Simmonds et al. 2005). In this study, 100 ambulatory patients (78 male and 22 female) were subjected to a battery of physical performance tests wherein the time taken or the distance reached or walked was measured. These subjects were compared with an age-matched control group without HIV infection. Results showed that physical performance in patients with HIV was compromised in a task-specific manner. The compromise in physical performance was apparently a result of pain (in 50% of subjects at the time of testing) and fatigue (98% of subjects).

In another study, exercise performance was investigated in 32 patients with a clinical diagnosis of AIDS with dyspnea on exertion and no evidence of significant cardiopulmonary or other complicating medical disorder. Subjects and an age, weight,

and height-matched control were subjected to an incremental physical exercise test to exhaustion during which cardiopulmonary variables were measured. Results and conclusions from the study were that patients with documented AIDS had significantly impaired exercise capacity thought to be a result of a central cardiac limitation. The possibility of a direct effect of the HIV infection or its complications on muscle function was not considered.

In another study, exercise testing was included as part of a clinical trial evaluating the effectiveness of corticosteroids on *Pneumocystis carinii* pneumonia in AIDS patients (Montaner et al. 1990). In this study, AIDS patients with *Pneumocystis* pneumonia were randomly allocated to either an experimental (receiving corticosteroids) or a control (receiving placebo) group and then monitored for 4 weeks. A maximal incremental exercise test was performed on days 0, 3, 7, 14, and 30. Effort tolerance was very poor in both groups on day 0. After treatment, the exercise tolerance improved sevenfold in the treatment group whereas it remained the same in the control group. This positive effect was attributed to the prevention of early clinical deterioration by the administration of corticosteroids in the treatment group. It is obvious that this study was not primarily aimed at investigating effort tolerance in these patients. However, the results do indicate that physical work is severely impaired in AIDS patients with associated *Pneumocystis* infection and that this can be improved by appropriate therapy.

In summary, the few studies on the effect of HIV infection on exercise performance show that physical performance in these patients is impaired but the precise mechanism is unclear.

Effect of training on physical performance in the HIV infected athlete

Fewer studies have looked at the effect of exercise training on physical performance in patients with HIV infection. The use of both aerobic and resistance exercise has been shown to improve physiologic parameters such as strength, endurance, time to fatigue, and body composition in the HIV infected population (Dudgeon *et al.* 2004).

Another study examined the effect of aerobic exercise on physiologic fatigue (measured by time on treadmill), dyspnea measured by rate of perceived exertion (RPE), forced expiratory volume in 1 second (FEV_1), weight, and body composition in the HIV-infected individual (Smith *et al.* 2001). Sixty subjects were randomized into two groups, an experimental group who completed a 12-week supervised aerobic exercise program, and a control group who continued their usual activities from baseline to week 12, after which they were enrolled into an exercise program. The experimental group was able to exercise longer on the treadmill, lost weight, showed a decreased body mass index (BMI), subcutaneous fat, and abdominal girth when compared with controls. The improvement in weight and body composition occurred without a decrease in kilocalories consumed.

The use of anabolic steroids has been shown to improve the benefits of resistance training in individuals with AIDS wasting syndrome (AWS; Mulligan *et al.* 2005). This will have legal and ethical implications in sport and the need to apply for a therapeutic use exemption (TUE) would have to be considered against the need for patient confidentiality. For a TUE to be granted there needs to be full disclosure by the applicant. The conclusion that can be drawn from these studies is that the compromised exercise performance in the HIV infected athlete can be improved by aerobic and resistance exercise training.

Effect of regular physical activity or exercise on the clinical outcome of HIV infection

It is a well-documented fact that HIV infection affects the immune system directly. If exercise has an effect on the immune system, it can be deduced that exercise and the HIV infection will both have a concomitant effect which may either have a beneficial or deleterious effect on the immune system. In general, exercise that is of moderate intensity and duration stresses the immune system less than more prolonged and intense exercise bouts. It appears that the function of neutrophils is suppressed during periods of heavy exercise training. Fewer studies have documented the response to long-term effects of exercise training. The only documented effect of long-term exercise training is the elevation of NK cell activity.

Changes in the lymphocyte subset show a greater increase in B cells than T cells and a greater increase in T4 cells than T8 cells, thereby decreasing the T4 : T8 ratio. This has implications in HIV infected athletes. Of importance is the response of the CD4 : CD8 ratio to exercise training. Researchers have recently concentrated on the effects of regular exercise training on the clinical outcome of HIV infection. However, there is a paucity of studies that have documented the effect of exercise on the long-term clinical outcome of HIV infection. However, it appears that moderate physical activity may be beneficial in the HIV infected person by slowing down disease progression.

Studies have shown that the use of both aerobic an anaerobic resistance exercise improve such physiologic parameters as strength, endurance, time to fatigue, and body composition in the HIV infected athlete. Exercise has also been used to treat psychologic conditions such a depression and anxiety common among those with HIV infection (Dudgeon *et al.* 2004). Although the effects of exercise on the immunologic parameters have shown varied results, it appears that exercise may result in an increase in the CD4+ T-cell count. This is seen mostly with an exercise regimen of interval aerobic training of at least 20–30 min duration, performed at least three times per week for 4 weeks. More benefit is seen in sustained exercise programs (Nixon *et al.* 2005). It has also been shown that exercise may have a beneficial role in viral load in those with HIV infection. An inverse relationship has been shown between physical activity and viral load (Bopp *et al.* 2004).

Table 10.12 Potential beneficial effects of exercise in the HIV infected athlete.

Stage I
Increased CD4 cells
Possible delay in onset of symptoms
Increase in muscle function and size

Stage II
Increase in CD4 cells (lesser magnitude of change)
Possible diminished severity and frequency of some
  symptoms

Stage III
Effects on CD4 cells are not known
Effects on symptoms are inconclusive

There are very few data available on the effects of exercise in patients on highly active anti-retroviral therapy (HAART). Work in this area is severely limited by the small sample sizes and the high dropout rate from studies. However, exercise has been listed as a popular adjunctive therapy to counteract adverse effects of HAART such as nausea, fatigue, pain, anxiety, and depression (Table 10.12; Ciccolo *et al.* 2004).

The effects of exercise on the clinical outcome of HIV infection and the effects of HIV infection on physical performance have practical implications in athletes with HIV infection. The challenge is to achieve a balance between maintaining optimum physical fitness and performance without advancing the progression of the disease. A basic understanding of these effects will help in developing guidelines for exercise prescription in those with HIV infection.

GUIDELINES FOR EXERCISE PARTICIPATION IN THE HIV INFECTED ATHLETE

General guidelines

All HIV infected athletes, regardless of age, sex, or stage of disease, must have a comprehensive PPE before exercise prescription or any advice on a training program. Baseline and serial immune monitoring tests should be carried out to assess the severity and monitor progression of the disease. The PPE must also be used to counsel the athlete on the HIV infection.

Ideally, an integrated cardiopulmonary exercise test with gas exchange measurements should be performed before an exercise prescription in any HIV infected individual to exclude subtle cardiopulmonary markers of occult infection, anemia, myopathies, etc., and should be performed before designing an exercise prescription. American College of Sports Medicine (ACSM) guidelines on physical testing and exercise prescription should always be complied with.

During training and sports participation, guidelines on prevention should always apply. For example, all open bleeding wounds and septic sores to be appropriately treated before contact with others.

Specific guidelines

These guidelines are discussed according to the different stages in HIV disease (Stages I–III).

Stage I – Asymptomatic At this stage there is no need to restrict sports participation and competition. The only consideration would be the health and well-being of the athlete, fellow team mates, supportive staff, fans, followers, and admirers. The challenge would be to ensure that the disease is contained and not spread to others, stable, and not accelerated by participation in sports. The PPE should include counseling, education, and life skills mentoring. Nutrition should be assessed and, where indicated, appropriate supplements should be recommended or prescribed.

Even though training is unrestricted, it is important that athletes try by all means to avoid overtraining. It is at this stage that the clinician must have cooperation and empathy from the coach or trainer. All training and exercise prescriptions should be discussed with the trainer or coach. The athlete's right to strict confidentiality should always be respected. This right to confidentiality will always be a challenge to the physician, especially when having to advise against too much high intensity training and/or overtraining with the trainer or coach.

In summary, guidelines for this stage are:
• Unrestricted training or competition;
• Close monitoring of the disease process; and
• Avoid overtraining.

Stage II – Early symptomatic Exercise at this stage should be limited by symptoms. Strenuous exercise, at intensities more than 80% of maximum heart rate, should be avoided at all costs. Athletes may have to reconsider participation in competitive sports as training and sports participation at this level is often strenuous. All training should be curtailed or stopped during periods of acute illness. Athletes should only resume normal training after clearance by the team physician. This would normally be after complete resolution of the illness with no residual symptoms. Individuals with HIV-associated muscle wasting may benefit from treatment with anabolic steroids (Mulligan *et al.* 2005). The use of these agents in professional sports persons requires a TUE. There are very few data available on exercise in those on ARV therapy. However, the following are adverse effects or signs of toxicity that may potentially negatively affect performance:

- Nausea, vomiting, diarrhea;
- Myopathy/peripheral neuropathy;
- Anemia;
- Lactic acidosis;
- Light headedness, anxiety, depression; and
- Severe rash (Steven–Johnson's)
  In summary, guidelines for Stage II are:
- Continue exercise on a symptom-limited basis;
- Curtail or stop exercise during periods of acute illness; and
- Avoid strenuous exercise;

Stage III – Full-blown AIDS Sports participation at this end-stage of the disease is not possible. Individuals are advised to remain physically active on a symptom-limited basis. Strenuous exercise should be avoided at all costs. There should be no exercise during periods of acute illness.

Infections of the central nervous system

Meningitis

Bacterial meningitis is a serious and potentially fatal infection that is associated with a high rate of neurologic complications (75%) and generally poor outcome despite treatment with appropriate antibiotics. Even in healthy individuals and athletes, untreated bacterial meningitis can rapidly progress to a fatal outcome. Aseptic meningitis is generally associated with a more benign course but unusual etiologies such as *Mycobacterium tuberculosis* and herpes simplex virus are associated with greater morbidity (Hosey & Rodenberg 2005).

The majority of the reported cases of meningitis outbreaks amongst sporting groups or at sports gatherings have been aseptic. These have generally been confined to team sports such as soccer and American football where individuals share infected water sources such as water bottles, ice, or liquid containers. Two outbreaks of *Neisseria meningitis* have been reported at an international soccer tournament and in a group of rugby players from a rugby club (Turbeville *et al.* 2006).

The primary pathogens responsible for aseptic meningitis are the enteroviruses (echoviruses 5, 9, 16 and 24; coxsackie A, B1, B2, B4 and B5 viruses; polio viruses; and enteroviruses). Of these, the enteroviruses are responsible for the majority of infections, are the most commonly isolated pathogen, and cause infections during the summer and early autumn months. Other viral causes of aseptic meningitis (e.g., measles, mumps, rubella, herpes viruses, HIV) and non-viral causes including fungal infections (*Cryptococcus*, histoplasmosis, blastomycosis, coccidiomycosis), protozoal and other bacterial etiologies (*Rickettsia*, *Mycobacterium*, *Mycoplasma*, *Lysteria monocytogenes*, and *Brucella*) should be considered in aseptic cases (Hosey & Todenberg 2005; Turbeville *et al.* 2006).

The patient's history may reveal clues to the possible etiology and should include age, exposure to cases of meningitis and tuberculosis (TB), traveling history and exposure to arthropod vectors, medical history, and use of medications. Pretreatment of bacterial meningitis with antibiotics may result in vague symptoms and an indolent course. The patient may present with the classic triad of fever, headache, and neck stiffness but this triad of symptoms may only be present in half of patients older than 16 years (Hosey & Todenberg 2005). Other non-specific symptoms include nausea, vomiting, pharyngitis, diarrhea, photophobia, and focal neurologic signs.

Table 10.13 Cerebrospinal fluid (CSF) characteristics in meningitis (From Longmore *et al.* 2004, p. 364.)

	Septic	Aseptic	TB meningitis
WCC	>1000·mm^{-3}	50–1500·mm^{-3}	10–1500·mm^{-3}
WC characteristics	Polymorphonuclear	Mononuclear/ polymorphonuclear	Mononuclear/ polymorphonuclear
CSF/serum glucose	<50%	>60%	<50%
Protein	>1.5 g·L^{-1}	<1.5 g·L^{-1}	1–5 g·L^{-1}

TB, tuberculosis; WC, white (blood) cell; WCC, white cell count.

Physical examination may reveal a febrile patient with varying alterations in level of consciousness and a characteristic rash specific to the offending agent. There may be focal neurologic signs as a result of encephalitis or mass shifts. Specific signs of meningeal irritation include Brudzinski's and Kernig's signs.

Cerebrospinal fluid (CSF) should be sent for analysis to distinguish between aseptic and septic causes of meningitis. Absolute indications for neuroimaging prior to lumbar puncture include depressed or deteriorating level of consciousness, papilloedema, focal neurologic signs, or unstable blood pressure and heart rate. Blood cultures should be obtained and treatment with age-appropriate broad-spectrum antibiotics should commence prior to neuroimaging.

CSF analysis should include cell counts, protein, glucose, Gram stain, culture, and sensitivity screening. Additional investigations include polymerase chain reaction studies for specific viral and bacterial etiologies. Previously, an overemphasis has been placed on the mononuclear CSF pleocytosis in aseptic meningitis. In a recent study, over 50% of cases with aseptic meningitis had a polymorphonuclear predominance at 24 h post-presentation. The presence of polymorphonuclear white cells should therefore not be used as a sole criterion in distinguishing bacterial from aseptic meningitis (Negrini *et al.* 2000). CSF findings for specific etiologies are summarized in Table 10.13.

Specific treatment of meningitis is based on the etiology. Age-appropriate broad-spectrum empiric antibiotics should not be discontinued until a bacterial etiology has been ruled out. Herpes simplex virus meningitis is treated with IV acyclovir. Non-viral causes of aseptic meningitis are treated as dictated by the specific etiology (TB, *Cryptococcus*). Treatment for other viral causes of aseptic meningitis is supportive (Hosey & Rodenberg 2005).

Athletes traveling to areas of the world where meningococcal infection is endemic should consider vaccination with the meningococcal quadrivalent vaccine, MPSV-4 (Menomune; A,C,Y,W-135). In addition, individuals with asplenia or terminal complement deficiency or individuals living in dormitories should also consider vaccination. Prevention of viral aseptic meningitis should include good handwashing practice and reducing shared water or fluid sources (Hosey & Rodenberg 2005).

Genitourinary tract infections

A detailed discussion of sexually transmitted infections is beyond the scope of this chapter; however, team physicians need to be aware that localized infections of the genitourinary tract can occur in athletes, in particular female athletes. The correct choice of underwear is important to prevent infections such as vaginitis or urethritis. Localized vaginitis without signs of pelvic inflammatory disease can be treated by local or topical application of antimicrobial agents. Full athletic activity can be continued throughout the treatment period. In the case of more regional infections such as cystitis or pelvic inflammatory disease systemic, antimicrobial agents are indicated and athletic activity should be restricted until full resolution of symptoms.

Immunization in athletes

There are a number of important considerations with respect to vaccinations in athletes. First, it is important that all athletes are properly vaccinated when traveling to countries for competition; vaccination against cholera and yellow fever are particularly important. Second, all athletes, in particular those participating in contact sports, must be vaccinated against tetanus and hepatitis A and B. Athletes should also be well educated about HIV transmission. Finally, athletes must be aware that it is advisable to restrict athletic activity for 2–3 days after vaccination because of minor systemic inflammation.

References

Auwaerter, P.G. (2004) Infectious mononucleosis: return to play. *Clinics in Sports Medicine* **23**, 485–497, xi.

Baj, Z., Kantorski, J., Majewska, E., Zeman, K., Pokoca, L., Fornalczyk, E., *et al.* (1994) Immunological status of competitive cyclists before and after the training season. *International Journal of Sports Medicine* **15**, 319–324.

Beck, C.K. (2000) Infectious diseases in sports. *Medicine and Science in Sports and Exercise* **32**, S431–S438.

Bopp, C.M., Phillips, K.D., Fulk, L.J., Dudgeon, W.D., Sowell, R. & Hand, G.A. (2004) Physical activity and immunity in HIV-infected individuals. *AIDS Care* **16**, 387–393.

Brenner, I., Shek, P.N., Zamecnik, J. & Shephard, R.J. (1998) Stress hormones and the immunological responses to heat and exercise. *International Journal of Sports Medicine* **19**, 130–143.

Chao, C.C., Strgar, F., Tsang, M. & Peterson, P.K. (1992) Effects of swimming exercise on the pathogenesis of acute murine *Toxoplasma gondii* Me49 infection. *Clinical Immunology and Immunopathology* **62**, 220–226.

Ciccolo, J.T., Jowers, E.M. & Bartholomew, J.B. (2004) The benefits of exercise training for quality of life in HIV/AIDS in the post-HAART era. *Sports Medicine* **34**, 487–499.

Dorman, J.M. (2000) Contagious diseases in competitive sport: what are the risks? *Journal of American College Health* **49**, 105–109.

Dudgeon, W.D., Phillips, K.D., Bopp, C.M. & Hand, G.A. (2004) Physiological and psychological effects of exercise interventions in HIV disease. *AIDS Patient Care and STDS* **18**, 81–98.

Friman, G. & Wesslen, L. (2000) Special feature for the Olympics: effects of exercise on the immune system – infections and exercise in high-performance athletes. *Immunology and Cell Biology* **78**, 510–522.

Gani, F., Passalacqua, G., Senna, G. & Mosca, F.M. (2003) Sport, immune system and respiratory infections. *Allergie et Immunologie (Paris)* **35**, 41–46.

Gleeson, M. & Pyne, D.B. (2000) Special feature for the Olympics: effects of exercise on the immune system – exercise effects on mucosal immunity. *Immunology and Cell Biology* **78**, 536–544.

Gleeson, M., Pyne, D.B. & Callister, R. (2004) The missing links in exercise effects on mucosal immunity. *Exercise and Immunology Reviews* **10**, 107–128.

Harrington, D.W. (2000) Viral hepatitis and exercise. *Medicine and Science in Sports and Exercise* **32**, S422–S430.

Ho-Yen, D.O. & Martin, K.W. (1981) The relationship between atypical lymphocytosis and serological tests in infectious mononucleosis. *Journal of Infection* **3**, 324–331.

Hosey, R.G. & Rodenberg, R.E. (2005) Training room management of medical conditions: infectious diseases. *Clinics in Sports Medicine* **24**, 477–506, vii.

Jeans, A.K. (2003) Tropical infections in athletes: malaria, schistosomiasis and African tick bite fever. ISMJ **4**. http://www.ismj.com

Kordi, R. & Wallace, W.A. (2004) Blood borne infections in sport: risks of transmission, methods of prevention, and recommendations for hepatitis B vaccination. *British Journal of Sports Medicine* **38**, 678–684.

Lakier, S.L. (2003) Overtraining, excessive exercise, and altered immunity: is this a T helper-1 versus T helper-2 lymphocyte response? *Sports Medicine* **33**, 347–364.

Longmore, M., Wilkinson, I.B. & Rajagopalan, S.R. (2004) *Oxford Handbook of Clinical Medicine*, 6th edn. Oxford University Press, Oxford.

Mackinnon, L.T. (2000) Special feature for the Olympics: effects of exercise on the immune system – overtraining effects on immunity and performance in athletes.

Immunology and Cell Biology **78**, 502–509.

Mackinnon, L.T. & Hooper, S. (1994) Mucosal (secretory) immune system responses to exercise of varying intensity and during overtraining. *International Journal of Sports Medicine* **15** (Supplement 3), S179–S183.

Mackinnon, L.T. & Jenkins, D.G. (1993) Decreased salivary immunoglobulins after intense interval exercise before and after training. *Medicine and Science in Sports and Exercise* **25**, 678–683.

Malm, C. (2004) Exercise immunology: the current state of man and mouse. *Sports Medicine* **34**, 555–566.

Montaner, J.S., Lawson, L.M., Levitt, N., Belzberg, A., Schechter, M.T. & Ruedy, J. (1990) Corticosteroids prevent early deterioration in patients with moderately severe *Pneumocystis carinii* pneumonia and the acquired immunodeficiency syndrome (AIDS). *Annals of Internal Medicine* **113**, 14–20.

Mulligan, K., Zackin, R., Clark, R.A., Alston-Smith, B., Liu, T., Sattler, F.R., *et al.* (2005) Effect of nandrolone decanoate therapy on weight and lean body mass in HIV-infected women with weight loss: a randomized, double-blind, placebo-controlled, multicenter trial. *Archives of Internal Medicine* **165**, 578–585.

Negrini, B., Kelleher, K.J. & Wald, E.R. (2000) Cerebrospinal fluid findings in aseptic versus bacterial meningitis. *Pediatrics* **105**, 316–319.

Nehlsen-Cannarella, S.L., Nieman, D.C., Fagoaga, O.R., Kelln, W.J., Henson, D.A., Shannon, M., *et al.* (2000) Saliva immunoglobulins in elite women rowers. *European Journal of Applied Physiology* **81**, 222–228.

Nieman, D.C. (2000) Special feature for the Olympics: effects of exercise on the immune system – exercise effects on systemic immunity. *Immunology and Cell Biology* **78**, 496–501.

Nieman, D.C. (2003) Current perspective on exercise immunology. *Current Sports Medicine Reports* **2**, 239–242.

Nixon, S., O'Brien, K., Glazier, R.H. & Tynan, A.M. (2005) Aerobic exercise interventions for adults living with HIV/AIDS. *Cochrane Database System Review* CD001796.

Pedersen, B.K. (2000) Special feature for the Olympics: effects of exercise on the immune system – exercise and cytokines. *Immunology and Cell Biology* **78**, 532–535.

Pedersen, B.K. & Ullum, H. (1994) NK cell response to physical activity: possible mechanisms of action. *Medicine and Science in Sports and Exercise* **26**, 140–146.

Roland, P.S. & Marple, B.F. (1997) Disorders of the external auditory canal. *Journal of the American Academy of Audiology* **8**, 367–378.

Shephard, R.J. (2000) Special feature for the Olympics: effects of exercise on the immune system – overview of the epidemiology of exercise immunology. *Immunology and Cell Biology* **78**, 485–495.

Shephard, R.J., Kavanagh, T., Mertens, D.J., Qureshi, S. & Clark, M. (1995) Personal health benefits of Masters athletics competition. *British Journal of Sports Medicine* **29**, 35–40.

Simmonds, M.J., Novy, D. & Sandoval, R. (2005) The differential influence of pain and fatigue on physical performance and health status in ambulatory patients with human immunodeficiency virus. *Clinical Journal of Pain* **21**, 200–206.

Smith, B.A., Neidig, J.L., Nickel, J.T., Mitchell, G.L., Para, M.F. & Fass, R.J. (2001) Aerobic exercise: effects on parameters related to fatigue, dyspnea, weight and body composition in HIV-infected adults. *AIDS* **15**, 693–701.

Tomasi, T.B., Trudeau, F.B., Czerwinski, D. & Erredge, S. (1982) Immune parameters in athletes before and after strenuous exercise. *Journal of Clinical Immunology* **2**, 173–178.

Turbeville, S.D., Cowan, L.D. & Greenfield, R.A. (2006) Infectious disease outbreaks in competitive sports: a review of the literature. *American Journal of Sports Medicine* **34**, 1860–1865.

Chapter 11

Gastrointestinal System and Exercise: A Clinical Approach to Gastrointestinal Problems Encountered in Athletes

MARTIN P. SCHWELLNUS AND JOHN WRIGHT

Exercise helps to throw down wind from the bowels and attenuates the contents of the stomach. It also serves as an evacuant, and a diversion by which artifices the humours are put into condition of flying off without the danger of bringing on spasms.

A Treatise of the Science of Muscular Action
(John Puch, 1794)

Many athletes have experienced the extreme frustration of a poor performance in an important sports event as a result of gastrointestinal (gastrointestinal tract) symptoms. Others have experienced the inability to train optimally because of a chronic gastrointestinal tract problem. The team physician is often the person that a frustrated athlete consults to alleviate such a so-called "trivial" problem. The aim of this chapter is to review normal gastrointestinal physiology, the pathophysiology of gastrointestinal distress in athletes, the epidemiology of gastrointestinal symptoms in athletes, and the clinical approach to the diagnosis and management of these symptoms in athletes.

Normal gastrointestinal physiology

In order to understand the pathophysiology of gastrointestinal symptoms in athletes, a basic review of normal gastrointestinal physiology is essential. It is important to understand that physiologic systems

The Olympic Textbook of Medicine in Sport, 1st edition. Edited by M. Schwellnus. Published 2008 by Blackwell Publishing, ISBN: 978-1-4051-5637-0.

in humans have been in place for over 3 million years. The eating habits of an athlete and the stresses on the gastrointestinal tract during maximum physical performance are two important components that can alter gastrointestinal physiology, and be responsible for symptoms.

Normal physiology of digestion

A brief review of the physiology of digestion starts with the understanding that at the thought of eating, salivation and gastric acid production starts. This is a short-lived reflex if no food is ingested. If food is swallowed, the lower section of the stomach – the antrum – secretes the hormone gastrin, while the first section of the duodenum secretes the hormones secretin and cholecystokinin. The plasma concentrations of these hormones peak at about 30 min after the meal starts. Gastrin increases gastric acid output, while the duodenal hormones stimulate the pancreas and the liver, causing the gallbladder to contract. In addition, there is a secondary action on the colonic motility resulting in an urge to defecate.

During food ingestion and throughout a 24-h period gastric contents continuously reflux into the esophagus. Physical factors such as gastric distension and posture (bending forwards), can increase this reflux. As soon as this reflux is detected, salivary glands produce saliva and swallowing occurs. Swallowing washes the esophageal content back into the stomach and neutralizes the acid component. However, during swallowing air is always included in the salivary "bolus," and while the air

365

is normally absorbed by the gastrointestinal tract, excessive swallowing can take place, in which case air is "belched" back out again. This can occur under conditions of emotional stress or when there is constant irritation of the distal esophagus by acid.

Once the acidified food leaves the stomach the process of digestion takes place. Minimal digestion would have taken place in the stomach as the digestive enzymes made by the stomach are destroyed by the gastric acid. One exception is alcohol, and 20% of the ingested alcohol may by metabolized by alcohol dehydrogenase in the gastric mucosa. The rate that food (now called chyme) leaves the stomach depends on a number of factors, including gastric volume, osmolarity, fat content, and the size of food particles. Energy concentration is also monitored so that the absorptive capacity of the small bowel is not overwhelmed.

Normal physiology of absorption

The three food components of carbohydrate, fat, and protein are digested and absorbed by different mechanisms. Complex carbohydrates (starches) are broken down to their constituent molecules by enzymes in the intestinal wall. The components (glucose, fructose, and lactose) are then absorbed across the gut wall by specific processes. These are often potentiated by the presence of salt. Generally, carbohydrate is absorbed in the first 50 cm of the 300 cm small bowel. If for some reason carbohydrate is not absorbed in the small bowel, there is no built-in control features to prevent this carbohydrate entering the colon where it will be fermented by colonic bacteria.

Fat absorption is more complex and tightly controlled. Enzymes from the pancreas and bile from the liver are added to the chyme. Bile is the main "waste product" of metabolism and is secreted from the liver. It contains bile salts, the breakdown products of cholesterol, which has a vital final function to render fats miscible. Fats are then broken down by pancreatic enzymes to fatty acids which are absorbed into the lymphatic ducts. Medium-chain fatty acids are absorbed directly into the villi without "digestion." Fat absorption can be a slow process and the full length of the small bowel may

be needed to absorb a fatty meal. If undigested fat should reach the end of the small bowel, the hormone motilin is released with the specific role of preventing fat loss. This hormone decreases gastric emptying, delays small bowel motility, and stimulates colonic emptying.

Protein absorption relies heavily on the enzymes secreted by the pancreas. Trypsinogen and other enzymes reduce proteins to their component peptides and amino acids which are then rapidly absorbed in the first few centimeters of the small intestine. Protein malabsorption is rare, unless the pancreatic enzymes are deficient.

It is important to note that the pancreas has a central role in the absorption of all food types except for the base component parts such as monosaccharides (glucose, lactose, and fructose), amino acids and fatty acids (excluding medium-chain fatty acids). However, the pancreas secretes large amounts of digestive enzymes, and there has to be a reduction in enzyme secretion of approximately 90% before clinical malabsorption occurs. This is a rare and serious condition most often seen following pancreatitis induced by excessive alcohol consumption over a period of time.

The absorption of vitamins and trace elements takes place throughout the small bowel. If intake is adequate, absorption is quick and efficient. The only exceptions are iron and vitamin B_{12}. Iron absorption requires an acid environment in the stomach to change the iron from the ferrous to ferric ion. Vitamin B_{12} also requires carrier molecules from the stomach and pancreas to prepare it for absorption from the last few centimeters of the terminal ileum.

In general, 3–4 L of food and liquid are normally consumed a day, and to this volume the upper gastrointestinal tract adds 6–7 L. The small bowel absorbs 9 of the 10 L, leaving 1 L to enter the colon. The colon in turn absorbs about 900 mL water and electrolytes, leaving 100 mL of stool to be passed daily. The main function of the colon is to redigest the chyme entering the colon and to extract residual energy, water, and electrolytes. In order to perform this function, bacteria in the colon metabolize the residual carbohydrate to hydrogen, methane and short-chain fatty acids. These products are then absorbed by the colonic mucosa and enter the energy chain. It is of interest to note that in hindgut fermenters (e.g., horses and elephants) most of their energy is absorbed by this route but in humans only up to 10% of the energy is absorbed via the colon.

Normal physiology of defecation

Defecation normally takes place on rising in the morning and again after dinner before retiring in the evening. Colonic motility follows a diurnal rhythm, and peristalsis starts between 4 and 5 o'clock in the morning, reaching its most active phase at about 6–8 o'clock in the morning. This corresponds to the first desire to pass stool on rising in the morning. The second stool is usually passed after the main meal of the day, which for most individuals (including athletes) is in the evening. These intervals correspond roughly to the "normal" transit time of 12 h. The passage of flatus indicates a mismatch between gas production and absorption. The amount of normal stool produced per day depends on the number of bacteria in the colon. This is because 90% of stool volume is simply bacteria. The remaining 5–10% is food residue, mainly fiber, bile, and cellular debris from the colon.

Effects of exercise on gastrointestinal tract physiology

The most important function of the gastrointestinal tract is to provide the nutrition needed for the body to perform at maximum efficiency. The potential effects of an acute bout of exercise on gastrointestinal physiology is briefly reviewed. This is important, as these effects form the basis of the proposed mechanisms to explain the pathophysiology of the development of gastrointestinal symptoms during exercise.

The first effect of exercise on gastrointestinal physiology relates to bodily movement. The onset of bodily movement stimulates the sigmoid to empty (e.g., a horse defecates on leaving the paddock gate). Although many athletes report that as long as they exercise they have normal bowel function, the evidence that regular physical exercise decreases total gastrointestinal transit time is not conclusive (Rao *et al.* 2004). However, it is known that stress and anxiety can stimulate defecation and on occasion diarrhea. Many athletes therefore find it unusually easy to pass stool on rising before a big race. It has been documented that under severe physical stress, such as participation in an ultramarathon, defecation during the run can occur in as many as 40–50% of runners (Priebe *et al.* 1984; Worobetz & Gerrard 1985).

The second effect of exercise on gastrointestinal tract physiology relates to posture. In upright sports such as running and walking, gastric emptying should be enhanced, while in more horizontal sports, cycling and board surfing, esophageal reflux might be expected. Although not substantiated by well-conducted research studies, these generalizations are observed clinically.

The third effect of exercise on functions of the gastrointestinal tract has to be considered in the context of the overall "stress" response during high intensity and/or prolonged physical exercise. There are three main known effects of high intensity and/or prolonged physical exercise on the gastrointestinal tract. Acute, intense, or prolonged physical exercise can result in:

1 *A decrease in intestinal blood flow* The normal blood supply to the gut is via the superior and inferior mesenteric arteries. During high intensity or prolonged exercise sessions, there is shunting of blood away from the gut, leading to relative ischemia. There is an added danger to the gut as the ischemia is caused by the end-artery supply to the gut mucosa. Particularly vulnerable areas are the stomach and the colon. In the stomach, hemorrhagic gastritis and acute gastric ulcers may occur, while a diffusely ulcerated, bleeding mucosa may be seen in the colon. However, there is rectal sparing because of a systemic blood supply to this area.

2 *Delayed gastric emptying* This has been associated with nausea and even vomiting in some athletes.

3 *Mass peristalsis of the colon* This can cause abdominal cramping and even defecation with great urgency. It should be noted that in other functional disorders of the gastrointestinal tract, delayed gastric emptying, early satiety, and mass peristalsis are important causes of functional dyspepsia and irritable bowel syndrome, respectively.

It is important to note that exercise performed at a lower intensity or for a shorter duration is associated with a decrease in these symptoms. Furthermore, regular exercise training can also ameliorate these effects. Finally, the role of ischemia in the etiology of runner's anemia is unclear as 40% of runners finishing a marathon may have increased fecal blood loss on occult blood testing of the stool. Anecdotal evidence suggests that athletes who have noticed small amounts of blood in the stool but do not necessarily experience any symptoms, may have surprisingly widespread areas of colonic mucosal hemorrhage at colonoscopy. This disproportionate colonic damage suggests that ischemia may occur in many other runners without major symptoms developing. Further research to determine the extent of gastrointestinal ischemia during intense prolonged exercise is required.

Epidemiology of gastrointestinal distress in athletes

It is common to classify gastrointestinal tract symptoms into those that are likely to originate from the upper gastrointestinal tract, and those that are likely to originate from the lower gastrointestinal tract. Surveys on gastrointestinal tract symptoms in athletes have mostly been conducted by administering questionnaires to groups of athletes at specific race events including runners (Simons & Kennedy 2004), cyclists, triathletes, swimmers, aerobic dancers, and canoeists (Schwartz et al. 1995). The type and frequency (number of athletes with a particular symptom) of gastrointestinal tract symptoms have been recorded (Schwartz et al. 1995). A summary of the combined results from a number of these surveys is depicted in Table 11.1.

A number of observations can be made from the results in Table 11.1. First, it is obvious that athletes experience a wide variety of symptoms. Second, there is a wide variation in the frequency of the different types of symptoms experienced and, finally, it appears that lower gastrointestinal tract symptoms are by far more frequent than upper gastrointestinal tract symptoms. There is also a wide spectrum of symptoms ranging from less severe symptoms (belching and nausea) to

Table 11.1 The frequency of gastrointestinal symptoms associated with exercise (Brouns et al. 1987; Halvorsen et al. 1990; Riddoch & Trinick 1988; Sanchez et al. 2006; Schwartz et al. 1995).

Symptom	Frequency (%)
Upper gastrointestinal tract	
Loss of appetite	12–50
Heartburn	8–11
Belching	12–36
Nausea	4–21
Vomiting	4–31
Lower gastrointestinal tract	
Abdominal cramps	25–67
Urge to defecate	30–63
Bowel movement	13–51
Diarrhea	10–30
Rectal bleeding	2–12

potentially life-threatening symptoms (frank rectal bleeding).

Although the incidence of gastrointestinal symptoms appears to be very high, many athletes do not develop any symptoms at all, and of those who do, most are accepted as being minor impediments to performance. However, some athletes have possible risk factors for the development of gastrointestinal tract symptoms (Table 11.2). Some of these factors need to be taken into account when planning for events.

Pathophysiology of gastrointestinal distress in athletes

The potential effects of an acute exercise bout on gastrointestinal physiology have been reviewed (Casey et al. 2005; Gil et al. 1998; Halvorsen & Ritland 1992; Larson & Fisher 1987; Moses 1990; Murray 2006; Peters et al. 1995; Putukian & Potera 1997; Sullivan 1984). For the clinician who consults with an athlete complaining of gastrointestinal distress, it is important to note:

1 It is most unlikely that there is one single cause for gastrointestinal tract symptoms during exercise; and

2 Gastrointestinal tract symptoms during exercise may be brought about by normal causes of gastrointestinal pathology that are totally unrelated to exercise.

Table 11.2 Possible risk factors that have been associated with the development of gastrointestinal symptoms during exercise.

Female gender
Younger age
Poorly conditioned athletes
Running or jumping sports
Downhill running
High intensity exercise
Diet
Dehydration
Lactose intolerance
Previous abdominal surgery
Medication

These causes include infections, cancers, gastric or duodenal ulcers, and a variety of other well-documented gastrointestinal tract diseases. Disregarding these conditions and continuing with exercise is irresponsible to the athlete concerned as well as to family and other team members.

As previously discussed, for symptoms that are only related to exercise and not to organic disease, a number of possible etiological mechanisms have been proposed (Table 11.3). First, exercise is associated with alterations in esophageal motility, reduced gastric emptying, and increased gastroe-sophageal reflux. In addition, blood is diverted away from the gastrointestinal tract to the contracting muscle during high intensity or prolonged exercise, which may result in a relative ischemia of the mucosal lining of the gastrointestinal tract. This may be the cause of rectal bleeding in some athletes. Altered orocecal transit time may be associated with changes in posture and mechanical movement or "bouncing" of the small and large intestines, particularly during running or jumping, and this may cause lower gastrointestinal tract symptoms. This is particularly common in athletes with concomitant irritable bowel syndrome. It has also been suggested that high intensity or prolonged exercise is associated with the release of a number of specific gastrointestinal tract hormones, which may have a role in the development of gastrointestinal symptoms during exercise.

Finally, it is important to note that there are documented potential benefits of regular exercise training on the gastrointestinal tract. These benefits have been reviewed (Peters *et al.* 2001) and include the potential benefit of regular training in reducing the risk of gastrointestinal cancers, cholelithiasis, gastrointestinal hemorrhage, inflammatory bowel disease, and constipation (Peters *et al.* 2001).

Table 11.3 Changes in gastrointestinal physiology in response to an acute exercise bout.

Change in the physiologic parameter	Possible mechanism(s)
Esophageal dysmotility (Simons & Kennedy 2004)	During exercise, esophageal contractions become weaker, less frequent, and shorter
Reduced gastric emptying (Murray 2006)	Increased exercise intensity Dehydration Hyperthermia Volume, type, and temperature of gastric content (ingested fluid and nutrients)
Increased gastroesophageal reflux (Murray 2006)	Reduced gastric emptying Decreased lower esophageal sphincter tone
Decreased splanchnic blood flow (Moses 2005; Murray 2006)	Mental stress of competition High intensity exercise Hyperthermia Dehydration Hypoglycemia
Altered orocecal transit time (increased or decreased) (Murray 2006)	Decreased colonic activity during exercise Mechanical movement of the colon during running sports High-fiber meals prior to exercise

Diagnostic approach to common gastrointestinal tract symptoms in athletes

The frequency, clinical features, causes and risk factors, and management principles of upper and lower gastrointestinal complaints during exercise are summarized in Tables 11.4 and 11.5, respectively. In any diagnostic process, it is important to first ascertain whether the symptoms or signs are, or can become, very serious or even life-threatening and, second, to identify which physiologic system is disturbed and therefore what the causes of the symptoms and signs are.

Serious events involving the gastrointestinal tract include vomiting blood and rectal bleeding, particularly of large volumes of blood, and abdominal pain that prevents further exercise. A physician needs to assess the athlete before any exercise is continued.

The analysis of symptoms to determine their physiologic origin applies to all presentations:
• Heartburn is invariably related to prolonged acid exposure to the esophageal mucosa as a result of gastroesophageal reflux (Parmelee-Peters & Moeller 2004; Yazaki *et al.* 1996).
• Tight retrosternal pain that is not cardiac in origin is usually caused by esophageal spasm, and may be associated with heartburn, but not necessarily so (Casey *et al.* 2005; Moses 1990; Parmelee-Peters & Moeller 2004; Worobetz & Gerrard 1985).
• Vomiting may be associated with a variety of causes, including anxiety, non-specific gastric irritation caused by NSAIDs or other drugs, and metabolic abnormalities (e.g., dehydration, overhydration, hypoglycemia, and electrolyte disturbances; Casey *et al.* 2005; Simons & Kennedy 2004).
• Abdominal pain and/or cramps are usually caused by colonic spasm and characteristically are relieved by the passage of stool or flatus. These pains are usually related to the irritable bowel syndrome and can prevent the athlete completing the event (Casey *et al.* 2005; Moses 1990; Simons & Kennedy 2004).
• Diarrhea implies intestinal hurry and can be caused by hypertonic fluid ingestion, gut ischemia, or a toxic food poisoning or infection (Boggess 2007; Casey *et al.* 2005).

• Rectal bleeding may result from lower gastrointestinal tract pathology (if bright red), or upper gastrointestinal pathology (if black and tarry in color). The association of diarrhea with blood may be caused by serious gut ischemia or a severe colonic infection (Casey *et al.* 2005; Moses 1990; Sullivan 1986).

In all cases, management should be aimed at identifying and treating the cause rather than just treating the symptom itself. Frequently, reassurance and not medical treatment is the appropriate response in spite of an athlete requesting a specific treatment.

Management of common gastrointestinal tract symptoms in athletes

In the first instance, management will depend on establishing the correct diagnosis (Swain 1994). Once the diagnosis is confirmed, treatment options are generally either non-pharmacologic or pharmacologic.

Non-pharmacologic management of gastrointestinal symptoms in athletes

If the symptom is attributed only to exercise and not to any organic disease, general practical advice can be given to the athlete based on their symptoms (Table 11.6).

Pharmacologic management of gastrointestinal symptoms in athletes

The use of medication to manage gastrointestinal symptoms in athletes has not received much attention by the research community. However, there are three important general considerations in the prescription of medication for an athlete who presents with gastrointestinal symptoms. First, a clear diagnosis must be established so that underlying pathology is not missed. This is most important, particularly in the older athlete. The diagnosis will obviously also determine what medication should be prescribed.

Second, any medication that is prescribed to an elite athlete must not contain substances in the banned list of drugs. In most cases, medication for

Table 11.4 Upper gastrointestinal complaints in athletes.

Condition	Frequency	Clinical features	Possible causes/risk factors	Management principles
Gastroesophageal reflux disease (GERD) (Jozkow et al. 2006; Parmelee-Peters & Moeller 2004; Shawdon 1995; Simons & Kennedy 2004)	Very common	Occurs in about 60% of athletes Occurs more frequently during exercise than at rest Presents with heartburn, chest pain, belching, nausea, or vomiting Aggravated by consumption of a meal before exercise Aggravated by meals high in fat, protein and fiber Associated upper respiratory symptoms may be present	Altered gastrointestinal motor function (decreased lower esophageal sphincter tone) Aerophagia (air swallowing) during exercise Diet (type of food, caffeine, increased food volume) Decreased splanchnic blood flow Neuroendocrine changes Mechanical effects (increased intra-abdominal pressure)	Establish correct diagnosis and treat appropriately Decrease exercise intensity Avoid postprandial exercise for 3 h Avoid high calorie, high fat and high protein meals before exercise During exercise, colder solutions contain <10% carbohydrate may decrease risk of GERD Topical antacids and antireflux medication may be considered Specialist referral and endoscopy may be required
Dyspepsia (including peptic ulcer disease and gastritis) (Casey et al. 2005)	Common	Vague upper gastrointestinal symptoms that may include epigastric pain, nausea, vomiting, bloating, indigestion, abdominal discomfort, or early satiety Common feature is mucosal damage	Decreased splanchnic blood flow during exercise Use of NSAIDs before and during exercise Factors similar to those related to GERD Consider *Helicobacter pylori* infection Consider other causes such as diabetes, thyroid disease, and lactose intolerance	Establish correct diagnosis and treat appropriately Specialist referral and endoscopy may be required
Dysphagia (esophageal) (Casey et al. 2005)	Rare	Difficulty with swallowing solids and liquids Occurs several seconds after swallowing Pain in the chest (retrosternal)	Gastroesophageal reflux (esophagitis secondary to acid reflux) Bilious vomiting Drugs (NSAIDs, tetracyclines, alendronate) Other (cancers, achalasia, scleroderma)	Establish correct diagnosis and treat appropriately
Dysphagia (oropharyngeal) (Casey et al. 2005)	Very rare	Greater difficulty in swallowing liquids compared with solids Repeated attempts to swallow accompanied by choking sensation Pain localized in the neck (painful variety)	Thyromegaly Upper respiratory tract infections (tonsillitis, laryngitis, cervical adenitis) Retropharyngeal abscess Anaphylaxis (consider exercise-induced) Neuromuscular disorder of oropharynx (painless variety) secondary to cancers, Guillian–Barré syndrome	Establish correct diagnosis and treat appropriately

GERD, gastro-esophageal reflux disease; NSAIDs, non-steroidal anti-inflammatory drugs.

Table 11.5 Lower gastrointestinal complaints in athletes.

Condition	Frequency	Clinical features	Possible causes/risk factors	Management principles
Diarrhea (Casey et al. 2005; Simons & Kennedy 2004)	Very common (runners and female athletes)	Abnormally frequent, semi-solid to watery bowel movements (>3 per day) Acute or chronic May be complicated by vomiting, malena, hematochezia, dehydration	Enteric fluid and electrolyte imbalances Decreases splanchnic blood flow causing mesenteric ischemia Mechanical trauma Neuroendocrine Endotoxins Infections (viral gastroenteritis) Toxic (food poisoning)	Establish correct diagnosis and treat appropriately Oral fluid and electrolyte solution No exercise in the acute phase (infective variety or if dehydration present) Avoid caffeine, NSAIDs Antidiarrheal medication can be considered but with caution (may cause depression of central nervous system, and affect heat dissipation) Chronic diarrhea requires diagnostic work-up
Irritable bowel syndrome (IBS) (Casey et al. 2005)	Common (females)	Diarrhea-predominant and constipation-predominant varieties described Cramping abdominal pain relieved by defecation Altered stool frequency, altered stool form, altered stool passage, sense of incomplete stool evacuation, abdominal distension following meals	Increased motor reactivity to various stimuli (stress, food, cholecystokinin) Impaired transit of bowel gas Visceral hypersensitivity Altered immune function Autonomic dysfunction	Establish correct diagnosis and treat appropriately Reassurance Stress reduction Small frequent meals during the day High fiber diet Avoid lactose-containing foods Continue with regular exercise Medication may be considered
Abdominal pain (Casey et al. 2005; Simons & Reynolds 2004)	Less common	Pain can be acute or more chronic Pain can be vague or localized "Side-stitch" can also be considered in this group	There are a variety of causes Consider hepatic, biliary, pancreatic, small bowel, large bowel, pelvic and retroperitoneal causes Hernia (umbilical, inguinal, "sportsman's" hernia) must be considered	Establish correct diagnosis and treat appropriately
Gastrointestinal bleeding (Casey et al. 2005; Rudzki et al. 1995; Simons & Kennedy 2004; Sullivan 1986)	Frank bleeding – rare Transient occult bleeding – more common	Occult bleeding often asymptomatic and athletes develop gradual onset iron deficiency (other causes of iron deficiency need to be considered) Frank rectal bleeding during or after exercise	Mesenteric ischemia from decreased splanchnic blood flow NSAID use Mechanical trauma Dehydration	Establish correct diagnosis and treat appropriately Stool test for occult blood Reduce exercise intensity and duration Maintain hydration during exercise Iron supplementation Specialist referral and endoscopy may be required

Table 11.6 Summary of general practical advice for an athlete with gastrointestinal symptoms.

Heartburn
Avoid large meals 2–3 h before training/racing
Use a topical antacid if necessary

Nausea/vomiting
Avoid large meals 2–3 h before training/racing
Avoid high intensity or prolonged exercise, particularly if you are not well trained
The use of anti-emetics before an event is not encouraged because they have some very unpleasant side effects and their
   effect on performance is unknown

Abdominal cramps
Be well trained for races
Avoid training at too high intensities if you are not accustomed to it
Avoid dehydration during training/racing
The use of anti-spasmodics before an event is not encouraged because they have side effects and their effect on
   performance is unknown

Urge to defecate/diarrhea
Avoid dehydration during training/racing
Attempt to stimulate a bowel movement before training/racing (caffeine can be used, e.g., a cup of tea or coffee)
Avoid hill running or running at high intensities
If severe and persistent, think about switching to gliding sports (e.g., cycling, swimming)
The use of non-prescribed anti-diarrheals before an event is not encouraged because they can have prolonged effects and
   their effect on performance is unknown

gastrointestinal tract symptoms are not on the banned list and can therefore safely be prescribed. Notable exceptions are, for example, appetite suppressants because they contain stimulants.

Third, medication should not interfere with the athlete's ability to perform optimally. There are very few studies that have examined the relationship between gastrointestinal tract medication and exercise performance. In one unpublished study, loperamide was shown not to affect exercise performance (endurance performance and isokinetic muscle strength). Anecdotal evidence suggests that topical antacids, H_2 antagonists, and proton pump inhibitors, which are all used to control heartburn, do not affect exercise performance. However, the use of medications to control nausea, such as prochlorperazine, cyclizine, and metoclopramide, can cause drowsiness as a side effect and therefore may impair sports performance. However, this has not been studied scientifically.

Whenever a sports physician consults with an athlete presenting with gastrointestinal symptoms, the possibility of serious underlying disease needs to be considered. These alarm symptoms include the following:

- Weight loss;
- Pyrexia;
- Bleeding;
- Symptoms unrelated to normal gastrointestinal functions, such as eating or defecation; or
- Initial development of symptoms in an athlete over 40 years of age (Swain 1994).

Foregut symptoms, such as heartburn, nausea and indigestion, are usually gastric acid related. If symptoms persist, in spite of the use of local antacids, or there are alarm symptoms, a gastroscopy is recommended to make a diagnosis.

Hindgut symptoms, such as abdominal pain without alarm symptoms, are usually caused by an irritable bowel syndrome. An essential observation is the improvement in symptoms after the passage of flatus or stool and a tendency to constipation as defined in the first section of this chapter. There is no universally useful drug medication other than prokinetic agents. Most athletes will improve on normalizing bowel function with the use of adequate dietary fiber (30–40 g·day^{-1}) and the addition of rough particles, such as whole nuts, large seeds (e.g., sunflower seeds) and corn kernels. The use of fruit to improve bowel function is analogous to a mild laxative and does not help in the medium to long term. Gassy foods, such as cauliflower and broccoli, usually add to the gas load in the gut with no real other advantage.

Conclusions

In summary, gastrointestinal symptoms in athletes are common, with hindgut (lower gastrointestinal tract) symptoms being more common. Although most symptoms are mild, life-threatening bleeding can occur which requires urgent medical treatment. The pathophysiology of these gastrointestinal symptoms during exercise is not completely understood, but factors associated with these symptoms include dietary, mechanical, ischemic, and neurohormonal factors. The diagnosis of the underlying cause is essential, and underlying gastrointestinal pathology must be excluded, particularly in the older athlete. Management of these symptoms is, in the first instance, non-pharmacologic. If medication is required it is important to make sure that the diagnosis is confirmed, that the medication does not violate doping regulations, and that the medication will not negatively affect exercise performance.

References

Boggess, B.R. (2007) Gastrointestinal infections in the traveling athlete. *Current Sports Medicine Reports* **6**, 125–129.

Brouns, F., Saris, W.H. & Rehrer, N.J. (1987) Abdominal complaints and gastrointestinal function during long-lasting exercise. *International Journal of Sports Medicine* **8**, 175–189.

Casey, E., Mistry, D.J. & MacKnight, J.M. (2005) Training room management of medical conditions: sports gastroenterology. *Clinics in Sports Medicine* **24**, 525–540, viii.

Gil, S.M., Yazaki, E. & Evans, D.F. (1998) Aetiology of running-related gastrointestinal dysfunction: how far is the finishing line? *Sports Medicine* **26**, 365–378.

Halvorsen, F.A., Lyng, J., Glomsaker, T. & Ritland, S. (1990) Gastrointestinal disturbances in marathon runners. *British Journal of Sports Medicine* **24**, 266–268.

Halvorsen, F.A. & Ritland, S. (1992) Gastrointestinal problems related to endurance event training. *Sports Medicine* **14**, 157–163.

Jozkow, P., Wasko-Czopnik, D., Medras, M. & Paradowski, L. (2006) Gastroesophageal reflux disease and physical activity. *Sports Medicine* **36**, 385–391.

Larson, D.L. & Fisher, R. (1987) Management of exercise-induced gastrointestinal problems. *Physician and Sportsmedicine* **15**, 112–126.

Moses, F.M. (1990) The effect of exercise on the gastrointestinal tract. *Sports Medicine* **9**, 159–172.

Moses, F.M. (2005) Exercise-associated intestinal ischemia. *Current Sports Medicine Reports* **4**, 91–95.

Murray, R. (2006) Training the gut for competition. *Current Sports Medicine Reports* **5**, 161–164.

Parmelee-Peters, K. & Moeller, J.L. (2004) Gastroesophageal reflux in athletes. *Current Sports Medicine Reports* **3**, 107–111.

Peters, H.P., Akkermans, L.M., Bol, E. & Mosterd, W.L. (1995) Gastrointestinal symptoms during exercise: the effect of fluid supplementation. *Sports Medicine* **20**, 65–76.

Peters, H.P., De Vries, W.R., Vanberge-Henegouwen, G.P. & Akkermans, L.M. (2001) Potential benefits and hazards of physical activity and exercise on the gastrointestinal tract. *Gut* **48**, 435–439.

Priebe, W.M. & Priebe, J.A. (1984) Runners' diarrhea: prevalence and clinical symptomatology. *American Journal of Gastroenterology* **79**, 827–828.

Putukian, M. & Potera, C. (1997) Don't miss gastrointestinal disorders in athletes. *Physician and Sportsmedicine* **25**, 80–94.

Rao, K.A., Yazaki, E., Evans, D.F. & Carbon, R. (2004) Objective evaluation of small bowel and colonic transit time using pH telemetry in athletes with gastrointestinal symptoms. *British Journal of Sports Medicine* **38**, 482–487.

Riddoch, C. & Trinick, T. (1988) Gastrointestinal disturbances in marathon runners. *British Journal of Sports Medicine* **22**, 71–74.

Rudzki, S.J., Hazard, H. & Collinson, D. (1995) Gastrointestinal blood loss in triathletes: its etiology and relationship to sports anaemia. *Australian Journal of Science and Medicine in Sport* **27**, 3–8.

Sanchez, L.D., Corwell, B. & Berkoff, D. (2006) Medical problems of marathon runners. *American Journal of Emergency Medicine* **24**, 608–615.

Schwartz, P.A., Schwellnus, M.P. & Koorts, A.S. (1995) The incidence and risk factors of gastrointestinal symptoms in six endurance sports. *South African Journal of Sports Medicine* March, 17–24.

Shawdon, A. (1995) Gastro-oesophageal reflux and exercise: important pathology to consider in the athletic population. *Sports Medicine* **20**, 109–116.

Simons, S.M. & Kennedy, R.G. (2004) Gastrointestinal problems in runners. *Current Sports Medicine Reports* **3**, 112–116.

Sullivan, S.N. (1984) The effect of running on the gastrointestinal tract. *Journal of Clinical Gastroenterology* **6**, 461–465.

Sullivan, S.N. (1986) Gastrointestinal bleeding in distance runners. *Sports Medicine* **3**, 1–3.

Swain, R.A. (1994) Exercise-induced diarrhea: when to wonder. *Medicine and Science in Sports and Exercise* **26**, 523–526.

Worobetz, L.J. & Gerrard, D.F. (1985) Gastrointestinal symptoms during exercise in Enduro athletes: prevalence and speculations on the aetiology. *New Zealand Medical Journal* **98**, 644–646.

Yazaki, E., Shawdon, A., Beasley, I. & Evans, D.F. (1996) The effect of different types of exercise on gastro-oesophageal reflux. *Australian Journal of Science and Medicine in Sport* **28**, 93–96.

Chapter 12

Exercise and the Kidney

BRIAN RAYNER AND MARTIN P. SCHWELLNUS

The major functions of the kidneys are the excretion of end-products of metabolism, the homeostasis of water and electrolytes, maintenance of acid–base balance, the control of blood pressure (BP), regulation of calcium metabolism through the activation of vitamin D, and the control of red cell mass through the secretion of erythropoietin. Despite these important physiologic functions the effect of exercise on the kidney has received little attention. This chapter reviews the normal physiology of the kidney and its response to exercise; exercise-induced acute renal failure (ARF); proteinuria, hematuria, and hyponatremia; and exercise in patients with chronic renal insufficiency.

Basic structure and function of the nephron

Each human kidney contains approximately 1,200,000 nephrons, which are the functional units of the kidney. Each nephron consists of a glomerulus and a long tubule. Blood enters the glomerulus through an afferent arteriole, forms a network of capillaries, and then leaves via an efferent arteriole. The network of capillaries is covered by epithelial cells which are encased in a capsule (Bowman's capsule). Glomerular filtrate enters the proximal tubule, then the thin descending and thick ascending loop of Henle, and finally the distal convoluted tubule and collecting ducts.

The Olympic Textbook of Medicine in Sport, 1st edition. Edited by M. Schwellnus. Published 2008 by Blackwell Publishing, ISBN: 978-1-4051-5637-0.

Most of the blood from the efferent arteriole flows through a capillary network that surrounds the cortical portions of the tubules. However, a proportion of the blood from the efferent arterioles (particularly from the juxtamedullary glomeruli) flows into straight capillary loops (known as the vasa recta) that extend downward into the medulla and envelop the thin segments of the loop of Henle.

Glomerular filtration rate, renal blood flow, and autoregulation

Glomerular filtration rate

The glomerular filtrate is the fluid that filters through the glomerulus into Bowman's capsule. The glomerular membrane differs from ordinary endothelial membranes because it is 100–1000 times more permeable despite having three layers (capillary epithelium, basement membrane, epithelial cells of Bowman's capsule). This permeability is imparted to the glomerular membrane by: (i) fenestrae in the capillary endothelium; and (ii) "slit pores" in the epithelium of Bowman's capsule. The fenestrae prevent filtration of particles greater than 160 A°, and the basement membrane prevents particles greater than 110 A°. The "slit pores" prevent filtration of particles greater than 70 A°. Albumin, the smallest plasma protein, is just too large to pass through the glomerular membrane. This means that for practical purposes there is filtration of all contents of plasma except proteins. The glomerular filtrate therefore contains no red blood cells, 0.03% protein, and similar electrolyte and solute composition to plasma. Because of the paucity of negatively charged proteins in the filtrate, the concentrations of anions (chloride, bicarbonate) and cations are 5% higher.

The volume of filtrate formed each minute is the glomerular filtration rate (GFR). This is normally about 125 mL·min^{-1}·1.73 m^{-2}. The following equation determines the GFR:

$$GFR = K_f [(P_{GC} - P_T) - (\pi_{GC} - \pi_T)]$$

where K_f is filtration coefficient, P_{GC} is the mean hydrostatic pressure in the glomerular capillaries, π_{GC} is the oncotic pressure in the glomerular capillaries, and π_T is the oncotic pressure in the tubules. In a given individual, K_f and $\delta\gamma$ oncotic pressure are relatively constant and the P_{GC} is the major determinate of changes in GFR. P_{GC} is determined by the renal blood flow, systemic BP, and afferent and efferent arteriolar tone.

GFR may be estimated using creatinine clearance, but this is impractical in the clinical setting and most clinicians use an estimated GFR based on the serum creatinine using the MDRD equation (Levey *et al.* 1999):

Estimated GFR (mL·min^{-1}·1.73 m^{-2})
    $= 1.86 \times (Scr)^{-1.154} \times (Age)^{-0.203} \times (0.742$ if female$)$
    $\times (1.210$ if black$)$.

Laboratories are now including this result in routine reports to improve recognition of early renal disease.

Normal renal blood flow at rest

Normal renal blood flow at rest in humans is about 20% of the cardiac output, and therefore is about 1200 mL·min^{-1}. This can vary from 12% to 30%. Each nephron receives its blood supply from the afferent arteriole. There are two capillary beds in each nephron. The first is the glomerular capillary bed which is separated from the peritubular capillary bed by the efferent arteriole. The efferent arteriole is an important regulator of pressure and therefore separates a high pressure capillary bed (glomerulus) from a low pressure capillary bed (peritubular). The vasa recta receives only 1–2% of the total renal blood flow, and therefore the tubules particularly in the

renal medulla are at risk for ischemic injury during times of stress.

The blood vessels of the kidney receive their nerve supply mainly from the sympathetic nervous system (12th thoracic to 2nd lumbar segments), which mainly cause vasoconstriction. This is an important mechanism for reduction of renal blood flow during exercise.

Control of renal blood flow at rest

The mean hydrostatic pressure in the glomerular capillaries (P_{GC}) is the major determinant of GFR, and it is critical for the kidney maintain intraglomerular pressure within a prescribed pressure range (autoregulation). Excessive intraglomerular pressure in the long term (as seen in patients with diabetes or systemic hypertension) causes damage to the glomerulus, while too low a pressure causes a reduction in GFR. The juxtaglomerular (JG) apparatus has a critical role in autoregulation of glomerular pressure (hence GFR) by controlling the efferent and afferent arteriolar tone.

The JG apparatus is formed by the close contact of specialized cells of the thick ascending loop of Henle (or macula densa), and JG cells between the early part of the distal tubule and the afferent and efferent arteriole. A decrease in renal blood flow and P_{GC} reduces delivery sodium to the JG apparatus. First, this causes afferent arteriolar dilatation via tubuloglomerular feedback mediated by prostaglandin and nitric oxide. Second, the JG cells release renin, which converts angiotensinogen to angiotensin I. Angiotensin I is then converted into angiotensin II via angiotensin-converting enzyme (ACE), which has the following effects:

1 Vasoconstriction of the efferent arterioles to increase glomerular pressure;

2 Vasoconstriction of the systemic arterioles to increase blood pressure; and

3 Aldosterone release to increase blood volume and blood pressure.

The net effect is to raise systemic BP and increase glomerular pressure and thus restore GFR. This mechanism helps explain the vulnerability of the kidney to ARF following the ingestion of non-steroidal anti-inflammatory drugs (NSAIDs) in the presence of a reduction in renal blood flow.

Control of renal blood flow during exercise

A number of researchers have examined the effect of exercise on renal blood flow. In most studies, the clearance of para-aminohippuric acid (PAH) was used as the measure of renal plasma flow (RPF). In general, the findings of most researchers are consistent and show that renal plasma flow decreases during exercise, and that exercise intensity is the most important determinant of the magnitude of this reduction.

In one study, a linear reduction ($r = -0.89$) in renal plasma flow was demonstrated with exercise performed at increasing heart rates (90% of resting RPF at 80 beats·min^{-1}; 35% of resting RPF at 190 beats·min^{-1}). Similarly, a reduction in the renal fraction of the cardiac output was demonstrated with increasing oxygen consumption (17% of CO at 15% of $\dot{V}o_{2max}$; 3% of CO at 80% $\dot{V}o_{2max}$; Grimby 1965). In this study the RPF returned to normal within 60 min post exercise.

The role of hydration and exercise on RPF have also been investigated. Overhydration only slightly minimized the effect of exercise on decreases in RPF (Castenfors 1967). Dehydration (4% and 8% reduction of body weight) resulted in a significantly greater reduction in RPF than in normally hydrated individuals.

In general, high intensity exercise results in a reduction in renal blood flow caused by a redistribution flow to the muscle, heart, and lungs mediated by the sympathetic nervous system, This is exacerbated by dehydration, a consequence of prolonged exercise. The renal tubules increase energy consumption because maximal sodium and water absorption is needed to restore intravascular volume, and renal autoregulation maintains GFR by dilating the afferent constricting the efferent arteriole, which further reduces renal blood flow to the tubules, particularly to the medulla. The combined effect is to make the kidney vulnerable to ischemic tubular injury and ARF, particularly if exercise is prolonged and is associated with dehydration, rhabdomyolysis, and the use of NSAIDs.

Urinary water excretion

Normal urinary water excretion at rest

The ability of the kidney to vary the amount of water in which a given amount of solute is excreted is fundamental to the maintenance of body water balance. The normal human kidney is able to vary the osmolality of urine 50–1400 mOsm·kg^{-1}. This enables the kidney to minimize fluid loss during prolonged exercise while maintaining GFR.

The normal osmolality of the filtrate that enters the proximal tubule is 300 mOsm·L^{-1}. Because the proximal tubule is permeable to water, the absorption of osmotically active substances from the proximal tubule is accompanied by movement of water and this will not affect osmolality.

The interstitial fluid in the medulla of the kidney that surrounds the descending and ascending loops of Henle becomes is very hyperosmolar because:
1 Active transport of NaCl from the lumen of the ascending limb of the loop of Henle into the interstitium;
2 Diffusion of urea from its high concentration in the collecting duct into the interstitium; and
3 The slow removal of NaCl and urea from the interstitium by the vasa recta.
Because the descending limb of the loop of Henle is permeable to water, water moves from the lumen into the interstitium. This results in a progressive increase in the osmolality of the fluid in the descending limb of the loop of Henle. The ascending limb of the loop of Henle is impermeable to water and the active transport of NaCl out of the lumen into the interstitium causes the osmolality to decrease again. This mechanism is known as the counter-current "multiplier" of the loop of Henle and its main function is to increase the osmolality of the interstitium.

Beyond the loop of Henle, the osmolality of the tubular fluid depends on the absorptive processes of the distal and collecting tubules as well as on the presence or absence of antidiuretic hormone (ADH). In the absence of ADH there is almost no water reabsorption from the collecting duct, and urine output can exceed 20 L. ADH increases the permeability of the luminal border of the epithelial cells to water. Water then passes readily into the interstitium along the strong osmotic gradient and the urine becomes concentrated.

FACTORS AFFECTING WATER EXCRETION

The principal regulatory site for water balance is the osmoreceptors of the hypothalamus. Maintenance of osmotic balance is critical for the normal function of the brain. Rapid increases or decreases in osmolality may lead to demyelination (central pontine myelinolysis) and cerebral edema respectively, both of which may be fatal. If water intake is in excess of body requirements, the serum osmolality (principally determined by serum sodium) decreases. The osmoreceptors respond by suppressing thirst and reducing ADH secretion from the hypothalamus. This makes the collecting ducts impermeable to water and excess water is excreted by the kidney. Conversely, in states of limited water intake, serum osmolality rises resulting in release of ADH and stimulation of thirst causing increased permeability of the collecting ducts and reabsorption of water, and increased water intake.

In general, this mechanism enables the body to maintain osmolality in a very tight range. However, under certain pathophysiologic situations ADH stimulation may occur in the absence of osmotic stimuli. Important causes of non-osmotic ADH release are stress, pain, prolonged exertion, intercurrent illness, drugs (e.g., tricyclic antidepressants) and a fall in systemic BP. This results in a falling serum osmolality or sodium in the face of continued water intake. The rapid fall in osmolality results in the movement of water into the brain as the brain needs several days to adjust to a lower serum osmolality. The net result in severe cases is cerebral edema, seizures, coma, and finally death.

Urinary water excretion during exercise

Exercise is usually associated with a reduction in urine flow. This may be an appropriate response to preserve water balance in individuals who are dehydrated. However, it has become increasingly clear that exercise, particularly strenuous exercise, may result in non-osmotic release of ADH that may, in the face of liberal water intake in excess of perspiration and insensible loss, lead to hyponatremia.

There is general agreement that exercise exerts an antidiuretic effect. This can lead to an anuric state after severe exercise. However, the degree, duration, and rate of this decrease in urine flow cannot be predicted accurately and factors such as degree of hydration, emotional state, and interindividual variability can affect urine flow (Poortmans 1984).

Hyperhydration prior to mild intensity exercise does not prevent a small decrease in free water clearance or urine flow (Castenfors 1967). In high intensity exercise, hyperhydration does not prevent the substantial decrease in urine flow (80%) associated with exercise (Poortmans 1984). Even if hyperhydration continued after exercise, the urine flow was still decreased after 80 min (Poortmans 1984).

The same factors that determine urine flow at rest also influence urine flow during exercise. The relative contributions of each of these during exercise is difficult to determine. However, it seems that the decrease in urine flow is mainly caused by increases in ADH levels during exercise. Early workers have documented that moderate intensity exercise does not increase plasma levels of ADH substantially, but that high intensity exercise increases plasma ADH concentration threefold (Kozlowski et al. 1967).

This could explain the significant decrease in urine flow at high intensity but not moderate or low intensity exercise. However, more recent work has shown a linear correlation ($r = 0.60$) between plasma ADH levels and work intensity (Wade et al. 1980). It also appears that the response of ADH to exercise depends on the state of hydration of the individual and the duration of exercise. Furthermore, the plasma ADH concentration during exercise may also be altered by the rate of breakdown of ADH in the kidney and liver. This rate is influenced by renal and hepatic blood flow which in turn is influenced by exercise intensity, duration, and the state of hydration of the individual (Wade & Claybaugh 1980).

Urinary electrolyte excretion

Urine electrolyte excretion at rest

The sodium concentration in the glomerular filtrate is approximately the same as plasma (142 mmol·L^{-1}). In the proximal tubule, sodium is transported actively out of the tubule. Chloride and water follow passively along the electrochemical and osmotic gradient, respectively. This results in a slight decrease in the sodium concentration in the proximal tubule. In the descending limb of the loop of Henle, sodium and chloride diffuse into the tubule, followed by water. In the ascending limb, sodium is actively transported out of the tubule into the interstitium, followed by chloride. However, the ascending limb is impermeable to water; therefore, the sodium concentration falls in this portion of the loop of Henle (20–30% of the original concentration in the glomerular filtrate).

The reabsorption of sodium in the distal tubule and collecting ducts is variable and depends largely on the presence or absence of aldosterone, and dietary intake of sodium. Aldosterone is secreted from the adrenal cortex and is responsible for the active reabsorption of sodium from the distal tubule and collecting ducts. This is coupled by transport of potassium out of the cell into the tubule.

Potassium is transported through the epithelium of the proximal tubule and the loop of Henle in almost a parallel fashion to sodium. By the time the tubular fluid reaches the distal tubule, more than 90% of the potassium that was filtered has been reabsorbed. In the distal tubule, potassium is actively secreted (coupled with sodium absorption) by the action of aldosterone. In the absence of aldosterone, potassium is reabsorbed in the distal tubule along an electrical gradient.

Urine electrolyte excretion during exercise

In general, strenuous exercise decreases the excretion of urinary electrolytes (Castenfors 1967; Grimby 1965; Raisz et al. 1959). A reduction of urinary sodium excretion has been well documented after exercise. In one study, a 60% reduction in urinary sodium excretion was observed following a 20-km run (Poortmans et al. 1994). The mechanism of the reduction in sodium excretion is not well documented, but it is probably related to an increased tubular reabsorption of sodium. An increased aldosterone concentration in the plasma (possibly secondary to increased renin release) is related to exercise intensity and duration and may well be responsible for the decreased urinary sodium excretion during exercise. Disturbances in sodium balance are seldom seen during exercise, and changes in serum sodium are mainly brought about by changes in water balance (i.e., dehydration [hypernatremia] and water intoxication [hyponatraemia]).

The effects of exercise on urinary potassium excretion during exercise are variable. In well-hydrated subjects who performed supine exercise, no changes in potassium excretion were observed. However, in high intensity prolonged exercise, urinary potassium excretion was increased. Changes in serum potassium are not a feature of exercise, but if an athlete has rhabdomyolysis and ARF, life-threatening hyperkalemia may occur.

Exercise-induced hyponatremia

Prevention of dehydration in ultradistance athletes has been important in the prevention of ARF. However, the overemphasis of maintenance of hydration at all costs led to several reports of severe and sometimes life-threatening hyponatremia in the early 1980s (Noakes et al. 1985). Initially, these reports were poorly understood, but it is now realized that intense and prolonged exercise causes non-osmotic release of ADH (as outlined above), which in the face of hyperhydration may lead to exercise-induced hyponatremia. Hyponatremia may be further exacerbated by salt loss from sweat, particularly in hot and humid conditions (Patel et al. 2005). In fact, up to 30% of long distance runners may develop hyponatremia in the range 125–135 mmol·L^{-1}. This is usually asymptomatic or may be associated with lethargy, nausea, and vomiting, but greater drops can have very serious repercussions. Severe hyponatremia leads to cerebral edema, seizures, coma, and, in rare instances, death (Hsieh 2004; Noakes 2002; Palmer *et al.* 2003). It is no longer tenable to promote unlimited water intake in ultra-distance athletes, and fluid recommendations need to be adjusted to the individual, length of the race, and climatic conditions.

Exercise-associated proteinuria

In humans there is a normal daily excretion of protein in the urine of about 40–80 mg (usually <150 mg). A number of researchers have observed that strenuous exercise can be associated with an increased protein excretion in the urine.

Animal studies have shown that substantially more protein appears in the glomerular filtrate than that which is eventually excreted. This means that protein absorption must occur in the tubules of the kidney. The amount and type of protein that can be detected in the urine will therefore depend on a number of factors:

1 Glomerular permeability to proteins;
2 Plasma concentration of the protein;
3 Tubular reabsorption of protein; and
4 Tubular secretion of protein.

However, protein should not be detected on standard dipstick tests and persistent proteinuria is almost always an indicator of renal disease. It is recommended that all athletes undergo routine dipstick examination of the urine prior to participation in exercise to avoid the problems of interpreting proteinuria after exercise.

Incidence

The first report of exercise-associated proteinuria (EAP) was documented in military recruits in 1878. Subsequent to that report, many researchers have observed proteinuria following exercise. The incidence is variable and depends on:

1 Sensitivity of the testing;
2 Type, intensity, and duration of the exercise; and
3 Considerable interindividual variation.

However, studies have shown an incidence varying from 11% to 100% after a bout of strenuous exercise (Poortmans *et al.* 1994).

Severity

The severity of EAP can be expressed as the protein excretion rate post exercise in $\mu g \cdot min^{-1}$ (150 mg·day^{-1} = 104 $\mu g \cdot min^{-1}$). Protein excretion rates have been documented for a variety of types of exercise at different intensities and duration. These post-exercise excretion rates vary considerably and values ranging from 86 $\mu g \cdot min^{-1}$ (123 mg·day^{-1}) to 5100 $\mu g \cdot min^{-1}$ (7.34 g·day^{-1}) have been documented. Although most studies indicate significant rises in excretion rates after exercise, the actual excretion rates rarely exceed 400 $\mu g \cdot min^{-1}$ (576 mg·day^{-1}).

The maximal protein excretion rate occurs in the first 20–30 min after stopping exercise. The decline in protein excretion rate after exercise and the return back to normal takes a few hours (approximately 4 h). This seems to be independent of the degree of dehydration.

Factors affecting exercise-associated proteinuria

A number of factors appear to influence the development of EAP.

TYPE OF EXERCISE

At similar intensities of exercise, running appears to result in higher urinary protein excretion rates than swimming or cycling (Poortmans 1984).

INTENSITY OF EXERCISE

In general, a relationship between the increased protein excretion rate and the high intensity of exercise can be observed (Poortmans & Labilloy 1988; Poortmans *et al.* 1996). In one study, protein excretion rates correlated with the blood lactate levels ($r = 0.85$; Poortmans *et al.* 1988).

TRAINING

There was some evidence from early studies that lack of conditioning is associated with EAP. Repeated exercise on five successive days showed a decline in proteinuria over the training days, being scarcely detectable on day 5 (Taylor 1960). This finding has been confirmed by others who tested athletes over longer periods of training (50 days; Cantone & Cerretelli 1960). However, it has been shown that if exercise is performed at the same absolute intensity, the rate of protein excretion is not affected (Poortmans 1984).

GENETIC PREDISPOSITION

In one study, protein excretion during exercise was documented in 73 pairs of monozygotic and dizygotic twins. Protein excretion rates correlated well in monozygotic but not dizygotic twins. This indicates that there may be a genetic predisposition to the development of EAP.

Protein electrophoretic pattern

The protein electrophoretic pattern of EAP reveals the following main findings (Poortmans 1984):
• A prominent albumin peak;
• A very intensive B1 peak which is constituted mainly by transferrin; and
• Immunoglobulin components similar to normal urinary immunoglobulins.
Furthermore, both high molecular weight (mainly from glomerular filtration) and low molecular weight proteins (resulting from impaired tubular reabsorption) can be demonstrated in EAP. This indicates that EAP is a mixed glomerular–tubular proteinuria, the glomerular type being predominant (Poortmans 1984).

Mechanisms

The mechanisms responsible for this reversible proteinuria of exercise are not known. However, a number of hypotheses have been put forward.

METABOLIC ACIDOSIS

It has been postulated that the metabolic acidosis that is associated with high intensity exercise may be responsible for EAP. It is known that acidosis can increase glomerular permeability.

RENAL HYPOXIA

Hypoxia resulting from decreased renal blood flow during exercise has also been suggested as a possible cause for the EAP.

RENAL VASOCONSTRICTION

Increased sympathetic stimulation during high intensity exercise can cause vasoconstriction of the renal arterioles. The reduced renal plasma flow and GFR will result in an increased filtration fraction of protein. This may enhance the diffusion of macromolecules into the glomerulus.

RENIN

It is well recognized that renin injection can cause proteinuria in an experimental animal. It has therefore been proposed that the increased renin activity during exercise may be responsible for EAP.

LOSS OF NEGATIVE CHARGE ON THE GLOMERULAR MEMBRANE

There is some evidence in experimental animals (running dogs) that exercise may be associated with a loss of negative charge on the glomerular membrane. This loss of the negative charge would facilitate the passage of negatively charged proteins across the glomerular membrane, resulting in proteinuria.

Clinical approach

An athlete will usually not present with symptoms of proteinuria. Proteinuria will usually be detected incidentally by dipstick test during a preseason medical assessment. Alternatively, it may be detected by dipstick test within 24–48 h after strenuous exercise. In most cases, proteinuria observed in otherwise healthy athletes after strenuous exertion that is not associated with the use of potentially nephrotoxic drugs (e.g., NSAIDs) resolves completely within 24–48 h, is benign, and has no long-term effects. However, persistent proteinuria requires

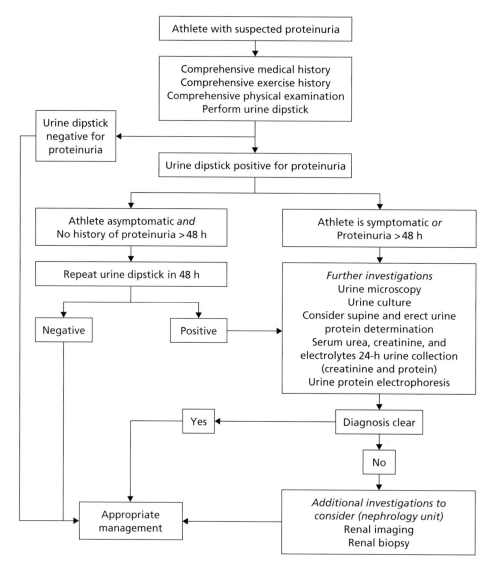

Fig. 12.1 Evaluation of the athlete with suspected proteinuria.

a sound clinical approach to rule out more serious renal disease (Fig. 12.1).

It is important to take a detailed medical history and perform a physical examination to exclude clinical evidence of renal or systemic disease. In particular, it is important to obtain a detailed exercise history including the intensity, duration, and type of exercise. Furthermore, the fluid intake, environmental conditions, and previous history of proteinuria is important. Finally, it is important to

note the time span between the last exercise bout and the urine dipstick examination. The presence of hematuria associated with proteinuria is usually not benign.

On physical examination, it is important to find evidence of associated renal or systemic disease such as hypertension, edema, or anemia. If there is clinical evidence of renal or systemic disease, further blood tests, renal function tests, renal imaging, and eventually a renal biopsy may be required to establish the diagnosis. These are best performed by a nephrologist.

If there is no clinical evidence of renal or systemic disease, qualitative tests for proteinuria should be repeated 2–3 times. If no proteinuria is detected in well-concentrated urine specimens, the proteinuria can be ascribed to transient or EAP proteinuria. The patient can be reassured and no further tests are required.

If proteinuria is detected each time during repeat tests, further investigation is required. This would include the following:

• Serum urea, electrolytes, and creatinine;
• Urinalysis for detection of casts;
• Estimated creatinine clearance based on serum creatinine;
• Protein : creatinine ratio (multiply ratio by 10 to give approximate estimate of 24-h proteinuria); and
• Renal ultrasound.

If the renal function and renal ultrasound tests are normal, the patient can be followed up annually, except if:

1 Proteinuria becomes persistent (in which case further investigation is required);
2 Proteinuria is associated with hematuria; or
3 The estimated proteinuria is more than 1 g·day^{-1}. Referral to a specialist renal unit for further investigation and management is advised in these circumstances.

Exercise-associated hematuria

Athletes may present to a sports physician with a complaint of "dark urine" or even frank blood in the urine after activity. The sports physician requires a thorough understanding of the possible causes and the approach to management of this problem.

Incidence

Both gross and microscopic hematuria have been reported in association with a variety of sports. Hematuria has been described in both trained and novice athletes. The incidence of exercise-associated hematuria (EAH) is variable and depends on the type, intensity, and duration of the sport as well the sensitivity of the techniques that were used to diagnose hematuria. In general, hematuria is more common after high intensity or prolonged exercise.

The prevalence of hematuria on positive dipstick tests in athletes participating in the 1974 Commonwealth Games was 11.4% (Bailey *et al.* 1976). In marathon runners, the incidence of hematuria after a standard marathon (Boston Marathon) was reported as 18% (Siegel *et al.* 1979), and after the Comrades Marathon it was 63% (Dancaster & Wheeat 1971).

Etiology and mechanisms

The precise etiology of EAH is not known. It is likely that EAH can be caused by a number of different pathologies at different sites in the renal tract (Table 12.1).

The earliest reports implicated the kidney as the source of the hematuria. The decrease in renal blood flow, particularly to the vessels supplying the renal papillae, has been implicated in EAH. This hypothesis is supported indirectly by the finding that exercise of increasing intensity and duration (possibly associated with dehydration) is more commonly associated with EAH (Kachadorian & Johnson 1971).

Mechanical trauma to the kidney has also been implicated in EAH. In one case report, jogging was described as a cause of nephroptosis in a patient

Table 12.1 Possible causes of exercise-associated hematuria (EAH). (After Goldszer 1991).

Site of pathology	Cause
Kidney	Ischemia
	Acute renal failure
	Increased vascular fragility
	Trauma
	Nephroptosis
	Calculi
Ureter	Calculi
Bladder	Contusion
	Calculi
	Infections
Urethra	Contusion
	Calculi
	Infection
	Trauma
	Cold

with weak ligamentous attachments of the kidney. It was suggested that jogging causes excessive displacement of the kidney with resultant trauma. Furthermore, in contact sports, direct trauma to the kidney has been implicated as the cause of the so-called "athletic pseudonephritis" which is a triad of hematuria, proteinuria, and casts in the urine post exercise (Gardner 1956). However, this is unlikely the only cause of this clinical picture as it also occurs in non-contact sports such as swimming and rowing (Alyea & Parish 1958).

Currently, the consensus of opinion is that the lower urinary tract is the most likely site of pathology in benign EAH. Runners with hematuria after a 10,000-m race were examined by cystoscopy and found to have contusions of the bladder mucosa (mostly in the intraureteric bar and the posterior rim of the internal meatus). Contrecoup lesions were demonstrated in the lower posterior bladder and the trigone (Blacklock 1977). It was postulated that the cause for hematuria in these athletes was repetitive trauma of the anterior bladder mucosa against the fixed posterior wall.

Clinical approach to post-exercise hematuria

EAH is benign in most cases, but is important to establish that the "dark" urine or positive dipstick test is not caused by pigments such as myoglobin or hemoglobin which may cause a false positive test. It is essential to perform microscopic examination of the urine to confirm the presence of red blood cells, and in their absence myoglobinuria resulting from rhabdomyolysis, or hemoglobin caused by "march" hemoglobinuria must be considered. In addition, certain glomerulonephritides (e.g., IgA nephropathy) may be asymptomatic and exacerbated by exercise.

EAH resolves spontaneously after 24–48 h. However, more sinister renal disease must be excluded, particularly if any of the following are present:
• Progressive symptoms: colic or flank pain;
• Persistent hematuria or proteinuria after 48 h;
• Presence of urinary casts: red cell, white cell, pigmented;
• Positive urine culture;
• Oliguria after prolonged strenuous exercise (longer than 12 h).

The evaluation of the athlete who presents with EAH is depicted in Fig. 12.2. Initial investigation should first include a comprehensive history, in particular to identify:
1 Type, duration, and frequency of exercise;
2 Fluid intake during exercise;
3 History of medication use;
4 Family history of renal disease; and
5 Systemic medical disease.

Second, the athlete should undergo a systematic physical examination including a urinalysis. If there are no identifiable causes for the EAH, the athlete should be reassessed after 48 h. If the hematuria has cleared and there are no other abnormalities on examination, the athlete can be followed up once more in 6 months.

If the repeat urinalysis is abnormal, further investigations are required. These include an intravenous pyelogram (IVP) and a cystoscopy. Further renal function tests are also indicated (Fig. 12.2) and even referral to a nephrologist.

Acute renal failure and exercise

ARF is the most serious renal complication that may occur after exercise and, if unrecognized, can be fatal because of hyperkalemia. The sports physician must understand the pathophysiology of this condition, recognize and manage it appropriately, and be able to give sound advice on its prevention.

Incidence

The precise incidence of ARF during exercise is not known. It is likely to be very variable, and the risk of ARF during exercise will depend on such factors as:
1 Different type of exercise;
2 Intensity and duration of exercise;
3 Environmental conditions;
4 The state of hydration of the participant; and
5 The use of medication during exercise.

Etiology and pathogenesis

ARF in the setting of exercise can be precipitated by a number of factors: dehydration, hyperpyrexia, myoglobinuria, hemoglobinuria, and the use of

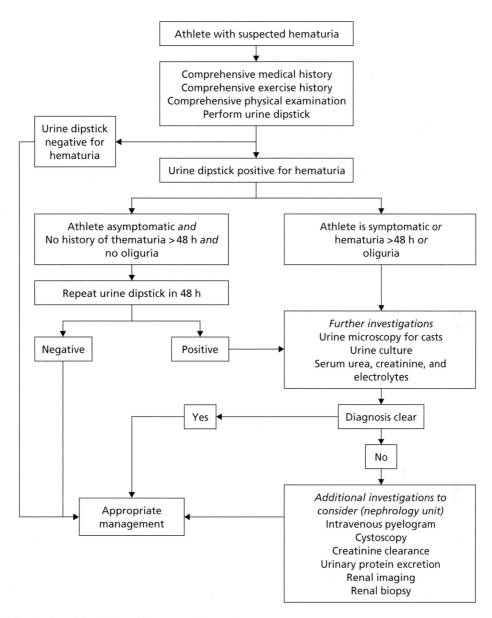

Fig. 12.2 Evaluation of the athlete with suspected hematuria.

nephrotoxic medications during exercise. Recreational drugs such as amphetamines may predispose to rhabdomyolysis and hyperpyrexia, while ingestion of alcohol may predispose to the development of rhabdomyolysis. ARF during exercise is seldom caused by one factor alone but is usually multifactorial.

DEHYDRATION

The magnitude and duration of dehydration during exercise and its effect on the physiologic reduction in renal blood flow during exercise have already been discussed. In severe dehydration, the reduction in renal blood flow can be very profound and result in renal ischemia and acute tubular necrosis.

HYPERPYREXIA

Strenuous exercise that is performed in hot humid environmental conditions can cause hyperpyrexia, particularly in athletes who are not heat acclimatized. Hyperpyrexia can cause damage to a variety of organ systems. In particular, it can cause skeletal muscle damage directly or indirectly by decreasing blood flow to muscles resulting in ischemia, and by aggravating the physiologic muscle damage that occurs, particularly with eccentric muscle contraction. Skeletal muscle damage (rhabdomyolysis) is associated with the release of nephrotoxic substances, in particular myoglobin. Furthermore, hyperpyrexia can also be associated with intravascular hemolysis and resultant hemoglobinemia.

MYOGLOBINURIA

Skeletal muscle damage (rhabdomyolysis) is associated with the release of myoglobin. Myoglobin is a globin chain containing a haem pigment. In acidic media such as during metabolic acidosis and during bicarbonate absorption in the proximal tubule, globin dissociates from this ferrihemate compound. This ferrihemate compound is directly nephrotoxic by interfering with renal tubular transport mechanisms.

HEMOGLOBINURIA

Hemoglobin has less dramatic effects on the kidney. Intravascular hemolysis can occur during exercise as a result of mechanical trauma to red cells (which is more severe if there are red cell abnormalities) or hyperpyrexia. The release of hemoglobin in the blood has a less profound effect on the kidney because it binds irreversibly to haptoglobin in the plasma, and it is a larger molecule than myoglobin and therefore less hemoglobin is filtered by the glomerulus. Filtered hemoglobin is also toxic to the renal tubule by a mechanism similar to that of myoglobin (acid medium dissociation). As with myoglobinuria, clinical experience indicates that hemoglobinuria compromises renal function only in the presence of other factors such as volume depletion, acidosis, or hypotension.

NEPHROTOXIC DRUGS

NSAIDs are commonly used by athletes, particularly during ultradistance running events. The use of these medications should be strongly discouraged because they may compromise renal function during exercise and may even lead to acute renal failure. The mechanisms by which NSAIDS interfere with normal renal function are: (i) to inhibit the synthesis of prostaglandins, which are important renal vasodilators, protecting renal blood flow, particularly in the presence of a pre-renal state; and (ii) acute allergic interstitial nephritis.

OTHER FACTORS

Other factors that may cause renal failure during rhabdomyolysis are as follow:

1 Disseminated intravascular coagulopathy and fibrin deposition in the glomeruli;
2 Intravascular volume depletion secondary fluid movement into damaged muscle; and
3 Release of purines resulting in a sudden increase in uric acid production.

Clinical experience suggests that rhabdomyolysis leads to myoglobinuric renal failure only when other factors such as intravascular volume depletion, hemoconcentration, renal vasoconstriction, or exposure to other nephrotoxins are present.

Clinical approach to the athlete who has not produced urine post exercise

Oliguria is defined as a urine volume of less than $400 \, \text{mL·day}^{-1}$ or less than $20 \, \text{mL·h}^{-1}$. On initial presentation of an athlete complaining that he or she has not passed any urine after exercise, the following steps should be taken.

HISTORY

A comprehensive history must be obtained, concentrating on the following:

• Type, duration, intensity at time of completion of exercise;
• Environmental conditions, fluid intake (type, volume, frequency);
• Time of last urination with approximate volume and color;
• Use of medications during race; and
• Systematic medical history including past history and relevant family history.

PHYSICAL EXAMINATION

A complete physical examination must be carried out. In particular, evidence of the following must be sought:
• Intravascular volume depletion (increased heart rate, decreased supine and erect blood pressure, reduced skin turgor, decreased jugular venous pressure, dryness of the axillae); and
• Increased core temperature.

If possible, a urine sample and a blood sample must be obtained. This will provide valuable information regarding the differential diagnosis of pre-renal and renal failure (Table 12.2).

If the athlete has not passed urine in the period 0–12 h post exercise, encourage increased fluid intake, particularly if there is evidence of intravascular volume depletion. Intravenous fluids may be indicated if this depletion is severe.

If the athlete presents 12 h or longer after exercise, further investigation (in addition to the above) is required. This would include the following:
• Hospitalization for investigation and observation;
• Urine examination (microscopy and electrolytes);
• Blood tests including serum urea, creatinine and electrolytes; and
• Renal ultrasound.

Prevention

Athletes must be made aware of the measures to decrease the risk of developing renal failure after exercise. The following are general guidelines for athletes:
• Drink enough fluid during exercise particularly in hot, humid environmental conditions;
• Acclimatize to hot, humid environmental conditions if possible;
• Do not use any form of medication during exercise unless advised by your doctor;
• Do not use any painkillers or anti-inflammatory drugs at least 48 h before prolonged strenuous exercise;
• Do not ignore blood in the urine after exercise;
• Make sure that you drink enough fluid in the first few hours after exercise;
• Seek medical advice urgently if you have not passed any urine 12 h after exercise.

Exercise and advanced chronic kidney disease

Although exercise should be encouraged in patients with chronic kidney disease (CKD) for improvement in well-being and cardiovascular status, it poses potential hazards in patients with stage 4 (GFR 15–29 mL·min⁻¹) or 5 disease (GFR <15 mL·min⁻¹) or those receiving dialysis. Exercise capacity is impaired for a variety of reasons.

Limitations and hazards of exercise in patients with chronic kidney disease

Patients with CKD are usually in poor physical condition. This is because of poor nutrition, prolonged illness, chronic anemia resulting from decreased erythropoietin production by the kidney,

Table 12.2 Urinary findings in pre-renal and acute renal failure.

Laboratory test	Pre-renal failure	Acute renal failure
Urine osmolality (mOsm·kg⁻¹)	>500	<400
Urine Na⁺ (meq·L⁻¹)	<20	>40
Urine : plasma creatinine	>40	<20
Urine sediment	Normal or occasional granular casts	Brown granular casts, cellular debris

uncontrolled hypertension, chronic fluid overload, cardiac dysfunction, electrolyte and acid–base disorders, obesity, side effects of multiple medications, muscle weakness, renal osteodystrophy, and peripheral neuropathies.

Exercise may be hazardous to the patient with CKD. Patients with stage 4 disease often have an inability to concentrate urine and prolonged exercise in hot weather without adequate fluids may precipitate renal failure. Conversely, excessive fluid intake may precipitate pulmonary edema as the kidney is unable to respond rapidly to increased intake. Patients are also at high risk for cardiovascular events and uncontrolled hyperkalemia may be fatal. Fractures resulting from renal bone disease and injury to peritoneal dialysis catheters or arteriovenous fistulae are further concerns.

Evaluation of a patient with chronic kidney disease prior to exercise

It is essential that a patient with CKD undergo full evaluation by a nephrologist before embarking on exercise. In general, the patient should have well-controlled BP, their fluid state needs to be optimized, and electrolytes – particularly potassium – should be in the normal range. Anemia must be corrected with erythropoietin and/or hematinics. All patients with CKD are at high risk for coronary heart disease and effort stress testing is recommended in most to detect asymptomatic ischemic heart disease. The type of exercise needs to be evaluated for each individual, but in general most centers accept that swimming, tennis, badminton, cycling, field hockey, sailing, canoeing, netball, cricket, track

athletics, golf, skiing, and rowing are reasonable choices (Patel *et al.* 2005). In the long term, a successful renal transplant is the key to returning to a relatively normal exercise capacity.

Exercise recommendations in athletes with solitary or polycystic kidneys

The prevalence of a congenital or acquired single solitary kidney is estimated to be 1 in 1500 persons. The loss or injury to a single kidney during contact sport almost invariably raises anxiety, and up to 68% of urologists recommend avoidance of contact sports (Sharp *et al.* 2002). The loss or injury to a solitary kidney despite its larger size is in reality a theoretical concern, and is much more likely to occur after motor vehicle accidents. In over 30 years at the Groote Schuur Hospital Renal Unit, not a single case of a patient requiring chronic dialysis after losing a single kidney during contact sport has been encountered. Current recommendations suggest that persons with a single kidney be allowed to compete in contact sport after explanation of the possible dangers (Holmes *et al.* 2003). In reality, common sense should prevail and persons with a normally functioning single kidney should be encouraged to exercise and this may include contact sports. More caution should be exercised if sports with the potential to cause serious injury are undertaken.

Autosomal dominant polycystic kidney disease is a common genetic form of kidney disease. The kidneys are very large, protrude from the abdomen, and are prone to injury. Contact sports should be discouraged as the risk for renal trauma is high.

References

Alyea, E.P. & Parish, H.H. Jr. (1958) Renal response to exercise: urinary findings. *JAMA* **167**, 807–813.

Bailey, R.R., Dann, E., Gillies, A.H., Lynn, K.L., Abernethy, M.H. & Neale, T.J. (1976) What the urine contains following athletic competition. *New Zealand Medical Journal* **83**, 309–313.

Blacklock, N.J. (1977) Bladder trauma in the long-distance runner: "10,000 metres haematuria". *British Journal of Urology* **49**, 129–132.

Cantone, A. & Cerretelli, P. (1960) Effect of training on proteinuria following muscular exercise. *Internationale Zeitschrift für Angewandte Physiologie* **18**, 324–329.

Castenfors, J. (1967) Renal function during exercise: with special reference to exercise proteinuria and the release of renin. *Acta Physiologica Scandinavica Supplement* **293**, 1–44.

Dancaster, C.P. & Whereat, S.J. (1971) Renal function in marathon runners.

South African Medical Journal **45**, 547–551.

Gardner, K.D. Jr. (1956) Athletic pseudonephritis; alteration of urine sediment by athletic competition. *JAMA* **161**, 1613–1617.

Goldszer, R.C. (1991) Renal abnormalities during exercise. In *Sports Medicine* (Strauss, R.H., ed.) W.B. Saunders, Philadelphia: 156–166.

Grimby, G. (1965) Renal clearances at rest and during physical exercise after injection of bacterial pyrogen. *Journal of Applied Physiology* **20**, 137–141.

Holmes, F.C., Hunt, J.J. & Sevier, T.L. (2003) Renal injury in sport. *Current Sports Medicine Reports* **2**, 103–109.

Hsieh, M. (2004) Recommendations for treatment of hyponatraemia at endurance events. *Sports Medicine* **34**, 231–238.

Kachadorian, W.A. & Johnson, R.E. (1971) The effect of exercise on some clinical measures of renal function. *American Heart Journal* **82**, 278–280.

Kozlowski, S., Szczepanska, E. & Zielinski, A. (1967) The hypothalamo-hypophyseal antidiuretic system in physical exercises. *Archives Internationales de Physiologie et de Biochimie* **75**, 218–228.

Levey, A.S., Bosch, J.P., Lewis, J.B., Greene, T., Rogers, N. & Roth, D. (1999) A more accurate method to estimate glomerular filtration rate from serum creatinine: a new prediction equation. Modification of Diet in Renal Disease Study Group. *Annals of Internal Medicine* **130**, 461–470.

Noakes, T. (2002) Hyponatremia in distance runners: fluid and sodium balance during exercise. *Current Sports Medicine Reports* **1**, 197–207.

Noakes, T.D., Goodwin, N., Rayner, B.L., Branken, T. & Taylor, R.K. (1985) Water intoxication: a possible complication during endurance exercise. *Medicine and Science in Sports and Exercise* **17**, 370–375.

Palmer, B.F., Gates, J.R. & Lader, M. (2003) Causes and management of hyponatremia. *Annals of Pharmacotherapy* **37**, 1694–1702.

Patel, D.R., Torres, A.D. & Greydanus, D.E. (2005) Kidneys and sports. *Adolescent Medicine Clinics* **16**, 111–119, xi.

Poortmans, J.R. (1984) Exercise and renal function. *Sports Medicine* **1**, 125–153.

Poortmans, J.R. & Labilloy, D. (1988) The influence of work intensity on postexercise proteinuria. *European Journal of Applied Physiology and Occupational Physiology* **57**, 260–263.

Poortmans, J.R., Mathieu, N. & De Plaen, P. (1996) Influence of running different distances on renal glomerular and tubular impairment in humans.

European Journal of Applied Physiology and Occupational Physiology **72**, 522–527.

Poortmans, J.R. & Vanderstraeten, J. (1994) Kidney function during exercise in healthy and diseased humans: an update. *Sports Medicine* **18**, 419–437.

Raisz, L.G., Au, W.Y. & Scheer, R.L. (1959) Studies on the renal concentrating mechanism. III. Effect of heavy exercise. *Journal of Clinical Investigation* **38**, 8–13.

Sharp, D.S., Ross, J.H. & Kay, R. (2002) Attitudes of pediatric urologists regarding sports participation by children with a solitary kidney. *Journal of Urology* **168**, 1811–1814.

Siegel, A.J., Hennekens, C.H., Solomon, H.S. & Van Boeckel, B. (1979) Exercise-related hematuria: findings in a group of marathon runners. *JAMA* **241**, 391–392.

Taylor, A. (1960) Some characteristics of exercise proteinuria. *Clinical Science* **19**, 209–217.

Wade, C.E. & Claybaugh, J.R. (1980) Plasma renin activity, vasopressin concentration, and urinary excretory responses to exercise in men. *Journal of Applied Physiology* **49**, 930–936.

Chapter 13

Obstetrics and Gynecology

RAUL ARTAL AND SUSAN HOFFSTETTER

The cardiopulmonary benefits of exercise are well recognized but not limited to other benefits including maintenance of muscle tone, strength, endurance, and a positive effect upon energy level, mood, and self-image. Physical fitness and conditioning are important to recreational athletes and essential to competitive female athletes. Often, women athletes are unaware of the potential risks of prolonged training and competitive activities on their reproductive and gynecologic health. This chapter reviews the benefits and risks of exercise during pregnancy and the postpartum period, as well as exercise prescriptions for both. Clinical approaches to the assessment and management of menstrual abnormalities, bone health, and osteoporosis in the female athlete are also discussed.

Benefits and risks of maternal exercise during pregnancy

Participation in a wide range of exercise is considered safe during pregnancy, and regular exercise has overall health benefits for the mother. The American College of Obstetricians and Gynecologists (ACOG) published recommendations and guidelines for exercise during pregnancy and the postpartum period in 2002 (American College of Obstetricians and Gynecologists 2002). The American Diabetes Association has previously endorsed exercise as "a helpful adjunctive therapy" for gestational diabetes

The Olympic Textbook of Medicine in Sport, 1st edition. Edited by M. Schwellnus. Published 2008 by Blackwell Publishing, ISBN: 978-1-4051-5637-0.

(Jovanovic-Peterson & Peterson 1996). In the absence of medical or obstetric complications, pregnant women can adopt the recommendations of the Centers for Disease Control and Prevention (CDC) and American College of Sports Medicine (ACSM) for exercise. These recommendations, aimed at improving the health and well-being of non-pregnant individuals, suggest that an accumulation of 30 min or more of moderate exercise a day should occur on most if not all days of the week (American College of Sports Medicine 2000). Absolute and relative contraindications to aerobic exercise during pregnancy as determined by ACOG are listed in Tables 13.1 and 13.2.

Nutrition and weight gain

Pregnancy is associated with profound anatomic and physiologic changes. The most obvious is maternal weight gain. Weight gain guidelines during pregnancy, established by the Institute of Medicine (IOM), are specific to pregravid maternal body mass index (BMI; in $kg \cdot m^{-2}$): BMI <19.8 = 9.07–18.14 kg, BMI 19.8–26 = 11.34–15.88 kg, BMI 26.1–29 = 6.80–11.34 kg, and BMI >29 = 6.80 kg (Institute of Medicine Subcommittee on Nutritional Status and Weight Gain During Pregnancy 1990). The primary goals of the IOM weight gain recommendations are to improve infant birth weight along with fetal and maternal outcomes. However, critics argue that the IOM's recommendations, which are higher than previous guidelines, are unlikely to improve fetal outcome and may actually result in increased adverse maternal and fetal outcomes (Johnson &

Table 13.1 Absolute contraindications for exercise in pregnancy. From American College of Obstetricians and Gynecologists (2002) with permission.

Hemodynamically significant heart disease
Pre-eclampsia/pregnancy-induced hypertension
Restrictive lung disease
Incompetent cervix/cerclage
Multiple gestation at risk for premature labor
Premature labor during the current pregnancy
Placenta previa after 26 weeks' gestation
Persistent second or third trimester bleeding
Ruptured membranes

Table 13.2 Relative contraindications to exercise during pregnancy. From American College of Obstetricians and Gynecologists (2002) with permission.

Severe anemia
Unevaluated maternal cardiac arrhythmia
Chronic bronchitis
Intrauterine growth restriction in current pregnancy
Extreme underweight with body mass index (BMI) <12
Poorly controlled type 1 diabetes
Extreme morbid obesity
Poorly controlled hyperthyroidism
Poorly controlled seizure disorder
Orthopedic limitations
Poorly controlled hypertension
History of extremely sedentary lifestyle
Heavy smoker

Yancey 1996). These recommendations are based upon historical concerns about the effects of dieting or famine on fetal growth retardation. We believe that weight gain recommendations for pregnancy should be individualized to the patient (Artal 2003).

After 13 weeks' gestation, an extra 1.2 MJ (300 kcal) are required to meet the metabolic demands of pregnancy (American Dietetic Association 2002; Clapp 1990). This energy requirement is increased further when daily energy expenditure is increased through exercise. In weight-bearing exercise (e.g., walking), the energy requirement progressively increases with the increase in weight during the course of the pregnancy. A related consideration to nutrition and exercise during pregnancy is adequate carbohydrate intake. Pregnant women use carbohydrates at a greater rate both at rest and during exercise than do non-pregnant women (Clapp *et al.* 1988;

Soultankis *et al.* 1996). It also appears that during non-weight-bearing exercise in pregnancy there is a preferential use of carbohydrates, possibly because of the anaerobic component of this type of activity (Romen *et al.* 1991).

Musculoskeletal system

The musculoskeletal system undergoes change as a result of increased maternal weight and hormonal influences during pregnancy. The growing uterus displaces the woman's center of gravity, resulting in progressive lumbar lordosis and rotation of the pelvis on the femur. For the pregnant woman to maintain balance and stability, the center of gravity must shift back over the pelvis to prevent a forward fall using the muscles and ligaments of the vertebral column for support (Romen *et al.* 1991). The very high prevalence of low back pain in pregnancy (50% occurrence) can be attributed to lordosis (Artal & O'Toole 2005). Increased maternal weight during pregnancy may significantly increase the forces across joints such as hips and knees by as much as 100% during weight-bearing exercise (Karzel & Friedman 1991). Such large forces can cause discomfort to normal joints and increase damage to arthritic or previously unstable joints. Additionally, abduction of the shoulders leads to increased paresthesias over the ulnar and/or median nerve (Crisp & DeFrancesco 1964). In the third trimester, reduced mobility of the ankle and wrists may occur because of water retention, mainly in the ground substance of the connective tissue, and visible ankle edema and paresthesias in the hands and carpel tunnel syndrome may develop (Tobin 1967; Votik *et al.* 1983).

The increase in the relaxation of the ligaments secondary to the increased release of relaxin and estrogens occurs early in pregnancy. Theoretically, this would predispose pregnant women to increased incidence of strains and sprains; however, there are no reports in the literature to confirm such occurrences. Softening of the cartilage and increase in synovial fluid widens the pelvic joint resulting in increased joint mobility and an unstable pelvis contributing to a waddling gait. Similar changes occur in other joints and muscles.

Cardiovascular system

Pregnancy induces multiple physiologic adaptations in maternal hemodynamics causing increases in blood volume, heart rate, stroke volume, and cardiac output and a decrease in systemic vascular resistance (Clark *et al.* 1989; Lund & Donovan 1967; Wolfe *et al.* 1989). Alterations in maternal cardiac output show an increase of 30–50% by mid pregnancy compared to non-pregnant values (Fig. 13.1; Morton 1991). Increased blood volume is a result of an increase in plasma volume of up to 50% and an increase in red cell volume of up to 20% (Fig. 13.2). This dilutional effect creates a reduction in hematocrit, a "physiologic anemia," without a subsequent interference with oxygen distribution (Romen *et al.* 1991). After the first trimester, the supine position results in relative obstruction of venous return and decreased cardiac output. In addition, motionless standing is associated with a significant decrease in cardiac output and symptomatic hypotension in approximately 10% of all pregnant women. For this reason, both the supine and motionless standing positions should be avoided as much as possible during pregnancy (Clark *et al.* 1991). Stroke volume increases by 10% at the end of the first trimester are followed by a 20% increase in heart rate during the second and third trimesters (Fig. 13.3; Morton *et al.*

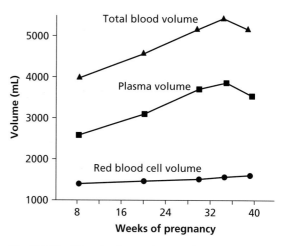

Fig. 13.2 Total blood volume, plasma volume, and red cell volume in normal pregnancy. Data from Shnider & Levinson (1993).

1985; Pivaranik 1996). Mean arterial pressure decreases 5–10 mmHg by the middle of the second trimester and then gradually increases back to prepregnancy levels. The decreased mean arterial pressure occurs as a result of the increased uterine vasculature and uteroplacental circulation and decrease in the vascular resistance of the skin and the kidney (Pivaranik 1996). These hemodynamic changes appear to establish a circulatory reserve necessary to provide nutrients and oxygen to both mother and fetus at rest and during moderate activity, but is limited in providing reserves during strenuous physical activity (Artal & O'Toole 2005). Therefore, strenuous physical activity in pregnancy should be limited to prevent potential adverse effects for the mother and fetus.

Respiratory changes

Pregnancy is associated with significant respiratory changes including minute ventilation increases to almost 50%, largely as a result of increased tidal volume (Artal *et al.* 1986; Prowse & Gaensler 1965). This results in an increase in arterial oxygen tension to 106–108 mmHg in the first trimester, which then decreases to a mean of 101–106 mmHg by the third trimester (Templeton & Kelman 1976). There is an associated increase in oxygen uptake, and a 10–20%

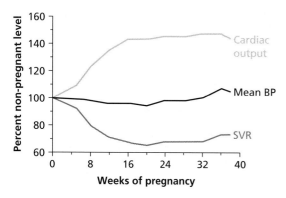

Fig. 13.1 Hemodynamic changes in normal pregnancy. Normal pregnancy is characterized by an increase in cardiac output, a reduction in systemic vascular resistance (SVR), and a modest decline in mean blood pressure (BP). These changes are associated with a 10–15 beat·min^{-1} increase in heart rate. Data from Shnider & Levinson (1993).

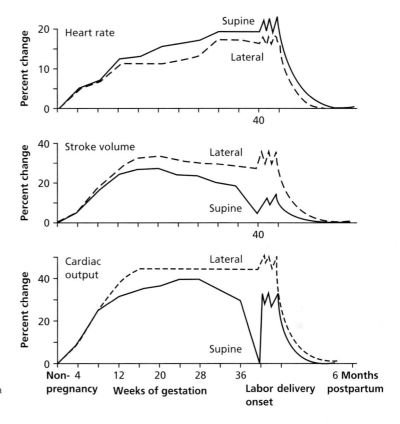

Fig. 13.3 Systemic hemodynamics during normal pregnancy. Data from Bonica & McDonald (1994).

increase in baseline oxygen consumption (Fig. 13.4). Physiologic dead space during pregnancy remains unchanged (Pivarnik *et al.* 1992; Prowse & Gaensler 1965; Sady *et al.* 1989). Changes in pulmonary function tests are noted during pregnancy (Fig. 13.5). Because of the increased resting oxygen requirements during pregnancy and the increased work of breathing caused by the pressure of the enlarging uterus on the diaphragm, there is decreased oxygen availability for the performance of aerobic exercise. Thus, both subjective workload and maximum exercise performance are decreased (Artal *et al.* 1986; Clapp 1990). During treadmill exercise in pregnancy, arteriovenous oxygen difference has been shown to be decreased (Pivarnik *et al.* 1990). However, in some fit women there appear to be no associated changes in maximum aerobic power or acid–base balance during exercise in pregnancy compared to non-pregnant controls (Pivarnik *et al.* 1992; Romen *et al.* 1991; Sady *et al.* 1989).

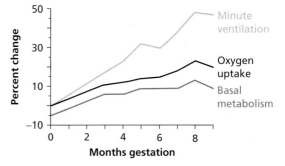

Fig. 13.4 Changes in ventilation during pregnancy. Time course of percent increases in minute ventilation, oxygen uptake, and basal metabolism during pregnancy.

Thermoregulation

During pregnancy, basal metabolic rate and therefore heat production are increased above non-pregnant

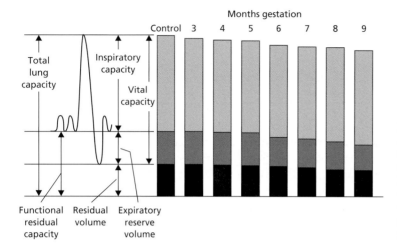

Fig. 13.5 Changes in pulmonary function tests during pregnancy. Serial measurements of lung volume compartments during pregnancy. Functional residual capacity decreases approximately 20% during the latter half of pregnancy, because of a decrease in both expiratory reserve volume and residual volume.

levels. A steady state of heat production versus heat dissipation is accomplished by the increased conductance of heat from the core to the periphery through the cardiovascular system as well as through evaporative cooling through sweat. If heat production exceeds heat dissipation capacity (e.g., during exercise in hot humid conditions or during very high intensity exercise), the core temperature will continue to rise. During prolonged exercise, loss of fluid as sweat may compromise heat dissipation. Therefore, maintenance of euhydration, and ultimately blood volume, is critical to heat balance (Artal & O'Toole 2005).

An increase in body temperature during exercise is directly related to the intensity and length of exercise. During moderate intensity aerobic exercise in thermo-neutral conditions, the core temperature of non-pregnant women rises an average of 1.5°C during the first 30 min of exercise and then reaches a plateau if exercise is continued for an additional 30 min (Soultankis *et al.* 1996). Fetal body core temperatures are about 1°C higher than maternal temperatures. It has been demonstrated that hyperthermia in animals can cause neural tube defects. Data from epidemiologic studies suggest that hyperthermia in excess of 39°C from 20–30 days after conception or 50 days from the last menstrual cycle may be teratogenic in humans (Latgering *et al.* 1991; Milunsky *et al.* 1992). However, there have been no reports to date linking hyperthermia with exercise and teratogenic effects in a human fetus.

Fetal responses

In the past, the main concerns of exercise in pregnancy were focused on the fetus, and any potential maternal benefit was thought to be offset by potential risks to the fetus. In the uncomplicated pregnancy, fetal injuries are highly unlikely. Most of the potential fetal risks are hypothetical (Artal 2003). One remaining concern is whether the selective redistribution of blood flow during regular or prolonged exercise in pregnancy interferes with the transplacental transport of oxygen, carbon dioxide, and nutrients and, if it does, what are the lasting effects, if any? The indirect evidence is that there are no lasting effects. However, given this concern, water exercise may be an excellent choice of exercise during pregnancy because a centripetal shift in blood volume occurs during immersion. The hydrostatic pressure of water exerts a force proportional to the depth of immersion. This pressure acts uniformly to push extravascular fluid into the vascular space resulting in a rapid expansion of the plasma volume. As the intravascular volume increases, a diuresis and natriuresis is initiated from hormonal signals. The diuresis may have positive effects on the pregnant woman who is affected by fluid retention (Katz *et al.* 1991).

Studies have examined the effects of immersion and exercise on pregnant women. Water aerobics – predominantly leg exercises – studied in pregnancy show that hemodynamic changes of immersion put less strain on uterine blood flow, decreased edema, and lowered heart rate than land exercises. Lack of increase in core body temperature is another benefit of water exercise as well as self-reported feelings of well-being (Katz *et al.* 1991).

It is well recognized that during obstetric events, transient hypoxia could result in fetal tachycardia and an increase in fetal blood pressure. These fetal responses are protective mechanisms allowing the fetus to facilitate transfer of oxygen and decrease the carbon dioxide tension across the placenta. Any acute alterations could result in fetal heart rate changes, whereas chronic effects may result in fetal intrauterine growth restriction. Despite reports of occasional fetal heart rate abnormalities, there are no reports to link such events with poor fetal oxygenation and maternal exercise (Artal & O'Toole 2005).

Responses of fetal heart rate to maternal exercise have been the focus of numerous studies (Artal 1990; Artal *et al.* 1986; Carpenter *et al.* 1988; Clapp 1985; Collings *et al.* 1983; Wolfe *et al.* 1988). Most studies show a minimum or moderate increase in fetal heart rate by 10–30 beats·min^{-1} over baseline during or after exercise, which would produce no lasting negative effects to the fetus. Fetal heart rate decelerations and bradycardia have been reported to occur with a frequency of 9.0% and speculation at the underlying etiology led to sporadic non-clinically relevant events, vagal reflex, umbilical cord compression, or fetal head compression. Studies that attempted to assess umbilical blood flow during maternal exercise are technically difficult and reliable data was obtained only before and after exercise by which time any possible changes could have returned to normal baseline (Artal & O'Toole 2005).

Epidemiologic studies have suggested a link between strenuous physical activity, deficient diets, and the development of fetal intrauterine growth restriction. This association appears to be true especially for the woman engaging in physical work. It has also been reported that mothers whose occupation requires long standing or repetitive strenuous physical work have a tendency to deliver earlier and have small for gestational age infants (Launer *et al.* 1990; McDonald *et al.* 1988; Naeye & Peters 1982). However, other studies fail to confirm these

associations (Ahlborg *et al.* 1990; Saurel-Cubizolles & Kaminshki 1987) suggesting that other factors or conditions such as deficient nutrition and socioeconomic status have to be present for strenuous activities to affect fetal growth.

In one study it was concluded that mean birth weight was substantially lower when women exercised at or above 50% of pre-conception levels compared with non-exercisers (Clapp & Capeless 1990). In another study (Sternfeld *et al.* 1995), no difference between the birth weights of the offspring of vigorous exercisers and those of sedentary women were found, and conversely one study found an increase in birth weight (Hatch *et al.* 1993). A high volume exercise program in mid to late pregnancy was found to decrease fetal growth as a result of reduction in fat rather than lean body mass (Clapp 1993). In a meta-analysis, differences in weighted mean birth weight for infants whose mothers exercised during pregnancy were minimal when compared with controls. However, women who continued to exercise vigorously during the third trimester were more likely to deliver infants who weighed 200–400 g less than comparable controls. Limiting factors in the analysis were low sample size, limited populations from varying socioeconomic levels, and lack of qualifying exercise by either caloric count or energy expenditure (Figs 13.6–13.11). Results based on studies stratified jointly by endurance level and period of exercise during pregnancy were supported by existing animal data, pregnant mice, rats, guinea-pigs, and sheep that exercised strenuously in the laboratory were more likely to produce smaller offspring (Leet & Flick 2003).

The information available in the literature is too limited to allow risk assignment for either fetal growth restriction or premature labor resulting from maternal recreational exercise or exercise habits of the elite athlete. Clinical observations indicate that women at risk of premature labor may have labor triggered by exercise. It appears that birth weight is not affected by exercise in women who have adequate energy intake. Reports on continuous physical training during pregnancy in athletes indicate that such activities carry very little risk (Erdelyi 1962). Links of exercise to deficient

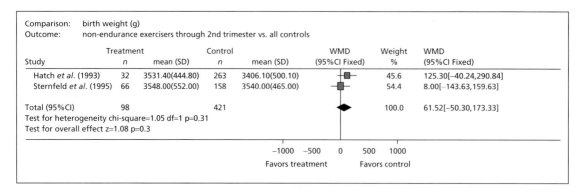

Fig. 13.6 Infant birth weight by maternal exercise status. From Leet & Flick (2003) with permission.

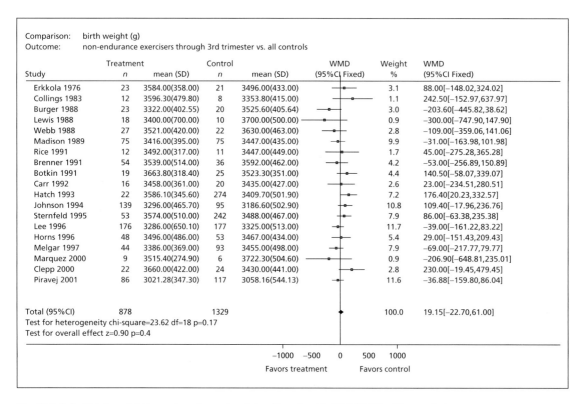

Fig. 13.7 Infant birth weight by maternal exercise status. From Leet & Flick (2003) with permission.

diets and fetal growth restriction should be the subject of further studies. Women who are diet conscious often do not receive the minimum required nutrients. The combined energy requirements of pregnancy and exercise coupled with poor weight gain may lead to fetal growth restriction.

Exercise prescription during pregnancy

The overall health, obstetric and medical risks should be reviewed before a pregnant woman is prescribed an exercise program. In the absence of contraindications, a pregnant woman should be

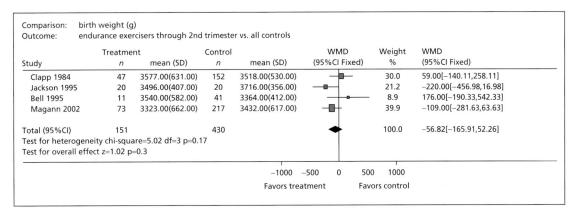

Fig. 13.8 Infant birth weight by maternal exercise status. From Leet & Flick (2003) with permission.

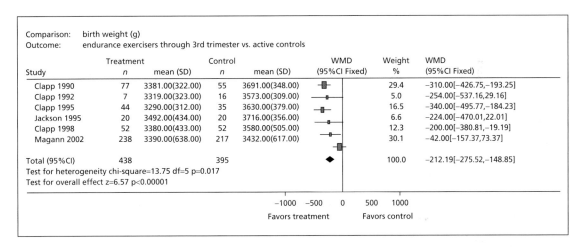

Fig. 13.9 Infant birth weight by maternal exercise status. From Leet & Flick (2003) with permission.

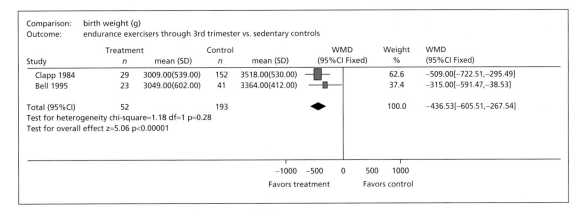

Fig. 13.10 Infant birth weight by maternal exercise status. From Leet & Flick (2003) with permission.

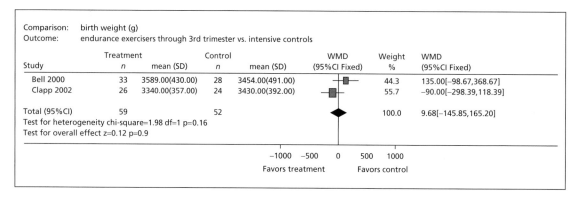

Comparison: birth weight (g)
Outcome: endurance exercisers through 3rd trimester vs. intensive controls

| | Treatment | | Control | | WMD | Weight | WMD |
Study	n	mean (SD)	n	mean (SD)	(95%CI Fixed)	%	(95%CI Fixed)
Bell 2000	33	3589.00(430.00)	28	3454.00(491.00)		44.3	135.00[−98.67,368.67]
Clapp 2002	26	3340.00(357.00)	24	3430.00(392.00)		55.7	−90.00[−298.39,118.39]
Total (95%CI)	59		52			100.0	9.68[−145.85,165.20]

Test for heterogeneity chi-square=1.98 df=1 p=0.16
Test for overall effect z=0.12 p=0.9

−1000   −500   0   500   1000
Favors treatment   Favors control

Fig. 13.11 Infant birth weight by maternal exercise status. From Leet & Flick (2003) with permission.

encouraged to engage in regular, moderate intensity physical activity to continue to derive the same associated health benefits during pregnancy as before pregnancy. However, pregnancy is not different than other phases of life; there are contraindications to exercise because of pre-existing or developing medical conditions. In addition, certain obstetric complications may develop in pregnant women regardless of the previous level of fitness, which could preclude them from continuing to exercise safely during pregnancy (e.g., premature labor, pre-eclampsia, fetal intrauterine growth restriction). The contraindications to exercise listed are suggested as guides to determining the appropriateness of exercise during pregnancy for individual women (Tables 13.1 & 13.2). If warning signs listed in Table 13.3 develop during pregnancy, exercise must be terminated.

An exercise prescription requires knowledge of potential risks and the assessment of physical ability

Table 13.3 Warning signs to terminate exercise during pregnancy. From American College of Obstetricians and Gynecologists (2002) with permission.

Vaginal bleeding
Dyspnea prior to exertion
Dizziness
Headache
Chest pain
Muscle weakness
Calf pain or swelling (rule out thrombophlebitis)
Preterm labor
Decreased fetal movement
Amniotic fluid leakage

to engage in various activities. The elements of an exercise prescription should be considered in every physical activity framework regardless of its purpose: basic health, recreational pursuits, or competitive activities. Consideration should be given to the type and frequency of exercise as well as to the duration and frequency of exercise sessions to balance the potential benefits and harmful effects. Additional attention should be given to progression in intensity over time (Artal & O'Toole 2005).

An exercise prescription for the development and maintenance of fitness in non-pregnant and pregnant women consists of activities to improve cardiorespiratory (aerobic exercise) and musculoskeletal (resistive exercise) status. Aerobic exercise can consist of any activity that uses large muscle groups in a continuous rhythmic manner: jogging, walking, hiking, dance, swimming, cycling, rowing, cross-country skiing, skating, rope skipping. Control of exercise intensity within rather precise limits is often desirable at the beginning of an exercise program. The most easily quantified activities such as walking or stationary cycling are useful. There are no data to support the restriction of pregnant women from participating in these activities, although some activities carry more risk than others. There are several activities that pose increased risks in pregnancy such as scuba diving and exertion in a supine position. Activities that increase the risk of falls (e.g., skiing) or those that may result in excessive joint stress (e.g., jogging and tennis) should be cautiously recommended for pregnant women and evaluated on an individual basis. Swimming is well tolerated and has the advantage of creating a buoyant condition that does not exert any biomechanical forces on joints or ligaments, thus preventing stress.

In addition to aerobic activities, activities that promote musculoskeletal fitness are part of an overall exercise prescription. These include both resistance training (weightlifting) and flexibility exercises. Limited information exists on strength training during pregnancy. It would be prudent to limit repetitive isometric or heavy resistance weightlifting and any exercises that result in a large pressure effect during pregnancy. Flexibility exercises should be used cautiously because of the increased relaxation of ligaments during pregnancy. Maintenance of normal joint range of motion, however, should not interfere with an exercise routine in pregnant women (Hall & Kaufmann 1987).

Intensity of exercise prescription

Intensity is the most difficult component of an exercise regimen to prescribe for pregnant women. To derive health benefits, non-pregnant women are advised to participate in at least moderate intensity exercise. In the combined CDC–ACSM recommendations for physical activity and health, moderate exercise is defined as exercise of 3–4 METS or any activity that is equivalent in difficulty to brisk walking (American College of Sports Medicine 2000; Pate *et al.* 1995). There is no reason to alter this recommendation for pregnant women with no medical or obstetric complications. The recommended intensity of physical activity for developing and maintaining physical fitness is somewhat higher. The ACSM recommends that intensity should be 60–90% of maximal heart rate or 50–85% of either maximal oxygen uptake or heart rate reserve. The lower end of these ranges (60–70% of maximal oxygen uptake) appears to be appropriate for most pregnant women who did not engage in regular exercise before pregnancy, and the upper part of these ranges should be used for those who wish to continue to maintain fitness during pregnancy. In a meta-analysis study of exercise and pregnancy, it was reported that no significant adverse effects were found with exercise intensities of 81% of heart rate maximum (American College of Sports Medicine 2000).

Conflicting evidence exists on maternal heart rate response to steady state submaximal exercise during pregnancy. Both blunted and normal responses to weight-bearing and non-weight-bearing exercise have been reported (McMurray *et al.* 1991; Pivarnik *et al.* 1990). Given the variability in maternal heart rate responses to exercise and its non-linear relationship in pregnancy to $\dot{V}o_2$, target heart rate cannot be used to monitor exercise in pregnancy (Artal & O'Toole 2005).

Ratings of perceived exertion have been found to be useful during pregnancy as an alternative to heart rate monitoring of exercise intensity (Pivarnik 1994). For moderate exercise, ratings of perceived exertion should be 12–14 (somewhat hard) on the 6–20 scale. Evidence of the efficacy of this approach is that, when exercise is self-paced, most pregnant women will voluntarily reduce their exercise intensity as pregnancy progresses (McMurray *et al.* 1993). Although an upper level of safe exercise intensity has not been established, women who were regular exercisers before pregnancy and who have uncomplicated healthy pregnancies should be able to engage in high intensity exercise programs, such as jogging and aerobics, with no adverse effects. The nutritional, cardiovascular, and musculoskeletal condition of the subject as well as fetal well-being should be periodically assessed during the prenatal visits in pregnant women undertaking high intensity exercise programs. Additional testing should be considered as clinically indicated, such as fetal heart rate non-stress testing and ultrasound to assess fetal growth. Dietary modification and changes in exercise routines should also be considered if clinically indicated. Routine prenatal care as advocated in the ACOG publications is sufficient for monitoring the exercise program (Artal & O'Toole 2005).

Duration of exercise prescription

Two concerns should be addressed before prescribing prolonged exercise (in excess of 45 min continuous exercise) regimens for pregnant women. The first is thermoregulation. Exercise should be performed, if possible, in a thermo-neutral environment or in controlled environmental conditions (air conditioning). Attention to proper hydration and subjective feelings of heat stress are essential. The second concern is energy balance. Energy costs of exercise should be estimated and balanced by appropriate energy intakes. Setting of limits to exercise durations is not possible because of the reciprocal relation between exercise intensity and duration. It should be noted that in studies in which exercise was self-paced and in a controlled environment, core temperatures rose less than 1.5°C over 30 min and stayed within safe limits (Soultankis *et al.* 1996). Accumulating the activity in shorter exercise periods, such as 15 min, may obviate concerns related to thermoregulation and energy balance during exercise sessions. ACSM recommends that non-pregnant women exercising to increase or maintain fitness may exercise for up to 60 min per exercise session (American College of Sports Medicine 2000).

Frequency of exercise

In the current CDC–ACSM recommendations for exercise aimed at health and well-being, the recommendations for non-pregnant women is that an accumulation of 30 min per day of exercise occur on most if not all days of the week. In the absence of either medical of obstetric complications, pregnant women could adopt the same recommendation.

Progression of exercise

Pregnant women who have been sedentary before pregnancy should follow a gradual progression of up to 30 min per day. This recommendation is not different from that for non-pregnant sedentary women who begin an exercise program. Pregnancy is not a time for greatly improving physical fitness. Therefore, women who have attained a high level of fitness through regular exercise prior to pregnancy should exercise caution about engaging in higher levels of fitness activities during pregnancy. Further, they should expect overall activity and fitness levels to decline somewhat as pregnancy progresses (McMurray *et al.* 1993).

Recreational activities

Most reports of participation in active recreational activities during pregnancy are anecdotal. In general,

participation in a wide range of recreational activities appears to be safe. The safety of each sport is largely determined by the specific movements required by the sport. Activities with a high risk of falling or those with a high risk of abdominal trauma should be considered undesirable (Artal 1999). Participation in recreational sports with a high potential for contact (e.g., ice hockey, soccer, and basketball) could result in significant trauma to both mother and fetus. Similarly, recreational activities with increased risk of falling such as gymnastics, horseback riding, downhill skiing, and vigorous racquet sports have inherent high risk of trauma in pregnant and non-pregnant women. Scuba diving should be avoided throughout pregnancy because the fetus is at increased risk of decompression sickness secondary to the inability of the fetal pulmonary circulation to filter bubbles formation (Camporesi 1996). As for exertion at altitude, reports are available for activities at less than 2500 m (6000 ft). In one study conducted at 2500 m, it was concluded that pregnant women may engage in periods of exercise and/or moderate physical tasks, but are limited in performing high intensity physical activities. No adverse fetal responses were recorded during this study (Artal *et al.* 1995). Other studies confirm the lack of adverse effects on the fetus at altitudes typically used for mountain sports such as hiking or skiing (<2500 m; Huch 1996). Avoidance of acute exposure (>3000 m) is recommended and intense exercise above 2500 m should be avoided. All women who are recreationally active should be aware of signs of altitude sickness, for which they should stop exercise, descend from altitude, and seek medical attention (Huch 1996). For symptoms of altitude sickness see Table 13.4.

Water exercise

The major effect of immersion is a redistribution of extravascular fluid into the vascular space, resulting in an increase in blood volume (Epstein 1984; Epstein *et al.* 1987). This effect occurs very rapidly and is proportional to the depth of immersion, leading to a decrease in systemic blood pressure (both systolic and diastolic). These changes are accompanied by a decrease in antidiuretic hormone, aldosterone, and plasma renin activity, while the

Table 13.4 Symptoms of acute mountain sickness. After Artal (1991).

Headache
Mild nausea/vomiting
Dyspnea
Anorexia/loss of appetite
Broken sleep patterns
Lethargy/weakness
Dizziness

If no descent, high altitude pulmonary edema or high altitude cerebral edema can develop; both can lead to coma and death.

atrial natriuretic factor decreases. The shift in blood volume leads to ventilatory changes with a decline in vital capacity, ventilation capacity, and expiratory reserve volume (Berry *et al.* 1989). Immersion is ideal for dissipating exercise-induced increases in temperature during exercise in pregnancy (McMurray *et al.* 1993).

In longitudinal studies of immersion exercise in pregnancy at 60% maximal oxygen consumption, it was found to be a safe activity, with advantageous effects on edema, thermal regulation, and buoyancy, thus minimizing the risk of joint injuries (Katz *et al.* 1988). Furthermore, no adverse effects on the fetus have been reported to occur during water exercise in pregnancy.

Exercise prescription for the pregnant elite athlete

Some competitive elite female athletes, as a result of their personal goals, continue intense training throughout the child-bearing years. Many female athletes defer pregnancy, but if they become pregnant, attempt to integrate training and competition schedules into the pregnancy with the recognition for potential maternal and fetal risks as for the general population. One study findings showed that elite athletes have less weight gain by the mother (4.6 kg), earlier deliveries (8 days), smaller babies (500 g), with shorter first and second stages of labor (Clapp & Dickstein 1984).

Pregnant elite athletes who intend to continue to train at a high level of intensity could lessen the risks by seeking closer obstetric supervision. The concerns of the pregnant competitive athlete fall into

two general categories: (i) the effects of pregnancy on competitive ability; and (ii) the effects of strenuous training and competition on pregnancy, particularly on the fetus.

Athletes often put themselves at higher risk for overuse injuries and often disregard body signals and continue to exercise despite discomforts. The degree of laxity in joints and ligaments in pregnancy will vary significantly from one individual to another and could prompt a change in training routine. The ability to stop and start or to change direction will progressively decrease. Attempts to substitute compensatory movements for finely tuned, skilled motor movements result in inefficient movements, a decrease in competitive ability, and an increase in the risk of injury for the athlete. Performance in sports in which endurance is important may be adversely affected by the physiologic anemia commonly associated with the increased blood volume of pregnancy. Physicians and trainers also need to realize that these women are accustomed to higher intensity training than recreational athletes and are better able to withstand heat stress (Hale & Artal 1991).

Often, the nutritional status of the competitive athlete is inadequate as a result of concerns about weight control. As assessment of the nutritional intake and need for vitamins and nutrients should be performed before pregnancy if possible. Many athletes alter their daily intake of carbohydrates, fats, and protein (Chen *et al.* 1989). Inadequate nutrition and weight gain has been associated with intrauterine growth restriction (IUGR) as a result of strenuous activities and deficient diet. IUGR occurs when the fetus weighs less than 10% for gestational age and is associated with an increased perinatal morbidity and mortality. Excessive intake of vitamins could potentially result in an increased incidence of human congenital malformations (Garcia *et al.* 1964).

There are no data to suggest that athletes have lower or higher rates of spontaneous abortion than non-athletes; the incidence of spontaneous abortion in the USA is about 16%. It is important to try to plan the pregnancy during the off-season because any threatened abortion would be a contraindication to physical activity. Other common first trimester symptoms include nausea, vomiting, and fatigue, which can have a serious impact on the athlete's ability to train or compete (Hale & Artal 1991), and put them at increased risk of dehydration.

Many athletes and trainers believe the myth that fluids are bad for an athlete during training. Dehydration must be prevented as this is the leading cause of an elevated core temperature (Hale & Milne 1996); the resultant hyperthermia may have deleterious effects on the mother and fetus. Hyperthermia in the first 30 days' gestation could cause neural tube defects (NTD). Thus, it is advisable that females do not engage in strenuous activities during this critical time. Activities that could raise the body core temperature above 39.2°C, the threshold for human teratogenesis are not recommended. Pregnant women should be instructed to take a minimum of one glass of fluid for every 15 min of workout or competition and to avoid elevation in body core temperature above 38.5°C. Fluid balance during and between exercise sessions can be monitored by weighing before and after the session. Any loss of weight is fluid which should be made up before the next session (1 lb weight loss = 1 pint of fluid; Artal & O'Toole 2005). Patients can also be instructed to observe their urine color. If it appears dark, the specific gravity of the urine should be tested.

It is extremely difficult for the athlete to participate in training beyond 20 weeks' gestation. Dependent upon the sport, this could be earlier, as the anatomic changes in posture, weight, and center of gravity affect the athlete's performance. The risk of direct fetal injury as pregnancy progresses is of significant concern. Blunt trauma or falls are more common types of injuries, with a penetrating trauma not likely during professional sports. A summary of the risks and guidelines for the elite professional athlete are found in Table 13.5.

Exercise prescription for special populations

Pregnant women with diabetes mellitus, morbid obesity, or chronic hypertension should have individualized exercise prescriptions. The information available in the literature is limited with regard to the role of physical activity for these women. The American Diabetes Association has endorsed exercise as "a helpful adjunctive therapy" for gestational diabetes when euglycemia is not achieved by diet alone (Javanovic 1998). Gestational diabetes is a state of altered insulin sensitivity; therefore exercise is a logical therapeutic intervention. A contracting skeletal muscle can increase its glucose uptake 35-fold. Following exercise, glucose tolerance is increased for variable periods, depending on both insulin and contractile activity. It appears that muscles help regulate the capacity for contraction stimulated glucose transport. Research suggests

Table 13.5 Risks of exercise in pregnancy for the elite athlete. From Artal (1991) with permission.

Risks	Guidelines
Maternal	
Musculoskeletal injuries	With evidence of joint and ligament laxity, individualize and modify training
Cardiovascular complications	Warning signs include palpitations and tachycardia at rest or any signs of orthostatic hypotension
Threatened abortion or premature labor	Stop training
Hypoglycemia	Prevent hypoglycemia by following proper nutritional guidelines
Fetal	
Fetal distress	Be alert to fetal movements/activity. In the presence of any complication, stop training and resume only after medical clearance
Intrauterine growth restriction	Stop training
Fetal malformations	Avoid hyperthermia and dehydration immediately after conception and weeks thereafter
Fetal injuries	Avoid sports in which there are a higher probability of blunt trauma after 16–20 weeks' gestation

that exercise may be beneficial in the prevention of gestational diabetes (GDM) especially in women with a BMI >33 kg·m^{-2}. In an unpublished study (Artal *et al.* 2005), moderate physical activity in obese and morbidly obese patients with GDM was beneficial when used in combination with an isocaloric or hypocaloric consistent carbohydrate diet to limit maternal weight gain during pregnancy. An exercise prescription for women who have traditional GDM can be applied to women with type 2 diabetes who become pregnant. An exercise program for pregnant women with type 1 diabetes may differ or be contraindicated because of exercise-related hypoglycemia and uncertain effects of previously injected insulin. An obstetrician with expertise in high risk obstetrics should be closely involved in the treatment of all patients who have GDM. Traditional care for women with GDM involves dietary changes and, if necessary, insulin therapy. Incorporating exercise, however, can reduce or eliminate the need for insulin (Artal 1996).

Currently, there is no information available on the effect of exercise on women with chronic hypertension. The current standard of care for women with pregnancy-induced hypertension is to limit physical activity.

Postpartum exercise prescription

Many of the physiologic and morphologic changes of pregnancy persist up to 4–6 weeks postpartum. Thus, exercise routines may be resumed gradually after pregnancy and should be individualized when physically and medically safe. This will certainly vary from one woman to another, with some being capable of engaging in an exercise routine within days of delivery.

Most women can resume their previous activities gradually during the postpartum period. However, there are no published studies to indicate that, in the absence of medical complications, rapid resumption of activities will result in adverse effects. No known maternal complications are associated with resumption of training (Pate *et al.* 1995). Failure to lose weight gained in pregnancy is a significant contributor to the obesity epidemic. One study showed that the amount of postpartum weight retention

increases with each subsequent pregnancy. Another study found that women who gained excessive weight during pregnancy and failed to lose it within 6 months postpartum were 8.3 kg heavier 10 years later. One reported study found that a weekly, structured exercise program plus diet in postpartum overweight women was much more effective in achieving weight loss after 12 weeks than a single 1-h education about diet and exercise (Artal 2003). Also, a return to physical activity after pregnancy has been associated with decreased postpartum depression, but only if the exercise is stress relieving and not stress provoking (Koltyen & Schultes 1997). Joints and ligaments may require as much as 3 months for return to their prepregnancy configuration. From the athlete's perspective, recovery from pregnancy, labor, and delivery is also overcoming a detraining period. The process of regaining complete physical fitness is a gradual one which includes restorative processes (Artal & Buckenmeyer 1995).

Moderate weight reduction while nursing is safe and does not compromise neonatal weight gain (McCrory *et al.* 1999). Failure of the infant to gain weight is associated with decreased milk production, which may be secondary to inadequate fluid or nutritional intake to balance training induced outputs. Fluid and nutritional status should be closely monitored in the athlete who is breastfeeding to ensure an adequate milk supply and that the proper nutritional quality is produced to maintain the health and growth of the infant. Nursing women should consider feeding their infants before exercising in order to avoid the discomfort of engorged breasts. (Kulpa 1994; Kulpa *et al.* 1987). In addition, nursing before exercise avoids the potential problems associated with increased acidity of milk secondary to any build-up of lactic acid.

Menstrual abnormalities in the female athlete

Women who are involved in strenuous recreational exercise, competitive athletics, and other forms of demanding activities have a significant incidence of delayed menarche, amenorrhea, and/or menstrual irregularities. It is impossible to predict what level of activity precedes these menstrual changes but once these changes occur, they may continue throughout her reproductive life (Hale 2004). Many athletes are not concerned with amenorrhea because menses are viewed as inconvenient and untimely for training and competition. Multiple sources have identified a phenomenon known as "the female athlete triad" which includes amenorrhea, eating disorder, and osteoporosis as a major concern among physically active females of all ages as well as elite athletes (American College of Sports Medicine 1997).

Frisch (1985) developed the critical weight hypothesis that states that the onset and regularity of menstrual function necessitates maintaining weight and body fat above a critical level (Frisch *et al.* 1981). The onset of menarche was believed to occur when a critical body weight declined to approximately 48 kg (106 lb). Some believe that the onset is determined by body composition; the ratio of fat : total body weight (Mishell *et al.* 1997). Accurate methods of determining body composition are available using hydrostatic weighing, considered to be the "gold standard" (Rosenbloom 1999), dual energy X-ray absorptiometry (DEXA), and air displacement plethysmography (Hoffman & Hildebrandt 2001).

Individuals who are moderately obese (20–30% above the ideal body weight) have an earlier onset of menarche than non-obese women. Malnutrition is known to delay the onset of menarche. In one study it was reported that ballet dancers, swimmers, and runners had menarche delayed to about age 15 if they began exercising strenuously before menarche. Girls engaged in athletic training before the onset of menarche had menarche delayed 0.4 years for each year of training or, as shown in other studies, had delays in menarche for up to 3 years, with a high incidence of menstrual irregularity (Speroff *et al.* 1999). Although the cause of delay in menarche is subject to debate, it does not seem to have an impact on future reproductive capability (Frisch *et al.* 1981).

Primary amenorrhea is defined as absence of any spontaneous menses in an individual older than 16.5 years. The incidence of primary amenorrhea is 0.1% (Mishell *et al.* 1997). Secondary amenorrhea is defined as the absence of periods for a length of time equivalent to a total of at least three of the previous cycle intervals or 6 months of amenorrhea in a person who has previously had spontaneous menstrual periods (Speroff *et al.* 1999). The incidence of secondary amenorrhea for women who do not exercise and for women who exercise for recreation is thought to be similar at 2–3%. For the woman who is involved in more strenuous training or where there is an emphasis on low body weight, the rate of occurrence increases (Drinkwater & Davajan 1991) and has been reported to be as high as 44% (American College of Sports Medicine 1997). It was also reported that the incidence of secondary amenorrhea in runners had a positive correlation with the number of miles run per week (Mishell *et al.* 1997). Prevalence rates vary by population, and type and level of activity (Table 13.6).

Etiology

The key to regular menstrual function lies in the production of gonadotropin-releasing hormone (GnRH) in the hypothalamus. As the critical body composition is reached with menarche, GnRH is secreted in greater amounts, causing pulsatile secretions of luteinizing hormone (LH), an increase of follicle-stimulating hormone (FSH), and activation of gonadatropin response to estradiol, resulting in ovulation and regular menses (Mishell *et al.* 1997).

Exercise is known to decrease gonadotropins and dependent upon the level of GnRH suppression, delayed menarche, inadequate luteal phase, anovulation, oligomenorrhea, secondary amenorrhea will develop (Speroff *et al.* 1999). Athletic amenorrhea is termed hypothalamic amenorrhea, based upon studies of the hypothalamic–pituitary–ovarian axis in eumenorrheic and amenorrheic athletes. Eumenorrheic women were found to have reduced LH pulsatile frequency, increased LH pulse amplitude, reduction in FSH response to GnRH stimulation, and a decrease in luteal function. This decrease in luteal function could potentially compromise fertility even in the presence of normal menses. In the amenorrheic woman, LH pulse frequency was reduced but the LH response to GnRH stimulation was increased (Drinkwater & Davajan 1991). It was

Table 13.6 Prevalence of secondary amenorrhea. From Artal (1991) with permission.

Population	Number	%	Definition of amenorrhea
Controls			
College	500	2.3	>2 months with no periods
Swedes	2000	3.3	<3 periods/year
Runners			
Cross-country	128	24.0	<3 periods/year
Cross-country	38	44.7	No periods for the last 3 months
>30 miles/week	89	24	0–5 periods/year
5–30 miles/week	22	14	0–5 periods/year
New York Marathon	270	1	<1 period for the last 10 months
Joggers	885	6	No definition provided
Marathon	237	25.7	<3 periods/year
Ballet dancers			
Students	69	18.8	At least 3 months with no period
Professional + students	34	44	At least 3 months with no period
Athletes			
College varsity	140	12.1	No periods for the last 3 months or <4 periods/year
Swimmers	197	12.3	<3 periods/year
Cyclists	33	12.1	<3 periods/year

reported that when training became more strenuous, LH and FSH levels fell significantly compared to those exercising at a moderate level (Mishell *et al.* 1997).

Exercise is also known to increase endorphins, growth hormone, testosterone, adrenocorticotropic hormone (ACTH), adrenal steroids, and prolactin as a result of both enhanced secretion and reduced clearance (Speroff *et al.* 1999). The arcuate nucleus area in the hypothalamus, the site of GnRH secretion, contains opioid receptors and produces endorphins. It has been shown that β-endorphins rise in response to acute exercise in non-athletes and that this response is augmented after training (Drinkwater & Davajan 1991). Women studied during a period of endurance conditioning demonstrated a steady increase in endorphin output after exercise. One study found that physical conditioning facilitates exercise-induced secretion of β-endorphin and its precursor β-lipoprotein in women (Mishell *et al.* 1997). There is evidence indicating that the endogenous opiate peptides inhibit the pulsatile gonadatropin secretion by suppressing hypothalamic GnRH (Drinkwater & Davajan 1991; Speroff *et al.* 1999).

Others question whether the observed increase in endogenous opiates is large enough to have a physiologic role in the etiology of athletic amenorrhea (Drinkwater & Davajan 1991).

Women with hypothalamic amenorrhea also demonstrate hypercortisolism supporting the hypothalamic–pituitary–ovarian and hypothalamic–pituitary–adrenal pathways in which stress interrupts reproductive function. Stress causes impaired activity of the opioid and serotonin neurotransmitters, resulting in multiple alterations in the hypothalamic control of the pituitary gland (Mishell *et al.* 1997). Eumenorrheic and amenorrheic athletes had no difference in ACTH response but cortisol levels were elevated in the amenorrheic group (Drinkwater & Davajan 1991; Mishell *et al.* 1997; Speroff *et al.* 1999).

Prolactin synthesis and release is controlled by the central nervous system neurotransmitters that act on the pituitary via the hypothalamus. The prolactin increases from exercise are variable, small in amplitude and short in duration, and do not occur in malnourished women. Insignificant differences occur in prolactin secretion when amenorrheic runners are compared with eumenorrheic runners or non-runners (Speroff *et al.* 1999). Therefore it is unlikely that the prolactin level contributes to the suppression of the menstrual cycle (Mishell *et al.* 1997).

Women athletes have elevated daytime melatonin levels, with amenorrheic athletes having an exaggerated nocturnal secretion of melatonin reflecting suppression of GnRH pulsatile secretion. Athletes can therefore expect to have more menstrual irregularities in the autumn and winter than in the spring or summer. Additionally, athletes have relatively low levels of T4 and amenorrheic athletes have been shown to have an overall suppression of all circulating thyroid hormones (Speroff *et al.* 1999).

Dietary intake can impact menstrual function by the caloric intake and nutritional content of the food. Various studies reported that amenorrheic athletes consume fewer calories than their eumenorrheic peers (Drinkwater & Davajan 1991), whereas others have reported no significant differences. An inadequate nutrient intake could theoretically affect neurotransmitter synthesis which could have an affect on hypothalamic function. However, there is no evidence to support a potential link (Drinkwater & Davajan 1991). In all of the studies, the caloric intake of the athletes was less than their predicted energy expenditure. The energy deficit could be enough for some women to initiate hormonal responses (elevated cortisol and depressed thyroid function) as seen in cachexia, starvation, or anorexia nervosa, causing interruption of the hypothalamic–pituitary–adrenal axis (Drinkwater & Davajan 1991). The role of body fat upon estrogen metabolism has been studied, with the suggestion that a suboptimal amount of body fat leads to an increased conversion of biologically active estrogens to inactive catecholestogens, with subsequent formation of 2-hydroxyestrone, an inactive metabolite. If true, this could interfere with feedback roles for estradiol in pituitary–ovarian interactions for athletic women (Speroff *et al.* 1999).

Exercising women often consciously make an effort to decrease body weight. Research shows the prevalence of eating disorders in exercising and elite female athletes ranging 1–62%, dependent upon the sport and measurement tool (Rosenbloom 1999). Rates of eating disorders in the general population range 0.5–1% for anorexia nervosa, 1–4% for bulimia nervosa with a ratio of 10:1 of women to men. Binge eating is the most common eating disorder, affecting 2% of all adults. Four stages of dieting behaviors have been defined: dieting for cosmetic reasons; dieting because of neurotic fixation on food intake and weight; the anorectic reaction; and true anorexia nervosa. Female athletes can develop an anorectic reaction consciously and voluntarily unlike true anorexia nervosa where misperception of reality and lack of insight exist (Speroff *et al.* 1999). Counseling and support can prevent the progression to anorexia nervosa.

Athletes participating in a sport where appearance, leanness, or weight classification is perceived to be a measure of their ability are at greater risk of developing an eating disorder. Restricting food or intake of fluids, increased exercise, and use of a sauna are common weight control measures used by athletes. Female gymnasts today weigh almost 20 lb less than their counterparts 20 years ago (Rosenbloom 1999). When women lose more than 15% of their ideal body weight, amenorrhea can occur as a result of CNS–hypothalmic dysfunction. When weight loss drops below 25% of ideal weight, pituitary gonadatropin function can also become abnormal (Mishell *et al.* 1997).

Weight gain may reverse the state of amenorrhea and the majority of women will resume ovulation when stress and exercise diminish. The response to GnRH, which is regained at approximately 15% below the ideal weight, must return to normal before the resumption of menses can occur (Speroff *et al.* 1999).

Evaluation and treatment

The patient who presents with amenorrhea requires a careful medical history, physical examination, pregnancy testing, and evaluation for psychologic dysfunction, emotional stress, family history of genetic anomalies, signs of a physical problem with focus on nutritional status, abnormal growth and development, the presence of a normal reproductive tract, and evidence for central nervous system disease. The diagnosis of delayed menarche versus primary amenorrhea should be determined by the clinician based on the presence of secondary sex characteristics and intact female genitalia. The initial steps in evaluating the patient with secondary amenorrhea, after excluding pregnancy, is to obtain a thyroid-stimulating hormone level, prolactin level, and a progestational challenge (Speroff *et al.* 1999). The purpose of the progestational challenge is to assess the level of endogenous estrogen and the competence of the outflow tract. The use of progestational agents such as medroxyprogesterone 10 mg for 12 days or progesterone 400 mg for 12 days are appropriate. Within 2–7 days of the progestational challenge, the patient will either bleed or not bleed. With a positive withdrawal bleed of any amount, the presence of estrogen is at least 40 $pg \cdot mL^{-1}$, minimal function of the ovary, pituitary, and CNS has been established and no further work-up is required (Speroff *et al.* 1999). Re-evaluation should occur in 3 months; in the absence of spontaneous menses, progesterone withdrawal should occur every 3 months.

If no withdrawal bleed occurs, a course of oral estrogen can be administered at a dosage of 0.625–1.25 $mg \cdot day^{-1}$ for 21 days followed by an additional progestational agent for the last 5 days. If no withdrawal bleed occurs, then additional laboratory studies are required to determine if the gonadatropin or follicular activities are functioning properly. A serum E2, FSH and mid-cycle LH can be drawn (Drinkwater & Davajan 1991; Speroff *et al.* 1999). Hormone therapy can be offered to counteract the hypoestrogenic state to provide protection for bone health. Treatment requires hormones used in a cyclic or continuous regimen in the form of oral contraceptives (the efficacy of transdermal or vaginal hormone rings remains to be proven). One retrospective study of amenorrheic runners compared hormonal therapy with placebo over 24–30 months. The regimen included either conjugated estrogen in a dosage of 0.625 $mg \cdot day^{-1}$ or an estradiol transdermal patch at 50 $\mu g \cdot day^{-1}$. Both were given in combination with medroxyprogesterone in a dosage of 10 $mg \cdot day^{-1}$ for 14 days per month. Patients receiving hormonal therapy showed a significant increase in bone mineral density, while those in the control group showed non-significant decreases of less than 2.5%. Small studies have supported the use of oral contraceptives in persons with athletic (hypothalamic) amenorrhea. Retrospective studies have shown that athletes with a history of oral contraceptive use may have decreased risk of stress fracture (Hobart & Smucker 2000).

If a hypoestrogenic woman refuses hormone therapy, counseling regarding the risk for developing premature osteoporosis should be offered. Minimally, treatment with calcium supplements of 1000–1500 $mg \cdot day^{-1}$ and 400–800 IU vitamin D to facilitate the absorption of calcium should be strongly encouraged. High calcium intake when combined with a high level of exercise is believed to be more effective in protecting the vertebral bone density than either exercise or calcium supplementation alone (Speroff *et al.* 1999).

Hypothalmic amenorrhea will not protect against pregnancy in the event that normal function unknowingly returns. It is reasonable to utilize a low dose oral contraceptive, vaginal ring, or transdermal patch to provide the missing estrogen. Athletes interested in avoiding menstruation can utilize these methods continuously every day/week/month (as appropriate for the chosen method), skipping the 1-week hormone-free interval. Breakthrough bleeding can result for some women on continuous therapy and athletes should be counseled about this potential side effect.

Women who exercise are more likely to develop dysmenorrhea than women who do not. Prostaglandin release resulting from exercise and the endometrium contribute to an increase in the strength of uterine contractions. Treatment with antiprostaglandin therapies or continuous combined estrogen–progesterone therapies can alleviate these symptoms (Clapp *et al.* 2000).

Exercise and bone health in the female athlete

There are two types of living bone found in the human skeleton: cortical and trabecular bone. Cortical bone is dense, used for structure and support, and makes up about 20% of the bone in our body. Trabecular bone is porous, forms the long and flat bones, and makes up approximately 80% of the human skeleton.

Living bone goes through a remodeling process in which osteoclasts dissolve bone mineral and digest bone matrix, and osteoblasts synthesize bone matrix. Approximately 40% of trabecular bone is recycled annually compared to only 10% of the cortical bone. This renewal process determines the strength of bone. Osteoblasts have estrogen receptors that increase the number of osteoblasts and osteoblast collagen production, increase nuclear progesterone receptors in osteoblasts, and increase the osteoblastic messenger RNA for transforming growth factor β. Estrogen also inhibits parathyroid hormone-related increase in cyclic adenosine monophospate (Notelovitz 1997).

Bone mass is maintained when the resorptive and formation phases are balanced. Accelerated bone loss is associated with enhanced osteoclast activity leading to osteoporosis; a skeletal disease characterized by low bone mass and microarchitectural deterioration of bone tissue. Osteoporosis is defined when the bone density is 2.5 standard deviations below the normal for the patient's age. Enhanced bone fragility with an increase in consequent increase fracture risk are hallmarks of the disease, which occurs more frequently in women after the menopause than in men (Notelovitz 1997).

Factors that affect peak bone mass include genetic make-up, nutrition, exercise, and hormonal status. Caucasian and Asian women as well as those with a family history of osteoporosis are at greater risk. Bone mineral densities of young women who are monozygotic are more similar than those of dizygotic twins. Vitamin D genetic defects are associated with reduced bone density.

Nutritional intake of calcium is essential to bone development. North American girls and women are often lacking the recommended calcium in their daily diets. Eating disorders such as bulimia and anorexia nervosa could lead to reduced bone mineral density. In 1997, the daily recommendations for calcium were increased for the first time since 1941. For adolescents aged 9–18 years, guidelines stipulate 1300 mg·day^{-1} calcium and adults aged 19–50 years need 1000 mg·day^{-1} (National Institutes of Health Consensus Development Panel on Optimal Calcium Intake 1994). Multiple studies of young girls showed the benefit of increasing calcium intake in daily diets. A 3-year study showed that 6- to 14-year-old girls enhanced the rate of bone mineral density by increasing their intake of calcium to 1600 mg·day^{-1} (Johnston 1992). A study in Utah with 9- to 13-year-old girls found similar results by increasing the intake of calcium to 1400 mg·day^{-1} (Chan 1995). No weight gain, body fat, or increase in total or saturated fat intake was noted. Twelve-year-old girls were given 1300 mg·day^{-1} calcium with significant increase of total and spinal bone density (Lloyd 1993).

Exercise is directly associated with the process of matrix remolding of the trabeculae and cortices of bone. Exercise initiates the bone remolding cycle because mechanical loading, muscular activity, and gravity stimulate the bone cells to differentiate and grow. Bone mineral maintenance depends upon the type of exercise, frequency of exercise, and use of gravity during exercise (Notelovitz 1997). The need for exogenous calcium to meet the increased demands may be a critical factor in maximizing exercise-induced osteogenesis. This may explain why exercising amenorrheic women have lower levels of trabecular but not cortical bone mineral when compared with menstruating women. The positive effect of exercise on bone mass may be related to an increase in muscle mass. Female tennis players were found to have greater overall bone mass than recreational tennis players and a 28.4% greater cortical thickness in the dominant arm (Notelovitz 1997).

Studies have shown that the earlier the age at menarche, the greater the subsequent bone mineral density (BMD) and, conversely, the later the age of menarche, the lower the BMD. Recent studies have indicated that peak bone mass occurs at a younger age than was previously described. Several studies have shown that the average age of peak bone mass is closer to 18–25 years rather than the currently accepted age of 30 years (Hobart & Smucker 2000).

Data indicate that exercising women with amenorrhea have a significant reduction in circulating estrogen levels (Hale 2004). Lack of estrogen triggers a dramatic increase in cytokines involved in bone remolding. Reduced BMD has been found in women with irregular menstrual cycles. In one study, bone mass was reduced by 12% in women who missed less than 50% of their expected menses and 31% in women who missed more than 50% of their expected cycles compared with women with normal monthly cycles. Women with asymptomatic anovulation and no associated amenorrhea have lower bone mass than normal ovulating women. Bone loss with anovulation was estimated in one study to be 4.2% (Notelovitz 1997). Prolonged amenorrhea was found to affect multiple axial and appendicular skeletal sites including those that were subjected to impact loading during exercise. In a study of young female athletes, persistent patterns of amenorrhea were found to have a linear correlation to measures of bone density (Hobart & Smucker 2000). Another study evaluated previously amenorrheic women who had resumed regular menses. After the first 14 months, their BMD increased by an average of 6%. However, this trend did not continue and the rate of increase slowed to 3% the following year. BMD reached a plateau at a level that was well below the normal level for their age (Hobart & Smucker 2000).

The prevention of osteoporosis starts with menarche. A combination of exercise, appropriate nutrition, and a healthy lifestyle maximizes bone mineral accrual and results in optimal peak bone mass. Normal ovarian function is essential to this process and it is generally recognized that exercise is essential to stimulate new bone formation. Adequate nutrition and calcium intake is essential to mineralize the newly formed osteoid and an estrogen replete state is necessary to modulate the rate of bone loss (Notelovitz 1997).

Treatments for osteoporosis with bisphosphonates and calcitonin have not been tested on younger women. However, all available treatment options should be considered in the athlete with osteoporosis on the basis of DEXA scanning (Hobart & Smucker 2000). Documentation of the bone loss may enhance patient compliance with recommendations for changes in eating behaviors, training regimens, and medical interventions as indicated.

Conclusions

Women are involved in recreational exercise or competitive athletics to improve both physical and mental health. Elite as well as recreational athletes must learn to balance both training and competitive activities to ensure gynecologic and reproductive function without the development of adverse consequences. Additionally, pregnancy and postpartum states present unique challenges for athletically active women and require careful monitoring to maintain maternal and fetal well-being. Conversely, pregnancy should not be a state of confinement. Women of all levels of physical activity should benefit from the awareness of issues affecting their gynecologic and reproductive health throughout their lifespan.

References

Ahlborg, G., Bodin, L. & Hagstedt, C. (1990) Heavy lifting during pregnancy: a hazard to the fetus? A prospective study. *International Journal of Epidemiology* **19**, 90–97.

American College of Obstetricians and Gynecologists (2002) Committee Opinion 267. *Exercise during Pregnancy and the Postpartum Period* **99**, No 1.

American College of Sports Medicine (1997) Position stand on the female athlete triad. *Medicine and Science in Sports and Exercise* **29**, i–ix.

American College of Sports Medicine (2000) *Guidelines for Exercise Testing and Prescription*, 6th edn. Lippincott,

Williams & Wilkins, Philadelphia: 133–173.

American Dietetic Association (2002) Position Statement: Nutrition and lifestyle for a healthy pregnancy outcome. *Journal of the American Dietetic Association* **102**, 1479–1483.

Artal, R. (1990) Exercise and diabetes mellitus: a brief review. *Sports Medicine* **9**, 261–265.

Artal, R. (1996) Exercise: an alternative therapy for gestational diabetes. *Physician and Sports Medicine* **24**, 54–61.

Artal, R. (1999) Exercise during pregnancy: safe and beneficial for most. *Physician and Sports Medicine* **27**, 51–60.

Artal, R. (2003) Make exercise recommendations a priority. *Obstetrics Gynecology News*, 48–49.

Artal, R. & Buckenmeyer, P. (1995) Exercise during pregnancy and postpartum. *Contemporary Obstetrics and Gynecology* **40**, 62–86.

Artal, R., Catanzara, R., Gavard, J., Mostello, D. & Friganza, J. (2007) Weight gain in pregnancy: comparison of a nutrition and physical activity intervention program for gestational diabetes. *Applied Physiology Nutrition Metabolism* **32**, 596–601.

Artal, R., Fortunator, V. & Welton, A. (1995) A comparison of cardiopulmonary adaptations to exercise in pregnancy at sea level and altitude. *American Journal of Obstetrics and Gynecology* **172**, 1170–1180.

Artal, R. & O'Toole, M. (2005) Guidelines of the American College of Obstetricians and Gynecologists for exercise during pregnancy and the postpartum period. *British Journal of Sports Medicine* **37**, 6–12.

Artal, R., Wiswell, R. & Roman, Y. (1986) Pulmonary responses to exercise in pregnancy. *American Journal of Obstetrics and Gynecology* **154**, 378–383.

Berry, M., McMurray, R. & Katz, V. (1989) Pulmonary and ventilatory responses to pregnancy, immersion and exercise. *Journal of Applied Physiology* **66**, 857–862.

Camporesi, E. (1996) Diving and pregnancy. *Seminar in Perinatology* **20**, 292–302.

Carpenter, M., Sady, S. & Hoegsberg, B. (1988) Fetal heart rate response to maternal exertion. *Journal of the American Medical Association* **259**, 3006–3009.

Chan, G. (1995) Effects of dairy products on bone and body composition in pubertal girls. *Journal of Pediatrics* **126**, 551.

Chen J., Wang, J. & Li, K. (1989) Nutritional problems and measures in elite and amateur athletes. *American Journal of Clinical Nutrition* **49**, 1084.

Clapp, J. III (1985) Fetal heart rate responses to running in mid-pregnancy and late pregnancy. *American Journal of Obstetrics and Gynecology* **153**, 251–252.

Clapp, J. III (1990) Exercise in pregnancy: a brief clinical review. *Fetal Medical Review* **161**, 1464–1469.

Clapp, J. III (1993) Exercise in Pregnancy, good, bad or indifferent? In: *Current Obstetric Medicine* (Lee, R., Garne, P. & Barron, W., eds.) CV Mosby, Chicago: 24–48.

Clapp, J. & Capeless, E. (1990) Neonatal morphometrics after endurance exercise during pregnancy. *American Journal of Obstetrics and Gynecology* **163**, 1805–1811.

Clapp, J. & Dickstein, S. (1984) Endurance exercise and pregnancy outcome. *Medicine and Science in Sports and Exercise* **16**, 556–562.

Clapp, J., Kim, H., Burciu, B. & Lopez, B. (2000) Continuing regular exercise during pregnancy: effect of exercise volume on feto-placental growth. *American Journal of Obstetrics and Gynecology* **183**, 1484–1488.

Clapp, J. III., Seaward, B. & Sleamakere, R. (1988) Maternal physiologic adaptations to early human pregnancy. *American Journal of Obstetrics and Gynecology* **159**, 1456–1460.

Clark, S., Colton, D. & Varnik, J. (1991) Position change and central hemodynamic profile during normal third trimester pregnancy and post-partum. *American Journal of Obstetrics and Gynecology* **164**, 883–887.

Clark, S., Cotton, D. & Lee, W. (1989) Central hemodynamic assessment of normal term pregnancy. *American Journal of Obstetrics and Gynecology* **161**, 1439–1442.

Collings, C., Curet, L. & Mulin, J. (1983) Maternal and fetal responses to a maternal aerobic exercise program. *American Journal of Obstetrics and Gynecology* **145**, 702–707.

Crisp, W. & DeFrancesco, S. (1964) The hand syndrome of pregnancy. *Obstetrics and Gynecology* **23**, 433.

Drinkwater, B. & Davajan. V. (1991) Amenorrheic athlete and conception. *Exercise in Pregnancy*, 2nd edn. Williams & Wilkins, Baltimore: 239–246.

Epstein, M. (1984) Water immersion and the kidney: implications for volume regulation. *Undersea Biomedical Research* **11**, 114–137.

Epstein, M., Loutzenhiser, R. & Friedland, E. (1987) Relationship of increased plasma atrial natriuretic factor renal sodium handling during immersion-induced central hypervolemia in normal humans. *Journal of Clinical Investigators* **79**, 738–745.

Erdelyi, G. (1962) Gynecological survey of female athletes. *Journal of Sports Medicine and Physical Fitness* **2**, 174–175.

Frisch R.E. (1985) Body fat, menarche and reproductive ability. *Seminars in Reproductive Endocrinology* **3**, 45.

Frisch, R., Gotz-Welbergen, A., McArthur, J., Albright, T., Witschi, J. & Bullen, B. (1981) Delayed menarche and amenorrhea of college athletes in relation to age of onset of training. *JAMA* **246**, 1559–1563.

Garcia, R., Friedman, W. & Kabascr, M. (1964) Idiopathic hypercalcemia and supravalvular stenosis: documentation of a new syndrome. *New England Journal of Medicine* **271**, 117–120.

Hale, R. (2004) American College of Obstetricians and Gynecologists. *Clinical Updates in Women's Health Care* **3**, No 3.

Hale, R. & Artal, R. (1991) Pregnancy in the elite and professional athlete: a stepwise approach. In *Exercise in Pregnancy* 2nd edn. Williams & Wilkins, Baltimore: 231–238.

Hale, R. & Milne, L. (1996) The elite athlete and exercise in pregnancy. *Seminars in Perinatology* **20**, 277–284.

Hall, D. & Kaufmann, D. (1987) Effects of aerobic and strength conditioning on pregnancy outcomes. *American Journal of Obstetrics and Gynecology* **157**, 1199–1203.

Hatch, M., Shu, X. & McLean, D. (1993) Maternal exercise during pregnancy, physical fitness and fetal growth. *American Journal of Epidemiology* **137**, 1105–1114.

Hobart, J. & Smucker, D. (2000) The female athlete triad. *American Academy of Family Physicians* **61**, 3357–3364.

Hoffman, C. & Hildebrandt, L. (2001) Use of air displacement plethysmograph to monitor body composition: a beneficial tool for dieticians. *Journal of the American Dietetic Association* **101**, 986–988.

Huch, R. (1996) Physical activity at altitude in pregnancy. *Seminars in Perinatology* **20**, 303–314.

Institute of Medicine Subcommittee on Nutritional Status and Weight Gain During Pregnancy (1990) *Nutrition During Pregnancy*. National Academy Press, Washington.

Javanovic, L. (1998) American Diabetes Association's Fourth International Workshop: conference on gestational diabetes mellitus summary and discussion. *Therapeutic interventions* **21** (Supplement 2), B131–B137.

Johnson, J. & Yancey, M. (1996) A critique of the new recommendations for weight gain in pregnancy. *American Journal of Obstetrics and Gynecology* **174**, 254–258.

Johnston, C.C. Jr., Miller, J.Z., Slemenda, C.W., Reister, T.K., Hui, S., Christian, J.C., *et al.* (1992) Calcium supplementation and increases in bone mineral density in children. *New England Journal of Medicine* **327**, 82–87.

Jovanovic-Peterson, L. & Peterson, C. (1996) Exercise and the nutritional management of diabetes during pregnancy. *Obstetric Gynecology Clinics of North America* **23**, 75–86.

Karzel, R. & Friedman, M. (1991) Orthopedic injuries in pregnancy. In *Exercise in Pregnancy*, 2nd edn. Williams & Wilkins, Baltimore: 123–132.

Katz, V., McMurray, R. & Berry M. (1988) Fetal and uterine responses to immersion and exercise. *Obstetrics and Gynecology* **72**, 325–330.

Katz, V., McMurray, R. & Cefalo, R. (1991) Aquatic exercise during pregnancy. In *Exercise in Pregnancy*, 2nd edn. Williams & Wilkins, Baltimore: 271–278.

Koltyen, K. & Schultes, S. (1997) Psychological effects of an aerobic exercise session and a rest session following pregnancy. *Journal of Sports Medicine Physical Fitness* **37**, 287–291.

Kulpa, P. (1994) Exercise during pregnancy and post-partum. In *Medical and Orthopedic Issues of Active and Athletic Women*. Hanley & Belfus, Philadelphia: 191–199.

Kulpa, P., White, B. & Visscher, R. (1987) Aerobic exercise in pregnancy. *American Journal of Obstetrics and Gynecology* **156**, 1395–1403.

Latgering, F., Van Doorn, M. & Strujik, P. (1991) Maximal aerobic exercise in pregnant women: heart rate, O_2 consumption, CO_2 production and ventilation. *Journal of Applied Physiology* **70**, 1016–1023.

Launer, L., Villar, J. & Kestler, E. (1990) The effect of maternal work on fetal growth and duration of pregnancy: a prospective study. *British Journal of Obstetrics and Gynecology* **97**, 62–70.

Leet, T. & Flick, L. (2003) The effect of exercise on birth weight. *Clinical Obstetrics and Gynecology* **46**, 423–431.

Lloyd, T. (1993) Calcium supplementation and bone mineral density in adolescent girls. *JAMA* **270**, 841.

Lund, C. & Donovan, J. (1967) Blood volume during pregnancy. *American Journal of Obstetrics andGynecology* **98**, 393.

McCrory, M., Nommsen-Rivers, L.A., Mole, P., Lonnerdal, B. & Dewey, K.G. (1999) Randomized trial of short-term effects of dieting compared with dieting plus aerobic exercise on lactation performance. *American Journal of Clinical Nutrition* **69**, 959–967.

McDonald, A., McDonald, J. & Armstrong, B. (1988) Prematurity and work in pregnancy. *British Journal of Industrial Medicine* **45**, 56–62.

McMurray, R., Hackney, A. & Katz, V. (1991) Pregnancy-induced changes in the maximal physiological responses during swimming. *Journal of Applied Physiology* **71**, 1454–1459.

McMurray R., Molttola, M. & Wolfe, L. (1993) Recent advances in understanding maternal and fetal responses to exercise. *Medicine and Science in Sports and Exercise* **25**, 1305–1321.

Milunsky, A., Ulcickas, M. & Rothman, K. (1992) Maternal heat exposure and neural tube defects. *Journal of the American Medical Association* **268**, 882–885.

Mishell, D., Stenchevere, M., Droegemueller, W. & Herbst, A., eds. (1997) *Comprehensive Gynecology*, 3rd edn. Mosby, Chicago: 1043–1067.

Morton, J., Paul, M. & Campass, G. (1985) Exercise dynamics in late gestation. *American Journal of Obstetrics and Gynecology* **152**, 91–97.

Morton, M. (1991) Maternal hemodynamics in pregnancy. In *Exercise in Pregnancy*, 2nd edn. Williams & Wilkins, Baltimore: 61–70.

Naeye, R. & Peters, E. (1982) Working during pregnancy, effects on the fetus. *Pediatrics* **69**, 724–727.

National Institutes of Health (1994) Consensus Development Panel on Optimal Calcium Intake. *JAMA* **272**, 1942.

Notelovitz, M. (1997) *Osteoporosis: Prevention, Diagnosis, and Management*, 2nd edn. Professional Communications Incorporated.

Pate, R., Pratt, M. & Blair, S. (1995) A recommendation from the Centers of Disease Control and Prevention and the American College of Sports Medicine. *JAMA* **273**, 402–407.

Pivarnik, J. (1994) Maternal exercise during pregnancy. *Sports Medicine* **18**, 215–217.

Pivaranik, J. (1996) Cardiovascular responses to aerobic exercise during pregnancy and postpartum. *Seminars in Perinatology* **20**, 242–249.

Pivarnik, J., Lee, W. & Clark, S. (1990) Cardiac output responses of primigravid women during exercise determined by the direct Fick technique. *Obstetrics and Gynecology* **75**, 954–959.

Pivarnik, J., Lee, W. & Spillman, T. (1992) Maternal respiration and blood gases during aerobic exercise performed at moderate altitude. *Medicine and Science in Sports and Exercise* **24**, 868–872.

Prowse, C. & Gaensler, E. (1965) Respiratory and acid–base changes during pregnancy. *Anesthiology* **26**, 381–392.

Romen, Y., Masaki, D., & Artal R. (1991) Physiological and endocrine adjustments to pregnancy. In *Exercise in Pregnancy*, 2nd edn. Williams & Wilkins, Baltimore: 9–29.

Rosenbloom, C., ed. (1999) *Sports Nutrition: A guide for the professional working with active people*. American Dietetic Association, Chicago: 445–462.

Sady, S., Carpenter, M. & Thompson, P. (1989) Cardiovascular response to cycle during and after pregnancy. *Journal of Applied Physiology* **66**, 336–341.

Saurel-Cubizolles, M. & Kaminshki, M. (1987) Pregnant women's working conditions and their changes during pregnancy: a national study in France. *British Journal of Industrial Medicine* **44**, 236–243.

Shnider, S.M. & Levinson, G. (1993) *Anesthesia for Obstetrices*, 3rd edn. Williams & Wilkins, Baltimore.

Soultankis, H., Artal R. & Wiswell R. (1996) Prolonged exercise in pregnancy: glucose homeostasis, ventilatory and cardiovascular responses. *Seminars in Perinatology* **20**, 315–327.

Speroff, L., Glass, R. & Kase, N. (1999) *Clinical Gynecologic Endocrinology and Infertility*, 6th edn. Lippincott, Williams & Wilkins, Baltimore: 401–456.

Sternfeld, B., Queensberry, C. Jr. & Eskenazi, B. (1995) Exercise during pregnancy and pregnancy outcome. *Medicine and Science in Sports and Exercise* **27**, 634–640.

Templeton, A. & Kelman, G. (1976) Maternal blood-gases (PaO2-PaO2) physiological shunt and VD/VT in normal pregnancy. *British Journal of Anesthesiology* **48**, 1001–1004.

Tobin, S. (1967) Carpel tunnel syndrome in pregnancy. *American Journal of Obstetrics and Gynecology* **23**, 493.

Votik, A., Mueller, J., Farlinger, D. & Johnson, R. (1983) Carpal tunnel syndrome in pregnancy. *Canadian Medical Association Journal* **128**, 277.

Wolfe, L., Lowe-Wydle, S. & Tranmer J. (1988) Fetal heart rate response during maternal static exercise. *Canadian Journal of Sports Medicine* **13**, 95–96.

Wolfe, L., Ohtake, P. & Mattola, M. (1989) Physiological interactions between pregnancy and aerobic exercise. *Exercise and Sport Sciences Reviews* **17**, 295–351.

Chapter 14

Neurologic Problems in Sport

PAUL MCCRORY

Neurologic conditions are common in sport and the effects of exercise on chronic neurologic conditions represent a relatively underinvestigated form of therapy. An understanding of common neurologic syndromes is therefore core knowledge for the practicing sports physician and all those involved in neurologic care need to be acquainted with the role that exercise can have in the overall management of such patients.

Headache and sport

Headache is one of the most common medical complaints and athletes are no exception to this. Few headaches fail to evoke some anxiety in the sufferer, which may in turn distort the clinical symptoms. Confronted by an athlete with exercise-related headache, the sports physician needs to be accurate in diagnosis, clear in the direction of treatment, and reassure the individual concerned (McCrory 2000).

History

The association between headache and exercise has been known since the time of Ancient Greece. In 450 BC, Hippocrates wrote: "One should be able to recognize those who have headaches from gymnastic exercises or running or walking or hunting or any other unseasonable labour or from immoderate venery" (Hippocrates 1849) By the first century AD,

The Olympic Textbook of Medicine in Sport, 1st edition. Edited by M. Schwellnus. Published 2008 by Blackwell Publishing, ISBN: 978-1-4051-5637-0.

Areteus of Cappadocia (30–90 AD) termed headache as heterocrania and this concept was further developed in the following century by Galen of Pergammon (138–201 AD) who was the first to use the term hemicrania from which the terms "megrim" and migraine were subsequently derived (Arateus 1856).

Epidemiology of sport-related headache

The prevalence of headache in different sports is largely unknown. In a study of collegiate athletes, headaches were reported by 35% of all respondents with no gender effect evident (Williams & Nukada 1994a,b). Their headache prevalence by headache type is set out in Table 14.1. The sports noted to cause headache included running/jogging, weights/gym, aerobics, and rugby football. Post-traumatic headaches were seen almost universally in males resulting from participation in rugby football.

Community studies also note exercise as a potent trigger of migraine and other forms of headache; however, the precise epidemiology of this phenomenon is unknown (Rasmussen 1995).

Table 14.1 Headache prevalence in athletes. After Williams & Nukada 1994a,b.

Headache type	Headache prevalence (%)
Effort migraine	9
Trauma-induced migraine	6
Effort/exertion headache	60
Post-traumatic headache	22
Miscellaneous	3

There have been anecdotal reports of migraine with aura in particular sports such as soccer (Mathews 1972) and rugby league (Gibbs 1994). In a recent study in Australian football, approximately 50% of players reported regular headaches, with 22% of all players fulfilling the International Headache Society (IHS) criteria for migraine (McCrory *et al.* 2005).

Causes of headache

Intrinsic to the understanding of the causation of headache are the intracranial pain pathways and their interconnections especially the trigemino-cervical pathway. The most important structures that register pain within the skull are the blood vessels. Neurotransmitter control in this pain pathway includes serotonin, peptides, and acetylcholine. These may provide the pharmacologic basis of drug therapy. For example, sumatriptan and methysergide both directly affect the serotonin receptor to modulate migraine. Recent advances in the field of molecular biology have suggested a causative role for other vasoactive agents in the genesis of headache which may have important treatment implications (Olesen 1988; Olesen *et al.* 1995).

Clinical approach to headache

The majority of cases do not require detailed radiologic investigations but rather a thorough history and physical examination. When seeing an athlete complaining of headache for the first time, a sports physician may follow the simple diagnostic clinical algorithm set out below:

1 Exclude possible intracranial causes on history and physical exam. If intracranial pathology is suspected then an urgent work-up is required which usually includes neuroimaging studies and/or laboratory investigations.

2 Exclude headaches associated with viral or other infective illness.

3 Exclude a drug-induced headache (see below) or headache-related to alcohol and/or substance abuse.

4 Consider an exercise (or sex-related) headache syndrome.

5 Differentiate between vascular, tension, cervicogenic, or other cause of headache.

Table 14.2 Commonly used drugs that may cause headache in athletes.

Alcohol	NSAIDs
Anabolic steroids	Nicotine
Analgesics	Nitrazepam
Antibiotics	Oral contraceptives
Anti-hypertensives	Sympathomimetics
Caffeine	Theophylline
Corticosteroids	Vasodilator agents
Dipyridamole	

NSAIDs, non-steroidal anti-inflammatory drugs.

Many commonly used drugs can provoke headaches. Some of these drugs such as non-steroidal anti-inflammatory drugs (NSAIDs) are in widespread use by athletes. If not recognized, this may be the reason for treatment failure. A list of commonly used drugs that can cause headaches in athletes is set out in Table 14.2.

A headful of symptoms

As with many aspects of clinical medicine, the history is the most important component of the assessment of the athlete with headache. Many headache syndromes such as migraine can be diagnosed with a degree of confidence on history alone. The typical qualities of the headache that should be sought on history are set out in Table 14.3. Particular emphasis should be placed on recent

Table 14.3 Clinical history of headache.

Age of onset of the headaches
Frequency and duration
Time of onset of headache
Mode of onset
Site of pain and radiation
Headache quality
Associated symptoms
Precipitating factors
Aggravating and relieving factors
Previous treatments
General health
Past medical history
Family history
Social and occupational history
Drug and medication use

changes in neurologic function such as the development of focal or systemic symptoms.

In all patients presenting with headache, a full neurologic and general physical examination is required. Particular attention should be paid to the cervical spine as a potential source of headache. The examination should consist of some or all of the following components of a focused and thorough neurologic examination, depending on the presence or absence of specific symptoms in the patient's history. The main examination points should include general appearance (including skin lesions), vital signs (pulse, blood pressure, and temperature), mental status and speech, gait, balance and coordination, cranial nerve and long tract examination, visual fields, acuity and ophthalmoscopic fundus examination, and skull palpation.

Key symptoms to flag

The majority of headaches are a result of benign causes. Nevertheless, certain symptoms may indicate the presence of more serious pathology, such as a mass lesion or infective process, and require urgent neurologic assessment. These new symptoms, which should be sought by specific questioning in all cases, are set out in Table 14.4.

Exercise-related headache syndromes

As in the general population, the common headache syndromes such as migraine, episodic tension-type

Table 14.4 Key symptoms of intracranial pathology.

Sudden onset of severe headache
Headache increasing over a few days
New or unaccustomed headache
Persistently unilateral headaches
Chronic headache with localized pain
Stiff neck or other signs of meningism
Focal neurologic symptoms or signs
Atypical headache/change in the usual pattern of headache
Headaches that wake the patient during the night or early morning
Local extracranial symptoms (e.g., sinus, ear, or eye disease)
Systemic symptoms (e.g., weight loss, fever, and malaise)

headache, and cervicogenic headache will occur in athletes. These are discussed briefly. Readers are referred to more general headache textbooks for a greater understanding of these syndromes (Dalessio 1987; Lance & Goadsby 1998). In addition, a group of headache syndromes unique to exercise need to be considered and are described in more detail.

MIGRAINE

Given that the prevalence of migraine is approximately 12–18% in community populations, it follows that migraine will be commonly seen in exercising athletes. Migraine is essentially an episodic headache that is usually accompanied by nausea and photophobia and may be preceded by focal neurologic symptoms. Symptoms vary considerably between individuals. Migraine represents an inherited tendency to headache with a lowered threshold of susceptibility to a variety of headache triggers such as exercise and head trauma. At present, there is no simple "cure" for migraine and an individualized management strategy needs to be developed for each patient. This may incorporate non-pharmacologic as well as pharmacologic strategies.

The accurate diagnosis of headache syndromes in sport has important treatment implications. (McCrory 1997). In elite athletes, there are specific management considerations related to the use of "banned" drugs. Many conventional headache medications (e.g., beta-blockers, caffeine, codeine-containing preparations, dextro-propoxyphene, narcotics, and opioids) are banned agents and their use, if detected, may result in severe penalties for the athlete concerned.

TENSION-TYPE HEADACHE

Tension-type headache results in a constant tight or pressing sensation which may initially be episodic and related to stress but can recur almost daily in its chronic form without regard to any obvious psychologic factors. In general, these headaches are distinguished from migraine by their milder severity and longer duration, although a precise separation may not always be possible. Treatment is usually multifactorial and by necessity includes psychologic and physical therapy, physiologic intervention, and pharmacologic treatment.

CERVICOGENIC HEADACHE

Abnormalities of the various structures within the neck have been implicated as the cause of cervicogenic headache. These structures include the synovial joints, the intervertebral disks, ligaments, muscles, nerve roots, and the vertebral artery (Bogduk et al. 1985; Bogduk & Marsland 1986). Cervicogenic headache shares many of the clinical features of chronic tension-type headache. It is usually occipital in onset and may radiate to the anterior aspect of the skull and face. The headache is usually constant in nature, lasts for days to weeks, and has a definite association with movement of cervical structures. Treatment usually involves physical or manipulative therapy to the cervical spine as well as consideration of anti-inflammatory drug therapy.

BENIGN EXERTIONAL HEADACHE

Benign exertional headache (BEH) has been recognized as a separate entity for over 50 years. In 1932, Tinel first described severe but short-lasting headaches following exercise and subsequent authors have characterized a clear-cut syndrome (Diamond & Medina 1982a,b; Diamond et al. 1998; Powell 1982; Tinel 1932).

The criteria for BEH include:
1 The headache is specifically brought on by physical exercise;
2 It is bilateral, throbbing in nature at onset, and may develop migrainous features in those patients susceptible to migraine;
3 It lasts from 5 min to 24 h;
4 It is prevented by avoiding excessive exertion; and
5 It is not associated with any systemic or intracranial disorder.

The onset of the headache is with straining and Valsalva type maneuvres such as seen in weightlifting. Clearly, the major differential diagnosis to be considered in this situation is a subarachnoid hemorrhage which needs to be excluded by the appropriate investigations. It has been postulated that exertional headache is caused by dilatation of pain-sensitive venous sinuses at the base of the brain as a result of increased cerebral arterial pressure caused by the exertion. Studies of weightlifters demonstrate that systolic blood pressure may reach levels above 400 mmHg and diastolic pressures above 300 mmHg with maximal lifts (MacDougall et al. 1985).

The implication that these headaches have a vascular basis is supported by the migrainous nature of the headache and one interesting study that utilized intravenous dihydroergotamine to relieve the headache (Hazelrigg 1986). A similar type of vascular headache is described in relation to sexual activity and has been termed benign sex headache or orgasmic cephalgia. It is worth noting, however, that despite their vascular nature, no convincing association with migraine is demonstrable.

Treatment strategies include NSAIDs such as indometacin at a dosage of 25 mg t.i.d. (Diamond & Medina 1982a,b). Other pharmacologic strategies that have anecdotal support include the prophylactic use of ergotamine tartrate, methysergide, or propranolol pre-exercise. In practice, the headaches tend to recur over weeks to months and then slowly resolve although some cases may be lifelong. In the recovery period, a graduated symptom-limited weightlifting program is appropriate.

Effort headache

In clinical practice, these types of headache can be seen as migraine-type headaches triggered by aerobic exercise. Effort headaches have been reported to be the most common type of headache in athletes (Williams & Nukada 1994a,b). These differ from exertional headaches in that they are not necessarily associated with a power or straining type exercise and a variety of sports have been associated with these headaches.

The clinical features of effort headache syndrome include:
1 Onset of mild to severe headache with aerobic type exercise;
2 More frequent in hot weather;

3 Vascular type headache (i.e., throbbing);

4 Short duration of headache (4–6 h);

5 Provoking exercise may be maximal or submaximal;

6 Patient may have prodromal "migrainous" symptoms;

7 Headache tends to recur in individuals with exercise;

8 Athlete may have a past history of migraine;

9 Normal neurologic exam and investigations.

These episodes of effort migraine are not necessarily benign, with at least one case of hemispheric cerebral infarction associated with an episode of effort headache (Seelinger *et al.* 1975). Treatment strategies for effort headaches are anecdotal and include the use of indometacin or various antimigraine preparations. In the author's experience, prophylactic NSAIDs are effective if given prior to exercise, although in the headaches that occur in hot weather these drugs seem to have reduced efficacy. Graduated exercise programs have also been studied as a means of preventing such headaches with limited success (Lambert & Burnett 1985).

Conclusions

The treatment of exercise-related headaches in athletes can be potentially rewarding for the sports physician as well as the athlete. While the common headache syndromes seen in the general population must be considered, recognition of the diversity of these sport-related headache syndromes provides the basis for good clinical care.

Stroke and sport

The occurrence of stroke in sport is a rare phenomenon. Most sports participants tend to be young and unlike older age groups, where stroke represents one of the most common neurologic diseases, stroke in young people is an uncommon event. Of course, both young and older athletes, whether performing at a recreational or elite level, may develop the same stroke syndromes as non-athletes. In some cases, the athlete may have unsuspected risk factors that increase the risk of stroke during exercise, whereas in other cases the sporting activity itself may confer an intrinsic stroke mechanism. A

sports physician therefore needs a background knowledge of stroke risk factors at all ages as well as specific knowledge of stroke syndromes associated with sport.

Epidemiology of stroke

Stroke is the third leading cause of death the Western world. In the USA alone, at least 500,000 people experience a new stroke each year and, of these, 150,000 die. The prevalence of stroke according to the US National Health Interview Survey is 720 per 100,000 in the white population and 910 per 100,000 in the non-white population (McCrory 1999). Community studies demonstrate that the annual incidence rate of stroke is 102 per 100,000 population. In the 15–44 year age group, the overall incidence of stroke is nine cases per 100,000 population (Stern & Wityk 1994, 1998).

Etiology of stroke in young patients

Ischemic strokes can be caused by intrinsic vascular occlusions (thrombus) or an occlusion of a vessel from material that originates elsewhere in the vascular system (embolism). An overview of published studies of ischemic stroke in young people suggests that the common causes of stroke are large artery atherosclerosis, migraine, lacunae (small vessel, deep infarctions), and cardiac embolism. Less commonly, hematologic disease and illicit drug abuse is recognized. Finally, in many patients the cause of the stroke remains undefined (van den Berg & Limburg 1993). There are a number of rarer cause of stroke in young populations that also may need to be considered (Table 14.5).

When considering stroke in sport, there are approximately 70 published case reports in the medical literature where stroke occurs in this setting (McCrory 1999). These reports demonstrate that arterial dissection is the predominant pathophysiologic mechanism of sport-related stroke occurring in approximately 80% of cases.

Pre-participation physical examination

Recognition that a variety of underlying conditions may predispose to stroke means that the team or

Table 14.5 Rare causes of stroke in the young. After van den Berg & Limburg 1993.

System	Disease
Cardiac emboli	Endocarditis
	Atrial fibrillation or flutter
	Recent myocardial infarction
	Dilated cardiomyopathy
	Intracardiac thrombus
	Valvular vegetations
	Prosthetic valve
	Mitral valve prolapse
	Atrial septal defect
Hematologic disorders	Sickle cell disease
	Hemoglobin SC disease
	Polycythemia
	Thrombocytosis
	TTP
	DIC
	Antiphospholipid antibodies
	Protein C & S, AT III deficiency
	Disorders of fibrinolysis
Hereditary diseases	Neurofibromatosis
	MELAS syndrome
	Homocysteinemia
	Sneddon's syndrome
	Williams' syndrome
Medication related	Proximal myotonic myopathy
	L-asparaginase
	i.v. immunoglobulin
	Methotrexate
	Interferon
Inflammatory diseases	Rheumatoid arthritis
	Systemic lupus erythematosus
	Scleroderma
	Polymyositis
	Polyarteritis nodosa
	Wegener's granulomatosis
	Sarcoidosis
Infectious diseases	Neuroborreliosis
	HIV infection
	Neurocysticercosis
	Herpes zoster
	Chlamydia pneumoniae
	Hepatitis C virus
	Hydatid cyst embolism
Malignant disease	Tumor emboli
	Malignant angioendotheliomatosis
	Illicit drugs
	Cocaine
	Methamphetamine
	MDMA (ecstasy)
	Ephedrine
	Phenylpropanolamine
	Methylphenidate
	Heroin
	Anabolic steroids

AT III, Anti-thrombin III; DIC, disseminated intravascular coagulation; MDMA, 3,4-methylene-dioxymethamfetamine; MELAS, mitochondrial myopathy, encephalopathy, lactoacidosis, and stroke; SC, sickle cell; TTP, thrombotic thrombocytopenic purpura.

family physician is ideally placed to perform routine pre-participation physical examination (PPPE) and look specifically for these risk factors. In sporting populations, the causes of stroke fall into a relatively small group of risk factors which should be specifically sought on the PPPE:

1 Trauma to the extracranial cerebral arterial tree;
2 Exercise-induced hypertension;
3 Pre-existing cardiac or vascular disease;
4 Environmental injuries (e.g., hyperthermia, decompression illness);
5 Drug and stimulant abuse.

A detailed history, physical examination, and the judicious use of investigations should assist the physician in determining the risk profile of the athlete being examined.

HISTORY

A history of recurrent syncope or loss of consciousness associated with exercise raises the possibility of occult cardiac disease. Approximately 15% of cases of sudden death in sport are associated with prior syncopal or pre-syncopal episodes (Maron *et al.* 1980). The traditional cardiac ischemic symptoms of chest pain or dyspnea with exercise should also be sought as well as a history of congenital heart disease or cardiac valve infection (Driscoll 1985).

The athlete should be asked about a history of headache. Migraine is extremely common, with a prevalence of 15–20% in community populations. The incidence of migrainous cerebral infarction symptoms is extremely low; however, this mechanism represents one of the causes of stroke in young people occurring in 2–18% of cases (van den Berg & Limburg 1993). Congenital intracranial aneurysms occur with an incidence of 2000 per 100,000 population and have a rate of rupture of 12 per 100,000 per year (Phillips *et al.* 1980). As many as 50% of patients describe a severe "sentinel" warning headache prior to rupture (Gillingham 1967). Differentiating these from other headache syndromes may be extremely difficult. The presence of an unexplained severe headache, particularly in patients with no headache history or with a family history of aneurysmal rupture, should prompt further investigation.

A history of drug, alcohol, and stimulant abuse must be specifically sought. A variety of medications and illicit drugs have been associated with stroke in this age group (Table 14.5). Similarly, a history of brain trauma, environmental exposure to altitude, extremes of heat, or scuba diving would raise suspicion of these mechanisms of cerebral injury.

EXAMINATION

On general appearance, a marfinoid body habitus should raise the possibility of cardiac valvular disease. The skin should be examined for lesions suggestive of an underlying vascular disease, such as Osler–Rendu–Weber syndrome. A full cardiovascular examination should be performed in all patients. Detailed guidelines for pre-participation examination in young athletes have been published elsewhere (Brukner & Khan 2006; Driscoll 1985).

INVESTIGATIONS

The role of investigations should be limited to those where the history or examination findings are suggestive of an underlying disease. If cardiac disease is suspected then chest X-ray, electrocardiogram (ECG), and echocardiogram are the usual initial screening investigations. If ischemic heart disease is suspected then an exercise ECG test or thallium scan may be performed. If an intracerebral aneurysm is suspected, then a cerebral computed tomography (CT) or magnetic resonance (MR) scan should be performed with MR angiography. This is considerably less invasive and carries less morbidity than carotid and vertebral angiography. Coagulopathic disease, bleeding diathesis, hyperviscosity syndromes, or auto-immune disease can be detected on appropriate hematologic and serologic work-up. A drug screen may be necessary in some situations.

Specific stroke syndromes in sporting populations

Stroke in athletes is commonly associated with dissection of the extracranial vessels, presumably secondary to arterial trauma either caused by neck movement or through a blow to the region. Far less commonly, other pathophysiologic mechanisms such as hyperviscosity states, hemodynamic compromise, exercise-induced hypertension, drug-induced stroke, or atherosclerotic small vessel disease has been noted.

VERTEBRAL ARTERIAL DISSECTION

Vertebral arterial dissection (VAD) is an uncommon and incompletely understood condition. The precise incidence is unknown (Hart 1988). Approximately 25 cases have been reported to occur in sport (McCrory 1999). Most patients are healthy without predisposing risk factors for stroke (Pryse-Phillips 1989). Failure to make the diagnosis and institute appropriate therapy may result in long-term neurologic sequelae or death, although spontaneous resolution of the condition does occur (Sturznegger 1994). The initiating factor for this condition is thought to be a tear in the arterial intima with subsequent formation of *in situ* thrombosis. The pathologic injury may only involve the arterial intima or may extend to involve the tunica media. More rarely, the adventitial layer is breached with bleeding outside the vessel wall. Spontaneous dissections are rare and reported cases are often related to associated disease states such as cystic medial necrosis, Behçets syndrome, rheumatoid arthritis, giant cell arteritis, osteogenesis imperfecta, and fibromuscular dysplasia (Showalter *et al.* 1997).

A great deal of discussion revolves around the relationship of cervical movement to vertebral artery compression. Anecdotally, the presence of cervical abnormalities such as zygapophyseal joint osteophytes, fractures, dislocations, and rheumatoid arthritis may potentially cause symptomatic vertebrobasilar ischemia with head turning. From a pathophysiologic standpoint, in order for vertebrobasilar ischemia to occur there must be contralateral vertebrobasilar artery hemodynamic restriction either from stenosis, atherosclerotic disease, or hypoplasia (Biousse *et al.* 1995; Mas *et al.* 1987, 1989).

Cases of vertebral artery dissection related to trauma are more commonly reported, often in the presence of major cervical spinal trauma such as vertebral fracture or subluxation (Willis *et al.* 1994).

However, most recognized cases occur following a seemingly trivial traumatic event such as sneezing, coughing, riding a roller-coaster, horse riding, visiting a hairdresser, or performing yoga exercises. Interestingly, in all of these cases the arteriographic appearance of the contralateral vertebrobasilar arteries were normal.

A wide variety of clinical neurologic deficits are found in relation to VAD, perhaps related to the variable pathologic mechanisms (thrombosis or embolism), the complexity of neural structures supplied by the posterior circulation, and the variability of the vascular architecture. The most common initial symptoms in VAD are neck pain and occipital headache which may precede the onset of neurologic symptoms from seconds to weeks. It was noted that headache symptoms in the majority of cases were ipsilateral to the vascular injury and that the pain usually radiated to the temporal region, frontal area, eye, or ear. None of the reported cases had cervical tenderness or objective restriction of neck movement although a subjective exacerbation of pain did occur with neck movement (Sturznegger 1994).

The typical course of untreated VAD is progression in a stuttering fashion over hours to days. This progression is thought to result either from propagation of the thrombus or from distal embolization. This is the rationale for the use of anticoagulation in the treatment of extracranial VAD.

From the standpoint of early recognition of this condition, the combination of unilateral neck pain or headache of abrupt onset following a history of neck trauma should lead to the suspicion of VAD even in the face of seemingly trivial trauma. The clinical suspicion of VAD should be investigated by either transcranial Doppler ultrasound, vertebral artery angiography, or magnetic resonance angiography (MRA) after neurologic opinion is sought. The history or detection of major neurologic findings such as vertigo, diplopia, ataxia, dysarthria, cranial nerve palsies, or altered mental function should be an absolute indication for urgent neurologic consultation and hospital admission. It is important to emphasize that the neurologic findings may be delayed days or weeks after the onset of neck pain and optimal management of this condition should involve early recognition, appropriate investigation, and institution of anticoagulation where indicated. A clinical algorithm for the emergency department management of VAD has been recently published (Showalter et al. 1997).

CAROTID ARTERIAL DISSECTION

Direct trauma to the head or neck during sport can potentially injure the carotid arteries. In addition, forcible hyperextension or lateral rotation may similarly cause arterial injury (Fields 1981a,b; Noelle & Clavier 1994). Hypertrophy of the posterior belly of the digastric muscle leading to compression of the internal carotid artery and causing transient ischemic episodes with neck rotation has been reported in a retired professional football player (Etheridge et al. 1984). Non-penetrating neck trauma has been reported to cause thrombosis of both the external carotid and more importantly the internal carotid artery with associated ischemic hemispheric injury. Fields (1981a,b) distinguishes four types of traumatic carotid arterial injury:

1 A blow to the head causing forceful compression of the ipsilateral carotid artery (ICA) with intimal rupture;

2 A direct blow to the anteromedial neck leading to atherosclerotic plaque rupture and thrombosis;

3 Skull fracture leading to thrombosis of the intrapetrous ICA; and

4 Blunt intra-oral trauma with ICA thrombosis.

Clinically, apart from the history of trauma and ipsilateral hemispheric stroke symptoms, tenderness of the carotid vessels, oculomotor palsies, and an ipsilateral Horner's syndrome may alert the examiner to the carotid injury. In addition to stroke episodes, trauma to the carotid arteries may induce a severe unilateral headache associated with profound autonomic symptoms. This entity is known as traumatic dysautonomic cephalgia which may be successfully treated with propranolol.

Anecdotally, about half of all carotid dissections result in stroke which is in keeping with the age profile of most cases and presumably an intact collateral circulation. Recurrence is unusual and does not typically affect the same segment or artery as the initial presentation. Most authors recommend anticoagulation therapy for carotid dissection although there are no prospective trials demonstrating the efficacy of such treatment.

SUBCLAVIAN ARTERY STENOSIS

One case of subclavian artery stenosis has been reported in a baseball pitcher who developed an acute hemispheric stroke as a result of propagated thrombus into the carotid artery. The putative lesion was thought to be caused by compression of the subclavian artery at the level of the thoracic outlet and first rib (Fields 1981a,b). More typically, subclavian vessel disease causes acute upper limb ischemia (as may be seen with dissections of the aortic arch), subclavian vein thrombosis (reported in racket sports and in throwing athletes), and subclavian artery stenosis causing the so-called subclavian "steal" phenomenon.

MIGRAINE

Migraine is often an etiologic consideration in young stroke patients. Because there is no diagnostic marker for migraine, the clinician must rely on the patient's history. Because exercise-related headache is common to many sports, differentiating migrainous events from other causes of headache can be clinically difficult.

Migraine without aura is associated with a three-fold increase in stroke in young women and a six-fold increase for migraine with aura. In addition, the risk of stroke in migrainous women is markedly increased in those using oral contraceptives (odds ratio 14) or those who are heavy smokers (odds ratio 10). Oral contraceptives have been implicated in some studies as a cause of stroke although this remains extremely controversial (World Health Organization 1996).

A conservative approach is to limit the diagnosis of migrainous stroke to patients with a history of migraine who have a stroke during a typical episode of headache and have no other identifiable cause for stroke. In some patients, angiography at the time of the event can show segmental narrowing of intracranial arteries suggestive of vasospasm. Subsequent angiography is typically normal, confirming the reversible nature of the lesion. It is important not to assign a diagnosis of migrainous stroke until after a thorough evaluation because many conditions may have a history of migraine-like headaches.

CARDIOGENIC EMBOLISM

Cardiac diseases that predispose to stroke syndromes are listed in Table 14.1. In most cases, these are extremely rare phenomena. Cardiogenic emboli leading to focal cerebral ischemia may occur during activity-induced cardiac dysrhythmias. Sinus bradyarrhythmias in athletes have been associated with atrial fibrillation and thrombus formation with secondary embolization to the brain (Abdon *et al.* 1984). Athletes who experience stroke episodes secondary to cardiogenic embolism or arrhythmias are at risk from repeated episodes unless the underlying problem can be corrected. In many cases this is not possible and long-term anticoagulation may be considered as a preventative therapy; however, this form of treatment may preclude athletes from participation in contact and collision sports.

STIMULANT AND DRUG ABUSE

Stroke can occur during the first minutes of acute intoxication with a drug, in the hours following ingestion, or weeks following intoxication (Kaku & Lowenstein 1990). Recognition of the role of drug use in the pathogenesis of stroke requires familiarity with the acute effects of commonly used recreational drugs and a high index of suspicion. The signs and symptoms of a stroke are not different in the user of recreational drugs unless the user is acutely intoxicated. The physician must question for a history of substance abuse from the patient, friends, and family. Suspicion of drug use can be confirmed through prompt urine toxicology screening.

Stroke can occur as both a direct and an indirect medical complication of the recreational use of several drugs. The direct complications related to cerebrovascular disease are either ischemic stroke, intracerebral hemorrhage, or subarachnoid hemorrhage. The drugs typically associated with these complications include cocaine, methamphetamine, 3,4-methylene-dioxymethamfetamine (MDMA or 'ecstasy'), ephedrine, phenylpropanolamine, methylphenidate, and heroin (Bendixen 1998).

Indirect complications are related to the means of its administration or to contaminants mixed in with the drug. For example, cardioembolic stroke can be secondary to bacterial endocarditis in an intravenous drug user who employs unsterile needles. Additionally, cocaine has been reported to cause myocardial infarctions and cardiomyopathies, creating the potential for cardioembolic stroke. Similarly, several drugs intended for intravenous use are mixed with talc or cornstarch. These substances have been found to occlude arteries, leading to a stroke (Brust & Richter 1977).

Strokes have also been reported several bodybuilders who were consuming anabolic steroids (Akhter & Hyder 1994; Jaillard & Hommel 1994). The duration of anabolic use in these cases ranged from 6 weeks to 4 years. Clinical presentations included hemispheric stroke and sagittal sinus thrombosis. Stroke has also been reported in patients using the same agents for medical indications, suggesting that this risk is not wholly unexpected (Ferenchick 1990).

Drug use should be suspected in any young person who presents with a stroke. It should be remembered that drug use encompasses not only illegal substances such as cocaine, methamphetamine, and heroin, but also diet pills, over-the-counter decongestants, methylphenidate (Ritalin), and asthma medications. A detailed history should be sought from the patient, friends, and family and urine toxicology screens used where necessary.

FAT EMBOLISM

Fat embolism is a common complication of severe bone trauma, particularly to the extremities, occurring in up to 15% of such cases (Lepisto & Alho 1975). Given that long bone trauma is common in many contact and collision sports, this entity needs to be considered in this setting. Plugging of small intracerebral blood vessels by lipid particles and fibrin clots leads to brain infarction. The neurologic presentation may be delayed by hours to days after trauma. The onset of neurologic symptoms such as hemiparesis, altered mental status, seizures, and coma is usually acute. Associated hypoxia secondary to pulmonary infarction may complicate the presentation. The treatment of fat embolism is improvement of the oxygen-carrying capacity by correction of hypoxia and, if necessary, red blood cell (RBC) transfusion. Even in cases of coma, the patient may still recover completely.

INTRACRANIAL HEMORRHAGE

Systolic blood pressure increases during exercise and the peak pressure rise correlates with the intensity of the exercise, the age of the patient, and inversely with their fitness (Carlstein & Grimby 1966). Where a vascular malformation or arterial wall defect such as an aneurysm exists, then the risk of rupture is increased during exercise. Given the high peak arterial pressures that occur with sports such as weightlifting, with systolic pressures exceeding 400 mmHg and diastolic pressures above 300 mmHg, it is surprising that intracranial hemorrhage (ICH) does not occur more frequently (MacDougall *et al.* 1985). In cases of stroke, approximately 50% of patients with aneurysms and 25% of those with vascular malformation present with bleeding during physical exertion or emotional strain (Department of Health and Human Services Task Force 1992; van den Berg & Limburg 1993; van Gijn & van Dongen 1980). Alcohol intoxication has been reported as an additional risk factor for aneurysm rupture (Vijayan 1977; Vijayan & Dreyfus 1975). In addition, two cases have been reported of bleeding into occult intracerebral tumours while jogging (Welch & Levine 1990).

Conclusions

Immediate recognition of a CNS injury, institution of cardiopulmonary support where required, and immobilization of the head and neck are the cornerstones of initial management of sport-related neurologic injury. More definitive investigation and treatment of specific stroke syndromes requires an understanding of the etiology, underlying pathogenesis, and temporal profile of the various causes of stroke in sport. The understanding of stroke risk factors in an athletic population may assist the clinician in instituting an appropriate pre-participation screening program to minimize the occurrence of such conditions.

Epilepsy and sport

Convulsive episodes when they occur in sport are rare but dramatic events. Traditionally, these episodes have been assumed to represent a form of epilepsy; however, recent studies have demonstrated that most, if not all, post-traumatic convulsive episodes seen acutely in a sporting situation are non-epileptic in nature (McCrory & Berkovic 1998).

In addition, individuals with epilepsy are encouraged to participate in sport and sports physicians need to understand the medical issues in relation to epilepsy, particularly drug therapy, in order to advise these individuals correctly. Details of epilepsy management are best sought in any of the published reference books available (Duncan *et al.* 1995; Engel & Pedley 1998).

Epidemiology and nomenclature

Epilepsy affects approximately 2% of the population. In three-quarters of these cases, the diagnosis is made before the age of 21 years. Thus, epilepsy is a relatively common condition that may affect individuals during the years of sport participation.

Epilepsy is a neurologic disorder of the brain characterized by recurrent (more than two) seizures. It has been estimated that approximately 10–30% of the population will have a seizure at some time in their lives (Sander & O'Donoghue 1997; Sander *et al.* 1990). However, neither single episodes of seizures during adolescence or adult life nor febrile convulsions in infancy constitute a diagnosis of epilepsy.

The terms "seizure," "epilepsy," "convulsion," and "fit" are often used interchangeably. For the purpose of this chapter, the term seizure will refer to an epileptic seizure and the term convulsion will be used to describe the movements during an episode without implying a specific etiology.

Pathology

A seizure usually occurs suddenly and is the result of an abnormal electrical discharge within the brain. In the vast majority of cases, the cause of the electrical disturbance in the brain is unknown. In a small percentage, either specific genetic inheritance or structural anatomic abnormalities can induce seizures. Cortical scars related to head injuries, stroke, and other intracranial injuries may also cause seizures. During the seizure there may be an initial prodromal stage ("aura"), followed rapidly by disturbances in movement and alterations in consciousness.

Epilepsy can be classified by criteria developed by the International League Against Epilepsy (ILAE 1989). This classification utilizes the electroclinical features of the seizure to make a syndromal or etiologic diagnosis, which then has important implications for management. In the broadest sense, the ILAE classification breaks down seizures into generalized or focal (depending on the origin of the seizure), and complex or partial (depending upon whether consciousness is preserved during the episode). Outside of neurologic practice, the specific epilepsy subtype may be difficult to quantify and subjects are often simply reported to have a generalized seizure. This type of seizure was previously known as "grand mal" but this term has fallen out of favor and should be avoided.

Generalized tonic–clonic seizure

In the generalized tonic–clonic seizure, the patient usually falls to the ground and goes through a "tonic" phase of muscle stiffness followed by a "clonic" phase of muscle twitches prior to resolution of the attack. After the attack the patient is usually sleepy, confused, and may have a headache. The average length of the seizure is usually no more than 30 s, although most people who have witnessed someone having a seizure feel that the attack seems to last much longer.

Convulsions that are not caused by epilepsy

In addition to the true epilepsy seizures described above, there are other situations where convulsions may occur. These may superficially resemble epilepsy although the etiology of such syndromes is distinctly different. These have the potential to cause confusion for non-neurologists and the eyewitness history usually provides the basis of the diagnosis. The two most common situations are:

1 Concussive convulsions, where a convulsion may be a manifestation of the concussive impact. Although usually brief and limited to tonic posturing, they may occasionally result in a prolonged convulsion over several minutes. These are benign phenomena and require no specific management beyond that of the underlying concussion (McCrory & Berkovic 1998, 2000);

2 Convulsive syncope, where convulsive movements (including generalized movements, tongue biting, and incontinence) occur in the setting of a syncopal faint.

In both situations, the convulsive movements result from reflex phenomena, not epileptic discharge.

Diagnosis of epilepsy

The diagnosis of epilepsy relies primarily upon the clinical history and on the nature of the electroencephalogram (EEG) changes. The most important and useful diagnostic consideration is history from an eyewitness who has seen and can describe the attack, particularly the onset and offset of the seizure. Any patient observed to have a seizure should be referred to a neurologist for assessment.

Investigations

In most cases of a seizure, a neurologist would order an EEG as well as neuroimaging studies (usually MRI). If the EEG is performed within 24 h of a seizure, its diagnostic sensitivity is increased from 30% to 50% and this may be further improved by performing a "sleep-deprived" EEG study. MRI is the investigation of choice to image the brain in this circumstance. Specific MRI protocols are necessary to obtain diagnostic information in these cases. Where necessary, these investigations would be supplemented by blood tests to rule out other causes of seizures, such as hypoglycemia, hypernatremia or hyponatremia, and hypercalcemia.

Treatment

The role of specific treatment in patients with a single seizure or recurrent seizures (epilepsy) requires an understanding of the nature of the seizure disorder and its natural history as well as individual patient consideration. In some situations, drug treatment should begin after a single seizure. Consideration of lifestyle factors in the overall management is paramount. Specific factors that may lower seizure threshold include sleep deprivation, alcohol, and use of recreational drugs. Patients must be specifically counseled about such lifestyle issues when they begin pharmacologic therapy.

More than half of the individuals taking antiepileptic medication for idiopathic generalized epilepsy can expect to be seizure-free with minimal restriction on their lifestyle. Approximately one-third may have only an occasional seizure, which usually does not greatly limit their lifestyle. The other 20% will have seizures frequently enough to restrict their lifestyle to some extent.

The medications used in the treatment of epilepsy can cause a number of side effects, including tiredness, poor concentration, impairment of coordination, and cognitive impairment. In some cases, medication (e.g. phenytoin) toxicity may result in permanent neurologic symptoms.

Exercise prescription in epilepsy

Regular physical activity is advocated for individuals with epilepsy (Nakken *et al.* 1990). In general, people with epilepsy report better seizure control when exercising regularly. Occasionally, some individuals will have more seizures with exercise and hence every case must be treated individually. Persons with epilepsy have no higher injury rate in sport than those without epilepsy and sport participation does not affect serum drug levels (Nakken *et al.* 1990).

In a sample of over 200 patients with epilepsy in Norway, exercise patterns were similar to that of the average population (Nakken *et al.* 1990). In the majority of the patients, physical exercise had no adverse effects, and over one-third of patients claimed that regular exercise contributed to better seizure control. In 10% of patients, exercise appeared to be a seizure precipitant and this applied particularly to those with symptomatic partial epilepsy (i.e. underlying structural brain lesion).

There are a number of important considerations when counseling the individual who has epilepsy and wishes to exercise. Patients having frequent seizures must be discouraged from activities such as scuba diving, cycling, horseback riding, or rock climbing. Sports where any impairment in split-second neuromuscular timing is dangerous (e.g. motor-racing or downhill ski racing) should also be avoided. Patients with epilepsy will not be affected adversely by indulging in contact sport provided the normal safeguards for participation are followed.

The frequency of seizures is important when considering activities such as swimming, where the potential for serious injury exists if a seizure were to occur. Generally, swimming is allowed under supervision (e.g. with a "buddy"). Swimming with a companion is a sensible rule for all swimmers, not just those with epilepsy.

The physical and psychologic well-being of the individual also requires attention. In children, particularly adolescents, participation in activities is important in establishing a good self-image and gaining peer group acceptance. Therefore, it is important to allow the child with epilepsy to pursue many activities. Absolute and relative contraindications to sporting activities are shown in Table 14.6.

Management of a seizure

Observing a seizure can be a frightening experience. For an observer, there is often an overwhelming feeling of helplessness and concern that the patient may die during the seizure. It is important to remember that seizures always terminate spontaneously and that rarely is a seizure life-threatening. Furthermore, the patient experiencing the seizure usually does not feel pain or remember the event.

Any individual observing or supervising an epileptic patient should remember two things when confronted by a seizure. First, the individual must be protected from injury. Second, the seizure must be closely observed in order to give an accurate description to the patient's physician. The long-standing convention of trying to put a knotted sheet or spoon in the patient's mouth should be discouraged and the patient should not be physically restrained under most circumstances.

It is important to remember that the shaking will cease spontaneously after a period of time. At the end of this time, the patient breathes normally and appears sleepy. The patient should then be managed as for an unconscious patient (e.g. Chapter 18).

Conclusions

Overall, people with epilepsy are able to participate in sport with few limitations. Occasionally, it is appropriate to restrict certain physical activities. A person with epilepsy must meet certain legal obligations when driving a car. The individual with epilepsy must take his/her medication correctly and ensure a well-balanced eating and sleeping schedule. Family, friends, team mates, and coaches must be aware of the epilepsy and understand what to do in the event of a seizure. All these factors will contribute to removing unnecessary barriers to a normal active lifestyle in those with epilepsy.

Table 14.6 Solo sporting activities contraindicated in people with epilepsy.

Absolute	Relative (with supervision)
Rock climbing	Swimming
Flying	Cross-country skiing
Hang-gliding	Backpacking
Pistol shooting	Cycling
Scuba diving	
Archery	
Sky diving, parachuting	
Motor racing	

Other neurolologic conditions and exercise

Multiple sclerosis

The clinical presentation of multiple sclerosis (MS) is characterized by a plethora of neurologic signs and symptoms such as fatigue, motor weakness, and poor balance. These episodes may be "relapsing and remitting" or "progressive" in nature. Specific episodes, particularly spinal cord lesions, often result in persistent problems such as lower limb spasticity, muscle spasms, or sphincteric disturbance.

In addition, MS symptoms may lead to physical inactivity associated with the development of secondary diseases and/or muscular deconditioning (Slawta *et al.* 2002). Although exercise prescription is gaining favor as a therapeutic strategy to minimize the loss of functional capacity in chronic diseases, it remains underutilized as an intervention strategy in the MS population. However, a growing number of studies indicate that exercise in patients with mild to moderate MS provides similar fitness and psychologic benefits as it does in healthy controls with minimal adverse effects (White & Dressendorfer 2004).

Despite the often unpredictable clinical course of MS, exercise programs designed to increase cardiorespiratory fitness, muscle strength, and mobility provide benefits that enhance lifestyle activity and quality of life while reducing risk of secondary disorders.

Parkinson's disease

Parkinson's disease is characterized by a progressive failure of dopaminergic function in the midbrain and manifest by the clinical triad of resting tremor, muscular rigidity, and bradykinesia. In addition, postural instability is a characteristic finding. Interestingly, higher levels of physical activity in early adulthood seems to be protective against the development of Parkinson's disease (Chen *et al.* 2005). The mechanism for this is unclear.

As a consequence, the physical deconditioning that accompanies advancing disease in combination with the clinical signs makes the individual particularly prone to falls and injury. Exercise programs and balance training improves the functional status and independence of patients with Parkinson's disease (Hirsch *et al.* 2003) as well as improving overall quality of life (Baatile *et al.* 2000).

Alzheimer's disease

The role of exercise and other non-pharmacologic therapy in aging and dementia has received considerable interest in recent times. Although epidemiologic studies are conflicting, it would seem that physical activity may help preserve (and possibly improve) cognitive function and decrease overall dementia risk. These benefits are seen even with relatively low intensity exercise programs (Bragin *et al.* 2005; Larson & Wang 2004; Petrovitch & White 2005; Rovio *et al.* 2005). The role of exercise in the overall management of dementia needs to be studied further.

By contrast, concern has been raised that either repeated sport-related concussions or repeated head impact can predispose to chronic brain injury and conditions such as Alzheimer's dementia (McCrory 2003), although the evidence for this is far from compelling at present. In boxing, where repetitive brain trauma does occur, the so-called "punch drunk syndrome" or chronic traumatic encephalopathy is seen at extremes of trauma or in conjunction with specific genotypes suggesting a multifactorial basis (Jordan 2000).

Motoneuron disease (amyotrophic lateral sclerosis)

Concern has been raised that either repeated concussions or repeated head impact can predispose to chronic brain injury and conditions such as Alzheimer's dementia (McCrory 2003) and motoneuron disease (McCrory 2005).

Chio *et al.* (2005) reported from Italy that there was an increased risk of developing motoneuron disease (MND) amongst Italian soccer players. In this retrospective cohort study, there were five diagnosed MND cases in a subpopulation of 7435 soccer players of the top two Italian divisions who played in the period 1970–2001. Although only small numbers of MND patients were identified, this exceeded the statistical likelihood of developing MND in this population.

This paper adds to the growing body of concern in regard to the risk of developing this condition from sport. Previously, a judicial report from the Italian soccer leagues raised similar concerns. A 4-year study commissioned by a local magistrate looked at every player in Serie A and B between 1960 and 1997. Of the total of 24,000 calciatori, eight were found to have died from MND. A further follow-up of those who were dead or who had fallen ill since 1997 found a further 32 cases (McCrory 2005).

The *Guardian* newspaper in England has reported that MND has claimed a number of former players in England in recent years including Don Revie, Rob Hindmarch of Derby and Sunderland, Middlesbrough's Willie Maddren, and the former Celtic winger Jimmy Johnstone (Fotheringham 2003).

Compared to individuals with other neurologic disease, patients with amyotrophic lateral sclerosis (ALS) are more likely to have a history of being athletic and slim, according to Scarmeas *et al.* (2002).

Such a somatotypic linkage has been suggested by the development of MND in athletes. In the USA, boxer Ezzard Charles, baseball player Catfish Hunter, and baseball icon Lou Gehrig died of MND. Three players from the San Francisco 49ers were diagnosed with MND in the 1980s, and Glenn Montgomery of the Seattle Seahawks lost his life to MND in 1998. It is likely that the pathogenesis of MND reflects a complex interaction between environmental factors, exercise, and specific susceptibility genes (Majoor-Krakauer *et al.* 2003).

References

Abdon, N., Lasdin, K. & Johansson, B.W. (1984) Athlete's bradycardia as an embolising disorder. *British Heart Journal* 52, 660–666.

Akhter, J. & Hyder, S. (1994) Cerebrovascular accident associated with anabolic steroid use in a young man. *Neurology* 44, 2405–2406.

Arateus, C. (1856) *The extant works of Areteus the Cappadocian.* The Sydenham Society, London: 45.

Baatile, J., Langbein, W., Weaver, F., Maloney, C. Jost, M.B. (2000) Effect of exercise on perceived quality of life of individuals with Parkinson's disease. *Journal of Rehabilitation Research Developments* 37, 529–534.

Bendixen, B. (1998) Stroke associated with drug abuse. In: *Neurobase* (Gilman, S., Goldstein, G. & Waxman, S., eds.) Arbor Publishers, San Diego.

Biousse, V., Chabriat, H., Amarenco, P. & Bousser, M.G. (1995) Roller-coaster induced vertebral artery dissection. *Lancet* 346, 767.

Bogduk, N., Corrigan, B., Kelly, P., Schneider, G. Farr, R. (1985) Cervical headache. *Medical Journal of Australia* 143, 202, 206–207.

Bogduk, N. & Marsland, A. (1986) On the concept of third occipital headache. *Journal of Neurology, Neurosurgery and Psychiatry* 49, 775–780.

Bragin, V., Chemodanova, M., Dzhafarova, N., Bragin, I., Czerniawski, J.L. & Aliev, G. (2005) Integrated treatment approach improves cognitive function in demented and clinically depressed patients. *American Journal of Alzheimer's Disease and Other Dementias* 20, 21–26.

Brukner, P. & Khan, K.M. (2006) *Clinical Sports Medicine.* McGraw-Hill, Sydney: 22–87.

Brust, J. & Richter, R. (1977) Stroke assciated with cocaine abuse. *New York State Journal of Medicine* 77, 1473–1475.

Carlstein, A. & Grimby, G. (1966) *The Circulatory Response to Muscular Exercise in Man.* Charles C. Thomas, Springfield, IL: 45–51.

Chen, H., Zhang, S.M., Schwarzschild, M.A., Hernán, M.A. & Ascherio, A. (2005) Physical activity and the risk of Parkinson's disease. *Neurology* 64, 664–669.

Chiò, A., Benzi, G., Dossena, M., Mutani, R. & Mora, G. (2005) Severely increased risk of amyotrophic lateral sclerosis among Italian professional football players. *Brain* 128, 472–476.

Dalessio, D., ed. (1987) *Wolff's Headache and Other Head Pain.* Oxford University Press, Oxford.

Department of Health and Human Services Task Force. (1992). *US Department of Health and Human Services Task Force on Black and Minority Health, 1984–1985. National Health Interview Survey.* US Department of Health and Human Services, Washington, D.C.: 1–81.

Diamond, S., Elkind, A., Jackson, R.T., Ryan, R., DeBussey, S. & Asgharnejad, M. (1998) Multiple-attack efficacy and tolerability of sumatriptan nasal spray in the treatment of migraine. *Archives of Family Medicine* 7, 234–240.

Diamond, S. & Medina, J. (1982a) Prolonged benign exertional headache. In: *Headache: Pathophysilogical and Clinical Concepts* (Critchley, M., ed.) Raven Press, New York: 145–149.

Diamond, S. & Medina, J. (1982b) Prolonged benign exertional headache and response to indomethacin. *Advances in Neurology* 33, 145–149.

Driscoll, D. (1985) Cardiovascular evaluation of the child and adolescent before participation in sports. *Mayo Clinic Proceedings* 60, 867–873.

Duncan, J., Shorvon, S. & Fish, D.R. (1995) *Clinical Epilepsy.* Churchill-Livingstone, London.

Engel, J. & Pedley, T., eds. (1998). *Epilepsy: A Comprehensive Textbook.* Lippincot-Raven, Philadelphia.

Etheridge, S., Effeney, D., *et al.* (1984) Symptomatic extrinsic compression of the cervical carotid artery. *Archives of Neurology* 41, 672–673.

Ferenchick, G. (1990) Are anabolic steroids thrombogenic? *New England Journal of Medicine* 322, 476–477.

Fields, W. (1981a) Neurovascular syndromes of the neck and shoulders. *Seminars in Neurology* 1, 301–309.

Fields, W. (1981b) Non-penetrating trauma of the cervical arteries. *Seminars in Neurology* 1, 284–290.

Fotheringham, W. (2003) Club doctor fears Italian study could lead to a legal nightmare. *The Guardian* (newspaper). Published January 16, 2003. http://football.guardian.co.uk/News_Story/0,1563,879069,00.html

Gibbs, N. (1994) Common rugby league injuries. Recommendations for treatment and preventative measures. *Sports Medicine* 18, 438–450.

Gillingham, F. (1967) The management of ruptured intracranial aneurysms. *Scottish Medical Journal* 12, 377–383.

Hart, R. (1988) Vertebral arterial dissection. *Neurology* 38, 987–989.

Hazelrigg, R. (1986) Intravenous DHE relieves exertional cephalgia. *Headache* **26**, 52–55.

Hippocrates (1849) *The Genuine Works of Hippocrates*. The Sydenham Society, London: 110.

Hirsch, M., Toole, T., Maitland, C.G. & Rider, R.A. (2003) The effects of balance training and high-intensity resistance training on persons with idiopathic Parkinson's disease. *Archives of Physical Medicine and Rehabilitation* **84**, 1109–1117.

International League Against Epilepsy (ILAE). (1989) Commission on the classification and terminology of the International League Against Epilepsy: A revised proposal for the classification of the epilepsies and epileptic syndromes. *Epilepsia* **30**, 389–399.

Jaillard, A. & Hommel, M. (1994) Venous sinus thrombosis associated with androgens in a healthy young man. *Stroke* **25**, 212–213.

Jordan, B. D. (2000) Chronic traumatic brain injury associated with boxing. *Seminars in Neurology* **20**, 179–185.

Kaku, D. & Lowenstein, D. (1990) Emergence of recreational drug abuse as a major risk factor for stroke in young adults. *Annals of Internal Medicine* **113**, 821–827.

Lambert, R. & Burnett, D. (1985) Prevention of exercise induced migraine by quantitative training. *Headache* **25**, 317–319.

Lance, J. & Goadsby, P. (1998) *Mechanism and Managment of Headache*. Butterworth-Heinemann, Oxford.

Larson, E. & Wang, L. (2004) Exercise, aging, and Alzheimer disease. *Alzheimer Disease and Associated Disorders* **18**, 57–64.

Lepisto, P. & Alho, A. (1975) Diagnostic features of the fat embolism syndrome. *Acta Chiropractica Scandanavica* **141**, 245–250.

MacDougall, J., Tuxen, D., Sale, D.G., Moroz, J.R. & Sutton, J.R. (1985) Arterial blood pressure response to heavy resistance exercise. *Journal of Applied Physiology* **58**, 785–790.

Majoor-Krakauer, D., Willems, P. & Hofman, A. (2003) Genetic epidemiology of amyotrophic lateral sclerosis. *Clinical Genetics* **63**, 83–101.

Maron, B., Roberts, W., McAllister, H.A., Rosing, D.R. Epstein, S.E. (1980) Sudden death in young athletes. *Circulation* **62**, 218–229.

Mas, J., Bousser, M., Hasboun, D. & Laplane, D. (1987) Extra-cranial vertebral artery dissections: a review of 13 cases. *Stroke* **18**, 1037–1047.

Mas, J., Henin, D., Bousser, M.G., Chain, F. & Hauw, J.J. (1989) Dissecting aneurysm of the vertebral artery and cervical manipulation. *Neurology* **39**, 512–515.

Mathews, W. (1972) Footballers migraine. *British Medical Journal* **2**, 326–327.

McCrory, P. (1997) Exercise related headache. *Physician and Sportsmedicine* **25**, 33–43.

McCrory, P. (1999). Stroke in athletes. In: *Neurologic Athletic Head and Spine Injuries* (Cantu, R., ed.) W.B. Saunders, Philadelphia: 200–210.

McCrory, P. (2000) Headaches and exercise. *Sports Medicine* **30**, 221–229.

McCrory, P. (2003) Brain injury and heading in soccer. *British Medical Journal* **327**, 352–352.

McCrory, P. (2005) A cause for concern? *British Journal of Sports Medicine* **39**, 249.

McCrory, P. & Berkovic, S. (1998) Concussive convulsions: incidence in sport and treatment recommendations. *Sports Medicine* **25**, 131–136.

McCrory, P. & Berkovic, S. (2000) Videoanalysis of the motor and convulsive manifestations of concussion in acute sport related head injury. *Neurology* **54**, 1488–1492.

McCrory, P., Heywood, J. & Coffey, C. (2005) Prevalence of headache in Australian footballers. *British Journal of Sports Medicine* **39**, e10–11.

Nakken, K., Bjorholt, P.G., Johanessen, S.I., Loyning, T. & Lind, E. (1990) Effect of physical training on aerobic capacity, seizure occurrence and serum level of anticonvulsant drugs in adults with epilepsy. *Epilepsia* **31**, 88–94.

Noelle, B. & I. Clavier (1994) Cervicocephalic arterial dissections related to skiing. *Stroke* **24**, 526–527.

Olesen, J. (1988) Classification and diagnostic criteria for headache disorders, cranial neuralgias and facial pain. *Cephalgia* **8** (Suppl. 7), 9–96.

Olesen, J., Thomsen, L., Lassen, L.H. & Olesen, I.J. (1995) The nitric oxide hypothesis of migraine and other vascular headaches. *Cephalgia* **15**, 94–100.

Petrovitch, H. & White, L. (2005) Exercise and cognitive function. *Lancet Neurology* **4**, 705–711.

Phillips, L., Whisnant, J., O'Fallon, W.M. & Sundt, T.M. (1980) The unchanging pattern of subarachnoid haemorrhage in the community. *Neurology* **30**, 1034–1040.

Powell, B. (1982) Weightlifters cephalgia. *Annals of Emergency Medicine* **11**, 449–451.

Pryse-Phillips, W. (1989) Infarction of the medulla and cervical cord following fitness exercises. *Stroke* **20**, 292–294.

Rasmussen, B. (1995) Epidemiology of headache. *Cephalgia* **15**, 45–68.

Rovio, S., Kareholt, I., Hekala, E.L., Viitanen, M., Winblad, B., Tuomilehto, J., *et al.* (2005) Leisure-time physical activity at midlife and the risk of dementia and Alzheimer's disease. *Lancet Neurology* **4**, 690–691.

Sander, J.W.A.S. & O'Donoghue, M.F. (1997) Epilepsy: getting the diagnosis right. All that convulses is not epilepsy. *British Medical Journal* **314**, 158–159.

Sander, J., Hart, Y., Johnson, A.L. & Shorvon, S.D. (1990) The National General Practice Study of Epilepsy: newly diagnosed epileptic seizures in a general population. *Lancet* **336**, 1267–1271.

Scarmeas, N., Shih, T., Stern, Y., Ottman, R. & Rowland, L.P. (2002) Premorbid weight, body mass, and varsity athletics in ALS. *Neurology* **59**, 773–775.

Seelinger, D., Coin, G.C. & Carlow, T.J. (1975) Effort headache with cerebral infarction. *Headache* **15**, 142–145.

Showalter, W., Esekogwu, V., Newton, K.I. & Henderson, S.O. (1997) Vertebral artery dissection. *Academic Emergency Medicine* **4**, 991–995.

Slawta, J., McCubbin, J., Wilcox, A.R., Fox, S.D., Nalle, D.J. & Anderson, G. (2002) Coronary heart disease risk between active and inactive women with multiple sclerosis. *Medicine in Science Sports and Exercise* **34**, 905–12.

Stern, B. & Wityk, R. (1994) Stroke in the young. In: *Current Diagnosis in Neurology* (Feldmann, E., ed.) Mosby-Wilkins, St. Louis, MO: 43–77.

Stern, B. & Wtiyk, R. (1998) Stroke in young adults. In: *Neurobase* Gilman, S., Goldstein, G. & Waxman, S., eds.) Arbor Publishing, San Diego.

Sturznegger, M. (1994) Headache and neck pain: the warning symptoms of vertebral artery dissection. *Headache* **34**, 187–193.

Tinel, J. (1932) La cephelee a l'effort, syndrome de distension des vienes intracraniences. *La Medicine* **13**, 113–118.

van den Berg, J. & Limburg, M. (1993) Ischemic stroke in the young: influence of diagnostic criteria. *Cerebrovascular Disorders* **3**, 227–230.

van Gijn, J. & van Dongen, K. (1980) Computed tomography in subarachnoid haemorrhage: difference between patients with and without aneurysms on angiography. *Neurology* **30**, 538–539.

Vijayan, N. (1977) A new post traumatic headache syndrome: clinical and therapeutic observations. *Headache* **17**, 19–22.

Vijayan, N. & Dreyfus, P. (1975) Posttraumatic dysautonomic cephalalgia: clinical observations and treatment. *Archives of Neurology* **32**, 649–652.

Welch, K. & Levine, S. (1990) Migraine-related stroke in the context of the International Headache Society classification of head pain. *Archives of Neurology* **47**, 458–462.

White, L. & Dressendorfer, R. (2004) Exercise and multiple sclerosis. *Sports Medicine* **34**, 1077–1100.

Williams, S. & Nukada, H. (1994a) Sport and exercise headache. Part 1: Prevalence amongst university students. *British Journal of Sports Medicine* **28**, 90–95.

Williams, S. & Nukada, H. (1994b) Sport and exercise headache. Part 2: Diagnosis and classification. *British Journal of Sports Medicine* **28**, 96–100.

Willis, B., Greiner, F., Orrison, W.W. & Benzel, E.C. (1994) The incidence of vertebral artery injury after mid-cervical fracture or subluxation. *Neurosurgery* **34**, 435–441.

World Health Organization. (1996). WHO Collaborative Study of Cardiovascular Disease and Steroid Hormone Contraception. Ischaemic stroke and combined oral contraceptives: results of an international, multicentre, case–control study. *Lancet* **348**, 498–505.

Chapter 15

Medical Care of the Disabled Athlete

DOUGLAS B. MCKEAG AND CHRIS KLENCK

Able-bodied athletes often encounter many obstacles throughout their careers. However, few of these athletes face as many challenges as their disabled counterparts. Despite these challenges, the number of disabled athletes competing in sports has substantially increased over the years. The Summer Paralympic Games has grown from 400 athletes from 23 countries in Rome in 1960, to 3806 athletes from 136 countries in Athens in 2004 (www.paralympic.org 2006). This growth requires sports medicine professionals to become more proficient in dealing with this unique population.

The increased number of disabled athletes may partly be a result of federal legislation that requires equal opportunity and access to individuals with disabilities. The Federal Rehabilitation Act of 1973 "prohibits the exclusion of otherwise qualified individuals from participation in federally funded programs." Furthermore, the Americans with Disabilities Act (1990) expanded the law to include the private sector (Nichols 1996). According to this legislation, a disabled individual is defined as one who has a physical or mental impairment that significantly limits one or more of his or her activities of daily living (Halpern *et al*. 2001; Nichols 1996).

The World Health Organization also offered terminology and definitions regarding disabled individuals. It defines impairment as any loss or abnormality of psychologic, physical, or anatomic structure or function. Disability is regarded as any restriction or lack of an ability to perform an activity in the manner or within the range considered normal for a human being. Finally, a handicap is described as a disadvantage for a given individual, resulting from an impairment or a disability that limits or prevents the fulfillment of a role that is normal for that individual based on age, sex, and social and cultural factors (Halpern *et al*. 2001).

With better access and opportunities, more disabled athletes are benefitting from regular physical activity. Disabled athletes tend to possess higher self-esteem, better satisfaction in life, and less depressive symptoms than their non-athletic counterparts (Halpern *et al*. 2001). One study evaluated the effects of aerobic exercise in adults with physical disabilities compared with a control group of inactive adults with physical disabilities. Not only did the physically active disabled adults achieve increased aerobic capacity as measured by $\dot{V}o_{2max}$, but they also displayed decreased depressive symptoms, decreased somatic complaints, and improved positive affect (Coyle & Santiago 1995). Just as in able-bodied people, regular exercise also diminishes the risks of cardiopulmonary disease, hypertension, and type 2 diabetes in disabled individuals (Halpern *et al*. 2001).

History

Individuals with disabilities have been involved in sports for more than 100 years. Sports clubs for deaf individuals were in existence in 1888 in Berlin, and

The Olympic Textbook of Medicine in Sport, 1st edition. Edited by M. Schwellnus. Published 2008 by Blackwell Publishing, ISBN: 978-1-4051-5637-0.

429

the World Organization of Sport for the Deaf was established in 1922. The deaf still organize their own World Games (www.paralympic.org 2006).

Sports for people with physical disabilities began shortly after World War II in an effort to rehabilitate injured veterans, women, and civilians. In 1944, Ludwig Guttmann established a spinal injuries center at Stoke Mandeville Hospital in England. Guttmann utilized sports as a means for treatment and rehabilitation for his patients with spinal cord injuries. This form of rehabilitation quickly led to recreational sport followed by competitive sport. On July 28, 1948, the Opening Ceremony of the 1948 Olympic Games in London was held. On this day, Guttman organized the first competition for wheelchair athletes called the Stoke Mandeville Games. The games expanded in 1952 to include Dutch ex-servicemen and the International Stoke Mandeville Games Committee (ISMGF) was founded (www.paralympic.org 2006). In 1948, the National Wheelchair Basketball Association (NWBA) was formed in the USA to govern the sport of wheelchair basketball. The National Wheelchair Athletic Association (NWAA) was subsequently formed in 1956 to govern sports other than basketball for disabled athletes. This organization is now called Wheelchair Sports USA (Halpern *et al.* 2001).

The first Paralympic Games was held in Rome, Italy in 1960 following the Olympic Games. It involved 400 athletes from 23 countries. The event continued every 4 years, usually in the same country that hosted the Olympic Games. The first Paralympic Winter Games took place in 1976 following the merger of several disability groups (Halpern *et al.* 2001; www.paralympic.org 2006).

In 1960, the International Working Group on Sport for the Disabled was established to study the problems associated with sports for disabled athletes. It led to the creation of the International Sport Organization for the Disabled (ISOD) in 1964. This organization provided opportunities to athletes with disabilities who could not affiliate to ISMGF. These athletes included amputees, visually impaired, and those with cerebral palsy. However, other organizations representing disabled athletes were also established including the Cerebral Palsy International Sports and Recreation Association (CP-ISRA) in 1978 and the International Blind Sport Federation (IBSA) in 1980. The international organizations together formed the International Coordinating Committee Sports for the Disabled in the World in 1982 which in turn led to the formation of the International Paralympic Committee (IPC; www.paralympic.org 2006).

The Special Olympics was established in 1968 to provide athletic competition to children and adults with intellectual disabilities. Eunice Kennedy Shriver organized the First International Summer Games at Soldier Field in Chicago, Illinois in 1968. The concept began in the early 1960s when Shriver started a day camp for individuals with intellectual disabilities. These individuals were noted to be much more capable of athletic competition than most experts thought. Since 1968, more than 1.7 million athletes have been involved in the Special Olympics from more than 150 countries. The organization offers year-round training and competition in 26 Olympic-type sports (www.specialolympics.org 2006).

Classification

To ensure fair competition between disabled athletes, a classification system is utilized. This system originally focused on muscle testing typically related to the level of spinal cord lesion. However, as more disability types were included, the classification system evolved into a functional classification system in 1992. This system relies more on the movements required for a sport. The goal is to ensure fair competition between athletes with a similar degree of disability (White 2002).

Athletes are divided into one of six disability categories for international competition in the Paralympic Games (www.bbc.co.uk 2000; White 2002).

1 *Wheelchair athletes* This category includes those with spinal cord injuries or disease that results in the loss of spinal cord function. Usually, the athlete must have at least a 10% loss of function of the lower limbs. Examples include paraplegia, quadriplegia, and poliomyelitis. Amputees and cerebral palsy athletes may also be included in this category (Fig. 15.1).

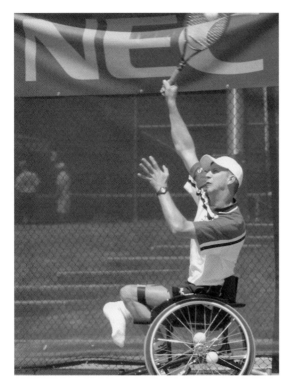

Fig. 15.1 Wheelchair athlete. Figures 15.1–15.3 illustrate various examples of disabled athletes.

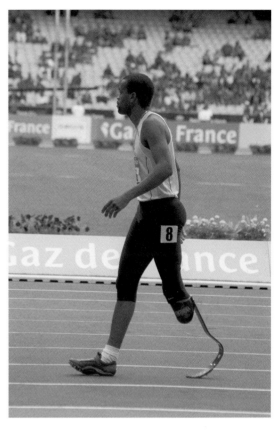

Fig. 15.2 Amputee athlete. Figures 15.1–15.3 illustrate various examples of disabled athletes.

2 *Amputee* These athletes have at least one major joint in a limb missing. This disability may be congenital or a result of trauma or disease. Examples of joints include elbow, knee, wrist, or ankle. Some of these athletes may be categorized as wheelchair athletes depending on the sport (Fig. 15.2).

3 *Cerebral palsy* This category involves those athletes with a disorder of "movement and posture due to damage to an area, or areas, of the brain that control and coordinate muscle tone, reflexes, posture, and movement." This group also includes athletes with cerebrovascular accidents, cerebral trauma, quadriplegia, and paraplegia with spasticity, ataxia, and/or athetosis.

4 *Visually impaired* This group includes athletes with any condition that results in visual loss.

5 *Intellectual disability* Athletes in this category have substantial intellectual functioning limitations in two or more adaptive skill areas. These areas are communication, self-care, home living, social skills, community use, self-direction, health and safety, functional academics, leisure, and work. The athlete must have acquired their condition before age 18 (Fig. 15.3).

6 *Les autres* (French, meaning "the others") This group includes all athletes with conditions that do not fit into other groups. Examples include dwarfism, osteogenesis imperfecta, muscular dystrophy, and arthrogryposis.

Deaf athletes are not included in this functional classification system as they typically have similar motor development and physical fitness levels as their counterparts. A possible exception includes those hearing-impaired athletes who have had concomitant injury to the semicircular canal system or vestibular apparatus resulting in equilibrium deficits. The governing body for deaf athletes is the

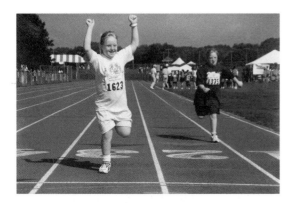

Fig. 15.3 Intellectually impaired athlete. (Special Olympics New York volunteer. Photographer Joe Putrock.) Figures 15.1–15.3 illustrate various examples of disabled athletes.

International Committee of Silent Sports which organizes and hosts the World Games for the Deaf.

After being placed in a category, disabled athletes are further subdivided into classes according to their differing levels of impairment. The classes differ between different sports and disabilities. Table 15.1 lists the various classification schemes for some of the specific sports included in the Paralympic Games.

Preparticipation examination

The preparticipation examination (PPE) is a critical component of injury prevention. Most organizations require athletes to complete a PPE to be eligible to compete. The examination for disabled athletes should not be significantly different to that performed for their able-bodied counterparts. However, it should also consider issues that may be unique to an athlete with a specific disability (Boyajian-O'Neill et al. 2004). The primary objectives of the PPE are to recognize issues that may need further evaluation and treatment prior to participation, require close monitoring during competition, or increase likelihood of injury. Other objectives include the assessment of general health, counseling to improve safe competition, and referrals for athletes who need specialized care for specific conditions (Malanga 2005). The traditional station method for PPE should be avoided for disabled athletes as they often have difficulty with mobility.

Each athlete's complete medical history must be obtained in order to make appropriate recommendations. The history should include lists of past injuries or illnesses, risks for future injuries, and current allergies and medications. Pertinent questions applicable to athletes without disabilities should also be asked of disabled athletes. In addition, several areas that should be emphasized in the history are listed in Table 15.2 (Boyajian-O'Neill et al. 2004).

In addition to the history, a thorough physical examination should be performed for each athlete. Again, the elements of the examination should be similar to that for athletes without disabilities. Close attention should be paid to visual screening and cardiovascular function including blood pressure, pulse, and presence of cardiac murmurs. Neurologic evaluations should focus on peripheral nerve entrapments as well as the presence of ataxia, muscle weakness, spasticity, and sensory dysfunction. An extensive dermatologic examination should be conducted to evaluate for blisters, abrasions, skin irritations, or ulcers which commonly occur in wheelchair athletes and amputees. Athletes with pressure ulcers should not be allowed to participate until the wound is healed. Finally, a musculoskeletal evaluation should include screening for strength and flexibility in commonly injured areas, such as upper extremities in wheelchair athletes and lower extremities and back in amputees and blind athletes (Boyajian-O'Neill et al. 2004).

Diagnostic imaging is not typically indicated in the PPE of disabled athletes. However, athletes with Down's syndrome often have atlantoaxial instability. These athletes with symptoms of instability should have cervical spine radiographs consisting of lateral cervical spine with flexion and extension views to determine the severity of the problem. The Special Olympics requires that all Down's syndrome athletes who participate in high-risk sports (e.g., judo, gymnastics, diving, soccer) must obtain screening cervical spine radiographs (Fig. 15.4a,b). The presence of instability subsequently disqualifies the athlete from participation in these sports (Boyajian-O'Neill et al. 2004). The

Table 15.1 Selected sport specific classifications for Paralympic Games (www.bbc.co.uk 2000; www.eis2win.co.uk 2006; www.paralympic.org 2006).

Archery
W1: spinal cord and cerebral palsy with impairment in all four limbs
W2: wheelchair athletes with full arm function
Standing: no disability in arms but some disability in legs (i.e., amputees, les autres and standing cerebral palsy)

Athletics
Includes all disability groups. Divided into groups by letters (F, field, T, track) and numbers (type of disability)
11–13: track and field athletes with visual impairments
20: track and field athletes with intellectual disabilities
31–38: track and field athletes with cerebral palsy
41–46: track and field athletes with amputations and les autres
T 51–56: wheelchair track athletes
F 51–58: wheelchair field athletes

Basketball
Open to wheelchair athletes. Classified according to physical ability using a point system ranging from 1 (most disabled) to 4.5 (least disabled). Each team has five players but total points for team must not be greater than 14 at any point in the game

Boccia
Open to cerebral palsy athletes using wheelchairs. Two categories:
1: depend on an electric wheelchair
2: poor functional strength in all extremities but can propel wheelchair

Cycling
Open to cerebral palsy, visual impaired, les autres, and amputees
Cerebral palsy have four categories, with class 4 being least disabled
Visual impaired compete together and ride with sighted guide
Amputee, spinal cord injury, les autres:
LC1: riders with upper limb disabilities
LC2: riders with disability in one leg but can pedal normally
LC3: riders with disability in one leg and use only one leg to pedal
LC4: riders with disability affecting both legs

Equestrian
Open to all groups and divided into four groups:
Grade 1: severe disability with cerebral palsy, spinal cord injury, les autres

Grade 2: reasonable balance and abdominal control, including amputees
Grade 3: good balance, leg movement, and coordination, includes blind
Grade 4: able to walk independently with impaired vision or limb function

Football (soccer) (visual impaired)
Open to visual impaired with three categories:
B1: blind
B2: ability to recognize hand shape to visual acuity of 2/60 and/or visual field of less than 5°
B3: visual acuity above 2/60 to acuity of 6/60 and/or visual field of more than 5° and less than 20°
Goalkeepers may be sighted

Football (soccer) (cerebral palsy)
Open to athletes with cerebral palsy and divided into categories from 5–8 (category 8 are athletes least impaired). Each team must include at least one member from class 5 or 6. All athletes must be ambulatory

Goalball
Open to visual impaired athletes with classification as for football

Judo
Open to visual impaired athletes and divided by weight with classification as for football

Powerlifting
Open to all disability groups and divided by weight with no classification

Sailing
Open to all disability groups. Point system assigned similar to basketball with maximum point value for team being 14

Shooting
SH1: pistol and rifle competitors who do not require a shooting stand
SH2: rifle competitors who require a shooting stand
SH3: rifle competitors with visual impairment (not included in Paralympics)

Swimming
S1–S10: physical impaired (low numbers with most severe disability)
S11–S13: visual impaired (S11 with no sight to S13 for legally blind)

Table tennis
1–5: wheelchair athletes (5, least disability)
6–10: competes standing (10, least disability)
11: intellectual disability (not included in Paralympics)

Table 15.2 Medical history questions pertinent to disabled athletes (Boyajian-O'Neill *et al.* 2004).

History of seizures, hearing loss, or visual loss?	Commonly seen in Special Olympic athletes
History of cardiopulmonary disease?	Cardiac defects commonly seen in Down's syndrome
History of renal disease?	Renal anomalies commonly seen in Down's syndrome
History of atlantoaxial instability?	Potential risk for athletes with Down's syndrome
History of heatstroke or heat exhaustion?	Athletes with spinal cord injuries are often at increased risk secondary to impaired thermoregulation
History of fractures or dislocations?	Down's syndrome athletes often have ligamentous laxity and joint hypermobility
Use of prosthetic devices or special equipment during competition or training?	Especially important in wheelchair athletes and amputees
Use of indwelling urinary catheter or need for intermittent catheterization of the bladder?	Common in athletes with spinal cord injuries
History of pressure sores or ulcers?	Especially important in wheelchair athletes and amputees
History of autonomic dysreflexia?	Seen in spinal cord injured athletes at level T6 or above

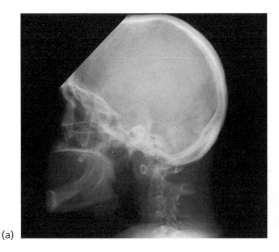
(a)

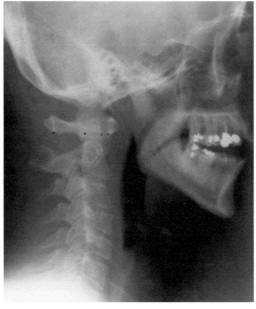
(b)

Fig. 15.4 (a) Atlantoaxial instability. (b) Normal cervical spine.

American Academy of Pediatrics (AAP) previously supported radiographic screening of individuals with Down's syndrome. However, in 1995, the AAP retracted that support stating that cervical spine films are of "unproven value in detecting patients at risk for developing spinal cord injury during sports participation" (Committee on Sports Medicine and Fitness 1995).

Common medical problems in the disabled athlete

Overview

Based on current epidemiologic studies, disabled athletes have similar injury rates and patterns as their able-bodied counterparts (Ferrara & Peterson

2000). This observation was noted by the British team's medical staff during the 1992 Paralympic Games in Barcelona. During the competition, the medical staff noted that most of the injuries and illnesses sustained by the disabled athletes were essentially the same as those encountered by athletes in able-bodied sports (Reynolds *et al.* 1994).

Some injuries and/or illnesses are more common in certain disability types than others (Ferrara & Peterson 2000). A cross-disability retrospective survey conducted by Ferrara *et al.* (1992) in 1989 analyzed injury rates and patterns in 426 disabled athletes participating in the national competition of the NWAA, US Association for Blind Athletes (USABA), and the UA Cerebral Palsy Athletic Association (USCPAA; Ferrara *et al.* 1992). They found that 32% of the responding athletes reported at least one injury resulting in limitation of sport participation lasting at least 1 day. Injuries to the shoulder and arm/elbow accounted for 57% of injuries to NWAA athletes, while 53% of the injuries to the USABA athletes involved the lower extremities, with ankle injuries being the most common. Athletes with cerebral palsy most commonly sustained injuries to the knee (21%) followed by shoulder, forearm/wrist, and leg/ankle. Comparing this data with non-disabled athletes in similar sports, they found approximately the same percentage of injury. Analysis of soft tissue injuries to USA Paralympians at the 1996 Summer Games in Atlanta, Georgia revealed similar injury patterns (Nyland *et al.* 2000). Nyland *et al.* (2000) compared injuries to athletes from Disabled Sports USA (DSUSA), USABA, USCPAA, and Wheelchair Sports USA (WSUSA). The results showed USABA athletes accounted for a greater number of lower extremity and cervicothoracic injuries, while WSUSA athletes had a greater number of upper extremity injuries.

Wheelchair athletes

Many disabled athletes rely on wheelchairs to compete in a variety of sports. The etiology of the disability varies from one athlete to another. Perhaps the most common cause of disability for wheelchair athletes is spinal cord injury (SCI). A SCI results

from damage of cells in the spinal cord. The level at which the injury occurs may result in either paraplegia or quadriplegia. Paraplegia results from injury below the first thoracic vertebra while quadriplegia results from injury in the cervical vertebra (Halpern *et al.* 2001). An athlete who is paraplegic typically experiences loss of sensation and movement of the lower body and extremities. A quadriplegic athlete may have loss of sensation and movement in both the upper and lower extremities, or any area below the neck. Athletes with other disabilities may also compete as wheelchair athletes. While a survey of wheelchair athletes published in 1985 by Curtis & Dillon (1985) showed that 65% of respondents had spinal cord injuries, other disabilities included polio or postpolio syndrome (12%), congenital disorders (9%), amputees (3%), and neuromuscular and musculoskeletal disorders (10%). The focus of this section is on wheelchair athletes with SCI while some of the other disability groups are discussed in later sections.

EXERCISE PHYSIOLOGY

Wheelchair athletes with SCI are physiologically different depending on the level of injury when compared to their able-bodied counterparts. An example of this difference can be seen in the maximum rate at which an individual can consume oxygen during exercise, also known as $\dot{V}o_{2max}$. This rate is especially important for competitions that require endurance. Important components of an individual's $\dot{V}o_{2max}$ are the delivery of oxygen to tissues and the utilization of oxygen by those tissues, particularly skeletal muscle mass. Athletes with SCI have 10–25% decrease in cardiac output and 15–30% lower stroke volume than able-bodied athletes (Halpern *et al.* 2001). In addition, quadriplegic athletes with injuries occurring above the level of sympathetic outflow typically have hypotension, limitations in maximum heart rates, and increased venous pooling further worsening cardiac output and stroke volume (Dec *et al.* 2000; Jacobs & Nash 2004). Both decreased cardiac output and stroke volume impairs oxygen delivery. Furthermore, athletes with SCI have less effective muscle mass than non-injured athletes. The amount of muscle available depends on the level of injury, with paraplegics typically having more effective muscle mass than quadriplegics (Halpern *et al*. 2001; Jacobs & Nash 2004). Reduced effective muscle mass impairs oxygen utilization. Therefore, mean $\dot{V}o_{2max}$ in paraplegic athletes are typically only comparable to sedentary able-bodied individuals while they are generally higher than quadriplegic athletes (Bhambhani 2002; Halpern *et al*. 2001).

MEDICAL ISSUES AND INJURIES

Wheelchair athletes are susceptible to several medical problems and injuries by virtue of their disability. The sports medicine professional must be familiar with these issues in order to both prevent and treat their occurrence.

Autonomic dysreflexia

Autonomic dysreflexia is a medical emergency that requires prompt recognition and treatment by medical professionals. This condition is usually seen in individuals with SCI at the T6 level or above. The estimated incidence is thought to be 50–70% (Bycroft *et al*. 2005; Dec *et al*. 2000). It is a condition that results in an uncontrolled sympathetic response which is precipitated by some noxious stimulus below the SCI level such as a fracture, distended bladder, urinary tract infection, or pressure sores. Common symptoms associated with autonomic dysreflexia include hypertension, headache, and flushing, as well as sweating typically above the level of injury. Other possible symptoms include blurred vision, bradycardia, nasal congestion, spasms, and "gooseflesh" below the level of the lesion (Fig. 15.5; Bycroft *et al*. 2005).

Initial treatment should include sitting the athlete upright to promote an orthostatic decrease in blood pressure. Careful monitoring of blood pressure should be employed while searching for the presence of a precipitating stimulus. Once identified, the stimulus should be removed, if possible. This may include emptying the bladder, removing a fecal mass, or removing a urinary catheter (Bycroft *et al*. 2005; Dec *et al*. 2000). If hypertension persists, the administration of an antihypertensive agent is indicated.

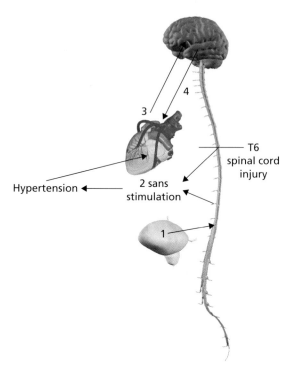

Fig. 15.5 Autonomic dysreflexia. 1, Distended bladder; 2, sympathetic autonomic nervous system stimulation; 3, baroreceptor stimulation in carotid sinuses and aortic arch; 4, brainstem stimulation of heart via vagus nerve resulting in bradycardia and vasodilation above the level of injury.

Either nitrates or nifedipine tends to be the most commonly used medications because of their rapid onset and short duration. Sublingual nifedipine 10 mg offers a rapid reduction of blood pressure but has been associated with adverse effects especially in the elderly and those with coronary artery disease (Grossman *et al*. 1996). Another popular method of administration is to "bite and swallow" the capsule (Blackmer 2003). There have been no reported adverse events from the use of nifedipine in the treatment of autonomic dysreflexia to date. Nitrates should be avoided in athletes who also use sildenafil for erectile dysfunction. Other potential agents include captopril and hydralazine. Finally, prevention of autonomic dysreflexia is paramont and includes counseling about bowel and bladder maintenance as well as skin care (Blackmer 2003; Bycroft *et al*. 2005).

Despite the danger associated with autonomic dysreflexia, some athletes attempt to induce it for competitive advantage. This practice is referred to as "boosting." Methods by which an athlete may self-induce autonomic dysreflexia include overdistending the bladder, sitting on sharp objects, or use of tight leg straps. Theoretically, the elevated blood pressure increases the cardiac output and results in better racing performance. One study documented a 10% improvement in wheelchair racing times in elite male wheelchair marathon racers who participated in "boosting" prior to the race (Bhambhani 2002). Given the dangers and unfair advantage this practice provides, it is considered "unethical and illegal" by the IPC. Therefore, sports medicine professionals must be able to recognize athletes with signs or symptoms consistent with "boosting" so that they may be withdrawn from competition if indicated.

Thermoregulation

Athletes with SCI often have difficulty regulating body temperature during training or competition in both warm and cold environments. This difficulty relates primarily to paralysis of skeletal muscle and loss of autonomic nervous system control (Halpern et al. 2001). The level of the spinal cord lesion has a role in the individual's thermoregulation. Paraplegics typically have larger increases in core body temperature when compared to able-bodied individuals. In addition, paraplegics with lesions at T6 or below show smaller increases in body temperature than do paraplegics with lesions above T6. Quadriplegic individuals tend to have the most difficulty with thermoregulation (Price & Campbell 2003).

Hyperthermia is a significant risk for athletes with SCI. Sweating and control of peripheral blood flow is often impaired below the level of the lesion (White 2002). Therefore, less surface area (i.e., upper extremities and trunk) is available for cooling via evaporation (Dec et al. 2000). Hyperthermia increases when competition is held in hot dry environments because 80–90% of heat loss occurs via evaporative sweat loss under these conditions (Bhambhani et al. 2005). Other factors contributing

to the risk of hyperthermia include dehydration and medications commonly used in SCI such as medications for bladder dysfunction, pain, and depression (Halpern et al. 2001; Malanga 2005). Prevention is key to avoiding complications of hyperthermia. Athletes should compete and train in cool environments such as early morning or evening whenever possible. Heat acclimatization should be undertaken with caution. Adequate fluid hydration is essential with approximately 1 L fluid consumed for each kilogram of body weight lost. Loose and lightweight clothing, as well as cooling towels and spraying water, may also assist in reducing hyperthermia (Bhambhani 2002; Halpern et al. 2001). Cooling devices have been studied in the past and have been felt to be ineffective. However, a recent study of six spinal cord injured subjects showed that a foot cooling device significantly reduced body temperature after exercise in hot environments (Hagobian et al. 2004). Webborn et al. (2005) found that pre-cooling and cooling during training or competition using an ice vest reduced core body temperatures compared with no cooling in eight quadriplegic athletes. Finally, signs of heat illness secondary to hyperthermia must be recognized in a timely manner: fatigue, weakness, lightheadedness, headache, vomiting, and/or myalgias. Treatment includes clothing removal, moving to a cool environment, external cooling, and administration of oral and/or intravenous fluids. Athletes with severe heat illness should be transported to an emergency department (Halpern et al. 2001).

Spinal cord injuries also predispose to hypothermia. These athletes have reduced skeletal muscle mass and activity as well as loss of autonomic nervous system control. The result is the inability to generate body heat by shivering (Dec et al. 2000; Halpern et al. 2001). Hypothermia is especially a concern in those athletes who train and compete in cold environments such as swimmers or skiers. In addition, athletes with sensation loss may be unaware of damp clothing which further increases heat loss. Prevention is again essential in avoiding complications associated with hypothermia. Athletes should wear appropriate layered clothing, remove wet clothing, and maintain adequate nutrition. Individuals with signs of hypothermia such as confusion, apathy, or clumsiness should undergo rewarming with transfer to a emergency room facility if indicated (Halpern *et al.* 2001).

Pressure sores

Pressure sores can be a significant problem for wheelchair athletes. They typically arise because of prolonged pressure over the skin resulting in disruption in skin integrity (Malanga 2005). The sores are often staged 1–4 depending on the depth of the sore (Fig. 15.6). Areas most affected include the sacrum and ischial tuberosities secondary to prolonged pressure over these areas during training and competition. Use of sports wheelchairs further increase the likelihood of pressure sores in these areas because they are designed to keep knees higher than the buttocks (Halpern *et al.* 2001). Vigilant skin care is essential in preventing pressure sores and includes weight shifts to relieve pressure, use of padding and moisture-wicking clothing, and careful monitoring of the skin (Halpern *et al.* 2001; Malanga 2005).

Neurogenic bladder

Athletes with SCI must often deal with neurogenic bladder or bladder dysfunction as a result of their injury. The bladder dysfunction predisposes these individuals to increased risks of urinary tract infections (UTI) from incomplete voiding, elevated intravesical pressure, and/or catheter use (Garcia & Esclarin De Ruz 2003). Common methods for bladder drainage include indwelling urethral catheters and intermittent catheterization. Indwelling catheters typically have the highest incidence of UTI. Typical signs and symptoms of UTI may be absent in athletes with SCI. The sports medicine practitioner must be able to recognize subtle indications that suggest UTI such as fever, discomfort over the kidney or bladder, urinary incontinence, increased spasticity, autonomic dysreflexia, malaise, lethargy, or sense of unease (Garcia & Esclarin De Ruz 2003). Prevention of UTI includes proper hydration, routine bladder emptying, and antiseptic methods of bladder catheterization (Halpern *et al.* 2001). Because many spinal cord injured individuals

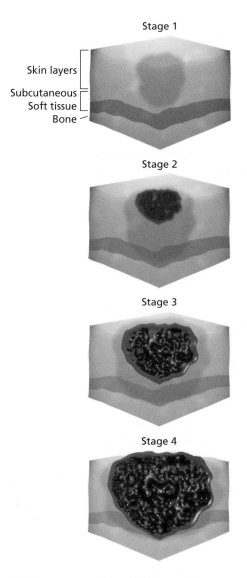

Fig. 15.6 Pressure sores. Stage 1, skin intact; Stage 2, extends into epidermis; Stage 3, extends through dermis and into subcutaneous tissue; Stage 4, extends to muscle and bone.

have bacteriuria, many experts do not recommend routine antibiotic treatment if the individual is asymptomatic because of the increased risk of developing drug-resistant bacteria. However, symptomatic athletes require antibiotic treatment for 10–14 days (Garcia & Esclarin De Ruz 2003).

Premature osteoporosis

The risk of osteoporosis is increased in athletes with SCI. These athletes often develop premature osteoporosis and subsequent fractures in lower extremities. Sports that increase the likelihood of contact or falls such as basketball have especially high risks of fractures (White 2002). The exact etiology for premature osteoporosis is unclear but appears to be because of both disuse and neural factors. During the first 24 months following a SCI, areas below the lesion level experience increased demineralization especially in weight-bearing sites such as the distal femur and proximal tibia (Jiang et al. 2006; Maimoun et al. 2006). Because these athletes may have impaired sensation, they may not recognize when fractures occur. Therefore, careful observation for signs of fractures after practice or games is critical, noting any areas with swelling or deformities (White 2002).

Managing premature osteoporosis in SCI can be challenging. One approach involves applying mechanical stimulus to the bones of the lower extremity by standing or walking with orthotic aides or functional electrical stimulation. Another approach involves the use of medications such as calcium supplements, calcitonin, and/or bisphosphonates (Maimoun et al. 2006). A recent study compared the effect of alendronate in combination with calcium with calcium alone on bone mineral density in SCI patients. The results showed that patients treated with alendronate showed increases from baseline in 9 of 12 densitometric parameters with statistical significance in two of those parameters over a 6-month course. The calcium-only group showed an increase in only one parameter with either no change or decrease in the remaining 11 parameters (Moran de Brito et al. 2005).

Peripheral nerve entrapment syndromes

Wheelchair athletes commonly present with symptoms of peripheral nerve entrapment. The two most common conditions are carpal tunnel syndrome (CTS) involving the median nerve and ulnar nerve entrapment either at the wrist or the elbow. The prevalence of CTS in manual wheelchair users has been estimated to be 49–73% (Boninger et al. 1996). Many experts believe the high incidence is partly caused by repetitive trauma to carpal tunnel structures from manual propulsion of the wheelchair. Repetitive pressure over the soft tissue structures of the carpal tunnel are also thought to contribute to the development of CTS (Halpern et al. 2001). Ulnar neuropathy is commonly seen at Guyon's canal in the wrist and less commonly at the cubital tunnel. As in CTS, etiology is believed to be brought about by repetitive pressure from the wheelchair at this area. In addition, repetitive contraction of the flexor carpi ulnaris muscle for wheelchair propulsion increases the likelihood of entrapment at the cubital tunnel (Halpern et al. 2001).

Because wheelchair athletes invest many hours in training and competition, some believe they may be at increased risk of peripheral nerve entrapments. However, recent studies have shown that the incidence of entrapments are no greater in the wheelchair athlete than in their non-athletic counterparts. Furthermore, incidence of nerve condition abnormalities correlated with duration of disability (Boninger et al. 1996; Burnham & Steadward 1994).

Prevention of peripheral nerve entrapments include the use of padded gloves to protect the volar surface of the wrist and maintaining wheelchairs in good condition. Treatment of CTS and ulnar neuropathy is similar to in able-bodied athletes. Use of wrist splints and non-steroidal anti-inflammatory agents may be beneficial. Surgery should be considered for those athletes who do not respond to conservative treatment.

Musculoskeletal injuries

Upper extremity injuries are the most common musculoskeletal injuries sustained by wheelchair athletes. The shoulders tend to function as weight-bearing joints for wheelchair propulsion and transfer. Therefore, overuse injuries involving the muscles and tendons of the shoulders as well as the elbows, wrists, and hands are common concerns for wheelchair users (Halpern et al. 2001; White 2002). Finley & Rodgers (2004) conducted a recent study of athletic versus non-athletic wheelchair users with shoulder pain and found that bicipital tendonitis and rotator cuff impingement were the most common pathologies. With training and competition, wheelchair athletes would seem to be at greater risk for overuse injuries. However, this study showed that athletic involvement did not appear to increase or decrease the risk of shoulder pain (Finley & Rodgers 2004). Other studies have reported that non-athletic wheelchair users actually have higher risks of shoulder pain than their athletic peers (Fullerton *et al.* 2003).

Contributing to the development of shoulder pain in wheelchair athletes is muscular imbalance. Wheelchair athletes typically have stronger shoulders than similar able-bodied athletes. However, abduction strength tends to be greater than both adduction and internal–external rotation. Muscles involved in scapulothoracic stabilization also tend to be weak. This imbalance leads to superior displacement of the humeral head and a reduced subacromial space (Burnham *et al.* 1993; Halpern *et al.* 2001).

Treatment of these injuries can often be difficult. Resting the shoulder is usually impractical as these athletes must rely on their upper extremities for routine activities of daily living. Therefore, acute pain should be managed with ice and non-steroidal anti-inflammatory agents. Subacromial corticosteroid injections may also provide some benefit. Finally, physical therapy should be initiated concentrating on flexibility of anterior shoulder musculature and strengthening muscles of adduction, internal–external rotation, and scapulothoracic stabilization (Curtis *et al.* 1999).

Athletes with cerebral palsy

Cerebral palsy is a disorder of movement and posture caused by damage to the brain. The damage may occur before, during, or shortly after birth. Some affected individuals may also have visual defects, deafness, seizures, or intellectual disabilities. The degree of disability varies with approximately half relying on wheelchairs for mobility. This group is often subdivided into eight different classes based on degree of disability. Some athletes have severe spastic symptoms involving all extremities and rely on motorized wheelchairs for mobility (class 1), while other athletes have only minor problems with balance and coordination (class 8).

EXERCISE PHYSIOLOGY

Athletes with cerebral palsy often have significant difficulty with ambulation secondary to spasticity. Those individuals who are ambulatory have reduced mechanical efficiency and increased energy requirements when compared to able-bodied individuals. In fact, children with cerebral palsy have been shown to have increased energy expenditures by nearly threefold compared to healthy controls at a given walking speed (Unnithan *et al.* 1998). Higher oxygen uptake, oxygen pulse, and respiratory exchange ratios have been documented in studies comparing cerebral palsy subjects with controls (Rose *et al.* 1993). Subnormal values for peak anaerobic power and muscular endurance of the upper and lower limbs are also seen in cerebral palsy.

MEDICAL ISSUES AND INJURIES

Injuries to athletes with cerebral palsy often affect both upper and lower extremities and depend greatly on ambulatory status. The common finding of spasticity in this group predisposes the athletes to injuries. Ferrara *et al.* (1992) found that cerebral palsy athletes most frequently sustained injuries to the knee, followed by the shoulder, forearm/wrist, and leg/ankle.

Knee injuries commonly involve the patellofemoral joint. Patellofemoral pain may be precipitated secondary to spasm of muscle groups surrounding the joint. Both quadriceps and hamstring muscles often have increased tightening leading to increased tension across the joint (Halpern *et al.* 2001).

Foot and ankle injuries can also be problematic. Individuals with cerebral palsy frequently have deformities of the ankle and foot including equinas, eqinovarus, and valgus deformities. These deformities may leave the athlete at increased risk for injuries including metatarsalgia, ankle instability, calluses, and pressure sores (Halpern *et al.* 2001).

Prevention and treatment of injuries to athletes with cerebral palsy typically include a combination of physical therapy, medications, and bracing. Attention should be given to an appropriate stretching program. Warm-ups and cool-downs must be included for training and competition. Administration of medications such as benzodiazepines may also help decrease muscle tone. The use of braces on affected extremities can also aid in reducing tone and improving ambulation (Malanga 2005). Finally, strength training has been controversial because it has been thought to increase spasticity. If strength training is undertaken, the athlete must be monitored closely for tone balance.

Amputee athletes

Amputee athletes have at least one joint missing in a limb. The amputation may be brought about by a congenital defect or trauma. These athletes frequently use a variety of prostheses to assist them in competition. They compete in several different categories depending on the number and site of amputations and the resulting degree of disability.

Stump injuries are common concerns for athletes with amputations. The stump is subjected to skin abrasions, pressure sores, blisters, and rashes. Improperly fitted prostheses increase the likelihood of these complications. In addition, athletes who compete in warm environments typically have issues with moisture predisposing to rashes and skin irritation. Ensuring prostheses and other assistive devices are fitted properly will help prevent many of these conditions. In addition, appropriate skin care including talcum powder and cool clothing to combat sweating will reduce risks of stump irritation. Appropriate rest of the stump must be encouraged whenever possible.

Altered biomechanics may increase the risk of many musculoskeletal injuries in amputee athletes. Cervical and thoracic spine injuries are commonly seen in individuals with upper extremity amputations because of imbalance and unequal movements in upper limbs during training and competition (White 2002). Likewise, lower extremity amputees often have low back pain as a result of excessive lumbar spine lateral flexion and extension to compensate for poor joint flexion at prosthetic sites (Halpern *et al.* 2001). Therapy focusing on back strengthening and flexibility can assist in minimizing these problems.

Increased injuries to the intact limb are also a concern. The athlete may increase the stress applied to the intact limb resulting in overuse injuries such as plantar fascitis or Achilles tendonitis, as well as the development of stress fractures. Increased rates of degenerative joint disease may also be seen. Close assessment of running and walking gaits by sports medicine professionals should be performed on these athletes. Based on this assessment, appropriate physical therapy and prosthetic devices must be employed to minimize the risk of injuries.

Blind athletes

Visually impaired athletes compete in many different sports either independently with the use of assistive devices (e.g., beeping balls, clap sticks) or with the help of normally sighted companions. The degree of visual impairment varies from no light perception to poor visual acuity and limited visual fields. Athletes are divided into appropriate categories based on their visual impairment. While exercise physiology of blind athletes does not differ significantly from able-bodied individuals, their disability does predispose them to injury.

Proprioception in blind individuals tends to be worse than those with partial vision and worse in those with acquired versus congenital visual impairment. Lower extremities are usually more profoundly affected. Poor proprioception can, in turn, result in abnormal gait and biomechanics. The result is increased incidence of overuse injuries of the lower extremities (White 2002).

Blind athletes most commonly sustain injuries to the lower extremities, especially the ankle (Ferrara *et al.* 1992; Nyland *et al.* 2000). Ankle sprains and contusions to shins are frequent complaints. Competing in unfamiliar environments with the lack of guides or assistive devices predispose these athletes to injury. Treatment of the injuries does not differ from able-bodied athletes. However, special attention should be taken to prevent injuries by providing adequate guidance and support to the athletes, especially when competing in new environments.

Deaf athletes

Deaf individuals often are able to compete in sports with non-disabled peers. They typically do not differ significantly from their peers with respect to motor function and fitness levels. However, some athletes with hearing impairment also have sustained injury to the semicircular canal or vestibular apparatus which results in equilibrium deficits. The primary barrier to competition is communication and emphasis must be placed on the use of physical cues. Therefore, caution must be taken to avoid the use of equipment, braces, or bandages that may limit their ability to interpret such cues.

Athletes with intellectual disabilities

Injuries sustained by athletes with intellectual disabilities are not significantly different than those seen in able-bodied athletes. However, these athletes often have comorbid illnesses that require special attention from sports medicine professionals. Some of these conditions include visual loss, congenital heart disease, and atlantoaxial instability.

Ocular and visual defects are quite common in athletes with intellectual disabilities. A recent study by Woodhouse *et al*. (2004) evaluated 505 Special Olympic athletes for visual defects. The results showed that 19% of athletes had significant refractive error, 32% had ocular anomalies, and 6% were visually impaired. Of these athletes, 15% had never had an optometric eye examination. Among the most common visual problems identified are poor visual acuity, refractive errors, astigmatism, and strabismus (Bouajian-O'Neill *et al*. 2004). Therefore, team physicians must be aware of the risks of visual impairments in this population and ensure routine visual screening to minimize complications associated with poor vision.

Congenital heart disease is frequently seen in intellectually impaired athletes, especially in those with Down's syndrome. Atrioventricular septal defects, ventricular septal defects, atrial septal defects, and other complex congenital heart diseases are examples of possible heart defects in this group. Careful history and physical examination as well as possible echocardiograms are indicated to screen for these disorders. Athletes who have these disorders will likely require treatment and clearance to participate from a cardiologist skilled in the management of these conditions.

In addition to cardiac defects, atlantoaxial instability is a concern for athletes with Down's syndrome. Approximately 15% of individuals with Down's syndrome have atlantoaxial instability. Atlantoaxial instability allows increased mobility at the first and second cervical vertebrae. Most of these individuals are asymptomatic but a small number may show symptoms. Symptoms of atlantoaxial instability include easy fatigue, walking difficulty, neck pain, torticollis, clumsiness, sensory deficits, hyperreflexia, sensory deficits, and other upper motoneuron and posterior column signs or symptoms. Radiographs may be normal initially but abnormal on follow-up or, more commonly, may be abnormal initially and normal on follow-up (Committee on Sports Medicine and Fitness 1995). While the need for yearly cervical spine radiographs is controversial, athletes with evidence of atlantoaxial instability should be restricted from competing in any sport that requires excessive neck flexion or extension (Malanga 2005).

Conclusions

Growing numbers of individuals with disabilities are training and competing in sporting events. The benefits of competition not only improve physical health but also self-esteem and mental well-being. As the number of disabled athletes continues to grow, so do the challenges and responsibilities to care for this group. Sports medicine professionals, along with a multidisciplinary team, must be ready to accept this responsibility. Continued research and maintenance of a working knowledge of the unique illness and injuries associated with disabilities will dramatically improve the outcomes of these athletes.

References

Bhambhani, Y. (2002) Physiology of wheelchair racing in athletes with spinal cord injury. *Sports Medicine* **32**, 23–51.

Blackmer, J. (2003) Rehabilitation medicine: autonomic dysreflexia. *Canadian Medical Association Journal* **169**, 931–935.

Boninger, M.L., Robertson, R.N., Wolff, M., *et al.* (1996) Upper limb nerve entrapments in elite wheelchair racers. *American Journal of Physical Medicine and Rehabilitation* **75**, 170–176.

Boyajian-O'Neill, L., Cardone, D., Dexter, W., *et al.* (2004) The preparticipation examination for the athlete with special needs. *Physician and Sportsmedicine* **32**, 13–9, 42.

Burnham, R.S., May, L., Nelson, E., *et al.* (1993) Shoulder pain in wheelchair athletes: the role of muscle imbalance. *American Journal of Sports Medicine* **21**, 238–242.

Burnham, R.S. & Steadward, R.D. (1994) Upper extremity peripheral nerve entrapments among wheelchair athletes: prevalence, location, and risk factors. *Archives of Physical Medicine and Rehabilitation* **75**, 519–524.

Bycroft, J., Shergill, I.S., Choong, E.A.L., *et al.* (2005) Autonomic dysreflexia: a medical emergency. *Postgraduate Medical Journal* **81**, 232–235.

Committee on Sports Medicine and Fitness (1995). Atlantoaxial instability in Down syndrome: subject review. *Pediatrics* **96**, 151–154.

Coyle, C.P. & Santiago, M.C. (1995) Aerobic exercise training and depressive symptomatology in adults with physical disabilities. *Archives of Physical Medicine and Rehabilitation* **76**, 647–652.

Curtis, K.A. & Dillon, D.A. (1985) Survey of wheelchair athletic injuries: common patterns and prevention. *Paraplegia* **23**, 170–175.

Curtis, K.A., Tyner, T.M., Zachary, L., *et al.* (1999) Effect of a standard exercise protocol on shoulder pain in long-term wheelchair users. *Spinal Cord* **37**, 421–429.

Dec, K.L., Sparrow, K.J., McKeag, D.B. (2000) The physically-challenged athlete: medical issues and assessment. *Sports Medicine* **29**, 245–258.

Ferrara, M.S., Buckley, W.E., McCann, B.C., *et al.* (1992) The injury experience of the competitive athlete with a disability: prevention implications. *Medicine and Science in Sports and Exercise* **24**, 184–188.

Ferrara, M.S. & Peterson, C.L. (2000) Injuries to athletes with disabilities: identifying injury patterns. *Sports Medicine* **30**, 137–143.

Finley, M.A. & Rodgers, M.M. (2004) Prevalence and identification of shoulder pathology in athletic and nonathletic wheelchair users with shoulder pain: a pilot study. *Journal of Rehabilitation Research and Development* **41**, 395–402.

Fullerton, H.D., Borckardt, J.J. & Alfano, A.P. (2003) Shoulder pain: a comparison of wheelchair athletes and nonathletic wheelchair users. *Medicine and Science in Sports and Exercise* **35**, 1958–1961.

Garcia, M.E. & Esclarin De Ruz, A. (2003) Management of urinary tract infection in patients with spinal cord injuries. *Clinical Microbiology and Infection* **9**, 780–785.

Grossman, E., Messerli, F.H., Grodzicki, T., *et al.* (1996) Should a moratorium be placed on sublingual nifedipine capsules given for hypertensive emergencies and pseudoemergencies? *JAMA* **276**, 1328–1331.

Hagobian, T.A., Jacobs, K.A., Kiratli, B.J., *et al.* (2004) Foot cooling reduces exercise-induced hyperthermia in men with spinal cord injury. *Medicine and Science in Sports and Exercise* 36, 411–417.

Halpern, B.C., Boehm, R. & Cardone, D.A. (2001) The disabled athlete. In *Principles and Practice of Primary Care Sports Medicine* (Garrett, W.E., Kirkendall, D.T. & Squire, D.L., eds.) Lippincott Williams & Wilkins, Philadelphia: 115–129.

History of Sport for Persons with a Disability. http://www.paralympic.org. Accessed January 29, 2006.

Jacobs, PL, Nash MS. (2004) Exercise recommendations for individuals with spinal cord injury. *Sports Medicine* **34**, 727–751.

Jiang, S.D., Dai, L.Y. & Jiang, L.S. (2006) Osteoporosis after spinal cord injury. *Osteoporosis International* **17**, 180–192.

Maimoun, L., Fattal, C., Micallef, J.P., Peruchon, E. & Rabisching, P. (2006) Bone loss in spinal cord-injured patients: from physiopathology to therapy. *Spinal Cord* **44**, 203–210.

Making sense of the categories. http://news.bbc.co.uk/sport1/hi/olympics2000/paralympics/959701.stm. Accessed January 29, 2006.

Malanga, G.A. (2005) Athletes with disabilities. emedicine. http://www.emedicine.com

Moran de Brito, C.M., Battistella, L.R., Saito, E.T., *et al.* (2005) Effect of alendronate on bone mineral density in spinal cord injury patients: a pilot study. *Spinal Cord* **43**, 341–348.

Nichols, A.W. (1996) Sports medicine and the Americans with Disabilities Act. *Clinical Journal of Sports Medicine* **6**, 190–195.

Nyland, J., Snouse, S., Anderson, M., *et al.* (2000) Soft tissue injuries to USA paralympians at the 1996 summer games. *Archives of Physical Medicine and Rehabilitation* **81**, 368–373.

Paralympic Games. http://www.paralympic.org. Accessed January 29, 2006.

Price, M.J. & Campbell, I.G. (2003) Effects of spinal cord lesion level upon thermoregulation during exercise in the heat. *Medicine and Science in Sports and Exercise* **35**, 1100–1107.

Reynolds, J., Stirk, A., Thomas, A., *et al.* (1994) Paralympics: Barcelona 1992. *British Journal of Sports Medicine* **28**, 14–17.

Rose, J., Haskell, W.L. & Gamble, J.G. (1993) A comparison of oxygen pulse and respiratory exchange ratio in cerebral palsied and nondisabled children. *Archives of Physical Medicine and Rehabilitation* **74**, 702–705.

Special Olympics History. http://www.specialolympics.org. Accessed January 29, 2006.

Sport Specific Classification. http://www.paralympic.org Accessed January 29, 2006.

Understanding Paralympic Classification. http://www.eis2win.co.uk/gen/news_paraclassification100903.aspx. Accessed January 29, 2006.

Unnithan, V.B., Clifford, C. & Bar-Or, O. (1998) Evaluation by exercise testing of the child with cerebral palsy. *Sports Medicine* **26**, 239–251.

Webborn, N., Price, M.J., Castle, P.C., *et al.* (2005) Effects of two cooling strategies on thermoregulatory responses of tetraplegic athletes during repeated intermittent exercise in the heat. *Journal of Applied Physiology* **98**, 2101–2107.

White, S. (2002) The disabled athlete. In *Clinical Sports Medicine*, 2nd edn. (Brukner, P. & Khan, K., eds.) McGraw-Hill, Australia: 705–709.

Woodhouse, J.M., Adler, P. & Duignan, A. (2004) Vision in athletes with intellectual disabilities: the need for improved eyecare. *Journal of Intellectual Disability Research* **48**, 736–745.

Chapter 16

Environmental Sports Medicine

TIMOTHY D. NOAKES, TAMARA HEW-BUTLER AND ROSS TUCKER

A remarkable feature of the human species is our great capacity to adapt to different environmental conditions. These capacities are frequently taxed to the limit in the pursuit of different sporting goals, most especially by international athletes who travel the world and compete in environmental conditions different from those to which they are accustomed. Obvious recent examples are the 2004 Athens Olympic Games, the 2006 Soccer World Cup, and the 2007 Cricket World Cup, all of which were held in unusually hot conditions and which would have favored athletes born in the warmer parts of the world.

This chapter reviews the physiologic challenges posed to athletes by altitude, atmospheric pollution, heat, cold, and intercontinental travel and discusses some techniques that may enhance performance under those conditions.

Exercise at high altitude

Besides the obvious risks of falling with often fatal consequences, high altitude poses two distinct physiologic challenges for the human body. The first is caused by the progressive reduction, as one ascends from sea level, in the amount of oxygen present in any volume of air. The second is posed by the cold and wind. Fortunately, high altitude is usually dry, so that it is easier to keep clothes dry than in the cold and wet conditions that predominate at lower altitudes. However, the presence

The Olympic Textbook of Medicine in Sport, 1st edition. Edited by M. Schwellnus. Published 2008 by Blackwell Publishing, ISBN: 978-1-4051-5637-0.

of high winds at altitude markedly increases the coldness of the environment by increasing the wind-chill factor. The issues of exercise in the cold are discussed below (see p. 467).

As the altitude above sea level increases the barometric pressure falls; this causes the distance between oxygen molecules in the air to increase and the partial pressure of oxygen (Po_2) in the inspired air to fall. Consequently, the arterial (Pao_2) partial pressure of oxygen falls as a function of the elevation above sea level. While a number of physiologic adaptations restrict the extent to which the Pao_2 falls with increasing altitude, ultimately each human being will reach an altitude at which they will no longer be able to survive, because their Pao_2 will have fallen below that value necessary for sustaining those brain functions necessary for life. As Reinholdt Messner, who, with Peter Habeler was the first climber to reach the summit of Mount Everest without the use of supplemental oxygen, has written: "The most dangerous part of climbing Mount Everest is the reduced partial pressure of oxygen in the summit region, which dulls judgment, appreciation, and indeed one's ability to feel anything at all" (Messner 1979).

In order to partially compensate for the progressive fall in Pao_2, humans breathe more often and more deeply as they ascend to higher altitudes. In addition, if they acclimatize by gradually increasing the altitudes at which they exercise and sleep for periods of some weeks, humans also develop a marked increase in red cell mass, causing increased circulating hemoglobin concentrations. Despite these adaptations, the lowest Pao_2 compatible with sustained life is reached at altitudes of about 7000 m in most humans. That some humans have reached the summit of Mount Everest (8840 m) without supplemental oxygen attests to a phenomenal biology that allows such unique humans to sustain much higher than expected Pao_2 at these extreme altitudes.

Interest in the challenge of climbing high mountains has led to a greater understanding of the factors that regulate exercise performance at such altitudes. This information has important practical consequences. There is now clear evidence that exercise at altitude is regulated by the brain to ensure that only those exercise intensities that will not lower the Pao_2 to the point at which consciousness is lost, are allowed. This novel interpretation comes from studies, discussed subsequently, showing that the maximal blood and muscle lactate concentrations, as well as the maximal cardiac output, are all lower at exhaustion during exercise at altitude than they are at sea level. This contrasts to the traditional idea that exercise must always terminate with very high muscle and blood lactate concentrations caused by increasing anaerobic conditions in the exercising muscles and which must be amplified during maximal exercise at altitude. However, the lower muscle and blood lactate concentrations and cardiac output during maximal exercise at altitude are more elegantly explained if the number of muscle fibers (motor units) that the brain chooses to activate at altitude is reduced in proportion to the fall in Pao_2 specifically to ensure that exercise always terminates before a fatally low Pao_2 is reached.

According to this model, an altitude will ultimately be reached at which the brain will finally choose not to activate enough motor units to allow continued exercise; hence the climber will appear to be paralyzed. Under these circumstances, the only actions that will save the climber's life are those that increase his or her Pao_2, either the provision of oxygen or the immediate descent to lower altitudes.

Some of the original studies of exercise at altitude that support this theory were undertaken by a US research group led by Dill (1938) from the Fatigue laboratory at Harvard University. Their research established two crucial findings. First, that peak blood lactate concentrations during maximum exercise fell with increasing altitude, a phenomenon labeled the "lactate paradox." This finding is paradoxical because, according to the traditional understanding, exercise at altitude should cause an increased skeletal muscle anaerobiosis so that exercise at altitude must always terminate with higher, not lower, blood lactate concentrations than at sea level.

The second unexpected finding was that the maximum heart rate and cardiac output were likewise lower at altitude than at sea level. This is paradoxical because the popular understanding is that the principal responsibility of the cardiovascular system during exercise is to maximize blood and oxygen delivery to the muscles in order to delay the development of an inevitable skeletal muscle anaerobiosis at exhaustion. In which case the maximum cardiac output during exercise at increasing altitude must either be the same or even higher than at sea level in order to supply as much oxygen-depleted blood to the exercising muscles, whose demand for oxygen is the paramount requirement, for the fulfillment of which the cardiovascular system exists.

Yet, the evidence from numerous studies is now absolutely clear; the heart makes exactly the opposite adjustment so that the maximum cardiac output falls with increasing altitude. Hence, the conclusion has to be that some unrecognized mechanism must be acting to ensure that neither the heart nor the skeletal muscles of healthy humans ever become "anaerobic" during maximal exercise at any altitude – from sea level to the summit of Mount Everest.

Dill's colleague, Edwards (1936), was the first to suggest a possible solution: "The inability to accumulate large amounts of lactate at high altitudes suggests a protective mechanism preventing an already low arterial saturation from becoming markedly lower. . . . It may be that the protective mechanism lies in an inadequate oxygen supply to essential muscles, e.g. the diaphragm or the muscles." A half century later Bigland-Ritchie and Vollestadt (1988) (see also: Noakes 2004c) provided this remarkable insight:

> Why should hypoxia have such a profound effect on limb muscle performance, while work capacity of respiratory muscles seemed

unaffected when both muscle groups were performing similar types of dynamic exercise? . . . It is essential for survival that somehow respiratory muscles must avoid the extremes of fatigue experienced by limb muscles . . . This could be achieved if CNS strategy involves some kind of reciprocal inhibition between the motor drive to limb and respiratory muscles, with that from the respiratory system dominating . . . Thus fatigue developed under these conditions may have been caused more by a reduced motor drive than by peripheral factors [so that] . . . taken together, these observations support the concept that the motor drive to limb muscles is reduced when the metabolic demand of skeletal muscle exceeds that which the respiratory muscles can supply.

These studies and interpretations invite two precise conclusions. First, that the oxygen demands of the skeletal muscles are not the cardinal priority and hence are not the "protected" variable during maximum exercise at extreme altitude. Second, neither the skeletal muscles nor the heart become "anaerobic" during maximal exercise under conditions of severe hypoxia. The sole conclusion must be that some type of regulator along the lines suggested by Bigland-Ritchie and Vollestadt must exist to limit maximum exercise at altitude. Furthermore, this raises the possibility that a similar control mechanism may also regulate maximum exercise at sea level.

These unexpected findings can best be explained by the presence of a "governor," probably in the central nervous system (CNS), the function of which is likely to prevent the Pao_2 from dropping too low for the normal function of one or more organs, most probably the brain but also perhaps the heart as also proposed by Dill (1938): "The capacity of the heart, as has already been suggested, is restricted at high altitude because of the deficiency in supply of oxygen to it." The same governor could serve a similar overall function at sea level, although the Pao_2 is clearly not the defended variable because it remains high during maximum exercise at sea level. Thus, the precise variables that are "protected" during maximal exercise at sea level remain uncertain.

However, the important point is that at both sea level and altitude, exercise terminates before the development of an oxygen deficiency or any other evidence for a failure of homeostatic regulation in any bodily function. Accordingly, we have proposed that the governor works in the following manner. From calculations made early in exercise on the basis of previous experience and of feedback from multiple body organs, the brain calculates the intensity that can be safely sustained for the expected duration of the exercise without causing homeostatic failure in any organ. The brain achieves this regulation by controlling the number of motor units (muscle fibers) that are recruited in the exercising muscles. As a result, the work output of the body is always limited to rates that can be safely sustained without threatening homeostasis under the conditions specific to each exercise.

Confirmation for the action of this theoretical governor during exercise at altitude comes from the work of Kayser et al. (1994). They showed that the amount of skeletal muscle recruited by the brain at peak exercise, as measured by skeletal muscle electromyographic (EMG) activity, is less at altitude (5050 m) than at sea level. However, the provision of 100% oxygen at the point of exhaustion reversed the fatigue, allowing exercise to continue to high work rates at altitude. EMG activity increased concurrent with this increase in work rate. The authors concluded that "During chronic hypobaric hypoxia, the central nervous system may play a primary role in limiting exhaustive exercise and maximum accumulation of lactate in blood." More recently, Kayser has concluded that exercise "begins and ends in the brain" (Kayser et al. 1994; Kayser 2003).

Interestingly, had the human body been designed to function according to the traditional theory, which requires that anaerobiosis must first develop in the exercising skeletal muscles before maximal exercise is terminated, no climber would ever have reached the summit of Mount Everest or any other high mountain, even with the use of supplemental oxygen. Rather, all would have succumbed to a combination of myocardial ischemia and cerebral hypoxia while their skeletal muscles were exercising vigorously and unrestrainedly, in pursuit of that homeostatic failure caused by skeletal muscle anaerobiosis which, according to the traditional theory, must occur before the exercise terminates.

In summary, studies of maximal exercise performance at extreme altitude confirm the hypothetical existence and action of a "governor" in the CNS, the function of which is to ensure that no bodily system ever reaches its absolute maximal functional capacity (Noakes *et al.* 2004a,c, 2005b; St Clair Gibson & Noakes 2004). Rather, exercise must always terminate while there is still functional reserve. Thus, before the absolute physiologic limits are reached, the CNS increases the perception of fatigue and discomfort to such high levels that the athlete makes the conscious decision to succumb to his or her discomfort. As a result, the extent of skeletal muscle recruitments either fails to rise further or it falls, limiting the work output of the body, thereby insuring that homeostasis is maintained.

That it is the brain and not the muscles that determine performance at high altitude would seem to be confirmed by the recollections of Professor Tom Hornbein, formerly Chairman of Anesthesiology at the University of Washington Medical School and member of the first team to reach the summit of Mount Everest by the West Ridge in 1963: "Without oxygen, each step at great heights is virtually a maximal effort; there is no reserve with which to face the unexpected. With oxygen there is a striking sensation of release, a spring in the step, a capacity to make a rapid movement, a desire to gaze elsewhere than at the slow alternate plod of each foot" (Hornbein 1980).

Note Hornbein's reference to the "sensation of release." From the effects of a central governor?

Practical relevance

ADVICE TO PERSONS WISHING TO CLIMB TO VERY HIGH ALTITUDES

Mount Everest, once the planet's supreme climbing challenge reserved for only the world's best climbers has, in the past decade, become just another commodity within the reach of the most affluent, regardless of their mountaineering abilities or lack thereof – the "apex of vanity" according to Messner (1979). These nouveaux climbers are perhaps less likely to show intellectual insight and restraint when they begin to feel tired a few hundred meters below the summit of Everest.

Indeed, the tragedies that occurred on Everest on May 9, 1996 (Krakauer 1997) could have been avoided if the professional guides had understood that when their clients begin to slow down at high altitude it was not because their muscles had been "poisoned" by lactic acid. The lactic acid/fatigue model, apparently believed by those guides, predicts that a period of rest will allow each to recover, after which it would be possible to climb yet higher. Rather, the onset of very slow climbing indicates that the affected climber is approaching the lowest arterial $P\text{ao}_2$ values compatible with continued survival. Climbing higher will lead ultimately to a state of complete paralysis from which the only escape is a rapid descent.

ROLE OF TRAINING AT ALTITUDE

Interestingly, the presence of a "governor" preventing the development of anaerobiosis in brain, heart, or skeletal muscle during exercise at medium altitude (1600–2900 m above sea level) has interesting implications for theories of how exercise training at altitude might improve athletic performance at sea level. For the principal action of the governor is to ensure that skeletal muscle anaerobiosis does not occur during exercise. Thus, any beneficial effect of altitude training cannot result from repeated exposure of either the brain, heart, or exercising skeletal muscles to greater levels of "anaerobiosis" than can be theoretically achieved during maximal exercise at sea level.

This might explain why there is still no convincing evidence that training at medium altitude improves athletic performance at sea level. At present there is some evidence that living at medium altitude but training at a lower altitude (live high, train low) may enhance athletic performance (Levine & Stray-Gundersen 2005), but the mechanism for this effect remains unclear (Noakes 2005). However, this effect cannot simply be caused by variables that increase oxygen delivery to muscle because the types of exercise for which such training may prove beneficial (e.g., foot races of 5000 m) are not limited by an inadequate oxygen delivery to the exercising muscles. Rather, it is not impossible that training at altitude alters the perception of fatigue during subsequent exercise at sea level, allowing a superior performance.

Exercise and atmospheric pollution

Atmospheric pollutants have a clearly detrimental effect on the ability to perform exercise. Despite these known health risks, exercise should not be actively discouraged but conversely *encouraged* during suitable times and in locations in which the environmental pollution is the least.

Environmental air pollution

Confirmed hazards of both acute and chronic exposure to ambient pollution include a reduction in lung function; increased risk of acute asthma attacks; increased prevalence of acute and chronic bronchitis; and increased risk of stroke, high blood pressure, and congenital heart defects, the latter caused by disturbance of cellular processes that provoke local and systemic inflammation, disrupt cardiac autonomic control, and induce vascular dysfunction (Zanobetti *et al.* 2004; Campbell *et al.* 2005). Individuals most at risk for chronic respiratory and cardiovascular sequelae include children, the elderly, and patients with diabetes, asthma, or other pre-existing heart and lung conditions.

Environmental air pollution is quantified with the Air Quality Index (AQI). The AQI is a standardized assessment of air quality in a given location and is described in parts per billion. Generally, six major air pollutants contribute to the AQI: ground level ozone (O_3), sulfur dioxide (SO_2), nitrogen dioxide (NO_2), carbon monoxide (CO), lead (Pb), and particulate matter (PM) (excluding pollen counts). The AQI is exacerbated by high temperatures, temperature inversion, and stagnant airflow. Many other gaseous and particulate pollutants that may be harmful, or even carcinogenic, exist in the atmosphere (such as CO_2, HNO_3, H_2SO_4, graphite, carbon, and peroxyacetyl nitrate) but these are not included in the AQI.

Different environmental agencies use different AQI standards to define "unhealthy air." The standards established by the US Environment Protection Agency (EPA) are more liberal than are those of the Meteorological Service of Canada (MSC) (Table 16.1).

An example of how such guidelines are followed is provided by the controls present in Malaysia. The air quality in Malaysia is determined by the Air Pollution Index (API – micrograms per cubic centimeter). When an API of >500 is measured, a state of emergency is usually declared and all non-governmental services are suspended, all ports in the immediate area are closed, and a prohibition of private sector commercial and industrial activities is enforced.

Exercise and air pollution

Regular physical activity has become a public health priority as such activity lowers the risk of cardiovascular disease, diabetes, osteoporosis, obesity, and mental heath problems. However, exercise increases pulmonary ventilation, which multiplies the inhaled dose (the product of concentration, time, and ventilation rate) of pollutants and their

Table 16.1 Standards to define healthy air adopted by the US Environmental Protection Agency (EPA) and the Meteorological Service of Canada (MSC).

EPA	MSC
0–50: Good (green)	0–25: Good (green)
51–100: Moderate (yellow)	26–50: Moderate (yellow)
101–150: Unhealthy for sensitive groups (orange)	51–100: Poor (orange/red)
151–200: Unhealthy (red)	101+: Very poor (purple)
201–300: Very unhealthy (purple)	
301–500: Hazardous (maroon)	

distribution through the oropharynx and respiratory tract. As a result, five times more particular matter is deposited in the lungs during moderate exercise than at rest. This raises concerns about the long-term health consequences and hence the wisdom of performing physical activity in polluted environments.

To minimize the adverse physiologic and potential long-term health consequences of air pollution while maximizing the health benefits of regular physical activity, an appreciation of the diurnal variation and distribution of environmental pollutants is essential.

Because environmental pollution results primarily from the combustion of fossil fuels, it is advised that physical activity should be undertaken in areas farthest away from congested and industrialized areas. The higher the concentration of air pollutants, the greater the concentration of gas and particulate matter inhaled during exercise. Thus, if outdoor activity is to be undertaken for prolonged periods, in order to minimize the exposure to pollution, special effort should be made to find recreational areas, such as parks or quiet roads, that are away from traffic.

Diurnal variation in the concentration of SO_2, CO, NO_2, O_3, and PM have been documented in Toronto, with PM showing the least variation. That study (Campbell *et al.* 2005) showed that the concentrations of CO, NO_2, and PM were highest when traffic flow was at its peak, whereas the concentrations of SO_2 and O_3 peaked for the period from midday to afternoon when the ambient temperature was the highest. The greatest percentage of "unhealthy" air days occurred during the summer months, when concentrations of O_3 and PM were the highest. Conversely, SO_2 and NO_2 levels were highest during the winter months when "unhealthy" air was reported less frequently. Therefore, the lowest concentrations of most environmental pollutants occur in the early morning or late evening. Physical activity at those times would be the least hazardous.

Effects of air pollution on exercise performance

Ozone levels as low as 0.08 ppm reduced the forced expiratory volume in 1 second (FEV_1) after 5 h of intermittent exercise at 30–45% $\dot{V}o_{2max}$ (Horstman *et al.* 1990) but the magnitude of the effect was subject-dependent. Although the duration of exposure produced a dose-dependent reduction in FEV_1, the concentration of O_3 in the inhaled air had a greater effect. Interestingly, trained athletes exposed to exercise on 4 consecutive days with an air O_3 content of 0.35 ppm O_3 showed a progressive improvement in performance and in $\dot{V}o_{2max}$ with a corresponding decrease in subjective symptoms when compared to the initial day of exposure (Foxcroft & Adams 1986). The results of this and other studies suggest a "habituation effect" to O_3 exposure that may be of pulmonary or central origin. Bronchial reactivity is significantly altered for up to 1 day following exposure to O_3, but this increased reactivity is readily reversible.

Conversely, there is a significant decrease in maximal exercise performance during exposure to CO at concentrations that are normally encountered in heavily polluted environments or after cigarette smoking (Aronow & Cassidy 1975). A carboxyhemoglobin concentration [COHb] of 4–6% may impair maximal exercise performance by increasing the probability that tissue hypoxia will occur. A dose-dependent relationship exists between increased [COHb] with both the onset of angina pectoris and electrocardiographic ST segment depression occurring at lower exercising work rates with increasing [COHb] with decrements first appearing at [COHb] of 2% (Allred *et al.* 1989).

Exposure to 1.0 ppm SO_2 in the inspired air induces pulmonary functional changes that are up to 22 times greater than at rest. Pulmonary function decrements have been documented during exercise at SO_2 concentrations as low as 0.1 ppm. However, the effects of these SO_2 concentrations on exercise performance have not been adequately documented.

Children and asthma

Asthma is the most common chronic disease of childhood. The increased incidence of asthma and wheeze in children in developing countries has been linked to urbanization. The incidence of exercise-induced bronchospasm (EIB) in children is also on the increase, perhaps as the result of a combination of increased awareness of the condition, improved diagnostic techniques, and increased exposure to environmental pollutants. Acute exposure to environmental pollutants, especially O_3, exacerbates asthma, which may account for some of the increase in the incidence of EIB over the past few decades.

In a large-scale prospective study conducted in six high- and six low-pollution communities in southern California, children aged 9–16 years who played three or more team sports and lived in communities exposed to higher levels of air pollution showed a 3.3-fold increased risk of developing asthma compared to children living in a low-pollution area (McConnell *et al.* 2002). Children with no history of wheeze had a relative risk of 4.4 of developing asthma if they lived in a high-pollution community, whereas time spent out-of-doors was associated with asthma in communities exposed to high but not to low levels of pollution.

When exposed to different levels of air pollution Finnish children with chronic respiratory symptoms displayed decrements in baseline lung function with increasing levels of air pollution (Timonen *et al.* 2002). There were no significant differences in bronchial responsiveness to the differing levels of ambient pollution, however, suggesting that the respiratory function is compromised before exercise commences in more polluted environments (Timonen *et al.* 2002).

EIB is more prevalent in children living in urban compared to rural areas in Kenya, South Africa, Ghana, and Zimbabwe, but not in Scotland. The reason for this disparity is currently unclear (Austin *et al.* 1994; Ng'ang'a *et al.* 1998).

Summary and conclusions

Vigorous physical activity should be scheduled during early morning or late evening hours, and performed in quiet areas away from traffic and areas of industrial activity. The intensity and duration of outdoor activity should be reduced when the air quality is regarded as "unhealthy" or when individual symptoms present. Symptoms resulting from the adverse cellular disruption caused by exposure to harmful air pollutions include coughing, wheezing, chest tightness, difficulty breathing, and chest pain. If any of these symptoms occur during outdoor activity, physical activity should cease and medical attention should be sought. Exercising indoors, preferably in a smoke-free, air-conditioned environment, is advised during "unhealthy" air days, particularly for those who are the most sensitive to the ill-effects of environmental pollution.

Heatstroke and hypothermia during exercise

In order to survive, humans are required to regulate their core body temperatures between 35 and 41°C. This temperature, the variation in which depends on the time of day, the amount of exercise undertaken, and the environmental conditions, represents a balance between the rate of heat production by and heat loss from the body. Hence, changes in the rates of either heat production or heat loss, or more commonly both, determine whether an abnormal rise in body temperature, leading to heat stroke, or an excessive fall causing hypothermia is likely to develop and under what conditions.

During exercise, the chemical energy stored in the muscles in the form of adenosine triphosphate (ATP) is converted into the mechanical energy of motion. However, this process is inefficient, so that only 25% of the chemical energy used by the muscles produces motion; while the remaining 75% is released as heat that must be lost from the body if the body temperature is to be safely regulated within the homeostatic range.

This phenomenon inspired the Norwegian Roald Amundsen, leader of the first expedition to reach the South Pole in 1911, to remark that: "The human body is a furnace." The furnace burns only more fiercely during exercise. Indeed, the rate at which the body produces heat is a linear function of speed when running (at any velocity) and when walking at speeds below 7 km·h^{-1}. At higher walking speeds, energy production rises as an exponential function of walking speed, as is also the case in cycling. Thus, in both cycling and very fast walking, it requires increasingly more energy to move just that little bit faster, with the result that more heat is also produced.

When ultramarathon runners run at an average pace of about 16 km·h^{-1} during races of 90–100 km, they use about 56 kJ energy every minute, or about 18,480 kJ in the 5.5 h that they require to complete these races. However, of the total amount of kilojoules used, only about 4000 kJ actually transports them from the start to the finish of the race. The remaining 14,480 kJ serves only to overheat the runners' bodies. To prevent their temperatures from rising to over 43°C and causing heatstroke, these athletes have to lose more than 90% of the heat they produce.

Therefore, the challenge when exercising in warm conditions is to lose heat fast enough to ensure that the body temperature does not rise too far causing heatstroke. In fact, the human brain regulates the exercise intensity "in anticipation" specifically to ensure that the body temperature does not rise excessively (Tucker *et al.* 2004, 2006). Thus, the real challenge for the body, especially during competitive exercise in the heat, is to lose heat fast enough to allow the highest possible exercise intensity at which thermal homeostasis can still be achieved without progressive heat accumulation leading to heatstroke. Conversely, the challenge when exercising, especially in cold and wet environmental conditions, is to retain that heat in order to prevent the development of hypothermia.

In order to transport heat from muscles to skin, as exercise begins, the blood flow to the muscles is increased. Not only does the heart pump more blood, but blood is preferentially diverted from non-essential organs toward the working muscles and skin. As it passes through the muscles, the blood is heated and distributes the added heat throughout the body, particularly to the skin. As a result, heat is conducted to the skin surface. Heat conduction to the skin is also achieved by direct transfer of heat from the site of heat production in the muscles lying close to the skin. The rate at which this heat will be lost by conduction from the body will, in turn, be determined by the magnitude of the temperature gradient – the steeper the gradient, the greater the heat loss – and the rapidity with which the cooler air in contact with the skin is replaced by colder air. Continual replacement of warmed air by cooler air causes loss of heat from the body, by

means of convection. Convection is simply the transfer of heat energy into the surrounding air; the body heats up the air surrounding it, thereby transferring heat to the environment. Convective heat loss rises as an exponential function of the speed at which air courses across the body, in effect the prevailing wind speed.

Wind of increasing speed dramatically increases the "coldness" of any environmental temperature, in effect reducing the effective temperature to which the body is exposed and thereby increasing the rate of heat loss from the body. This is known as the wind-chill factor. As the rate of heat loss by convection is determined by the rate of air movement across the body, it is greatly increased in athletes who move at fast speeds (e.g., cyclists on the descent stages of the major cycling tours and downhill skiers). In contrast, the velocity of air movement is low, for example, on the ascents of large mountain stages in cycling tours or when running or cycling slowly in wind-still conditions or with a tail wind that exactly matches the rate of forward movement.

Any nearby object, whose surface temperature is greater than that of the surface of the body (33°C), will attract this heat, which travels by electromagnetic waves in a form of energy transfer known as radiation. In contrast, when surrounding objects are hotter than the body (e.g., hot tar roads), heat is transferred by radiation from those objects to the runner's body.

Surface heat is also lost when the sweat produced by the sweat glands in the skin evaporates. Sweating itself does not cause heat loss; it is the evaporation of the sweat into the atmosphere as a vapor that causes heat to be lost from the body. The humidity of the air determines the extent to which heat can be lost to the environment in the form of sweat and, to a lesser extent, in the vapor from the respiratory membranes. This evaporation is the predominant source of heat loss in exercising humans, especially in the heat, because each gram (mL) of water so evaporated removes 1.8 kJ from the body. Only sweat that evaporates from the skin actively contributes to heat loss; sweat that drips from the skin fails to cool the body. As the humidity of the air rises, the efficiency of heat loss by evaporation falls so that the ease of maintaining heat balance becomes increasingly difficult as the humidity rises above 60–70%.

As a result of the high rates of heat production during exercise, with only minor changes in their clothing, humans are able to regulate their body temperatures very effectively during exercise in a wide range of environmental temperatures. For example, a human running at 16 km·h^{-1}, will maintain a normal body temperature even at external temperatures as low as 0°C when wearing clothing that provides only one clothing unit (CLO) of insulation. This clothing equates to normal business attire. At lower temperatures, especially in wet and windy conditions, humans can maintain thermal balance only by wearing progressively more layers of clothing with the external garment being completely water-repellent. Failure to wear properly water-repellent clothes when exposed to wet conditions will eliminate the insulating properties of clothing, thereby increasing the rate of heat loss from the body and predisposing it to hypothermia.

In contrast, humans have increasingly more difficulty exercising at higher environmental temperatures and humidity, especially in wind-still conditions. When the air temperature is above 33°C, it exceeds the temperature at the skin surface. As a result the skin absorbs heat from the environment. Under these conditions, sweating becomes the only avenue for heat loss. However, as the humidity of the air rises, the effectiveness of heat loss by the evaporation of sweat is reduced and becomes ineffective as the air humidity approaches 100%.

Thus, the limiting environmental conditions, above which it is not safe to exercise at anything other than low exercise intensities, are air temperatures above 33°C, air humidity above about 70–80%, and wind-still conditions. The closer to these limiting conditions, the lower the exercise intensity the brain will allow so that thermal homeostasis can still be maintained. Fortunately, the central governor in the brain takes note of all these environmental constraints and usually makes the correct calculation to ensure that the optimum exercise intensity is chosen, specific for those exact environmental conditions (Tucker *et al*. 2004, 2006).

Whereas air is a poor conductor of heat and hence a good *insulator*, water conducts heat approximately 25-fold faster than does air and is hence a very poor insulator. Thus, the thin layer of air trapped next to the skin by clothing is rapidly heated to the skin temperature, thereby producing a layer of insulation. However, the saturation of clothing with water removes this insulating layer and exposes the skin to whatever is the external temperature. This loss of insulation caused by water explains why saturated, wet clothing, or alternatively, swimming in cold water, predisposes to the development of hypothermia. Under these conditions, the exposed human must either find dry, warm clothing and a warm shelter, or warm all the air in the entire planet or, if swimming, the water in all the oceans, to 33°C, or die from hypothermia. There is no other alternative. All deaths from hypothermia occur as an inevitable consequence of these fundamental laws of physics.

Elevated body temperatures of up to 41.5°C are frequently found in healthy winners of short distance (5–15 km) running events contested in hot, humid, windless environmental conditions (Byrne *et al*. 2006). Such high body temperatures occur because of the fast rates at which elite athletes produce heat when running at their maximum pace and the reduced capacity of hot humid environments to absorb that heat. Fortunately, the brain has evolved protective mechanisms that reduce the allowable rate of energy production (exercise intensity/speed) during exercise in the heat. Thus, as a result of feedback from sensors throughout the body to a central regulator in the brain, the postulated central governor (Noakes *et al*. 2005b) monitors both the extent of the environmental stress to which the body is exposed, as well as the rate at which the body stores heat during exercise in those environmental conditions. Because it is safe to exercise only to a body temperature of less than 42°C, on exposure to the prevailing environmental conditions at the onset of exercise, and on the basis of the rate at which heat will be stored and the expected duration of the exercise, the brain calculates the rate at which work can be safely performed under those specific environmental conditions (Tucker *et al*. 2006). The central governor therefore pre-sets the number of motor units in the active muscles that can be recruited in order to ensure that a safe rate of heat production is allowed for the expected duration of the exercise. At the same time, the brain pre-sets the rate at which the perception of effort increases during the exercise bout so that the perceived effort of continuing to exercise becomes intolerable *before* the body temperature is elevated to dangerous levels.

In this way, the brain ensures that heatstroke occurs uncommonly during exercise. However, drugs that interfere with this central control mechanism, and, in particular, with the perception of effort during exercise, make heatstroke more likely. So it is that some of the classic cases of heatstroke in famous athletes, including the tragic death of British cyclist, Tom Simpson on the Mount Ventoux stage of the 1967 Tour de France, were clearly caused by the use of amphetamines or other centrally acting stimulants that override this usually effective safety mechanism. As a result, incidences of severe heat injury (heatstroke) are remarkably uncommon in sport despite the frequency with which vigorous sporting activities are undertaken in severe environmental conditions.

Low body temperatures of 35°C or lower (hypothermia) occur in swimmers exposed to cold water temperatures for many hours (e.g., in (English) Channel swimmers, or in mountaineers caught in cold, wet and windy conditions). In both conditions, hypothermia occurs because the human body exposed to a body of water or wet clothing that is colder than the skin temperature is unable to produce heat as rapidly as it is lost through conduction to the surrounding water. Wearing more appropriate clothing, in particular, drysuits or wetsuits in swimming, or clothing that remains dry in exercise on land, maintains a layer of insulating water or air heated to body temperature next to the skin. This is the only way to prevent the ultimate development of a fatal hypothermia (low body temperature) when exposed to cold water or cold, wet, windy conditions on land for any prolonged period.

Regulating body temperature during exercise

Because "the human body is a furnace," and the brain has evolved to ensure that thermal homeostasis is maintained during exercise, regardless of the environmental conditions, the real challenge for humans during athletic competition is not to lose heat sufficiently fast to prevent heatstroke. Rather, the challenge is to maximize rates of heat loss so that thermal balance can be maintained at the highest possible rates of heat production (and hence the greatest levels of athletic endeavor).

Fortunately, of all mammals, humans have the greatest capacity to exercise in hot, humid conditions. Thus, in the words of Schmidt-Nielsen (1964) "The human is an excellent thermal regulator." This superior capacity results from the human's capacity to mount a prodigious sweating response during exercise in hot, humid, environmental conditions.

SWEATING: A HUMAN ADAPTATION OF PROFOUND EVOLUTIONARY SIGNIFICANCE

During exercise, there is a loss of body water in the form of sweat from the body. Evaporation of this sweat from the skin surface removes heat from the body. Sweat is purely a dilute concentration of plasma and therefore contains mainly water with a low concentration of sodium chloride (salt). The concentration of salt is least in those who have trained in the heat and who ingest a low salt diet and is highest in those who are less heat-acclimatized but who ingest diets with a high salt content.

The total volume of water in the body is regulated in order to ensure that the osmolality of all the tissues is homeostatically regulated within a narrow range. This means that fluid balance in the body is regulated in relationship to the whole body electrolyte content. Replacement of the electrolytes lost in sweat is necessary before there is complete restoration of fluid balance. Fortunately, the human diet usually contains a gross excess of salt – daily intakes of 5–8 g are common, whereas daily human salt requirements are closer to 1 g except in those who exercise daily for many hours in the heat – and an adequate intake of potassium. Sweat salt losses help to maintain salt balance in humans currently living on diets that contain excessive amounts of salt.

However, the crucial point is that it is the tissue osmolality and not the body weight that is homeostatically regulated during exercise (Hew-Butler *et al.* 2006). Tissue osmolality must be regulated in order to control cellular volume. As the osmolality increases, the cells shrink, whereas the opposite occurs when the osmolality falls. Indeed, it is the loss of some weight during exercise that allows the tissue osmolality to remain within the normal homeostatic range. A failure to lose weight or worse, to gain weight, reduces tissue osmolality causing the potentially fatal condition of exercise-associated hyponatremic encephalopathy (EAHE), which results from excessive swelling of the (hypo-osmolar) brain cells.

Rates of body weight loss during exercise have been used to calculate sweat rates during exercise, as well as the rates at which fluid should be replaced during exercise. However, these calculations represent an approximation because the weight lost during exercise does not comprise only sweat losses, but also weight lost as a result of the fuel stores that are irreversibly oxidized to provide the chemical energy for the exercise. In addition, an unknown amount of water is stored in muscle and liver in association with carbohydrate (glycogen) stored in those organs. Because this fluid is released as the glycogen is used during exercise, it follows that this weight loss does not contribute to a real water loss during exercise. The size of this water reserve is not known but may be as large as 1–2 kg. Thus, it is possible that a sizable weight loss during prolonged exercise may come from sources that do not contribute to a water loss and hence to "dehydration," and so do not need to be replaced during exercise. As a result, levels of "dehydration" determined solely on the extent of weight loss during exercise overestimate the true extent to which the total body water content has been reduced (Kozlowski & Saltin 1964).

However, using this imprecise methodology it has been found that sweat rates in humans during exercise may increase to ~1.8 L·h^{-1} in 60–70 kg runners racing and training in the humid summer heat of the southern USA (Millard-Stafford *et al.* 1995). Even higher rates of up to 2.5 L·h^{-1} may occur in 150 kg professional American football players during training in the heat. One result is that one man (and his dog) were able to survive exposure to a temperature of 105°C for 15 min, sufficient to cook

some eggs and a piece of raw steak (Kenney *et al.* 2004). Why would humans ever require such a remarkable capacity to lose heat?

One possibility is that through the process of natural selection, successful early human ancestors (hominids) developed the capacity to run long distances in the midday heat even though they had no immediate access to water. This ability may then have provided a profound biologic advantage for the subsequent evolution of humans (Heinrich 2001; Noakes 2006a). This theory proposes that the ancestral hominids developed the capacity to sweat and hence to become dehydrated during exercise, specifically to *protect* themselves from developing heatstroke when exercising in the heat. The development of this physiologic feature then allowed hominids to either scavenge or hunt other nutritionally dense mammals such as antelope. The extra energy and nutrients provided by those high protein, high fat diets then allowed the growth and development of those higher brain centers on which superior human intelligence depends.

Perhaps University of Vermont biologist, Heinrich (2001) is the scientist most responsible for the formulation of this (Heinrich) theory:

> The fact that we, as savanna-adapted, animals have such hypertrophied sweating responses implies that, if we are naturally so profligate with water, it can only be because of some very big advantage. The most likely advantage was that it permitted us to perform prolonged exercise in the heat. A sweating response is not needed to outrun predators, because that requires relatively short, fast sprinting, where accumulating a heat load is, like a lactic acid load, acceptable. What is needed in sweating is to *sustain* running in the heat of the day – the time when most predators retire into the shade.

Heinrich also notes that modern hunter-gatherers, like the !Kung Bushmen of Southern Africa "carry no food or water with them (on 30 km hunts in the heat) because that hinders their ability to travel." That the human musculoskeletal structure also appears to have evolved specifically to allow locomotion over long distances at moderate velocities has also recently been proposed (Bramble & Lieberman 2004).

According to the Heinrich theory, it is the capacity to sweat that allows humans to exercise in the heat by protecting them from developing heatstroke. Indeed, it is the inability to sweat, of those humans born with the congenital absence of sweat glands, that greatly increases their risk for developing heatstroke (Hopkins & Ellis 1996).

Until 1969, the advice given to athletes mirrored this historical understanding of how humans evolved this exceptional capacity to lose heat during exercise. Human athletes were advised *not* to drink during exercise (Noakes 1993, 1995). This advice seems to have worked, because those athletes who followed this guideline repeatedly established world records at all running distances without any evidence that their lives were at unusual risk. Indeed, the retrospective investigation of those few well-remembered cases in which elite athletes suffered serious ill-health during exercise reveals that factors other than an inability to cope with hot exercise conditions usually caused the medical problem (Table 16.2). Rather, illicit drug use was usually involved.

Indeed, the immediate reason why doping control was introduced into world sport after 1968 was specifically to protect athletes from the risk of dying as a result of doping. This decision was taken on the basis of perhaps 2–3 high profile deaths in major international competitions (Table 16.2). Had an equal or greater number of athletes died because they had failed to ingest sufficient fluid during exercise, one must presume that the same authorities who chose to remove doping from world sport on the basis of two doping-related deaths in cyclists, would surely have acted decisively at the same time. History has shown that it is, after all, somewhat easier to encourage athletes to drink more during exercise (Noakes & Speedy 2006) than to discourage their use of performance-enhancing drugs (Noakes 2004c). This evidence alone suggests that, prior to 1969, there could not have been a substantial number of medical complications or deaths in athletes who drank little or nothing during exercise.

However, after 1969, the idea that humans could safely exercise without drinking was replaced with an opposite theory, specifically that exercise could only be safely undertaken, especially in the heat, by those who ingested fluid at high rates (Noakes 2007). Sweating was no longer regarded as the singular physiologic adaptation that had allowed the evolution of fragile hominids into robust modern

Table 16.2 Famous cases of collapse or death in athletes associated with the ingestion of alcohol or drugs. Reproduced with permission from Noakes (2006b).

Event	Precipitating factors	Reference
1 Thomas Hicks finishes the 1904 St. Louis Olympic Games Marathon in an advanced state of distress	Hicks received two tablets of 1/60th grain strychnine sulfate during the race as well as brandy and eggs	Martin & Glynn (2000)
2 Collapse of Dorando Pietro at the finish line of the 1908 London Olympic Games Marathon	Gargling with chianti and reportedly sharing a bottle of wine with his coach "just outside the stadium", "Dorando was already suffering from heat exhaustion and the effect of the wine knocked him bow-legged." Seems his victory celebration was somewhat premature!	Bryant (2005)
3 Danish cyclist, Knut Jensen, collapses and dies during the 100 km road race in the 1960 Rome Olympic Games	Jensen had ingested the amphetamine, Ronicol, before the race	Todd & Todd (2001)
4 Tom Simpson dies from heatstroke on Mount Ventoux during the 13th stage of the 1967 Tour de France	Amphetamines found in Simpson's clothing at the time of his death. He had also ingested brandy at the start of the climb up Mount Ventoux	Fotheringham (2002)

humans. Rather, by reducing the total body water and hence producing "dehydration," sweating was now projected as a significant threat to the health of exercising humans. Surprisingly, this new attitude arose shortly after the development, in Florida, of the world's first sports drink. Some might suggest that this close temporal relationship is not purely coincidental (Noakes 2004a, 2006a,b; Noakes & Speedy 2006, 2007).

These novel ideas about the dangers that continuous sweating at high rates pose for human survival led to a series of novel dogmas about how the body temperature is regulated during exercise, in particular the role of fluid ingestion and fluid loss on that regulation, and the factors that are homeostatically regulated during exercise.

Dogma 1: The level of dehydration is the most important determinant of the rectal temperature during exercise so that high rates of fluid ingestion during exercise are required to prevent heatstroke

Perhaps the first comprehensive study of the factors that influence the temperature during exercise was performed by Nielsen (1938). This article is written in German and so has not been widely read. There were at least two key findings of that study that have essentially been removed from modern thinking.

The first finding was that the body temperature during exercise is homeostatically regulated in proportion to the rate at which the work is being performed – the metabolic rate. Nielsen found that the rectal temperature rose during the initial portion of the exercise, before stabilizing at a constant temperature, dependent on the exercise intensity, for the rest of the activity. Thus, the greater the work rate, the higher the value at which the rectal temperature stabilized.

Second, Nielsen found that, at any work rate, the level at which the rectal temperature stabilized was the same regardless of the environmental conditions – unless conditions were extremely hot. Thus, the exercising work rate, not the environmental conditions, determined the extent to which the rectal temperature rose. In warmer conditions, the body responded by increasing heat loss so that the

rectal temperature at the same work rate was the same whether the work was conducted in hot or cool conditions.

The next influential finding arose from a series of studies occasioned by the World War II and the exposure of Allied troops to either dry heat in the desert warfare in North Africa, or the humid heat of the jungles of South East Asia. These studies established that subjects who ingested fluid during exercise were more likely to complete any exercise task, particularly if it was prolonged. In addition, fluid ingestion lowered the rectal temperature during exercise. However, even in those who did not drink during exercise, the rectal temperature remained well below values measured in patients with heatstroke (Nielsen 1938; Pitts *et al.* 1944; Rothstein & Towbin 1947; Ladell 1955). It was these findings that would ultimately lead to the novel dogmas that: (i) the level of dehydration, offset by the extent of fluid ingestion during exercise, and not the exercising work rate, is the prime determinant of the rectal temperature response during exercise; and (ii) high rates of fluid ingestion during exercise, sufficient to prevent any weight loss, are essential to optimize athletic performance (Armstrong *et al.* 1996; Convertino 1996; Casa *et al.* 2000).

Perhaps the classic study that accelerates the adoption of these novel ideas was the study of Wyndham and Strydom (1969). These South African scientists of considerable international eminence studied a group of Johannesburg runners who participated in three 32-km races over a period of about 3 months. Although the primary goal of the study was to establish whether or not adding sugar to the habitual diet improved athletic performance (which it did), the authors also found that the post-race rectal temperatures of the subjects who lost more than 3% of their body weight during exercise were increased as a linear function of their level of "dehydration." Accordingly, the authors concluded that the level of dehydration was the principal determinant of the rectal temperature response during exercise. The idea that the failure to drink adequately during exercise would place an athlete at increased risk for the development of heatstroke arose. They therefore concluded that preventing athletes from drinking freely during exercise was "criminal folly." The reasons why Wyndham and Strydom's conclusions were not evidence-based have been argued previously (Noakes *et al.* 1988; Noakes 1995, 2004a).

The other significant event was the development of the world's first sports drink, Gatorade, by Cade in Florida (Rovell 2005) in the early 1960s. The drink was developed to assist football players at the University of Florida to complete, with reduced distress, matches and practices in the humid heat of Florida. Gatorade's success soon outstripped these modest goals as the drink quickly became a cultural icon in the USA. An ignored component of the phenomenal success of this product was the associated marketing hubris that produced a novel interpretation of human physiology, one that owed much to Dr Cade's private biases. Those biases were already apparent in his earliest writings.

For example, in one of his first studies, completed when Gatorade was already on its way to iconic status, Dr Cade and his group studied a group of athletes completing a 7-mile (11-km) run (Cade *et al.* 1972). They found that fluid ingestion reduced the ~2°C rise in rectal temperature by 0.2–0.5°C. They concluded that: "The amelioration of temperature rise by ingestion of a hypotonic saline solution or even more strikingly by the saline-glucose solution surely recommends the use of such solutions to decrease the likelihood (sic) of heatstroke when exercise must be performed in a hot clime." In an earlier study, Cade *et al.* (1971) proposed, without supporting evidence, that the fluid loss from sweating during exercise causes a loss of circulating blood volume which "adversely affects the ability of the body to dissipate heat . . . and may, indeed, be of major importance in the genesis of heatstroke."

These ideas then led to his "hyperthermia/volume-reduction hypothesis" for the development of heatstroke (Cade *et al.* 1992; Cheuvront *et al.* 2003) which I have since renamed the Cardiovascular Model of Thermoregulation during Exercise (Noakes 2006a) and which is a predictable extension of the Cardiovascular/Anaerobic/Catastrophic model of exercise physiology (Noakes & St. Clair Gibson 2004c) that currently dominates teaching in our discipline.

Perhaps Dr Cade's bias came from his contact with the writings of other influential heat researchers of that period. For example, Buskirk *et al.* (1958) had proposed that: "Acute dehydration apparently limits man's ability to work, largely through impaired cardiovascular function (Adolph 1947a)," whereas Nadel *et al.* (1980) had written that "The excessive hyperthermia that occurs in hypohydrated individuals during exercise in the heat is due to modifications in the control of skin blood flow . . . A reduction in maximal attainable skin blood flow limits heat transfer during prolonged exercise."

More recently, Cheuvront *et al.* (2003) have described their interpretation of this model: "Body water deficits will increase cardiovascular strain as indicated by increased heart rate and decreased stroke volume during exercise in temperate or hot environments. If heat strain is present during exercise, the athlete may be unable to sustain cardiac output (Sawka *et al.* 1979). Body water deficits reduce cardiac filling because of the reduced blood volume often accompanied by increased skin blood flow and compliance (from increased heat strain) . . . Dehydration mediated core temperature elevations reduce exercise performance by augmenting cardiovascular strain." Yet the authors conclude that: "The exact mechanisms by which the cardiovascular strain translates into reduced performance are unclear."

Similarly, current employees of the company that Dr Cade's invention created, have written:

> Cardiac output is reduced, the increase in skin blood flow is attenuated, and core temperature rises at an accelerated rate with progressive dehydration and continued exercise (Montain & Coyle 1992). Hypohydration, a chronic fluid deficit, also has negative consequences on cardiovascular function and thermoregulation (Sawka *et al.* 1985) and can reduce or eliminate the protection offered by heat acclimatization (Sawka *et al.* 1983, 1998). Hypohydration in athletes could have similar adverse outcomes in the field and put the athletes at higher risk for heat exhaustion or heatstroke, the latter being a potentially catastrophic event (Binkley *et al.* 2002).

(Stover *et al.* 2006)

The crucial point is that the writings of Dr Cade and his scientific progeny have developed a novel model of how the body temperature is regulated during exercise. This model predicts that cardiovascular function, in particular cardiac output, is the principal determinant of the body's ability to thermoregulate during exercise because it determines the adequacy of the skin blood flow. Any factor that impairs cardiovascular function must therefore reduce the skin blood flow and, as a consequence, the sweat rate, leading to heat retention and ultimately heatstroke. Because, according to this model, it reduces the total body water and the circulating blood volume, sweating, rather than preventing heatstroke (as in the Heinrich "sweating allows humans to exercise in the heat" hypothesis), must ultimately cause heatstroke by reducing the filling pressure of the heart, and hence the stroke volume, cardiac output, and skin blood flow, and hence the capacity to lose heat by either convection or evaporation.

According to this novel model, any sweating that is uncorrected by fluid ingestion during exercise must inevitably induce a vicious cycle of increasing heat gain, terminating ultimately in heatstroke. Therefore, the central prediction of this novel Cardiovascular Model of Thermoregulation is that, by impairing cardiovascular function, dehydration caused by sweating becomes the most important determinant of the body temperature during exercise and ultimately the key determinant of exercise performance in the heat. Indeed, this is the interpretation that has been applied universally (Gisolfi 1996; Sawka & Montain 2000) to the findings of Wyndham and Strydom (1969).

Of course, this is the complete reversal of the Heinrich hypothesis which holds that humans developed the capacity to sweat, specifically to *protect* them from the development of heatstroke during exercise in the heat. Thus, according to the Heinrich model, the capacity to sweat extensively and to become markedly dehydrated allowed early hominids to hunt or scavenge food at midday on the hot African plains at the precise time that their competitor predators, larger, more furry, horizontally aligned and unable to sweat, were incapacitated by the heat.

The outstanding challenges faced by this Cardiovascular Model of Thermoregulation are that: (i) it conflicts with a historical reality; (ii) it has no logical physiologic basis, and (iii) it fails to explain what actually happens.

In the first place, sweating is the most important mechanism of heat loss in out-of-water exercise (Winslow *et al.* 1937) and is regulated independently of skin blood flow (Shibasaki *et al.* 2003). Thus, the capacity to lose heat (by sweating) is essentially independent of the cardiovascular response to exercise but requires an intact neural supply to the sweat glands (Hopkins & Ellis 1996). Second, although fluid loss during exercise does cause the body temperature to be regulated at a slightly higher body temperature – about 0.2°C for each 1% body weight loss – there is no evidence that this is caused by a reduced sweat rate. All the classic studies show that sweat rates are maintained in dehydration (Eichna *et al.* 1945; Adolph 1947b; Ladell 1955; Costill *et al.* 1970). Indeed, Ladell (1955) wrote that: "Abstention from water had no effect on the sweat rate, until water deficits of more than 2.5 L had been incurred." In one of the original classic industry-funded studies, Costill *et al.* (1970) wrote that even when they did not drink during 2 h of exercise in the heat, "the runners' skin was sufficiently wetted by sweat to permit maximal evaporation." Third, Nielsen *et al.* (1971) showed that the modestly higher equilibrium (esophageal) temperatures in subjects who drank less than they lost as sweat was not the result of a reduced cardiac output during exercise. Although stroke volume was lower in the dehydrated state because of a reduced plasma volume, the higher heart rate compensated to maintain an unchanged cardiac output. The plateau value was linearly related to the serum osmolality.

The authors concluded that: "It seems that the observed changes in esophageal temperature during work cannot be ascribed to central circulatory failure." Rather, they attributed the higher plateau temperatures when exercising in a mildly dehydrated state to a "direct effect of plasma osmolality on the activity of cells in hypothalamic temperature centers via a reflex from adjacent osmoreceptors in the anterior hypothalamus, or the osmolality effect may be the result of a peripheral inhibition of the sweat gland function."

The conclusion must be that the elevated temperature in those who do not drink during exercise is not caused by a dehydration-induced failure of sweating and skin blood flow secondary to cardiovascular failure, as predicted by the Cardiovascular Model, but must be caused by some other effect, perhaps related to changes in serum osmolality.

There is no evidence for any loss of thermal homeostasis in those who do not drink during exercise; the body temperature is simply regulated at a higher absolute temperature. This is most clearly shown in the industry-funded study of Montain and Coyle (1992), the very study on which the American College of Sports Medicine (ACSM) guidelines to drink either 1.2 L·h^{-1} or "as much as tolerable" are based (Armstrong *et al.* 1996). Despite an absence of adequate convective cooling (Saunders *et al.* 2005) and even though they did not drink, subjects were able to exercise in hot conditions (32°C; relative humidity 50%) for 2 h at 62% of their maximum oxygen consumption without developing any evidence for heat illness. Furthermore, the final rectal temperatures of these dehydrated athletes were well below values measured in patients with heatstroke. The final (2 h) rectal temperatures of subjects who did not drink at all was 39.2 (± 0.2°C) compared to 38.3 (± 0.1°C) when they drank "to replace all their sweat losses during exercise." Patients with heatstroke usually have rectal temperatures in excess of 42°C.

Paradoxically the *absence* of serious consequences in these dehydrated athletes who had not drunk at all during 2 h of vigorous exercise in moderately severe heat was subsequently used by the ACSM as evidence for the need for all to drink "as much as tolerable" during exercise. This logic appears strangely perverse.

As a consequence of the universal adoption of this novel Cardiovascular Model of Thermoregulation, the historic teaching that the body temperature is homeostatically regulated (Nielsen 1938) and that weight loss as a result of sweating is an essential component of that regulation, has been removed from the modern literature. Now, as a consequence of the paradigm shift occasioned by Dr Cade and the development of the world's first sports drink, it is assumed that body weight is *the* critical variable that must be defended at all costs during exercise (Baker *et al.* 2005; Dugas 2006; Noakes 2006b).

This explanation is naturally most attractive to the sports drink industry driven by the need to increase profits by insuring that humans always drink "as much as tolerable" of their product in order to prevent any level of dehydration during exercise. However, there is no convincing evidence that subjects do not perform optimally if they ingest fluid *ad libitum* during exercise (Noakes 2003a, 2007) or that, when environmental conditions are appropriate and not artificial (e.g., in the laboratory with inadequate convective cooling) (Saunders *et al.* 2005), fluid ingestion at excessively high rates greater than *ad libitum* are necessary to ensure that the rise in rectal temperature during exercise is not excessive.

This evidence should be interpreted as proof that, although increasing levels of dehydration are associated with somewhat higher rectal temperatures during exercise, these levels remain homeostatically regulated, perhaps as a function of the serum osmolality, and are well below temperatures measured in athletes who develop heatstroke during exercise. Furthermore, the rate of heat production, determined by the exercising work rate, is probably the most important determinant of the rectal temperature during exercise. The easiest way to ensure that athletes do not develop heatstroke during exercise in the heat, is simply to ensure that they exercise less vigorously; not that they drink more.

CONCLUSIONS

The dogma that the level of dehydration is the most important factor determining the core temperature response during exercise is, in the authors' opinion, an unfortunate byproduct of the development of the sports drink industry after the mid-1960s and the marketing hubris used to sell this novel and soon-to-be iconic product (Noakes & Speedy 2007). Thus, either as a deliberate marketing strategy or as a fortuitous consequence, the sports drink industry was instrumental in the marketing of a novel model of the physiology of heat regulation during exercise.

This novel model, termed the Cardiovascular Model of Thermoregulation (Noakes & Speedy 2006; Noakes 2007), predicts that the human body is able to regulate its body temperature during exercise only if optimal cardiovascular function is maintained. By producing a state of "dehydration" that supposedly impairs cardiovascular function leading to dehydration-induced circulatory failure, this novel model predicts that sweating must ultimately cause the death of each athlete exercising in the heat unless each drinks "as much as tolerable."

This model is wrong because sweating is regulated by neural mechanisms that are largely independent of the adequacy of the cardiovascular system. Furthermore, sweating continues unabated at high rates, even in athletes who have lost at least 2.5 kg fluid from sweating. Thus, there is no evidence that the levels of dehydration usually encountered in modern endurance athletes (<4%) impairs their sweating response during exercise and that this causes an excessive and dangerous rise in their body temperatures. As a consequence, drinking either too little or too much is not the factor that will either cause or prevent heatstroke during exercise. The pathophysiology of heatstroke is somewhat more complex, as discussed subsequently.

Dogma 2: Athletes who collapse after exercise are suffering from dehydration and hyperthermia and must be treated urgently with intravenous fluids

If dehydration causes hyperthermia as a result of circulatory failure, according to the Cardiovascular Model of Thermoregulation, and if athletes with heatstroke collapse during and after exercise, then it is quite "logical" to assume that all athletes who collapse after exercise must be dehydrated and hyperthermic, and in need of immediate correction of their "dehydration-induced cardiac failure" with intravenous (IV) fluids. The personal experience of running 70 marathons or longer distance races, and of being the Medical Director at other such races, intermittently since 1975, has led the author to suspect that this theory is wrong. Thus, after the mid-1980s, our research group began actively to study this question.

During this period our key findings have been the following:

1 Collapsed ultramarathon runners are no more hyperthermic than are non-collapsed (control) runners (Holtzhausen *et al.* 1994). Furthermore, we now know that core temperatures in excess of 41°C are frequently present in athletes who are completely without symptoms (Byrne *et al.* 2006). Thus, a failure of heat dissipation with excessive body heat storage cannot explain why some athletes collapse with body temperatures that are substantially lower. By extension of reasoning, if dehydration causes hyperthermia (according to the Cardiovascular Model of Thermoregulation), then collapsed athletes with body temperatures below the heatstroke range of >42°C can also not be more dehydrated than are non-collapsed runners. Even if they are more dehydrated, then this model is still unable to explain why they collapse.

2 Eighty-five percent of collapsed runners finished these races before they collapsed (Holtzhausen *et al.* 1994). The act of stopping especially after prolonged exercise in the heat must cause the condition. However, such collapse could not be caused by dehydration because, according to the Cardiovascular Model, dehydration must first cause circulatory collapse during exercise when the stress on the cardiovascular system is the greatest. Dehydration-induced circulatory failure cannot explain collapse that occurs on the cessation of exercise when the demands on the cardiovascular system are rapidly reducing.

3 Collapsed ultramarathon runners were not in a state of cardiovascular shock because, although they had clear evidence for postural hypotension (as shown by a sharp drop in systolic blood pressures to <85 mmHg on standing), on lying supine their blood pressures were usually >100 mmHg and their heart rates below 90 beats·min^{-1} (Holtzhausen & Noakes 1995, 1997). Heart rates below 100 beats·min^{-1} are not compatible with a diagnosis of shock resulting from dehydration-induced circulatory failure.

Rather, these are features of a very low peripheral vascular resistance, associated with a high cardiac output, the classic cardiovascular features of exertional heatstroke (O'Donnell & Clowes 1972), and of the syncope that occurs in unacclimatized persons on first exposure to exercise in the heat (Eichna *et al.* 1945; Eichna & Horvath 1947).

On the basis of these findings, the authors have concluded that athletes collapse after exercise because they are unable to maintain their blood pressures when standing. This is caused by the continuation into recovery of a state of high cardiac output and low peripheral vascular resistance with high rates of blood flow to the dependent limbs including the skin. By suddenly stopping exercise, athletes remove the action of the lower limb muscle pump – the second heart – the function of which is to maintain the central blood volume and the right atrial filling pressure and the stroke volume, even when the peripheral vascular resistance is low and the cardiac output is high, as occurs during the first few minutes after stopping exercise. This is complicated by the effects of any sudden reduction in atrial pressure that occurs on exercise cessation. This aggravates the already low peripheral vascular resistance by inducing an additional but atavistic vasodilatation in the exercising limbs – the Barcroft–Edholm reflex (Noakes 2003c).

According to this theory, the treatment of collapsed runners must aim to increase the central blood volume and the right atrial pressure by reducing the volume of blood displaced into the dependent limbs. The authors therefore began to experiment by treating collapsed athletes in the head-down position, with their feet elevated above the level of the heart, so that venous return to the heart and therefore right atrial pressure would be immediately increased. The results were quite remarkable and very rapidly caused the blood pressures of collapsed athletes to stabilize with reversal of their hypotensive symptoms.

Consequently, the authors now advise that all conscious athletes with post-exercise collapse must be nursed with their legs elevated so that venous return to the heart is increased (Holtzhausen & Noakes 1997; Noakes 2000b) leading to an increase in right atrial pressure. Only if there is no immediate and sustained improvement in symptoms following the adoption of this simple therapy does it become necessary to look for an alternate cause for the condition. Using this technique the authors have

essentially eliminated the need to use IV fluids in the treatment of post-exercise collapse. Thus, no IV fluids were given to any collapsed finishers in the 2000 and 2001 South African triathlons at which the first author was the Medical Director. In general, this approach has been adopted by the medical teams directing many marathon and ultra-distance endurance events in South Africa.

PRACTICAL CONCLUSIONS

Most cases of post-exercise collapse in athletes who are conscious but have low blood pressures in the standing position are brought about by the persistence into recovery of the state of high cardiac output/low peripheral vascular resistance that occurs during exercise. The most important treatment option is to elevate the affected athlete's legs above the level of the heart. This increases the venous return and the central blood volume, leading to an increase in right atrial pressure, rapidly reversing symptoms in those with more severe degrees of postural hypotension. However, complete recovery, shown by the ability to stand without the development of postural hypotension, may still take 1–2 h, because this requires the return of the normal vascular reactivity, in particular vasoconstriction, in the lower limb and splanchnic arterioles. Delayed recovery of such vascular reactivity is probably a sign of excellent health, because it indicates a remarkable capacity for arteriolar vasodilatation, presumably mediated by local vasodilatory substances, such as nitric oxide.

Dogma 3: Exertional heatstroke always occurs in athletes who exercise in environmental conditions that are so hot that they are unable to lose heat sufficiently rapidly to prevent progressive heat accumulation

Recently, a legal case in the USA involved a professional sportsman who had died within 12 h of collapsing from "heatstroke." The prosecution's argument was that the player must have died because he had not drunk sufficient fluids during and before practice which was clearly held in conditions that were too hot to be safe. Thus, his heatstroke was due to "dehydration" and the coaching staff had been negligent in allowing the practice to take place in such conditions. It was also argued that the doctors who had treated the player were also culpable because they had not reduced his body temperature sufficiently rapidly to prevent the widespread organ damage that led ultimately to his death from cardiac arrest.

The problem with these legal arguments was that they were the converse of the facts. The subject had been drinking voraciously both before and during the fatal practice, so much so that he had vomited clear fluid at the time of hospital admission. The vomiting of clear fluid is substantive evidence for the presence of unabsorbed fluid in the bowel as a result of high rates of fluid ingestion.

Furthermore, the player's serum sodium concentration on hospital admission was well below the normal range, indicating the presence of hyponatremia resulting from fluid overload (Hew-Butler *et al.* 2005). In addition, the day was hot but no hotter than many such days on which generations of professional sportsmen have trained without developing heatstroke. He was also the first professional player in the more than 100-year history of his particular sport ever to die from heatstroke. Finally, and perhaps most importantly, he had exercised for only 8 min at the time he first collapsed.

This latter finding is especially surprising because the simple laws of physics indicate that to heat a body from 37 to 42°C, the temperature at which heatstroke occurs, requires the retention of an enormous amount of heat. It would be impossible to produce that much heat during the 8-min of exercise he undertook on that fatal day. Other factors must have been at work in this case and perhaps also in other similar cases. What might those factors be?

First, the development of heatstroke requires a sufficient period during which the rate of heat production by the body exceeds the rate of heat loss, leading to heat accumulation and a progressive rise in body temperature. Importantly, rapid body cooling begins the moment the exercise terminates so that, for example, the body temperatures of marathon runners will return to pre-race values within about 30 min of stopping exercising and without the need for any specific cooling interventions. For

heatstroke to occur, the activity must be sustained in order that high rates of heat production are maintained to drive the body temperature to those very high values necessary to cause the condition according to this conventional explanation. In addition, according to the finding that the body temperature normally falls when the exercise terminates, heatstroke cannot first occur in otherwise healthy subjects, only *after* exercise when the source of heat production – the contraction of the exercising muscles – has ceased.

Second, the athlete's brain is, or should be, the ultimate determinant of whether or not heatstroke occurs during exercise, because the brain regulates the rate of heat production by the body during exercise. Only the brain can determine how many skeletal muscle motor units, and hence muscle fibers, it will choose to recruit at any time or for any duration during exercise. It is the activity of the muscle fibers, voluntarily recruited by the brain, that theoretically generates the excessive heat necessary to cause heatstroke. Thus, a large number of muscle fibers must be recruited continually for a substantial period for heatstroke to happen.

Third, it seems illogical that the brain would ever "choose" heatstroke as an exercise outcome because, without correct treatment, the final outcome of heatstroke will always be the death of the brain itself. Rather, it seems more probable that the brain should have some protective mechanisms to ensure that it regulates the rate of heat accumulation by the body specifically so that it eliminates the risk that heatstroke will develop, thereby sparing itself from what is, in effect, suicide.

Indeed, the body appears to use at least two such mechanisms to ensure that heatstroke is not the usual outcome during exercise in unfavorable environmental conditions. First, it appears to set the work rate during exercise according to the rate at which body heat is accumulating (Tucker *et al.* 2004). The brain regulates the rate of heat production by modifying the number of motor units and, hence, muscle fibers that are recruited. This appears to be an anticipatory response, the function of which may be to ensure that exercise should always terminate before a dangerously high core temperature is reached. The mechanism of control appears to be by pre-setting the rate at which the perception of fatigue (rating of perceived exertion, RPE) rises during exercise, as seems also to be the case during prolonged exercise when there is a risk that muscle glycogen depletion will occur. As a result, a limiting RPE is reached before a fatal temperature elevation occurs.

The second control mechanism appears to be the near-total inhibition of muscle recruitment, so that no further work can be performed when a certain ("critical") body temperature is reached (Nybo & Nielsen 2001). As a result, the rate of active heat production ceases and passive whole-body cooling will commence. Interestingly this "critical" temperature is much lower during laboratory exercise than during competitive sport out-of-doors (Byrne et al. 2006).

Speculative evidence for this latter mechanism comes from Englishwoman Paula Radcliffe's experience during the 2004 Olympic Marathon in Athens, which was run in unacceptably extreme conditions (35°C). She stopped running at 36 km, apparently "paralyzed" by the action of the central mechanisms described above (St. Clair Gibson & Noakes 2004) but *before* she developed heatstroke. Her control mechanisms to prevent heatstroke were clearly intact. Indeed, the surprising observation, made already in 1957, is how effective these mechanisms are – heatstroke is so uncommon and appears not to have occurred during either of the Athens Olympic Marathons. As Ladell (1957) wrote: "Whenever one's body temperature rises, even for physiologic reasons, we enter into danger and anything that interferes with physiological cooling, or adds to the internal heat load, exacerbates that danger. The wonder is, not that anyone gets hyperpyrexia, but that so few of us do." For heatstroke to occur, both of these mechanisms have to fail and, as suggested by Ladell, this happens remarkably infrequently.

For a state of elevated body temperature to be sustained for longer than a few minutes in an athlete who has collapsed and is therefore no longer actively contracting his or her muscles and so generating metabolic heat at a fast rate, there must be a source of continued heat production at a high rate somewhere in the body. The most logical candidate must be the previously active muscles, even though they are no longer visibly contracting and producing external work. If this is correct, then there must be a primary or secondary abnormality in the muscles causing them to continue producing heat after exercise, even though they are not producing external work. The evidence is that some humans are susceptible to this abnormal response which can be genetically determined and may be induced by agents such as drug use or fasting (Hopkins & Ellis 1996; Muldoon et al. 2004).

Perhaps the point is that heatstroke is not the normal response to exercise. Applying the "normal" precautions that are usually prescribed (e.g., drinking more before, during, and after exercise, and even avoiding exercise in extreme heat), will never be totally effective if the real causes are a failure of brain regulatory mechanisms associated with a range of skeletal muscle biochemical abnormalities, some of which are probably genetically based. Rather, we should perhaps look for the obscure explanations for most cases of heatstroke. These would include skeletal muscle metabolic abnormalities and other unusual environmental influences (Hopkins & Ellis 1996; Muldoon et al. 2004). If skeletal muscle abnormalities are present, the drug dantrolene may be effective, because it acts to reduce calcium release from the ryanodine receptor of the sarcoplasmic reticulum, a possible site of some of the skeletal muscle abnormalities associated with malignant hyperpyrexia and probably exertional heatstroke (Hopkins & Ellis 1996; Muldoon et al. 2004).

Perhaps if we taught that heatstroke is brought about by pathology somewhere in the body and is not simply caused by normal physiology that is overwhelmed by unusually severe environmental demands, we might better understand:

1 Why the condition is so uncommon;

2 Why apparently "logical" preventive measures are not always effective; and

3 Why whole-body cooling does not always prevent massive rhabdomyolysis leading to renal and cardiac failure and death in some heatstroke patients.

Perhaps in such patients, more attention needs to be paid to methods that would reverse the ongoing heat production in the affected muscles.

PRACTICAL CONCLUSIONS

It seems highly improbable that the majority of cases of especially fatal heatstroke are simply the result of abnormal heat retention in otherwise healthy humans. Rather, it seems far more likely that heatstroke occurs as a result of accelerated thermogenesis in the skeletal muscles of a few genetically susceptible individuals and which continues even after collapse. This thermogenesis must be so great that it overwhelms the heat-losing mechanisms of the immobile human. Such accelerated thermogenesis most probably originates in the skeletal muscles as a result of genetic predisposition and the action of agents toxic to muscle. Such agents are likely to include drugs and latent viral infections amongst many others.

Persons with a variety of genetic disorders of skeletal muscle metabolism, known collectively as the malignant hyperthermia disorders, may be at risk of developing heatstroke during exercise. When exposed to a variety of different stressors which may include:

1 Exercise, whether or not it is in the heat;
2 Anesthesia with specific drugs;
3 Fasting; or alternatively;
4 Eating a low carbohydrate diet while continuing to exercise vigorously; or
5 The use of certain recreational drugs, including amphetamines or the ephedra compounds
the muscles of affected persons undergo a rapid and apparently irreversible breakdown (rhabdomyolysis) associated with an uncontrolled metabolic activity that generates inordinate amounts of heat (malignant hyperthermia). Toxic substances released from dying muscle further complicate the disease because they cause kidney and ultimately heart failure, leading to death. When this condition occurs in predisposed persons during exercise, it should be labeled exercise-induced malignant hyperthermia (EIHM) to differentiate it from the condition of environmentally and exercise-induced heatstroke (EEIH) that would, by definition, occur only in otherwise healthy athletes (without such muscle disorders) who exercise in environmental conditions that are too hot. The condition of EIHM explains why some athletes can develop what

appears to be typical heatstroke (EEIH) even when exercising in relatively cool environmental conditions.

The practical point is that this accelerated thermogenesis may not be the biologic event that kills the patient, because most hospitalized heatstroke patients die with normal body temperatures. Rather, it may be that the rhabdomyolysis that accompanies this accelerated thermogenesis releases toxic biochemicals into the circulation, and it is these chemicals that cause the multiorgan failure characteristic of heatstroke and which includes disseminated intravascular coagulation, acute renal failure, respiratory distress and, ultimately, cardiac failure and cardiac arrest.

Hence, treating the elevated temperature treats merely one of the symptoms of this condition. The interventions that will save lives are those that reverse the rhabdomyolysis and that prevent the leakage of toxic molecules from skeletal muscles into the circulation. Yet, to my knowledge, this is never considered to be an important goal in the treatment of heatstroke.

Conclusions

In this section we have presented some of the current dogmas that direct how athletes are advised to conduct themselves during exercise and how clinicians believe they should treat those who collapse or who develop heatstroke during or after exercise. Our central argument is that humans evolved to exercise in the heat for prolonged periods with little or no fluid replacement. When athletes followed that practice, up to 1969, there was no evidence that they placed themselves at increased risk of serious medical consequences.

However, either indirectly or as the result of a covert marketing plan, the development of the sports drink industry led to the acceptance of a novel dogma that holds that fluid loss from sweating during exercise poses a significant health risk that can be prevented only by ensuring that no weight is lost during exercise; that is, by drinking either "as much as tolerable" or to "replace all the weight lost during exercise." The inevitable corollary was that athletes who collapse during or after exercise are "dehydrated" and suffering from circulatory failure that requires immediate correction with copious amounts of fluids given intravenously as a matter of great urgency.

Rather, we argue that the levels of dehydration that develop in athletes who drink according to the dictates of their thirst pose no risk to their health or to their exercise performance. In fact, all the evidence shows that drinking to thirst optimizes exercise performance and reduces the risk that fluid overload, leading to exercise-associated hyponatremia (EAH), will develop. In contrast, some athletes who have drunk "as much as tolerable" have died from EAHE (Noakes 2003b, 2004a).

Furthermore, the available evidence shows that athletes collapse after exercise because they develop postural hypotension immediately they stop running. Because IV fluids cannot reverse this state of low peripheral vascular resistance, it follows that treatment with IV fluids is not the logical first line of therapy. Certainly, there is no evidence from controlled randomized clinical trials to establish that IV fluids are essential for the treatment of post-exercise collapse in those with postural hypotension. Rather, we have found that elevating the legs above the level of the heart rapidly reverses the symptoms of postural hypotension and expedites recovery in this condition.

Finally, we argue that the condition currently defined as exertional heatstroke (EEIH) is not likely caused by a simple failure of heat loss during excessively vigorous exercise in extreme heat. Rather, it is probable that some component of excessive thermogenesis must be involved in at least some of these cases. Thus, it seems probable that cases of heatstroke, in which there is sustained thermogenesis and extensive rhabdomyolysis, must be caused by some inherited aberration and cannot be caused simply by a failure of the heat-losing mechanism or inappropriate or inadequate treatment. We also argue that rhabdomyolysis and not hyperthermia is the probable cause of the multiorgan failure that leads to death in this condition. If this is the case, greater effort should be expended to understand the biologic basis for this rhabdomyolysis and how best it should be treated.

In summary, our contentions are as follow:

1 All the published evidence supports the belief that health and performance during exercise are optimized by drinking according to the dictates of thirst (*ad libitum*) (Noakes 2007).

2 The brain sets both the work rate and the rectal temperature during exercise specifically to ensure that heatstroke will almost never occur in otherwise healthy humans. As a result, the rectal temperature is determined principally by the exercising work rate, influenced by serum osmolality.

3 Post-exercise collapse in athletes who remain conscious is caused by a low peripheral vascular resistance to which dehydration makes essentially no contribution.

4 Heatstroke is more likely caused by an exaggerated and explosive thermogenesis that develops in genetically predisposed individuals on exposure to exercise and other triggering environmental factors. We also suggest that the skeletal muscles are the site of this florid thermogenesis and that the leakage of toxic proteins into the circulation from damaged muscles, and not the hyperthermia, is the more likely cause of the multiorgan failure that typifies fatal heatstroke.

Even if heatstroke is more likely caused by internal rather than external factors, there are a number of changes in the conduct of sport over the past 20 years that have most likely reduced the risk that the condition will occur. The more important of these changes are the following:

1 Sporting events, most especially running races longer than 3 km, are no longer held in the heat of the day, as was the case before about 1970. Rather, those events in which high rates of energy expenditure and hence heat production are required over prolonged periods are now usually scheduled in the cooler conditions of the early morning or late evening. This is not universally true. Certainly, the Woman's 2004 Athens Olympic Marathon was contested in unacceptable environmental conditions.

2 Athletes have become aware of the need to pre-acclimatize by training in the heat if they are to compete in the heat.

3 Athletes are now more aware that it is not safe to run at a maximum effort when the environmental conditions are unfavorable.

4 The facilities for providing the athletes with fluid replacement during exercise have greatly improved. Currently, refreshment stations are provided every 2–3 km and often more frequently at the most popular marathon foot races. There is no independent evidence that such fluid replacement has contributed to the prevention of heatstroke. However, when fluids are available in excess and large numbers of athletes take more than 5 h to complete endurance events such as marathon races and are encouraged to drink "as much as tolerable", the probability is increased that EAH and EAHE will develop (Noakes *et al.* 2005a; Noakes & Speedy 2006).

Finally, optimum exercise performance in long-distance running events occurs at an environmental temperature of about 11–13°C. At higher environmental temperatures, athletes generate heat too rapidly for the achievement of an optimum heat balance. As a consequence, the regulatory centers in the brain ensure that only a pace that will allow safe heat balance will be allowed.

In contrast, the reason why exercise performance is impaired at environmental temperatures below about 10°C is unknown, because logic suggests that higher rates of energy expenditure that is at higher exercise intensities could be sustained without the risk that heat injury would develop. Perhaps feedback from temperature sensors in the skin and the respiratory tract detect the coldness of the environment and the inspired air and regulate the speed of movement and the rate of breathing specifically to ensure that cold injury to either the skin or the respiratory tract does not occur during exercise in extremely cold conditions.

Exercise performance and intercontinental travel

Intercontinental travel

There are few studies of the effects of intercontinental travel on athletic performance so much opinion is based on anecdotal experiences. Rapid air travel across three or more time zones produces a condition commonly referred to as "jet-lag." This condition is widely recognized but poorly understood.

The disruption of normal circadian rhythm by more than 3 h causes physiologic asynchrony; leading to non-specific symptoms such as general malaise, headaches, sleepiness at inappropriate times and, conversely, insomnia, dizziness, lack of concentration, and gastrointestinal distress.

Air travel from north to south, without crossing more than three time zones, leads to generalized fatigue and decreased psychomotor performance. However, there are minimal alterations in physiologic rhythms with north to south flight. Furthermore, studies confirm that such flights do not elicit any significant disruptions in sleep; this includes total hours slept, total REM sleep, sleep onset latency or REM latency (O'Connor & Morgan 1990).

Transmeridian flight across three or more time zones, however, causes significant disturbances in physiologic rhythms. Circadian rhythms in heart rate and rectal temperature remain out of phase for 4–8 days following such flights. Furthermore, sleep patterns are significantly altered following transmeridian flight; with decreases in both sleep onset latency and total REM sleep.

Disturbances in physiologic rhythms primarily result from "phase shifts" which occur when physiologic rhythms become asynchronous with the day–night cycle at the new location. These phase shifts are shown by alterations in the timing of the minimal and maximal rectal temperatures and encompass changes within the cardiovascular, endocrine, and renal systems. Circadian rhythms adapt faster to phase delays following westward flights compared to phase advances produced by eastward flights; with resynchronization following east to west flights occurring 30–50% more rapidly than following west to east flights. These phase shifts are transient in nature, with complete resynchronization occurring 3–11 days following west to east travel and 2–6 days following east to west travel. The more time zones that are crossed, the longer time required for complete resynchronization to occur.

Transient psychologic impairment has also been documented following transmeridian flights. Studies utilizing standardized psychometric instruments have documented that state anxiety, as measured by the State-Trait Anxiety Inventory, was significantly elevated during travel and persisted for 48 h post flight. State anxiety returned to pre-flight levels only 72 h after arrival. This same time-frame of changes was noted in mood states as measured by the Profile of Mood States Inventory (O'Connor & Morgan 1990).

Performance decrements have been documented in volleyball and netball players traveling across time zones (O'Connor & Morgan 1990; Bishop 2004). These studies were not well controlled, however, and caution should be used when extrapolating these findings. Soldiers crossing six time zones displayed performance decrements of 8–12% in both the 270 m sprint and 2.8 km run. Significant reductions in elbow flexor strength (but not leg strength or endurance) were also noted immediately following transmeridian flights. More than 50% of these soldiers reported increased sleepiness and fatigue, and more than 40% reported weakness.

Transmeridian flights have a negative impact on physical activity, mood, and performance which must be considered when planning intercontinental travel and competition. The number of time zones crossed, plus the direction of travel must be considered when determining the time period required for physiologic acclimatization after arrival at the new locations. Athletes must be allowed time to completely resynchronize to the day–night cycle at the new location if maximum athletic performance is desired.

Exercise in the cold

The maintenance of a normal body temperature depends on a balance between heat loss and heat production. Heat loss occurs via conduction, convection, radiation, and evaporation, while heat gain is greatly increased during exercise. Normally, this increased rate of heat production challenges the body's ability to lose the heat sufficiently rapidly so that the brain will allow an exercise intensity appropriate to the competitive desires of the athlete. However, when environmental conditions are particularly cold, for example: (i) during winter conditions at latitudes above about 50° in either hemisphere; (ii) when cold is associated with windy and especially wet conditions; or (iii) when the athlete exercises in cold water for prolonged periods,

the risk arises that the athlete will lose heat faster than he or she can produce it. Under these conditions, the body may be unable to maintain its core body temperature, which may fall progressively, leading to hypothermia (core temperature <35°C) and the risk of death from the exposure–exhaustion syndrome.

Incidents of hypothermia during exercise in cold, wet, and windy conditions on land

Hypothermia has long been recognized as a serious condition, often with fatal consequences, for mountain hikers, fell runners, and high-altitude mountain climbers. For example, three hikers died when taking part in the 1964 Four Inns Walking Competition in Derbyshire (Pugh 1966, 1967, 1971). Temperatures during the competition were estimated at between 0 and 4°C, with wind speeds in excess of 25 knots. Characteristics common to all three fatalities were the following:
• Clothing was inadequate, as none had waterproof outer garments, such as oilskins. Therefore their clothing would have provided no insulation when wet (Pugh 1966, 1971).
• Subjects were lean with little subcutaneous fat. When the insulating effect of clothing is lost, the subcutaneous fat and muscle become the sole remaining insulators.
• All subjects had collapsed within 1.5–2 h after becoming progressively fatigued, and had started to walk more slowly. In contrast, those who finished the event were able to maintain high rates of energy expenditure (and hence high rates of heat production) for the duration of the event.

Hypothermia has also been encountered in long-distance runners. The first, recently documented case of hypothermia in a marathon runner was that of Ledingham et al. (1982), who reported a rectal temperature of 34.4°C in a runner who collapsed in the Glasgow Marathon, which was run under dry but cold conditions (dry bulb temperature 12°C) with a strong wind of 16–40 km·h^{-1}. In a 56 km ultramarathon held in cool conditions (19.8°C, rain, and wind speed of 30 km·h^{-1}), 28% of runners who were treated in the medical tent had rectal temperatures below 37°C, with one thin elite runner reaching 35°C after collapsing during the race (Sandell *et al.* 1988).

Factors predisposing to the development of hypothermia during exercise on land

A normal body temperature of 36–37°C is maintained by the balance between heat loss and heat production. In cold, wet, and windy conditions, heat loss is greatly increased, and so heat gain must also be substantially increased to prevent the onset of hypothermia. The rate at which heat is produced increases as a linear function of exercise intensity, and so vigorous exercise attenuates the reduction in rectal temperature in cold conditions. For this reason, incidents of hypothermia occur when hikers, climbers, or runners become fatigued and stop running, climbing, or walking altogether.

Environmental factors also have a major role in the development of hypothermia, for they affect the degree of heat loss that occurs for a given level of heat production. Heat loss is greatly increased when the air temperature is reduced, as this increases the gradient for heat loss by means of conduction and convection. Convective cooling is further increased when the movement of air over the skin is increased, because this continually replaces air in contact with the skin with cooler air. High wind speeds therefore dramatically increase the risk of hypothermia. The presence of water increases the risk of hypothermia, because water conducts heat approximately 25 times faster than air. The normal insulation provided by the thin layer of air which is heated and then trapped between the skin and clothing is removed when the clothing becomes wet, and the athlete must either find dry, warm conditions, or warm clothing.

Aesthetic reasons apart, the usual reason for wearing clothes is to trap a thin layer of air next to the body. As air is a poor conductor of heat (and hence a good insulator), this thin layer rapidly heats up to body temperature and acts as an insulator, reducing heat loss from the body. Clearly, during exercise, especially in the heat, any clothing that is worn must be designed to achieve the opposite effect: promoting heat loss.

The ability of clothing to retain body heat, known as the insulating capacity of clothing, is expressed in clothing (CLO) units. One CLO unit is equivalent to the amount of insulation provided by ordinary business apparel, which provides comfort at temperatures of 21°C when both wind speed and humidity are low. The clothing of the Eskimo provides 10–12 CLO units and is essential for life in polar conditions. However, because of the considerable heat production during exercise, clothing that will provide 1 CLO unit of insulation is all that is required when running in temperatures as low as –22°C, provided there is little or no wind or rain. As soon as there is any wind, convective cooling increases as an exponential (non-linear) function of the wind speed. Hence, more clothing providing greater CLO units must be worn whenever conditions are windy. In contrast, substantially less clothing needs to be worn during exercise in cold conditions than is the case when one is at rest in the same environmental conditions.

Whereas a resting human needs to wear 12 CLO units to maintain body temperature at –50°C, when running at 16 km·h⁻¹ at the same temperature the same person would be adequately protected by only 1.25 CLO units. However, clothing with at least four times more insulation is required to maintain body temperature at rest in wind still conditions at an air temperature of 0°C as when running at 16 km·h⁻¹ at the same temperature. Changing from exercising to resting in the same environmental conditions requires that substantially more clothing be worn. A problem is that clothing able to provide 4 CLO units may weigh as much as 10–15 kg and few hikers, for example, would be prepared to carry the extra weight of clothing on the off-chance that they might suddenly need the extra clothing to maintain heat balance in the same, cold environmental conditions were they forced, for any reason, to stop exercising. A water-resistant down jacket is one lightweight solution.

Allowance must always be made for clothing that becomes wet, because wetness reduces the insulating properties of clothing because, unlike air, which is a good insulator, water is an excellent conductor of heat. Studies of the three young hikers who died of hypothermia/exposure during the 1964 Four Inns Walking Competition in Derbyshire established that the insulating properties of the wet clothing found on those who died was only 0.2 CLO units or about one-tenth the insulating capacity of that same clothing when dry (Pugh 1966, 1967). In practice, sweating alone will not cause clothing to lose its insulating properties completely, especially when running in cold, dry conditions. Problems will arise in athletes who exercise in drenching rain with strong facing winds for periods exceeding 1–2 h. The rain will saturate the clothing destroying its insulating properties as occurred in the Four Inns Walking disaster. Under such conditions, an impervious wind- and water-resistant jacket should be worn. In all other conditions, garments that breathe by allowing sweat to vaporize through pores in the material are more comfortable as they keep the garments closer to the skin drier for somewhat longer. Alternatively, polar explorers have learned to regulate their exercise intensity specifically so that they do not sweat because the risk is that their wet clothes will freeze.

The point is that as a natural consequence of the high rates of heat production by humans during exercise, when exercising in cold conditions even modest amounts of clothing will ensure that the body temperature will be maintained. However, as a general rule, people who continue to move are at low risk of developing hypothermia. Once the subject becomes too exhausted to continue, his or her rate of heat production falls sharply and the risk is high that fatal hypothermia will develop. The important practical point is that the change from running to walking, for example, has a marked effect on the clothing needed to maintain body temperature, even at relatively mild temperatures. Clothing with at least four times more insulation is required to maintain body temperature at rest at an effective air temperature of 0°C than when running at 16 km·h^{-1}. Extra (dry) clothing should always be available if there is any possibility that fatigue will develop when exercising in cold conditions.

If the insulating properties of the clothing are removed as a result of saturation, then insulation can still be provided by non-perfused muscle and adipose tissue. During exercise, muscle blood flow increases, and so the muscle becomes a conductor and loses its insulating properties, leaving adipose tissue as the sole insulator. It is for this reason that those athletes who have hypothermia during exercise are often lean and have a relatively small muscle mass (Pugh 1966, 1971; Sandell et al. 1988).

In order to maintain thermal homeostasis, heat loss must be limited and heat production maximized. This requires that as much of the skin as feasible is covered and that clothing is kept as dry as possible in order to preserve the insulating properties of the clothing. The exercise intensity must be maintained as high as possible. Increased adiposity also protects against the reduction in core temperature that would occur under these conditions. However, if fatigue develops, causing a reduction in running or walking speed, for example, and the clothing becomes wet, then the athlete must either be removed from the environment or provided with dry clothing in order to continue safely.

The key to safe exercise in the cold is to be properly clothed and to remain dry because this ensures that the insulating layer of air next to the skin is equal to the skin temperature. However, if the clothing becomes saturated, the insulating layer is lost and the rate of heat loss to the environment is dramatically increased. It follows that the only adaptation most exercisers require in order to ensure that they can exercise safely in cold conditions, is not primarily a physiologic adaptation in bodily function. Rather, it is to ensure that they purchase and use the clothing that is appropriate to all the possible environmental conditions that they might experience. When these conditions include wet, very cold, and windy conditions, it is imperative that the outer layer of the clothing is totally water-resistant (e.g., an oilskin raincoat or jacket).

Treatment of developing hypothermia

Once the climber or runner becomes too tired to continue exercising in cold, wet, and windy conditions, either because he or she is already developing hypothermia or because of the onset of exhaustion, the development of hypothermia will only be prevented if most of the following steps are taken:
• The athlete must be taken to buildings or geographic features that provide shelter from the wind and rain and where there is an external source of heat.

• A change into dry, water-repellent clothes must be provided. Because the athlete has stopped exercise at this point, the rate of heat production will decrease and so more clothing is required than was needed during exercise. For example, at an air temperature of 0°C, four times more clothing is needed to maintain body temperature at rest than when running at 16 km·h⁻¹.

• Food must be given to the athlete, because this aids in the generation of heat, providing energy so that shivering thermogenesis can occur.

Hypothermia during exercise in cold water

During exercise in cold water, the rate of heat loss is substantially higher than during exercise on land at a similar temperature, for the reasons described earlier. Long-distance, especially (English) Channel swimmers face the challenge that they are unable to wear appropriately insulating clothing to retard the rate of heat loss to the water which is always colder than their skin temperatures. Because no swimmer has yet been able to heat all the oceans of the world to the human's skin temperature (33°C), the body temperatures of all swimmers must ultimately fall to the temperature of the water in which they are swimming. Therefore, the risk of hypothermia is great when prolonged exercise is undertaken in cold water and a progressive fall in body temperature is inevitable at all water temperatures below 30°C. However, Channel swimmers have shown that it is possible to swim in cold (<15.5°C) water for prolonged periods, longer than 8 h.

Initially, it was thought that the success of certain individuals in cold water was because of their ability to achieve very high rates of heat production, and advice was given that people should "swim or struggle as hard as they can for as long as they can" (Glaser 1950). However, it has since been shown that in relatively lean individuals, the rectal temperature drops more rapidly during exercise in cold water than when they are at rest (Pugh & Edholm 1955). This occurs because exercise increases blood flow to the muscle, and perfused muscle loses its insulating properties.

Interestingly, in a fatter individual, the rectal temperature actually rose during exercise (Pugh & Edholm 1955). This difference in the response to exercise in the cold water may be because of the increased adipose tissue of the fatter individual, which provides sufficient insulation to prevent a fall in body temperature. On the basis of those findings, it was concluded that:

• Increased subcutaneous body fatness explained why Channel swimmers were better able to maintain heat balance when exposed to cold water.

• When immersed in cold water, fatter swimmers were better able to maintain their body temperatures when they increased their rates of heat production by swimming.

• In contrast, when they swam in cold water, thinner non-swimmers were unable to maintain their body temperatures as their rates of cooling increased more than did their rates of body heat production. This effect is a result of the loss of insulation induced by exercising the arms in persons with little other forms of insulation (adipose tissue) in their arms.

It must be noted that physical discomfort was much higher in the thinner individual when he lay still in the cold water, indicating that the muscle temperature also contributes to the discomfort. That individual also had to be lifted out of the water after 33 min exposure because his muscles had become so rigid that he was unable to perform any voluntary movements. It is therefore debatable whether it is in fact wise to remain still in cold water, because the loss of muscle function and physical incapacitation would predispose to drowning, even though the body temperature may be higher than if the individual swam in the cold water for the same duration. Therefore, remaining still in the water confers a thermoregulatory advantage, which may be negated by the loss of function caused by peripheral muscle cooling.

In summary, one of the more important physiologic adaptations to cold water swimming is to increase the muscle and fat mass to improve insulation. It is also likely that other subtle adaptations occur in blood flow distribution patterns in those who train repeatedly in cold water, thereby increasing the insulating capacity and reducing the rate of heat loss from actively contracting muscles. There are also likely to be other subtle whole-body changes that increase the capacity to exercise for longer before a critically low body temperature is reached.

Physiologic response to cold water immersion

The physiologic responses to immersion in cold water have been classified into four different categories:

1 Initial responses to immersion (0–3 min);
2 Short-term immersion (3–15 min);
3 Long-term immersion (>30 min); and
4 Post-immersion (Tipton 1989).

The nature and extent of the physiologic responses and the duration of survival are determined principally by the water temperature.

INITIAL RESPONSE TO IMMERSION: THE COLD SHOCK RESPONSE

Immersion in cold water induces an immediate peripheral vasoconstriction, tachycardia, and an increased cardiac output. As a result, systolic blood pressure may rise to 180 mmHg and heart rate to 120 beats·min^{-1}. Such changes do not pose a risk to healthy individuals. However, in susceptible individuals, these changes may activate cardiac dysfunction which precipitates drowning.

In healthy individuals, it is the respiratory and musculoskeletal responses that pose the greatest risk to life and which explain why the majority (>60%) of fatalities in open water occur within 3 m of safety, even in persons considered to be good swimmers (Tipton 1989). Immersion in cold water induces an immediate and uncontrollable hyperventilation, with both the tidal volume and breathing rate increasing. Hyperventilation results in a loss of the normal coupling of respiration and locomotor activity, in which one or two breaths are taken for each cycle of muscular activity, be it in swimming, running, or rowing. Such high ventilation rates disturb this normal coupling, resulting in the likely inhalation of water. A 70-kg man, for example, requires approximately 1.5 L sea water and 3.0 L fresh water to drown – the equivalent of one large inhalation. Swim failure also occurs within a few minutes, even in competent swimmers.

Also, hyperventilation causes a respiratory alkalosis, which may lead to a reduction in cerebral blood flow and disorientation and confusion.

The magnitude of the cold shock response is similar at all temperatures between 5°C and 15°C. It is primarily determined by the extent of the surface area exposed to the cold water, with the greatest response occurring when the back and trunk are exposed. The cold shock can be reduced by up to 50% with repeated cold water immersions (Tipton & Golden 1998). Thus, cold habituation is important in individuals wishing to swim in cold water. It does not appear that adiposity influences the magnitude of the cold shock response.

FACTORS INFLUENCING SURVIVAL TIMES IN COLD WATER

Water temperature

Survival times in very cold (<15°C) water are short because of the cold shock response already described, and because of the increased risk of cardiac arrhythmias as a result of the return of cold blood from the peripheries to the heart. In warmer water (>15°C), survival times are greatly increased because the magnitude of the cold shock is reduced. Also, the temperature gradient between the warmer body core and water is reduced and so heat loss is lower. It has been found that the rectal temperature decreases at a rate inversely proportional to the water temperature.

Clothing

Clothing decreases the rate at which the body temperature falls during exposure to cold water. It does this by maintaining higher skin and therefore higher body temperatures. For example, people working unclothed in water at 5°C for 20 min reduced their body temperature by 1.6°C, whereas when clothed the fall was only 0.6°C in the same time. In contrast, if they remained inactive in the water when fully clothed, the fall in temperature was reduced to 0.3°C (Keatinge et al. 1969).

The use of a drysuit or wetsuit obviously reduces the rate of cooling the most effectively, with a sixfold increase in survival time when using a wetsuit. If a drysuit is used, in which air, not water, is in contact with the skin, survival time increases 10-fold (Noakes 2000a).

Body fat content

The effect of increasing body fat content is similar to that already described for exercise on land. Increasing body fatness reduces the rate of body cooling by providing additional insulation. Pugh *et al.* (1960) calculated that each 1 mm increase in the thickness of the subcutaneous fat layer effectively raises the water temperature by 1.5°C.

Metabolic rate

When exposed to cold water a thin person will begin to shiver, thereby increasing the metabolic rate in order to increase heat production. However, this shivering response also has the effect of causing vasodilatation in the arterioles supplying the shivering muscles. As a result, muscle blood flow increases. The effect is that shivering reduces the insulating effect normally provided by the thickness and mass of the inactive muscles. A similar phenomenon explains why rectal temperatures decline more rapidly when exercising in cold water than when at rest. There is therefore an increase in both the rate of heat production and the rate of heat loss as a result of shivering or exercise in cold water, and the effect on the whole-body temperature will be determined by the water temperature, the person's body fatness, the intensity of the shivering or exercise, and the nature of the activity undertaken.

Nature of activity

Toner *et al.* (1984) showed that the rate of cooling during immersion in cold water at 20, 26, or 33°C was always greatest for arm exercise compared with either leg exercise alone or arm and leg exercise at the identical metabolic rate. They concluded that heat loss was greater from the arms than from the legs when either muscle group was exercised at the same absolute metabolic rate. Other studies have similarly concluded that the arms are an important source of heat loss during exercise in cold water (Golden & Tipton 1987). As a result, exercise involving only the leg muscles can attenuate the decline in rectal temperature, whereas exercise with the arms will accelerate the rate at which hypothermia develops.

Habituation

Swimmers who train frequently in cold water develop a habituation so that they become better able to maintain higher temperatures and to swim for longer before they fatigue. This occurs because the magnitude of the cold shock response is reduced, enabling improved coordination of the swimming stroke, as well as an improved non-shivering thermogenic capacity. Thus, habituated individuals are better able to produce heat from non-shivering sources, as a result of the effects of the hormones thyroxine, epinephrine, norepinephrine, adenocorticotropic hormone (ACTH), and cortisol.

Practical conclusions for exercise in the cold

In conclusion, hypothermia is less common during exercise on land than in water at the same temperature because still air is a good insulator whereas cold water is an excellent heat conductor. In addition, there is the opportunity to wear layers of dry clothing on land. Exercise reduces the clothing requirements and improves survival at any cold air temperature on land whereas the opposite applies in swimming as exercise reduces the insulating capacity, especially on the muscles of the upper limbs, thereby increasing heat loss from the body. The key for survival during exercise in extreme conditions on land (as in water) is to maintain a high metabolic rate and to stay dry. In water this is achieved by wearing either a wetsuit or a drysuit, both of which should cover the arms.

When exposed accidentally to ice-cold water, the initial crisis is to survive the cold shock response. It is also unlikely that most people will be able to cover more than 50–100 m should they attempt to swim to land. The prospect of survival is determined almost entirely by the speed with which dry land is reached. Any delay increases the probability that drowning by inhalation, secondary to physical incapacitation, will occur.

If the accidental exposure is to warmer water, the survival time may be substantially prolonged. The popular advice under these conditions remains that given by Nadel *et al.* (1974): "The choice between vigorous swimming and floating would depend upon the water temperature, the resistance to heat flow provided by clothing or fatty tissue and the length of time one could tolerate heavy exercise."

Clinical guidelines for fluid intake during exercise

The idea that an athlete should drink during exercise, especially in marathon running, is of recent origin. Joseph Forshaw, USA, who finished fourth in the 1908 Olympic Marathon and tenth in the 1912 Olympic Marathon, wrote: "I know from actual experience that the full race can be covered in creditable time without so much as a single drop of water being taken or even sponging of the head." Similarly, advice given to marathon runners of the early 1900s included the following caveats: "Don't get into the habit of drinking and eating in a marathon race; some prominent runners do, but it is not beneficial."

As recently as 1957, Englishman Jim Peters, who set the world marathon record on four occasions and who may have been the greatest marathon runner of all time, expressed a similar belief: "[In the marathon race] there is no need to take any solid food at all and every effort should also be made to do without liquid, as the moment food or drink is taken, the body has to start dealing with its digestion, and in so doing some discomfort will almost invariably be felt."

The development of the world's first sports drink in Florida in 1965, and the landmark scientific study of two South African physiologists, Cyril Wyndham and Nick Strydom in 1969, were crucial factors in reversing those beliefs. For the originator of that sports drink, Dr Robert Cade, was convinced that his product would prevent heat illnesses during exercise. The result was that his perception was adopted and became the platform for a global marketing exercise that fundamentally changed the

common understanding of human physiology (see p. 457) to one in which it was assumed that the level of "dehydration" developed during exercise was the principal factor regulating the body temperature during exercise (Noakes 2006a; Noakes & Speedy 2006). As a result, athletes were encouraged to drink "as much as tolerable" during exercise even though there was no evidence that such high rates of fluid ingestion were necessary or beneficial (Noakes 2007).

This novel interpretation received crucial support from the study of Wyndham and Strydom (1969) (see p. 456), which led to the incorrect conclusion that the weight loss that develops during exercise is detrimental because it causes the body temperature to rise excessively, leading ultimately to heatstroke. This conflicted with the popular teaching that it is the rate of doing work (the exercise intensity or the metabolic rate) that determines the extent to which the body temperature rises during exercise (Nielsen 1938; Noakes *et al.* 1991). Thus, it is in short-distance running events, in which very high rates of heat production are maintained for relatively short periods of time and in which significant dehydration is unlikely to occur, that are likely pose the greatest risk that heatstroke will occur (Noakes 1982). Indeed, if this is not what is found, then some other unrecognized factor must be operative during prolonged exercise in which the rate of energy production is low. This other unrecognized factor must be an endogenous factor present in the individuals and which makes them unusually susceptible to the condition.

Nevertheless, the 1969 South African study was of great practical significance, for it drew attention to the potential dangers of the International Amateur Athletic Federation's Rule No. 165.5, which stipulated that marathon runners could drink no fluids before the 11 km mark of a 42 km marathon and thereafter could only drink every 5 km. This ruling was an improvement of the 1953 rule that stated that: "Refreshments shall (only) be provided by the organizers after 15 km. No refreshments may be carried or taken by a competitor other than that provided by the organizers." These early rulings discouraged marathon runners from drinking during races and promoted the idea that drinking was unnecessary and a sign of weakness.

From the results of their original study, Wyndham and Strydom concluded that marathon runners should aim to drink 250 mL fluid every 15 min during exercise to give a total of 1000 mL·h^{-1}, a value that matched their sweat rates. In time this advice was extended so that currently the ACSM (Armstrong *et al.* 1996), the International Olympic Committee (Coyle 2004a,b), the Nutrition and Athletic Performance Joint Position Stand (ACSM *et al.* 2000), and the National Athletic Trainers Association (Casa *et al.* 2000) all propose that athletes should drink either "as much as tolerable" or to replace all the sweat lost during exercise in order to optimize performance especially in the heat. Are these ideas evidence-based (Noakes 2007)? Or is it possible that humans evolved specifically to be able to regulate their body temperatures effectively during exercise without the need for excessive fluid ingestion according to the Heinrich hypothesis (see p. 454)?

The first study to address the role of dehydration on marathon running performance was that of Buskirk and Beetham (1960), performed in New England in 1959. They concluded that:

> Weight loss in the marathon runners varied from 2.5 to 7.4%, yet a performance decrement in these men apparently did not occur. Running speed (pace) was maintained essentially constant by each man in all races – there was no let down in pace near the end of the race. In fact, a sprint finish was frequently attempted . . . post-race rectal temperature was, in most cases, within limits that suggest successful maintenance of thermoregulation during the latter stages of the race. Thus, well-conditioned men running in a cool environment seem to tolerate a 3–7% dehydration rather well.

In fact, the authors even proposed that "dehydration" might provide certain physiologic benefits.

The next study from the UK (Pugh *et al.* 1967) showed that the top finishers in an English marathon run in cool conditions were both the hottest and the most dehydrated and drank only about 100 mL·h^{-1} during the race. The authors concluded that marathon runners are apparently immune to the effects of dehydration and hyperthermia: "Successful marathon runners . . . can tolerate exceptionally high rectal temperatures . . . Another condition of success seems to be a high tolerance to fluid loss."

Essentially the same findings were reported by Wyndham and Strydom, although they failed to interpret their identical findings in the same words. Those authors reported that the individual, who won the two 32-km races that they studied, finished with the highest body temperature and the greatest level of dehydration. Yet their conclusion was the opposite of that advanced by both Buskirk and Beetham (1960) and Pugh *et al.* (1967). Rather, Wyndham and Strydom concluded that: "The present practice of marathon runners drinking only small quantities of water is dangerous. The danger to health, and even of death, of not drinking adequate amounts of water has been emphasized." Any independently minded marathon runners considering these conflicting theories would surely have concluded that the avoidance of drinking during exercise was clearly beneficial because this was what the winners were doing. So how could it possibly be incorrect?

Similarly, Muir *et al.* (1970) reported that the winner of the 1970 Edinburgh Commonwealth Games Marathon, PhD chemist Dr Ron Hill, in a then world-best time (for an out-and-back course) of 2:09:28, did not drink during the race, losing 2.3 kg (3.9% of his pre-race body weight of 59.4 kg). They wrote: "This degree of dehydration (>2.5 kg), which must have been greatly exceeded by some of the Edinburgh competitors, might be expected to give rise to symptoms and also signs of physiological inefficiency. That it does not do so is indicated by the fact that in Edinburgh few runners took the trouble to correct it by drinking during the race. Perhaps their arduous training protects them in some way against the adverse effects of dehydration." Perhaps these runners were simply doing that for which athletic humans were designed – running long distances in the heat with little or no fluid replacement according to the Heinrich hypothesis.

More recently, Cheuvront *et al.* (2003) have reported a linear relationship between the average running speed and the level of dehydration of

42 km marathon runners so that those athletes who became the most dehydrated ran the fastest. The authors caution that: "This should not be wrongly interpreted as support for an ergogenic effect of dehydration," but they do not explain why it is inappropriate even to consider the heinous possibility that dehydration might aid performance in weight-bearing activities such as long-distance running. Rather, they allow their own biases, however ingrained, to determine their interpretation. Yet they note that: "The question of how competitive runners perform so well when dehydrated still remains."

Our own studies confirmed exactly the same findings. We also found a linear relationship between the speed of completing the race and the level of dehydration in athletes completing the South African Ironman Triathlon. As a result, increasing levels of dehydration were associated with faster finishing times (Sharwood *et al.* 2002, 2004).

However, our more recent analysis of all the studies that have evaluated the effects of fluid ingestion on performance during exercise reveals the following (Noakes 2007):

1 Compared with any amount of fluid ingestion during exercise, not drinking is more likely to be associated with impaired performance during any exercise lasting more than 1 h, especially if performed in the heat. Thus, there is clear scientific support for the view that ingesting any fluid during exercise, especially in the heat, is likely to enhance performance.

2 The fluid must be ingested (i.e., swallowed) because simply rinsing the mouth with water does not prevent the deterioration of performance found in those who do not ingest any fluid during exercise (Dugas *et al.* 2006).

3 There is no evidence that drinking "as much as tolerable" improves performance more that does drinking to the dictates of thirst, so-called *ad libitum* drinking. Furthermore, drinking "as much as tolerable" during exercise may impair exercise performance (Robinson *et al.* 1995). It has been associated with an increased prevalence of symptoms, usually in the gastrointestinal tract (Glace *et al.* 2002a,b; Noakes & Glace 2004b) and may, on occasion, cause death (Noakes 2003b).

4 There is no evidence that either drinking nothing, some, or "as much as tolerable" influences the probability that athletes will develop either heatstroke or any of the other inappropriately termed "heat illnesses" during exercise (Noakes 1995, 2004a, 2007). This is because there are no randomized controlled clinical trials (RCTs) that specifically address this question. However, cross-sectional studies give not the slightest indication that this effect is likely (Sharwood *et al.* 2002, 2004) so that there appears little evidence as to why such RCTs are necessary. Paradoxically, only the sports drink industry has the financial muscle to fund such trials but they seemingly lack the desire because their focus is on other outcomes. As Goldman (2001) has written: "Unfortunately, the late-20th century marketing success of 'sports drinks,' which contain large (sic) amounts of electrolytes and glucose, seems certain to continue to provide funds to (i) support research *proving* (author's emphasis) the benefits of such drinks, and (ii) attempt to convince the military that purchase of such drinks would be beneficial to troops. These commercial marketing attempts may well prevail."

In summary, a sober, independent review of the published evidence indicates that provided subjects drink according to the dictates of thirst (*ad libitum*), their athletic performance will be optimized. Because *ad libitum* drinking is associated with varying levels of dehydration, this finding suggests that it is not the level of dehydration that impairs exercise performance in those who drink either nothing or too little during exercise. Rather, it could be that increased sensations of thirst in those who drink too little during exercise may impair their performance through the action of a central governor (Noakes *et al.* 2005b).

Unfortunately, the novel drinking dogma that athletes should drink "as much as tolerable" during exercise, occasioned by the ACSM guidelines and as championed by the Gatorade Sports Science Institute (GSSI), happened at the very moment that marathon running, particularly in the USA, underwent its most fundamental change since 1976.

Prior to 1976, there were few runners in marathon races and most were usually well trained and quite able to finish the 42 km in less than 3.5 h. Since 1996 this had changed so that the majority of the current generation of marathon runners in the USA requires 4–5 h or more to complete the marathon distance (Dugas 2006). Encouraging less well-conditioned athletes traveling at slow speeds (8–9 km·h⁻¹) for prolonged periods (>4.5 h) to drink "as much as tolerable" to prevent a condition, heatstroke, that occurs infrequently in such slow runners, very quickly produces an unexpected, but entirely predictable consequence (Noakes *et al.* 1985; Frizzell *et al.* 1986; Dugas 2006).

That tragic consequence was the development of deaths from EAHE in US marathon runners and army personnel. Fortunately, the US Army took action by quickly identifying the cause of the problem and issuing contradictory guidelines requiring their soldiers to drink much less during exercise (Gardner 2002; Noakes & Speedy 2006; Noakes 2007). As a result, the incidence of this condition fell rapidly in the US Army. Sadly, this action of the US Army (Gardner 2002) occurred at the very moment that the ACSM and the GSSI were advocating the opposite, namely, that athletes should drink "as much as tolerable during exercise."

Practical conclusions

Athletes should be encouraged to drink according to the dictates of thirst during exercise. This will reduce (but not absolutely exclude) the possibility that EAHE will develop, because some slow runners in marathon and ultramarathon races still considered drinking "as much as tolerable" as *ad libitum* drinking. Drinking *ad libitum* will also optimize their exercise performance (Noakes 2007). There is no evidence from properly designed and correctly conducted RCTs to show that drinking any volume of fluid during exercise alters the risk that either heatstroke or "heat illness" will develop. Thus, there is no reason to believe that drinking *ad libitum* will place athletes at risk of developing specific medical complications during exercise.

However, non-elite joggers and walkers are quite capable of drinking fluid at such high rates because they travel so slowly and have ample time to stop and drink as often as they desire during "competition." Because such high rates of fluid ingestion

exceed the real fluid requirements of persons sweating little because they are exercising at such low intensities, these high rates of fluid ingestion will cause the development of EAHE if sustained for more than 3–4 h. Indeed, runners in Wyndham and Strydom's study drank only about 100 mL·h⁻¹, which is probably similar to the current practices of world-class runners in races of 5–42 km.

In general, most studies show that the voluntary rates of fluid intake during exercise are usually 250–1000 mL·h⁻¹. By comparison, sweat rates may range from 200–2500 mL·h⁻¹. The lowest rates will be found in those who exercise slowly in cool conditions, for example, recreational joggers or walkers who take 4 h or more to complete 42 km marathon races, or in those involved in ultra-distance running events held in cold conditions (e.g., in Alaska or other venues at high latitudes). The highest sweat rates will be found in those with high rates of energy expenditure because they are either exercising very vigorously in hot and especially humid conditions, or because they are unusually large (>130 kg), such as American football players. Typical examples of vigorous exercisers would be 10 km runners competing in hot, humid conditions in the southern states of North America or in many Asian countries, or cyclists in the Tour de France. Because they are exercising at a high intensity, in particular because their rates of breathing are high, it is not possible for these athletes to consume fluid at the same rate at which they are sweating. As a result, they develop varying degrees of weight loss during these events. Provided the events are relatively short (e.g., 10 km races), the degree of water loss is relatively small and of no proven consequence. However, the body weight of leading competitors in 224 km Ironman Triathlons may fall by up to 6–8 kg during such races, of which at least 4–6 kg is likely to be a result of water loss. Whether or not such high levels of fluid deficit (dehydration) either aid or impair the performances of such athletes has yet to be established. That the winners of these races are usually amongst the most "dehydrated" finishers suggests that many of the presumptions of the "dangers" of dehydration are overstated.

Perhaps the best practical advice is that drinking according to the personal dictates of thirst (*ad libitum*) appears to be both safe and effective. *Ad libitum* rates of fluid intake typically range 400–800 mL·h^{-1} in most forms of recreational and competitive exercise: less for slower, smaller athletes exercising in mild environmental conditions; more for superior athletes competing at higher intensities in warmer environments. To ensure they do not develop EAHE, subjects exercising for prolonged periods in extreme cold may need to drink even less.

Finally, the full replacement of any fluid deficit incurred during exercise occurs only when food is eaten usually with the evening meal. Thus, the provision of adequate food and fluids, particularly at the evening meal, is required if athletes who exercise vigorously on a daily basis in the heat, are to maintain optimum fluid balance.

Consequences of drinking too much during exercise: Exercise-associated hyponatremia and exercise-associated hyponatremic encephalopathy

The hyponatremia of exercise was first recognized in a female South African ultramarathon runner competing in the 1981 90 km Comrades Marathon (Noakes *et al.* 1985). This condition is a truly modern complication of more prolonged exercise, usually lasting at least 4–5 h. It occurs when the total water content of the body increases as a consequence of an excessive fluid intake (water intoxication) causing a dilutional fall in the osmolality of the body fluids. As the body water content rises in persons who overdrink, the water moves from the blood stream into all the cells of the body. The organ at greatest risk from the falling whole-body osmolality is the brain, because it is encased in a rigid skull. Thus, as the water content of the brain increases, the pressure inside the skull and brain must rise. The rising pressure impairs normal brain functioning causing an altered level of conscious (EAHE) leading to confusion, epileptic seizures, coma, and ultimately death from cardiac or respiratory arrest, especially if the patient has received intravenous fluids for the incorrect diagnosis of "dehydration." The condition has become perhaps the most common serious complication of prolonged exercise with more than seven deaths and 250 cases of hospitalization

reported amongst runners, triathletes, hikers, and army personnel in the past 17 years (Noakes *et al.* 2005a; Noakes & Speedy 2006).

The condition occurs in subjects who ingest fluid at faster rates than they lose that fluid, either in sweat or urine during exercise. Common features of those who develop hyponatremic encephalopathy are that, with the exception of those occurring in the US Army, they are more likely to be females, especially marathon runners, who run those races at speeds slower than 8–9 km·h^{-1} (~5 miles·h^{-1}); they gain weight during exercise because they drink "the maximal amount that can be tolerated" both before and during exercise, sometimes in excess of 100 cups of fluid during the race (approximately 15 L fluid during 5–6 h exercise); they do not develop a marked sodium deficit (Noakes 2004b), but retain water because of a failure to suppress appropriately the secretion of the water-retaining hormone, arginine vasopressin (AVP; also known as antidiuretic hormone, ADH). In addition, they may fail to mobilize ionized sodium from the intracellular osmotically inactive sodium stores. Or else they may inappropriately inactivate circulating ionized sodium (Na^{+}), storing sodium in an osmotically inactive form, thereby exacerbating the hyponatremia and the hypoosmolality (Noakes *et al.* 2005a).

It is probable that affected athletes choose to drink too much because they have absorbed the prevailing, but unproven, doctrine of the dangers of dehydration – the "dehydration myth" (Noakes 1995, 2004a, 2006b; Noakes & Speedy 2006, 2007) – from other athletes, coaches, race organizers, well-meaning exercise scientists and sports physicians, and the sports media, including advertisements sponsored by the sports drinks industry, all of which take their direction from the apparently authoritative and widely circulated guidelines of the ACSM and other influential organizations, such as the International Olympic Committee. Currently, only the US Army has issued a firm directive distancing itself from the "the maximal amount that can be tolerated" dictum. Thus: "The dangers of drinking too much water (>1–1.5 quarts·h^{-1} [~900–1350 mL·h^{-1}]) in attempts to prevent exertional heat illness must be made known to all personnel of all services, particularly those involved in training" (Gardner 2002).

If further deaths from this preventable condition are to be avoided, most especially in the USA, more rational, evidence-based advice must be given to all exercisers but most especially to recreational marathon runners. In particular, all exercisers, but female marathon runners particularly, need to be warned that the overconsumption of fluid, either water or sports drinks, before, during, or after exercise, is unnecessary and can have a potentially fatal outcome. Perhaps the best advice is that drinking according to the personal dictates of thirst (*ad libitum*) appears to be both safe and effective.

Furthermore, there is a need to ensure that sports physicians do not assume that athletes collapse after exercise because they are dehydrated and are therefore in need of rapid intravenous fluid replacement. Rather, there is no evidence that dehydration contributes to post-exercise collapse in athletes and current guidelines emphasize that most such collapses are caused by the onset of post-exercise postural hypotension, for which the most appropriate treatment is simply nursing in the head-down position. Intravenous fluid therapy must be reserved only for those conditions for which there is valid proof that such treatment is beneficial.

References

Adolph, E.F. (1947a) *Physiology of Man in the Desert*. Interscience Publishers, New York.

Adolph, E.F. (1947b) Water metabolism. *Annual Review of Physiology* **9**, 381–408.

Allred, E.N., Bleecker, E.R., Chaitman, B.R., *et al.* (1989) Short-term effects of carbon monoxide exposure on the exercise performance of subjects with coronary artery disease. *New England Journal of Medicine* **321**, 1426–1432.

American College of Sports Medicine, American Dietetic Association and Dietitians of Canada (2000) Joint Position Statement: nutrition and athletic performance. *Medicine and Science in Sports and Exercise* **32**, 2130–2145.

Armstrong, L.E., Epstein, Y., Greenleaf, J.E., *et al.* (1996) American College of Sports Medicine position stand. Heat and cold illnesses during distance running. *Medicine and Science in Sports and Exercise* **28**, i–x.

Aronow, W.S. & Cassidy, J. (1975) Effect of carbon monoxide on maximal treadmill exercise. A study in normal persons. *Annals of Internal Medicine* **83**, 496–499.

Austin, J.B., Russell, G., Adam, M.G., Mackintosh, D., Kelsey, S. & Peck, D.F. (1994) Prevalence of asthma and wheeze in the Highlands of Scotland. *Archives of Diseases in Children* **71**, 211–216.

Baker, L.B., Munce, T.A. & Kenney, W.L. (2005) Sex differences in voluntary fluid intake by older adults during exercise. *Medicine and Science in Sports and Exercise* **37**, 789–796.

Bigland-Ritchie, B. & Vollestadt, N. (1988) Hypoxia and fatigue: How are they related? In: *Hypoxia: The Tolerable Limits* (Sutton, J.R., Houston, C.S. & Coates, G., eds.) Benchmark, Indianapolis, IL: 315–325.

Binkley, H.M., Beckett, J., Casa, D.J., Kleiner, D.M. & Plummer, P.E. (2002) National Athletic Trainers' Association Position Statement: Exertional Heat Illnesses. *Journal of Athletic Training* **37**, 329–343.

Bishop, D. (2004) The effects of travel on team performance in the Australian national netball competition. *Journal of Science and Medicine in Sport* **7**, 118–122.

Bramble, D.M. & Lieberman, D.E. (2004) Endurance running and the evolution of Homo. *Nature* **432**, 345–352.

Bryant, J. (2005) *The London Marathon: The History of the Greatest Race on Earth*. Hutchinson, London.

Buskirk, E.R. & Beetham, W.P.J. (1960) Dehydration and body temperature as a result of marathon running. *Medicina Sportiva* **14**, 493–506.

Buskirk, E.R., Iampietro, P.F. & Bass, D.E. (1958) Work performance after dehydration: effects of physical conditioning and heat acclimatization. *Journal of Applied Physiology* **12**, 189–194.

Byrne, C., Lee, J.K., Chew, S.A., Lim, C.L. & Tan, E.Y. (2006) Continuous thermoregulatory responses to mass-participation distance running in heat. *Medicine and Science in Sports and Exercise* **38**, 803–810.

Cade, J.R., Free, H.J., De Quesada, A.M., Shires, D.L. & Roby, L. (1971) Changes in body fluid composition and volume during vigorous exercise by athletes. *Journal of Sports Medicine and Physical Fitness* **11**, 172–178.

Cade, R., Packer, D., Zauner, C., *et al.* (1992) Marathon running: physiological and chemical changes accompanying late-race functional deterioration. *European Journal of Applied Physiology and Occupational Physiology* **65**, 485–491.

Cade, R., Spooner, G., Schlein, E., Pickering, M. & Dean, R. (1972) Effect of fluid, electrolyte, and glucose replacement during exercise on performance, body temperature, rate of sweat loss, and compositional changes of extracellular fluid. *Journal of Sports Medicine and Physical Fitness* **12**, 150–156.

Campbell, M.E., Li, Q., Gingrich, S.E., Macfarlane, R.G. & Cheng, S. (2005) Should people be physically active outdoors on smog alert days? *Canadian Journal of Public Health* **96**, 24–28.

Casa, D.J., Armstrong, L.E. & Hillman, S.K. (2000) National Athletic Trainers Association Position Statement: Fluid replacement for athletes. *Journal of Athletic Training* **35**, 212–224.

Cheuvront, S.N., Carter, R. III & Sawka, M.N. (2003) Fluid balance and endurance exercise performance. *Current Sports Medicine Reports* **2**, 202–208.

Convertino, V.A., Armstrong, L.E., Coyle, E.F., *et al.* (1996) American College of Sports Medicine position stand. Exercise and fluid replacement. *Medicine and Science in Sports and Exercise* **28**, I–vii.

Costill, D.L., Kammer, W.F. & Fisher, A. (1970) Fluid ingestion during distance running. *Archives of Environmental Health* **21**, 520–525.

Coyle, E.F. (2004a) Fluid and fuel intake during exercise. *Journal of Sports Sciences* **22**, 39–55.

Coyle, E.F. (2004b) Fluid and fuel intake during exercise. In: *Food, Nutrition and Sports Performance II* (Maughan, R.J., Burke, L.M. & Coyle, E.F., eds.) Routledge, London: 63–91.

Dill, D.B. (1938) *Life, Heat and Altitude*. Harvard University Press, Cambridge, MA.

Dugas, J.P. (2006) Sodium ingestion and hyponatraemia: sports drinks do not prevent a fall in serum sodium concentration during exercise. *British Journal of Sports Medicine* **40**, 372–374.

Dugas, J.P., Oosthuizen, V., Tucker, R. & Noakes, T.D. (2006) Drinking "ad libitum" optimises performance and physiological function during 80 km indoor cycling trials in hot and humid conditions with appropriate convective cooling. *Medicine and Science in Sports and Exercise* **38**, S176.

Edwards, H.T. (1936) Lactic acid in rest and work at high altitude. *American Journal of Physiology* **116**, 367–375.

Eichna, L.W., Bean, W.B., Ashe, W.F. & Nelson, N. (1945) Performance in relation to environmental temperature. *Bulletin of Johns Hopkins Hospital* **76**, 25–58.

Eichna, L.W. & Horvath, S.M. (1947) Post-exertional orthostatic hypotension. *American Journal of Medicine and Science* **213**, 641–654.

Fotheringham, W. (2002) *Put Me Back on my Bike: In Search of Tom Simpson*. Yellow Jersey Press, London, UK.

Foxcroft, W.J. & Adams, W.C. (1986) Effects of ozone exposure on four consecutive days on work performance and $\dot{V}o_{2max}$. *Journal of Applied Physiology* **61**, 960–966.

Frizzell, R.T., Lang, G.H., Lowance, D.C. & Lathan, S.R. (1986) Hyponatremia and ultramarathon running. *Journal of the American Medical Association* **255**, 772–774.

Gardner, J.W. (2002) Death by water intoxication. *Military Medicine* **167**, 432–434.

Gisolfi, C.V. (1996) Fluid balance for optimal performance. *Nutrition Reviews* **54**, S159–S168.

Glace, B., Murphy, C. & McHugh, M. (2002a) Food and fluid intake and disturbances in gastrointestinal and mental function during an ultramarathon. *International Journal of Sport Nutrition and Exercise Metabolism* **12**, 414–427.

Glace, B.W., Murphy, C.A. & McHugh, M.P. (2002b) Food intake and electrolyte status of ultramarathoners competing in extreme heat. *Journal of the American College of Nutrition* **21**, 553–559.

Glaser, E.M. (1950) Immersion and survival in cold water. *Nature* **166**, 1068.

Golden, F.S. & Tipton, M.J. (1987) Human thermal responses during leg-only exercise in cold water. *Journal of Physiology* **391**, 399–405.

Goldman, R.F. (2001) Introduction to heat-related problems in military operations. In: *Medical Aspects of Harsh Environments* (Pandolf, K.B. & Burr, R.E., eds.) Office of The Surgeon General Department of the Army, Washington DC: 3–49.

Heinrich, B. (2001) *Racing the Antelope*. Harper Collins, New York.

Hew-Butler, T.D., Almond, C.S., Ayus, J.C., *et al.* (2005) Consensus Document of the 1st International Exercise-Associated Hyponatremia (EAH) Consensus Symposium, Cape Town, South Africa 2005. *Clinical Journal of Sport Medicine* **15**, 207–213.

Hew-Butler, T.D., Verbalis, J.G. & Noakes, T.D. (2006) Defending plasma osmolality and plasma volume: Updated fluid recommendations from the International Marathon Medical Directors Association. *Clinical Journal of Sport Medicine* **16**, 283–292.

Holtzhausen, L.M. & Noakes, T.D. (1995) The prevalence and significance of post-exercise (postural) hypotension in ultramarathon runners. *Medicine and Science in Sports and Exercise* **27**, 1595–1601.

Holtzhausen, L.M. & Noakes, T.D. (1997) Collapsed ultraendurance athlete: proposed mechanisms and an approach to management. *Clinical Journal of Sport Medicine* **7**, 292–301.

Holtzhausen, L.M., Noakes, T.D., Kroning, B., de Klerk, M., Roberts, M. & Emsley, R. (1994) Clinical and biochemical characteristics of collapsed ultra-marathon runners. *Medicine and Science in Sports and Exercise* **26**, 1095–1101.

Hopkins, P.M. & Ellis, F.R., eds. (1996) *Hyperthermic and Hypermetabolic Disorders: Exertional Heat-Stroke, Malignant Hyperthermia and Related Syndromes*. Cambridge University Press, London.

Hornbein, T.F. (1980) *Everest: The West Ridge*. Mountaineers, Seattle.

Horstman, D.H., Folinsbee, L.J., Ives, P.J., Abdul-Salaam, S. & McDonnell, W.F. (1990) Ozone concentration and pulmonary response relationships for 6.6-hour exposures with 5 hours of moderate exercise to 0.08, 0.10, and 0.12 ppm. *American Review of Respiratory Disease* **142**, 1158–1163.

Kayser, B. (2003) Exercise starts and ends in the brain. *European Journal of Applied Physiology* **90**, 411–419.

Kayser, B., Narici, M., Binzoni, T., Grassi, B. & Cerretelli, P. (1994) Fatigue and exhaustion in chronic hypobaric hypoxia: influence of exercising muscle mass. *Journal of Applied Physiology* **76**, 634–640.

Keatinge, W.R., Prys-Roberts, C., Cooper, K.E., Honour, A.J. & Haight, J. (1969) Sudden failure of swimming in cold water. *British Medical Journal* **1**, 480–483.

Kenney, W.L., DeGroot, D.W. & Holowatz, L.A. (2004) Extremes of human heat tolerance: Life at the precipice of thermoregulatory failure. *Journal of Thermal Biology* **29**, 479–485.

Kozlowski, S. & Saltin, B. (1964) Effect of sweat loss on body fluids. *Journal of Applied Physiology* **19**, 1119–1124.

Krakauer, J. (1997) *Into Thin Air*. Villard, New York.

Ladell, W.S. (1955) The effects of water and salt intake upon the performance of men working in hot and humid environments. *Journal of Physiology* **127**, 11–46.

Ladell, W.S. (1957) Disorders due to heat. *Transactions of the Royal Society of Tropical Medicine and Hygiene* **51**, 189–207.

Ledingham, I.M., MacVicar, S., Watt, I. & Weston, G.A. (1982) Early resuscitation after marathon collapse. *Lancet* **2**, 1096–1097.

Levine, B.D. & Stray-Gundersen, J. (2005) Point: positive effects of intermittent hypoxia (live high: train low) on exercise performance are mediated primarily by augmented red cell volume. *Journal of Applied Physiology* **99**, 2053–2055.

Martin, D.E. & Gynn, R.W.H. (2000) *The Olympic Marathon*. Human Kinetics, Champaign, IL.

McConnell, R., Berhane, K., Gilliland, F., *et al.* (2002) Asthma in exercising children exposed to ozone: A cohort study. *Lancet* **359**, 386–391.

Messner, R. (1979) *Everest: Expedition to the Ultimate*. Kaye & Ward, London.

Millard-Stafford, M., Sparling, P.B., Rosskopf, L.B., Snow, T.K., DiCarlo, L.J. & Hinson, B.T. (1995) Fluid intake in male and female runners during a 40-km field run in the heat. *Journal of Sports Sciences* **13**, 257–263.

Montain, S.J. & Coyle, E.F. (1992) Influence of graded dehydration on hyperthermia and cardiovascular drift during exercise.

Journal of Applied Physiology **73**, 1340–1350.

Muir, A.L., Percy-Robb, I.W., Davidson, I.A., Walsh, E.G. & Passmore, R. (1970) Physiological aspects of the Edinburgh Commonwealth Games. *Lancet* **2**, 1125–1128.

Muldoon, S., Deuster, P., Brandom, B. & Bunger, R. (2004) Is there a link between malignant hyperthermia and exertional heat illness? *Exercise and Sport Sciences Reviews* **32**, 174–179.

Nadel, E.R., Fortney, S.M. & Wenger, C.B. (1980) Effect of hydration state on circulatory and thermal regulations. *Journal of Applied Physiology* **49**, 715–721.

Nadel, E.R., Holmer, I., Bergh, U., Astrand, P.O. & Stolwijk, J.A. (1974) Energy exchanges of swimming man. *Journal of Applied Physiology* **36**, 465–471.

Ng'ang'a, L.W., Odhiambo, J.A., Mungai, M.W., *et al.* (1998) Prevalence of exercise induced bronchospasm in Kenyan school children: an urban–rural comparison. *Thorax* **53**, 919–926.

Nielsen, B. (1938) Die regulation der körpertemperatur bei muskelarbeit. *Skandinavisches Archiv für Physiologie* **79**, 195–230.

Nielsen, B., Hansen, G., Jorgensen, S.O. & Nielsen, E. (1971) Thermoregulation in exercising man during dehydration and hyperhydration with water and saline. *International Journal of Biometeorology* **15**, 195–200.

Noakes, T.D. (1982) Letter: Heatstroke during the 1981 National Cross-Country Running Championships. *South African Medical Journal* **61**, 145.

Noakes, T.D. (1993) Fluid replacement during exercise. *Exercise and Sport Sciences Reviews* **21**, 297–330.

Noakes, T.D. (1995) Dehydration during exercise: what are the real dangers? *Clinical Journal of Sport Medicine* **5**, 123–128.

Noakes, T.D. (2000a) Exercise and the cold. *Ergonomics* **43**, 1461–1479.

Noakes, T.D. (2000b) Hyperthermia, hypothermia and problems of hydration in the endurance performer. In: *Endurance in Sport* (Shephard, R.J. & Astrand, P.O., eds.) Blackwell, London: 591–613.

Noakes, T.D. (2003a) Fluid replacement during marathon running. *Clinical Journal of Sport Medicine* **13**, 309–318.

Noakes, T.D. (2003b) Overconsumption of fluids by athletes. *British Medical Journal* **327**, 113–114.

Noakes, T.D. (2003c) The forgotten Barcroft/Edholm reflex: potential role in exercise associated collapse. *British Journal of Sports Medicine* **37**, 277–278.

Noakes, T.D. (2004a) Can we trust rehydration research? In: *Philosophy and Sciences of Exercise, Sports and Health* (McNamee, M., ed.) Taylor & Francis Books (UK), Abingdon, Oxfordshire, UK: 144–168.

Noakes, T.D. (2004b) Sodium ingestion and the intervention of hyponatraemia during exercise. *British Journal of Sports Medicine* **38**, 790–792.

Noakes, T.D. (2004c) Tainted glory: doping and athletic performance. *New England Journal of Medicine* **351**, 847–849.

Noakes, T.D. (2005) Comments on Point: Counterpoint "Positive effects of intermittent hypoxia (live high:train low) on exercise performance are/are not mediated primarily by augmented red cell volume." *Journal of Applied Physiology* **99**, 2453.

Noakes T.D. (2006a) Exercise in the heat: Old ideas, new dogmas. *International SportMed Journal*. Available from: http://www.ismj.com/default.asp?pageID=945606131.

Noakes, T.D. (2006b) Sports drinks: prevention of "voluntary dehydration" and development of exercise-associated hyponatremia. *Medicine and Science in Sports and Exercise* **38**, 193.

Noakes, T.D. (2007) Drinking guidelines for exercise: What is the evidence that athletes should either drink "as much as tolerable" or "to replace all the weight lost during exercise" or "ad libitum." *Journal of Sports Sciences* **25**, 781–796.

Noakes, T.D., Adams, B.A., Myburgh, K.H., Greeff, C., Lotz, T. & Nathan, M. (1988) The danger of an inadequate water intake during prolonged exercise. A novel concept re-visited. *European Journal of Applied Physiology and Occupational Physiology* **57**, 210–219.

Noakes, T.D., Calbet, J.A., Boushel, R., *et al.* (2004a) Central regulation of skeletal muscle recruitment explains the reduced maximal cardiac output during exercise in hypoxia. *American Journal of Physiology-Regulatory Integrative and Comparative Physiology* **287**, R996–R999.

Noakes, T.D. & Glace, B. (2004b) Letters to the Editors. *International Journal of Sports Nutrition and Exercise Metabolism* **14**, 249–254.

Noakes, T.D., Goodwin, N., Rayner, B.L., Branken, T. & Taylor, R.K. (1985) Water intoxication: a possible complication during endurance exercise. *Medicine and Science in Sports and Exercise* **17**, 370–375.

Noakes, T.D., Myburgh, K.H., du Plessis, J., *et al.* (1991) Metabolic rate, not percent dehydration, predicts rectal temperature in marathon runners. *Medicine and Science in Sports and Exercise* **23**, 443–449.

Noakes, T.D., Sharwood, K., Speedy, D., *et al.* (2005a) Three independent biological mechanisms cause exercise-associated hyponatremia: evidence from 2135 weighed competitive athletic performances. *Proceedings of the National Academy of Sciences of the USA* **102**, 18550–18555.

Noakes, T.D. & Speedy, D.B. (2006) Case proven: exercise associated hyponatraemia is due to overdrinking. So why did it take 20 years before the original evidence was accepted? *British Journal of Sports Medicine* **40**, 567–572.

Noakes, T.D. & Speedy, D.B. (2007) Lobbyists for the sports drink industry: an example of the rise of "contrarianism" in modern scientific debate. *British Journal of Sports Medicine* **41**, 107–109.

Noakes, T.D. & St. Clair Gibson, A. (2004c) Logical limitations to the "catastrophe" models of fatigue during exercise in humans. *British Journal of Sports Medicine* **38**, 648–649.

Noakes, T.D., St. Clair Gibson, A. & Lambert, E.V. (2005b) From catastrophe to complexity: a novel model of integrative central neural regulation of effort and fatigue during exercise in humans: summary and conclusions. *British Journal of Sports Medicine* **39**, 120–124.

Nybo, L. & Nielsen, B. (2001) Hyperthermia and central fatigue during prolonged exercise in humans. *Journal of Applied Physiology* **91**, 1055–1060.

O'Connor, P.J. & Morgan, W.P. (1990) Athletic performance following rapid traversal of multiple time zones. A review. *Sports Medicine* **10**, 20–30.

O'Donnell, T.F. Jr. & Clowes, G.H. Jr. (1972) The circulatory abnormalities of heat stroke. *New England Journal of Medicine* **287**, 734–737.

Pitts, G.C., Johnson, R.E. & Consolazio, F.C. (1944) Work in the heat as affected by intake of water, salt and glucose. *American Journal of Physiology* **142**, 253–259.

Pugh, L.G. (1966) Accidental hypothermia in walkers, climbers, and campers: report to the Medical Commission on Accident Prevention. *British Medical Journal* **5480**, 123–129.

Pugh, L.G. (1967) Cold stress and muscular exercise, with special reference to accidental hypothermia. *British Medical Journal* **2**, 333–337.

Pugh, L.G., Corbett, J.L. & Johnson, R.H. (1967) Rectal temperatures, weight losses, and sweat rates in marathon running. *Journal of Applied Physiology* **23**, 347–352.

Pugh, L.G. & Edholm, O.G. (1955) The physiology of channel swimmers. *Lancet* **269**, 761–768.

Pugh, L.G., Edholm, O.G., Fox, R.H., *et al.* (1960) A physiological study of channel swimming. *Clinical Science* **19**, 257–273.

Pugh, L.G.C.E. (1971) Deaths from exposure on Four Inns Walking Competition, March 14–15, 1964. In: *Exercise and Cardiac Death* (Jokl, E. & McClellan, J.T., eds.) University Park Press, Baltimore, MD: 112–120.

Robinson, T.A., Hawley, J.A., Palmer, G.S., *et al.* (1995) Water ingestion does not improve 1-h cycling performance in moderate ambient temperatures. *European Journal of Applied Physiology and Occupational Physiology* **71**, 153–160.

Rothstein, A. & Towbin, E.J. (1947) Blood circulation and temperature of men dehydrating in the heat. In: *Physiology of Man in the Desert*. Interscience Publishers, New York: 172–196.

Rovell, D. (2005) *First in Thirst. How Gatorade turned the science of sweat into a cultural phenomenon*. Amacom, New York.

Sandell, R.C., Pascoe, M.D. & Noakes, T.D. (1988) Factors associated with collapse during and after ultramarathon footraces: A preliminary study. *Physician and Sportsmedicine* **16**, 86–94.

Saunders, A.G., Dugas, J.P., Tucker, R., Lambert, M.I. & Noakes, T.D. (2005) The effects of different air velocities on heat storage and body temperature in humans cycling in a hot, humid environment. *Acta Physiologica Scandinavica* **183**, 241–255.

Sawka, M.N., Knowlton, R.G. & Critz, J.B. (1979) Thermal and circulatory responses to repeated bouts of prolonged running. *Medicine and Science in Sports* **11**, 177–180.

Sawka, M.N., Latzka, W.A., Matott, R.P. & Montain, S.J. (1998) Hydration effects on temperature regulation. *International Journal of Sports Medicine* **19** (Supplement 2), S108–S110.

Sawka, M.N. & Montain, S.J. (2000) Fluid and electrolyte supplementation for exercise heat stress. *American Journal of Clinical Nutrition* **72**, 564S–572S.

Sawka, M.N., Toner, M.M., Francesconi, R.P. & Pandolf, K.B. (1983) Hypohydration and exercise: effects of heat acclimation, gender, and environment. *Journal of Applied Physiology* **55**, 1147–1153.

Sawka, M.N., Young, A.J., Francesconi, R.P., Muza, S.R. & Pandolf, K.B. (1985) Thermoregulatory and blood responses during exercise at graded hypohydration levels. *Journal of Applied Physiology* **59**, 1394–1401.

Schmidt-Nielsen, K. (1964) *Desert Animals*. Oxford University Press, London.

Sharwood, K.A., Collins, M., Goedecke, J.H., Wilson, G. & Noakes, T.D. (2004) Weight changes, medical complications, and performance during an Ironman triathlon. *British Journal of Sports Medicine* **38**, 718–724.

Sharwood, K.A., Lambert, M.I., St. Clair, G.A. & Noakes, T.D. (2002) Changes in oxygen consumption during and after a downhill run in masters long-distance runners. *Clinical Journal of Sport Medicine* **12**, 308–312.

Shibasaki, M., Kondo, N. & Crandall, C.G. (2003) Non-thermoregulatory modulation of sweating in humans. *Exercise and Sports Science Reviews* **31**, 34–39.

St. Clair Gibson, A. & Noakes, T.D. (2004) Evidence for complex system integration and dynamic neural regulation of skeletal muscle recruitment during exercise in humans. *British Journal of Sports Medicine* **38**, 797–806.

Stover, E.A., Zachwieja, J., Stofan, J., Murray, R. & Horswill, C.A. (2006) Consistently high urine specific gravity in adolescent American football players and the impact of an acute drinking strategy. *International Journal of Sports Medicine* **27**, 330–335.

Timonen, K.L., Pekkanen, J., Tiittanen, P. & Salonen, R.O. (2002) Effects of air pollution on changes in lung function induced by exercise in children with chronic respiratory symptoms. *Occupational and Environmental Medicine* **59**, 129–134.

Tipton, M.J. (1989) The initial responses to cold-water immersion in man. *Clinical Science (London)* **77**, 581–588.

Tipton, M.J. & Golden, F.S.T.C. (1998) Immersion in cold water: Effects on performance and safety. In: *Oxford Textbook of Sports Medicine* (Harries, M., Williams, C., Stanish, W.D. & Micheli, L.J., eds.) Oxford University Press, Oxford: 241–254.

Todd, J. & Todd, T. (2001) Significant events in the history of drug testing and the Olympic movement: 1960–1999. In: *Doping in Elite Sport: The Politics of Drugs in the Olympic Movement*. Human Kinetics, Champaign, IL: 65–128.

Toner, M.M., Sawka, M.N. & Pandolf, K.B. (1984) Thermal responses during arm and leg and combined arm-leg exercise in water. *Journal of Applied Physiology* **56**, 1355–1360.

Tucker, R., Marle, T., Lambert, E.V. & Noakes, T.D. (2006) The rate of heat storage mediates an anticipatory reduction in exercise intensity during cycling at a fixed rating of perceived exertion. *Journal of Physiology* **574**, 905–915.

Tucker, R., Rauch, L., Harley, Y.X. & Noakes, T.D. (2004) Impaired exercise performance in the heat is associated with an anticipatory reduction in skeletal muscle recruitment. *Pflugers Archives* **448**, 422–430.

Winslow, C.E.A., Herrington, L.P. & Gagge, A.P. (1937) Physiological reactions of the human body to varying environmental temperatures. *American Journal of Physiology* **120**, 1–22.

Wyndham, C.H. & Strydom, N.B. (1969) The danger of an inadequate water intake during marathon running. *South African Medical Journal* **43**, 893–896.

Zanobetti, A., Canner, M.J., Stone, P.H., *et al.* (2004) Ambient pollution and blood pressure in cardiac rehabilitation patients. *Circulation* **110**, 2184–2189.

Chapter 17

Drugs in Sport

DON H. CATLIN, GARY GREEN AND CAROLINE K. HATTON

The beginnings

Since the very beginnings of competition, sport and doping have walked hand in hand. Ancient Olympians raised their achievement level by eating bread soaked in opium. The Incas chewed coca leaves to sustain an enormous work effort. Berserkers ate mushrooms containing muscarine before battle. Shortly after amphetamine, strychnine, and ephedrine became available as pharmaceuticals in the 1800s, there were reports of abuse by canal swimmers in the Netherlands and cyclists in America and Europe. To provide perspective on the issue, consider the following quote from a concerned scientist written almost 70 years ago: "There can be no doubt that stimulants are today widely used by athletes participating in competitions; the record-breaking craze and the desire to satisfy an exacting public play a more and more prominent role, and take higher rank than the health of the competitors itself" (Boje 1939). In today's world, daily doping headlines are the norm.

The International Olympic Committee (IOC) was in charge of doping matters until 1999 when it developed the World Anti-Doping Agency (WADA) to take over the operation of a worldwide year-round anti-doping program. There is a concerted effort led by WADA to harmonize the doping rules across sports and countries. Despite very complicated international issues and bewildering rules promulgated by dozens of sport organizations,

WADA is making excellent progress toward harmonization. It has found a prominent place in the family of world organizations. In large part this is likely because of the desperate need for order, brilliance, and organization in the field.

The physician and doping control

In the early days of doping control, the physician, and particularly the sports medicine physician, was the central figure. As drug use, drug testing, and doping control in sport became increasingly complicated, administrators became necessary. Nowadays anti-doping policies are set mostly by administrators. It is critical to refocus on the need for physician participation in this unique specialty. The more complicated the issues surrounding the use or abuse of medications become, the greater the need for medical expertise.

Physicians in general, including those in sports medicine, take responsibility for the overall medical management of their patients and make the ultimate health care recommendations. This arises from the physician–patient relationship where the physician's duty is to protect the health of the patient, who happens to be a competitive athlete. However, within the sports medicine environment there are issues relating to drug use that affect both the athlete and team physician that may strain the relationship. For example, short- and long-term health risks may not be of paramount importance to the athlete, who is only concerned with performance. However, a physician may serve a sports organization or team whose interests conflict with the athlete's health

The Olympic Textbook of Medicine in Sport, 1st edition. Edited by M. Schwellnus. Published 2008 by Blackwell Publishing, ISBN: 978-1-4051-5637-0.

needs. These are only some of the factors that complicate the relationship and, as a result, the physician has become one element of the doping control process, rather than the sole authority.

Some physicians who have provided athletes with banned substances, have used the doctor–patient relationship as a justification for their actions. Hoberman (2002) notes that some physicians have maintained that the doctor–patient relationship trumps any doping control regulations. This view is certainly losing ground but it would be unrealistic to expect that it would disappear.

Because physicians are inherently capable of aiding athletes to enhance their performance, the fact that they are asked to do so is nothing new. In Ancient Greece, where medicines were traditionally dispensed by physicians, they were approached by athletes to supply ergogenic aids. This is still the case today, as shown by the 2006 National Collegiate Athletic Association Survey of Use and Abuse Habits of Collegiate Athletes (Green *et al.* 2001b). For anabolic steroid users, physicians were the suppliers of anabolic androgenic steroids (AAS) in 13% of the cases.

Although team physicians are usually not the final authority with respect to drug use in athletes, they have a central role in the use and abuse of drugs by athletes. Physicians are critical educators, with unique insight into the patient and the science. In addition to the caring role, physicians act as medical directors, medical review officers for drug testing, and provide therapeutic use exemptions (TUEs). It is therefore imperative that physicians who serve as team physicians be familiar with the drugs used by athletes, their effects, doping control regulations, and ethical boundaries. The high profile nature of sports medicine is a dual-edged sword as mistakes are often magnified. At the 2000 Summer Olympics, a Romanian team physician inadvertently provided a gymnast with pseudoephedrine, which was banned at that time, leading to her disqualification and medal loss, as well as his own 4-year suspension. Although this chapter provides a current overview for the team physician, the rapidly changing landscape of drug use in sports necessitates constant attention to emerging trends and regulations.

Sports pharmacology and doping categories

WADA has established international standards for doping control, including an extensive prohibited list which is divided into the categories of drugs and methods shown in Table 17.1 (World Anti-Doping Agency 2006). While this is useful as a classification scheme and for drug testing, it has less utility for the clinician attempting to diagnose, treat, and prevent drug use in an athlete. Sports pharmacology classifies drugs according to their reason for use, rather than by their chemical structure, mechanism of action, or pharmacologic effects. For example, a traditional system would group all stimulant drugs together. In sports pharmacology, a drug is classified as ergogenic, recreational, or therapeutic depending on the main reason why the athlete has chosen to use it.

Ergogenic drugs are defined here as substances that are taken for the sole intention of increasing performance (e.g., a body builder taking anabolic steroids in order to increase muscle mass or a marathon runner transfusing a unit of blood just before a race). Although most ergogenic drugs have multiple uses, sports pharmacology classifies a drug according to the athlete's main reason for use. As an example, the 2005 NCAA Study asked anabolic steroid users their reasons for using AAS and the two leading responses were 51% for athletic performance enhancement and 16% to improve physical appearance (NCAA Study Staff 2006).

Recreational drugs are the next category. Athletes are similar to their non-athlete peers in their reasons for using these drugs: to relieve stress, to escape, as a social drug, or as a stimulant or depressant. Being an athlete does not create immunity from the physical or psychologic effects of these drugs, including addiction. For example, the 2005 NCAA survey regarding marijuana asked for the reason for use (NCAA Study Staff 2006). A whopping 93% answered for recreational purposes or to feel good, with only 0.9% using it to improve athletic performance.

The final category is therapeutic drugs and these are taken to treat an underlying condition (e.g., type 1 diabetic athlete using insulin). Although some of these drugs are banned by sports organizations,

Table 17.1 World Anti-Doping Agency (WADA) 2006 prohibited list. Adapted from World Anti-Doping Code (2006) Prohibited List. www.wada-ama.org/rtecontent/document/2006_LIST.pdf [Accessed August 25, 2006].

Prohibited substances

S1. Anabolic agents	1. Anabolic androgenic steroids (AAS)
	(a) Exogenous AAS
	(b) Endogenous AAS
	2. Other anabolic agents
	e.g., clenbuterol, zeranol, zilpaterol
S2. Hormones and related substances	1. Erythropoietin
	2. Growth hormone, insulin-like growth factor
	3. Gonadotropins
	4. Insulin
	5. Corticotrophins
S3. β_2-Agonists	
S4. Agents with anti-estrogenic activity	1. Aromatase inhibitors
	2. Estrogen receptor modulators
	3. Other anti-estrogenic substances
S5. Diuretics and other masking agents	
S6. Stimulants	
S7. Narcotics	
S8. Cannabinoids	
S9. Glucocorticosteroids	

Prohibited methods
M1. Enhancement of oxygen transfer
M2. Chemical and physical manipulation
M3. Gene doping

Substances prohibited in particular sports
P1. Alcohol
P2. Beta-blockers

TUEs are generally allowed if they meet certain criteria, which are discussed in this chapter. Although the distinction between therapeutic and ergogenic use is generally clear, the team physician may be involved in the resolution of complicated cases.

It is thus possible under sports pharmacology to classify a single drug in multiple categories depending on the rationale for use. For example, the central nervous system stimulants amphetamines can be used for many different purposes. They are used by athletes in endurance sports, such as cycling, as an ergogenic aid to increase alertness and delay fatigue. Amphetamines in the form of methamphetamine (often called meth, crystal meth, or ice) are used recreationally by athletes as a euphoriant and can lead to increasing use and addiction.

Amphetamines can be used therapeutically to treat attention deficit, hyperactivity disorder (ADHD) with drugs such as amphetamine/dextroamphetamine combinations or methylphenidate to help with concentration during school.

In this chapter we use the WADA Prohibited List as the major subchapter headings. Each category will be discussed in terms of the mechanism of action, performance effects, adverse reactions, and reasons for use. Although the basic pharmacology of a drug is certainly important, understanding whether a drug is being used for ergogenic, recreational, or therapeutic reasons is a critical distinction in order to comprehend fully the complicated issue of drug use in athletes. It is through this broad approach that strategies aimed at reducing drug use can be developed and implemented.

Classes of doping agents

Anabolic androgenic steroids

Anabolic androgenic steroids (AAS) in sport began with surreptitious use by weightlifters and body builders in the 1950s and have entered into the lexicon and become cultural icons. There is a paradox in that AAS are banned by sports organizations, yet they are used as an adjective to describe something that is powerful and appealing. This was evidenced by a US NASA spokesman in 2005, who in his description of a new spaceship being developed that will fly to the Moon, asked people to think of it as the Apollo [rocket] on steroids (Pae 2005). There are many examples of AAS being used in the lay press to convey positive qualities; however, an athlete who tests positive for AAS is shunned by the public and often savaged by the media for breaking the rules of sport.

Although they are commonly referred to as "steroids," it is more accurate to refer to them as anabolic androgenic steroids to indicate that they result in both anabolic (increasing protein synthesis) and androgenic (expressing male secondary sex characteristics) effects. This also distinguishes these drugs from other steroid drugs, such as estrogens and glucocorticosteroids. The latter are a separate category of drugs and will be discussed later in the chapter.

In the early years of AAS research it was thought that the anabolic and androgenic effects were mediated at two different receptors; however, only one receptor has been identified and the search for a pure androgen or pure anabolic agent has been abandoned. Although there is a body of literature on the topic arising from research on small animals (Hershberger et al. 1953), there is no human equivalent. Although some drugs have been touted as having relatively greater anabolic properties than their androgenic ones, it appears that all AAS have both anabolic and androgenic effects in humans. In fact, most consequences of AAS use are anabolic in nature and act through a single androgen receptor. Further, some authors have even described typical androgenizing effects, such as male sexual organ regulation, as essentially an anabolic effect on the sex organs (Catlin 2005). There was much debate on the existence of separate anabolic and androgen receptors, but that has largely been disproved by the demonstration to date of a single androgen receptor. Evidence for this comes from many sources, but the strongest proof derives from the fact that patients with complete testicular feminization have high levels of testosterone and when given AAS develop neither anabolic nor androgenic effects (Strickland & French 1969).

AAS affect almost every organ, and androgen receptors have been identified in such diverse tissues as the reproductive organs, brain, kidneys, liver, skin, skeletal and cardiac muscle, bone, larynx, thymus, hematopoietic system, and lipid tissue (Catlin 2005). Once an AAS has entered the cell, it binds to the androgen receptor, which is located in the cytoplasmic compartment. Following that is a dissociation process and translocation to the nucleus. This eventually modulates androgen-responsive genes which regulate the expression of various proteins (Jasuja et al. 2005). Muscle biopsies from AAS – using power lifters – have demonstrated increases in muscle size resulting from both hypertrophy and the formation of new muscle fibers (Kadi et al. 1999). The anabolic or androgenic expression is thus solely dependent on the nature of the response of the target organ.

EFFECTS OF AAS ON MUSCLE AND PERFORMANCE

AAS use in athletes has been documented since the 1950s and the effects on muscle building and performance are well known to athletes and body builders. The *Underground Steroid Handbook* (Duchaine 1989), a how-to book on the use of AAS, was first published in 1988 and became the "bible" of AAS use among strength athletes and body builders. However, the scientific community did not acknowledge the effects of AAS for many years. Three years after Ben Johnson tested positive for stanozolol at the 1988 Olympics, a review article on the effects of AAS on muscular strength concluded, "Anabolic steroids may slightly enhance muscle strength in previously trained athletes. No firm conclusion is possible concerning their efficacy in enhancing overall athletic performance" (Elashoff *et al.* 1991). The main reason for this statement was that randomized controlled trials of AAS tended to use physiologic replacement doses in untrained subjects. It was not until 1996 that the first study established an increase in muscle size using supraphysiologic doses of testosterone in combination with a high protein diet and weight training in previously trained subjects (Bhasin *et al.* 1996). This critical paper finally confirmed that AAS do in fact increase lean body mass in normal subjects.

While there is no debate on the fact that supraphysiologic doses of AAS can increase muscle mass, the effects on actual performance are less clear. In many sports, performance is difficult to measure as it is influenced by many factors other than strength alone. Despite the ubiquitous use of strength training in athletes, there is a paucity of data to support its positive effects on performance. Studies have been limited to obvious targets, such as weightlifting and measuring acceleration in sprinters (Carlock *et al.* 2004; Sleivert & Taingahue 2004). There is an enormous amount of anecdotal information supporting the efficacy of AAS. One fascinating but disturbing source is the androgenization program fomented by the former German Democratic Republic (GDR) (Franke & Berendonk 1997). Based on various reports, it is clear that whole teams, such as women's swimming, were being given large amounts of AAS. In 1972, prior to the beginning of the androgenization program, GDR female swimmers won two individual silver medals, two bronze medals, and did not set any Olympic or World Records. Four years later, in 1976, following the doping program, the GDR female swimmers won 10 of the 11 individual gold medals and set 10 Olympic or World Records. Following the unification of the German Democratic Republic and Germany and disbanding of the androgenization program, the unified German women's swimming team won one gold, two silver, and four bronze medals and did not set an Olympic or World Record at the 1992 Summer Olympics.

TYPES OF AAS

There are two types of AAS: exogenous and endogenous compounds. Endogenous AAS are those that are naturally produced by the body in some amounts and are problematic for drug testing because their chemical structure is identical to that of naturally occurring compounds. The most commonly used endogenous AAS is testosterone. As an ester it can be injected into muscle, absorbed through the skin using a patch or gel, or across the buccal mucosa in the form of a pellet. Natural testosterone precursors, such as androstenedione and androstenediol, were available for sale in the USA until 2005 as nutritional supplements. These drugs when taken orally were found to transiently increase testosterone levels (Leder *et al.* 2001). Although closely related to these other compounds, dehydroepiandrosterone (DHEA) was not included in the 2004 US Anabolic Steroid Control Act and is still legally available as a nutritional supplement in the USA. (It has been on the WADA/IOC list since 1987.)

Owing to their chemical structure being identical to that of natural compounds, endogenous AAS sometimes present problems for doping control. Since 1982 the traditional method of distinguishing endogenous from pharmaceutical testosterone has been to measure the testosterone : epitestosterone (T : E) ratio in urine (Catlin *et al.* 1997). The median T : E is about 1; however, the values in males who have not used testosterone range from 0.2 to 6.0. A few males have even higher natural ratios. The application of exogenous testosterone will cause the T : E to rise by increasing testosterone and suppressing epitestosterone. According to WADA, a ratio greater than 4 : 1 requires investigation. In many WADA laboratories, gas chromatography-combustion-isotope ratio mass spectrometry (GC-C-IRMS or IRMS) is used to confirm that a banned substance was used. This technique determines if the steroid that is causing the elevated testeosterone arises from natural or pharmaceutical sources (Aguilera *et al.* 1999). In addition, laboratories also quantify the amount of epitestosterone to deter athletes from simultaneously taking both testosterone and epitestosterone in order to simultaneously increase both the testosterone and epitestosterone and thereby maintain a normal T : E ratio. Epitestosterone levels above 200 ng·mL^{-1} urine constitute a doping offense.

The 19-norsteroids have also caused some confusion because trace amounts of the nandrolone metabolite, 19-norandrosterone, has been detected in the urine of both men and women who have not used any 19-norsteroids (Le Bizec *et al.* 1999). The complexity results from the fact that 19-norandrosterone and 19-noretiocholanolone are also metabolites of several exogenous AAS, including nandrolone (19-nortestosterone), 19-norandrostenedione, and 19-norandrostenediol. As opposed to purely synthetic AAS, for which any amount of drug is prohibited, WADA has set a cut-off for 19-norandrosterone of 2 ng·mL^{-1}. That this level could be exceeded by orally ingesting small amounts of 19-norandrostenedione complicated doping control, especially prior to 2005 when its classification in the USA changed from an over-the-counter nutritional supplement to a controlled AAS (Catlin *et al.* 2000). IRMS has potential application to this area, but it has not been easy to develop a method that would detect 2 ng·mL^{-1} urinary 19-norandrosterone.

The second major type of AAS is exogenous or xenobiotic. These are products developed by the pharmaceutical industry to treat patients with various androgen states and a few other conditions. None of these AAS are produced in the body. Examples include methandienone (former brand name, Dianabol; black market name, D-bol), methyltestosterone, and stanozolol. Stanozolol, boldenone, trenbolone, and other AAS are available as veterinary products.

ADVERSE EFFECTS OF AAS

Any discussion of the adverse effects associated with AAS is complicated by the fact that randomized controlled trials using the dosages and combinations employed by athletes would be unethical. Supraphysiologic doses are required for muscle building in normal adults, and most randomized controlled trials of AAS have utilized physiologic doses for relatively short periods of time and studied only one AAS. A 2005 survey of 207 AAS users revealed that they had used an average of 3.1 AAS during their most recent cycle of drugs (Perry *et al.* 2005). The average cycle was 5–10 weeks and

involved doses that averaged 5–29 times normal physiologic replacement doses. Owing to ethical limitations, it is necessary then to extrapolate from therapeutic administration studies (i.e., low-dose, long-term use) of AAS and anecdotal reports of athletes abusing AAS.

AAS affect virtually every organ in the body and their effects can be divided into organic systemic, psychologic, sex-specific, and potential effects on immature individuals. The two systems that have been most studied are the cardiovascular and gastrointestinal systems. AAS affect the cardiovascular system by increasing total cholesterol, low-density lipoprotein (LDL) cholesterol and blood pressure, while lowering high-density lipoprotein (HDL) cholesterol. When these are combined with the pro-thrombotic effects of AAS, the risk of coronary artery disease dramatically increases. This has led to anecdotal reports of relatively young AAS users suffering myocardial infarctions (Huie 1994; Fineschi *et al.* 2001). There have also been reports of AAS-induced cardiomyopathy following prolonged use of supraphysiologic doses of the drugs (Nieminen *et al.* 1996; Vogt *et al.* 2002).

The liver is the main target organ for gastrointestinal effects of AAS. There are many reports and series of cases with hepatocellular dysfunction and peliosis hepatis. In addition, several types of hepatic neoplasms are associated with AAS including hepatocellular adenoma and carcinoma (Ishak & Zimmerman 1987). Almost all reports of serious hepatic dysfunction with elevated levels of serum enzymes are the result of the 17-alpha alkylated AAS. Steroid chemists working in the pharmaceutical industry added a methyl group to C-17 in order to resist first pass metabolism and inactivation by the liver. These types of AAS have a much greater potential for hepatic damage than the endogenous AAS. Files from the GDR revealed three deaths secondary to liver failure and several cases of severe liver disease (Franke & Berendonk 1997).

There are several other bodily systems that are purportedly affected by AAS use such as the musculoskeletal system and skin. There are multiple case reports of tendon ruptures that have been associated with AAS use and some animal studies have demonstrated structural changes in tendons following AAS use. However, a comparison of ruptured tendons in AAS users and non-users revealed no differences in histologic character (Evans *et al*. 1998). It may be that AAS increase the risk of tendon rupture through muscle hypertrophy without a corresponding increase in tendon strength. Regardless of the mechanism, a thorough history of AAS use should be carried out in unusual cases of tendon rupture. The skin will often be the most obvious organ affected and will display acne, striae, and abscesses, with the latter the result of injectable use.

The psychologic effects of AAS have also garnered attention because of their propensity to cause personality changes, hyperaggressiveness, and addiction. The former is complicated not only by lack of controlled studies, but the potential for pre-existing mental illness. Despite these limitations and conflicting data, a 2005 review found that AAS could cause aggressiveness, rage, delirium, depression, psychosis, and mania (Hall *et al*. 2005). The psychiatric effects also appear to be dose-dependent. Dependence and withdrawal are also controversial, but one study determined that 75% of AAS users met the criteria for dependence (Brower *et al*. 1990). There have also been several cases reported in the media of teenagers who became severely depressed shortly after discontinuing AAS use and committed suicide.

The endocrinologic effects of AAS are mainly related to dose and gender. For example, males produce about 7 mg·day^{-1} testosterone and females about one-tenth of that amount. Excessive doses administered to men will cause oligospermia, azoospermia, gynecomastia, and many more effects. Females will experience all of the virilizing effects of AAS, including male pattern alopecia, clitoromegaly, hirsutism, breast atrophy, as well as menstrual disturbances (Catlin 2005). In addition to their effects on the pituitary–gonadal axis, there is some evidence that AAS also impair thyroid function (Deyssig & Weissel 1993).

ANABOLIC AGENTS

There are some pharmacologic agents whose effects and usage patterns merit a special category, despite their apparent chemical similarity to other drugs. This is true of clenbuterol, zilpaterol, zeranol, and tibolone, drugs that are often classified as anabolic agents but, except for tibolone, are chemically unrelated to AAS. The first two are β_2-agonists. Zilpaterol is used as a feed additive for livestock and clenbuterol has been used in the treatment of asthma since 1977 in several countries. Clenbuterol became of concern as an ergogenic drug about the time of the 1992 Summer Olympic Games. Six athletes tested positive for it while preparing for those Games. At high doses, clenbuterol is considered a repartitioning agent because of its apparent ability to increase muscle mass and decrease fat deposits in animals, such as livestock (Spann & Winter 1995). Clenbuterol appears to affect muscle through muscle hypertrophy, favoring type 2 fast-twitch muscle over slow-twitch muscle and increasing the glycolytic capacity (Zeman *et al*. 1988). Similar effects have not been demonstrated in humans. Owing to the supposition that this is most likely mediated through β-receptors, it is felt that other β_2-agonists may possess similar ability. However, it is likely that in order to act as a partitioning agent, β_2-agonists would need to be given in large oral doses. The significant adverse effects of β_2-agonists at high levels, such as anxiety, tremor, and palpitations, would likely limit the dosage. There have been case reports of various types of chronic nephrotoxicity resulting from prolonged use of high-dose clenbuterol (Chan 1999; Hoffman *et al*. 2001).

The two other drugs listed in this category, zeranol and tibolone, are non-AAS hormones with the potential for anabolic activity. Zeranol is a synthetic compound related to phytoestrogens that has significant estrogenic potency. It is used in some countries as an anabolic growth promoter in beef cattle and significant concerns have been expressed about its effects on the consumers of the beef (Leffers *et al*. 2001).

Tibolone is a synthetic steroid with estrogenic, progestogenic, and mild androgenic properties when given via the oral route. It is used in females as a treatment for post-menopausal symptoms. The results of strength gains in post-menopausal women have been mixed with some increases in hand grip strength, but lack of effect in explosive leg strength or endurance (Meeuwsen *et al.* 2002a,b). Although there are no efficacy (performance enhancement) studies in athletes with any of these four drugs, there are reports of athletes using them for their potential benefits. Given that these drugs have limited therapeutic indications at this time, it is understandable to place them on the prohibited list.

Hormones and related substances

This category of drugs is perhaps the most difficult to define, and testing is problematic. The body naturally produces all of the drugs in this section and all have legitimate therapeutic indications for often life-threatening conditions. This creates a great deal of difficultly, not only in detection, but in sanctions and appeals. As the detection of synthetic agents, such as AAS, improves, this area continues to present a major challenge to doping control. The drugs in this category are all peptide and glycopeptide hormones, and with one exception, must be taken parenterally to be effective.

ERYTHROPOIETIN AND DARBEPOETIN ALFA

Recombinant human erythropoietin (rHuEPO) is perhaps the most abused drug available to the athlete (Catlin *et al.* 2006). Natural EPO is produced by the kidneys in response to changes in oxygen tension. It stimulates the formation of proerythroblasts and reticulocyte release from the bone marrow and increases red blood cell mass. The release of rHuEPO in 1987 as a pharmaceutical has led to very significant and tremendous advances in the treatment of anemia, especially secondary to renal failure, cancer, chemotherapy, and HIV infection. Given that $\dot{V}o_{2max}$ is dependent on the oxygen-carrying capacity of hemoglobin and that blood transfusions have attendant risks, it is not surprising that athletes rapidly gravitated to rHuEPO soon after its introduction to the market. Indeed, the release of the drug darbepoetin alfa, a long-acting form of EPO, in late 2001, was followed by positive drug tests for three athletes at the 2002 Winter Olympics in February 2002 (Catlin *et al.* 2002b). The enhanced endurance that accompanies increasing the red blood cell mass is well known. Many clinical experiments have shown that transfusions increase human performance (Buick *et al.* 1980). While the number of studies on the effect of rHuEPO on endurance performance are limited, it is clear from the available placebo-controlled literature that rHuEPO increased $\dot{V}o_{2max}$ by 6.0% to 7.7% after 3–4 weeks of subcutaneous administration of 150 $IU \cdot kg^{-1} \cdot week^{-1}$ (Russell *et al.* 2002).

The use of rHuEPO is not without risk, but it is very difficult to obtain trustworthy data on the true incidence of adverse effects. The propensity of athletes to titrate their hematocrits to high levels and to take rHuEPO without adequate medical supervision, together with their risk for iron disorders and exercise-induced increased systolic pressure, make it likely that more adverse effects are occurring than are reported in the medical literature. This underreporting is inherent to the secretive nature of doping.

It has long been suspected that the unexplained deaths of 18 Dutch and Belgian cyclists between 1987 and 1990 were linked to the use of exogenous EPO (Adamson & Vapnek 1991). The suspicion has been that the increasing blood viscosity resulting from rHuEPO combined with dehydration from exercise will result in thrombosis. Indeed, renal patients receiving rHuEPO had a sixfold increase in thrombosis compared to controls (Muirhead *et al.* 1992). In addition, rHuEPO is noted to enhance platelet activation, increase endothelin production by the vascular endothelium, and augment vascular smooth muscle response to norepinephrine and angiotensin II, all of which increase the risk of thrombosis (Smith *et al.* 2003). There is one documented case report of a cyclist suffering a cerebral sinus thrombosis through misuse of rHuEPO (Lage *et al.* 2002).

Although suspicions of substantial use of rHuEPO began as soon as the drug was released in 1987, it is exceedingly difficult to document the amount of use. Most truly knowledgeable and conservative experts place the amount at very high levels. To some extent the drug seizures and arrests during the 1998 Tour de France and other races have confirmed the substantial use; however, it is the development of tests for detecting it that is beginning to provide data.

The first test for rHuEPO was an indirect blood test that used elevated red blood cell mass, in conjunction with increased of erythropoiesis and high EPO concentrations, to determine whether a sample is non-physiologic, resulting from rHuEPO use (Parisotto *et al.* 2000). Later a urine test (Lasne & de Ceaurriz 2000) was developed that actually looked for the presence of rHuEPO and is therefore a *direct* test. By means of separation in an electrical field and detection with a very sensitive and selective method, this test is widely accepted and considered validated by the doping community. The test reveals the isoform patterns of urinary EPO. The isoform pattern of rHuEPO is distinctively different from endogenous EPO and the test also determines if darbepoetin alfa is present. Although the duration of efficacy for rHuEPO exceeds its window of detection, an effective test for rHuEPO has been a major breakthrough in doping detection.

GROWTH HORMONE

The next major frontier in doping control is the detection of recombinant human growth hormone (rHuGH). Naturally occurring human growth hormone (hGH) is a polypeptide hormone of 191 amino acids that is produced in the anterior pituitary gland at a rate of 0.4–1.0 mg·day^{-1} in healthy adult males. Natural hGH is secreted as multiple isoforms with the predominant one being a 22-kD monomer and about 10% being the 20-kD form. This is in contrast to rHuGH, which contains only the 22-kD isomer. Parenteral administration of rHuGH peaks in 1–3 h and is imperceptible at 24 h. rHuGH seems to work as a *partitioning* agent, rather than a true anabolic agent. Under this mechanism, protein synthesis is favored over fat synthesis. However, insulin is required for this to occur, otherwise rHuGH would be a catabolic substance.

In humans, hGH stimulates the production of various markers, the most prominent being another substance in this category, insulin-like growth factor (IGF-1) or somatomedin-C. Although there is some debate about whether substances such as hepatic-produced IGF-1 are markers or mediators, hGH exerts most of its effects through receptors at target cells. Despite a great deal of debate and

marketing, there is little evidence that the commercially available IGF-1 products have any ability to increase IGF-1 levels or strength. It is also clear that while some controlled, albeit limited, studies of rHuGH have revealed increases in IGF-1 and changes in lean body mass, none have definitively demonstrated increases in strength or athletic performance (Deyssig *et al.* 1993).

The adverse effects of rHuGH are mainly obtained from extrapolation of studies of hGH-deficient patients, acromegalic patients, or anecdotal reports. Short-term use has been reported to cause fluid retention and muscle edema, while long-term use has resulted in arthralgias, diabetes, myopathies, carpal tunnel syndrome, and acromegaly (Sonksen 2001). This latter is worrisome in that patients with acromegaly may produce as little as 2 mg·day^{-1}, leaving a narrow therapeutic window. Although cadaveric hGH is not used clinically, there is still evidence of its availability on the black market and with it the risk of Creutzfeldt–Jakob disease.

Research on a test for human growth hormone in urine or blood began 10 years ago and is still an active area. Although no definitive test exists, lately there has been some progress. Of the two candidate methods, one uses immunoassays to estimate the amounts of the 20 and 22 kD isomers in the serum. The amount of 20 kD is suppressed when rHuGH (22 kD) is given; thus, a high ratio of 22–20 kD will indicate use of synthetic GH. This method has shown promise of detecting rHuGH but appears to have a short detection period within 24 h of the last dose (Wu *et al.* 1999). It cannot detect cadaveric hGH.

The second method relies on measuring a medley of markers in serum (Healy *et al.* 2003). Studies have shown that of the many markers of hGH use, IGF-1, and procollagen type III can consistently discriminate rHuGH users from non-users (Sonksen 2001). It remains to be seen whether this approach to drug testing would survive forensic challenges in a system that has traditionally relied on mass spectrometry and a *fingerprint* identification of the banned substance.

INSULIN

Insulin is another drug in this category, one of the most fascinating for physicians who have been trained to view insulin as a solely therapeutic drug. Perhaps influenced by the treatment of diabetics who are often resistant to insulin therapy, the medical community has been surprised by anecdotal cases of insulin overdoses by non-diabetic body builders (Evans & Lynch 2003). Indeed, a 2005 study of 500 AAS users revealed that 25% reported concurrent use of hGH and insulin (Parkinson & Evans 2006), while another study found 5% of AAS users also used insulin (Perry *et al.* 2005).

It is not obvious how insulin might enhance strength among body builders. One speculation is that insulin has inhibitory functions. It deters lipolysis, glycolysis, gluconeogenesis, proteolysis, and ketogenesis through its actions in the liver. When combined with an anabolic agent such as hGH or AAS, the protein-sparing effects of insulin produce a larger anabolic result. WADA has prohibited insulin, although currently there is no approved test for it. The combination of ineffective testing, potential anabolic effects, relative accessibility, and legitimate therapeutic usage ensure more reports of insulin abuse in the coming years.

GONADOTROPINS

Gonadotropins are anterior pituitary hormones that stimulate the gonads and control reproductive activity. Luteinizing hormone (LH) and human chorionic gonadotropin (HCG) are prohibited in women. Follicle-stimulating hormone (FSH) is not specifically banned by WADA.

Follitropin alfa and beta are FSH produced by recombinant processes. These drugs stimulate ovarian follicle growth and are used as fertility drugs in women. Follitropin alfa used in combination with HCG increases low sperm counts in males. Pergonal® (menotropins) contains both FSH and LH and is given parenterally to anovulatory women to stimulate the ovarian follicle maturation.

HCG is obtained from the urine of pregnant women. It mimics the action of LH, which controls the release of eggs from the ovary in women, and it controls the production of testosterone in men. Clinically, it is used to stimulate ovulation in infertile women after follicle development has been stimulated with FSH. In men, it is used in the management of delayed puberty, undescended testes, and oligospermia. The gonadotropins affect multiple cell types and elicit multiple responses from the target organs. LH stimulates the Leydig cells of the testes and the theca cells of the ovaries to produce testosterone. It has some ergogenic properties. FSH stimulates the spermatogenic tissue of the testes and the granulosa cells of ovarian follicles. FSH and HCG are sometimes used to stimulate the testes after being suppressed by a course of AAS.

ADRENOCORTICOTROPIC HORMONE

Adrenocortictropic hormone (ACTH) increases the secretion of glucocorticosteroids. It is presumed that the rationale for prohibiting it is because it releases another class of prohibited substances, glucocorticoids. There is some anecdotal suggestion that athletes combine ACTH with anabolic agents such as insulin or AAS.

β₂-Agonists

β_2-Agonists are a specific type of stimulant that deserves special mention because of their widespread use as a therapeutic drug in the treatment of asthma. The distinction between therapeutic and ergogenic uses of β_2-agonists crystallizes the discussion of this topic. Asthma and exercise-induced asthma (EIA) has been estimated to affect as many as 22% of Winter Olympic athletes (Weiler & Ryan 2000). The issue, however, is how many athletes have genuine asthma and how many use asthma as an excuse to use an ergogenic drug. For the past few Olympic Games the IOC has gradually required athletes to demonstrate or provide objective evidence of asthma. This testing has resulted in a reduction in the number of athletes seeking approval to use an inhaled β_2-agonist (Anderson *et al.* 2006). The IOC now requires that the diagnosis of asthma or EIA be established on the basis of eucapnic voluntary hyperpnea testing. In addition, in order to use these inhalers and compete at the Olympic Games, an independent medical advisory board must review the athlete's case and determine whether a legitimate medical condition exists.

β₂-Agonists are the mainstay of treatment for asthma. It has been well-established that their main effect on asthma is through smooth muscle relaxation and bronchodilatation via inhalation 15–30 min before athletic participation. β₂-Agonists are excellent examples of the contentious nature of drug use in athletes. When it was discovered that large numbers of winter sport athletes were requesting β₂-agonists, the authorities suspected they were seeking a competitive advantage. Another factor is that recent studies suggest that chronic exertion in low temperatures may cause persistent asthma, and breathing diesel exhaust in indoor ice arenas may produce bronchial hyperresponsiveness (Rundell *et al.* 2004). Although asthma is a complex disorder and its treatment adds to the complexity, there is good evidence that efforts to require athletes to undergo physiologic testing are bringing the problem under control.

Agents with anti-estrogenic activity

The anti-estrogens and aromatase inhibitors are a new class of substances to be prohibited by WADA. These drugs are immediately familiar to clinicians in the treatment of diseases such as breast cancer and infertility. What is surprising is that they are used by athletes for ergogenic gain. Males will use aromatase inhibitors, such as exemestane and anastrazole, to block the conversion of high doses of anabolic-androgenic steroids to estrogens. Reducing this conversion attenuates side effects, such as gynecomastia and impotence in males. The aromatase inhibitors are also used in conjunction with estrogen receptor modifiers (e.g. tamoxifen) to further lessen the estrogenic effects. In addition, fertility drugs with anti-estrogenic properties are used by males for their ability to stimulate LH and FSH. Drugs in this category, such as clomiphene, are sometimes used at the end of an AAS cycle to stimulate the testes to restart production of testosterone that had been suppressed by exogenous AAS.

While the use of these agents is fairly well known among male body builders, only recently has their use by women been recognized. Women use drugs such as tamoxifen to block the effects of estrogens, which leaves testosterone unopposed (Seehusen & Glorioso 2002). Healthy women taking tamoxifen experience reduced body fat, but commonly suffer from decreased breast mass, hot flashes, and night sweats. There is also the risk of bone density loss, teratogenic potential, and possible endometrial cancer. It is clear that physicians need to be aware of both male and female use of these types of drugs.

Diuretics and other masking agents

This broad classification encompasses different types of drugs that are all on the banned list, despite the fact that they generally do not increase performance. The use of these drugs is predictable given the cat-and-mouse game of drug detection. Diuretics are well known to physicians in the treatment of hypertension and fluid overload states, and are used by athletes for several reasons:

1 Dilute the urine and thus the concentration of a banned substance;
2 Reduce the excretion of a banned substance;
3 Reduce the fluid-retaining effects of a banned substance (e.g., AAS);
4 Eliminate fluid in order to reach a lower weight class in sports such as boxing or wrestling;
5 Lose weight in sports where thinness is an advantage (e.g., gymnastics).

These latter two reasons could technically improve performance, but the main focus on diuretics is as a masking agent.

Sports drug testing has developed protocols that discourage the use of diuretics as dilutants by requiring an athlete to produce a valid urine sample with a minimum specific gravity of 1.005. In addition, diuretics can be detected by a combination of liquid chromatography and tandem mass spectrometry (LC-MS-MS) that is able to detect diuretics for up to 4 days after ingestion. Diuretics can be used therapeutically in athletes in the treatment of hypertension, although the fluid and electrolyte disturbances exacerbated by exercise would make them a poor choice in athletes. In addition, volume loss would also predispose an athlete to heat injury. Despite these relative contraindications, a TUE can be applied with the caveat that there cannot be any other banned substances found in the urine sample. Certain masking agents can also be used to block the excretion of banned substances. For example, probenecid is used to extend the half-life of penicillin by preventing elimination of the drug, and is also used by athletes to prevent the presence of AAS in the urine.

Another masking agent, epitestosterone, further illustrates how an athlete's knowledge of drug testing results in specific methods to avoid detection. The detection of exogenous testosterone is usually determined by the measurement of the T : E ratio. In order to maintain a normal T : E in the face of administered testosterone, athletes may ingest epitestosterone. Epitestosterone is not available as a pharmaceutical but can be purchased in bulk from chemical supply companies. Epitestosterone is inactive and its role in the body is not known. It does not enhance performance, but it is used as an emergency means to quickly reduce an elevated T : E ratio or to camouflage the daily use of testosterone. The BALCO investigation reported that some athletes used dermatologic formulations of testosterone and epitestosterone designed to maintain their T : E below 4. The T : E ratio was originally developed to deter athletes from using exogenous testosterone. That began a cycle of athletes taking epitestosterone to avoid detection, and sports organizations eventually banned epitestosterone above 200 ng·mL^{-1} to close this loophole (Catlin *et al.* 1997).

Another class of masking agents with little ergogenic enhancement is plasma expanders, such as hydroxyethyl starch (HES) and albumin. Although volume expansion may improve performance in endurance events and help resist heat illness, the use of plasma expanders is mainly prohibited for its role in masking the use of illegal methods of red blood cell expansion. Blood doping and rHuEPO increase red cell mass, and some sports organizations conduct pre-competition blood tests with maximum cut-offs (e.g., 50% and 47% hematocrit for men and women, respectively) above which athletes are removed from competition. Such *health tests* protect athletes from the risks associated with a high hematocrit, while protecting sports organizations from the legal risks that would be associated with formal doping control tests and disqualifications. In this context, the use of plasma expanders would create a volume dilution and reduce

hematocrit. This provides the rationale for banning the use of these agents, and testing for agents such as HES is relatively simple (Thevis *et al.* 2000).

Prohibited methods

ENHANCEMENT OF OXYGEN TRANSFER

It has clearly been demonstrated that increasing oxygen delivery to muscles is of benefit to endurance athletes. There are many different methods of achieving this result and they exist on a continuum of prohibited and permissible techniques. For example, training at high altitude is easily accessible to most athletes, can increase red blood cell mass, and is a common practice. Blood doping, by infusing either autologous or heterologous red blood cells, is clearly prohibited as an artificial method of increasing oxygen-carrying capacity. Between these extremes would be sleeping in an artificial nitrogen tent that simulates high altitude. Currently, WADA is considering prohibiting nitrogen tents.

All forms of blood doping are prohibited. Autologous blood doping involves removing one's own red blood cells, waiting a few days or weeks for the natural processes to replace the cells, and then reinfusing the cells. There were many reports of this practice just before the 1984 Summer Olympics. The introduction of rHuEPO in the late 1980s allowed a much more efficient means of increasing red blood cell mass without the attendant risks of transfusions, and blood doping fell out of favor. Ironically, the advent of effective testing for rHuEPO and the related darbepoetin has again shifted the focus back to blood doping. One athlete, who competed in the 2004 Olympic Games, was found guilty of blood doping in a test conducted after the Games. Blood tests can be used to show that blood doping took place by providing evidence of different cell populations.

Athletes have also gone beyond red blood cell augmentation in their quest to increase oxygen-carrying capacity. Artificial non-heme oxygen carriers, such as perflurocarbons, have been abused for their ability to dissolve oxygen. There has also been interest in drugs that manipulate the delivery of oxygen to the tissues by shifting the oxygen dissociation curve to the right. The best known of these is efaproxiral (RSR-13), which modifies hemoglobin's affinity for oxygen and allows for oxygen to be unloaded at low tension. A detection method was developed for this agent even before it was added to the banned list. It is now formally prohibited (Breidbach & Catlin 2001).

CHEMICAL AND PHYSICAL MANIPULATION

Given the increasingly severe penalties for a positive drug test, it is not surprising that athletes will go to extraordinary measures to avoid testing positive. The simplest method is substituting a clean urine sample for one's own. Many of these ruses can be detected through the use of witnessed urine collection and testing urine for temperature; although women athletes have developed methods of concealment that have been difficult to detect. Male athletes have been caught using devices such as an artificial penis and bladder, or bulb-filled syringes that are inserted rectally and connected to tubing leading to the penis. Obviously, monitored urine collection should detect these practices. To circumvent these defenses, athletes have reportedly resorted to self-catheterization and instilling clean urine into their bladder just before a urine test. Owing to this, most in-competition drug protocols specify that a courier notifies the athlete of the drug test and accompanies him or her until they report to the drug testing station.

Athletes have also attempted to manipulate their samples by adding chemicals to their urine, usually alkalinizing agents. These can be hidden under a fingernail or applied to the skin, and the athlete will urinate on their fingers to wash off the chemical. This method is most effective in disguising the presence of alkaloids, such as cocaine. The pH of a specimen is usually measured at the time of sample collection. Samples with a pH greater than 7.5 are not considered valid and require a new sample collection. Athletes will also attempt to avoid a positive test by intentionally diluting their urine, either through the use of diuretics, or ingesting excessive free water. Most sports organizations test for specific gravity at the time of collection and if a sample is less than 1.005 by refractometer or less than 1.010 by test strip, it is considered invalid and the athlete must remain at the site until he or she produces an adequate sample.

This section illustrates that urine collection is a critical and integral part of the drug testing process. The laboratory is only as good as the collection process and the entire program can be compromised unless protocols are well-written and adhered to.

GENE DOPING

Genetic (gene) doping was included for the first time in the 2004 World Anti-Doping Code, which defines it as the non-therapeutic use of genes, genetic elements and/or cells that have the capacity to enhance athletic performance. As in the case of other medical discoveries that have improved the treatment of serious diseases (e.g., rHuEPO and rHuGH), athletes have seized upon these breakthroughs as means of improving their performance. It is inevitable that genetic alteration will be available some day and sport is attempting to prepare for this.

In the late 1990s, scientists attempted to transfer EPO genes into primates with the result being that their red blood cell counts doubled in 10 weeks. Unfortunately, EPO production continued unabated and the animals needed regular phlebotomies (Sweeney 2004). In other experiments, mice were injected with adeno-associated genes for IGF-1 that were placed into skeletal muscle. The mice developed much stronger muscles and elevated levels of IGF-1 (Sweeney 2004). There has also been extensive research into myostatin, a protein responsible for inhibiting the activation of satellite cells that reside in skeletal muscle. A deficiency of this protein leads to significant generalized muscle hypertrophy (Schuelke et al. 2004) and a technology that could induce this effect would be coveted by athletes.

The limiting factor in these designs has been the method of delivery. Inserting the genetic material correctly and controlling protein production has been problematic, as in the above example of EPO into primates. However, the potential to deliver protein hormones via an orally ingested DNA plasmid has been proposed for drugs such as insulin (Rothman et al. 2005). Under this method, the DNA plasmid is swallowed and encodes production of the drug by the cells in the small intestine for a short period of time. This manufactured protein would be "natural" and would therefore be difficult to detect.

Although the application of genetic alterations to the treatment human disease must surmount many hurdles before it is widely available, it appears that the use of this technology in sport may not be far off. The trial of a disgraced former East German coach in February 2006 revealed communications detailing the knowledge of the genetic drug Repoxygen (Deutsche Welle-World 2006). Repoxygen is an experimental drug that stimulates the body to produce additional red blood cells in response to low oxygen tension. In effect, this drug signals the body to make more EPO and thus raise hemoglobin. Although Repoxygen was developed for the treatment of anemia and is intended to work only when the red blood cell count and oxygen level is low, it is quite conceivable that an athlete could take Repoxygen and then induce hypoxemia through an artificial altitude tent or ascent to higher elevations. The chilling fact is that this drug has never been used in humans and its safety is unknown. This may signal that the use of genetic doping is quite near. While this technology seems quite ominous, the reality is that it is technically demanding, and there is still no practical gene therapy for any disease.

Stimulants

These are the oldest drugs known to have been abused by athletes. Indeed, some of the earliest reports of drug use in sports were secondary to stimulants, where several prominent sportsmen were alleged to have died secondary to stimulant overdoses, including cyclists Arthur Linton in 1896, Knud Jensen in 1960, and Tom Simpson in 1967 (Bahrke *et al.* 2002). Each of these tragic deaths reinforced the lure of stimulants in athletics.

Stimulants are a broad class of sympathomimetic amines and alkaloids related to epinephrine, which contain both central and peripheral effects. A testimony to their multiple purposes is reflected in the NCAA study of substance abuse and the reasons athletes gave as the main reason they used amphetamines. While only 7% used them specifically for athletic performance, 28% used them for more energy, and 4% to lose weight or as appetite suppressant. Interestingly, 32% stated they used it for the treatment of ADHD (NCAA Study Staff 2006). It is very clear that athletes employ stimulants for ergogenic, recreational, and therapeutic reasons.

Many of the stimulants are sympathomimetic amines that include amphetamines, MDMA, ephedrine, phenylpropanolamine, pseudoephedrine, phenylephrine, β_2-agonists, methylphenidate, and dextroamphetamine. The effects of these drugs depend on the particular receptor that is stimulated: alpha receptors mediate smooth muscle contraction and vasoconstriction; β_1-receptors mediate inotrophic and chronotrophic effects; and β_2-receptors mediate smooth muscle relaxation and bronchodilatation. These drugs act by means of several mechanisms that influence endogenous catecholamines which include increased liberation and reuptake, attenuation, displacement of bound catecholamines, as well as creation of false neurotransmitters and inhibition of monoamine oxidase.

The literature has conflicting studies regarding sympathomimetic amines and performance enhancement (Committee on the Judiciary 1973; Beckett & Cowan 1978; Green & Puffer 2002). Although amphetamines may improve activities that involve simple, repetitive tasks, they are likely to be ineffective (or even detrimental) in more complex endeavors. There is also a great deal of individual variation.

Cocaine is prohibited. It acts by blocking the neuronal reuptake of norepinephrine resulting in increased blood pressure and heart rate, as well as reduced threshold for seizures and ventricular arrhythmias. Cocaine also acts as a local anesthetic and although local anesthetics are permitted by WADA, cocaine is specifically excluded. Because of its effects on central thermoregulation, cocaine increases susceptibility to heat injury. It is likely that all stimulants would increase the risk of heat injury by increasing the metabolic rate and heat production. Stimulant use should be investigated in the case of heat injury in athletes.

There are three unusual stimulants that have been found in athletes under special circumstances. Several cases of bromantan were found in urine samples collected at the 1996 Summer Olympics in Atlanta, Georgia. The investigations suggested that it might modulate dopamine, serotonin, or norepinephrine, and thus affect perception of pain or fatigue or, alternatively, may have a thermoprotective effect. There is also some indication that it was developed as a masking agent because in most chromatographic systems, its retention time is close to that of epitestosterone.

Mesocarb is a CNS stimulant that augments dopamine and catecholamines in the manner of a stimulant; however, it may also affect the hypothalamic-pituitary-gonadal axis and influence LH and testosterone. Modafinil (and the related compound adrafinil) is a stimulant drug used to treat narcolepsy and multiple sclerosis which has recently turned up in the urine of several athletes not known to have narcolepsy.

Cannabinoids and narcotics

These two categories are grouped together because athletes mainly use them for recreational purposes and rarely for any potential ergogenic effect. Indeed, 94% of NCAA marijuana users stated their main reason for use was to make them feel good or for recreational purposes (NCAA Study Staff 2006). There was some debate over whether or not these drugs fit the traditional WADA reasons for prohibiting a substance; however, they were considered to have a health risk for the athlete and it was determined that they violate the "spirit of sport."

Cannabinoids refer to a class of compounds containing the active ingredient Δ-9-tetrahydrocannabinol (THC) and most sports organizations set a drug testing cut-off level of $15 \, \text{ng} \cdot \text{mL}^{-1}$ urine for a positive result. This level effectively excludes passive inhalation and recognizes the widespread use of marijuana within and outside of the athletic community. Indeed, athletic surveys have generally found that marijuana is the second most abused drug in athletes after alcohol (NCAA Study Staff 2006). Despite the extensive use by athletes, there are few studies on the effects of THC on exercise. Limited studies have found an attenuation of exercise capacity, lowered peak exercise performance,

a decreased maximum work capacity, and an increased metabolic rate following THC ingestion (Renaud & Cormier 1986). It is well known that acute THC ingestion causes a decrement in reaction time and the ability to perform psychomotor tasks that would significantly affect sports performance. The existing literature clearly demonstrates the ergolytic effects of marijuana.

Narcotic analgesics are also generally considered to have little positive effect on performance, although masking pain might be considered ergogenic. However, the sedating effect of most narcotics would likely obviate any particular gains in this area. A more significant risk is the athlete who initially uses the drugs to relieve sports-related pain and becomes physically dependent. Participation in sports does not preclude narcotic addiction, and practitioners should be trained in the recognition of the signs and symptoms of narcotic use and withdrawal and understand the treatment options in these cases.

Prohibited substances in particular sports

Certain substances are prohibited only in a limited number of sports where they would provide a therapeutic advantage. These are interesting from a pharmacologic perspective because some drugs in this category actually reduce performance in many sports. The best example in this group are the beta-blockers that are used therapeutically for hypertension and arrhythmias and are generally regarded by clinicians as contraindicated in the treatment of athletes because their negative chronotropic effects would severely attenuate endurance activity. However, this same effect turns out to be advantageous in certain sports, such as shooting events, in which fine motor control and a low heart rate are of benefit. Because of this, beta-blockers are prohibited in competition, specifically in sports such as archery, shooting, billiards, and chess, among others. In a remarkable display as to the specificity of effects from beta-blockers, they are banned in the sport of sailing, but only in the helmsman. There is no need to ban them in the other members of the crew because the drugs would decrease their ability to perform high-intensity tasks. It is therefore imperative for a physician treating elite athletes to be aware of the restrictions in each sport.

The other drug in this category is alcohol, the most abused drug in society. The major sports where alcohol is banned are generally those in which intoxication would present a danger to the athlete and the other competitors. These include archery, shooting, automobile racing, motorcycle racing, power boating, and karate, among others. There is some indication that small doses of ethanol actually improve shooting scores. Because of the limitations in urine testing, alcohol detection is usually conducted via breath and/or blood analysis. Obviously, the majority of alcohol use is for recreational purposes and not performance enhancement, and it is more likely that the team physician will be confronted by an athlete with an alcohol problem. It is therefore imperative that the team physician be aware of the signs and symptoms of alcohol abuse and have the appropriate treatment resources available.

Dietary supplements

In the late 1990s the entire field of drug testing was disturbed by the explosion onto the world market of dietary supplements. Largely fueled by the US Congress' 1994 Dietary Supplement Health and Education Act (DSHEA), this Act has provided the consumer with access to a host of unproven and unregulated drugs. Although DSHEA was ostensibly passed in order to improve consumer access to supplements, in the late 1990s two consequences have caused confusion among the public and massive profits for the supplement manufacturers. The entire supplement industry mushroomed after the passage of DSHEA and none more so than the sector of sports nutrition. It appears that athletes are extremely vulnerable to promises of increased muscle, energy, and endurance.

Unfortunately, this largely unregulated industry could not guarantee the purity of many of its products and multiple studies demonstrated both macro- and micro-contamination (Catlin *et al.* 2000; Green *et al.* 2001a; Geyer *et al.* 2004). Because of this, the cost to athletes is much greater than the average consumer who is not subject to drug testing.

Whether truthful or not, many athletes who test positive under sports drug testing place the blame for their positive test on a contaminated supplement. This defense has generally not been successful because of WADA's "strict liability." Even in cases where it has been proven that minuscule amounts of a contaminated substance were the reason for a positive test and the athlete had no knowledge of it, WADA has upheld the conviction because of strict liability. Given the plethora of claims of contamination by athletes testing positive, it is a rare occasion when an athlete will file a suit against the supplement manufacturer. Recently, an athlete was successful in bringing a legal action against a supplement manufacturer (Hunninghake 2005). The athlete was awarded several hundred thousand US dollars as compensation for causing his positive drug test and missing the 2004 Olympics. Given these circumstances, the message to athletes is clear: until DSHEA is reformed, dietary supplements are taken at the athlete's own risk. Athletes need to be informed of the facts and weigh any performance advantages in taking a supplement with the risk of a positive test and the negative career impact.

The sports medicine physician can take several approaches with respect to nutritional supplements. The first is as a resource for athletes to obtain accurate and informative advice. According to the 2005 NCAA survey, only 4% of athletes listed the team physician as a source for information about nutritional supplements (NCAA Study Staff 2006). They were much more likely to go to a friend, parent, or retail store than the team physician. In order to provide information, physicians must keep abreast of changing patterns of supplement use among athletes. Second, the physician can provide sound nutritional alternatives to supplements. The diet is underutilized as a source for nutrition and most items that athletes obtain from supplements, such as protein, are readily available in the diet. Frequently, it is the team physician who has knowledge of these products and it is paramount that the physician assumes leadership on this issue that can potentially affect an entire program. Third, the physician can recommend that the athlete only take supplements that have been tested (every batch) and found not to contain prohibited substances.

Therapeutic use exemption

A TUE allows athletes who need a prohibited medication for legitimate medical reasons to use it in a specific sport for a finite time period. The WADA International Standard (World Anti-Doping Agency 2006) for TUEs was developed to help harmonize the process of granting them across sports and countries, and its major tenets are summarized in Table 17.2.

The first criterion for granting a TUE is that the athlete and physician must apply for it before the competition in which it will be needed. Retroactive approval will be considered, but only in cases of emergency treatment of an acute condition or under exceptional circumstances.

The second criterion is that the athlete truly needs the medication. This may be obvious in some cases, such as a type 1 diabetic and insulin, or vague, as in some cases of an athlete with ADHD on methylphenidate. In the latter case, the impairments to mental health can be subtle. In such complex cases, the medical practitioner's written declaration, together with documentation of the diagnosis and medical history have a heightened influence on the TUE committee's recommendation to grant or deny the request.

The third criterion is that the athlete must not benefit from any performance-enhancing effect other than the return to a normal state of health. In some conditions (e.g., an asthmatic using a β_2-agonist), pulmonary function tests can clearly prove this point. However, other diseases cannot be evaluated by objective tests. Because of this, WADA specifically states that a TUE cannot be granted for treating "low-normal" levels of endogenous hormones. Given the wide range and individual variability of testosterone and growth hormone, this caveat closes what could have been a giant loophole.

The fourth criterion is that there is no reasonable therapeutic alternative. Although this is sound in theory, with diseases such as diabetes in which insulin is the standard treatment, it becomes more problematic in deciding how far an athlete should go in order to satisfy this condition. For example, in the treatment of ADHD, atomoxetine is approved for this condition and is not prohibited. Is it reasonable to require that every athlete with ADHD have a therapeutic trial of atomoxetine before being granted a TUE for methylphenidate?

The final criterion in Table 17.2 is that the need for the medication in question cannot be to treat a condition resulting from past non-therapeutic use of a prohibited substance. By adding this statement, WADA took special precautions to prevent an obvious approach to abusing the TUE process. For example, following the extended use of AAS, particularly long-acting compounds, the pituitary-gonadal axis will be impaired, often for several months. An athlete could apply for a TUE to use testosterone on the basis of subnormal testosterone levels. This TUE criterion makes it clear that an athlete could not receive a benefit after such use.

The WADA TUE standard outlines a reasonable method for distinguishing legitimate, therapeutic uses from ergogenic uses of prohibited substances. Although every case might not be clear-cut, at least there are guidelines to attempt harmonization and equitable handling of athletes. Physicians can do much to help achieve this by exercising their best professional judgment.

Table 17.2 Adapted World Anti-Doping Agency (WADA) criteria for granting a therapeutic use exemption (TUE). Adapted from World Anti-Doping Code. International Standard for Therapeutic Use Exemption. www.wada-ama.org/rtecontent/document/international_standard.pdf [Accessed August 25, 2006].

1 The TUE should be submitted no less than 21 days prior to an event

2 The athlete would experience a significant impairment to health if the prohibited substance were to be withheld in the treatment of a chronic medical condition

3 The TUE would produce no additional enhancement of performance other than the restoration to normal health from the treatment of a legitimate medical condition

4 There is no reasonable therapeutic alternative to the prohibited substance

5 The use of the prohibited substance cannot be a consequence of prior non-therapeutic use of any prohibited substance

Doping control procedures

The doping control procedure depends on whether the urine sample is collected in competition or out of competition. Substances such as stimulants, which enhance performance at the time of competition, are prohibited only in competition. Other substances, such as anabolic steroids or EPO, which are likely to be abused during training, are prohibited year-round in and out of competition.

Athlete selection is carried out according to the sport authority's written drug testing protocol. At the Olympic Games and in competition, the top four finishers are tested, as well as other randomly selected athletes. An official notifies them after they cross the finish line and escorts them through medal ceremonies and media interviews. The very first urine sample produced is the one that must be collected because it contains any substance present in the athlete's body during the competition. A stimulant would have to be present in non-negligible quantities to enhance performance, and therefore it is easy to detect. However, athletes determined to cheat can discontinue anabolic steroids some days before competition, eliminate the drugs completely, and pass the test, while perhaps still enjoying performance enhancement.

In out-of-competition tests, athletes are at risk for being tested at any date or time with short notice or no notice, and therefore they are deterred from using drugs at all times. Out-of-competition tests target anabolic and masking agents. Athletes subject to out-of-competition testing are responsible for making sure the sporting authority knows where to find them at all times. They do so by reporting their whereabouts in advance year-round. Typical programs allow a finite list of excuses for missing a test and allow only two missed tests before the third one triggers sanctions.

In either in-competition or out-of-competition testing, the athlete must present identification. Next, he or she selects a clean, plastic-wrapped beaker and goes into the restroom stall accompanied by one official observer of the same sex. The athlete strips from the armpits to the knees and allows the observer to check for the presence of any suspicious object. Then he or she urinates into the beaker and the official witnesses the flow. The official's job is to make sure that authentic urine from the correct individual is collected. To avoid contamination or sabotage, athletes are advised to drink only from sealed containers before providing the sample and never to leave their urine beaker unattended. The athlete brings the beaker of urine out of the stall to a table and chooses a clean pair of containers into which the urine is poured. The containers are identified only by a code number followed by the letter A or B. Only the athlete and the sporting authority know whose urine sample it is – not the drug testing laboratory. The paperwork that is filled out constitutes the beginning of the chain of custody documentation, a record of who has custody of the samples or where they are securely stored from this moment to shipment by commercial courier, to receipt at the laboratory, throughout all the laboratory work, until the time when the samples are ultimately discarded.

The laboratory screens the samples for all the substances on the relevant (in- or out-of-competition) list, "menu," or "panel." Screening determines whether a sample is certainly negative or might containing a prohibited substance. Screening data merely provide a preliminary indication, not full proof, that the substance is present. For example, laboratories might run one stimulant screen, two steroid screens, and one diuretic screen on a batch of a dozen or more test tubes (one tube for each athlete). If the screening data hint at a prohibited substance, a new portion (aliquot) of urine is worked up in order to attempt to confirm the finding.

Except for large molecules, such as EPO, a glycopeptide, most prohibited drugs and their metabolites are identified by gas chromatography-mass spectrometry (GC-MS), the workhorse of doping control laboratories. Identification is achieved by matching the analytical data between the unknown in the athlete's urine sample and an authentic reference standard, more specifically the chromatographic retention times and mass spectra. Identifying metabolites prove that the drug was administered to the athlete and was not just spiked into the urine sample.

Laboratory turnaround time is 1–2 weeks for year-round testing, and can be as short as 24 h for negative results during major games or championships. Confirmation takes longer. Games results are needed as soon as possible because the world is watching and some athletes compete more than once. If they have competed on a prohibited substance, they should be removed from competition.

When the laboratory reports the presence of a prohibited substance in a urine sample (identified only by a container number), most sporting authorities inform the athlete, then request that the sample be analyzed a third time before sanctions are applied. For this "B confirmation," the athlete has the right to come to the laboratory or send a representative of his or her choice, to examine the B sample, still sealed, exactly as the athlete last saw it, and witness its analysis.

All laboratory work must be carried out according to the Standard Operating Procedure (SOP), meet WADA Standards, be accompanied by an unbroken chain of custody, be kept confidential, and meet forensic standards in case substances are identified and reported, and legal activities result for years to come.

LABORATORY TESTING

Urinary steroids are identified by their chromatographic retention time and mass spectrum. These two characteristics are determined by various types of mass spectrometry. In the case of exogenous or xenobiotic AAS, the finding of the drug is usually sufficient to establish that doping has taken place. If the urine also contains metabolites of the drug, this confirms that the individual had ingested the AAS in question. After decades using GC-MS to prove the presence of AAS, the introduction of more sensitive technologies, such as high-resolution mass spectrometry (HRMS), ion trap mass spectrometry, and LC-MS-MS, has extended the period of detectability of xenobiotic AAS. One potential limitation of testing based on mass spectrometry is that there may not be known reference standards for newly produced "designer" AAS. Several new drugs have been "discovered" that have heretofore not been detected by WADA laboratories; for example, tetrahydrogestrinone (THG) (Catlin et al. 2004), norbolethone (Catlin et al. 2002a), and madol (Sekera

et al. 2005). There are likely to be several more of these drugs appearing on the market as the users attempt to thwart efforts at doping control.

Ethical issues and doping control

There are a variety of ethical issues that the sports medicine physician encounters in the field of doping control. Physicians enter into a variety of arrangements with athletes, including the traditional doctor–patient relationship, and these can influence the use and abuse of ergogenic drugs. In the typical doctor–patient arrangement, the physician is obligated to first do no harm and also to improve a patient's health. This often leads to a blurring between therapeutic and ergogenic usage of drugs.

A physician may be placed in difficult circumstances in which he or she is asked to balance competing interests, for example, an injured athlete that might benefit from a prohibited substance. Another scenario is a patient requesting prescription drugs so as to avoid safety issues associated with "black market" sources. Athletes will frequently "doctor shop" until they find a physician who will acquiesce to their requests and the physician must weigh the loss of patient income against ethical demands.

The physician–patient dynamic is further complicated when the physician has a relationship to a sports organization. Being a team physician for a high-profile sports team often has significant benefits to the physician in terms of prestige, finances, and community visibility. The position of team physician can be so desirous that a number of US professional teams have entered into "medical sponsorship" arrangements in which the role of team physician goes to the highest bidder (i.e., the physician compensates the team). The status that accrues to the physician and the desire to maintain that status creates the potential for conflict. A physician may be pressured by the athlete or employing organization to prescribe ergogenic drugs unethically. As the athlete is not paying the physician, this often confuses the traditional doctor–patient relationship.

These three issues – the desire to heal, altered doctor–patient relationship, and team physician status – can make the physician vulnerable to prescribing ergogenic drugs unethically. Given the tight control of drugs such as anabolic steroids, a physician might be tempted to make them available to patient-athletes for non-medical reasons or for monetary gain. Perhaps the most glaring examples of physician abuse were previously mentioned regarding the records of the GDR in which physicians played an integral part in the state-sponsored doping program (Franke & Berendonk 1997). It is also clear that physicians participated in the 1998 Tour de France doping scandal by monitoring the drug use of cyclists (Voet 2001).

On the positive side, physicians are involved with anti-doping efforts in virtually all international and national sport organizations. Very often they occupy pivotal positions. In the USA, physician involvement is required for all review panels of doping offenses. In addition, physicians may have a role in the treatment of the athletes who develop a dependency to ergogenic drugs.

Conclusions

Now that sports medicine is an established specialty for both orthopedic and primary care physicians, its practitioners have many roles in the care of athletes. At the same time, doping rules have become more complex and the list of prohibited substances is lengthening. Sports have become a huge revenue generator, and the amount of money that can be lost by a positive test is enormous. One only has to witness the havoc that follows the announcement of a positive AAS for a well-known athlete.

The sports medicine physician must be thoroughly familiar with the list, both to avoid inadvertently prescribing a prohibited substance and to educate the patient-athlete. Sometimes a physician might be tempted to assist an athlete to violate anti-doping efforts. Although these lines are often crossed unintentionally, the consequences are the same; the athlete has a positive test result and is sanctioned. In some cases the physician may be sanctioned. Physicians need to be judicious in their prescribing patterns. If prohibited drugs are prescribed, physicians must be aware of TUE requirements, as well as the medicolegal restrictions. With continuing diligence of the entire sports medicine community and particularly the sports medicine physician, the current trend to rid sports of performance-enhancing substances will flourish.

References

Adamson, J.W. & Vapnek, D. (1991) Recombinant erythropoietin to improve athletic performance. *New England Journal of Medicine* **324**, 698–699.

Aguilera, R., Catlin, D.H., Becchi, M., *et al.* (1999) Screening urine for exogenous testosterone by isotope ratio mass spectrometric analysis of one pregnanediol and two androstanediols. *Journal of Chromatography. B, Biomedical Sciences and Applications* **727**, 95–105.

Anderson, S.D., Sue-Chu, M., Perry, C.P., *et al.* (2006) Bronchial challenges in athletes applying to inhale a β2-agonist at the 2004 Summer Olympics. *Journal of Allergy and Clinical Immunology* **117**, 767–773.

Bahrke, M., Hinitz, D. & Yesalis, C.E. (2002) History of doping in sport. In: *Performance-Enhancing Substances in Sports and Exercise* (Bahrke, M., ed.) Human Kinetics, Champaign, IL: 1–20.

Beckett, A.H. & Cowan, D.A. (1978) Misuse of drugs in sport. *British Journal of Sports Medicine* **12**, 185–194.

Bhasin, S., Storer, T.W., Berman, N., *et al.*. (1996) The effects of supraphysiologic doses of testosterone on muscle size and strength in normal men. *New England Journal of Medicine* **335**, 1–7.

Boje, O. (1939) Doping: A study of the means employed to raise the level of performance in sport. *Bulletin of the Health Organization of the League of Nations* **8**, 439–469.

Breidbach, A. & Catlin, D.H. (2001) RSR13, a potential athletic performance enhancement agent: detection in urine by gas chromatography/mass spectrometry. *Rapid Communications in Mass Spectrometry* **15**, 2379–2382.

Brower, K.J., Eliopulos, G.A., Blow, F.C., Catlin, D.H. & Beresford, T.P. (1990) Evidence for physical and psychological dependence on anabolic androgenic steroids in eight weight lifters. *American Journal of Psychiatry* **147**, 510–512.

Buick, F.J., Gledhill, N., Froese, A.B., Spriet, L. & Meyers, E.C. (1980) Effect of induced erythrocythemia on aerobic work capacity. *Journal of Applied Physiology* **48**, 636–642.

Carlock, J.M., Smith, S.L., Hartman, M.J., *et al.* (2004) The relationship between vertical jump power estimates and weightlifting ability: a field-test approach. *Journal of Strength and Conditioning Research* **18**, 534–539.

Catlin, D.H. (2005) Anabolic steroids. In: *Endocrinology*, 5th edn. (DeGroote, L.J. & Jameson, L., eds.) W.B. Saunders, Philadelphia, PA: 3265–3282.

Catlin, D.H., Ahrens, B.D. & Kucherova, Y. (2002a) Detection of norbolethone, an anabolic steroid never marketed, in athletes' urine. *Rapid Communications in Mass Spectrometry* **16**, 1273–1275.

Catlin, D.H., Breidbach, A., Elliott, S. & Glaspy, J. (2002b) Comparison of the isoelectric focusing patterns of darbepoetin alfa, recombinant human erythropoietin, and endogenous erythropoietin from human urine. *Clinical Chemistry* **48**, 2057–2059.

Catlin, D.H., Hatton, C.K. & Lasne, F. (2006) Abuse of recombinant erthropoietins by athletes. In: *Erythropoietins and Erythropoiesis* (Molineux, G., Foote, M.A. & Elliott, S.G., eds.) Birkhauser Verlag, Basel, Boston, Berlin: 205–227.

Catlin, D.H., Hatton, C.K. & Starcevic, S.H. (1997) Issues in detecting abuse of xenobiotic anabolic steroids and testosterone by analysis of athletes' urine. *Clinical Chemistry* **43**, 1280–1288.

Catlin, D.H., Leder, B.Z., Ahrens, B., Hatton, C.K. & Finkelstein, J.S. (2000) Trace contamination of over-the-counter androstenedione and positive urine test results for a nandrolone metabolite. *Journal of the American Medical Association* **284**, 2618–2621.

Catlin, D.H., Sekera, M.H., Ahrens, B.D., Starcevic, B., Chang, Y.C. & Hatton, C.K. (2004) Tetrahydrogestrinone: discovery, synthesis, and detection in urine. *Rapid Communications in Mass Spectrometry* **18**, 1245–1249.

Chan, T.Y. (1999) Health hazards due to clenbuterol residues in food. *Journal of Toxicology and Clinical Toxicology* **37**, 517–519.

Committee on the Judiciary Subcommittee to Investigate Juvenile Delinquency of United States Congress. Senate (1973) *Proper and Improper Use of Drugs by Athletes*. US Government Printing Office, Washington, DC.

Deyssig, R., Frisch, H., Blum, W.F. & Waldhor, T. (1993) Effect of growth hormone treatment on hormonal parameters, body composition and strength in athletes. *Acta Endocrinolica (Copenhagen)* **128**, 313–318.

Deyssig, R. & Weissel, M. (1993) Ingestion of androgenic-anabolic steroids induces mild thyroidal impairment in male body builders. *Journal of Clinical Endocrinology and Metabolism* **76**, 1069–1071.

Duchaine, D. (1989) *Underground Steroid Handbook II*. HLR Technical Books, Venice, CA.

Deutsche Welle-World (2006) German coach suspected of genetic doping. http://www.dw-world.de/dw/article/0,2144,1890782,00.html. Accessed August 2006.

Elashoff, J.D., Jacknow, A.D., Shain, S.G. & Braunstein, G.D. (1991) Effects of anabolic-androgenic steroids on

muscular strength. *Annals of Internal Medicine* **115**, 387–393.

Evans, N.A., Bowrey, D.J. & Newman, G.R. (1998) Ultrastructural analysis of ruptured tendon from anabolic steroid users. *Injury* **29**, 769–773.

Evans, P.J. & Lynch, R.M. (2003) Insulin as a drug of abuse in body building. *British Journal of Sports Medicine* **37**, 356–357.

Fineschi, V., Baroldi, G., Monciotti, F., Paglicci, R.L. & Turillazzi, E. (2001) Anabolic steroid abuse and cardiac sudden death: A pathologic study. *Archives of Pathology and Laboratory Medicine* **125**, 253–255.

Franke, W.W. & Berendonk, B. (1997) Hormonal doping and androgenization of athletes: a secret program of the German Democratic Republic government. *Clinical Chemistry* **43**, 1262–1279.

Geyer, H., Parr, M.K., Mareck, U., Reinhart, U., Schrader, Y. & Schanzer, W. (2004) Analysis of non-hormonal nutritional supplements for anabolic-androgenic steroids: results of an international study. *International Journal of Sports Medicine* **25**, 124–129.

Green, G. & Puffer, J. (2002) Drugs and doping in athletes. In: *The Team Physician's Handbook*, 3rd edn. (Mellion M., Walsh W.M., Madden C., Putukian M. & Shelton G.L., eds.) Hanley & Belfus, Philadelphia, PA: 180–198.

Green, G.A., Starcevic, B. & Catlin, D.H. (2001a) Analysis of over-the-counter steroid supplements. *Clinical Journal of Sport Medicine* **11**, 254–259.

Green, G.A., Uryasz, F.D., Petr, T.A. & Bray, C.D. (2001b) NCAA study of substance use and abuse habits of college student-athletes. *Clinical Journal of Sport Medicine* **11**, 51–56.

Hall, R.C., Hall, R.C. & Chapman, M.J. (2005) Psychiatric complications of anabolic steroid abuse. *Psychosomatics* **46**, 285–290.

Healy, M.L., Gibney, J., Russell-Jones, D.L., *et al.* (2003) High dose growth hormone exerts an anabolic effect at rest and during exercise in endurance-trained athletes. *Journal of Clinical Endocrinology and Metabolism* **88**, 5221–5226.

Hershberger, L.G., Shipley, E.G. & Meyer, R.K. (1953) Myotrophic activity of 19-nortestosterone and other steroids determined by modified levator ani muscle method. *Proceedings of the Society for Experimental Biology and Medicine* **83**, 175–180.

Hoberman, J. (2002) Sports physicians and the doping crisis in elite sport. *Clinical Journal of Sport Medicine* **12**, 203–208.

Hoffman, R.J., Hoffman, R.S., Freyberg, C.L., Poppenga, R.H., & Nelson, L.S. (2001) Clenbuterol ingestion causing prolonged tachycardia, hypokalemia, and hypophosphatemia with confirmation by quantitative levels. *Journal of Toxicology and Clinical Toxicology* **39**, 339–344.

Huie, M.J. (1994) An acute myocardial infarction occurring in an anabolic steroid user. *Medicine and Science in Sports and Exercise* **26**, 408–413.

Hunninghake, S. (2005) Swimming: 20 questions with USA swimmings Kicker Vencill. USA Swimming http://www.usaswimming.org/USASWeb/ViewMiscArticle.aspx?TabId=280&Alias=Rainbow&Lang=en&mid=408&ItemID=1706. Accessed August 2006.

Ishak, K.G. & Zimmerman, H.J. (1987) Hepatotoxic effects of the anabolic/androgenic steroids. *Seminars in Liver Disease* **7**, 230–236.

Jasuja, R., Catlin, D.H., Miller, A., *et al.* (2005) Tetrahydrogestrinone is an androgenic steroid that stimulates androgen receptor-mediated, myogenic differentiation in C3H10T1/2 multipotent mesenchymal cells and promotes muscle accretion in orchidectomized male rats. *Endocrinology* **146**, 4472–4478.

Kadi, F., Eriksson, A., Holmner, S. & Thornell, L.E. (1999) Effects of anabolic steroids on the muscle cells of strength-trained athletes. *Medicine and Science in Sports and Exercise* **31**, 1528–1534.

Lage, J.M., Panizo, C., Masdeu, J. & Rocha, E. (2002) Cyclist's doping associated with cerebral sinus thrombosis. *Neurology* **58**, 665.

Lasne, F. & de Ceaurriz, J. (2000) Recombinant erythropoietin in urine. *Nature* **405**, 635.

Le Bizec, B., Monteau, F., Gaudin, I. & Andrae, F. (1999) Evidence for the presence of endogenous 19-norandrosterone in human urine. *Journal of Chromatography, B: Biomedical Sciences and Applications* **723**, 157–172.

Leder, B.Z., Catlin, D.H., Longcope, C., Ahrens, B., Schoenfeld, D.A. & Finkelstein, J.S. (2001) Metabolism of orally administered androstenedione in young men. *Journal of Clinical Endocrinology and Metabolism* **86**, 3654–3658.

Leffers, H., Naesby, M., Vendelbo, B., Skakkebaek, N.E. & Jorgensen, M. (2001)

Oestrogenic potencies of Zeranol, oestradiol, diethylstilboestrol, Bisphenol-A and genistein: implications for exposure assessment of potential endocrine disrupters. *Human Reproduction* **16**, 1037–1045.

Meeuwsen, I.B., Samson, M.M., Duursma, S.A. & Verhaar, H.J. (2002a) Muscle strength and tibolone: a randomised, double-blind, placebo-controlled trial. *British Journal of Obstetrics and Gynaecology* **109**, 77–84.

Meeuwsen, I.B., Samson, M.M., Duursma, S.A. & Verhaar, H.J. (2002b) Tibolone does not affect muscle power and functional ability in healthy postmenopausal women. *Clinical Science (London)* **102**, 135–141.

Muirhead, N., Laupacis, A. & Wong, C. (1992) Erythropoietin for anaemia in haemodialysis patients: results of a maintenance study (the Canadian Erythropoietin Study Group). *Nephrology Dialysis Transplantation* **7**, 811–816.

NCAA Study Staff (2006) National Collegiate Athletic Association 2005 Study of Substance Use Habits of College Student-Athletes. NCAA, Indianapolis. http://www.ncaa.org/library/research/substance_use_habits/2006/2006_substance_use_report.pdf. Accessed August 2006.

Nieminen, M.S., Ramo, M.P., Viitasalo, M., *et al.* (1996) Serious cardiovascular side effects of large doses of anabolic steroids in weight lifters. *European Heart Journal* **17**, 1576–1583.

Pae, P. (2005) Back to the moon via Apollo on steroids. *Los Angeles Times* September 20, 2005.

Parisotto, R., Gore, C.J., Emslie, K.R., *et al.* (2000) A novel method utilising markers of altered erythropoiesis for the detection of recombinant human erythropoietin abuse in athletes. *Haematologica* **85**, 564–572.

Parkinson, A.B. & Evans, N.A. (2006) Anabolic androgenic steroids: A survey of 500 users. *Medicine and Science in Sports and Exercise* **38**, 644–651.

Perry, P.J., Lund, B.C., Deninger, M.J., Kutscher, E.C. & Schneider, J. (2005)

Anabolic steroid use in weightlifters and bodybuilders: An internet survey of drug utilization. *Clinical Journal of Sport and Medicine* **15**, 326–330.

Renaud, A.M. & Cormier, Y. (1986) Acute effects of marihuana smoking on maximal exercise performance. *Medicine and Science in Sports and Exercise* **18**, 685–689.

Rothman, S., Tseng, H. & Goldfine, I. (2005) Oral gene therapy: a novel method for the manufacture and delivery of protein drugs. *Diabetes Technology and Therapeutics* **7**, 549–557.

Rundell, K.W., Spiering, B.A., Evans, T.M. & Baumann, J.M. (2004) Baseline lung function, exercise-induced bronchoconstriction, and asthma-like symptoms in elite women ice hockey players. *Medicine and Science in Sports and Exercise* **36**, 405–410.

Russell, G., Gore, C.J., Ashenden, M.J., Parisotto, R. & Hahn, A.G. (2002) Effects of prolonged low doses of recombinant human erythropoietin during submaximal and maximal exercise. *European Journal of Applied Physiology* **86**, 442–449.

Schuelke, M., Wagner, K.R., Stolz, L.E., *et al.* (2004) Myostatin mutation associated with gross muscle hypertrophy in a child. *New England Journal of Medicine* **350**, 2682–2688.

Seehusen, D.A. & Glorioso, J.E. (2002) Tamoxifen as an ergogenic agent in women body builders. *Clinical Journal of Sport of Medicine* **12**, 313–314.

Sekera, M.H., Ahrens, B.D., Chang, Y.-C., Starcevic, B., Georgakopoulos, C. & Catlin, D.H. (2005) Another designer steroid: discovery, synthesis, and detection of 'madol' in urine. *Rapid Communications in Mass Spectrometry* **19**, 781–784.

Sleivert, G. & Taingahue, M. (2004) The relationship between maximal jump-squat power and sprint acceleration in athletes. *European Journal of Applied Physiology* **91**, 46–52.

Smith, K.J., Bleyer, A.J., Little, W.C. & Sane, D.C. (2003) The cardiovascular

effects of erythropoietin. *Cardiovascular Research* **59**, 538–548.

Sonksen, P. (2001) Reflections from a 40 year journey with growth hormone and IGF-1. *Growth Hormone and IGF Research* **11**, 329–335.

Spann, C. & Winter, M.E. (1995) Effect of clenbuterol on athletic performance. *Annals of Pharmacotherapy* **29**, 75–77.

Strickland, A.L. & French, F.S. (1969) Absence of response to dihydrotestosterone in the syndrome of testicular feminization. *Journal of Clinical Endocrinology and Metabolism* **29**, 1284–1286.

Sweeney, H.L. (2004) Gene doping. *Scientific American* **291**, 62–69.

Thevis, M., Opfermann, G. & Schanzer, W. (2000) Detection of the plasma volume expander hydroxyethyl starch in human urine. *Journal of Chromatography, B: Biomedical Sciences and Applications* **744**, 345–350.

Voet, W. (2001) *Breaking the Chain: Drugs and Cycling: The True Story.* Yellow Jersey Press, UK.

Vogt, A.M., Geyer, H., Jahn, L., Schanzer, W. & Kubler, W. (2002) Cardiomyopathy associated with uncontrolled self medication of anabolic steroids. *Zeitschrift fur Kardiologie* **91**, 357–362.

Weiler, J.M. & Ryan, E.J. III (2000) Asthma in United States Olympic athletes who participated in the 1998 Olympic Winter Games. *Journal of Allergy and Clinical Immunology* **106**, 267–271.

World Anti-Doping Agency (2006) World Anti-Doping Code: Therapeutic use exemptions. http://www.wada-ama.org/rtecontent/document/international_standard.pdf. Accessed August 2006.

Wu, Z., Bidlingmaier, M., Dall, R. & Strasburger, C.J. (1999) Detection of doping with human growth hormone. *Lancet* **353**, 895.

Zeman, R.J., Ludemann, R., Easton, T.G. & Etlinger, J.D. (1988) Slow to fast alterations in skeletal muscle fibers caused by clenbuterol, a β_2-receptor agonist. *American Journal of Physiology* **254**, E726–E732.

Chapter 18

Emergency Sports Medicine

LUCY-MAY HOLTZHAUSEN AND CHRIS HANNA

Most competitive sporting events have medical personnel dedicated to the care of injured athletes at the event venue. Fortunately, life-threatening emergencies are rare at sports events; however, these personnel may occasionally be called upon to deal with medical emergencies in spectators, event officials, or injured athletes. In most circumstances these personnel rely heavily on the local emergency medical services (EMS) to provide transport for the seriously injured athlete or help with the emergency care of the spectators and officials. It is the responsibility of this medical team to ensure that they have ready access to sufficient health care personnel to assist in an emergency; appropriate medical supplies and emergency equipment; and immediate access to a telephone or other means of communication with the EMS system. Any health care practitioner who takes on this role should be fully certified in basic life support (BLS) and advanced cardiac life support (ACLS) and have a working knowledge of the injuries and conditions likely to be encountered at the event.

The expected type and number of casualties will vary depending on a number of variables related to the event, the participants, and the environment in which the sporting activity is held (Table 18.1). In the team sports setting, especially in contact or high-speed sports, medical personnel may encounter emergencies arising as a result of traumatic injury including head and neck trauma, cardiac contusion,

vascular disruption, and visceral organ disruption. In endurance sport, environmental and medical emergencies are more common than trauma. The most common presentation of athletic emergency is the sudden collapse of the athlete on the field of play or on the event course. This signifies an abrupt loss of postural tone with or without a loss of consciousness. The following section outlines a general approach to the collapsed athlete in a team and in an endurance sport setting.

General approach to the collapsed athlete

One member of the medical team is identified as the team leader who will direct all the emergency care. The team familiarize themselves beforehand with the expected types of casualties that may arise. Ideally, the team rehearses the management plan

Table 18.1 Variables affecting the expected casualties seen at sporting events.

Environmental factors (temperature, humidity, wind-chill factor, UV intensity)
Location of the event (site access, water availability, terrain, indoor vs. outdoor)
Duration of the event (hours, single day, multiday event)
Nature of the sport (contact, high-speed, endurance, multisport events)
Level of competition (recreational, amateur, professional)
Participants (number of competitors, age, level of fitness, and conditioning)
Spectators (number, seated or mobile, population demographics, drug or alcohol use)

The Olympic Textbook of Medicine in Sport, 1st edition. Edited by M. Schwellnus. Published 2008 by Blackwell Publishing, ISBN: 978-1-4051-5637-0.

for these conditions prior to the event. This will ensure rapid, effective evaluation and intervention in all scenarios.

When an athlete collapses the medical team rapidly establishes whether the collapse has been witnessed or not and whether it has been traumatic or atraumatic. The etiology of the collapse in a traumatic witnessed event is often apparent. In the case of atraumatic collapse, it cannot be assumed that trauma is not a factor, as head injury or intracranial bleeding resulting from recent, non-witnessed trauma may be the cause of the collapse. This is especially true when dealing with athletes in high-speed or contact sports. The necessary precautions when examining and transporting the athlete should thus be observed when there is any doubt as to the element of trauma. If the collapse has not been witnessed by the medical team then other officials or spectators may provide clues to the cause of the collapse.

Primary survey

The medical team leader rapidly ascertains whether the athlete is alert and responds to verbal or painful stimuli by calling to the athlete by name. It may be necessary to use loud and repeated verbal stimulation to evoke a response. If the athlete is unresponsive, serious neck injury is assumed and immediate care taken to stabilize the athlete's neck by placing a hand on either side of their head. The athlete's head or neck is not moved until it has been established that they do not have a serious neck injury. The medical team proceeds with basic life support using the "ABCDE" approach to resuscitation. This should occur where the athlete is found. If the athlete is in a prone position and unconscious or there is a problem performing basic life support then the athlete is log rolled to a supine position (Luke & Micheli 1999; Blue & Pecci 2002).

The log roll is a four-person technique in which the team leader is positioned at the athlete's head maintaining in-line head and neck immobilization, while the other three members of the team are controlling the torso, hips, and legs. The athlete is turned on the count of the team leader in the direction of the three assistants. A spine board is placed underneath the athlete.

If the athlete is wearing a helmet and or a padded vest and jersey these should not be removed as this can potentially cause additional spinal cord injury. The padded vest and helmet act together as a unit and removing either of them forces the neck out of the neutral plane (Gastel *et al.* 1998; Haight & Shiple 2001). Padding and sandbags should be placed around the helmet and shoulders. The hips and legs are immobilized. Face guards can be removed by cutting them away from the headgear to gain airway access. If the athlete is not wearing a helmet then a rigid cervical collar is applied with in-line immobilization of the cervical spine.

The athlete's airway is then secured. In an unconscious athlete the muscle tone decreases and the tongue and epiglottis may obstruct the pharynx. A foreign body such as a portion of a mouth guard, teeth, vomitus, or blood may also cause obstruction. The athlete's mouth is opened, the tongue and lower jaw grasped between the thumb and fingers and the mandible lifted (tongue-jaw lift). This action may be sufficient to dislodge a foreign body and if it can be seen one may retrieved with the fingers. Care should be taken not to force the foreign body further down the airway. If no foreign body is visible, perform the jaw-thrust maneuver without head tilt to open the airway. This maneuver is the safest in the case of suspected neck injury (American Heart Association 2000a). Manual suction may be used to remove blood, vomitus, or secretions which may contribute to the laryngospasm.

To assess breathing, the medical team leader observes the athlete's chest for symmetrical movements and listens and feels for air escaping from the mouth or nostrils. Reflex gasping respiratory efforts (agonal respirations) are a sign of inadequate compromised breathing and may signify serious brain or brainstem injury (American Heart Association 2000a; Bruzzone *et al.* 2000). If the medical team leader is not confident that respirations are adequate, the team should proceed immediately with rescue breathing.

In an unconscious patient who is breathing spontaneously but has a loss of gag reflex and is not maintaining their airway an oral airway may be used. More formal airway protection may be necessary if the athlete does not show signs of recovering spontaneously within 1–2 min. Depending on the experience of the medical team, options for securing the airway may include: an appropriate-sized endotracheal tube with laryngoscope placement; a cuffed tube that can be inserted blindly with inflation of the cuffs to isolate the trachea from the esophagus (e.g., Combitube); and a selection of laryngeal mask airways (LMAs). Some LMAs now have a double lumen which is designed to allow vomitus to bypass the LMA (e.g., LMA ProSeal). These are easy to insert with a little training and do not require the use of a laryngoscope. If the athlete is unconscious because of airway obstruction as in a severe laryngeal injury then a surgical airway should be provided. Needle cricothyroidotomy is useful if high pressure oxygen is available, otherwise a formal cricothyroidotomy is indicated. Cricothyroidotomy kits can be purchased for the sideline doctor's bag, and the technique is taught in ATLS courses.

While the medical team leader is attending to the athlete's airway another member of the team can check for circulation by feeling for the carotid or femoral pulse. If this is palpable the systolic blood pressure is likely to be greater than 60 mmHg and adequate for reasonable tissue perfusion. Pulse checking is no longer recommended as part of the cardiopulmonary resuscitation (CPR) protocol for the lay person, and for medical staff should take no longer than 10 s to do. If pulses are absent chest compressions are commenced. It is best to have one person perform the CPR protocol doing 15 chest compressions followed by 2 breaths and maintaining a rate of 100 compressions per minute and 10–12 breaths per minute (American Heart Association 2000a; Bruzzone et al. 2000). There is some evidence now emerging that in cardiac arrest and low-flow states the provision of overzealous (or even "normal") ventilatory rates with intermittent positive pressure ventilation can significantly diminish both systemic and coronary circulation, most likely through inhibition of venous return (Pepe et al. 2005).

Other medical team members can expose the athlete and check for torrential arterial bleeding and treat as described in the section below. Basic CPR continues until the athlete is stabilized and can be safely transported from the field or event course to a secluded area for secondary survey.

Secondary survey

If the airway is clear, strong rhythmical breathing is present, and the pulse is normal then the athlete who has experienced a traumatic injury should have their cervical spine stabilized while a more comprehensive regional examination is undertaken (Table 18.2). The Glasgow Coma Scale (GCS) is used to score the athlete's level of consciousness and to determine the grade of head injury if present (Table 18.3). In the event that the athlete has required resuscitation, has not recovered consciousness, or has a GCS <14 within 3 min of the collapse then the medical team leader should alert the EMS system and arrange transport to a hospital as soon as possible (Geffen et al. 1998). Other criteria for referral to hospital in the case of head or neck trauma are discussed under the section on head and neck injury.

The medical team then proceeds to a neurologic screening and mental status examination if the athlete has suspected peripheral nerve, spinal cord, or head injury, even if the loss of consciousness was brief or neurologic symptoms appear to have resolved (Tables 18.4 & 18.5). This is followed by a comprehensive physical examination to rule out any injuries that may require further management. A more detailed management protocol for specific traumatic injuries is outlined in the following section.

In the case of an endurance athlete whose collapse is atraumatic, the conditions giving rise to syncope and altered mental status are often unique to these endurance sporting events (Table 18.6). The athlete may collapse on the course and be brought into the finish line medical facility by ambulance personnel

Table 18.2 Regional assessment of injuries.

Evaluate the Glasgow Coma Scale
Check pupil size, symmetry, and reaction to light
Inspect and palpate the scalp for wounds and fractures
Check nose and ears for bleeding or clear fluid leakage
Inspect and palpate the face and anterior neck for soft
  tissue swelling, abrasions, and lacerations
Check along the cervical spinous processes for spine
  alignment, step-off defects, and tenderness
Inspect and palpate the trunk, abdomen, pelvis, and limbs
  for other injuries

Table 18.3 Glasgow Coma Scale – total score 3–15.

Eye opening		Best verbal response		Best motor response	
Spontaneous	4	Orientated	5	Obeys commands	6
To speech	3	Confused	4	Localizes pain	5
To pain	2	Inappropriate words	3	Withdraws from pain	4
None	1	Incomprehensible sounds	2	Abnormal flexion	3
		None	1	Extension	2
				None	1

Table 18.4 Neurologic screening examination.

Eyes	Examine pupil size and reflexes, visual acuity and fields, ocular movements and nystagmus
Reflexes	Test corneal, Hoffman's, and plantar reflexes and then upper and lower limb tendon reflexes
Power	Test upper and lower limbs for weakness and hypotonia
Coordination	Test finger–nose touching, rapid alternation of forearm supination and pronation, heel–toe walking

Table 18.5 Mental status examination for concussion. From Geffen *et al.* (1998).

Immediate memory	Five words read to the athlete and recalled on three successive trials, scored out of 15
Processing speed	Sentences read allowed for 2 min, number correctly identified as true or false. Scores less than 38 indicate impairment
Orientation	Ask about orientation for time, place and situation, scored out of 5
Retrograde amnesia	Query event recall prior to trauma, score out of 5
Delayed recall	Free recall of five items presented at immediate recall, scored out of 5

Table 18.6 Types of casualties expected at endurance events.

Exercise-associated collapse (postural hypotension)
Dehydration
Hyponatremia
Hypothermia
Exertional heat stroke
Gastrointestinal problems (vomiting, diarrhea, cramps)
Exertional hematuria
Trauma
   macrotrauma (fractures, dislocations, sprains, strains,
     contusions, skin abrasions, blisters)
   microtrauma (overuse injuries such as medial tibial
     stress syndrome, stress fractures, plantar fasciosis)
Life-threatening emergencies (cardiac arrest, respiratory
   distress – asthma and anaphylaxis, diabetic
   hyperglycemia or hypoglycemia, seizures)

or may collapse immediately on completing their event (Holtzhausen & Noakes 1997). Loss of consciousness is less common than feeling of dizziness and weakness and complaint of nausea. These athletes are often escorted into the medical facility supported by two aides looking an unhealthy shade of white or gray and feeling near-syncopal (Mayers & Noakes 2000).

The initial evaluation of the athlete should include a brief history if they are lucid and able to converse (Table 18.7). Athletes who collapse during the race are more likely to be suffering from heat stroke, hyponatremia, or a cardiac problem. Those who collapse on completion of their race are most likely to have profound postural hypotension and a condition known as exercise-associated collapse. The history may give clues to the hydration status of the athlete and other factors such as drugs or intercurrent illness that may be contributing to the problem (Table 18.7). Body weight change is a useful criterion to determine the athlete's hydration status and has been very successfully used in Ironman Triathlon events in South Africa, New Zealand, and some of the US races in directing the need for intravenous fluid therapy in these athletes.

Table 18.7 Helpful questions to ask the collapsed endurance athlete.

Where did your collapse occur? On the course or at the finish line?

Have you noticed your finger rings or forearm bracelets becoming tighter through the race?

How much and what have you drunk during the race?

How many times have you passed urine during the race?

Have you experienced vomiting and/or diarrhea before and during the race?

How much and what have you eaten before and during the race?

What medications have you taken before and during the race?

Have you experienced any recent intercurrent illness?

What specific race preparation and heat acclimatization did you do prior to the race?

What has your training volume and schedule been leading up to your race?

In most cases where the athlete is found to be conscious and stable, vital signs and key blood tests (Table 18.8) can be safely carried out and treatment delayed by a couple of minutes to allow for a specific diagnosis to be made and appropriate management instituted. The specific management protocols for life-threatening and potentially fatal conditions are expanded on in the sections below.

Immediate life-threatening conditions

Respiratory compromise

Respiratory arrest is rare in competitive organized sports but the attending medical team should be prepared to deal with this promptly. It is important to recognize airway obstruction and to distinguish it from other conditions that may present with similar symptoms (Table 18.9).

Foreign bodies may cause either partial or complete upper airway obstruction. With partial obstruction the athlete may be capable of "good" or "poor air exchange." With good air exchange the athlete is responsive and can cough forcefully. They may wheeze between coughs. As long as good air exchange occurs, encourage the athlete to continue spontaneous coughing and breathing efforts.

If breathing efforts deteriorate to poor air exchange the athlete becomes increasingly panicky, is unable to talk, and may give the universal "choke" sign. Little or no air movement may be felt through the oronasal passages. Significant accessory muscle use occurs and stridorous, wheezing, or snoring breath sounds are made. The athlete should be treated immediately as if they have complete airway obstruction.

Several techniques are used throughout the world to relieve foreign body airway obstruction in the responsive choking patient, and it is difficult to compare the effectiveness of any one method with another. Most resuscitation councils recommend either Heimlich abdominal thrusts, back blows, chest thrusts, or a combination of these. Abdominal thrusts can cause complications such as rupture or laceration of abdominal or thoracic viscera or regurgitation and aspiration of stomach contents (Orlowski 1987; Majumdar & Sedman 1998; Anderson & Buggy 1999). It is recommended that if

Table 18.8 Initial evaluation of a collapsed athlete.

	Not severe	Severe
Mental state	Conscious Alert Orientated	Unconscious Altered. Disorientated. Delirious Combative and aggressive
Rectal temperature	<40.5°C	>40.5°C
Systolic blood pressure	>100 mmHg	<100 mmHg
Heart rate	<100 beats·min^{-1}	>100 beats·min^{-1}
Blood glucose	4–10 mmol·L^{-1}	<4 or >10 mmol·L^{-1}
Serum sodium	135–148 mmol·L^{-1}	<135 or >148 mmol·L^{-1}
Body weight loss	0–5%	>10%
Body weight gain	<2%	>2%

Table 18.9 Causes of respiratory arrest.

Etiology	Specific examples
Upper airway obstruction	Loss of consciousness with occlusion of the airway by the athlete's tongue
	Foreign body such as a mouth guard, vomitus, blood or teeth secondary to maxillofacial trauma
	Direct trauma to the larynx with laryngeal fracture
	Laryngospasm directly from anterior neck trauma or reflexively from traumatic stimulation of visceral nerve endings in the thorax or abdomen
Acute respiratory failure; Po_2 <50 mmHg; hypoxia; hypercapnia	Exertional syncope secondary to intense prolonged exercise mainly in unconditioned individuals
	Brain or spinal cord injury
	Fractured ribs and flail chest
	Drug-induced; cocaine or narcotics
	Asthmatic attack
Pneumothorax	Traumatic: secondary to rib fracture or other penetrating wound injury
	Spontaneous: may be associated with exertion in a young, tall, thin individual
	Tension pneumothorax
Pulmonary embolism	Traumatic in lower limb fracture or from deep venous thrombosis
High-altitude pulmonary edema	Occurs in 1–2% of healthy individuals of any age ascending rapidly above 2500 m

the Heimlich maneuver is used that the patient be medically evaluated afterwards so as not to miss these complications. The thrusts are repeated until the object is expelled from the airway or the athlete becomes unresponsive.

If the athlete has lost consciousness perform a tongue-jaw lift maneuver in the supine position and try to visualize the foreign body. This can be also removed with instruments, such as Magill forceps, which should only be used if the foreign body is easily seen. Either a laryngoscope or tongue blade and flashlight can be used to permit better visualization. Care should be taken not to push the foreign body further down into the pharynx. Once removed, the airway is opened and assisted breathing begun. If the athlete's chest does not rise then reposition the head and try to ventilate again. If this fails then straddle the patient's thighs and perform the Heimlich maneuver from below (up to five times) in the supine position.

Chest compressions may also be effective for the relief of foreign body airway obstruction in the unresponsive patient. A recent study using cadaver subjects has shown that chest compressions create a peak airway pressure that is equal to or superior to that created by abdominal thrusts (Langhelle *et al.*

2000). An oral and/or nasal airway may be inserted as necessary thereafter and assisted breathing begun.

When maxillofacial trauma is present oral suctioning equipment is useful to help clear the airway of blood. The conscious athlete with facial trauma should be sat upright with the neck extended as this will help to keep the airway patent. Cricothyrotomy should only be performed by trained personnel authorized to perform this surgical procedure if all other attempts at establishing an airway have failed.

Blunt trauma to the anterior region of the neck may result in contusions and/or fractures of the trachea, larynx, and hyoid bone and cause serious airway compromise. Injuries of this nature are not uncommon in field and ice-hockey, rugby, fencing, netball, basketball, and lacrosse (McCutcheon & Anderson 1985; Storey *et al.* 1989). Several of these sports mandate that players wear a neck protection extension on masks to protect this vital area. Immediate symptoms of laryngeal injury may include hoarseness, dyspnea, coughing, difficulty swallowing, and pain. Subcutaneous emphysema, crepitus, and a palpable fracture may be evident on examination. *Laryngospasm* and acute respiratory distress may ensue. Soft tissue swelling is usually maximal within 6 h, but may occur as late as 24–48 h after injury necessitating that the athlete is watched carefully over this period as internal hemorrhage and local soft tissue swelling may compromise the airway at any time during this period. The sudden inability to breathe can produce immediate panic and anxiety in the athlete and make airway management difficult. The team doctor should reassure the athlete and maintain an open airway as a priority. In mild to moderate cases, sitting the athlete upright helps to maintain the airway. Applying ice gently to the injured area and administering nebulized adrenalin will limit swelling. In case of severe neck trauma or spasm, it is important to keep in mind an associated injury to the cervical spine. In these cases, carefully place and maintain the athlete's neck in a neutral position, and apply a rigid cervical collar. Perform the jaw-thrust maneuver as described above so as to pull the hyoid bone and surrounding soft tissues away from the vocal cords and open the airway. As the laryngospasm relaxes, usually within a minute, a loud inspiratory crowing sound may be heard (McCutcheon & Anderson 1985). If impending respiratory arrest persists following the jaw-thrust maneuver, nasotracheal or endotracheal intubation should be considered. If the laryngeal anatomy is disrupted and the cricothyroid membrane cannot be palpated then cricothyroidotomy is contraindicated, but if there is complete airway obstruction needle cricothyroidotomy and jet insufflation may be attempted. All patients with laryngeal injury should be referred for immediate specialist review and laryngoscopy (McCutcheon & Anderson 1985).

Pulmonary contusion is the most common intrathoracic injury in non-penetrating chest trauma although, like other serious internal complications, it rarely occurs as the result of sport participation. The condition may occur in contact or high-speed sporting accidents during forceful contact with another individual or a hard surface. Most injuries are not serious and go undetected except when the individual coughs up blood or has other underlying problems such as pneumothorax, rib fractures, or subcutaneous emphysema.

Direct blows or compression of the chest can lead to rib fractures, and rarely involve more than one or two ribs. In high-speed sporting activities, such as motor sports, multiple fractures can penetrate the lungs or intra-abdominal viscera leading to respiratory compromise and shock from internal bleeding.

Flail chest involves three or more consecutive ribs on the same side of the chest wall that are fractured in at least two separate locations. The upper four ribs are rarely fractured, because they are well-protected by the scapula and clavicle. The fifth through to the ninth ribs are most commonly fractured. The lower two ribs have greater movement, being attached only to the thoracic vertebrae, and are difficult to injure (Miles & Barrett 1991). A rib fracture results in intense local pain aggravated by deep inspiration so that the athlete is happier with shallow breathing and often attempts to splint the chest wall by flexing the trunk over the affected side.

In a flail chest, signs of paradoxical breathing may be seen with the flail segment moving out with expiration and in with inspiration. The flail segment should be stabilized with a hand or a sandbag and immediate transport of the athlete to the nearest hospital arranged. Oxygen is given by nasal canula or mask and analgesics administered as required. Underlying internal complications should be looked for and ruled out. Intercostal nerve blocks with local anesthetic (Marcaine) in experienced hands can be very useful to reduce severe pain.

Pneumothorax occurs when there is a breach of the visceral, parietal, or mediastinal pleura, and *tension pneumothorax* may develop when the pleural defect acts as a one-way valve resulting in increasing collapse of a portion of the lung by this pocket of air (Leigh-Smith & Harris 2005). It seldom occurs bilaterally. Direct chest trauma with fractured rib and lacerated lung tissue is the leading cause of pneumothorax. Fractured ribs may also rupture blood vessels within the chest cavity giving rise to loss of blood into the pleural cavity and *hemothorax*. The athlete with a traumatic severe pneumothorax or hemothorax presents with sudden onset of chest pain and difficulty with breathing. There may or may not be referred pain to the shoulder. On examination, the athlete displays tachypnea and tachycardia and has decreased breath sounds on auscultation of the chest, hyperresonance to percussion, and decreased vocal fremitus on the involved side.

Rarely, pneumothorax occurs spontaneously in a young, tall, and thin athlete during or following strenuous physical activity. Symptoms in severe cases are similar to traumatic pneumothorax, although 5% may have no symptoms. In some cases the chest pain can stop abruptly after onset, leading to delay in treatment. Spontaneous pneumothorax infrequently progresses to tension pneumothorax (Adelman & Spector 1989). These individuals should be closely observed for respiratory deterioration and transported to hospital as soon as possible for plain radiographs and further management.

Tension pneumothorax results in displacement of the mediastinum by the expanding air pocket to the opposite side, compressing the uninjured lung and compromising venous return to the heart. Signs and symptoms may include severe difficulty with breathing, tachypnea, tachycardia, and hyperresonance to percussion with absence of breath sounds on the affected side. Pre-terminal signs include decreasing respiratory rate, syncope, and hypotension. Tracheal deviation away from the affected side and distension of the neck veins are inconsistent signs (Leigh-Smith & Harris 2005). It is mandatory to recognize the onset of tension pneumothorax and to act immediately to relieve the air pressure in the pleural cavity on the affected side. A 14-gauge catheter over a needle is inserted into the second intercostal space in the mid-clavicular line. If the needle is correctly placed within the pleural space, air can be heard to release through the canula. The patient should be transported to hospital for plain radiographs and further management with possible intercostal drain placement. Any sucking chest wound should be sought and firmly sealed with a dressing. In the case of hemothorax the patient is treated for shock and transported as soon as possible to hospital for chest drain insertion.

Sudden death

Although sudden death is occasionally seen at sporting events in spectators or officials, it is a rare occurrence in athletes. When it does occur in a young athlete it often makes news headlines and has far-reaching effects on the local community. The question is raised by the media and concerned

Table 18.10 Classification of sudden death in the athlete.

Traumatic
Death from blunt force (e.g., cardiac contusion, head or neck trauma, intracranial bleeding, visceral organ disruption)
Death from penetrating trauma (e.g., vascular disruption with torrential bleeding)

Non-traumatic
Non-cardiovascular (e.g., hyperthermia, asthma, rhabdomyolysis, hyponatremia)
Cardiovascular (e.g., ischemic heart disease, cardiomyopathies)

family whether such a tragedy could have been foreseen and avoided – especially amongst young competitive athletes who are seen as the epitome of health and fitness. Table 18.10 categorizes the causes of sudden death in athletes and reiterates the point made earlier that witnessing the collapse and categorizing it as traumatic or non-traumatic makes it easier to assess and treat accurately.

In the general population and competitive athletes over the age of 35 years, atherosclerotic coronary artery disease accounts for the majority of sudden cardiac deaths. Non-coronary causes of sudden cardiac death in the mature athlete are rare and include acquired valvular disease, mitral valve prolapse, and hypertrophic cardiomyopathy (Maron *et al.* 1986; Burke *et al.* 1991; Quigley 2000). In younger athletes a broad spectrum of cardiovascular causes has been reported, including congenital and inherited disorders (Table 18.11; Van Camp *et al.* 1995; Maron *et al.* 1996; Corrado *et al.* 2003).

The risk of sudden death in a young athletic population is 2.5-fold higher than in a non-active population of the same age range (12–35 years) (Corrado *et al.* 2003). However, sports participation is not a cause of increased mortality per se but acts as a trigger of cardiac arrest upon underlying cardiovascular disease that predisposes to life-threatening ventricular arrythmias.

The incidence of sports-related sudden deaths has been difficult to quantify because of its rarity. Incidences differ slightly between different populations studied. This is thought in part to be due to differences in ethnicity, genetic factors, age ranges, and level of sport participation. Retrospective

Table 18.11 Cardiovascular causes of sudden death in young athletes (<35 years).

	Van Camp et al. (1995)	Maron et al. (1996a)	Corrado et al. (2003)
Hypertrophic cardiomyopathy	51 (38%)	48 (36%)	1 (2%)
Congenital coronary artery anomaly	16 (12%)	25 (19%)	6 (12%)
Increased cardiac mass	5 (4%)	14 (10%)	Not reported
Myocarditis	7 (5%)	4 (3%)	3 (6%)
Aortic rupture (Marfan's syndrome)	2 (1.5%)	6 (5%)	1 (2%)
Mitral valve prolapse	1 (0.7%)	3 (2%)	5 (10%)
Arrythmogenic RV cardiomyopathy	1 (0.7%)	4 (3%)	11 (22.4%)
Dilated cardiomyopathy	5 (4%)	4 (3%)	1 (2%)
Atherosclerotic coronary artery disease	3 (2%)	3 (2%)	9 (18.4%)
Conduction system abnormalities	1 (0.7)	1 (0.5%)	4 (8.2%)
Aortic valve stenosis	6 (4.3%)	5 (3%)	0

USA-based population studies have estimated sudden cardiac death in competitive sports at 0.75 and 0.13 deaths per 100,000 men and women per year, giving a risk of 1 per 133,000 men and 1 per 769,000 women (Van Camp et al. 1995). Quigley's (2000) recent study has also shown an overall incidence of sudden death in sport as 1 per 600,000 of the Irish population (genders combined) for all age ranges. From the Veneto region of Italy, Corrado et al. (2005a) have reported incidences of sudden death of 2.3 (2.62 in males and 1.07 in females) per 100,000 athletes per year from all causes, and of 2.1 per 100,000 athletes per year from cardiovascular diseases.

For exercise-related cardiac death in healthy non-competitive adults at any age in the USA the incidence still remains low at 5.4 deaths per 100,000 or a rate of 1 death for every 18,000 men (Siscovick et al. 1984). Maron et al. (1996b) calculated the risk of sudden cardiac death in marathon runners of all ages as 1 death per 50,000 runners, which works out as one-hundredth of the annual overall risk associated with living, either with or without heart disease. The benefits of exercise to the health of the general population still outweigh any increased risk those with heart disease may have while exercising.

There is a striking male predominance (male : female ratio of up to 9 : 1) of fatal events in competitive athletes. Male gender has been reported recently to be, in itself, a risk factor for sports-related sudden cardiac death as a consequence of the greater prevalence and phenotypic expression in young males of cardiac diseases at risk of arrhythmic cardiac arrest (Nava et al. 2000; Miura et al. 2002).

The highest rates of sudden death in the USA are seen in basketball and American football players, whereas in Europe they are recorded amongst soccer players (Corrado et al. 2003). Quigley's study confirmed golf and Gaelic football has having the highest rates of sudden death in Ireland (Quigley 2000). These rates reflect the number of participants in these sports rather than an increased risk of participation in a particular sport.

A comparison of the data from the Veneto region of Italy with Burke's USA data shows a similar prevalence of hypertrophic cardiomyopathy (HCM) in non-sport-related sudden cardiac death (1 in 500 individuals); but a strong difference (2 vs. 24%) in sports-related cardiac deaths (Burke et al. 1991; Corrado et al. 2001, 2003). The Italians attribute this difference to the systematic preparticipation screening protocol that they use to identify high-risk athletes. This includes a mandatory screening 12-lead electrocardiogram (ECG) investigation in every young athlete. Preparticipation cardiovascular screening recommended by the American Heart Association has traditionally relied on history (personal and family) and physical examination alone. The assumption has been that 12-lead ECG is not cost effective for screening a large population of young athletes because of its low specificity and high rate of false positives (Maron 2003). The Italians argue that because the ECG is abnormal in up to 95% of patients with HCM it has the potential to enhance the sensitivity of the screening process. In addition, they believe that it also offers the opportunity for detecting other potentially lethal cardiovascular conditions, such as arrythmogenic right ventricular cardiomyopathy, dilated cardiomyopathy, long QT syndrome, and Wolff–Parkinson–White syndrome which may be missed on history and examination (Corrado *et al.* 2005a,b).

Screening efforts carried out on smaller populations within the USA that have included routine ECG evaluation have had less productive results than the Italian model (Maron *et al.* 1987; Fuller *et al.* 1997). Some researchers believe that this reflects the heterogeneity and variable presentation of HCM in different population groups. False positive ECG results secondary to morphologic alterations in highly trained athletes remains an obstacle to use of ECG preparticipation screening (Maron 2003). It is recommended that suspected high-risk athletes are reviewed by a cardiologist experienced with highly trained athletes.

High-risk patients can now have a cardioverter-defibrillator implanted for the primary prevention of sudden cardiac death. This makes the identi fication of asymptomatic patients with genetic cardiac diseases of even greater importance. However, the presence of an implanted cardioverter-defibrillator is not a sufficient reason, in and of itself, to allow an athlete to return to high-intensity exercise (Maron 2000).

Participation guidelines for athletes with known cardiovascular abnormalities are detailed in the recommendations of the 26th Bethesda Conference papers (Maron & Mitchell 1994). These guidelines may be difficult to implement in high-profile athletes who do not fully appreciate the implications of the medical information presented to them and who may present medicolegal dilemmas to the consulting physician.

Although cardiac arrest from underlying heart disease can be immediately fatal, a number of cases of young athletes have been described in whom prompt recognition of the arrest and use of an automated external defibrillator (AED) has restored normal cardiac rhythm and saved their lives. If AEDs become more widely available for use by the general public at schools and athletic facilities they will undoubtedly result in the survival of more athletes who have cardiac arrest as a result of blows to the chest or "silent" cardiovascular disease (Maron 2003).

Acute coronary syndrome and cardiac arrest

Early recognition, intervention, and transport of athletes with suspected acute coronary syndrome (ACS) from the field to the hospital can substantially reduce morbidity and mortality (Larsen *et al.* 1993; Swor *et al.* 1995). Fibrinolytic agents and percutaneous coronary interventions (including angioplasty or stent) may reopen blocked coronary vessels that cause myocardial ischemia. To be most effective, these interventions must be administered within the first few hours of symptom onset. Delays in transport to hospital occur when the athlete, bystanders, or attending medical team fail to recognize the signs and symptoms of ACS and act in a timely manner (Weaver 1995).

The classic symptoms of ACS are dull, substernal discomfort, often described as a pressure or tightness, and pain radiating to the left arm, neck, or jaw. They may be associated with shortness of breath, palpitations, nausea, vomiting, or sweating and triggered by exercise or stress. The problem of recognizing ACS in athletes, especially those participating in endurance sports, is that these additional symptoms may be present for other medical reasons (hypoglycemia, hyponatremia, and hyperthermia). Symptoms of angina pectoris typically last less than 15 min, while symptoms of acute myocardial infarction are characteristically more intense and last for more than 15 min.

Older athletes, women, or people with diabetes may present with more vague complaint of atypical chest pain that is more diffuse, may radiate to the back, or be concentrated between the scapulae. These patients may feel light-headed, short of breath, nauseous or faint, or have a cold sweat (Solomon *et al.* 1989; Peberdy & Ornato 1992; Douglas & Ginsburg 1996).

Sudden collapse and immediate death may be the first sign that the more mature athlete has underlying coronary artery disease and is experiencing a significant myocardial infarct. In 17% of ACS patients, ischemic pain is the first, last, and only

Table 18.12 Assessing risk of acute coronary syndrome.

Current age greater than 60 years
Previous symptoms of chest pain, tightness, discomfort, breathlessness, or palpitations
Smoker or ex-smoker
Family history of cardiac event <55 years of age
Hypertension
Hypercholesterolemia
Diabetic or have relative with diabetes

symptom (Kannel & Schatzkin 1985). It should be recognized promptly and treated immediately.

In the athlete with new onset of chest discomfort the medical team first encourages the athlete to rest quietly while questions are asked about the athlete's risk of ACS (Table 18.12). If the chest discomfort lasts more than a few minutes then the team should call the local EMS system for transport of the athlete to the nearest hospital; start monitoring with an ECG machine (if this is available) to detect infarct changes or onset of potentially lethal cardiac arrhythmias; begin administering oxygen; establish an intravenous line at a low flow rate and administer basic drugs (Table 18.13).

Be prepared at all times to administer basic life support and rapid defibrillation (if a defibrillator or AED is available). If the athlete is in severe respiratory distress, advanced airway control and intubation may be necessary. The use of continuous positive airway pressure masks, employed in hospitals to avoid intubation in some cases of congestive heart failure, is currently under investigation in pre-hospital trials, with reported positive results (Perina & Braithwaite 2001).

When an ECG reading is obtained, most adults with sudden witnessed, non-traumatic cardiac arrest are found to be in ventricular fibrillation. For these patients the time from collapse to defibrillation is the single greatest determinant of survival (Calle *et al.* 1997; Mosesso *et al.* 1998). Therefore, recognition of potentially life-threatening arrhythmias and on-the-scene electrical counter-shock of ventricular fibrillation within 5 min of diagnosis is important. If the attending medical team does not have an ECG machine or a defibrillator to hand then chest compressions are initiated if signs of circulation are absent. CPR is continued until EMS personnel arrive on the scene with more equipment.

Blunt cardiac trauma

Non-penetrating chest trauma presents with a spectrum of injury from minor impact with superficial contusion of the chest wall in contact sports to more massive injury with possible catastrophic vessel rupture and contusion of the myocardium in high-speed sports. Myocardial contusion can lead to disturbances of the conduction system and sudden death. It is seen histologically as an abrupt demarcation between normal and contused tissue with patchy hemorrhage, lacerations, and cellular fragments within the contused area.

In contrast, the cardiac concussion syndrome, or *commotio cordis*, is a condition in which sudden death follows a low impact blow to the chest wall and in which no structural damage to the heart or overlying protective structures (sternum or ribs) can be seen. Mild soft tissue contusion of the left chest

Table 18.13 Therapy for acute coronary syndrome.

Drug/dosage	Comments
Nitroglycerin 1 tablet/1 spray	Administer at intervals of 5 min up to 3 occasions Monitor blood pressure after each administration
Aspirin 325 mg	Administer as a stat dose Inhibits coronary reocclusion and recurrent events after fibrinolytic therapy
Morphine 10 mg	Check blood pressure before administration Reduces pain, decreases myocardial oxygen requirements and left ventricular preload and afterload
Promethazine HCl 10 mg	Administer as stat dose to control nausea

wall is commonly found in commotio cordis (Maron *et al*. 1995). The precordial blow is often not perceived as unusual for the sporting event involved or deemed of sufficient magnitude to cause death. Cardiac arrest and sudden death intervenes when the precordial impact occurs at an electrically vulnerable phase of ventricular excitability. This may lead to conduction defects, especially ventricular dysrhythmias that are often resistant to conventional resuscitation techniques (Maron *et al*. 1995). In animal studies, the abnormal rhythms observed following experimentally induced chest wall trauma are sinoatrial nodal dysrythmia, atrial fibrillation, atrioventricular irregularities, right bundle branch block, and ventricular fibrillation (Crown & Hawkins 1997).

The frequency of commotio cordis during sporting events is not known but it may be a more common cause of fatality in younger athletes than many of the cardiovascular diseases known to cause cardiac arrest. It has been found to be the cause of sudden cardiac death in 20% of young athletes (Maron *et al*. 1996a). It is most common amongst male children (mean age of 13.6 years) who are engaged in competitive sport (62%). This age group has more compliant chest walls which may facilitate the transmission of the energy from the chest impact to the myocardium (Maron *et al*. 2002).

Precordial blows can be caused by sports projectiles (balls and pucks), players colliding with each other (outfielders chasing a ball), or being hit by an opponent in contact sports or the martial arts. Commotio cordis is not necessarily confined to organized competitive sport and has also been described as an accidental occurrence following a chest blow delivered in an effort to relieve hiccups or in friendly play. Preventive strategies, including the wearing of protective sports equipment and the use of softer balls, has been considered and tested under laboratory conditions. However, these do not provide absolute protection against sudden death (Maron *et al*. 1995, 2002).

Despite the poor response of efforts to resuscitate athletes with commotio cordis, it is important to attempt CPR and defibrillation within 4 min of the witnessed collapse in this condition. Rapid defibrillation could be greatly assisted by the ready availability of AEDs at sporting facilities. However, given the rarity of the occurrence of sudden death (1 per 180,000 per year), some argue that the need for AEDs at athletic facilities is less clear than at high-traffic public places (Hosey & Armsey 2003) or mass participation sporting events.

Anaphylactic shock

Anaphylaxis refers to the symptom complex resulting from an immunoglobulin E (IgE) mediated response to an allergen. Medical teams should be prepared to deal with anaphylactic reactions to insect bites, food ingestion (milk, eggs, fish, shellfish, nuts), drugs (aspirin, non-steroidal anti-inflammatory drugs [NSAIDs], penicillin) or exercise. The incidence of anaphylaxis in the general population is less than 1% and death is a rare occurrence (Yocum *et al*. 1999). The preparticipation physical examination is the ideal time to be made aware of potentially lethal allergic reactions in an athlete. High risk athletes with known significant allergies should be encouraged to carry a kit of self-injectable intramuscular adrenaline or epinephrine (0.5 mL of 1 : 1000) and to wear a Medic Alert tag or bracelet.

Anaphylaxis is a collection of symptoms affecting multiple systems in the body (Table 18.14). The location and concentration of the mast cells determine the organ(s) most affected. Typically two or more of the systems listed in Table 18.15 are involved. The sooner the reaction occurs after exposure, the more likely it is to be severe. The most dangerous symptoms include breathing difficulties and a drop in blood pressure or shock, which are potentially fatal (Ring & Behrendt 1999).

Exercise-induced anaphylaxis (EIA) is uncommon, and death resulting from an episode is rare. Most athletes with this problem either have mild symptoms or recognize life-threatening symptoms early and discontinue the exercise. Athletes may present in one of three ways: cholinergic urticaria, classic EIA, or variant EIA. Patients with cholinergic urticaria manifest with papules surrounded by an erythematous halo (2–5 mm) on the upper thorax and neck which may spread to the trunk and limbs. These lesions may appear in response to exercise, passive warming, or emotional stress. Classic EIA

Table 18.14 Clinical signs and symptoms of anaphylaxis.

Oral	Pruritus of lips, tongue, and palate and edema of lips and tongue Metallic taste in the mouth
Cutaneous	Flushing, pruritus, urticaria, angioedema, morbilliform rash, and pilor erecti
Gastrointestinal	Nausea, abdominal pain (colic), vomiting (large amounts of stringy mucus), and diarrhea
Respiratory	*Laryngeal* Pruritus, and "tightness" in the throat, dysphagia, dysphonia and hoarseness, dry "staccato" cough *Ears* Sensation of itching in the external auditory canal *Lungs* Shortness of breath, dyspnea, chest tightness, "deep" cough, and wheezing *Nose* Pruritus, congestion, rhinorrhea, and sneezing
Cardiovascular	Feeling of faintness, syncope, chest pain, dysrhythmia, hypotension

Table 18.15 Drugs useful for anaphylactic shock.

Drug/dosage/route of administration	Comments
Adrenaline (epinephrine) 0.3–0.5 mL of 1 : 1000 i.m.	Administered to all patients who have clinical signs of shock, airway swelling or definite breathing difficulty Shock may delay achievement of maximum plasma concentrations if the adrenaline is administered subcutaneously If patient profoundly shocked then administer intravenously
Diphenhydramine 1 mg/kg up to 75 mg i.m. H_2 blockers (cimetidine) 300 mg p.o. or i.m.	
Albuterol inhaled	If bronchospasm is a major feature Adrenaline should be administered before the albuterol if hypotension is present
Glucagon 1–2 mg every 10 min i.m.	For patients unresponsive to adrenaline, especially those receiving beta-blockers

manifests with urticaria, or angioedema, upper airway obstruction, and hypotension from vascular collapse. Symptoms can last from 30 min to 4 h after exercise. Patients with variant EIA present in much the same way as cholinergic urticaria but are generally only provoked by exercise and may progress to anaphylaxis (Volcheck & Li 1997).

Some patients have food-dependent exercise-induced anaphylaxis (FDEIA), in which exercise following ingestion of a specific food leads to anaphylaxis. Tomatoes, cereals, and peanuts seem to be the most common food triggers in FDEIA. Anaphylaxis can be avoided if exercise is prolonged up to 4 h after food ingestion.

Management of EIA is directed at modifying behavior and activities. Affected individuals should not exercise alone and should carry a self-injectable kit of adrenaline. They should not exercise within 4 h of eating. Athletes who develop prodromal symptoms of anaphylaxis, such as fatigue, undue feeling of warmth, or whole body itching, should stop exercising and self-administer adrenaline immediately if no medical personnel are to hand to help. Antihistamines are effective at preventing EIA.

Pre-hospital treatment of anaphylactic shock starts with placing the patient in a position of comfort. If hypotension is present, elevate the legs until replacement fluids and vasopressors restore the blood pressure. The patient's airway is managed according to ACLS principles and supplemental oxygen administered at high flow rates. Drugs useful for the management of anaphylactic shock are outlined in Table 18.15. Steroids are sometimes recommended but their value is debatable short term. However, they may minimize delayed recurrence. Start an intravenous line with isotonic crystalloid (normal saline) if hypotension is present and does not respond to adrenaline. A rapid infusion of 1–2 L may be needed initially (Sorensen *et al.* 1989).

The patient should be transported to a hospital for close observation up to 24 h after the attack. Many patients do not respond promptly to therapy, and symptoms may recur in up to 20% of patients within 1–8 h despite an intervening asymptomatic period.

Severe hemorrhage

Severe hemorrhage in an injured athlete can be internal or external in nature. It may be caused by bleeding from an internal organ, a major fracture (long bone or pelvis), or arterial disruption secondary to joint dislocation, fracture, or extreme deceleration as seen in motor sports.

Blood is a potential source of disease transmission and standard precautions should be taken when managing bleeding athletes (Garner 1996). Gloves should be worn by all coaching and medical staff and contaminated items disposed of appropriately or cleaned with a solution of bleach and detergent. An athlete with severe, life-threatening bleeding should be managed as outlined above (see p. 504) beginning with airway assessment, cervical spine stabilization, assisted breathing, and circulation assessment. Control of bleeding commences immediately. Documentation of neurologic status follows and the athlete is then fully exposed to ensure that no other significant source of bleeding is overlooked.

Despite its importance in trauma management, control of external bleeding has received relatively little attention in the medical literature. Basic management includes direct compression and, where possible, elevation of the limb above the level of the heart. If this fails then further compressive dressing should be applied. Recently, the use of elastic adhesive compression dressings has been reported as useful in difficult to control bleeding (Naimer *et al.* 2004a,b). With an exsanguinating arterial bleed, direct manual pressure on the artery, use of an artery clip, hemostat or suture holder, or ligation of the bleeding vessel can be lifesaving.

Management of internal bleeding follows the same basic life support principles, but immobilization becomes more important than direct pressure. This is essential in long bone and pelvic fractures where timely external stabilization of the fracture becomes the key to early stabilization of the patient (Heetveld *et al.* 2004). External compression may also have a role. Medical Anti Shock Trousers (MAST) can help to maintain central venous pressure in trauma patients. However, the quality of the available studies on the efficacy of MAST is poor and there is currently no good evidence that they reduce mortality. They may in fact prolong hospitalization (Dickinson & Roberts 2000). Often internal bleeding can only be controlled by surgery and there is good evidence to show that the sooner this occurs, the better the athlete's chance of survival (Clarke *et al.* 2002). This may explain why studies comparing on-site advanced life support with basic life support and transport to hospital ("scoop and run") have shown no benefit from more advanced care in the field (Liberman *et al.* 2000).

Once blood loss is controlled the severity of hypovolemia is then assessed as part of the secondary survey (Table 18.16). Excessive blood loss may result in *shock*, which is defined as a failure of cardiac output to provide adequate end organ perfusion. The athlete may be pale, cold, sweaty, and syncopal, with altered levels of consciousness or irritability. Quantifiable clinical signs of shock that can be assessed include increased respiratory rate, tachycardia, low systolic blood pressure, pulse pressure changes that may be elevated in the early stages and drop later, and reduced urine output (Table 18.17) (Shafi & Kauder 2004).

Management of hypovolemic shock includes hemostasis, supplemental oxygen, and fluid replacement. Traditionally, rapid and aggressive fluid resuscitation has been the standard of care. Current issues under debate include colloid vs. crystalloid fluid use and the role of permissive hypotension. Crystalloids are electrolyte and buffered solutions, such as normal saline and lactated Ringer's; while colloids are large molecular weight solutions that may be synthetic (dextrans, starches, and gelatins) or plasma derived (predominantly albumin).

Crystalloid solutions are cheaper and readily available; they have a longer shelf life and are relatively safe to administer. However, with crystalloid use only 20–25% of the solution remains in the intravascular space providing volume expansion

Table 18.16 Classification of shock. After Shafi & Kauder (2004).

Clinical signs	Class I	Class II	Class III	Class IV
Heart rate	<100	>100	>120	>140
Systolic blood pressure	Normal	Normal	Decreased	Decreased
Pulse pressure	Normal/increased	Decreased	Decreased	Decreased
Respiratory rate	14–20	20–30	30–40	>35
Urinary output (mL·h^{-1})	>30	20–30	5–15	Negligible
Mental status	Slightly anxious	Mildly anxious	Anxious, confused	Confused, lethargic
Percent blood volume loss	Up to 15%	15–30%	30–40%	>40%
Blood loss (mL)	Up to 750	750–1500	1500–2000	>2000

Table 18.17 Factors associated with increased risk of drowning.

Alcohol
Illicit drug use
Inability to swim
Fatigue or exhaustion
Hyperventilation
Hypothermia
Cerebrovascular accidents
Seizures
Myocardial infarctions
Trauma
Suicide
Child abuse or neglect

for 1–4 h compared to colloid use in which 70–100% expansion occurs lasting 12–24 h. Twenty five percent albumin solutions can provide up to 500% volume expansion (American Thoracic Society 2004). Not only do colloids remain in the intravascular compartment longer, but some may help to reduce vascular permeability. This coupled with the colloid oncontic pressure probably helps to reduce interstitial edema. Synthetic colloids have been associated with anaphylaxis, end organ damage, and coagulopathy in some patients. Albumin, being derived from blood products, carries the risk of disease transmission. A Cochrane Review comparing colloids with crystalloids has concluded that there is no current evidence of any advantage to the use of colloids in emergency fluid resuscitation and, as they are also more expensive, their utilization is hard to justify in this setting (Roberts *et al.* 2004). The American Thoracic Society (2004) in a consensus statement recommends that colloids are administered first in non-hemorrhagic shock and dialysis

patients and are avoided in patients with traumatic brain injury.

It is hypothesized that aggressive fluid replacement in a trauma setting impairs hemostasis by reducing the concentration of coagulation factors and by displacing initial fibrin clots through increased perfusion pressure and reduced blood viscosity. These factors may combine to increase bleeding and further need for volume expansion and thus lead to further hemodilution (Revell *et al.* 2003). The resultant drop in hematocrit lowers tissue oxygen tension, the key change in shock, despite good perfusion pressure. Additionally, the delay in transporting an injured patient while intravenous cannulation is attempted increases morbidity.

This hypothesis suggests a role for permissive hypotension in the acute management of trauma-induced shock. Research into the optimal field management of injured soldiers has recommended low volume resuscitation in hypovolemic shock. One suggested US protocol is the intravenous administration of up to two hypertonic fluid boluses of 250 mL depending on the injured soldier's vital signs and mental status (Rhee *et al.* 2003). Another protocol uses the presence of a palpable radial pulse as an indirect indicator in an adult of a systolic blood pressure of 80–90 mmHg and adequate perfusion (Revell *et al.* 2003). This group make the point that hemostasis is the priority. The presence of a central pulse indicates adequate perfusion for patients with penetrating chest trauma. Brachial pulses should be used to assess children younger than 1 year. They also recommend that transport of the patient should not be delayed by attempts at cannulation but that cannulation should be tried en route to the hospital and that only two attempts should be made. They recommend normal saline be given intravenously in boluses of 250 mL until the radial pulse can be palpated.

Scalp lacerations can be severe enough to cause significant blood loss and hypovolemic shock. They may be complicated by altered levels of consciousness caused by traumatic brain injury or the hypovolemia. This level of severity is generally only seen in motor vehicle accidents where the unrestrained patient is partially or fully ejected from the vehicle (Turnage & Maull 2000). Fortunately, in the sporting situation, blood loss from scalp wounds is easily controlled with direct pressure and elevation. Bleeding from full thickness scalp lacerations can be managed in the short term with simple sutures and approximation of the wound edges until such time as the wound can be assessed and managed formally. When managing a full thickness scalp laceration, the presence of a skull fracture should always be assessed by inspection and insertion of a gloved fingertip prior to closure, although neither technique is reliable.

Submersion

Submersion is defined as an emergency event in which a person experiences some swimming-related distress that is sufficient to require support in the field plus transportation to a hospital for further observation and treatment. A *water rescue* is an event in which the person is alert, experiences some distress while swimming, and receives help from others but displays minimal, transient symptoms, such as coughing, that clear quickly. This person is not transported to an emergency facility for further care as the individual is deemed well and recovered from the submersion.

Drowning is defined as death by suffocation from submersion in water where the patient suffers cardiopulmonary arrest and cannot be resuscitated. Death can be pronounced at the scene of the submersion, in the emergency department, or within 24 h of the event. If the death occurs after 24 h, the term drowning is still used as in *"drowning-related death."* Up until the time of drowning-related death, the patient is referred to as a submersion patient.

Although the term *"near-drowning"* has been extensively used in the past, the recent guidelines recommend that this term no longer be used (American Heart Association 2000b). It was defined as recovery, at least temporarily, after suffocation by submersion in water, and applied to patients who survived >24 h after the submersion event and required active intervention for one or more submersion complications. These could include pneumonia, acute respiratory distress syndrome, or neurologic sequelae. However, rescuers and emergency personnel find this definition irrelevant, because the drowning vs. near-drowning distinction often cannot be made for 24 h. The use of the term near-drowning also makes interpretation of mortality and morbidity data on submersion patients difficult.

The majority of deaths by drowning (85–90%) occur with aspiration of water into the lungs ("wet" drowning) (Weinstein & Krieger 1996; DeNicola *et al.* 1997). Some "wet" drowning cases are thought to be caused by pulmonary edema from marked intrathoracic pressures created during attempts at inhalation against a closed glottis. The remaining 10–15% of cases are "dry" drownings secondary to laryngospasm. The sequence of events that occur preceding death have been described as beginning with panic and struggle to stay above the water surface, followed by breath-holding, apnea, fluid swallowing, and either aspiration or laryngospasm ending in unconsciousness.

In the earlier literature distinction was made between saltwater and freshwater drowning. Although there have been shown to be differences in animal studies between the physiologic effects of saltwater and freshwater submersion, these differences are not clinically significant in humans (Olshaker 2004). The problem in both freshwater and saltwater immersion remains that of intrapulmonary shunting, decreased compliance, and ventilation–perfusion mismatch, leading to hypoxia. The most important factors that determine outcome of submersion are the duration of the submersion and the duration and severity of the hypoxia.

Drowning accounts for 4500 deaths each year in the USA and is one of the leading causes of injury among all age categories. Sports-related drownings account for 15% of this total, with the highest incidence amongst young adults. A number of factors are clearly associated with an increased risk of drowning (Table 18.17; Olshaker 2004).

Hyperventilation before underwater swimming significantly lowers the partial pressure of arterial carbon dioxide ($Paco_2$) while the partial pressure of arterial oxygen (Pao_2) does not change very much. Once submersed after hyperventilation, the individual's $Paco_2$ can decrease to 30–40 mmHg, reducing the stimulus to breathe and prolonging submersion to the point of oxygen deprivation sufficient to cause cerebral hypoxia and loss of consciousness ("shallow water blackout"). Drowning might then result during this period of blackout.

Submersion in very cold water can either be beneficial or disastrous. The potential benefits are that:
1 Hypothermia decreases the metabolic demands of the body helping to delay the adverse effects of hypoxia; and
2 Cold water can bring on the *diving reflex*. This reflex is a primitive one seen most often in children when blood is shunted from less vital organs to the heart and brain (Gooden 1992; Golden *et al.* 1997).
The problems encountered with hypothermia are arrhythmias and quick exhaustion with greater likelihood of submersion.

When attempting to rescue a submersion patient, the rescuer should get to the patient as quickly as possible, preferably by some floating conveyance (boat, raft, kayak, surfboard, or flotation device). In sporting activities that include endurance swim events it is vital to have experienced rescuers such as surf lifesavers in kayaks or on surfboards keeping abreast of the swimmers and vigilantly looking out for possible submersion in an athlete. This is particularly important in cold water conditions and prolonged swims with older race entrants who may take longer to complete the swim than the elite athletes.

It is ideal for the rescuer to extricate the athlete onto a firm surface, such as a surfboard or flat bottomed boat, so that CPR can be begun as soon as possible. Valuable time can be lost getting the patient to the water's edge. In-water resuscitation efforts should also not delay getting the patient out of the water. Spinal injury is particularly likely with

diving or boating accidents and should be assumed if the submersion episode has not been witnessed. Immobilization of the cervical and thoracic spine is important if injury to the cervical spine is suspected. Use should be preferentially made of the jaw-thrust maneuver without head tilt or chin lift to open the patient's airway in these cases.

Postural drainage maneuvers are of unproven benefit and not recommended (Rosen *et al.* 1995). Prompt initiation of rescue breathing has a positive association with survival. Even in the spontaneously breathing patient, 100% oxygen should be started at the scene of the submersion as soon as possible. Apneic patients or those with minimal respirations require bag mask ventilation or endotracheal intubation regardless of body temperature.

Vomiting is likely to occur when chest compressions or rescue breathing is performed, and will often complicate efforts to maintain a patent airway. In a 10-year study in Australia, vomiting occurred in half of submersion patients who required no interventions after removal from the water. Vomiting occurred in two-thirds of patients who received rescue breathing and 86% of patients who required compression and ventilation (Manolios & Mackie 1988). Log roll the vomiting patient to the side and if available remove the vomitus with manual suction.

Ninety-three percent of submersion patients who arrive at hospital with a spontaneous pulse survive without further medical problems, emphasizing the importance of instituting early, effective CPR. Approximately 10% of submersion survivors suffer permanent neurologic sequelae and about one-quarter admitted to hospital subsequently die. Patients who present awake and alert to hospital have good neurologic outcomes and the majority who present with altered mental status (obtunded, stuporous but arousable) ultimately do well neurologically. However, one-third of those who arrive unconscious with a GCS <5 will die, 55% will have normal survival, and 24% will survive with neurologic sequelae. Preventing cerebral injury and improving outcome for these patients remains a challenge. Because it is difficult to predict which of these patients will make a normal recovery, all submersion patients require aggressive resuscitation in the field and in the hospital setting (Lavelle & Shaw 1993; Weinstein & Krieger 1996).

Potentially life-threatening conditions

Head injury

Head injury in athletes can range from mild concussion to more severe injury with physical damage to the brain or the skull. Concussion is by definition transient and resolves with time. Head injuries may result in diffuse injury or focal lesions. Any athlete with a head injury should be managed as if the injury is severe until confirmation of the severity can be ascertained. If there is altered level of consciousness, then the presence of a cervical injury is assumed and appropriate immediate management instituted as described earlier.

Transient loss of consciousness does not appear to have any correlation with the severity of brain injury, but prolonged loss of consciousness should warrant evacuation to the nearest appropriate emergency department for further management. Similarly, the presence of brief post-traumatic seizure activity associated with concussion has been shown to have a poor correlation with concussion severity. Unremitting seizures lasting longer than 5 min or recurrent seizures indicate a more severe problem which is usually the result of the trauma but could be caused by a metabolic problem such as hypoglycemia. Therefore, checking blood glucose and correcting this with intravenous dextrose may be useful. The drug of choice for status epilepticus is lorazepam at a dose of 0.1 mg·kg^{-1} intravenously or intramuscularly (Marik & Varon 2004). Lorazepam is preferred over diazepam because it has a longer duration of action (Sirven & Waterhouse 2003). Some forms of recurrent post-traumatic seizure activity may be resistant to standard anti-epileptic medications and require specialist review (Hudak et al. 2004).

Intracranial bleeds may be present in any athlete with a head injury. Of these, acute subdural hematoma is most commonly seen in the sports person following inertial loading of the brain. Less common are epidural hematomas. These commonly result from rupture of the middle meningeal artery when the groove in which it runs along the inside of the temporal bone is fractured, but may occur from a tear of venous signs in the parieto-occipital region or posterior fossa. The classic description of a patient with an epidural hematoma is deterioration of the level of consciousness which follows an initial window of normality after a head injury. The symptomatic presentation may be delayed as is illustrated by one reported case in which the athlete had a normal computed tomography (CT) scan 80 min after his head injury and then subsequently deteriorated with evidence 8 h later on CT scan of an epidural hematoma (Bruzzone et al. 2000). Intracranial bleeds should be suspected in any athlete with prolonged loss of consciousness or deteriorating status following head injury. Other signs may include lateralizing neurology (altered muscle tone, primitive reflexes) or any indicators of imminent coning (single dilated pupil, loss of light reflex, and Cheyne–Stokes breathing). Immediate management includes attention to ABC, maintaining adequate blood pressure and possibly intubation and ventilation with high flow oxygen. Ultimately, imaging and specialist assessment is essential to categorize the patient into surgical or non-surgical treatment.

Traditionally, head injuries have been classified as "minor" if they have a GCS of 13–15, and "moderate" if the score is 9–12. There is now evidence that patients with a GCS of 13 are more likely to require surgical intervention than patients with a GCS of 14–15, and therefore should be considered as moderate injuries. They should be transported to a facility where urgent CT scanning, neurosurgical, and intensive care facilities exist (Stein 2001). Indications for imaging are listed in Table 18.18 (Murshid 1998; Stein 2001; Dunning et al. 2004; McCrory et al. 2005). When radiologic evaluation is indicated there is no benefit to doing plain skull films and CT scanning or magnetic resonance imaging (MRI) is preferable (Murshid 1998; Dunning et al. 2004).

When managing a patient with a suspected head injury, the mechanism of injury can be an important indicator of the severity of the injury. A high-speed fall while skiing or a motor-sport injury is more likely to have associated potentially life-threatening injuries that will affect the ability to accurately

Table 18.18 Indications for imaging the brain in head injury.

Glasgow Coma Scale ≤13
Glasgow Coma Scale <15 at 2 h after the injury
Any clinical suggestion of basal (or other) skull fracture
Focal neurologic signs
More than one episode of vomiting
Worsening symptoms
Ongoing amnesia lasting more than 30 min
Age greater than 65 years
Presence of coagulopathy
High risk mechanism of injury (pedestrian vs. car, fall
    more than 1 m)

assess the extent of the head injury, as opposed to a head clash in soccer or football, where the head and neck are most likely to be injured in isolation. Nonetheless, the standard primary and secondary survey described earlier will protect the athlete from oversight by the medical team.

In the first instance, the airway and cervical spine must be protected. In an unconscious patient, a rigid cervical collar and oral airway may be reasonable if the athlete is breathing spontaneously. More formal airway protection may be necessary if the athlete does not show signs of recovering within 1–2 min.

If the athlete is on the ground, and conscious enough to be attempting to get up, the team doctor encourages them to lie down for the primary survey and reassures them with an explanation of what has happened to cause the injury. Cooperation is more likely if the team doctor places his or her hand on the chest of the athlete and encourages the athlete to lie down. It is particularly useful if this management approach has been explained to the players in the preseason and they know what to expect. If there is any neck pain, tenderness, or signs of neurologic injury then the cervical spine must be stabilized and the athlete transported from the field for secondary survey.

If the athlete is standing unaided, talking appropriately, and there is no evidence of cervical injury, they should be escorted from the field of play to a quiet secluded area for the secondary survey. This is managed as described earlier. Sideline concussion assessment tools such as the SAC, SCAT, or Sideline ImPACT are available. They are only useful in

documenting immediate post-injury status if the athlete remains symptomatic. The Prague Guidelines (McCrory et al. 2005) recommend that no concussed athlete return to sport on the same day as the concussion; that all concussions require medical clearance before a graduated return to sport; and that no athlete should return to sport while there are ongoing symptoms. Ideally, all contact sport players should have baseline neuropsychometric testing performed preseason. After an episode of concussion the athlete can be retested and return to sport only permitted when these tests have returned to baseline and all symptoms have resolved (McCrory et al. 2005).

One of the main reasons for these strict return-to-play guidelines is that there have been cases reported in the literature suggesting that a head injury that occurs while an athlete is still symptomatic from a previous head injury may be associated with a condition called "second impact syndrome" where there is thought to be loss of cerebrovascular autoregulation with subsequent cerebral edema and brainstem herniation within seconds to minutes. Recommended treatment is immediate intubation and mild hyperventilation, administration of an osmotic diuretic (mannitol), and transport urgently to a hospital (Cantu 1995). The use of hyperventilation has been questioned as it may result in cerebral vasoconstriction and exacerbate cerebral hypoxic damage in head injury patients (Stocchetti et al. 2005). Despite aggressive treatment, mortality and morbidity remain high (Cantu 1998). Some clinicians have questioned the existence of this condition; but until second impact syndrome is disproved, current guidelines prohibiting return to sport until the head injury has resolved should be adhered to (McCrory & Berkovic 1998).

Athletes who have sustained a head injury in the absence of a team doctor must be assessed on the same day by a medical person. If concussion is diagnosed, the athlete should not be left alone for the next 24 h. Indications for admission to hospital for further treatment include any persisting alteration in GCS, neurologic deficit, post-traumatic seizure, any suspicion of skull fracture, deteriorating mental function, or absence of a competent person at home to monitor the athlete (Murshid 1998). Children, patients with hemophilia, or patients on anticoagulants should also be transported to hospital for further assessment. Any athlete who has been concussed but has no indication for hospital admission must be passed on to the care of a responsible adult. Advice is given on the warning signs of deterioration that indicate the need for further assessment in hospital. The SCAT Card has an example of suitable head injury information for patients and caregivers (McCrory *et al.* 2005). Concussed athletes should not drive themselves and should be examined again the following day with a full neurologic assessment in order to detect any developing intracranial lesion.

The Prague Guidelines (McCrory *et al.* 2005) divide concussion into simple and complex. Simple concussions settle within 7–10 days without complication. They can be managed by primary care physicians or athletic trainers working under medical supervision. Management includes rest until there is resolution of all symptoms, followed by a graduated return to training, progressing in intensity as symptoms allow. Complex concussions include athletes with persistent symptoms, concussive convulsions, loss of consciousness greater than 1 min, and prolonged cognitive changes. These require formal neuropsychologic assessment and usually also need imaging. They should be managed by an experienced multidisciplinary team (McCrory *et al.* 2005).

Neck injury

Sport and recreation is the second leading cause of spinal cord injury. The sports that account for the most admissions to spinal injury units are diving, rugby football, and equestrian sports. The catastrophic consequences of these injuries have led to enlightened preseason training programs for athletes in contact sports, better protective equipment, rule changes, and a higher index of suspicion for these injuries by medical staff attendant at sporting events. Such measures have dramatically reduced the severity of head and neck injuries associated with many sports. Nevertheless, transient neuropraxias occur frequently in contact sports and may be treated with less respect than they deserve by coaching staff and players.

Severe injuries to the neck region include airway injuries discussed above, vertebral column and spinal cord injuries. Any athlete in whom cervical spine or cord injury is suspected should have their cervical spine immobilized as part of the primary survey, followed by transportation with appropriate spinal precautions, including log-rolling, spine board or scoop stretcher, immobilization on the board, and transport to an appropriate center for further assessment. Any athlete who sustains a major injury elsewhere in the body must also be assessed carefully for cervical injury, and, if there is any doubt, immobilized with a cervical collar. Athletes in pain from some other injury may not be aware of the severity of their cervical injury. Indications for spinal immobilization are listed in Table 18.19.

If an athlete is down with a suspected cervical injury, begin with manual in-line immobilization followed by the primary survey as described above. If the athlete is responsive enquire how they feel and what they think happened to cause the injury. Ask if they have pain anywhere, particularly in the neck or arms. While maintaining cervical immobilization, their upper limb strength and sensation can be assessed. Next, the cervical spine is palpated for tenderness. In the hospital setting, with normal plain films, midline cervical tenderness is one indicator of possible significant injury. In the field setting, any tenderness raises a doubt, and as such needs to be treated as a significant injury until cleared with imaging. If there are no other distracting injuries and the assessment so far has been normal, the medical team may ask the athlete to move their head into flexion, extension, and

Table 18.19 Indications for cervical immobilization.

Loss of consciousness (or altered levels of consciousness resulting from trauma, hypoxia, hypovolemia, drugs or alcohol)
Cervical pain or tenderness
Athlete's concern about their neck
Neurologic symptoms (radicular pain, paraesthesia, numbness, weakness)
Restricted range of cervical spine movement
Presence of another major injury

rotation. If there is any pain the athlete should be immobilized (Table 18.19).

If all of the above is normal, and the athlete has no concerns about their neck, they should be moved to the side of the field for the secondary survey. Any abnormality should be treated as an unstable injury until imaging has been completed. Even if the suspected cervical spine injured athlete has no indication for immobilization or the diagnosis appears clear, he or she should still be assisted to the sideline for a more detailed cervical and neurologic examination as described in the previous section. Other injuries and shock related to spinal cord injury also need to be excluded in the secondary survey. Spinal cord shock produces loss of neuronal and reflex activity at and below the level of the cord lesion.

It is useful in the preseason to discuss with the players the medical team's standard on-field approach to suspected spinal injury. This reduces stress if the players have considered the situation and seen or even experienced, in the safety of the training room, a cervical collar being applied. It is essential that all members of the medical team who will be involved in the immobilization and transport of a player with a cervical injury rehearse the most likely scenarios before the event.

Severe cervical injury is fortunately a rare occurrence in sport, while transient nerve injuries known as "burners" or "stingers" are more commonly encountered. These are transient neuropraxias of the brachial plexus that occur either by traction, compression, or direct trauma (Vaccaro *et al.* 2002). They present as an immediate onset of burning pain radiating into the shoulder girdle or down the arm. It is usually unilateral and often associated with symptoms such as numbness, tingling as far as the fingers, muscle weakness, or temporary paresis. Motor signs are most common in the C5 and C6 myotomes. Symptoms generally settle within 10–15 min and players often continue to play, only presenting to the team doctor after the game. However, some of the symptoms can persist for up to 36 h. It should be borne in mind that the term "burner" describes a symptom complex and does not specify a specific diagnosis, severity, nerve injury, or prognosis.

Transient neuropraxia involving the cervical spinal cord usually leads to transient quadriplegia or quadriparesis with symptoms including paraesthesiae, pain, and weakness. These are more variable than the symptoms of brachial plexus involvement and can refer into the arms and/or the legs. Transient spinal cord or nerve injuries are more common in the presence of congenital or acquired cervical stenosis, kyphosis, congenital fusion, cervical instability, or cervical disc protrusion (Cantu *et al.* 1998). The association of transient cervical cord neurapraxia with these physical entities makes imaging essential on first presentation. While plain films may be useful for assisting with the diagnosis of injury or degenerative change, MRI or CT scan are required to formally assess for stenosis, disc or cord injury. Athletes who have had "stingers" that have been triggered by relatively minor collisions, are recurring despite complete resolution of symptoms and signs, or have symptoms lasting more than a brief period require MRI scanning.

Athletes may only return to contact sport after their first episode of transient quadriplegia if there is complete resolution of symptoms, full range of motion, and a normal cervical spinal curvature without evidence of spinal stenosis on MRI, CT, or myelography (Vaccaro *et al.* 2002). Athletes with their first episode of transient brachial neuropraxia may be able to return to sport on the same day provided their nerve sensation and power examine normally and they have a pain-free range of cervical spine motion. An extensive list of return-to-play criteria, along with relative and absolute contraindications, is given by Cuculino & DiMarco (2002).

Ophthalmologic injury

While eye injuries are not usually life-threatening, there are situations in which prompt appropriate management may help preserve vision. Examination of the eyes following suspected eye injury should include visual acuity, visual fields, the eyelids and periorbital bony structures, the surface of the globe (conjunctiva, sclera, cornea), the pupils (size, shape, reactivity), occular movements, and fundoscopic examination (Khaw *et al.* 2004).

Injuries such as isolated corneal abrasions and corneal foreign bodies are usually not emergencies. However, they should be assessed by a doctor with experience in this field, and assessment should include documentation of visual acuity as well as slit lamp examination with fluorescein dye. Ultra-violet light can cause corneal damage and may be seen in people visiting the snow for the first time or, on occasion, at aquatic venues. Treatment is as for corneal abrasion and consists of topical antibiotics, analgesia, and tetanus prophylaxis (Maus 2001).

The presence of an intraorbital foreign body, corneal laceration, or globe rupture is an indication for urgent specialist referral. The eye should not be firmly padded as external pressure may worsen the situation. A rigid eye cup should be placed over the injured eye. If the non-injured eye is also not covered, the patient will tend to look around causing the injured eye to move as well; so it may be helpful to cover both eyes with an explanation to the athlete why this is being done. Presence of a hyphema (blood in the anterior chamber) is an indication of an intraocular injury, the blood usually coming from the iris; and the athlete should be referred for further specialist management.

Eyelid lacerations, particularly full thickness lacerations, tears that involve the leading edge of the lid, or the medial end of either the upper or lower lids (and therefore, possibly involve the superior or inferior canaliculi) also require specialist attention. Lid injuries heal well, but require meticulous repair. Lacerations of the bulbar conjunctiva usually heal without difficulty, but the importance of their presence is that they may indicate a more significant bulbar injury such as a scleral laceration or a retinal contusion.

Fractures of the orbital walls or floor are thought to occur as a result of raised pressure when an object such as a ball or a fist forces the eyeball back into the orbit. There is some evidence that a buckle fracture of the floor may occur as a result of a direct blow to the inferior orbital rim (Khaw *et al.* 2004). The orbital floor and the medial wall are the weakest parts of the orbit. Indicators of orbital fracture include a history of trauma to the eye, diplopia, enophthalmos (difficult to assess in the early stages), ipsilateral nose bleed, and altered sensation in the infraorbital nerve distribution (lower lid, side of the nose, and gingiva of the upper jaw from the premolars forward to the midline) (Maus 2001). These

fractures often require reduction, particularly in young athletes (Khaw *et al.* 2004). Diplopia may settle conservatively.

Chemical eye injuries require urgent lavage with copious amounts of water or, if available, saline. Treatment should include "the three I's" – irrigation, irrigation, irrigation (Khaw *et al.* 2004). Chemical eye injuries are also potentially blinding and should be referred on for specialist review. Indications of severity include staining with fluorescein of more than one quarter of the cornea, grayness of the cornea, or staining of the opposing tarsal and bulbar conjunctiva.

Nasal injury

In the athletic population, nasal injuries do not tend to be emergencies. Epistaxis in sport is usually the result of a blow to the nose causing bleeding from Little's area, the mucosa lining the nasal septum located just inside the nostril. Basic principles of hemostasis apply – pressure and elevation. Compressing the soft tissue of the nose and getting the athlete to sit down quietly, leaning forward for a couple of minutes will usually control the bleeding. Helping the athlete to cool down and calm down will also reduce his or her hyperdynamic state and bleeding. In the sporting situation, where the athlete wishes to return to competition, it may be necessary to insert a nasal tampon. Calcium alginate, which promotes clot formation, is available in a nasal "rope."

Occasionally, epistaxis is not caused by a soft tissue injury and these measures do not work. Nasal fractures can be associated with significant bleeding. Unfortunately, while reduction may help control bleeding, it can also cause further bleeding. Orbital blow out fractures can also be associated with significant nasal bleeding (Maharaj *et al.* 2002). Uncontrollable nasal bleeding requires specialist review. Nasal bone fractures can often be reduced acutely without anesthetic; however, if the septal cartilage is dislocated, the bone fragments are unlikely to remain reduced. If the athlete presents late, then it is common to leave reduction for 7–10 days to allow the swelling to resolve. Reductions at this time usually require some form of anesthesia.

Septal hematomas are a complication of nasal trauma. A septal hematoma is a collection of blood between the mucosa of the septum and the septal cartilage. Its appearance is similar to a nasal polyp. There is a risk of infection in the hematoma and consequent long-term destruction of the nasal cartilage with significant cosmetic deformity. Management includes aspiration and nasal packing, with or without antibiotics. If the hematoma cannot be drained, antibiotics are essential.

Ear injury

As for nasal injuries, ear injuries do not tend to be emergencies. The exceptions to this rule are avulsions and barotraumas in scuba divers. There are a number of causes of balance alteration from influences on the inner ear in scuba divers, but the important concept to grasp is that these may be the only indicators present for decompression illness, and these patients may need urgent transfer to a hyperbaric chamber.

Contact sports in which head gear is not often worn can result in soft tissue injuries to the ear. An auricular hematoma is a subperichondral accumulation of blood that may arise following blunt trauma. If large enough and left to organize, these hematomas can cause bulky scar tissue that deforms the ear known as "cauliflower ear." Infection of the hematoma can result in destruction of the cartilage of the ear with significant cosmetic deformity. A small auricular hematoma may be ignored. Management of larger hematomas includes aseptic aspiration followed by packing of the ear. Collodion-soaked cotton wool will mould to the ear and can be strapped in place. A two-pot silicone rubber product is also available. It can be mixed and molded in a similar way, giving a more robust and more easily reused packing. A "through-and-through" suture tied over a bolster on each side of the ear can be used instead of packing to prevent reaccumulation of the hematoma. Oral antibiotics should be prescribed if this method is used to help prevent infection. Daily review with reaspiration and repacking as necessary is recommended. If an athlete presents late and the clot has organized such that it cannot be aspirated, incision and drainage may be necessary.

Tympanic membrane rupture occurs as the result of a blow to the ear in which the external auditory meatus is occluded and the pressure generated exceeds the ability of the tympanic membrane to withstand it. Athletes report the blow, followed by a change in their hearing, occasionally tinnitus and vertigo. They are unable to equalize ear pressure and hear a hissing sound when they try. There may be a small amount of blood from the external auditory meatus. Otoscopic examination reveals perforation of the membrane, limited usually to the pars flaccida of the membrane. Small perforations will heal well within 3 weeks with avoidance of any further impact to the ear and strict instructions to the athlete not to "pop" the ear or to get any water into it until healing is complete. In practice this can be facilitated by using soft ear plugs when showering. Athletes should not be permitted to submerse their heads under water in public swimming pools until cleared to do so. This type of water has a lower surface tension than pure water and may penetrate into the ear more easily. Pool water is also more likely to carry organisms and increase the risk of middle ear infection or failure of the tympanic membrane to close. Occasionally, a large disruption, particularly if there is involvement of the ossicles of the middle ear, will warrant otorhinolaryngology specialist intervention in the early stages. If there is any doubt as to the extent of middle ear injury onward specialist referral is recommended.

Abdominal injury

Abdominal injuries can be difficult to diagnose and catastrophic if overlooked. Disruption of a hollow viscus or solid intra-abdominal organ (kidney, spleen, or liver) can occur from either rapid deceleration, direct blunt trauma to the abdomen, or indirect trauma from a displaced lower rib fracture (Amaral 1997). Symptoms and signs may include abdominal pain, nausea and vomiting, abdominal wall tenderness and guarding, and signs of shock. The diagnosis cannot be confirmed on the sideline or in the changing room but must be ruled out with imaging and further specialist investigation. Therefore, all athletes with suspected abdominal injuries should be urgently transported to the nearest hospital with large bore venous access and nil by mouth. Ultrasound may be used in the trauma setting to diagnose some organ injuries and free intraperitoneal fluid. CT scanning is very good for diagnosing injuries to organs such as the liver and spleen. Diagnostic peritoneal lavage may be used to diagnose intra-abdominal bleeding in the absence of available imaging.

Rectus sheath hematomas can present with acutely painful swelling in the abdomen. They may be differentiated from intra-abdominal injuries with Carnett's sign (Amaral 1997). This is assessed by palpating the patient's abdomen; first, in a relaxed supine position and then with the patient's shoulders raised from the bed. If the pain is eliminated on palpation with the shoulders elevated then it is probably of an intra-abdominal source; but if it remains painful in both positions it is likely from within the abdominal muscle wall.

Genitourinary injury

Genitourinary injury can occur in both males and females and can involve the kidneys, ureters, bladder and urethra, or the external genitalia. These injuries seldom require immediate emergency intervention. Suspicion of genitourinary injury should be based on the mechanism of injury as well as on the presence and degree of hematuria (Herrmann & Crawford 2002).

Hematuria can be a presentation of injury to any part of the internal genitourinary tract. The history is important as blunt trauma to the flank may indicate renal damage, whereas a pelvic fracture may be associated with injury to the ureters, bladder, or urethra. However, one should keep in mind that injury to the kidney may be present without hematuria and that hematuria does not always signify significant renal injury. In the absence of trauma, hematuria in an endurance athlete is known as "runner's bladder." It is hypothesized to be brought about by the "slapping" of the posterior wall of the empty bladder on the trigone. As hematuria in the absence of trauma can be an indicator of malignancy, "runner's bladder" should be a diagnosis of exclusion and it should be fully investigated.

The urethra is rarely injured in the female because of its short course; whereas in the male injury resulting from direct trauma in a straddle-type fall (such as onto a bicycle frame) is more likely, although quite uncommon. Gross blood at the urethral meatus, a scrotal or perineal hematoma, and an absent or high riding prostate on rectal examination are all signs of urethral trauma and warrant further investigation with pelvic CT and retrograde urethrogram. In the male, blunt trauma to the external genitalia can cause contusions and ruptures of the penis and scrotum. Penile fractures require surgical exploration and repair. They are unlikely to present as on-field injuries because they only occur as a result of injury to the erect penis. Testicular fracture or rupture of the tunica albuginea does occur in contact sports. Signs include swelling, erythema, and significant tenderness and pain. A non-palpable testicle may indicate traumatic displacement of the testicle into the perineum or inguinal canal. Surgical intervention is required acutely as delayed repair carries a poor prognosis.

In females, straddle-type falls onto the perineum can give rise to labial or clitoral injury. Occasionally, tears of the perineum have been reported as a result of falls into the splits position (Wan & Bloom 2003). A fall while waterskiing can result in forced vaginal douche with injury to the reproductive tract. Women are therefore advised always to wear a wetsuit when waterskiing.

Testicular torsion is an emergency that may not have a preceding history of injury. Testicular torsion usually occurs in adolescents or young adults and presents with acute onset of severe pain in the scrotal area. It is the most common cause of testicular loss in this age group (Yuen et al. 2001). Detortion within 6 h is associated with a better outcome and delay beyond 12 h is usually associated with loss of the testicle. Urgent referral for emergency color flow Doppler ultrasound is thus mandatory to confirm the diagnosis and bring about early surgical treatment.

Musculoskeletal emergencies

Musculoskeletal injuries that require emergency management include joint dislocations, simple and compound fractures, crush injuries, deep lacerations, and any injury associated with neurovascular injury. Injuries to the skull, spine, and pelvis have been discussed above.

Dislocation of any joint requires urgent reduction in order to help restore normal function and prevent complication. Distal neurovascular function should always be assessed and documented prior to attempted reduction. In the upper limb, dislocation of the fingers and metacarpophalangeal joints may be attempted on the field. They sometimes require surgical reduction. Dislocations of the elbow or shoulder should be taken to a medical room for assessment and attempted reduction. Transport to a hospital may be necessary if there is significant pain, or the first attempt at reduction is unsuccessful. Simple, low stress techniques such as the Spaso technique (Gallagher & Hackett 2004) may allow relatively comfortable reductions without the need for muscle relaxants provided the attempt is made early. There is a risk of undiagnosed fracture, particularly in the older athlete. If there is any doubt of fracture presence, pre-reduction films should be obtained. Post-reduction assessment of neurovascular status should be repeated, and any deterioration is indication for immediate onward referral. Post-reduction plain films are indicated for all first dislocations to detect associated fractures.

In the lower limb, hip dislocations usually require heavy sedation or general anesthetic for reduction. Patellar dislocations can be reduced by gentle passive knee extension. A true knee dislocation is a major injury and may be reduced by gentle traction and extension of the knee. Because of the risk of intimal damage to the popliteal artery these should always be referred on for full assessment. Ankle and foot dislocations do best if reduced as early as possible. The patient is usually much more comfortable if splinted in the reduced position. This type of injury should always be assessed by a specialist in case internal fixation is required.

Fractures should be splinted, elevated, and transported to an appropriate facility. In cases where there is neurovascular compromise, or there will be a delay in transportation, reduction may be attempted. Compound fractures should be dressed with a moist, sterile gauze dressing and the extremity splinted with no attempts made to push the extruding bone or soft tissue back into the wound or reduce the fracture, unless neurovascular compromise is present.

In the event of a traumatic amputation, the proximal stump should be irrigated with a sterile solution and a sterile pressure dressing applied. A tourniquet should only be used for severe uncontrolled bleeding and other methods of bleeding control as described above tried first. The amputated portion should also be irrigated, wrapped in a sterile manner, placed in a bag, and put on ice with rapid transport to an appropriate medical facility. Crush injuries are uncommon in sports, but should be treated with the standard primary and secondary survey, compression, splinting, and transport for further assessment to a surgical hospital where compartment pressure may be monitored if necessary. Management of deep lacerations is discussed above.

Environmental emergencies

High-altitude pulmonary edema

The term *high-altitude illness* includes three unique cerebral and pulmonary conditions that develop over hours to days at high altitude as a result of acute exposure to hypobaric hypoxia: acute mountain sickness (AMS); high-altitude cerebral edema (HACE); and high-altitude pulmonary edema (HAPE). Although high-altitude illness is preventable, AMS and/or HACE and HAPE remain common consequences of rapid ascent above 2500 m for both unacclimatized and some acclimatized individuals. Whether high-altitude illness will develop in an individual depends on variables unique not only to the individual but also to each ascent: genetic differences in anatomy and individual physiology, the ascent rate, the maximum altitude attained, the barometric pressure, the elevation at which one sleeps, the duration at high altitude, exertion, temperature, pre-acclimatization, the altitude of residence, a prior history of high-altitude illness, and certain pre-existing illnesses and medications (ventilatory depressants) (Hackett & Rennie 1976).

The diagnosis of HAPE is made in the presence of at least two of the following symptoms – dyspnea at rest, cough, weakness or decreased performance, chest tightness or congestion; and two of the following signs – crackles or wheezing, central cyanosis, tachypnea or tachycardia. Early pulmonary edema may be inaudible and simply manifest as a decreased exercise tolerance and dry cough. This can progress over a period of hours to days to audible gurgling sounds, coughing up of blood-tinged sputum, marked respiratory distress and, in some cases, death (Yarnell *et al.* 2000). Early diagnosis is critical because HAPE accounts for the greatest number of deaths related to high-altitude illness (Hackett & Roach 2001).

In the setting of recent ascent, decreased exercise performance and dry cough should raise the suspicion of impending HAPE. It usually presents within 1–3 days of arrival at a new altitude and rarely after 4 days at that altitude (Gallagher & Hackett 2004). Alternative diagnoses such as pneumonia, cardiogenic pulmonary edema, pulmonary embolus, and spontaneous pneumothorax should be considered for respiratory distress if this presents beyond 4 days at the new altitude.

Pulmonary edema progression is accelerated by cold exposure, vigorous exertion, and continued ascent. Treatment of mild HAPE begins therefore with stopping further ascent, resting in a warm tent, and avoiding further strenuous activity. Mild illness may completely resolve in 1–2 days with this approach. Most cases of more severe HAPE respond rapidly to increasing inspired oxygen through actual descent, simulated descent (hyperbaric therapy), supplemental oxygen, or some combination of these (Gallagher & Hackett 2004) (Table 18.20).

Newer selective pulmonary vasodilating agents, such as nitric oxide, sildenafil, and prostacyclin in oral or inhaled forms, are currently under study and may be useful in more remote settings where supplemental oxygen is not available or immediate descent not practical (Tom *et al.* 1994). Although proper management immediately improves HAPE symptoms and prevents death, it may take a number of days to completely resolve and require careful monitoring to optimize care. Every effort should therefore be made to get the patient down from the high elevation and to the nearest field hospital for further monitoring and treatment.

Hypothermia

Hypothermia is a decrease in body temperature that renders the body unable to adequately generate sufficient heat to continue its normal functions. This decrease is classically defined as a core body temperature of less than 35°C. One would most expect to encounter hypothermia in winter sports participants, such as skiers, mountaineers, and snowmobilers. It can also occur in those sports where an athlete may be exposed to environmental temperatures lower than the normal core body temperature, including orienteering, hiking, whitewater rafting, swimming and running events (Blue & Pecci 2002). Medical personnel must anticipate the possibility of hypothermia in situations where it may not normally be expected, such as

Table 18.20 Management of high-altitude pulmonary edema.

Action/therapy	Comments
Oxygen	4–6 $L\cdot min^{-1}$ until improved then 2–4 $L\cdot min^{-1}$ to conserve supplies and maintain SaO_2 >90%
Descend/evacuate	>500–1000 m as soon as possible
Portable hyperbaric therapy	14–27 KPa continuously if descent or oxygen therapy not available
Nifedipine	10 mg p.o., then 30 mg SR p.o. b.i.d.
Salmeterol/albuterol inhaled	If HACE not present
Dexamethasone	Only if HACE develops. Does not improve HAPE
Expiratory positive airway mask	May be a useful temporizing measure when supplemental oxygen and descent not available

HACE, high-altitude cerebral edema; HAPE, high-altitude pulmonary edema; SR, extended release formulation.

Table 18.21 Classification of hypothermia. Data from Jolly & Ghezzi (1992).

Severity	Core temperature	Physiologic response and presentation
Mild	32–35°C	Conscious but may be confused and disorientated Shivering and dysarthriac Tachypnea and tachycardia
Moderate	28–32°C	Loss of shivering, diminished level of consciousness May be combative and uncooperative Depressed blood pressure, heart rate, and respiratory rate
Severe	<28°C	Comatose Loss of reflexes Muscles are rigid and areflexic Vital signs difficult to measure Prone to atrial and ventricular arrhythmias

long-distance events, when climate may change very rapidly over the course of the race (Jolly & Ghezzi 1992). Hypothermia should always be suspected in an athlete who presents with altered mental status and has had prolonged exposure to a cold environment. Additional predisposing factors include lack of appropriate clothing for the cold environment, wind chill, and precipitation.

Hypothermia should be assessed with a low-reading rectal thermometer, as oral, axillary, and tympanic standard body thermometers do not give accurate assessments of core temperature in moderate to severe cases. Hypothermia is classified by the degree to which the core temperature has dropped below the normal (Table 18.21) and the physiologic responses to this drop (Schneider 1992). In the absence of a low-reading thermometer, an initial estimate of the degree of hypothermia can be made by the level of consciousness and the presence or absence of shivering.

In the management of athletes with mild hypothermia, the chief aim is prevention of further heat loss. The athlete should be removed as soon as possible from the cold environment to a warm, sheltered place. Their wet clothing must be replaced with dry clothes and they must be passively, externally rewarmed by wrapping their body in layers of other dry blankets and, outside of that, an insulating "space" blanket. Their core temperature and cardiac rhythm are to be monitored regularly. They may be given warm fluids orally as required.

Patients with severe hypothermia have a marked drop in cerebral blood flow and oxygen requirement, show reduced cardiac output and decreased arterial pressure, and can appear clinically dead because of profound depression of their brain function (Sterz et al. 1991; Larach 1995; Holzer et al. 1997). Hypothermia can exert a protective effect on the brain and organs in cardiac arrest. If the patient cools rapidly without hypoxemia, decreased oxygen consumption and metabolism may precede the arrest and reduce organ ischemia (Schneider 1992; Gilbert et al. 2000). Full resuscitation with intact neurologic recovery is rare but can occur after hypothermic cardiac arrest and lifesaving procedures should therefore not be withheld purely on the basis of the clinical presentation (Nozaki et al. 1986). The lowest temperature recorded in an adult survivor has been 16°C (Steinman 1986).

In severe hypothermia, the patient's pulse and respiratory rate will be slow and peripheral vasoconstriction will make pulses difficult to feel. Therefore the resuscitation team should take at least 45 s to assess breathing and then pulse to confirm respiratory and cardiac arrest, or bradycardia profound enough to require CPR (Reuler 1978). Performing chest compressions on a hypothermic patient with a pulse may precipitate a fatal arrhythmia. Rescue breathing is initiated immediately if the athlete is not breathing. If possible, administer warmed (42–46°C) humidified oxygen during bag mask ventilation. Endotracheal intubation should be performed with care but not delayed as it enables the provision of more effective ventilation with warm, humidified oxygen and isolates the airway to reduce the likelihood of aspiration.

If the patient is without a pulse, with no detectable signs of circulation, start chest compressions immediately. Basic life support measures should not be withheld until the patient is rewarmed. The core temperature and cardiac rhythm are monitored regularly. If the patient's skin is extremely cold, it may not be possible to obtain an ECG or to monitor cardiac rhythm by use of adhesive electrodes. If necessary, needle electrodes may be used. Rough movement of the patient should be avoided as this may also precipitate ventricular fibrillation in moderate to severe hypothermia.

If ventricular tachycardia or fibrillation is present defibrillation may be attempted. Up to three shocks can be delivered to determine fibrillation responsiveness. If the athlete is unresponsive further defibrillation attempts should be deferred and CPR continued. The patient is then stabilized for immediate transport to the nearest hospital. If core temperature is <30°C, successful conversion to normal sinus rhythm may not be possible until rewarming has occurred (Larach 1995). The hypothermic heart may also be unresponsive to cardioactive drugs. Care should be taken when administering medications repeatedly in the severely hypothermic patient as these can accumulate to toxic levels in the peripheral circulation owing to their reduced rate of metabolism. Intravenous drugs should not be administered to patients with core temperatures <30°C. In those with core temperatures >30°C intravenous medications are administered at longer than standard intervals.

For patients with a core temperature <28°C or in cardiopulmonary arrest, passive rewarming alone will not be effective in raising the core temperature (Simon 1993). The patient should be transported as quickly as possible to a facility where active internal warming can be performed in a controlled environment by experienced personnel.

Prevention of hypothermia involves educating sport participants on appropriate dress for the environmental conditions and encouraging them to cover areas of the body that lose large amounts of heat such as the head, neck, legs, and hands. It also means allowing the medical personnel at an event to judge the risk to the athlete of the weather conditions and giving them the authority to call the event off or postpone it if the conditions become too risky.

EXERTIONAL HYPERTHERMIA AND HEAT STROKE

Under normal circumstances, body temperature is closely regulated by homeostatic control mechanisms within a narrow diurnal range of between 36°C and 37.5°C. An elevation of body temperature because of a failure of the balance between heat production and dissipation is termed *hyperthermia*. Hyperthermia may be caused by excessive body heat production, diminished body heat dissipation, and/or malfunction of the hypothalamic thermostat (Noakes 1993).

Exertional hyperthermia is a physiologic response to intense exercise and is brought about by excessive body heat production. When working at maximal intensity, skeletal muscles increase their energy consumption 20-fold. Because the body's efficiency is only about 25%, much of this energy is converted into heat and transferred to blood. The athlete's core temperature may be raised to 41°C in high-intensity exercise. This heat is then dissipated by cutaneous vasodilatation and sweating. Acclimated athletes seldom produce more than 1.2 L·h^{-1} of sweat during marathon pace racing. However, higher sweat rates (up to 1.7 L·h^{-1}) have been recorded when the environmental conditions are more severe (dry bulb temperature >25°C) or when the activity is held indoors without the benefit of adequate convective cooling (Noakes 1988; Holtzhausen *et al.* 1994; Holtzhausen & Noakes 1995, 1997). Exertional hyperthermia is usually asymptomatic and self-limited; the athlete's body adequately compensating for the increased heat production and adjusting the work load so as not to overload heat dissipation mechanisms. When exercise stops, the rate of heat production drops and the athlete begins cooling immediately with their elevated core temperature normalizing within 10–20 min of cessation of exercise.

An athlete who has overexerted themselves toward the end of their race may develop syncope if they stop abruptly at the finish line. This has variously been described in the early literature as "heat exhaustion," "heat strain," or "heat syncope." More recently, it has been shown that the majority of athletes who collapse following sudden cessation of exercise do so because of profound postural hypotension (a postural drop of >20 mmHg systolic blood pressure). This is postulated to occur as a result of blood pooling in the dilated capacitance veins of their lower limbs, loss of the pump action of their leg muscles in aiding venous return to the heart, and a blunted vasoconstrictor response to hypotensive stress brought about by training-induced adaptations in the autonomic system (Holtzhausen *et al.* 1994). The unfortunate use of the terms "heat exhaustion" and "heat syncope" has implied that the collapse is a mild form of heat stroke and is, in all cases, associated with raised body temperature and profound levels of dehydration. However, it has been subsequently demonstrated that those athletes who experience such syncope after stopping their running abruptly do not have abnormally elevated core body temperatures but demonstrate marked postural hypotension, and are also not necessarily more dehydrated than those who do not collapse while exercising under the same environmental conditions (Noakes 2000). The use of a rectal thermometer to measure core body temperature can distinguish those athletes who have exercise-associated collapse from those who truly have exertional heat stroke. The best treatment for this form of exercise-associated collapse is lying the athlete down in the supine position with the lower limbs and pelvis elevated above the level of the heart. Athletes can be encouraged to ingest oral fluids if they are mildly dehydrated while awaiting reduction of their postural hypotension which generally improves within 15–20 min (Simon 1993).

Exertional heat stroke may arise if the athlete's ability to dissipate their heat load generated during exercise is overwhelmed. Factors that control the rate of heat loss from the athlete's body include ambient temperature and humidity, the rate of wind movement across the athlete's body, solar radiation levels, and the rate of sweating. The rate of heat production is determined by the athlete's mass and work rate. Thus, the risk of heat stroke is greatest in those who run the fastest, have the highest work rates, weigh the most, and overexert themselves in hot, humid, windless conditions. Other minor factors that have not been well researched but could have a role in reducing heat dissipation include genetic susceptibility, unaccustomed drug use, or subclinical viral infection.

Most of the documented case series of exertional heat stroke are described in military recruits, miners, and endurance athletes. From these reports it would appear that exertional heat stroke occurs sporadically. Most of the reported cases are males, a reflection of their predominance in military and mining activities (Sandor 1997; Epstein *et al.* 1999). Exertional heat stroke is a medical emergency and should be looked for in any unconscious athlete who has been exercising in a hot, humid environment. However, heat-related illness can also occur in more temperate conditions, especially in unacclimatized novice runners who are mildly overweight and exercise at high intensity (Costrini *et al.* 1979).

Athletes with exertional heat stroke typically present with a rectal temperature >40.5°C and central nervous system dysfunction manifesting as aggressive combativeness, disorientation, and confusion or, in severe cases, with coma (Shibolet *et al.* 1976). Seizures may not initially be present but can manifest during cooling (Shibolet *et al.* 1976; Hanson & Zimmerman 1979; England *et al.* 1982; Shapiro & Seidman 1990). The athlete may have some prior warning of the hyperthermia, experiencing a sensation of dizziness, weakness, nausea, and headache. These symptoms are often ignored until the athlete collapses acutely (Noakes 2000).

Athletes are almost always found to be sweating and may or may not be dehydrated. Although some researchers believe that in classic heat stroke, dehydration and a relative state of fluid depletion may have a role in reducing the effectiveness of heat transfer, the significance of its role in exertional heat stroke remains controversial and unsubstantiated (Shapiro & Seidman 1990). Signs that accompany the hyperthermia include tachycardia, hypotension, and tachypnea. Vomiting and diarrhea are common, occurring in up to two-thirds of patients (Armstrong *et al.* 1996a).

Morbidity and mortality are directly related to the duration of elevated core temperature. When left untreated, heat stroke patients can progress rapidly to cardiac and hepatic necrosis, rhabdomyolysis, disseminated intravascular coagulation, adult respiratory distress syndrome, and renal failure. All patients suspected with even minor heat illness should therefore be assessed for the possibility of heat stroke and be monitored continuously for development of this. It is essential to begin cooling of the athlete as soon as possible.

The athlete is removed from the hot environment to a cool, shaded area. While further assessment of the patient is made all insulating clothing is removed and initial cooling is begun. Airway, breathing, and circulation are assessed, and CPR performed as necessary in the non-responsive athlete. The most effective way of rapidly cooling the body is whole-body ice water immersion (Lugo-Amador & Moyer 2004). Other methods include wrapping the individual in cool, wet towels, fanning the body, and applying ice packs to the neck, axillae, and groin. Evaporative techniques are limited in very humid conditions, but can be achieved in a moving vehicle with open ventilation or placing the patient within a helicopter downdraft (Shapiro & Seidman 1990; Armstrong *et al.* 1996b).

Core temperature is checked every 5 min during the cooling process until core temperature reaches 38°C. The athlete is then removed from the ice water, or other cooling methods are reduced, to ensure that the patient's temperature does not overshoot into hypothermia. Patients should be placed on a cardiac monitor and supplemental oxygen given if this is available. Hypotension can be treated with intravenous normal saline but most patients will probably not require more than 1 L of fluid. Seizures and excessive shivering can be treated with a benzodiazepine. Transportation to the nearest hospital is prudent in most severe cases as rebound hyperthermia may occur, and prolonged monitoring and correction of electrolyte abnormalities may be necessary.

Current heat stroke survival is reported to be 90–100% – greatly improved from a rate of about

Table 18.22 Risk factors for heatstroke.

Increased body heat production
Overexertion
Drugs (e.g., sympathomimetics, caffeine)

Increased environmental heat load
High ambient temperature
Lack of air movement
High UV radiation
Sun exposure time
High reflected temperature from the running surface

Decreased heat loss
Exogenous
   High humidity
   Low wicking, dark clothing
Endogenous
   Lack of acclimatization
   Overweight
   Inadequate fluid intake
   Concurrent illness (upper respiratory tract infection, gastroenteritis)
   Drugs (e.g., phenothiazines, antihistamines, alcohol)

20% documented early in the previous century (Royburt *et al.* 1993). This can be attributed to more prompt recognition of the problem and improved initial management with early and aggressive cooling measures. Recognition of predisposing risk factors (Table 18.22) would assist the medical team in discussing preventative measures with the athlete.

Athletes who have been patients of exertional heat stroke will be anxious to know if there are any long-term sequelae to the condition and if their risk can be reduced in future events. Royburt *et al.* (1993) have shown that in a case–control study of 21 young patients with exertional heat stroke who were subsequently followed up for 6 months and tested for heat tolerance and psychologic sequelae, none were found to have any subsequent clinical problems (Armstrong *et al.* 1996b).

Preventative measures that can be undertaken to reduce a future risk of developing heat illness include gradual acclimatization (8–10 days in adults, 10–14 days in children) in a hot, humid environment; wearing appropriate lightweight, loose-fitting clothing when training and racing; ensuring adequate fluid intake and rest periods during the exercise; and being realistic about the intensity of exercise relative to their fitness levels. The medical team and support personnel should be aware of the weather conditions and be prepared to cancel or postpone the athletic event if the risk of heat illness is too high. The American College of Sports Medicine (ACSM 1987) recommends canceling sporting events when the wet-bulb globe index is above 28°C (Irving *et al.* 1991; Speedy *et al.* 1999, 2000a).

Exercise-associated hyponatremia

Exercise-associated hyponatremia is the development of a low serum sodium concentration (<135 mmol·L^{-1}) during or immediately following endurance exercise. The hyponatremia, depending on its level, may be asymptomatic or symptomatic. Serum sodium values as low as 120 mmol·L^{-1} have been recorded in asymptomatic runners post race (L.M. Holtzhausen, unpublished finding). Current evidence indicates that athletes with this condition ingest fluid at unusually high rates during prolonged exercise and retain fluid inappropriately (Noakes 2000). Fluid is initially retained in the extracellular space, but osmotic forces eventually cause rapid diffusion into the intracellular space. The pathogenesis of this inappropriate fluid retention remains unknown, but it is postulated that in susceptible individuals the rate of urine production is markedly reduced during exercise of long duration (Irving *et al.* 1991; Speedy *et al.* 1999). Sodium deficits in hyponatremic runners are not significantly different from normonatremic controls, indicating that symptomatic hyponatremia is not brought about primarily by sodium losses in the sweat. There is also no evidence for elevated aldosterone or vasopressin concentrations in this condition (Hiller *et al.* 1985).

Estimates of the incidence of hyponatremia vary according to the endurance event and the serum sodium value used (<130 or <135 mmol·L^{-1}). The highest published incidence of hyponatremia has been 29% from the Hawaiian Ironman Triathlon. Holtzhausen *et al.* (1994) have shown that 10% of asymptomatic runners finishing a 56-km running race were hyponatremic. Conversely, Noakes *et al.* (1990) have reported data that suggest a very low

incidence (0.2%) of symptomatic hyponatremia at the 1986 and 1987 Comrades Ultramarathon (87 km). They have also reported a 2% incidence of asymptomatic hyponatremia in a 186 km triathlon but 0% incidence of symptomatic hyponatremia (Noakes 2000).

Athletes who collapse and are found to be unconscious during or immediately after an ultra-endurance event and whose rectal temperatures are not elevated should be considered to have symptomatic hyponatremia until measurement of the serum sodium concentration refutes the diagnosis (Speedy *et al.* 2001b). A useful sign of overhydration in an athlete is the development of tightness of rings, watches, or race bracelets that may have been loose at the start of the race. Symptoms of hyponatremia can range from non-specific lightheadedness, fatigue, nausea, and headache to those suggestive of cerebral edema including confusion, incoordination, disorientation, and delirium. Seizures, progressive coma, and death from respiratory or cardiac arrest may finally result if the fluid retention is not reversed (Noakes 1995; Holtzhausen & Noakes 1997; Mayers & Noakes 2000).

Appropriate management of symptomatic hyponatremia includes close clinical observation, with regular monitoring of serum sodium concentrations, while awaiting a spontaneous diuresis of the retained fluid. Provided the athlete is clinically stable and without significant symptoms or signs of cerebral or pulmonary edema, they can be managed at the finish line medical facility. These athletes should not be given intravenous fluids as they are already fluid overloaded. Intravenous access may be established with an intravenous cannula and Luer plug in case drug administration is required. The exact role of hypertonic saline in the treatment of exercise-associated hyponatremia is unclear as the only published data are case reports. Intravenous fluids should never be given to a collapsed ultra-endurance athlete before an accurate diagnosis has been made because of the risk of harm from exacerbation of an unrecognized hyponatremia resulting from fluid overload (Worthley & Thomas 1986).

Seizures and coma are life-threatening emergencies, and these patients require aggressive treatment with hypertonic saline (29.2%) to create an osmolar gradient of 10–20 mosmol·L^{-1} in order to rapidly mobilize brain water (Hammes *et al.* 1998). A bolus dose of 50 mL of a 4 mmol·L^{-1} concentration of sodium chloride (NaCl) can be injected into a large vein. This is then followed by a continuous infusion of 3% saline which should probably be instituted in a hospital setting where close monitoring of serum sodium can be performed regularly. A loop diuretic can also be given to encourage diuresis in severe cases. The amount of NaCl required for infusion must be calculated precisely to ensure sodium is not corrected too rapidly (ideally <25 mmol·L^{-1} in 48 h) (Cluitmans & Meinders 1990). There is a risk of inducing pontine myelinolysis with too rapid correction of serum sodium. However, this has not been encountered in the management of exercise-related hyponatremia, but rather in chronic long-standing hyponatremia cases (Noakes 1993).

Because hyponatremia is the result of overhydration, prevention should focus on educating novice ultra-endurance athletes on appropriate volumes of fluid ingestion and the dangers of drinking too much. Noakes (1993) has suggested that a fluid intake of no more than 600 mL·h^{-1} is appropriate for most non-competitive athletes during prolonged exercise in the heat (Burke 1993). Burke recommends a fluid intake of 500–1000 mL·h^{-1} in ultra-endurance events (Speedy *et al.* 2000a). These recommendations are lower than the ACSM's position statement that rates of fluid intake should be 600–1200 mL·h^{-1}. Douglas Casa has recently formulated a self-testing program for optimal hydration in which athletes are encouraged to calculate their expected fluid losses over a 1 h training run that simulates race pace and environmental conditions. This program can be accessed online at the USATF web page (www.usatf.org/groups/Coaches/library/hydration/USATFSelfTestingProgramForOptimalHydration.pdf). Educating athletes on the appropriate levels of fluid ingestion during an ultra-endurance event and reducing the availability of rehydration fluids at support stations has been shown by Speedy *et al.* to reduce the percentage of athletes requiring treatment for hyponatremia from 24% to 4% in an Ironman triathlon event (Rogers *et al.* 1997; Fallon *et al.* 1998; Speedy

et al. 2001b). Three studies have looked at the mean fluid intake of athletes during ultra-endurance exercise and these have shown levels to range from 540 to 737 L·h^{-1} (Speedy *et al.* 2000b). Some runners still develop hyponatremia at modest fluid intakes, and for slower athletes or those who are small or female fluid intakes should be at the lower end of the recommended range (Noakes 1995). There is no evidence that the mild dehydration (up to 4% body weight) found in the athletes who follow these guidelines is detrimental to their health or performance (Armstrong *et al.* 1996b).

Medical preparedness for sports events

The aim of this section is to provide a practical guideline on formulating an emergency medical care plan for team and endurance sporting events. Each of these event types has their own unique challenges in this regard.

Team sports

The key to providing comprehensive team sports medical coverage is preparation. Preparation starts with understanding the factors listed in Table 18.1, all of which may play a part in determining the number and type of expected casualties. This will then dictate how many people are required for adequate medical support. The support team may include other doctors, physiotherapists, sports trainers, massage therapists, trained first-aiders, ambulance staff, and coaching staff. At the grass roots level a minimum requirement would be at least one trained first-aider with each team. Coaching certification should ideally include BLS training and yearly recertification. This may obviate the need for further medical staff at the field side. In national level contact sport each team should have a doctor, physiotherapist, and a qualified trainer. For teams traveling internationally, the identification of a local doctor who can provide access to local specialists, including surgeons and radiologists, is very useful.

Once an appropriate medical team has been selected they should meet and agree on the hierarchy of command and the protocols for the management of a number of emergency situations. These may include the management of an unconscious athlete, approach to a head or spinal injury, and the transport of an athlete with a limb injury. Each of these protocols should be rehearsed regularly throughout the season. In some cases, the rules of the game will dictate who can enter the field of play and when they are permitted to do so. It is essential that these rules are understood in advance.

The opportunity should be taken, if possible, to assess the facilities at the event venue prior to the competition: suitable medical rooms assigned for management of bleeding players and the assessment of severely injured players; and the medical equipment provided at the venue, including waste disposal and sharps containers. Ideally, the equipment provided at the venue should also include a spinal board or scoop stretcher, oxygen, and AED. The changing and toilet areas should be assessed for safety and hygiene, and the playing surface and surrounding area evaluated for potential hazards. These may include poorly covered irrigation nozzles, pipe work or fencing that is too close to the boundaries of the playing field, and loose pieces of ground cover or turf. Enquiries must be made prior to the competition about the level of medical support that will be available; what emergency equipment will be provided at the venue; and the access to a telephone in the medical area. Ensure that a list of local emergency contact numbers is attached to the telephone and that the telephone is in working order.

Communication between the medical and coaching staff is very important and may require the use of radios or mobile telephones during the event. In the Australian National Rugby League events the rules do not permit entry of any individual with a two-way radio onto the field of play. Most medical teams in this situation use hand signals from the field to indicate the current status of the athlete. These are agreed on and revised prior to the event.

On arrival at the venue the team doctor should communicate with the opposition team's medical and support staff who may be called on to assist in case of an emergency. Doctors should agree on the chain of command and whether they will assist with the opposing team's seriously injured players. The home team doctor should make him or herself available to recommend an appropriate facility for transport in the event of severe injury. The team doctors should not assume that the emergency equipment provided at the ground is indeed present or functioning optimally and should double-check this prior to the event. As part of this preparation it is also important to decide in advance, amongst all the medical personnel, who will bring the equipment out and what signals will be used to indicate that they are needed. The team doctor should also identify him or herself to any local EMS personnel in attendance at the game and discuss with them the evacuation needs of seriously injured athletes. The team doctor must also establish what level of certification and support the EMS personnel can provide and which local hospitals they recommend for the different types of injury.

Prior to attending a game, doctors should review their medical kits, ensuring that they have adequate supplies for any emergency and fresh batteries for their handheld equipment. Drugs should be restocked and equipment checked for failures. At the venue, the team doctor must identify a suitable area for medical assessment and lay out any equipment that may be needed in an emergency. Security may be an issue. If a door is to be locked during the game, the team doctor should ensure that he or she knows how to get it unlocked. The team doctor should also be familiar with the evacuation plans of the event venue.

During the game gloves should be worn at all times and changed after each use. It is useful to have a plastic hazard bag on the sideline to dispose of blood-contaminated gloves, gauze, or towels. Blood on the skin or equipment of players should be washed off with a solution of household bleach (one part in 10), detergent (one part in 20) and water. This can be made up simply with 30 mL bleach, 15 mL detergent, and 250 mL water. It should be mixed up fresh for each game. If stored in a spray bottle it can be easily applied to skin, clothing, and equipment. Control of bleeding is essential and an elastic adhesive bandage over an occlusive dressing will control most wounds. Occasionally, scalp or facial wounds will need closing. In some cases it may be appropriate to close the wound and return the player to the game, but in the interests of optimal wound care, it is recommended that the doctor review the wound at the end of the game, and, if necessary, open it again and rinse thoroughly with saline before closing carefully.

Following the game, each player should be approached and questioned about any injury they may have incurred during the game. Injuries should be documented and follow-up management planned. Any players who required urgent transport from the venue during the game should be followed up at this stage. It is important to maintain good communication with the patient primarily and, with his or her permission, with their next-of-kin and the coaching staff.

In professional sports there is usually an injury review clinic on the day after the game allowing for players who may not be aware of injury concerns immediately after the match to be assessed and treated. This should be in a clinic setting where time can be taken, issues can be discussed confidentially, and the players have the space to express any concerns or ask any questions that they may not wish to ask in front of other members of the team. Following this clinic, player availability for training and the following game should be discussed with the coaching staff and rehabilitation plans laid out with the trainers and physiotherapists.

Documentation is essential and all requests for medical assistance from the team members or staff

and treatment provided, including medications dispensed, should be meticulously noted. Following a tour with a team, a medical report should be completed documenting rates and types of medical problems, advantages and disadvantages of venues attended, contact details for local medical specialists who provided useful services or information, and any issues that may be worth changing for future tours. This will provide useful information on estimates of medication and equipment requirements for the team management and new medical staff when planning future tours.

The medical equipment required will vary according to the requirements of the event and the expected casualties. Some basic kit lists have been formulated to assist the medical team in adequate equipment provision. These include a basic diagnostic equipment and stationery list (Table 18.23); an eye injury management kit (Table 18.24) that can be stored separately for quick access if required; a comprehensive wound management equipment list of items to be stored in the emergency room (Table 18.25); a simple side line wound management kit that can be carried in a pouch for attending to on field and side line minor injuries (Table 18.26); and a basic trauma kit for providing airway management and basic life support (Table 18.27). These lists should be tailored to suit the needs of the doctor and the team depending on sex, age, and whether on tour or at home. A list of suggested medications (Table 18.28) is provided as a guideline

Table 18.23 Basic diagnostic equipment and stationery.

Diagnostic	Stationery
Thermometer	Paper for medical notes (or dictaphone)
Stethoscope	Letterhead paper for referrals
Sphygmomanometer	Prescription pad
Diagnostic set (ophthalmoscope, otoscope)	Radiology request forms
Eye chart	Blood/laboratory request forms
Tendon hammer	Permits to travel with medications
Tongue depressors	Medications catalog
Cotton buds	Spare pens (ballpoint, permanent markers)
Tape measure	Copy of practicing certificate/medical qualification
Urine and blood glucose dipsticks	Envelopes
Sideline concussion assessment tool (SAC, SCAT, Sideline Impact)	

Table 18.24 Eye injury management kit.

Eye shield
Eye pads
Cotton buds
Normal saline
Tape
Fluorescein drops or strips
Cobalt blue light
Local anesthetic drops
Contact lens case
Mirror
Antibiotic eye ointment

Table 18.25 Wound management equipment.

Dressing packs	Small sharps container
Betadine or chlorhexadine	Antibiotic ointment
Sterile gloves	Occlusive dressings
Normal saline	Elastic adhesive bandages
Sterile scrub brush	Steri-strips
Suture kits	Band-aids
Sutures (including nylon and dissolving)	Strip adhesive dressings
Local anesthetic	Scissors
Needles and syringes	Spare gauze squares
Skin glue	Biohazard bags
Staple gun	Bleach and detergent solution in spray bottle

Table 18.26 Sideline wound management kit.

Tape (elastic adhesive, rigid, and electrician's tape)
Gauze squares
Normal saline sachets 200 mL
Antibiotic ointment
Scissors
Gloves
Nasal tampons
Spare salbutamol inhaler
Decongestant nasal spray

to what may be required in various emergency situations. Some of the medications are restricted in athletes who are competing at a level at which they may be drug tested. These medications need notification and approval before use in competition. Some of the medications may also be banned in competition, but athletes who need them are usually not able to compete so the question of prior notification is not that urgent.

Endurance sports

Endurance sporting activities such as marathons, triathlons, and multisports events have become increasingly popular and many of them attract sufficient numbers of participants and spectators to constitute a mass gathering (>1000 people). Medical coverage for these events requires careful pre-event planning and the cooperation and coordination of many individuals within the local community on race day. The primary goal of the medical team is to ensure the safety of the competitors and to help relieve the burden of casualties on the local public services. Being mass gatherings there is a risk of mass casualty and the medical team need to have put in place a disaster plan to cover such an eventuality.

A race medical director is appointed as a member of the race organizing committee to oversee the organization of all the medical personnel, facilities, and provisions and to advise on any safety issues. Ideally, this person should have experience in the sports medicine field and have a good knowledge of the types of conditions encountered in endurance events. Depending on the size and complexity of the event, the race director may elect a committee of medical and non-medical volunteers to assist with the pre-race organization. The medical chain of command should be clear to the other race organizers and volunteer staff prior to race day. All medical queries pertaining to the competitors and event should be passed on to the medical director prior to and during the event to ensure uniformity of care.

The type of event, number of participants, course peculiarities, and environmental conditions are all important factors to take into consideration when determining the extent of medical coverage required for an endurance event (Holtzhausen & Noakes 1997). In most well-established events, records will have been kept by previous medical teams on the number and type of casualties and the

Table 18.27 Suggested staffing numbers per 1000 athletes in an endurance event.

Medical doctors	5–8	Inclusive of one emergency medicine specialist and some doctors familiar with conditions presenting in endurance athletes
Nurses	8–10	Ideally, some of these nurses should be familiar with working in emergency rooms with resuscitation equipment
First aid personnel	1–2 per aid station	They should be familiar with basic first aid treatment protocols and with treating minor injuries
Administrative assistants	10–12 at the finish line facility	These volunteers need not be medically trained personnel. They can assist with stretchering collapsed athletes from the finish line to the medical facility, spotting athletes who appear to be in distress or unwell on the course, assist with keeping medical records and with communication between facilities
Advanced paramedics	2	To man a rapid response vehicle or ambulance. Ideally, conversant with the local road system
Physiotherapists	2–4	It is useful for these personnel to have an area they can work in apart from but adjacent to the main finish line medical facility
Podiatrists	2–4	To help with foot injuries and blisters

Table 18.28 Trauma kit.

Stiff neck cervical collar	Spacer (or nebulizer) for salbutamol
Oral airways	Salbutamol inhaler or ampoules
Cuffed endotracheal tubes	Giving sets
Laryngeal masks	Tape
Combitube	Sterile gloves
Manual suction	Cricothyroidotomy kit and/or large-bore cannula
Laryngoscope	10 mL syringe
McGill forceps	Lubricant
Bag mask	Alcohol swabs
IV fluid	Scalpel handle
Cannulae	Disposable #11 blades

weather conditions on race day. This greatly assists the new team in predicting the casualties and preparing adequately for the next event (Mayers & Noakes 2000).

Pre-event planning

The key areas that the medical director needs to be involved in during the planning stages of the race include the following.

SCHEDULING OF THE EVENT

The race medical director can help in choosing an event time of year, location, and time of day to optimize weather conditions and avoid risk of environmental hazards. Weather conditions that may warrant event cancellation, alteration, or postponement can be predetermined and contingency plans instituted by the organizing committee prior to race day.

LAYOUT OF THE COURSE

The medical director must ensure that the course is safe for both the participants and spectators. Often this is furthest from the minds of race organizers who are dealing with competing priorities of sponsors, media personnel, and spectators. Biking, swimming, and skiing events carry additional risk elements such as water safety and trauma potential associated with high speeds (Reid *et al.* 2004). Water temperature, sea and road conditions, transition, acceleration and deceleration areas, and protective equipment requirements all need to be carefully evaluated and policy discussed based on these variables. Emergency vehicles need to have quick and easy access to all parts of the course for removal of injured athletes or spectators. Medical facilities and personnel need to be placed at appropriate support and transition stations and at the finish line to ensure adequate medical coverage. Support (drink) stations need to be positioned at 2.5–3 km intervals along the course to minimize risk of over- or underhydration of the competitors (Roberts 1989). The race director needs to ensure that the sponsored rehydration fluid provided is reconstituted to the correct concentration on race day by the support station volunteers and appropriate foods supplied for energy and mineral needs.

PREDICTING THE NUMBER OF CASUALTIES

Injury rates for various events have been reported in the literature and summarized by Roberts (1989), Hiller *et al.* (1987) and Holtzhausen & Noakes (1997). These vary from 5% of race participants in cycling and standard distance triathlon events to 30% in ultradistance running and multisport events. Injury rates increase with increased distance, environmental temperature, and humidity (Maron *et al.* 1996b). Previous years' experience and keeping of good medical records for each casualty is very helpful in planning for subsequent events. Similar events held in the same weather conditions can be used in the initial medical planning and preparation stages for new events. Table 18.6 lists the types of casualties that can be expected at ultra-endurance events. Documented cardiac fatalities in marathons suggest that approximately 1 per 50,000 runners risks fatal arrhythmia or myocardial infarction, with most episodes occurring during the event – not at or after the finish line (Laird 1989). The risk for exertional death in endurance events is thus fortunately rare.

MEDICAL COVER OFFERED AT THE EVENT

The race medical director will have to decide what level of care will be made available on the course and at the finish line medical facility. This will often depend on what local emergency facilities are available within the vicinity of the race, how prepared these facilities are for dealing with the expected emergencies, and how remote the course is. The aid stations on the course may provide primary first aid care and basic life support while relying on emergency response vehicles to provide advanced life support. If the local hospital or emergency facility is too far away for timely evacuation of an urgent case or lacks the personnel or equipment to deal with the expected casualties then this may have to be provided for at the race finish line medical tent.

Coordination with the local EMS, emergency departments, and hospitals is mandatory to ensure appropriate medical coverage of the event. Areas that may require discussion with these groups include the optimum management protocols for each type of casualty, the usage and type of intravenous fluids, availability of oxygen, medications, and advanced cardiac and trauma life support equipment.

Quick effective response to emergencies is best provided by motorbike, kayak, or EMS rapid response vehicles (Noakes 2000). The medical director should determine in advance the transfer protocols for each type and severity of casualty so that aid station volunteers and EMS workers can evacuate the athlete without unnecessary delays. Suggested automatic transfers to a well-equipped local hospital or emergency facility may include those not responding to usual treatment protocols, severe multitrauma casualties not responding rapidly, cardiac and respiratory arrest patients requiring advanced airway and life support, hyperthermia or hyponatremia patients with seizure or coma, and severe hypothermia patients.

A decision needs to be made by the medical director on what medications will be made available on the course, at the first aid stations, and at the finish line facility. It is recommended that these be tightly controlled and all medical personnel and competitors made aware of what will be available. Athletes with chronic medical conditions, such as asthma, diabetes, and hypertension, should be forewarned about carrying their own medications and wear a Medic Alert bracelet or tag during the event.

Race registration forms should include a brief medical questionnaire on the participant's past and present medical conditions, current medications, and known allergies. This information greatly assists the provision of optimal care in the case of emergency. In some conditions it can be very helpful in making the right diagnosis.

Competitors and emergency medical staff should be familiar with the "impaired competitor" policy of the race. This involves deciding prior to the event how to handle the injured athlete and what medical criteria will be used to pull the athlete from the competition. Clinical criteria should be used to determine if the athlete is unfit to continue the race and when they would be putting their life at risk by continuing the race. If the individual is orientated for time and place, and demonstrates appropriate competitive posture and is able to proceed in a straight line along the course, they should be left to continue their race. If there is any doubt as to the athlete's fitness to continue they should be watched intermittently along the course by designated spotters or first aid personnel. Some races elect to institute cut-off times by which the athlete must have completed a specific distance or leg of the race. This has been reported to considerably reduce the number of casualties seen (Cianca et al. 2001). The impaired competitor policy should be well publicized before the event so that all parties are aware of it and it does not become a contentious issue on race day.

EDUCATION OF THE PARTICIPANTS

The number of casualties can be greatly reduced by educating the athletes prior to the event about adequate training; acclimatization for the expected weather conditions; wearing of appropriate clothing for the event; prevention of injuries and illness; recognition of conditions that may result in health risks (including intercurrent upper respiratory tract infections and gastroenteritis) and precautions to avoid these risks. This information can be provided through the race website, handouts that accompany the race pick-up packet, and seminars. During the pre-race briefing the medical director can also provide information on location of the medical aid

stations on the course and available first aid services in these areas, as well as the "impaired competitor" policy of the event. Race day information regarding weather conditions and health warnings have been used with success at numerous events (Holtzhausen & Noakes 1997).

STAFFING NEEDS AND TRAINING

Staffing requirements will vary and may be unique to each event, but a suggested minimum number and type of medical personnel required per 1000 participants is listed in Table 18.27. About 60% of these staff should be positioned at the finish line medical facility, 10% at the finish line itself, 20% at the support stations out on the course, and 10% patroling the course in rapid response vehicles. Medical and paramedical staff should be easily identified on race day with a brightly colored armband or bib, or a clearly marked T-shirt. They should be provided with access passes to all areas of the course and finish line necessary to their support role.

Medical volunteers are gathered from diverse backgrounds and experience levels and most of them are probably better versed at providing medical care within a hospital or private clinic setting. They may not have experience with managing the conditions peculiar to endurance sports. An education session prior to race day is therefore ideal to review with these volunteers the medical plan, chain of command, and level of care expected. Triage and treatment protocols specific for the event, course maps, availability of parking, proximity to water, food and support stations, communication and transportation plans need to be provided in written form to these personnel.

COMMUNICATIONS ON RACE DAY

Rapid, clear, and effective communication on race day between the race director, medical director, and other race volunteers is essential. This can be achieved by means of a communications network that includes mobile phones, ham- and hand-held radios. The system should be tested before the event and personnel given an opportunity to become conversant in its use. A back-up system must be available in case of failure on race day. A plan outlining how EMS will be requested and dispatched, where injured athletes will be transported to, and when to contact the medical director will reduce race day chaos and delayed response to emergencies. It is best to have a central base from which to coordinate all dispatch requests manned by an advanced paramedic who can triage and assess all emergency calls. This communication base is best situated adjacent to the finish line medical facility. It is useful in large races to consider providing a publicly displayed board or computer screen with the list of athletes who have retired from the race because of illness or injury and are being treated within the medical facility. This greatly reduces the anxiety of the supporters and the number of people attempting to gain access to the medical facility looking for their athlete.

FINISH LINE MEDICAL FACILITY AND FIRST AID STATIONS

The main medical facility should ideally be positioned within line of site of the finish line. This may need to be a large tent if an existing field side building is not available. It should not be positioned too far away from the finish line so as to make transporting collapsed athletes time-consuming and back-breaking work. The race finish line is often very noisy with public address system announcements, music, and cheering spectators. This may make it impossible to ausculate a patient's chest or heart if the medical facility is positioned too close to the finish line.

This facility should be large enough to partition off into four separate areas to serve as a triage zone, a massage and physiotherapy area, minor illness and treatment areas, and an emergency treatment zone. Thought should be given to the flow of athletes through this facility so as not to create chaos and bottlenecks at the time of peak casualty rates. Peak rates tend to occur in the middle of the race when athletes are attempting to make the finish line under a certain personal best time or toward the end of the race when they are endeavoring to make the finish line cut-off time.

If a tent needs to be constructed, thought will also have to be given to how:
• Good ventilation can be maintained during the heat of the day within the facility;
• Adequate warmth can be created in the evening if the event is longer than 12 h;
• Adequate lighting, a power source, and water supply can be provided safely to the facility;
• Storage space and cooling facilities can be made available within the tent for equipment and medications;
• The facility can be made easily accessible to stretchers and ambulances.

The aid stations should be positioned close to the drink stations – ideally at intervals of 2.5–3 km for races longer than 10 km. These should provide a sheltered secluded area where athletes with minor problems can be treated in privacy or collapsed athletes awaiting transfer can be safely observed. This can take the form of a small tent, mobile caravan, or convenient roadside building. Provision of plastic disposable raincoats to hand out to athletes in case of inclement weather can greatly reduce the number of patients with hypothermia should wind chill, rain, or snow become a concern.

EQUIPMENT REQUIREMENTS

The equipment requirements for the central medical facility are listed in Tables 18.23–18.26, 18.28 and 18.29, respectively. Specific quantities are not given but can be determined based on the previous year's usage. It is therefore important to have one person in charge of documenting the equipment needs of the medical team, keeping track of the stores, having an emergency supplier on hand to contact should any important item run out, and taking an inventory at the end of the day of what has been used and most needed.

Race day management of casualties at the finish line medical facility

Race day should not be chaotic, with the pre-event planning well organized and each volunteer conversant with their role and tasks. However, with large fields of participants the number of

Table 18.29 Medications.

Emergency	Adrenaline (epinephrine), atropine, prochlorperazine, metoclopramide, promethazine, glugagon injection, diazepam (rectal and i.v.), dexamethasone, 10 mL 50% dextrose solution, frusemide, inhaled fentanyl, GTN spray or tablets (spray has a longer shelf-life)
Pain	Paracetamol/acetaminophen, non-steroidal anti-inflammatory drugs, tramadol, morphine or pethidine, naloxone, local anesthetic for nerve blocks, sumatriptan
Ear/eyes/nose/ throat/respiratory	Salbutamol, inhaled corticosteroid prednisone, corticosteroid nasal spray, loratadine, nasal spray decongestant, Sofradex ear drops, chloramphenicol, eye ointment, throat lozenges, cough lozenges, Vicks Vaporub or eucalyptus oil, antibiotics
Gastrointestinal	Metoclopramide, loperamide, coloxyl ranitidine, Gaviscon, hyoscine N-butyl, bromide, magnesium hydroxide enema, hemorrhoid cream and suppositories
Skin	Lamisil cream, corticosteroid cream, combined antifungal and corticosteroid cream, antibiotic sunscreen
Genitourinary	Condoms, contraceptive pill (morning after), urinary alkalinizer, antifungal cream, antibiotics
Other	Zopiclone, melatonin, triamcinolone for injection

GTN, glyceryl trinitrate.

collapsed athletes presenting to the medical facility at peak finishing times during the race can exceed 30 athletes per hour. This can overwhelm even the optimally planned and organized medical facility. In our experience, it is important to have a triage area in which athletes can be sat down for a couple of minutes while they catch their breath and get over the overwhelming emotions of having completed their event successfully. This allows time for a number of doctors and experienced nursing staff to elicit a good history from these athletes and establish if the athlete requires further medical management and/or admission to the main medical facility (Holtzhausen *et al.* 1994; Holtzhausen & Noakes 1995). Medical conditions such as exercise-associated collapse, heat stroke, chest pain, and hyponatremia can be triaged from muscle cramps, blisters and injuries, and directed to the appropriate treatment areas. The majority of cases of collapsed athletes who have experienced syncope

on completion of their race will be found to have exercise-associated collapse and can be safely treated conservatively with elevation of their pelvis and lower limbs as discussed above. For more severe cases, where the athlete is brought in on a stretcher from the course or finish line and has altered mental status, the individual can be admitted directly to a high-care emergency area for immediate attention.

Post-race tasks

A scheduled post-race feedback session is very helpful to determine from volunteers what worked and how the medical care plan can be improved for the next event. The problems and protocols that worked well should be documented in a medical director's report which is submitted to the race director for discussion and action before the next event.

References

Adelman, D.C. & Spector, S.L. (1989) Acute respiratory emergencies in emergency treatment of the injured athlete. *Clinics in Sports Medicine* **8**, 71–79.

Amaral, J.F. (1997) Thoracoabdominal injuries in the athlete. *Clinics in Sports Medicine* **16**, 739–753.

American College of Sports Medicine (1987) Position stand on the prevention of thermal injuries during distance running. *Medicine and Science in Sports and Exercise* **19**, 529–533.

American Heart Association in collaboration with the International Liaison Committee on Resuscitation

(2000a) Guidelines 2000 for Cardiopulmonary Resuscitation and Emergency Cardiovascular Care. Part 3: Adult basic life support. *Circulation* **102** (Supplement): 122–159.

American Heart Association in collaboration with the International Liaison Committee on Resuscitation

(2000b) Guidelines 2000 for Cardiopulmonary Resuscitation and Emergency Cardiovascular Care. Part 8: Advanced challenges in resuscitation: Section 3: Special challenges in ECC. *Circulation* **102** (8 Supplement): 1229–1252.

American Thoracic Society (2004) Evidence-based colloid use in the critically ill: American Thoracic Society Consensus Statement. *American Journal of Respiratory and Critical Care Medicine* **170**, 1247–1259.

Anderson, S. & Buggy, D. (1999) Prolonged pharyngeal obstruction after the Heimlich manoeuvre. *Anaesthesia* **54**, 308–309.

Armstrong, L.E., Crago, A.E., Adams, R., *et al.* (1996a) Whole-body cooling of hyperthermic runners: Comparison of two field therapies. *American Journal of Emergency Medicine* **14**, 355–358.

Armstrong, L.E., Epstein, Y., Greenleaf, J.E., *et al.* (1996b) American College of Sports Medicine position stand. Heat and cold illnesses during distance running. *Medicine and Science in Sports and Exercise* **28**, i–x.

Blue, J.G. & Pecci, M.A. (2002) The collapsed athlete. *Orthopedic Clinics of North America* **33**, 471–478.

Bruzzone, E., Cocito, L. & Pisani, R. (2000) Intracranial delayed epidural hematoma in a soccer player: A case report. *American Journal of Sports Medicine* **28**, 901–903.

Burke, A.P., Farb, A., Virmani, R., Goodin, J. & Smialek, J.E. (1991) Sports-related and non-sports-related sudden cardiac death in young adults. *American Heart Journal* **121**, 568–575.

Burke, L. (1993) *Fluid and food intake during training and competition. State of the art review.* Australian Sports Commission, Canberra.

Calle, P.A., Verbeke, A., Vanhaute, O., Van Acker P., Martens, P. & Buylaert, W. (1997) The effect of semi-automatic external defibrillation by emergency medical technicians on survival after out-of-hospital cardiac arrest: An observational study in urban and rural areas in Belgium. *Acta Clinica Belgica* **52**, 72–83.

Cantu, R.C. (1995) Second impact syndrome: A risk in any contact sport. *Physician and Sportsmedicine* **23**, 27–34.

Cantu, R.C. (1998) Second-impact syndrome. *Clinics in Sports Medicine* **17**, 37–44.

Cantu, R.C., Bailes, J.E. & Wilberger J.E. Jr. (1998) Guidelines for return to contact or collision sport after a cervical spine injury. *Clinics in Sports Medicine* **17**, 137–146.

Cianca, J.C., Roberts, W.O. & Horn, D. (2001) *Distance Running: Organization of the Medical Team.* McGraw-Hill, New York.

Clarke, J.R., Trooskin, S.Z., Doshi, P.J., Greenwald, L. & Mode, C.J. (2002) Time to laparotomy for intra-abdominal bleeding from trauma does affect survival for delays up to 90 minutes. *Journal of Trauma* **52**, 420–425.

Cluitmans, F.H. & Meinders, A.E. (1990) Management of severe hyponatremia: Rapid or slow correction? *American Journal of Medicine* **88**, 161–166.

Corrado, D., Basso, C., Schiavon, M. & Thiene, G. (2003) Does sports activity enhance the risk of sudden death in adolescents and young adults? *Journal of the American College of Cardiologists* **42**, 1959–1963.

Corrado, D., Basso, C. & Thiene, G. (2001) Sudden cardiac death in young people with apparently normal heart. *Cardiovascular Research* **50**, 399–408.

Corrado, D., Pelliccia, A., Bjornstad, H.H., *et al.* (2005a) Cardiovascular pre-participation screening of young competitive athletes for prevention of sudden death: proposal for a common European protocol. Consensus Statement of the Study Group of Sport Cardiology of the Working Group of Cardiac Rehabilitation and Exercise Physiology and the Working Group of Myocardial and Pericardial Diseases of the European Society of Cardiology. *European Heart Journal* **26**, 516–524.

Corrado, D., Pelliccia, A., Bjornstad, H.H. & Thiene, G. (2005b) Cardiovascular pre-participation screening of young competitive athletes for prevention of sudden death. Proposal for a common European protocol: reply. *European Heart Journal* **26**, 1804–1805.

Costrini, A.M., Pitt, H.A., Gustafson, A.B. & Uddin, D.E. (1979) Cardiovascular and metabolic manifestations of heat stroke and severe heat exhaustion. *American Journal of Medicine* **66**, 296–302.

Crown, L.A. & Hawkins, W. (1997) Commotio cordis: Clinical implications of blunt cardiac trauma. *American Family Physician* **55**, 2467–2470.

Cuculino, G.P. & DiMarco, C.J. (2002) Common opthalmologic emergencies: a systematic approach to evaluation and management. *Emergency Medical Report* **23**, 163–178.

DeNicola, L.K., Falk, J.L., Swanson, M.E., Gayle, M.O. & Kissoon, N. (1997) Submersion injuries in children and adults. *Critical Care Clinics* **13**, 477–502.

Dickinson, K. & Roberts, I. (2000) Medical anti-shock trousers (pneumatic anti-shock garments) for circulatory support in patients with trauma. *Cochrane Database System Reviews* **2**, CD001856.

Douglas, P.S. & Ginsburg, G.S. (1996) The evaluation of chest pain in women. *New England Journal of Medicine* **334**, 1311–1315.

Dunning, J., Batchelor, J., Stratford-Smith, P., *et al.* (2004) A meta-analysis of clinical correlates that predict significant intracranial injury in adults with minor head trauma. *Journal of Neurotrauma* **21**, 877–885.

England, A.C. 3rd, Fraser, D.W., Hightower, A.W., *et al.* (1982) Preventing severe heat injury in runners: suggestions from the 1979 Peachtree Road Race experience. *Annals of Internal Medicine* **97**, 196–201.

Epstein, Y., Moran, D.S. & Shapira, Y. (1999) Exertional heat stroke: A case series. *Medicine and Science in Sports and Exercise* **31**, 224–228.

Fallon, K.E., Broad, E., Thompson, M.W. & Reull, P.A. (1998) Nutritional and fluid intake in a 100-km ultramarathon. *International Journal of Sport Nutrition* **8**, 24–35.

Fuller, C.M., McNulty, C.M., Spring, D.A., *et al.* (1997) Prospective screening of 5,615 high school athletes for risk of sudden cardiac death. *Medicine and Science in Sports and Exercise* **29**, 1131–1138.

Gallagher, S.A. & Hackett, P.H. (2004) High-altitude illness. *Emergency Medical Clinics of North America* **22**, 329–355.

Garner, J.S. (1996) Guideline for isolation precautions in hospitals. The Hospital Infection Control Practices Advisory Committee. *Infection Control and Hospital Epidemiology* **17**, 53–80. [Erratum appears in *Infection Control and Hospital Epidemiology* 1996, **17**, 214.]

Gastel, J.A., Palumbo, M.A., Hulstyn, M.J., Fadale, P.D. & Lucas, P. (1998) Emergency removal of football equipment: a cadaveric cervical spine injury model. *Annals of Emergency Medicine* **32**, 411–417.

Geffen, L.G.G., Geffen, S. & Hinton-Bayre, A.D. (1998) On site assessment and management of head injury. In: *Oxford Handbook of Sports Medicine* (Sherry, E. & Wilson, S.F., eds.) Oxford University Press, Oxford: 167.

Gilbert, M., Busund, R., Skagseth, A., Nilsen, P.A. & Solbo, J.P. (2000) Resuscitation from accidental hypothermia of 13.7 degrees C with circulatory arrest. *Lancet* **355**, 375–376.

Golden, F.S., Tipton, M.J. & Scott, R.C. (1997) Immersion, near-drowning and drowning. *British Journal of Anaesthesia* **79**, 214–225.

Gooden, B.A. (1992) Why some people do not drown. Hypothermia versus the diving response. *Medical Journal of Australia* **157**, 629–632.

Hackett, P.H. & Rennie, D. (1976) The incidence, importance, and prophylaxis of acute mountain sickness. *Lancet* **2**, 1149–1155.

Hackett, P.H. & Roach, R.C. (2001) High-altitude illness. *New England Journal of Medicine* **345**, 107–114.

Haight, R.R & Shiple, B.J. (2001) Sideline evaluation of neck pain. *Physician and Sportsmedicine* **29**, 45–62.

Hammes, M., Brennan, S. & Lederer, E.D. (1998) *Severe Electrolyte Disturbances.* McGraw-Hill.

Hanson, P.G. & Zimmerman, S.W. (1979) Exertional heatstroke in novice runners. *Journal of the American Medical Association* **242**, 154–157.

Heetveld, M.J., Harris, I., Schlaphoff, G. & Sugrue, M. (2004) Guidelines for the management of haemodynamically unstable pelvic fracture patients. *Australian and New Zealand Journal of Surgery* **74**, 520–529.

Herrmann, B. & Crawford, J. (2002) Genital injuries in prepubertal girls from inline skating accidents. *Pediatrics* **110**, e16.

Hiller, D.B., Massimino, F., Hiller, R.E. & Laird, R.H. (1985) Plasma electrolyte and glucose changes during the Hawaiian Ironman Triathlon. *Medicine and Science in Sports and Exercise* **17** (Supplement), 219.

Hiller, W.D., O'Toole, M.L., Fortess, E.E. *et al.* (1987) Medical and physiological considerations in triathlons. *American Journal of Sports Medicine* **15**, 164–167.

Holtzhausen, L.M. & Noakes, T.D. (1995) The prevalence and significance of post-exercise (postural) hypotension in ultramarathon runners. *Medicine and Science in Sports and Exercise* **27**, 1595–1601.

Holtzhausen, L.M. & Noakes, T.D. (1997) Collapsed ultraendurance athlete: Proposed mechanisms and an approach to management. *Clinical Journal of Sport Medicine* **7**, 292–301.

Holtzhausen, L.M., Noakes, T.D., Kroning, B. *et al.* (1994) Clinical and biochemical characteristics of collapsed ultra-marathon runners. *Medicine and Science in Sports and Exercise* **26**, 1095–1101.

Holzer, M., Behringer, W., Schorkhuber, W., *et al.* (1997) Mild hypothermia and outcome after CPR. Hypothermia for Cardiac Arrest (HACA) Study Group. *Acta Anaesthesiologica Scandinavica Supplement* **111**, 55–58.

Hosey, R.G. & Armsey, T.D. (2003) Sudden cardiac death. *Clinics in Sports Medicine* **22**, 51–66.

Hudak, A.M., Trivedi, K., Harper, C.R., *et al.* (2004) Evaluation of seizure-like episodes in survivors of moderate and severe traumatic brain injury. *Journal of Head and Trauma Rehabilitation* **19**, 290–295.

Irving, R.A., Noakes, T.D., Buck, R., *et al.* (1991) Evaluation of renal function and fluid homeostasis during recovery from exercise-induced hyponatremia. *Journal of Applied Physiology* **70**, 342–348.

Jolly, B.T. & Ghezzi, K.T. (1992) Accidental hypothermia. *Emergency Medical Clinics of North America* **10**, 311–327.

Kannel, W.B. & Schatzkin, A. (1985) Sudden death: lessons from subsets in population studies. *Journal of the American College of Cardiology* **5** (Supplement), 141B–149B.

Khaw, P.T., Shah, P. & Elkington, A.R. (2004) Injury to the eye. *British Medical Journal* **328**, 36–38.

Laird, R.H. (1989) Medical care at ultraendurance triathlons. *Medicine and Science in Sports and Exercise* **21** (Supplement), S222–225.

Langhelle, A., Sunde, K., Wik, L. & Steen, P.A. (2000) Airway pressure with chest compressions versus Heimlich manoeuvre in recently dead adults with complete airway obstruction. *Resuscitation* **44**, 105–108.

Larach, M.G. (1995) Accidental hypothermia. *Lancet* **345**, 493–498.

Larsen, M.P., Eisenberg, M.S., Cummins, R.O. & Hallstrom, A.P. (1993) Predicting survival from out-of-hospital cardiac arrest: A graphic model. *Annals of Emergency Medicine* **22**, 1652–1658.

Lavelle, J.M. & Shaw, K.N. (1993) Near drowning: Is emergency department cardiopulmonary resuscitation or intensive care unit cerebral resuscitation indicated? *Critical Care Medicine* **21**, 368–373.

Leigh-Smith, S. & Harris, T. (2005) Tension pneumothorax: time for a re-think? *Emergency Medical Journal* **22**, 8–16.

Liberman, M., Mulder, D. & Sampalis, J. (2000) Advanced or basic life support for trauma: Meta-analysis and critical review of the literature. *Journal of Trauma* **49**, 584–599.

Lugo-Amador, N.M. & Moyer, R.T. (2004) Heat-related illness. *Emergency Medical Clinics of North America* **22**, 315–327.

Luke, A. & Micheli, L. (1999) Sports injuries: Emergency assessment and field-side care. *Pediatric Reviews* **20**, 291–301; quiz 302.

Maharaj, D., Ramdass, M., Teelucksingh, S., Perry, A. & Naraynsingh, V. (2002) Rectus sheath haematoma: A new set of diagnostic features. *Postgraduate Medical Journal* **78**, 755–756.

Majumdar, A. & Sedman, P.C. (1998) Gastric rupture secondary to successful Heimlich manoeuvre. *Postgraduate Medical Journal* **74**, 609–610.

Manolios, N. & Mackie, I. (1988) Drowning and near-drowning on Australian beaches patrolled by life-savers: A 10-year study, 1973–1983. *Medical Journal of Australia* **148**, 165–167, 170–171.

Marik, P.E. & Varon, J. (2004) The management of status epilepticus. *Chest* **126**, 582–591.

Maron, B.J. (2000) Ventricular arrhythmias, sudden death, and prevention in patients with hypertrophic cardiomyopathy. *Current Cardiology Reports* **2**, 522–528.

Maron, B.J. (2003) Sudden death in young athletes. *New England Journal of Medicine* **349**, 1064–1075.

Maron, B.J. & Mitchell, J.H. (1994) Twenty-sixth Bethesda Conference: recommendations for detecting eligibility for competition in athletes with cardiovascular abnormalities. *Journal of American College of Cardiology* **24**, 845–899.

Maron, B.J., Bodison, S.A., Wesley, Y.E., Tucker, E. & Green, K.J. (1987) Results of screening a large group of intercollegiate competitive athletes for cardiovascular disease. *Journal of the American College of Cardiology* **10**, 1214–1221.

Maron, B.J., Epstein, S.E. & Roberts, W.C. (1986) Causes of sudden death in competitive athletes. *Journal of the American College of Cardiology* **7**, 204–214.

Maron, B.J., Gohman, T.E., Kyle, S.B., Estes, N.A. 3rd & Link, M.S. (2002) Clinical profile and spectrum of commotio cordis. *Journal of the American Medical Association* **287**, 1142–1146.

Maron, B.J., Poliac, L.C., Kaplan, J.A. & Mueller, F.O. (1995) Blunt impact to the chest leading to sudden death from cardiac arrest during sports activities.

New England Journal of Medicine 333, 337–342.

Maron, B.J., Poliac, L.C. & Roberts, W.O. (1996b) Risk for sudden cardiac death associated with marathon running. *Journal of the American College of Cardiology* 28, 428–431.

Maron, B.J., Shirani, J., Poliac, L.C., *et al.* (1996a) Sudden death in young competitive athletes. Clinical, demographic, and pathological profiles. *Journal of the American Medical Association* 276, 199–204.

Maus, M. (2001) Update on orbital trauma. *Current Opinions on Ophthalmology* 12, 329–334.

Mayers, L.B. & Noakes, T.D. (2000) A guide to treating Ironman triathletes at the finish line. *Physician and Sportsmedicine* 28, 35–50.

McCrory, P., Johnston, K., Meeuwissw, W., *et al.* (2005) Summary and agreement statement of the 2nd International Conference on Concussion in Sport, Prague 2004. *British Journal of Sports Medicine* 39, 196–204.

McCrory, P.R. & Berkovic, S.F. (1998) Second impact syndrome. *Neurology* 50, 677–683.

McCutcheon, M.L. & Anderson, J.L. (1985) How I manage sports injuries to the larynx. *Physician and Sportsmedicine* 13, 100–112.

Miles, J.W. & Barrett, G.R. (1991) Rib fractures in athletes. *Sports Medicine* 12, 66–69.

Miura, K., Nakagawa, H., Morikawa, Y., *et al.* (2002) Epidemiology of idiopathic cardiomyopathy in Japan: results from a nationwide survey. *Heart* 87, 126–130.

Mosesso, V.N. Jr., Davis, E.A., Auble, T.E., Paris, P.M. & Yealy, D.M. (1998) Use of automated external defibrillators by police officers for treatment of out-of-hospital cardiac arrest. *Annals of Emergency Medicine* 32, 200–207.

Murshid, W.R. (1998) Management of minor head injuries: admission criteria, radiological evaluation and treatment of complications. *Acta Neurochirurgica (Wien)* 140, 56–64.

Naimer, S.A., Anat, N., Katif, G., and the Rescue Team. (2004a) Evaluation of techniques for treating the bleeding wound. *Injury* 35, 974–979.

Naimer, S.A., Nash, M., Niv, A. & Lapid, O. (2004b) Control of massive bleeding from facial gunshot wound with a compact elastic adhesive compression dressing. *American Journal of Emergency Medicine* 22, 586–588.

Nava, A., Bauce, B., Basso, C., *et al.* (2000) Clinical profile and long-term follow-up of 37 families with arrhythmogenic right ventricular cardiomyopathy. *Journal of the American College of Cardiology* 36, 2226–2233.

Noakes, T.D. (1988) Why marathon runners collapse. *South African Medical Journal* 73, 569–571.

Noakes, T.D. (1993) Fluid replacement during exercise. *Exercise and Sport Science Reviews* 21, 297–330.

Noakes, T.D. (1995) Dehydration during exercise: What are the real dangers? *Clinical Journal of Sport Medicine* 5, 123–128.

Noakes, T.D. (2000) *Hyperthermia, Hypothermia and Problems of Hydration.* Blackwell Science, Oxford.

Noakes, T.D., Norman, R.J., Buck, R.H., *et al.* (1990) The incidence of hyponatremia during prolonged ultraendurance exercise. *Medicine and Science in Sports and Exercise* 22, 165–170.

Nozaki, R., Ishibashi, K., Adachi, N., Nishihara, S. & Adachi, S. (1986) Accidental profound hypothermia. *New England Journal of Medicine* 315, 1680.

Olshaker, J.S. (2004) Submersion. *Emergency Medical Clinics of North America* 22, 357–367, viii.

Orlowski, J.P. (1987) Vomiting as a complication of the Heimlich maneuver. *Journal of the American Medical Association* 258, 512–513.

Peberdy, M.A. & Ornato J.P. (1992) Coronary artery disease in women. *Heart Disease and Stroke* 1, 315–319.

Pepe, P.E., Roppolo, L.P. & Fowler, R.L. (2005) The detrimental effects of ventilation during low-blood-flow states. *Current Opinions in Critical Care* 11, 212–218.

Perina, D. & Braithwaite, S. (2001) Acute myocardial infarction in the prehospital setting. *Emergency Medical Clinics of North America* 19, 483–492.

Quigley, F. (2000) A survey of the causes of sudden death in sport in the Republic of Ireland. *British Journal of Sports Medicine* 34, 258–261.

Reid, S.A., Speedy, D.B., Thompson, J.M., *et al.* (2004) Study of hematological and biochemical parameters in runners completing a standard marathon. *Clinical Journal of Sport Medicine* 14, 344–353.

Reuler, J.B. (1978) Hypothermia: pathophysiology, clinical settings, and management. *Annals of Internal Medicine* 89, 519–527.

Revell, M., Greaves, I. & Porter, K. (2003) Endpoints for fluid resuscitation in hemorrhagic shock. *Journal of Trauma* 54 (Supplement), S63–S67.

Rhee, P., Koustova, E. & Alam, H.B. (2003) Searching for the optimal resuscitation method: Recommendations for the initial fluid resuscitation of combat casualties. *Journal of Trauma* 54 (Supplement), S52–62.

Ring, J. & Behrendt, H. (1999) Anaphylaxis and anaphylactoid reactions. Classification and pathophysiology. *Clinical Review of Allergy and Immunology* 17, 387–399.

Roberts, I., Alderson, P., Bunn, F., *et al.* (2004) Colloids versus crystalloids for fluid resuscitation in critically ill patients. *Cochrane Database Systematic Reviews* 4, CD000567.

Roberts, W.O. (1989) Exercise-associated collapse in endurance events: A classification system. *Physician and Sportsmedicine* 17, 49–57.

Rogers, G., Goodman, C. & Rosen, C. (1997) Water budget during ultra-endurance exercise. *Medicine and Science in Sports and Exercise* 29, 1477–1481.

Rosen, P., Stoto, M. & Harley, J. (1995) The use of the Heimlich maneuver in near drowning: Institute of Medicine report. *Journal of Emergency Medicine* 13, 397–405.

Royburt, M., Epstein, Y., Solomon, Z. *et al.* (1993) Long-term psychological and physiological effects of heat stroke. *Physiology and Behavior* 54, 265–267.

Sandor, R. (1997) Heat illness: on-site diagnosis and cooling. *Physician and Sportsmedicine* 25, 35–40.

Schneider, S.M. (1992) Hypothermia: from recognition to rewarming. *Emergency Medical Reports* 13, 1–20.

Shafi, S. & Kauder, D.R. (2004) Fluid resuscitation and blood replacement in patients with polytrauma. *Clinical Orthopaedics and Related Research* 422, 37–42.

Shapiro, Y. & Seidman D.S. (1990) Field and clinical observations of exertional heat stroke patients. *Medicine and Science in Sports and Exercise* 22, 6–14.

Shibolet, S., Lancaster, M.C. & Danon, Y. (1976) Heat stroke: A review. *Aviation, Space and Environmental Medicine* 47, 280–301.

Simon, H.B. (1993) Hyperthermia. *New England Journal of Medicine* 329, 483–487.

Sirven, J.I. & Waterhouse, E. (2003) Management of status epilepticus. *American Family Physician* 68, 469–476.

Siscovick, D.S., Weiss, N.S., Fletcher, R.H. & Lasky, T. (1984) The incidence of primary cardiac arrest during vigorous exercise. *New England Journal of Medicine* **311**, 874–877.

Solomon, C.G., Lee, T.H., Cook, E.F., *et al.* (1989) Comparison of clinical presentation of acute myocardial infarction in patients older than 65 years of age to younger patients: The Multicenter Chest Pain Study experience. *American Journal of Cardiology* **63**, 772–776.

Sorensen, H.T., Nielsen, B. & Ostergaard Nielsen, J. (1989) Anaphylactic shock occurring outside hospitals. *Allergy* **44**, 288–290.

Speedy, D.B., Noakes, T.D., Rogers, I.R., *et al.* (1999) Hyponatremia in ultradistance triathletes. *Medicine and Science in Sports and Exercise* **31**, 809–815.

Speedy, D.B., Noakes, T.D., Kimber, N.E., *et al.* (2001a) Fluid balance during and after an ironman triathlon. *Clinical Journal of Sport Medicine* **11**, 44–50.

Speedy, D.B., Noakes, T.D. & Schneider, C. (2001b) Exercise-associated hyponatremia: A review. *Emergency Medicine (Fremantle)* **13**, 17–27.

Speedy, D.B., Rogers, I.R., Noakes, T.D., *et al.* (2000a) Diagnosis and prevention of hyponatremia at an ultradistance triathlon. *Clinical Journal of Sport Medicine* **10**, 52–58.

Speedy, D.B., Rogers, I.R., Noakes, T.D., *et al.* (2000b) Exercise-induced hyponatremia in ultradistance triathletes is caused by inappropriate fluid retention. *Clinical Journal of Sport Medicine* **10**, 272–278.

Stein, S.C. (2001) Minor head injury: 13 is an unlucky number. *Journal of Traumatology* **50**, 759–760.

Steinman, A.M. (1986) Cardiopulmonary resuscitation and hypothermia. *Circulation* **74**, IV29–32.

Sterz, F., Safar, P., Tisherman, S., Radovsky, A., Kuboyama, K. & Oku, K. (1991) Mild hypothermic cardiopulmonary resuscitation improves outcome after prolonged cardiac arrest in dogs. *Critical Care Medicine* **19**, 379–389.

Stocchetti, N., Maas, A.I., Chieregato, A. & van der Plas, A.A. (2005) Hyperventilation in head injury: a review. *Chest* **127**, 1812–1827.

Storey, M.D., Schatz, C.F. & Brown, K.W. (1989) Anterior neck trauma. *Physician and Sportsmedicine* **17**, 85–96.

Swor, R.A., Jackson, R.E., Cynar, M., *et al.* (1995) Bystander CPR, ventricular fibrillation, and survival in witnessed, unmonitored out-of-hospital cardiac arrest. *Annals of Emergency Medicine* **25**, 780–784.

Tom, P.A., Garmel, G.M. & Auerbach, P.S. (1994) Environment-dependent sports emergencies. *Medical Clinics of North America* **78**, 305–325.

Turnage, B. & Maull, K.I. (2000) Scalp laceration: an obvious 'occult' cause of shock. *Southern Medical Journal* **93**, 265–266.

Vaccaro, A.R., Klein, G.R., Ciccoti, M., *et al.* (2002) Return to play criteria for the athlete with cervical spine injuries resulting in stinger and transient quadriplegia/paresis. *Spine Journal* **2**, 351–356.

Van Camp, S.P., Bloor, C.M., Mueller, F.O., Cantu, R.C. & Olseon, H.G. (1995) Nontraumatic sports death in high school and college athletes. *Medicine and Science in Sports and Exercise* **27**, 641–647.

Volcheck, G.W. & Li, J.T. (1997) Exercise-induced urticaria and anaphylaxis. *Mayo Clinic Proceedings* **72**, 140–147.

Wan, J. & Bloom, D.A. (2003) Genitourinary problems in adolescent males. *Adolescent Medicine* **14**, 717–731, viii.

Weaver, W.D. (1995) Time to thrombolytic treatment: factors affecting delay and their influence on outcome. *Journal of the American College of Cardiology* **25** (Supplement), 3S–9S.

Weinstein, M.D. & Krieger, B.P. (1996) Near-drowning: epidemiology, pathophysiology, and initial treatment. *Journal of Emergency Medicine* **14**, 461–467.

Worthley, L.I. & Thomas, P.D. (1986) Treatment of hyponatraemic seizures with intravenous 29.2% saline. *British Medical Journal (Clinical Research Education)* **292**, 168–170.

Yarnell, P.R., Heit, J. & Hackett, P.H. (2000) High-altitude cerebral edema (HACE): the Denver/Front Range experience. *Seminars in Neurology* **20**, 209–217.

Yocum, M.W., Butterfield, J.H., Klein, J.S., *et al.* (1999) Epidemiology of anaphylaxis in Olmsted County: A population-based study. *Journal of Allergy and Clinical Immunology* **104**, 452–456.

Yuen, M.C., Yap, P.G., Chan, Y.T. & Tung, W.K. (2001) An easy method to reduce anterior shoulder dislocation: The Spaso technique. *Emergency Medical Journal* **18**, 370–372.

Chapter 19

Genetics and Sports Participation

KYRIACOS I. ELEFTHERIOU AND HUGH E. MONTGOMERY

It is the shared inheritance of 30,000 genes spread over 23 pairs of chromosomes that defines our species, and each of us as "human." What defines us as individuals, however, is a personal unique combination of small variations, or polymorphisms, within each gene (our "genotype") and its interaction with our environmental experiences. This interaction determines our physical characteristics, or "phenotype": our aptitudes, capabilities, vulnerabilities, and even our behavior, are all shaped in this way.

This influence of genotype extends to every phenotypic characteristic studied so far; it is a general rule that at least 30% of the variance in any human characteristic can be accounted for by genetic factors. It should not surprise us that this is also true of sporting prowess. An array of rodent studies demonstrate the influence of genetic inheritance on mammalian performance (Dohm *et al.* 1994; Houle-Leroy *et al.* 2000; Koch & Britton 2001). Amongst our own species, a role for genes is directly apparent from our earliest childhood years, when we recognize the "gifted" athlete of similarly gifted parents. Recent advances in the science of genetics and its related technologies have made it possible not only to quantify the magnitude of such genetic influences on performance, but also to identify some of the responsible individual genetic loci (and their variants).

Such loci are likely to be both diverse and numerous. Physical performance is determined by the complex interaction of wide-ranging anatomic, biochemical, and physiologic components and systems: we might think almost immediately of a vast number of such factors – from stature and limb length to cardiac size and contractility, lung function, and muscle bulk. Each of these phenotypes will be under the influence of a large number of individual genes. However, each of these broader phenotypes is comprised of a spectrum of other phenotypes. Thus, skeletal form is not just about long-bone length; it is about joint geometry, cartilage depth and constitution, bone volumes and density, and matrix composition. Each of these lesser phenotypes is itself influenced by diverse other processes (appetite, calcium absorption and renal loss, vitamin D activity) and cell types (renal tubules, gut epithelium, chondrocytes, osteoblasts, osteoclasts).

Each of these numerous genetic factors will, in turn, interact with diverse environmental stimuli (such as diet) to determine our final form and function. This will also be true of the training stimulus: while one range of genetic factors may impact on our aptitude for exercise, others may influence the response to such exercise.

The study of the genetic influences on sporting performance may be of great value to humanity as a whole: through the study of exercise-related health, we can better learn to understand the processes of disease. However, this also raises issues of wider importance to society: we may soon enter an era when genetic screening will assist in the

The Olympic Textbook of Medicine in Sport, 1st edition. Edited by M. Schwellnus. Published 2008 by Blackwell Publishing, ISBN: 978-1-4051-5637-0.

identification of the "potentially elite" sports person (and the rejection of those less likely to succeed). Meanwhile, emerging "gene therapy" technologies may be utilized to modify the genetic constitution of the individual athlete in order to achieve higher levels of performance.

Role of genes in determining sports performance

Quantifying the magnitude of genetic influence on sporting phenotypes

The influence of genetic factors on any given phenotype may be expressed in a number of different ways. The heritability (h^2) is the proportion of the total variation of a phenotype that can be attributed to genetic effects. It can be expressed as a fraction, or converted to a percentage which ranges from 0 to 100%, with heritability near zero indicating a phenotype where genetic factors have little influence, and values approaching 100% being consistent with a central role for genetic factors in determining the trait. It is important to note that heritability is dependent on the relative influence and interaction of genetic and environmental factors and is therefore both population- and time-specific; in a population in which the environment is very similar, the heritability will increase.

With families sharing the same genes, but also much the same environment, the two main strategies used to estimate heritability are family studies and twin studies, both of which allow not just easier

statistical analysis of the degree of inheritance, but can also provide an estimate for the upper limit of heritability for that trait. In family studies, the similarities between parents and children, and between siblings, are observed and analyzed to estimate heritability. In twin studies, both monozygotic (MZ) and digozygotic (DZ) twins are studied. The former, also known as identical twins, share an identical genetic background, while DZ twins share 50% of the same genes. For a trait influenced by genetic factors, the similarity in MZ twins is expected to be higher than in DZ twins; using various statistical analyses and modeling the heritability for that trait can be calculated. Heritability estimates for a number of sporting and performance traits have been estimated in a number for twin or family studies, some of which are summarized in Table 19.1.

The role of genetic factors can be sought in their contributions to phenotypes such as the ones listed above (Table 19.1), which themselves might influence sporting activity (intermediate phenotypes). These may be anatomic (e.g., variables related to skeletal structure or muscle mass), physiologic (e.g., anaerobic threshold), biochemical (insulin sensitivity), or even behavioral (willingness to train). Thus, the heritability of systemic arterial blood pressure (BP) has been recognized since the mid-1960s (Schlager 1965), and confirmed over subsequent decades (McIlhany et al. 1975; Wang et al. 1990; Boomsma et al. 1998; Rotimi et al. 1999; Atwood et al. 2001). While blood pressure per se may be unrelated to human physical performance, its strong heritability suggests that underlying

Table 19.1 Heritability (h^2) estimates for various performance phenotypes: Genetic influence on intermediate phenotypes.

Performance trait	h^2 Estimate (%)	References
$\dot{V}O_{2max}$	20–66	Bouchard et al. (1998) Frederiksen & Christensen (2003)
Static strength (e.g., hand grip, arm pull)	14–83	Bouchard et al. (1997) Beunen & Thomis (2004)
Dynamic strength (e.g., standing, vertical jumps)	22–85	Bouchard et al. (1997) Beunen & Thomis (2004)
Muscular endurance	40–75	Bouchard et al. (1997) Beunen & Thomis (2004)
Sports participation	38–62	Frederiksen & Christensen (2003)

physiological pathways – such as cardiac contractility and output, and the form and function of the peripheral vasculature – may also be genetically influenced. Indeed, a strong genetic influence on heart rate has been demonstrated in rodents (Kreutz *et al.* 1997) and confirmed in humans, where it accounts for up to 23% of variability (Singh *et al.* 1999). Meanwhile, although initially debated (Klissouras 1971; Adams *et al.* 1985; Landry *et al.* 1985; Harshfield *et al.* 1990; Bielen *et al.* 1991), human left ventricular mass (LVM) is influenced by genetic determinants. In a study of 110 adult twin pairs, heritability was estimated to be 0.69 (Swan *et al.* 2003), while a study of 341 twin pairs suggested genetic variation to be responsible for over 60% of the variance of LVM (Verhaaren *et al.* 1991). Thus, diverse cardiovascular phenotypes are genetically influenced, and it would seem only a matter of time before those more directly involved in athletic performance – such as peak cardiac output – are demonstrated to be similarly influenced.

Another intermediate phenotype that is more likely to influence human physical performance is that of strength, and the genetic influences on this have been reviewed extensively (Bouchard *et al.* 1997; Beunen & Thomis 2004). Some heritability estimates are shown in Table 19.1. Using sibling correlations for grip strength and pull and push, heritability was estimated to vary from 0.44 to 0.58 (Beunen & Thomis 2004), while h^2 ranged from 0.14 to 0.83 in 15 twin studies (Beunen & Thomis 2004). Significant genetic influences have also been shown for explosive strength (or power) as measured with standing vertical jump or broad jump. Overall, h^2 estimates were higher from twin studies than family studies, genetic influences appear to be stronger for static strength and power than for muscular endurance, and possibly such influences appear to be stronger in males than females (Bouchard *et al.* 1997). The results of other twin studies are also suggestive that such genetic influences are stronger during the growth process, and in younger adults compared to older adults (Frederiksen *et al.* 2003; Beunen & Thomis 2004; Tiainen *et al.* 2004), with evidence that different genes may exert an influence at the different times of childhood, adolescence, and adulthood (Maes *et al.* 1996).

Such a strategy may also be applied to measures of performance within a sporting discipline, and the magnitude of genetic influence sought.

Identifying genetic factors of influence

Thus, one might take a "general" approach, in which the overall contribution of genetic factors to variance in phenotypic expression is sought. However, one might also seek to identify specific genetic factors associated with "direct" sporting phenotypes (such as reaction time), with elite participation in a given sport, or with measures of performance within that sporting discipline itself. Two main methodologies are utilized to achieve this: linkage analysis studies and candidate allelic association studies.

LINKAGE ANALYSIS

In linkage analysis, the whole or a large part of the genome is analyzed and highly variant DNA markers identified that are regularly placed throughout the genome. Various parametric and non-parametric analyses are then employed to assess whether a marker at a certain location is co-transmitted (i.e., is in linkage) with a gene linked to the phenotype assessed in a family. That gene or genetic position is termed a quantitative trait locus (QTL). A significant linkage (usually taken as a Lod score ≥3) is suggestive of a significant linkage between that marker and a locus associated with the phenotype. Certainly, an advantage of such methods is that a likely physiologic mechanism is not required to identify possible QTLs. For a model-based analysis of family data, the mode of inheritance is needed. This is a problem for sporting phenotypes, which are not only determined by environmental factors, but also by a number of genes of unknown inheritance. Although a number of non-parametric (model-free) methods are available, these have a number of disadvantages with regards to their power and interpretation. Furthermore, the identified QTLs are often quite large in size, and may contain a number of possibly related genes. Finally, such studies can at times generate "false positive" loci. In practice, the use of linkage analysis, although helpful in identifying areas or genes of interest, is not as straightforward as it first appears.

ALLELIC ASSOCIATION STUDIES

The second group of methodologies involves studying the influence of a specific polymorphism (variation), usually within a candidate gene, and assessing whether there are measurable differences in the level of the phenotype/trait studied in groups of different genotypes for that allelic polymorphism. To explain this further let us consider protein A, thought to influence human skeletal muscle growth and encoded for by gene A. Gene A is not on a sex chromosome, and exhibits variation in one single base pair ("single nucleotide polymorphism" or SNP) which influences the transcription of that gene: allelic variant A_1 is associated with enhanced gene transcription when compared with allele A_2. Within the population under examination, individuals will carry two A_1 alleles (A_1 homozygotes), two A_2 alleles (A_2 homozygotes) or an A_1 and an A_2 allele (heterozygotes). Let us now apply a uniform training stimulus, designed to promote muscle hypertrophy, to all individuals in our population sample. If protein A is indeed a mediator of skeletal muscle growth, the degree of skeletal hypertrophy observed is expected to be associated with the carriage of the A_1 allele: thus, those of A_1A_1 genotype will exhibit a greater growth response than those of A_2A_2 genotype. However, such studies are not without caveats. The A_1 allele may in fact be in linkage disequilibrium (i.e., occurring in association) with an unrecognized functional variant in a nearby gene which is, in reality, the true mediator of the observed effect. In many cases, numerous polymorphisms within one or more genes are assessed and, rather than testing for an association with each polymorphism separately, haplotypes – sets of multiple SNPs along a genomic region – are analyzed and associations of a specific haplotype with a specific trait (such as increased strength) are assessed. Such a strategy can also be applied using case–control studies, in which the occurrence of a specific allele in a group of people with a particular trait is assessed and compared with a group of control subjects. One might, for instance, seek an increasing allele frequency amongst athletes compared with controls, or within athlete groups with increasing distance running. An advantage of such strategies is that they do not require subjects to come from the same family, and tend to be powerful – especially when individuals of homogeneous race and sex are studied.

In general, these two groups of strategies complement one other. While allelic association studies are often easier to perform, allow unrelated subjects to be studied, and may detect much smaller gene effects compared to linkage analysis, their results may be challenged by the possible mediation of observed effect being through a neighboring (linked) site. On the other hand, linkage analyses necessitate the study of a very large number of related individuals and may only provide evidence for an association with large segments of the genome with rather strong effects on that trait, and segments that may contain a large number of possible genes. Nevertheless, they can confirm the findings of allelic association studies, and also be suggestive of candidate genes that can be studied using the latter approach.

Specific genetic influences associated with performance

$\dot{V}o_{2MAX}$

Maximum oxygen uptake ($\dot{V}o_{2max}$) during physical exercise is a measure of the integrated performance of the cardiopulmonary, circulatory, and muscle units in delivering and utilizing oxygen for aerobic work. Genetic factors are likely to influence each of these components, and thus a substantial genetic contribution to variance in $\dot{V}o_{2max}$ is to be expected. Indeed, up to 40% of the interindividual variance $\dot{V}o_{2max}$ seems due to genetic factors (Bouchard et al. 1986).

Polymorphic variation in mitochondrial DNA has been associated with baseline $\dot{V}o_{2max}$ in sedentary young males, and also with its response to training (Dionne et al. 1991). Meanwhile, sarcolemmal sodium-potassium-ATPase has an important role in maintaining electrolyte gradients across the cell membrane. Sarcolemmal action balance may be important for endurance capacity, especially in younger individuals (Gambert & Duthie 1983). Sodium-potassium-ATPase activity increases during exercise, and the surpassing of its functional capacity during high-intensity exercise may limit maximal muscle activity (Clausen *et al.* 1998). In keeping with such a hypothesis, a rise in $\dot{V}_{O_{2max}}$ over a 20-week endurance training program has been associated with an α-subunit isoform 2 exon 21-22 marker of the Na^+-K^+-ATPase gene (Rankinen *et al.* 2000a).

Meanwhile, the skeletal muscle isozyme of creatine kinase (CKMM) is involved in generating ATP in muscle fibers; change in $\dot{V}_{O_{2max}}$ after training was found to be CKMM (*NcoI* polymorphism) genotype-dependent (Rivera *et al.* 1997). It is estimated that this variation may account for as much as 9% of the observed change in $\dot{V}_{O_{2max}}$ (Rivera *et al.* 1997). This polymorphism is found in a non-coding region of the gene, and has thus been suggested to be in linkage disequilibrium with another locus or gene in the region which has yet to be identified.

Bouchard *et al.* (2000) have used genome-wide scanning to find loci of association with the change in $\dot{V}_{O_{2max}}$ with exercise training in white two-generation families in the HERITAGE Family Study. Having assessed 289 markers covering the 22 autosomal chromosomes and adjusting for a number of covariates, baseline $\dot{V}_{O_{2max}}$ was "suggestively linked" with chromosomal locations 4q12, 8q24.12, 11p15.1, and 14q21.3 ($P < 0.01$). "Potentially useful linkages" were seen in another 18 loci ($0.01 < P < 0.05$). A number of genes have been identified and mapped to these regions and include the β- and γ-sarcoglycans, the sulfonylurea receptor (involved in regulating the secretion of insulin), syntrophin β-1 and dystrophin-associated glycoprotein-1 of the dystrophin–glycoprotein complex, and lamin A/C. The dystrophin–glycoprotein complex of skeletal muscle is believed to be involved in providing stability to the myofiber membrane and to link the intracellular actin cytoskeleton with the extracellular basement membrane. Another five chromosomal loci exhibited "suggestive linkages" with the *increase* in $\dot{V}_{O_{2max}}$ after exercise training, including 1p11.2, 2p16.1, 4q26, 6p21.33, and 11p14.1 ($P < 0.01$),

while another 21 loci showed "potentially useful linkages" ($0.01 < P < 0.05$). Genes mapped in these areas include the voltage-gated K^+-channel, the long QT syndrome locus, fatty acid binding protein 2, pancreatic co-lipase, calmodulin 2, calcineurin B, cardiac calsequestrin and 3β-hydroxysteroid dehydrogenase. It was the authors' conclusion that these genes are involved in "cardiac contractility, long-chain fatty acid absorption, calcium signaling in cardiac and skeletal muscle, and steroid hormone synthesis," which all provide biologically plausible mechanisms that could influence the $\dot{V}_{O_{2max}}$ changes elicited with exercise training (Bouchard *et al.* 2000).

More recently, other investigators have associated the Gln carriers of the adrenergic receptor β2 (ADRB2) Gln27Glu genotype with higher values of $\dot{V}_{O_{2max}}$ in post-menopausal women (McCole *et al.* 2004). The Trp64Arg polymorphism of the adrenergic receptor β3 (ADRB3) gene was also investigated and the Trp/Arg genotype group was associated with higher $\dot{V}_{O_{2max}}$ compared with the Trp/Trp homozygotes in the same group (McCole *et al.* 2004).

LEFT VENTRICULAR MASS

Cardiac size may influence physical performance, at least in racehorses (Buhl *et al.* 2005; Young *et al.* 2005). The association of pathologic left ventricular (LV) hypertrophy with excess cardiovascular mortality (Levy *et al.* 1990; Koren *et al.* 1991; Vakili *et al.* 2001) has led to extensive investigation into the genetic factors that influence LV growth responses. Perhaps the human angiotensin 1-converting enzyme (ACE) I/D polymorphism is the best example, discussed in detail later in the text. At this point, it is important to note that the deletion (D) rather than the insertion (I) polymorphic variant of the ACE gene is associated with greater LV ACE activity (Danser *et al.* 1995) and growth response (Myerson *et al.* 2001), is an effect that may be mediated through increased synthesis of the growth factor angiotensin II, or the degradation of growth-inhibitory kinins (Murphey *et al.* 2000). With regards to the latter, a polymorphic variant of the bradykinin 2 receptor (B2BKR) gene exists where the absence (–) rather than the presence (+) of a

9-bp deletion in the gene is associated with greater concentrations of receptor mRNA (Lung *et al.* 1997). Brull *et al.* (2001) explored the hypothesis that if ACE does indeed regulate cardiac growth through kinin modulation, LV growth in response to an environmental stimulus would be influenced by both ACE and B2BKR genotypes, and they showed that in a group of 109 military recruits undergoing their training, the two genotypes interacted biologically in an additive way as expected.

An important metabolic adaptation of the hypertrophied heart is an increase in the utilization of glucose with a corresponding decrease in fatty acid oxidation (FAO) attributable to the downregulation of FAO enzyme mRNA levels (Sack *et al.* 1996). Substrate utilization appears to be important in the pathogenesis of ventricular hypertrophy as suggested by the findings that inhibition of FAO in animal models is associated with cardiac hypertrophy (Binas *et al.* 1999; Chiu *et al.* 2001), and defects in mitochondrial FAO enzymes cause childhood mitochondrial cardiomyopathy (Kelly & Strauss 1994). Peroxisome proliferator-activated receptor α (PPARα) is a ligand-activated transcription factor (Issemann & Green 1990) and regulator of genes that are involved in fatty acid uptake and oxidation, lipid metabolism, and inflammation (Fruchart *et al.* 1999). It is downregulated in cardiac hypertrophy *in vitro* and *in vivo* (Barger *et al.* 2000) with PPARα knockout mice having significantly reduced FAO, and exhibiting cardiac lipid accumulation and fibrosis (Watanabe *et al.* 2000), and dying on inhibition of mitochondrial fatty acid uptake (Djouadi *et al.* 1998). With this background, the role of PPARα in LV growth was investigated in 144 young male British Army recruits undergoing a 10-week physical training program (Jamshidi *et al.* 2002). A G/C polymorphism in intron 7 of the PPARα gene had a significant influence on the LV growth response to exercise ($P = 0.009$); LV mass increased by 6.7 ± 1.5 g in G allele homozygotes but was significantly greater in those heterozygous for the C allele (11.8 ± 1.9 g) and in the CC homozygotes (19.4 ± 4.2 g). As part of the this study, the same association was investigated in a group of 578 men and 564 women participating in the echocardiographic substudy of the third MONICA Augsburg survey (Schunkert *et al.* 1999; Jamshidi *et al.* 2002); the C allele homozygotes had significantly higher LV mass, which was greater still in hypertensive subjects. It was therefore concluded that variation in the PPARα gene influences human LV growth in response to exercise and hypertension, indicating that maladaptive cardiac substrate utilization can have a causative role in the pathogenesis of LV hypertrophy (Jamshidi *et al.* 2002).

Other loci have also been identified that seem to be associated with LV hypertrophic responses to pathologic stimuli (Table 19.2). However, the parallel association with exercise-related (physiologic) hypertrophy has yet to be demonstrated for these responses.

SKELETAL MUSCLE

Genetic factors appear to strongly influence skeletal muscle mass, being responsible for half of the total variance of lean body mass in a cohort of post-menopausal women (Arden &Spector 1997) and as much as much as 80% of the variance in human skeletal muscle mass in a group of younger individuals (Seeman *et al.* 1996). To date, QTLs have been identified in mice on chromosomes 7, 9, 11, 13, and 17, which together account for only a small proportion (19.2%) of such variance (Masinde *et al.* 2002). A number of genetic factors have been investigated that may influence both basal (untrained) body habitus and skeletal mass and the hypertrophic response to training, some of which are discussed below.

Normal thyroid function is essential for the normal growth and development of many tissues, including muscle (Weiss & Refetoff 1996), with the effects of thyroid hormone on growth explained by its ability to promote the secretion of growth hormone (GH) and its necessity for normal GH expression both *in vitro* (Crew & Spindler 1986; Ceda *et al.* 1992) and *in vivo* (Shapiro *et al.* 1978). The anabolic effects of GH are themselves mediated by insulin-like growth factor 1 (IGF-1) with *free* IGF-1 being the major biologically active hormonal form (Janssen *et al.* 2003). Nevertheless, the effects of thyroid hormone on the IGF-1 system are not all mediated by GH as thyroid hormone also interacts

Table 19.2 Candidate genes and polymorphisms investigated for possible association with left ventricular (LV) mass.

Gene	Function and theoretical link with LV mass	Polymorphism investigated	Association shown
GNB3-s (3 subunit of the heterotrimeric Gi-protein)	Key role in signal transduction. May have a role in arterial wall vascular smooth muscle cell proliferation	C825T SNP	No association in 2 studies (Sedlacek et al. 2002; Shliakhto et al. 2003), but 825T allele associated with increased LV mass index in another study (Semplicini et al. 2001)
IL-6	Inflammatory cytokine that may be involved in LV hypertrophy	−174G>C	C allele associated with larger LV mass index in end-stage renal disease patients (Losito et al. 2003)
Adducin	Cytoskeleton protein involved in assembly of actin fibers	Gly460Trp of alpha-adducin	Associated with increased LV mass (Winnicki et al. 2002)
ENOS (endothelial nitric oxide ynthase)	Endothelial NO production associated with various cardiovascular diseases	Glu298Asp	No association found (Karvonen et al. 2002)

with IGF-1 with T_4 shown to be able to stimulate IGF-1 activity in the absence of GH (Gaspard et al. 1978; Burstein et al. 1979; Chernausek et al. 1982). An association of two polymorphisms of the type 1 deiodinase (D1) gene with serum iodothyrodine levels has been demonstrated (Peeters et al. 2003), the D1 haplotype 2 allele (aT-bA) showing lower, and haplotype 3 allele higher activity (aC-bG, respectively). The same investigators then went on to show that amongst 350 elderly men, carriers of the D1a-T variant had higher lean body mass ($P = 0.03$), as well as higher isometric grip strength ($P = 0.047$) and maximum leg extensor strength ($P = 0.07$), suggestive that this polymorphism is associated with increased muscle mass through the associated decreased D1 activity and increase in IGF-1 levels concurrently shown in the study (Peeters et al. 2005).

Insulin-like growth factor 2 (IGF-2) is a broad-spectrum potent mitogen with important roles both in fetal growth, as well as in the development of cancer and given its involvement in satellite cell proliferation (Haugk et al. 1995), and the age-associated decrease in IGF-2 gene expression secondary to muscle damage (Marsh et al. 1997), it is possible that IGF-2 could influence the ability of muscle to regenerate in aging and influence rates of age-associated losses in muscle mass and strength in humans. It has

recently been shown that the A/A ApaI polymorphism of the IGF-2 gene was associated with lower total body fat-free mass (FFM) compared with the G/G group at various time intervals within a longitudinal study group. The difference between the genotype groups is maintained at age 65 and across the adult age span, supporting the hypothesis that variation within this gene, known to influence developing muscle, may affect muscle mass in later life (Schrager et al. 2004).

Glucocorticoids are also known to have a significant role in determining body composition. A polymorphism (ER22/23K) of the glucocorticoid receptor gene (in codons 22 and 23) has previously been shown to be associated with relative glucocorticoid resistance, as well as low cholesterol levels and increased insulin sensitivity (van Rossum et al. 2002). In a cohort of 350 subjects observed from age 13 to 36 years, non-carriers and carriers (27 individuals, 8%) of the ER22/23EK variant were compared for anthropometric parameters, body composition, and muscle strength, as measured by arm pull tests and high jump from a standing position (van Rossum et al. 2004). In the males, at 36 years of age, ER22/23EK carriers were found to be taller, to have more lean body mass, greater thigh circumference, and more muscle strength in arms and legs, but no differences in body mass index or fat mass. The female ER22/23EK carriers at the age of 36 years had smaller waist and hip circumferences, but again no differences in their body mass index. The investigators concluded that the ER22/23EK polymorphism is associated "with a sex-specific, beneficial body composition at young adult age, as well as greater muscle strength in males" (van Rossum *et al.* 2004).

Other genetic loci that have been associated with FFM amongst other related phenotypes include the C174T polymorphism in the ciliary neurotrophic factor receptor (CNTFR) gene (see below) (Roth *et al.* 2003a), while the G174C promoter polymorphism of interleukin-6 (IL-6) – an inflammatory cytokine associated with skeletal muscle wasting in animal models (Goodman 1994; Tsujinaka *et al.* 1996) and with lower muscle mass and strength in healthy older individuals (Visser *et al.* 2002) – was shown to be significantly associated with FFM in men but not women (Roth *et al.* 2003b).

IL-15 is an anabolic cytokine produced in skeletal muscle that has direct effects on muscle anabolism in both animal and *in vitro* models (Quinn *et al.* 1995, 1997; Carbo *et al.* 2000). In another study, the influence of genetic variations in the IL-15 receptor-α gene (IL15RA) on muscle responses to 10 weeks of resistance exercise training in young men and women was examined (Riechman *et al.* 2004). A single nucleotide polymorphism in exon 7 of IL15RA was strongly associated with muscle hypertrophy and accounted for 7.1% of the variation in regression modeling. A polymorphism in exon 4 was also independently associated with muscle hypertrophy and accounted for an additional 3.5% of the variation in hypertrophy. Such results are suggestive that IL-15 may be an important mediator of the muscle mass response to resistance exercise training in humans, with genetic variation in IL15RA being accountable for a significant proportion of the variability in this response (Riechman *et al.* 2004).

Genetic factors influence not only skeletal muscle mass, but function. Grip strength and pull and push heritability was estimated to vary from 0.44 to 0.58 (Beunen & Thomis 2004), while h^2 ranged from 0.14 to 0.83 in 15 twin studies (Beunen & Thomis 2004) (Table 19.1). Also, genetic influences appeared to be stronger on static strength and power compared to muscular endurance, with these influences being possibly stronger in males than females (Bouchard *et al.* 1997), and during the growth process in younger compared to older adults (Frederiksen *et al.* 2003; Beunen & Thomis 2004; Tiainen *et al.* 2004), with evidence that different genes may be influencing at the different times of childhood, adolescence, and adulthood (Maes *et al.* 1996).

The achievement of optimal muscle mass and strength is central to the training programs of the majority of athletes. Myostatin is a member of a superfamily of related molecules called transforming growth factors β (TGF-β). It is rather better known through its relationship with the cattle industry, where the particular big beefy breeds of Belgian Blue and Piedmontese cattle have been shown to have inherent mutations of their myostatin gene (Kambadur *et al.* 1997; McPherron & Lee 1997) (Fig. 19.1). Similarly, interference with this gene in mice was associated with a generalized increase in skeletal mass, suggesting that myostatin has an inhibitory effect on skeletal muscle growth (McPherron *et al.* 1997; Szabo *et al.* 1998). Polymorphisms of the gene in humans have been associated with hip flexion strength in older women (Seibert *et al.* 2001) and the amount of muscle wasting with human immunodeficiency virus (HIV) infection (Gonzalez-Cadavid *et al.* 1998).

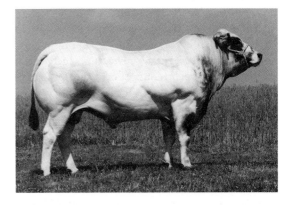

Fig. 19.1 The "beefy" Piedmontese breed of cattle have been shown to have inherent mutations of their myostatin gene. Figure reproduced with permission from Anaborapi, Str. Trinità 32/A, 12061 Carrù (CN), Italy.

The association of IGF-2 genotype with body FFM has already been mentioned. The IGF-2 genotype has been associated with grip strength in middle-aged men (Sayer et al. 2002), but neither the serum IGF levels correlated with the latter, nor was there a linear relationship with the three genotypes, suggesting that the difference seen may be a manifestation of another gene locus linked to the IGF-2 gene variant (Payne & Montgomery 2004). According to Schrager et al. (2004), isokinetic arm strength was also measured and found to be lower in A/A men than in G/G men ($P <0.05$). In women, the G/G genotype group, compared with the A/A group, had lower total lower isokinetic arm and leg strength at the time of first visit, and lower values at age 35 years ($P <0.05$). Furthermore, this difference between the genotype groups was maintained at age 65 and across the adult age span ($P <0.05$).

Collagen includes a group of connective tissue proteins, of which type I is a triple-stranded fibrillar protein containing two α1 polypeptide chains and one α2 chain encoded by the collagen type I α1 (COL1A1) and α2 (COL1A2) genes, respectively. It is the major collagen of skin, tendon and bone, but is also found in the epimysium and (less so) in the perimysium of skeletal muscle (Jarvinen et al. 2002). Slow muscles have more type I collagen, with type III collagen being more abundant in fast muscle (Miller et al. 2001). Both types serve as a supportive structure in the muscle tissue where they attach myocytes and muscle bundles to each other through their presence in this tissue (Jarvinen et al. 2002). Through this function, but also through their intimate association between muscle and other connective tissues (e.g., tendon and bone), the collagen fiber network of skeletal muscle has been shown to be a major contributor to the integrity and tensile strength of the latter (Han et al. 1999; Takala & Virtanen 2000). A polymorphic binding site of the Sp1 transcription factor in the gene encoding for the α1 chain of type I collagen exists, and the s (vs. the S) allele of this polymorphism, has been associated with lower grip and biceps strength on the dominant side, with the difference between the two homozygous genotype groups amounting to 21% and 30%, respectively (Van Pottelbergh et al. 2001).

The ciliary neurotrophic factor (CNTF) is a member of the IL-6 family, with a well-documented neurotrophic role (Siegel et al. 2000; Giehl 2001; English 2003), but there is accumulating evidence for CNTF having protective and/or trophic effects on skeletal muscle through nerve-mediated influences and through effects on muscle proteins and enzymes (Vergara & Ramirez 2004). CNTF treatment was shown to have a partially protective effect on the soleus muscle of rats after denervation of the sciatic nerve (Helgren et al. 1994), and to increase cross-sectional areas of innervated soleus muscle fibers (Guillet et al. 1999). Similarly, CNTF administration affects expression of several muscle proteins (Boudreau-Lariviere et al. 1996). The association between its receptor gene (CNTFR) and FFM has already been mentioned (Roth et al. 2003a), but of note is that the A allele of the G>A polymorphism of the CNTF gene was also associated with higher peak torque of both knee extensor and flexor muscle groups (Roth et al. 2001).

Vitamin D receptors (VDRs) are expressed in skeletal muscle (Costa et al. 1986), where they appear to have non-traditional vitamin D dependent actions (i.e., other than those involved with the regulation of the homeostasis of minerals). Although significant vitamin D deficiency can lead to a severe myopathy in keeping with the relevant abnormalities in mineral ion levels, in vitro studies have shown that 1,25-dihydroxyvitamin D can have rapid effects on muscle through phosphorylation and activation of secondary messengers (Buitrago et al. 2001). VDR-null 3-week-old mice (at a time when they still have normal levels of mineral ions and vitamin D metabolites) have smaller muscle fibers and a persistently high expression of markers of early muscle differentiation, such as myogenein, Myf5, and neonatal myosin heavy chain (Endo et al. 2003). In keeping with such effects, polymorphic variation in the VDR gene has been associated with skeletal muscle function in both post-menopausal (Geusens et al. 1997) and more recently in pre-menopausal women (Grundberg et al. 2004). The presence of the BsmI SNP in the VDR gene was shown to be associated with quadriceps muscle and grip strength in healthy post-menopausal elderly females (Geusens et al. 1997), with these findings being consistent with those found by Grundberg *et al.* (2004) in pre-menopausal women, in which those with shorter (ss) polyadenosine A repeat, and/or BB BsmI genotype of the VDR had higher hamstring strength compared with those with a longer poly A repeat (LL) and/or the presence of the linked BSmI restriction site (bb genotype).

BONE MINERAL DENSITY

The development of stress fractures is a major problem in the world of athletics. Although, in the elderly, the risk of fragility fracture is closely related to bone mineral density (BMD) (Kiel *et al.* 1997), this relationship has not been conclusively shown in younger adults (Giladi *et al.* 1991; Jones *et al.* 2002). Nevertheless, BMD is used a surrogate for bone strength, a complex phenotype especially in the younger adult athletes, where other properties of bone, such as elasticity and anatomic features, are also of considerable importance.

Rodent studies initially suggested a strong genetic influence on skeletal form and function. A study of 12-week-old female mice of different strains suggested a heritability of some 35% for BMD (Klein *et al.* 1998). More recently, such findings have been extended to humans, where heritability estimates for BMD at the lumbar spine and femoral neck range 57–92% (Smith *et al.* 1973; Pocock *et al.* 1987). Significant correlations have also been observed in the fragility fracture rates of female members of the same family (Cummings *et al.* 1995; Torgerson *et al.* 1996).

Studies investigating BMD are inherently problematic for a number of reasons: the regulation of BMD is modified by sex, race, age, and environmental factors, but also depends on the area of the skeleton measured. It is therefore essential that any associations are assessed in a homogeneous manner, as any effect may be specific to various subgroups of the population (Rizzoli *et al.* 2001). As an exemplar, the active form of vitamin D (calcitriol) is strongly involved in the regulation of calcium and phosphate metabolism, and its effects are mediated through a specific VDR (Christakos *et al.* 1996). VDR BsmI genotype seems associated with BMD in children (Sainz *et al.* 1997), but not in pre-menopausal women (Ferrari *et al.* 1998). Such subgroup-specific associations may account for the presence of only non-significant trends for significance of association of BsmI genotype with BMD in a meta-analysis of 16 studies (Cooper & Umbach 1996). Further studies and meta-analyses, however, suggest that VDR genotypes associated with reduced receptor function may be associated with increased osteoporosis risk (Gong *et al.* 1999; Thakkinstian *et al.* 2004; Ferrari & Rizzoli 2005).

Caution must also be extended in the assumption that the association of a polymorphism with skeletal structure is mediated through direct effects on the bone itself: a polymorphism that influences muscle performance will have effects on bone through alterations in delivered mechanical load. Thus, any effect of VDR genotype on skeletal composition may in part be mediated through changes in skeletal muscle performance, given the expression of such receptors in such tissues (see above).

Nonetheless, a number of polymorphic variants have been associated with static BMD and its change in response to a variety of environmental stimuli. These include genes related to calcium/phosphate handling, such as calcitonin receptor (Zhao *et al.* 2003), parathyroid hormone (Hosoi *et al.* 1999), aromatase enzyme (Salmen *et al.* 2003; Van Pottelbergh *et al.* 2003), and estrogen receptor alpha (Kobayashi *et al.* 1996; Mizunuma *et al.* 1997), as well as other messengers/molecules that are involved in bone metabolism, such as IL-6 (Feng *et al.* 2003; Ferrari *et al.* 2003) and α2-HS glycoprotein (Liu *et al.* 2003). An overview of such gene polymorphisms and gene loci that have been examined is summarized in Table 19.3.

While the impact of genetic variation on BMD is thus clear, the role of such influences in the determination of bone strength is less well-explored – partly as BMD is not the sole determinant of bone mechanical properties. Indeed, factors such as bone shape and elasticity may be of greater importance. Neither can associations with BMD be extended to infer an association with athletic performance, or risk of injury-related skeletal injury. Finally, associations of polymorphic variation with risk of fragility fracture in the elderly cannot be assumed to extend similarly to stress failure in the younger athlete.

Table 19.3 Gene polymorphisms and loci associated with bone mineral density (BMD).

Gene	Polymorphisms	Comments
Calcium-handling regulating genes		
Vitamin D receptor (VDR)	3'UTR *Bsm1, Apa1, Taq1* (Morrison *et al.* 1994; Riggs *et al.* 1995) *Fok1* (Gross *et al.* 1996)	Meta-analyses of a number of VDR studies suggest that VDR genotypes associated with reduced receptor function may be associated with increased osteoporosis risk (Gong *et al.* 1999; Thakkinstian *et al.* 2004; Ferrari & Rizzoli 2005)
Parathyroid hormone (PTH)	*BstB1*	In Japanese post-menopausal women (Hosoi *et al.* 1999)
Estrogen receptor (ESR)-α	*PvuII, XbaI*	In post-menopausal (Kobayashi *et al.* 1996) and pre-menopausal (Mizunuma *et al.* 1997) Asian women. A meta-analysis of 22 studies was also suggestive of such an association (Ioannidis *et al.* 2002)
Estrogen receptor (ESR)-β	CA repeat (18–32)	Shown in post-menopausal Japanese women (Ogawa *et al.* 2000), but also in men and women from the Framingham Osteoporosis Study (Shearman *et al.* 2004)
Androgen receptor	(ACG)n repeat (exon1)	Shown in 261 pre- and perimenopausal women of the Michigan Bone Health (MBH) Study (Sowers *et al.* 1999)
Calcitonin	CA repeat (12–20)	As found in Japanese post-menopausal women (Miyao *et al.* 2000)
Calcitonin receptor (CALCR)	*AluI* (Taboulet *et al.* 1998) and *TaqI* (Masi *et al.* 1998)	In another study CALCR genotypes were associated with femoral neck BMD in post- but not pre-menopausal women (Zhao *et al.* 2003)
Glucocorticoid receptor	Codon 363 variant	(Huizenga *et al.* 1998)
Bone matrix protein and components		
Osteocalcin	*HindIII*	In post-menopausal Japanese (Dohi *et al.* 1998) and Chinese (Chen *et al.* 2001) women
Osteonectin	CA repeat	Shown in women of the MBH Study (Willing *et al.* 1998)
Osteopontin	CA repeat	Shown in women of the MBH Study (Willing *et al.* 1998)
Osteoprotegerin	Sequence variations in the gene promoter	Shown in European (Arko *et al.* 2002) and Japanese women but not men (Yamada *et al.* 2003b)
Collagen type I α1 (COLIA1)	*Sp1 (intron 1)* (Grant *et al.* 1996), *MnlI* (Willing *et al.* 1998), *RsaI* (Baker *et al.* 1991)	The overall results are suggestive that the COLIA1 Sp1 polymorphism is likely to be a variant with negative effects on bone structure and strength (Ralston 2002). It may also be an important marker of the risk of an osteoporotic fracture as it predicts fractures independent of BMD (McGuigan *et al.* 2001)
Collagen type α2 (COLIA2)	*RsaI* & *PvuII* (Willing *et al.* 1998), (ACT)n VNTR (Pepe 1993)	

Local messengers and cytokines

Interleukin-6 (IL–6)	−174G > C −572 G > C −634G	The −174G and/or the −572C alleles have been linked with low bone mass and other indices of bone fragility in elderly women (Feng *et al.* 2003; Ferrari *et al.* 2003; Nordstrom *et al.* 2004), the −174GG genotype in younger men and women (Lorentzon *et al.* 2000; Garnero *et al.* 2002). In Japanese women the −634G polymorphism has been associated with low BMD (Yamada *et al.* 2003a). The 174G > C genotype has also been associated with the BMD response to HRT in post-menopausal women (James *et al.* 2004)
IGF-1	CA repeat (promoter)	Shown in Japanese post-menopausal women (Miyao *et al.* 1998)
Interleukin-1β (IL-1β)	C/T (exon 4)	Found in osteoporotic patients (Langdahl *et al.* 2000)
IL-1 receptor antagonist	86VNTR	In early post-menopausal women (Keen *et al.* 1998)
Transforming growth factor β1	T/C-Prol/Leu (exon 1) (Yamada *et al.* 1998), 713-8delC (Langdahl *et al.* 1997)	

Others

Apolipoprotein E	E2, E3, E4	The E4 allele has been associated with reduced bone density in a number of studies (Shiraki *et al.* 1997; Sanada *et al.* 1998; Dick *et al.* 2002; Pluijm *et al.* 2002)
Low-density lipoprotein receptor related protein 5 (LRP5)	Polymorphisms in exons 9 and 18	A QTL for BMD was mapped at the LRP5 locus (Koller *et al.* 1998; Carn *et al.* 2002) and a number of studies have shown an association between LRP5 polymorphisms and BMD (Ferrari *et al.* 2004; Mizuguchi *et al.* 2004; Urano *et al.* 2004)
Microsomal triglyceride transfer protein (MTP)	−493G > T	Shown in premenopausal Japanese women (Yamada *et al.* 2005)
Very low density lipoprotein receptor (VLDLR)	CGG repeat	Shown in Japanese men (Yamada *et al.* 2005)
Peroxisome proliferators-activated receptor γ (PPARγ)	−161C > T	In Japanese (Ogawa *et al.* 1999) and Korean (Rhee *et al.* 2005) women
Cytochrome p450 (CYP) 19 aromatase	(TTTA)n repeat (intron 4)	Gennari *et al.* (2004)
CYP17A1	−34C > T	In post-menopausal Japanese women (Yamada *et al.* 2005)
Methylentetrahydrofolate reductase (MTHFR)	MTHFR A/V	In post-menopausal Japanese women (Miyao *et al.* 2000)

Rather than concentrating on individual determinants of performance, some researchers have sought association of specific polymorphic variants with *elite* athletic status per se. In this way, variation in the α-actinin 3 (ACTN3) gene has been associated with elite endurance athletic performance (Yang *et al.* 2003). α-Actinin 3 is a member of the family of actin-binding proteins that are found in skeletal muscle. They seem to have a role in coordinating myofiber contraction, in view of their involvement in myofibrillar architecture. In humans, there are two α-actinin genes: ACTN-2, expressed in all fibers, and ACTN-3, which is specifically expressed in fast twitch (type 2) myofibers involved in generating force at high speed. There is a common deficiency of α-actinin 3 in the general population because of homozygosity for a common stop-codon polymorphism in the ACTN3 gene (R577X) (North *et al.* 1999). Nevertheless, in the normal population this does not appear important, most likely because of its compensation by the homologous protein, α-actinin 2 (North *et al.* 1999). However, Yang *et al.* (2003) hypothesized that at extremes of performance this deficiency may be disadvantageous. In their study of 436 controls, 107 sprinters, and 194 endurance athletes, both male and female elite sprint athletes were found to have significantly higher frequencies of the 577R allele than controls. There was also a genotype association in female sprint and endurance athletes, with higher than expected numbers of 577RX heterozygotes among sprinters and lower than expected among endurance athletes. This was not seen in males, suggesting that the effect of the ACTN3 genotype may be sex-dependent (Yang *et al.* 2003).

Other genetic loci that have been investigated with no association shown include three mitochondrial DNA (mtDNA) polymorphisms (Rivera *et al.* 1998). Here the investigators examined the association between elite endurance athlete status and three mtDNA restriction fragment polymorphisms (RFLPs) in the 5 subunit of the nicotinamide adenine dinucleotide (NADH) dehydrogenase locus and one in the D-loop region in 125 Caucasian males compared with 65 sedentary controls. With one polymorphism not being present in their sample population, analysis of the other three mtDNA polymorphisms found no association between the other three loci and elite endurance athlete status (Rivera *et al.* 1998).

Circulating and tissue renin-angiotensin systems

The first gene for which a polymorphic variant was associated with human physical performance was the human ACE gene (Montgomery *et al.* 1998). Since that time, the ACE gene has become by far the best-studied locus in this regard, and warrants more detailed specific discussion.

As a component of the circulating or endocrine renin-angiotensin system (RAS), the renally derived aspartyl protease renin cleaves the hepatically synthesized α_2-globulin angiotensinogen to yield decapeptide angiotensin I. Acted upon by the peptidyl dipeptidase ACE, this generates the octapeptide angiotensin II (Ang II) whose effects are, in turn, mediated through two receptors: AT_1 and AT_2 (Timmermans & Smith 1994). There is also a third receptor (AT_4 receptor), which is more sensitive to the degradation product angiotensin IV. It is still unclear what the exact roles of the AT_2 and AT_4 receptors are in relation to circulating RAS, but stimulation of the AT_1 receptor by Ang II induces vasoconstriction and adrenal aldosterone release, leading with a consequent pressor effect.

Tissue kallikreins are a family of proteases that cleave kininogen to form the decapeptide bradykinin. ACE is a potent kininase, and bradykinin levels are thus inversely related to ACE activity. Bradykinin activates two main receptor classes, BK_1 and BK_2, and action on the latter leads to vasodilatation. Increasing ACE activity therefore promotes hypertension (increased AT_1 receptor activation) and reduces hypotensive responses (reduced BK_2 receptor activation). It also has an axial role in the regulation of human blood pressure and salt and water balance (Kem & Brown 1990). However, local paracrine RAS are now also well-described in human tissues as diverse as the vasculature, heart, kidney, brain, uterus and placenta, skin, ovary and testis, adipose tissue, and skeletal muscle (Dzau 1988; Lee *et al.* 1992; Hagemann *et al.* 1994; Jonsson *et al.* 1994; Harris & Cheng 1996; Buikema *et al.* 1997; Jones & Woods 2003). Here, they subserve a variety of functions related to the regulation of tissue growth and injury responses.

A polymorphism of the ACE gene has been identified in which the absence (deletion "D" allele) rather than the presence (insertion "I" allele) of a 287-bp marker in intron 16 is associated with raised circulating (Rigat *et al.* 1990) as well as tissue (Costerousse *et al.* 1993; Danser *et al.* 1995) ACE activity.

ACE I/D POLYMORPHISM AND EXERCISE-INDUCED LEFT VENTRICULAR HYPERTROPHY

Local myocardial RAS may have an important role in the regulation of LV growth responses. RAS components, including ACE, are expressed in the myocardium (Danser *et al.* 1999). Such expression increases with cardiac growth (Schunkert *et al.* 1990), while ACE inhibition attenuates such growth (Lievre *et al.* 1995) – as it does in a variety of animal models. Furthermore, the administration of ACE inhibitors to humans may lead to a greater regression in LV mass than is seen with other similarly hypotensive agents (Cruickshank *et al.* 1992; Schmieder *et al.* 1996, 1998). Such hypertrophic effects may, in part, be mediated through increased synthesis of Ang II (Beinlich *et al.* 1991; Liu *et al.* 1998). Ang II causes hypertrophy of cardiomyocytes (Liu *et al.* 1998; Wollert & Drexler 1999), an effect that seems mediated by activation of the AT_1 receptor (Liu *et al.* 1998). Meanwhile, kinins may exert a growth-inhibiting effect on myocardial tissue (Linz & Scholkens 1992), and increased ACE activity may therefore promote cardiac growth through an increase in kinin degradation (Murphey *et al.* 2000; Brull *et al.* 2001).

Exercise is a significant stimulus to LV growth, with studies showing as much as 40% increase in baseline LV mass after either isometric or endurance training programs (DeMaria *et al.* 1978; Zeldis *et al.* 1978; Kanakis & Hickson 1980; Wieling *et al.* 1981). If local ACE expression were to be important in modulating or transducing such growth, then we might anticipate the ACE D allele to be associated not only with raised ACE activity but also with greater LV growth in response to a uniform hypertrophic stimulus. Several studies suggest this to be the case. The first such study examined the LV growth response to 10 weeks of identical physical training amongst 140 Caucasian male military recruits (Montgomery *et al.* 1997). Echocardiographically determined LV dimensions and mass ($n = 140$) were compared at the start and end of this training period. Both septal and posterior wall thicknesses increased with training, with LV mass increasing by 18% ($P < 0.0001$). More importantly, the magnitude of the response was strongly associated with ACE I/D genotype, with mean LV mass changing by +2.0, +38.5, and +42.3 g in the II, ID, and DD groups, respectively ($P < 0.0001$). In addition, the prevalence of electrocardiographically defined left ventricular hypertrophy (LVH) also increased significantly only among those of *DD* genotype ($P < 0.01$). This association of the ACE D allele with an increased physiologic growth response has since been confirmed using cardiac magnetic resonance imaging (MRI) (Myerson *et al.* 2001). In this study, 141 British Army recruits homozygous for the ACE gene (79 DD and 62 II) were randomized to receive losartan at a subhypotensive dose or placebo throughout a similar 10-week training program. In the placebo group, MRI-determined LVM increased with training (8.4 g, $P < 0.0001$ overall; 12.1 vs. 4.8 g for DD vs. II genotype in the placebo limb, $P = 0.022$) with a similar LV growth seen in the group taking losartan (11.0 vs. 3.7 g for DD vs. II genotypes; $P = 0.034$). The LV growth was abolished in the II group, whereas it remained in the DD subjects (−0.022 vs. 0.131 g kg^{-1}, respectively; $P = 0.0009$) when indexed to lean body mass, thus confirming that exercise-induced LVH is ACE I/D dependent. The absence of an influence by AT_1 receptor antagonism in those taking losartan was also suggestive that the greater LV growth in those homozygous for the D allele may be caused by the effects of angiotensin II on other angiotensin receptors or a reduced level of degradation of growth-inhibitory kinins (Myerson *et al.* 2001).

Results from such gene–environment interaction studies have since been confirmed in studies of LVM amongst athletes as diverse as wrestlers (Kasikcioglu *et al.* 2004), soccer players (Fatini *et al.*

2000), and endurance athletes (Hernandez *et al.* 2003). Further, the ACE genotype also seems associated with pathologic LVH, in conditions as diverse as hypertension (Kuznetsova *et al.* 2000), diabetes (Estacio *et al.* 1999), hypertrophic cardiomyopathy (Yoneya *et al.* 1995), and aortic stenosis (Dellgren *et al.* 1999). Evidently LVM is determined by the interaction of genes with diverse environmental hypertrophic stimuli. It is thus of some note that those studies that have demonstrated a role for the ACE genotype in the determination of LVM have examined population samples exposed to growth stimuli of uniform nature and (often) scale. The variety of studies that have failed to identify such associations have generally studied populations of diverse age, sex and race, or those exposed to a variety of different hypertrophic stimuli over variable periods of time (Lindpaintner *et al.* 1996; Staessen *et al.* 1997; Karjalainen *et al.* 1999; Wu *et al.* 2000; Yildiz *et al.* 2000; Gruchala *et al.* 2003; Wang *et al.* 2003).

Evidently, the impact of ACE genotype on the cardiac growth response to exercise might be mediated through altered synthesis of (growth-promoting) Ang II, or the increased degradation of (growth-inhibiting) bradykinin. The administration of non-hypotensive doses of antagonists to the AT_1 receptor seem to have little impact on physiologic (exercise-driven) LV growth as previously mentioned (Myerson *et al.* 2001). Meanwhile, other studies implicate altered kinin action at the bradykinin BK2 receptor in the mediation of these associations of ACE genotype. A polymorphism in the bradykinin 2 receptor (BK2R) gene exists in which the presence of a 9-bp insertion (+9) rather than its absence (−9) is associated with lower gene transcription (Braun *et al.* 1996) and receptor response (Houle *et al.* 2000). In a group of 109 male army recruits, both ACE and B2BKR genotypes were determined and the physiologic LV growth response to a 10-week physical training program was assessed (Brull *et al.* 2001). Mean LV growth was 15.7 g (standard error, SE 3.5) in those homozygous for the ACE D and B2BKR +9 genotypes, but −1.37 g (SE 4.1) in those homozygous for ACE I and B2BKR genotype −9 ($P = 0.003$ for trend across genotypes), suggestive that some of the effects of ACE on LV growth are mediated by kinins which

themselves appear to regulate LV growth (Brull *et al.* 2001).

ACE genotype and $\dot{V}o_{2MAX}$

Any putative association of ACE genotype with $\dot{V}o_{2max}$ remains contentious. In a study of 85 female and 62 male US Army recruits undergoing an 8-week basic training program, Sonna *et al.* (2001) identified no significant association between ACE genotype and peak oxygen uptake (or other measures of performance as assessed on the Army Physical Fitness Test), although heterogeneity in the study population makes reliable interpretation hard. Such a view was confirmed by Bouchard *et al.* (2000) using a genomic scan covering all 22 pairs of autosomes on the Caucasian families of the HERITAGE Family Study (Bouchard *et al.* 1995). No evidence of linkage was observed on chromosome 17 (which includes the ACE locus on 17q23) for either baseline $\dot{V}o_{2max}$ or its change after a 20-week standardized endurance training program. In another study, Woods *et al.* (2002b) similarly identified no significant association when assessing the response to training in 58 army recruits. By contrast, a small ($n = 60$) study purported to demonstrate an association of the ACE I allele with $\dot{V}o_{2max}$ amongst post-menopausal women (Hagberg *et al.* 1998), with similar findings in patients with heart failure (Abraham *et al.* 2002).

ACE genotype and skeletal muscle function

Skeletal muscle RAS might, in theory, influence muscle function through Ang II genesis, or kinin degradation. First, Ang II is a recognized trophic agent for vascular smooth muscle (Berk *et al.* 1989) and also cardiac muscle (Liu *et al.* 1998; Wollert & Drexler 1999). It is thus perhaps unsurprising that it has been implicated in skeletal muscle growth where it may indeed have a key role in transducing mechanical load to yield growth responses (Gordon *et al.* 2001). Thus, increased ACE expression, as marked by the ACE D allele, might be expected to be associated with skeletal muscle hypertrophy in response to exercise. Ang II also has a metabolic role; Ang II infusion leads to a cachexia in rodent models, a component of which is not attributable to an anorexic effect (Brink *et al.* 2001) and weight loss (Brink *et al.* 1996). Meanwhile, bradykinin also has metabolic effects, influencing glycogen levels, lactate concentration (Linz *et al.* 1996), the availability of glucose-free fatty acid substrate (Wicklmayr *et al.* 1980), and the expression of the GLUT-4 glucose transporter (Taguchi *et al.* 2000). RAS expression also has an important role in the regulation of fat storage in adipocytes (Shenoy & Cassis 1997; Ailhaud 1999).

Whether through such mechanisms or others, the ACE genotype is associated with differences in skeletal muscle form and function. In conditions of intensive training and high calorie expenditure, a relative anabolic response was observed to be associated with the ACE I allele amongst military recruits (Montgomery *et al.* 1999). The I allele was similarly associated with greater increases in adductor pollicis muscle strength gain in response to hormone replacement therapy (HRT) in postmenopausal women (Woods *et al.* 2001). In young Caucasian military recruits, the maximum duration of standardized repetitive elbow flexion with a 15-kg barbell was studied before and after 10 weeks of military training. While pre-training performance was independent of ACE genotype, exercise duration increased significantly for the 66 individuals of either II or DD genotype (79.4 ± 25.2 and 24.7 ± 8.8 s; $P = 0.005$ and 0.007, respectively) but not for the 12 DD homozygotes (7.1 ± 14.9 s; $P = 0.642$), showing an 11-fold greater improvement for the II homozygotes compared to those with the DD genotype ($P = 0.001$) (Montgomery *et al.* 1998). 'Delta efficiency' (DE) is the ratio of external mechanical work to internal work performed by skeletal muscle, which increased significantly over a period of training for young Caucasian military recruits of II genotype when compared to those of DD genotype (Williams *et al.* 2000).

Meanwhile, quadriceps muscle strength is D-allele-associated in patients with chronic obstructive pulmonary disease (Hopkinson *et al.* 2004), and gains in quadriceps muscle strength in response to strength training seem D-allele-associated in young adult men (Folland *et al.* 2000).

Thus, although some variable data exist, it generally seems that the ACE I allele is associated with fatigue resistance, and the D allele with strength gain, at least amongst males and in response to training. Such associations are supported by the association of ACE genotype with elite sporting disciplines (see below). It may be that some of these effects are mediated through alterations in skeletal muscle fiber type. The I allele may be associated with a higher proportion of type 1 fibers, and DD genotype with a lower proportion of type 2b (Scott *et al.* 2001).

ACE GENOTYPE AND ELITE PERFORMANCE

ACE genotype is thus associated with a variety of sporting intermediate phenotypes. From these (above), we might generally anticipate an association of the I allele with endurance sports, and the D allele with strength- and/or power-dependent sports.

An excess of the I allele (compared with controls) was found in Australian national rowers (Gayagay *et al.* 1998), Russian athletes (Nazarov *et al.* 2001), and elite long-distance cyclists (Alvarez *et al.* 2000). Similarly, amongst British Olympic-standard runners, I allele frequency increased with the distance run: for the three distance groups 200, 400–3000, and 5000 m, the I allele frequency was 0.35, 0.53, and 0.62 ($P = 0.009$ for linear trend) (Myerson *et al.* 1999). A number of other studies have linked ACE genotype with various elite performance groups. Tsianos *et al.* (2004) investigated elite swimmers and showed data suggestive of the ACE I allele being associated with shorter distance swimmers, with the D allele linked with swimming shorter distances, while in another study Collins *et al.* (2004) showed an association of the I allele with endurance performance in the fastest 100 South African-born finishers during the South African Ironman Triathlons. Furthermore, I allele frequency is greater amongst elite UK mountaineers than amongst controls (Montgomery *et al.* 1998). If conferring a survival advantage, one might expect an I allele excess amongst high-altitude populations compared to those living in low altitude; Rupert *et al.* (2003), testing this hypothesis in the Native American population, showed no such evidence in five such polymorphisms including the ACE I/D variant. Tsianos *et al.* (2005), meanwhile, identified an association of the I allele with success in rapid ascent to high altitude. Such effects may be dependent upon I-allele-associated gains in $\dot{V}o_{2max}$, or in metabolic efficiency (see above). However, the ACE I allele may also be associated with an enhanced ventilatory drive to acute hypoxia (Patel *et al.* 2003), and thus with preserved arterial oxygenation at high altitude (Woods *et al.* 2002a).

However, conflicting data do exist. These are generally explained by the study of heterogeneous (often mixed race and sex, and sporting discipline) subject groups (Karjalainen *et al.* 1999; Taylor *et al.* 1999; Rankinen *et al.* 2000b; Woods *et al.* 2000; Sonna *et al.* 2001; Montgomery & Dhamrait 2002). Some of these effects may, in part, be mediated through alterations in bradykinin metabolism. The presence (+9) rather than absence (−9) of a 9-bp fragment in the gene for the BK2R is associated with lower gene transcription (Braun *et al.* 1996) and receptor response (Houle *et al.* 2000). Williams *et al.* (2004) investigated whether this variant is associated with DE (as previously defined) in 115 healthy men and women, or with running distance in 81 Olympic-standard track athletes. DE was shown to be highly significantly associated with B2BKR genotype (23.84 ± 2.41 vs. 24.25 ± 2.81 vs. 26.05 ± 2.26% for those of +9/+9 vs. +9/−9 vs. −9/−9 genotype; $P = 0.0008$). There was also evidence for an interaction with ACE I/D genotype, with those who were of ACE II and B2BKR −9/−9 genotype having the highest baseline DE and significantly associated with endurance (predominantly aerobic) among the elite athletes, suggestive that at least part of the associations of ACE and fitness phenotypes is via higher kinin activity (Williams *et al.* 2004).

Relationship between genes and the risk of sports injuries

Sporting injuries are heterogeneous in character and in cause, making the identification of genetic factors associated with such risk difficult. Nevertheless, such studies are likely to prove fruitful.

Genes and musculoskeletal injury

Genetic factors account for up to 50–70% in the variance of BMD (Rizzoli *et al.* 2001). However, BMD has been shown to be a major determinant in the risk for developing an osteoporotic fracture (Marshall *et al.* 1996). It is therefore not surprising that a significant heritability component has been found for the risk of sustaining an osteoporotic fracture (McKay *et al.* 1994; Seeman 1994; Seeman *et al.* 1994), with genetic factors contributing up to one-third of such cases (MacGregor *et al.* 2000). Collagen type I is the major extracellular organic component of bone and has been shown to affect its mechanical properties (Burr 2002), while vitamin D receptors have a major involvement in mineral ion homeostasis. Calcium is usually obtained from dairy products which contain lactose, the main sugar of milk, which is broken down by lactase in the bowel wall. Lactose is metabolized to glucose and galactose by the lactase enzyme (LCT) in the intestinal wall. Whether lactase activity has any effect on calcium absorption is controversial: some studies have reported reduced absorption of calcium in lactase-deficient subjects (Cochet *et al.* 1983), while others have shown the opposite (Debongnie *et al.* 1979; Tremaine *et al.* 1986). Polymorphisms of the COL1A1 (Uitterlinden *et al.* 1998), vitamin D receptor (Garnero *et al.* 2005), and lactase genes (Enattah *et al.* 2005) have all been associated with an increased risk of fragility fractures. However, while BMD is a major determinant of the risk of developing an osteoporotic fracture, it is only of one of the determinants of what can be called bone strength. In this regard, a number of macro- and microstructural properties (including bone shape, mineralization pattern, and elasticity) all have a role. In the younger athlete, such factors as these, and the general preservation in BMD, may explain the difficulty in identifying an association of BMD with stress fracture risk (Giladi *et al.* 1991; Jones *et al.* 2002). The association of genetic elements with both BMD and fragility fracture does not thus imply a similar association with stress fracture risk, although associations may exist: just as IL-6 genotype may be associated with bone remodeling in response to exercise (Dhamrait *et al.* 2003), it is also associated with BMD in osteoporotic women (James *et al.* 2004). To date, candidate gene-association studies in stress fractures have proven few, and underpowered (Enattah *et al.* 2004; Valimaki *et al.* 2005).

Similarly, one could anticipate that the risk of developing a ligamentous injury, and resultant outcome, would have a genetic component. A familial predisposition toward tearing the anterior cruciate ligament has been shown (Flynn *et al.* 2005), but there have been no studies looking at specific genes and their influence of the risk; likely candidate genes would include those coding for components of ligament structure such as collagen.

Genes and the risk of cardiac problems and sudden death

Sudden cardiac death is not uncommon, and although an overall incidence rate of 1 in 100,000 persons per year has been documented, a much higher proportion occurs among athletes (2.3 in 100,000 per year) compared with non-athletes (0.9 in 100,000 per year) – usually in one's early twenties, with males being more commonly affected (Corrado *et al.* 2003). While it is often the case that a definitive diagnosis is not made, several inherited diseases are known to be implicated: hypertrophic cardiomyopathy, long-QT syndrome, Marfan's syndrome, and arrhythmogenic right ventricular cardiomyopathy. Such conditions contribute to about 80% of non-traumatic sudden deaths in young athletes (Firoozi *et al.* 2002), with hypertrophic cardiomyopathy contributing 40–50% to this and affecting approximately 1 in 500 young adults (Maron *et al.* 1995). Such conditions have been shown to have (at least partly) a genetic component and a number of genetic loci have been identified as summarized in Table 19.4. In addition, phenotypic expression (and arrhythmic incidence) is likely to be influenced by polymorphic variation in other so-called "modifier" genes.

Genes and the risk of brain damage

Boxers are at risk of chronic traumatic brain injury (CTBI), which occurs in about 1 in 5 professional boxers (Jordan 2000) who exhibit varying degrees of motor, cognitive, and behavioral impairment associated with various pathologic findings, such as tearing of the septum pellicidum with gliosis of the thalamus; inferior cerebellar folia also tend to atrophy, with loss of pigmented neurones in the substantia nigra and the presence of neurofibrillary tangles in the temporal lobes, as is the case with Alzheimer's disease (Moseley 2000).

Apolipoproteins are a group of plasma proteins that function as carrier molecules for lipids, cholesterol, and other related molecules, both in the circulation but also at a local level in various tissues. There is ample evidence to suggest that apolipoprotein E (apoE) may have an active role in the response to brain injury. It is synthesized by astrocytes reacting to injury and its function is to transport lipids to regenerating neurons and to promote the repair and construction of new cell membranes and synapses (Nathan *et al.* 1994; Poirier 1994; Mahley *et al.* 1995) with associated upregulation of the apoE-mediated lipid-transport system seen after acute brain injury (Pluta *et al.* 1994; Pluta 2000). The three isoforms of apoE (E2, E3, and E4) have significant effects on its function, with apoE4 being associated with reduced growth and branching of neurites in cell culture (Nathan *et al.* 1994; Holtzman *et al.* 1995; Mahley *et al.* 1995). ApoE4 also tends to bind less strongly to various cytoskeletal proteins (Strittmatter *et al.* 1994), but more so to amyloid β-protein, enhancing the aggregation of amyloid β-protein into amyloid fibrils (Ma *et al.* 1994). ApoE ε-4 (apoE-ε4), a susceptibility gene for late-onset familial and sporadic Alzheimer's disease (Corder *et al.* 1993; Saunders *et al.* 1993), has been associated with an increased risk of CTBI in boxers (Jordan *et al.* 1997). In a group of 30 boxers with high exposure to the sport, those who had an apoE-ε4 allele showed greater neurologic dysfunction than those without such an allele. Furthermore, all the boxers who had severe impairment had an apoE-ε4 allele. Further evidence supporting a genetic predisposition to the risk of traumatic brain injury comes from Teasdale *et al.* (1997), who have reported a significant association between apoE-ε4 polymorphism and morbidity outcomes following acute traumatic brain injury in non-boxers.

Table 19.4 Conditions associated with sudden cardiac death in athletes and their genetic component.

Condition	Clinical implications	Genetic influence
Long QT syndrome	QT interval prolongation associated with ventricular tachyarrhythmias, syncope and sudden cardiac death	Both autosomal dominant (Romano–Ward) and recessive forms (Jervell and Lange–Nielsen) have been described (Priori *et al.* 2003). A number of genetic loci and genes have been identified and associated with the syndrome: KCNQ1 gene on chromosome 11 (LQT1) (Wang *et al.* 1996) KCNH2 gene on chromosome 7 (LQT2) (Curran *et al.* 1995) SCN5A gene on chromosome 3 (LQT3) (Wang *et al.* 1995) KCNE1 and KCNE2 genes on chromosome 21 (LQT 5 & 6) (Splawski *et al.* 1997) These genes code for ion-channel subunits that influence cardiac myocyte excitability (Priori *et al.* 2003) Genetic testing is only successful in 55–65% of affected patients (Splawski *et al.* 2000; Priori *et al.* 2003) suggestive of the presence of other relevant genes
Catecholaminergic polymorphic ventricular tachycardia	Associated with bi-directional polymorphic ventricular tachycardia which is uniform and can be induced by exercise leading to syncope but sometimes also to cardiac death	The pattern of inheritance appears to mainly be autosomal dominant (Leenhardt *et al.* 1995) Mutations of the cardiac ryanodine receptor (RyR2) gene identified onchromosome 1 have been associated with the syndrome (Priori *et al.* 2001) which is involved in the release of Ca^{2+} during the Phase 2 of the action potential A less common recessive form has been linked to the *CASQ2* gene on chromosome 1 which encodes for calsequestrin, which serves as a Ca^{2+} reservoir in the heart and is linked to RYR2 and compatible with the less common recessive form of the syndrome (Lahat *et al.* 2001)
Brugada syndrome	Characterized by elevation of the ST segment in leads V_1–V_3, right bundle branch block and susceptibility to arrhythmias. Thought to be more common in the Far East (known as sudden unexplained nocturnal death syndrome) (Priori *et al.* 2003)	Associated with mutations in the cardiac sodium channel gene (SCN5A), but is likely that other mutations contribute to the syndrome (Chen *et al.* 1998; Priori *et al.* 2002, 2003)
Hypertrophic cardiomyopathy	There are several patterns, which are characterized by varying degrees of myocardial hypertrophy, gross disorganization of muscle bundles and cardiac microstructural architecture which predispose to arrhythmias and sudden death (Firoozi *et al.* 2002)	Hypertrophic cardiomyopathy usually displays an autosomal dominant pattern of inheritance and a number of causative or contributing genes have been identified which are involved in coding for proteins involved in cardiac muscle architecture such as actin, myosin heavy and light chains, cardiac troponin I, α-tropomyosin and myosin-binding protein C (Firoozi *et al.* 2002). What is also accepted is that environmental and other genes may modify the expression of the disease which varies even within members of the same family

Thus, genetic factors strongly influence body form and physiology and, as a consequence, both human physical performance and risk of injury. The identification of specific genetic elements of risk will lead to a greater understanding of the mechanisms through which physiologic performance is regulated, and how the health benefits of exercise are derived. They may also help us understand the mechanisms predisposing to risk of sports-related injury in athletes, as well as to disease states in more sedentary individuals.

Gene therapy and genetic testing in elite sports: what does the future hold?

Many genes associated with performance have been identified through the study of human physiology or disease, without the specific intent of influencing sporting performance. The science of gene therapy involves the transfer of genetic material to human cells for the *treatment* of a disease or disorder. Such technology has been developed for the benefit of patients. However, in future, this technology might be applied so as to enhance an athlete's performance.

Gene therapy – the technology

Gene therapy is based on the ability to deliver genetic material to a cell, so as to modify its function. In patients, such a process is generally intended to offer compensation for the defective expression of a specific protein. The extra genetic material is usually introduced into the cell using a vector. This might be a virus which has been changed and so is no longer harmful (such as a retrovirus or adenovirus), or a lipid molecule (such as a liposome). The introduction of the extra DNA material can be carried out either by directly injecting into the tissue or organ (or its blood supply) that one needs to modify (or by inhalation in the case of the lungs) or by treating cells removed from the patient, treating them in the laboratory, and reintroducing them back to the patient. These modified cells can then start producing the new protein which can then act both locally or throughout the body through the circulation.

To date, the technology has been used successfully in patients with X-linked severe combined immunodeficiency disease (Hacein-Bey-Abina *et al.* 2002) and hemophilia B (Kay *et al.* 2000). In addition, the use of gene technology has been used to block the replication of cytomegalovirus (CMV) eye infections using anti-sense oligonucleotides (ISIS 13312 and ISIS 2922 [Isis Pharmaceuticals, Inc., Carlsbad, CA]) (Henry *et al.* 2001; Orr 2001).

Gene therapy and the athlete

The use of such technologies by athletes (so-called "gene doping") may offer some immediate attraction. Indeed, several candidate genes have already been suggested (Haisma 2004):

ERYTHROPOIETIN

Erythropoietin (Epo) is a naturally occurring hormone that drives red cell production. This increases oxygen carriage, but also increases viscosity of the blood. Epo is often used in clinical practice in the treatment of patients with kidney failure, in whom Epo levels (and thus red cell mass) is low. However, it has been increasingly used amongst athletes in an effort to increase oxygen transport, and thus performance. Of historical interest is the case of Eero Mäntyranta, the 1964 Olympic Gold Medalist Finnish skier; he was later diagnosed to have a natural mutation of his Epo gene, giving him more oxygen-carrying red blood cells and a natural advantage (Sweeney 2004). In the future, gene therapy may be used to create such advantages in the same way. This has been carried out successfully in monkeys and mice (Zhou *et al.* 1998) using adenoviral delivery to increase hematocrit by up to 80%.

MYOSTATIN

Myostatin is an inhibitor of muscle growth. Natural mutations that reduce its inhibitory function have been documented for some time in the big beefy breeds of Belgian Blue and Piedmontese cattle (Kambadur *et al.* 1997; McPherron & Lee 1997), but the first natural mutation documented in humans was recently published and associated with gross muscle hypertrophy in a child (Schuelke *et al.* 2004). Although there have been rumors that such mutations may have given a natural advantage to weightlifting champions in the past, this is undocumented (Sweeney 2004). The potential of using gene therapy, to negate the inhibitory effect of myostatin either directly, or through the production of its inhibitors such as follistatin, is of concern, while at the same time research into such technology would be of great interest and possibly of great benefit to those patients with muscular dystrophies (Bogdanovich *et al.* 2002).

RISKS OF GENE DOPING

To some athletes, the introduction of genetic material into their bodies represents a risk-free means to improve their performance without the worry of detection. However, such a concept is misguided at a number of levels:

1 Human performance relies upon the complex integration of multiple physiologic pathways. It is perhaps naive to think that altering the expression of a single gene is likely, of itself, to alter performance radically.

2 Increased activity of one biologic component alone may be detrimental. Thus, increasing muscle strength by itself may lead to an increase in tendon injury or bony stress fracture, if these elements are stressed beyond their adaptive limit.

3 There are difficulties in introducing a gene to only one tissue in one anatomic area.

4 The regulation of gene expression is highly complex and still poorly understood. It is unlikely that one would wish to introduce a gene causing, for example, muscle hypertrophy, unless one were able to ensure that its expression only occurred in response to a training stimulus or to some other control element. Unrestricted muscle growth would clearly not be to the advantage of the athlete.

5 Abnormal expression of growth factors may have long-term risks. Such expression is associated with the development of cancers, while increased Epo production and its association with higher hematocrit (thicker blood) increases the risk of clot-related problems, including myocardial infarction and stroke.

6 Viral vectors may themselves prove hazardous. Being themselves antigenic, influenza-like symptoms are commonly reported by patients treated with gene therapy.

7 Although, theoretically, the new gene would code for a protein that would be naturally produced in the body, any small changes or variations may induce the body to recognize that protein as foreign, and instigate an autoimmune response against this, with possibly detrimental effects to the athlete. Perhaps for this reason, Epo gene delivery has been associated with the development of severe autoimmune anemia in a simian model (Gao *et al.* 2004). Other reported problems from the utilization of the technology in humans include the development of a leukemoid condition in patients cured for immunodeficiency disease (Hacein-Bey-Abina *et al.* 2003) and the development of chronic liver disease and vector overdosing (Hacein-Bey-Abina *et al.* 2003).

TESTING FOR GENE DOPING

The international sports organizations have not only recognized the potential of the use of the technology, but also the problems related to detecting athletes who may use gene doping to improve their performance (WADA 2003, 2005; Haisma 2004). A number of difficulties have been recognized regarding detection:

1 The transferred genetic material is usually of human origin, and by becoming part of an athlete's genome, it could be difficult to detect.

2 In a number of cases, gene therapy would be confined to a specific area or tissue (e.g., muscle) and therefore would be undetected unless that tissue is directly analyzed.

3 The transferred or modified gene would, in the majority of cases, encode natural proteins expressed only at a local level. These would prove hard to detect.

4 A number of forms of genetic doping would not require the treatment to take place at the natural site of where these genes are usually expressed, but can be used at other sites in the body (e.g., in the case of the Epo gene) from where it can be transferred to the acting site via the bloodstream.

5 Detection techniques may include the need for tissue biopsy; asking a competing athlete to accept

having a biopsy taken of his or her muscle during the period of competition would be very difficult.

At first glance, all these issues may be of encouragement to those athletes who may be considering gene doping in the future in that they will not be "caught", and proceed with such treatment (despite being aware of the risks involved). Although difficult, the various anti-doping bodies have already recognized the potential of the technology and have not only included gene doping and therapy in their list of banned technologies (WADA 2003), but have already started the fight against it, by funding research into detection technologies (WADA 2005) and warning athletes that "detection is possible and probable." This might be accomplished through the detection of the actual DNA transferred, the vectors used, the expression of the gene and the protein produced, the effects of the new gene and, finally, effects on other gene functions.

Conclusions

Human form and function are dictated by the interaction of genes with environmental stimuli. Thus, variations in environmental exposures will strongly influence phenotype. However, although our core genetic inheritance is common to all humans, common small functional variations exist in these genes which dictate that our responses to environmental challenge will differ between individuals.

Such genetic variations influence sporting performance through associated differences in anatomy and physiology, and their response to training stimuli. The study of genetics and sport thus offers us a means to explore human functional biology, and the mechanisms through which sporting activity improves health. In addition, such studies may help us to understand the mechanisms of injury and disease amongst sports persons and the sedentary population alike.

Our increased understanding of genetics and sport does, however, bring concerns. It may yet prove possible to "genetically screen" individuals to identify those most likely to perform well in a given discipline, as well as those at greater risk of injury. This brings with it the potential for "primary exclusion" of individuals from selection for further training. It also offers the potential for "gene doping" of athletes, with a significant subtended risk.

References

Abraham, M.R., Olson, L.J., Joyner, M.J., Turner, S.T., Beck, K.C. & Johnson, B.D. (2002) Angiotensin-converting enzyme genotype modulates pulmonary function and exercise capacity in treated patients with congestive stable heart failure. *Circulation* **106**, 1794–1799.

Adams, T.D., Yanowitz, F.G., Fisher, A.G., *et al.* (1985) Heritability of cardiac size: an echocardiographic and electrocardiographic study of monozygotic and dizygotic twins. *Circulation* **71**, 39–44.

Ailhaud, G. (1999) Cross talk between adipocytes and their precursors: relationships with adipose tissue development and blood pressure. *Annals of the New York Academy of Sciences* **892**, 127–133.

Alvarez, R., Terrados, N., Ortolano, R., *et al.* (2000) Genetic variation in the renin-angiotensin system and athletic performance. *European Journal of Applied Physiology and Occupational Physiology* **82**, 117–120.

Arden, N.K. & Spector, T.D. (1997) Genetic influences on muscle strength, lean body mass, and bone mineral density: A twin study. *Journal of Bone and Mineral Research* **12**, 2076–2081.

Arko, B., Prezelj, J., Komel, R., Kocijancic, A., Hudler, P. & Marc, J. (2002) Sequence variations in the osteoprotegerin gene promoter in patients with postmenopausal osteoporosis. *Journal of Clinical Endocrinology and Metabolism* **87**, 4080–4084.

Atwood, L.D., Samollow, P.B., Hixson, J.E., Stern, M.P. & MacCluer, J.W. (2001) Genome-wide linkage analysis of pulse pressure in Mexican Americans. *Hypertension* **37**, 425–428.

Baker, R., Lynch, J., Ferguson, L., Priestley, L. & Sykes, B. (1991) PCR detection of five restriction site dimorphisms at the type I collagen loci COL1A1 and COL1A2. *Nucleic Acids Research* **19**, 4315.

Barger, P.M., Brandt, J.M., Leone, T.C., Weinheimer, C.J. & Kelly, D.P. (2000) Deactivation of peroxisome proliferator-activated receptor-alpha during cardiac hypertrophic growth. *Journal of Clinical Investigation* **105**, 1723–1730.

Beinlich, C.J., White, G.J., Baker, K.M. & Morgan, H.E. (1991) Angiotensin II and left ventricular growth in newborn pig heart. *Journal of Molecular and Cellular Cardiology* **23**, 1031–1038.

Berk, B.C., Vekshtein, V., Gordon, H.M. & Tsuda, T. (1989) Angiotensin II-stimulated protein synthesis in cultured vascular smooth muscle cells. *Hypertension* **13**, 305–314.

Beunen, G. & Thomis, M. (2004) Gene powered? Where to go from heritability (h^2) in muscle strength and power? *Exercise and Sport Sciences Reviews* **32**, 148–154.

Bielen, E., Fagard, R. & Amery, A. (1991) The inheritance of left ventricular structure and function assessed by imaging and Doppler echocardiography. *American Heart Journal* **121**, 1743–1749.

Binas, B., Danneberg, H., McWhir, J., Mullins, L. & Clark, A.J. (1999) Requirement for the heart-type fatty acid binding protein in cardiac fatty acid utilization. *FASEB Journal* **13**, 805–812.

Bogdanovich, S., Krag, T.O., Barton, E.R., *et al.* (2002) Functional improvement of dystrophic muscle by myostatin blockade. *Nature* **420**, 418–421.

Boomsma, D.I., Snieder, H., de Geus, E.J. & van Doornen, L.J. (1998) Heritability of blood pressure increases during mental stress. *Twin Research* **1**, 15–24.

Bouchard, C., Daw, E.W., Rice, T., *et al.* (1998) Familial resemblance for $\dot{V}o_{2max}$ in the sedentary state: the HERITAGE family study. *Medicine and Science in Sports and Exercise* **30**, 252–258.

Bouchard, C., Leon, A.S., Rao, D.C., Skinner, J.S., Wilmore, J.H. & Gagnon, J. (1995) The HERITAGE family study. Aims, design, and measurement protocol. *Medicine and Science in Sports and Exercise* **27**, 721–729.

Bouchard, C., Lesage, R., Lortie, G., *et al.* (1986) Aerobic performance in brothers, dizygotic and monozygotic twins. *Medicine and Science in Sports and Exercise* **18**, 639–646.

Bouchard, C., Malina, R.M. & Perusse, L. (1997) *Genetics of Fitness and Physical Performance.* Human Kinetics, Champaign, IL: 24–26.

Bouchard, C., Rankinen, T., Chagnon, Y.C., *et al.* (2000) Genomic scan for maximal oxygen uptake and its response to training in the HERITAGE Family Study. *Journal of Applied Physiology* **88**, 551–559.

Boudreau-Lariviere, C., Sveistrup, H., Parry, D.J. & Jasmin, B.J. (1996) Ciliary neurotrophic factor: regulation of acetylcholinesterase in skeletal muscle and distribution of messenger RNA encoding its receptor in synaptic versus extrasynaptic compartments. *Neuroscience* **73**, 613–622.

Braun, A., Kammerer, S., Maier, E., Bohme, E. & Roscher, A.A. (1996) Polymorphisms in the gene for the human B2-bradykinin receptor. New tools in assessing a genetic risk for bradykinin-associated diseases. *Immunopharmacology* **33**, 32–35.

Brink, M., Price, S.R., Chrast, J., *et al.* (2001) Angiotensin II induces skeletal muscle wasting through enhanced protein degradation and down-regulates autocrine insulin-like growth factor I. *Endocrinology* **142**, 1489–1496.

Brink, M., Wellen, J. & Delafontaine, P. (1996) Angiotensin II causes weight loss and decreases circulating insulin-like growth factor I in rats through a pressor-independent mechanism. *Journal of Clinical Investigation* **97**, 2509–2516.

Brull, D., Dhamrait, S., Myerson, S., *et al.* (2001) Bradykinin B2BKR receptor polymorphism and left-ventricular growth response. *Lancet* **358**, 1155–1156.

Buhl, R., Ersboll, A.K., Eriksen, L. & Koch, J. (2005) Changes over time in echocardiographic measurements in young Standardbred racehorses undergoing training and racing and association with racing performance. *Journal of the American Veterinary Medical Association* **226**, 1881–1887.

Buikema, H., Pinto, Y.M., van Geel, P.P., *et al.* (1997) Differential inhibition of plasma versus tissue ACE by utibapril: biochemical and functional evidence for inhibition of vascular ACE activity. *Journal of Cardiovascular Pharmacology* **29**, 684–691.

Buitrago, C., Vazquez, G., De Boland, A.R. & Boland, R. (2001) The vitamin D receptor mediates rapid changes in muscle protein tyrosine phosphorylation induced by 1,25(OH)(2)D(3). *Biochemical and Biophysical Research Communications* **289**, 1150–1156.

Burr, D.B. (2002) The contribution of the organic matrix to bone's material properties. *Bone* **31**, 8–11.

Burstein, P.J., Draznin, B., Johnson, C.J. & Schalch, D.S. (1979) The effect of hypothyroidism on growth, serum growth hormone, the growth hormone-dependent somatomedin, insulin-like growth factor, and its carrier protein in rats. *Endocrinology* **104**, 1107–1111.

Carbo, N., Lopez-Soriano, J., Costelli, P., *et al.* (2000) Interleukin-15 antagonizes muscle protein waste in tumour-bearing rats. *British Journal of Cancer* **83**, 526–531.

Carn, G., Koller, D.L., Peacock, M., *et al.* (2002) Sibling pair linkage and association studies between peak bone mineral density and the gene locus for the osteoclast-specific subunit (OC116) of the vacuolar proton pump on chromosome 11p12-13. *Journal of Clinical Endocrinology and Metabolism* **87**, 3819–3824.

Ceda, G.P., Fielder, P.J., Donovan, S.M., Rosenfeld, R.G. & Hoffman, A.R. (1992) Regulation of insulin-like growth factor-binding protein expression by thyroid hormone in rat GH3 pituitary tumor cells. *Endocrinology* **130**, 1483–1489.

Chen, H.Y., Tsai, H.D., Chen, W.C., Wu, J.Y., Tsai, F.J. & Tsai, C.H. (2001) Relation of polymorphism in the promotor region for the human osteocalcin gene to bone mineral density and occurrence of osteoporosis in postmenopausal Chinese women in Taiwan. *Journal of Clinical Laboratory Analysis* **15**, 251–255.

Chen, Q., Kirsch, G.E., Zhang, D., *et al.* (1998) Genetic basis and molecular mechanism for idiopathic ventricular fibrillation. *Nature* **392**, 293–296.

Chernausek, S.D., Underwood, L.E. & Van Wyk, J.J. (1982) Influence of hypothyroidism on growth hormone binding by rat liver. *Endocrinology* **111**, 1534–1538.

Chiu, H.C., Kovacs, A., Ford, D.A., *et al.* (2001) A novel mouse model of lipotoxic cardiomyopathy. *Journal of Clinical Investigation* **107**, 813–822.

Christakos, S., Raval-Pandya, M., Wernyj, R.P. & Yang, W. (1996) Genomic mechanisms involved in the pleiotropic actions of 1,25-dihydroxyvitamin D3. *Biochemical Journal* **316**, 361–371.

Clausen, T., Nielsen, O.B., Harrison, A.P., Flatman, J.A. & Overgaard, K. (1998) The Na+,K+ pump and muscle excitability. *Acta Physiologica Scandinavica* **162**, 183–190.

Cochet, B., Jung, A., Griessen, M., Bartholdi, P., Schaller, P. & Donath, A. (1983) Effects of lactose on intestinal calcium absorption in normal and lactase-deficient subjects. *Gastroenterology* **84**, 935–940.

Collins, M., Xenophontos, S.L., Cariolou, M.A., *et al.* (2004) The ACE gene and endurance performance during the South African Ironman Triathlons. *Medicine and Science in Sports and Exercise* **36**, 1314–1320.

Cooper, G.S. & Umbach, D.M. (1996) Are vitamin D receptor polymorphisms associated with bone mineral density? A meta-analysis. *Journal of Bone and Mineral Research* **11**, 1841–1849.

Corder, E.H., Saunders, A.M., Strittmatter, W.J., *et al.* (1993) Gene dose of apolipoprotein E type 4 allele and the risk of Alzheimer's disease in late onset families. *Science* **261**, 921–923.

Corrado, D., Basso, C., Rizzoli, G., Schiavon, M. & Thiene, G. (2003) Does sports activity enhance the risk of sudden death in adolescents and young adults? *Journal of the American College of Cardiology* **42**, 1959–1963.

Costa, E.M., Blau, H.M. & Feldman, D. (1986) 1,25-Dihydroxyvitamin D3 receptors and hormonal responses in cloned human skeletal muscle cells. *Endocrinology* **119**, 2214–2220.

Costerousse, O., Allegrini, J., Lopez, M. & Alhenc-Gelas, F. (1993) Angiotensin I-converting enzyme in human circulating mononuclear cells: genetic polymorphism of expression in T-lymphocytes. *Biochemical Journal* **290**, 33–40.

Crew, M.D. & Spindler, S.R. (1986) Thyroid hormone regulation of the transfected rat growth hormone promoter. *Journal of Biological Chemistry* **261**, 5018–5022.

Cruickshank, J.M., Lewis, J., Moore, V. & Dodd, C. (1992) Reversibility of left ventricular hypertrophy by differing types of antihypertensive therapy. *Journal of Human Hypertension* **6**, 85–90.

Cummings, S.R., Nevitt, M.C., Browner, W.S., *et al.* (1995) Risk factors for hip fracture in white women. Study of Osteoporotic Fractures Research Group. *New England Journal of Medicine* **332**, 767–773.

Curran, M.E., Splawski, I., Timothy, K.W., Vincent, G.M., Green, E.D. & Keating, M.T. (1995) A molecular basis for cardiac arrhythmia: HERG mutations cause long QT syndrome. *Cell* **80**, 795–803.

Danser, A.H., Schalekamp, M.A., Bax, W.A., *et al.* (1995) Angiotensin-converting enzyme in the human heart. Effect of the deletion/insertion polymorphism. *Circulation* **92**, 1387–1388.

Danser, A.H.J., Saris, J.J., Schuijt, M.P. & van Kats, J.P. (1999) Is there a local renin-angiotensin system in the heart? *Cardiovascular Research* **44**, 252–265.

Debongnie, J.C., Newcomer, A.D., McGill, D.B. & Phillips, S.F. (1979) Absorption of nutrients in lactase deficiency. *Digestive Diseases and Science* **24**, 225–231.

Dellgren, G., Eriksson, M.J., Blange, I., Brodin, L.A., Radegran, K. & Sylven, C. (1999) Angiotensin-converting enzyme gene polymorphism influences degree of left ventricular hypertrophy and its regression in patients undergoing operation for aortic stenosis. *American Journal of Cardiology* **84**, 909–913.

DeMaria, A.N., Neumann, A., Lee, G., Fowler, W. & Mason, D.T. (1978) Alterations in ventricular mass and performance induced by exercise training in man evaluated by echocardiography. *Circulation* **57**, 237–244.

Dhamrait, S.S., James, L., Brull, D.J., *et al.* (2003) Cortical bone resorption during exercise is interleukin-6 genotype-dependent. *European Journal of Applied Physiology and Occupational Physiology* **89**, 21–25.

Dick, I.M., Devine, A., Marangou, A., *et al.* (2002) Apolipoprotein E4 is associated with reduced calcaneal quantitative ultrasound measurements and bone mineral density in elderly women. *Bone* **31**, 497–502.

Dionne, F.T., Turcotte, L., Thibault, M.C., Boulay, M.R., Skinner, J.S. & Bouchard, C. (1991) Mitochondrial DNA sequence polymorphism, $\dot{V}o_{2max}$, and response to endurance training. *Medicine and Science in Sports and Exercise* **23**, 177–185.

Djouadi, F., Weinheimer, C.J., Saffitz, J.E., *et al.* (1998) A gender-related defect in lipid metabolism and glucose homeostasis in peroxisome proliferator-activated receptor alpha-deficient mice. *Journal of Clinical Investigation* **102**, 1083–1091.

Dohi, Y., Iki, M., Ohgushi, H., *et al.* (1998) A novel polymorphism in the promoter region for the human osteocalcin gene: The possibility of a correlation with bone mineral density in postmenopausal Japanese women. *Journal of Bone and Mineral Research* **13**, 1633–1639.

Dohm, M.R., Richardson, C.S. & Garland, T. Jr. (1994) Exercise physiology of wild and random-bred laboratory house mice and their reciprocal hybrids. *American Journal of Physiology* **267**, R1098–1108.

Dzau, V.J. (1988) Tissue renin-angiotensin system: physiologic and pharmacologic implications. Introduction. *Circulation* **77**, 11–13.

Enattah, N., Valimaki, V.V., Valimaki, M.J., Loyttyniemi, E., Sahi, T. & Jarvela, I. (2004) Molecularly defined lactose malabsorption, peak bone mass and bone turnover rate in young Finnish men. *Calcified Tissue International* **75**, 488–493.

Enattah, N.S., Sulkava, R., Halonen, P., Kontula, K. & Jarvela, I. (2005) Genetic variant of lactase-persistent C/T-13910 is associated with bone fractures in very old age. *Journal of the American Geriatrics Society* **53**, 79–82.

Endo, I., Inoue, D., Mitsui, T., *et al.* (2003) Deletion of vitamin D receptor gene in mice results in abnormal skeletal muscle development with deregulated expression of myoregulatory transcription factors. *Endocrinology* **144**, 5138–5144.

English, A.W. (2003) Cytokines, growth factors and sprouting at the neuromuscular junction. *Journal of Neurocytology* **32**, 943–960.

Estacio, R.O., Jeffers, B.W., Havranek, E.P., Krick, D., Raynolds, M. & Schrier, R.W. (1999) Deletion polymorphism of the angiotensin converting enzyme gene is associated with an increase in left ventricular mass in men with type 2 diabetes mellitus. *American Journal of Hypertension* **12**, 637–642.

Fatini, C., Guazzelli, R., Manetti, P., *et al.* (2000) RAS genes influence exercise-induced left ventricular hypertrophy: an elite athletes study. *Medicine and Science in Sports and Exercise* **32**, 1868–1872.

Feng, D., Ishibashi, H., Yamamoto, S., *et al.* (2003) Association between bone loss and promoter polymorphism in the IL-6 gene in elderly Japanese women with hip fracture. *Journal of Bone and Mineral Metabolism* **21**, 225–228.

Ferrari, S.L., Ahn-Luong, L., Garnero, P., Humphries, S.E. & Greenspan, S.L. (2003) Two promoter polymorphisms regulating interleukin-6 gene expression are associated with circulating levels of C-reactive protein and markers of bone resorption in postmenopausal women. *Journal of Clinical Endocrinology and Metabolism* **88**, 255–259.

Ferrari, S.L., Deutsch, S., Choudhury, U., *et al.* (2004) Polymorphisms in the low-density lipoprotein receptor-related protein 5 (LRP5) gene are associated with variation in vertebral bone mass, vertebral bone size, and stature in whites. *American Journal of Human Genetics* **74**, 866–875.

Ferrari, S.L. & Rizzoli, R. (2005) Gene variants for osteoporosis and their pleiotropic effects in aging. *Molecular Aspects of Medicine* **26**, 145–167.

Ferrari, S.L., Rizzoli, R., Slosman, D.O. & Bonjour, J.P. (1998) Do dietary calcium and age explain the controversy surrounding the relationship between bone mineral density and vitamin D receptor gene polymorphisms? *Journal of Bone and Mineral Research* **13**, 363–370.

Firoozi, S., Sharma, S., Hamid, M.S. & McKenna, W.J. (2002) Sudden death in young athletes: HCM or ARVC? *Cardiovascular Drugs and Therapy* **16**, 11–17.

Flynn, R.K., Pedersen, C.L., Birmingham, T.B., Kirkley, A., Jackowski, D. & Fowler, P.J. (2005) The familial predisposition toward tearing the anterior cruciate ligament: a case–control study. *American Journal of Sports Medicine* **33**, 23–28.

Folland, J., Leach, B., Little, T., *et al.* (2000) Angiotensin-converting enzyme genotype affects the response of human skeletal muscle to functional overload. *Experimental Physiology* **85**, 575–579.

Frederiksen, H., Bathum, L., Worm, C., Christensen, K. & Puggaard, L. (2003) ACE genotype and physical training effects: a randomized study among elderly Danes. *Aging Clinical and Experimental Research* **15**, 284–291.

Frederiksen, H. & Christensen, K. (2003) The influence of genetic factors on physical functioning and exercise in second half of life. *Scandinavian Journal of Medicine and Science in Sports* **13**, 9–18.

Fruchart, J.C., Duriez, P. & Staels, B. (1999) Peroxisome proliferator-activated receptor-alpha activators regulate genes governing lipoprotein metabolism, vascular inflammation and atherosclerosis. *Current Opinion in Lipidology* **10**, 245–257.

Gambert, S.R. & Duthie, E.H. Jr. (1983) Effect of age on red cell membrane sodium–potassium dependent adenosine triphosphatase (Na⁺-K⁺ ATPase) activity in healthy men. *Journal of Gerontology* **38**, 23–25.

Gao, G., Lebherz, C., Weiner, D.J., *et al.* (2004) Erythropoietin gene therapy leads to autoimmune anemia in macaques. *Blood* **103**, 3300–3302.

Garnero, P., Borel, O., Sornay-Rendu, E., *et al.* (2002) Association between a functional interleukin-6 gene polymorphism and peak bone mineral density and postmenopausal bone loss in women: the OFELY study. *Bone* **31**, 43–50.

Garnero, P., Munoz, F., Borel, O., Sornay-Rendu, E. & Delmas, P.D. (2005) Vitamin D receptor gene polymorphisms are associated with the risk of fractures in postmenopausal women, independently of bone mineral density. The OFELY study. *Journal of Clinical Endocrinology and Metabolism* **90**, 4829–4835.

Gaspard, T., Wondergem, R., Hamamdzic, M. & Klitgaard, H.M. (1978) Serum somatomedin stimulation in thyroxine-treated hypophysectomized rats. *Endocrinology* **102**, 606–611.

Gayagay, G., Yu, B., Hambly, B., *et al.* (1998) Elite endurance athletes and the ACE I allele: the role of genes in athletic performance. *Human Genetics* **103**, 48–50.

Gennari, L., Masi, L., Merlotti, D., *et al.* (2004) A polymorphic CYP19 TTTA repeat influences aromatase activity and estrogen levels in elderly men: effects on bone metabolism. *Journal of Clinical Endocrinology and Metabolism* **89**, 2803–2810.

Geusens, P., Vandevyver, C., Vanhoof, J., Cassiman, J.J., Boonen, S. & Raus, J. (1997) Quadriceps and grip strength are related to vitamin D receptor genotype in elderly nonobese women. *Journal of Bone and Mineral Research* **12**, 2082–2088.

Giehl, K.M. (2001) Trophic dependencies of rodent corticospinal neurons. *Reviews in the Neurosciences* **12**, 79–94.

Giladi, M., Milgrom, C., Simkin, A. & Danon, Y. (1991) Stress fractures. Identifiable risk factors. *American Journal of Sports Medicine* **19**, 647–652.

Gong, G., Stern, H.S., Cheng, S.C., *et al.* (1999) The association of bone mineral density with vitamin D receptor gene polymorphisms. *Osteoporosis International* **9**, 55–64.

Gonzalez-Cadavid, N.F., Taylor, W.E., Yarasheski, K., *et al.* (1998) Organization of the human myostatin gene and expression in healthy men and HIV-infected men with muscle wasting. *Proceedings of the National Academy of Sciences of the United States of America* **95**, 14938–14943.

Goodman, M.N. (1994) Interleukin-6 induces skeletal muscle protein breakdown in rats. *Proceedings of the Society for Experimental Biology and Medicine* **205**, 182–185.

Gordon, S.E., Davis, B.S., Carlson, C.J. & Booth, F.W. (2001) ANG II is required for optimal overload-induced skeletal muscle hypertrophy. *American Journal of Physiological Endocrinology and Metabolism* **280**, E150–159.

Grant, S.F., Reid, D.M., Blake, G., Herd, R., Fogelman, I. & Ralston, S.H. (1996) Reduced bone density and osteoporosis associated with a polymorphic Sp1 binding site in the collagen type I alpha 1 gene. *Nature Genetics* **14**, 203–205.

Gross, C., Eccleshall, T.R., Malloy, P.J., Villa, M.L., Marcus, R. & Feldman, D. (1996) The presence of a polymorphism at the translation initiation site of the vitamin D receptor gene is associated with low bone mineral density in postmenopausal Mexican-American women. *Journal of Bone and Mineral Research* **11**, 1850–1855.

Gruchala, M., Ciecwierz, D., Ochman, K., *et al.* (2003) Left ventricular size, mass and function in relation to angiotensin-converting enzyme gene and angiotensin-II type 1 receptor gene polymorphisms in patients with coronary artery disease. *Clinical Chemistry and Laboratory Medicine* **41**, 522–528.

Grundberg, E., Brandstrom, H., Ribom, E.L., Ljunggren, O., Mallmin, H. & Kindmark, A. (2004) Genetic variation in the human vitamin D receptor is associated with muscle strength, fat mass and body weight in Swedish women. *European Journal of Endocrinology* **150**, 323–328.

Guillet, C., Auguste, P., Mayo, W., Kreher, P. & Gascan, H. (1999) Ciliary neurotrophic factor is a regulator of muscular strength in aging. *Journal of Neuroscience* **19**, 1257–1262.

Hacein-Bey-Abina, S., Le Deist, F., Carlier, F., *et al.* (2002) Sustained correction of X-linked severe combined immunodeficiency by *ex vivo* gene therapy. *New England Journal of Medicine* **346**, 1185–1193.

Hacein-Bey-Abina, S., von Kalle, C., Schmidt, M., *et al.* (2003) A serious adverse event after successful gene therapy for X-linked severe combined immunodeficiency. *New England Journal of Medicine* **348**, 255–256.

Hagberg, J.M., Ferrell, R.E., McCole, S.D., Wilund, K.R. & Moore, G.E. (1998) $\dot{V}o_{2max}$ is associated with ACE genotype in postmenopausal women. *Journal of Applied Physiology* **85**, 1842–1846.

Hagemann, A., Nielsen, A.H. & Poulsen, K. (1994) The uteroplacental renin-angiotensin system: A review. *Experimental and Clinical Endocrinology* **102**, 252–261.

Haisma, H.J. (2004) *Gene Doping*. Netherlands Centre for Doping Affairs (NECEDO), the Netherlands.

Han, X.Y., Wang, W., Myllyla, R., Virtanen, P., Karpakka, J. & Takala, T.E. (1999) mRNA levels for alpha-subunit of prolyl 4-hydroxylase and fibrillar collagens in immobilized rat skeletal muscle. *Journal of Applied Physiology* **87**, 90–96.

Harris, R.C. & Cheng, H.F. (1996) The intrarenal renin-angiotensin system: a paracrine system for the local control of renal function separate from the systemic axis. *Experimental Nephrology* **4** (Supplement 1), 2–7.

Harshfield, G.A., Grim, C.E., Hwang, C., Savage, D.D. & Anderson, S.J. (1990) Genetic and environmental influences on echocardiographically determined left ventricular mass in black twins. *American Journal of Hypertension* **3**, 538–543.

Haugk, K.L., Roeder, R.A., Garber, M.J. & Schelling, G.T. (1995) Regulation of muscle cell proliferation by extracts from crushed muscle. *Journal of Animal Science* **73**, 1972–1981.

Helgren, M.E., Squinto, S.P., Davis, H.L., *et al.* (1994) Trophic effect of ciliary neurotrophic factor on denervated skeletal muscle. *Cell* **76**, 493–504.

Henry, S.P., Miner, R.C., Drew, W.L., *et al.* (2001) Antiviral activity and ocular kinetics of antisense oligonucleotides designed to inhibit CMV replication. *Investigative Ophthalmology and Visual Science* **42**, 2646–2651.

Hernandez, D., de la Rosa, A., Barragan, A., *et al.* (2003) The ACE/DD genotype is associated with the extent of exercise-induced left ventricular growth in endurance athletes. *Journal of the American College of Cardiology* **42**, 527–532.

Holtzman, D.M., Pitas, R.E., Kilbridge, J., *et al.* (1995) Low density lipoprotein receptor-related protein mediates apolipoprotein E-dependent neurite outgrowth in a central nervous system-derived neuronal cell line. *Proceedings of the National Academy of Sciences of the USA* **92**, 9480–9484.

Hopkinson, N.S., Nickol, A.H., Payne, J., *et al.* (2004) Angiotensin converting enzyme genotype and strength in chronic obstructive pulmonary disease. *American Journal of Respiratory and Critical Care Medicine* **170**, 395–399.

Hosoi, T., Miyao, M., Inoue, S., *et al.* (1999) Association study of parathyroid hormone gene polymorphism and bone mineral density in Japanese postmenopausal women. *Calcified Tissue International* **64**, 205–208.

Houle, S., Landry, M., Audet, R., Bouthillier, J., Bachvarov, D.R. & Marceau, F. (2000) Effect of allelic polymorphism of the B(1) and B(2) receptor genes on the contractile responses of the human umbilical vein to kinins. *Journal of Pharmacology and Experimental Therapeutics* **294**, 45–51.

Houle-Leroy, P., Garland, T. Jr., Swallow, J.G. & Guderley, H. (2000) Effects of voluntary activity and genetic selection on muscle metabolic capacities in house mice Mus domesticus. *Journal of Applied Physiology* **89**, 1608–1616.

Huizenga, N.A., Koper, J.W., De Lange, P., *et al.* (1998) A polymorphism in the glucocorticoid receptor gene may be associated with and increased sensitivity to glucocorticoids *in vivo*. *Journal of Clinical Endocrinology and Metabolism* **83**, 144–151.

Ioannidis, J.P., Stavrou, I., Trikalinos, T.A., *et al.* (2002) Association of polymorphisms of the estrogen receptor alpha gene with bone mineral density and fracture risk in women: a meta-analysis. *Journal of Bone and Mineral Research* **17**, 2048–2060.

Issemann, I. & Green, S. (1990) Activation of a member of the steroid hormone receptor superfamily by peroxisome proliferators. *Nature* **347**, 645–650.

James, L., Onambele, G., Woledge, R., *et al.* (2004) IL-6-174G/C genotype is associated with the bone mineral density response to oestrogen replacement therapy in post-menopausal women. *European Journal of Applied Physiology and Occupational Physiology* **92**, 227–230.

Jamshidi, Y., Montgomery, H.E., Hense, H.W., *et al.* (2002) Peroxisome proliferator-activated receptor alpha gene regulates left ventricular growth in response to exercise and hypertension. *Circulation* **105**, 950–955.

Janssen, J.A., van der Lely, A.J. & Lamberts, S.W. (2003) Circulating free insulin-like growth-factor 1 (IGF-1) levels should also be measured to estimate the IGF-1 bioactivity. *Journal of Endocrinological Investigation* **26**, 588–594.

Jarvinen, T.A., Jozsa, L., Kannus, P., Jarvinen, T.L. & Jarvinen, M. (2002) Organization and distribution of intramuscular connective tissue in normal and immobilized skeletal muscles. An immunohistochemical, polarization and scanning electron microscopic study. *Journal of Muscle Research and Cell Motility* **23**, 245–254.

Jones, A. & Woods, D.R. (2003) Skeletal muscle RAS and exercise performance. *International Journal of Biochemistry and Cell Biology* **35**, 855–866.

Jones, B.H., Thacker, S.B., Gilchrist, J., Kimsey, C.D. Jr. & Sosin, D.M. (2002) Prevention of lower extremity stress fractures in athletes and soldiers: a systematic review. *Epidemiologic Reviews* **24**, 228–247.

Jonsson, J.R., Game, P.A., Head, R.J. & Frewin, D.B. (1994) The expression and localisation of the angiotensin-converting enzyme mRNA in human adipose tissue. *Blood Press* **3**, 72–75.

Jordan, B.D. (2000) Chronic traumatic brain injury associated with boxing. *Seminars in Neurology* **20**, 179–185.

Jordan, B.D., Relkin, N.R., Ravdin, L.D., Jacobs, A.R., Bennett, A. & Gandy, S. (1997) Apolipoprotein E ε4 associated with chronic traumatic brain injury in boxing. *Journal of the American Medical Association* **278**, 136–140.

Kambadur, R., Sharma, M., Smith T.P. & Bass, J.J. (1997) Mutations in myostatin (GDF8) in double-muscled Belgian Blue and Piedmontese cattle. *Genome Research* **7**, 910–916.

Kanakis, C. & Hickson, R.C. (1980) Left ventricular responses to a program of lower-limb strength training. *Chest* **78**, 618–621.

Karjalainen, J., Kujala, U.M., Stolt, A., *et al.* (1999) Angiotensinogen gene M235T polymorphism predicts left ventricular hypertrophy in endurance athletes. *Journal of the American College of Cardiology* **34**, 494–499.

Karvonen, J., Kauma, H., Kervinen, K., *et al.* (2002) Endothelial nitric oxide synthase gene Glu298Asp polymorphism and blood pressure, left ventricular mass and carotid artery atherosclerosis in a population-based cohort. *Journal of Internal Medicine* **251**, 102–110.

Kasikcioglu, E., Kayserilioglu, A., Ciloglu, F., *et al.* (2004) Angiotensin-converting enzyme gene polymorphism, left ventricular remodeling, and exercise capacity in strength-trained athletes. *Heart and Vessels* **19**, 287–293.

Kay, M.A., Manno, C.S., Ragni, M.V., *et al.* (2000) Evidence for gene transfer and expression of factor IX in haemophilia B patients treated with an AAV vector. *Nature Genetics* **24**, 257–261.

Keen, R.W., Woodford-Richens, K.L., Lanchbury, J.S. & Spector, T.D. (1998) Allelic variation at the interleukin-1 receptor antagonist gene is associated with early postmenopausal bone loss at the spine. *Bone* **23**, 367–371.

Kelly, D.P. & Strauss, A.W. (1994) Inherited cardiomyopathies. *New England Journal of Medicine* **330**, 913–919.

Kem, D.C. & Brown, R.D. (1990) Renin: from beginning to end. *New England Journal of Medicine* **323**, 1136–1137.

Kiel, D.P., Myers, R.H., Cupples, L.A., *et al.* (1997) The BsmI vitamin D receptor restriction fragment length polymorphism (bb) influences the effect of calcium intake on bone mineral density. *Journal of Bone and Mineral Research* **12**, 1049–1057.

Klein, R.F., Mitchell, S.R., Phillips, T.J., Belknap, J.K. & Orwoll, E.S. (1998) Quantitative trait loci affecting peak bone mineral density in mice. *Journal of Bone and Mineral Research* **13**, 1648–1656.

Klissouras, V. (1971) Heritability of adaptive variation. *Journal of Applied Physiology* **31**, 338–344.

Kobayashi, S., Inoue, S., Hosoi, T., Ouchi, Y., Shiraki, M. & Orimo, H. (1996) Association of bone mineral density with polymorphism of the estrogen receptor gene. *Journal of Bone and Mineral Research* **11**, 306–311.

Koch, L.G. & Britton, S.L. (2001) Artificial selection for intrinsic aerobic endurance running capacity in rats. *Physiology Genomics* **5**, 45–52.

Koller, D.L., Rodriguez, L.A., Christian, J.C., *et al.* (1998) Linkage of a QTL contributing to normal variation in bone mineral density to chromosome 11q12-13. *Journal of Bone and Mineral Research* **13**, 1903–1908.

Koren, M.J., Devereux, R.B., Casale, P.N., Savage, D.D. & Laragh, J.H. (1991) Relation of left ventricular mass and geometry to morbidity and mortality in uncomplicated essential hypertension. *Annals of Internal Medicine* **114**, 345–352.

Kreutz, R., Struk, B., Stock, P., Hubner, N., Ganten, D. & Lindpaintner, K. (1997) Evidence for primary genetic determination of heart rate regulation: Chromosomal mapping of a genetic locus in the rat. *Circulation* **96**, 1078–1081.

Kuznetsova, T., Staessen, J.A., Wang, J.G., *et al.* (2000) Antihypertensive treatment modulates the association between the D/I ACE gene polymorphism and left ventricular hypertrophy: a meta-analysis. *Journal of Human Hypertension* **14**, 447–454.

Lahat, H., Eldar, M., Levy-Nissenbaum, E., *et al.* (2001) Autosomal recessive catecholamine- or exercise-induced polymorphic ventricular tachycardia: Clinical features and assignment of the disease gene to chromosome 1p13-21. *Circulation* **103**, 2822–2827.

Landry, F., Bouchard, C. & Dumesnil, J. (1985) Cardiac dimension changes with endurance training. Indications of a genotype dependency. *Journal of the American Medical Association* **254**, 77–80.

Langdahl, B.L., Knudsen, J.Y., Jensen, H.K., Gregersen, N. & Eriksen, E.F. (1997) A sequence variation: 713-8delC in the transforming growth factor-beta 1 gene has higher prevalence in osteoporotic women than in normal women and is associated with very low bone mass in osteoporotic women and increased bone turnover in both osteoporotic and normal women. *Bone* **20**, 289–294.

Langdahl, B.L., Lokke, E., Carstens, M., Stenkjaer, L.L. & Eriksen, E.F. (2000) Osteoporotic fractures are associated with an 86-base pair repeat polymorphism in the interleukin-1: receptor antagonist gene but not with polymorphisms in the interleukin-1beta

gene. *Journal of Bone and Mineral Research* **15**, 402–414.

Lee, M.A., Paul, M., Bohm, M. & Ganten, D. (1992) Effects of angiotensin-converting enzyme inhibitors on tissue renin-angiotensin systems. *American Journal of Cardiology* **70**, 12C–19C.

Leenhardt, A., Lucet, V., Denjoy, I., Grau, F., Ngoc, D.D. & Coumel, P. (1995) Catecholaminergic polymorphic ventricular tachycardia in children. A 7-year follow-up of 21 patients. *Circulation* **91**, 1512–1519.

Levy, D., Garrison, R.J., Savage, D.D., Kannel, W.B. & Castelli, W.P. (1990) Prognostic implications of echocardiographically determined left ventricular mass in the Framingham Heart Study. *New England Journal of Medicine* **322**, 1561–1566.

Lievre, M., Gueret, P., Gayet, C., *et al.* (1995) Ramipril-induced regression of left ventricular hypertrophy in treated hypertensive individuals. HYCAR Study Group. *Hypertension* **25**, 92–97.

Lindpaintner, K., Lee, M., Larson, M.G., *et al.* (1996) Absence of association or genetic linkage between the angiotensin-converting-enzyme gene and left ventricular mass. *New England Journal of Medicine* **334**, 1023–1028.

Linz, W. & Scholkens, B.A. (1992) A specific B2-bradykinin receptor antagonist HOE 140 abolishes the antihypertrophic effect of ramipril. *British Journal of Pharmacology* **105**, 771–772.

Linz, W., Wiemer, G. & Scholkens, B.A. (1996) Role of kinins in the pathophysiology of myocardial ischemia. *In vitro* and *in vivo* studies. *Diabetes* **45** (Supplement 1), S51–58.

Liu, X.H., Liu, Y.J., Jiang, D.K., *et al.* (2003) No evidence for linkage and/or association of human alpha2-HS glycoprotein gene with bone mineral density variation in Chinese nuclear families. *Calcified Tissue International* **73**, 244–250.

Liu, Y., Leri, A., Li, B., *et al.* (1998) Angiotensin II stimulation *in vitro* induces hypertrophy of normal and postinfarcted ventricular myocytes. *Circulation Research* **82**, 1145–1159.

Lorentzon, M., Lorentzon, R. & Nordstrom, P. (2000) Interleukin-6 gene polymorphism is related to bone mineral density during and after puberty in healthy white males: A cross-sectional and longitudinal study. *Journal of Bone and Mineral Research* **15**, 1944–1949.

Losito, A., Kalidas, K., Santoni, S. & Jeffery, S. (2003) Association of interleukin-6 -174G/C promoter polymorphism with hypertension and left ventricular hypertrophy in dialysis patients. *Kidney International* **64**, 616–622.

Lung, C.C., Chan, E.K. & Zuraw, B.L. (1997) Analysis of an exon 1 polymorphism of the B2 bradykinin receptor gene and its transcript in normal subjects and patients with C1 inhibitor deficiency. *Journal of Allergy and Clinical Immunology* **99**, 134–146.

Ma, J., Yee, A., Brewer, H.B. Jr., Das, S. & Potter, H. (1994) Amyloid-associated proteins alpha 1-antichymotrypsin and apolipoprotein E promote assembly of Alzheimer beta-protein into filaments. *Nature* **372**, 92–94.

MacGregor, A., Snieder, H. & Spector, T.D. (2000) Genetic factors and osteoporotic fractures in elderly people. Twin data support genetic contribution to risk of fracture. *British Medical Journal* **320**, 1669–1670; author reply 1670–1671.

Maes, H.H., Beunen, G.P., Vlietinck, R.F., *et al.* (1996) Inheritance of physical fitness in 10-year-old twins and their parents. *Medicine and Science in Sports and Exercise* **28**, 1479–1491.

Mahley, R.W., Nathan, B.P., Bellosta, S. & Pitas, R.E. (1995) Apolipoprotein E: impact of cytoskeletal stability in neurons and the relationship to Alzheimer's disease. *Current Opinion in Lipidology* **6**, 86–91.

Maron, B.J., Gardin, J.M., Flack, J.M., Gidding, S.S., Kurosaki, T.T. & Bild, D.E. (1995) Prevalence of hypertrophic cardiomyopathy in a general population of young adults. Echocardiographic analysis of 4111 subjects in the CARDIA Study. Coronary Artery Risk Development in (Young) Adults. *Circulation* **92**, 785–789.

Marsh, D.R., Criswell, D.S., Hamilton, M.T. & Booth, F.W. (1997) Association of insulin-like growth factor mRNA expressions with muscle regeneration in young, adult, and old rats. *American Journal of Physiology* **273**, R353–358.

Marshall, D., Johnell, O. & Wedel, H. (1996) Meta-analysis of how well measures of bone mineral density predict occurrence of osteoporotic fractures. *British Medical Journal* **312**, 1254–1259.

Masi, L., Becherini, L., Colli, E., *et al.* (1998) Polymorphisms of the calcitonin receptor gene are associated with bone mineral density in postmenopausal Italian women. *Biochemical and*

Biophysical Research Communications **248**, 190–195.

Masinde, G.L., Li, X., Gu, W., Hamilton-Ulland, M., Mohan, S. & Baylink, D.J. (2002) Quantitative trait loci that harbor genes regulating muscle size in (MRL/MPJ × SJL/J) F(2) mice. *Functional Integrational Genomics* **2**, 120–125.

McCole, S.D., Shuldiner, A.R., Brown, M.D., *et al*. (2004) Beta2- and beta3-adrenergic receptor polymorphisms and exercise hemodynamics in postmenopausal women. *Journal of Applied Physiology* **96**, 526–530.

McGuigan, F.E., Armbrecht, G., Smith, R., Felsenberg, D., Reid, D.M. & Ralston, S.H. (2001) Prediction of osteoporotic fractures by bone densitometry and COLIA1 genotyping: a prospective, population-based study in men and women. *Osteoporosis International* **12**, 91–96.

McIlhany, M.L., Shaffer, J.W. & Hines, E.A. Jr. (1975) The heritability of blood pressure: an investigation of 200 pairs of twins using the cold pressor test. *Johns Hopkins Medical Journal* **136**, 57–64.

McKay, H.A., Bailey, D.A., Wilkinson, A.A. & Houston, C.S. (1994) Familial comparison of bone mineral density at the proximal femur and lumbar spine. *Bone and Mineral* **24**, 95–107.

McPherron, A.C., Lawler, A.M. & Lee, S.J. (1997) Regulation of skeletal muscle mass in mice by a new TGF-beta superfamily member. *Nature* **387**, 83–90.

McPherron, A.C. & Lee, S.J. (1997) Double muscling in cattle due to mutations in the myostatin gene. *Proceedings of the National Academy of Sciences of the USA* **94**, 12457–12461.

Miller, T.A., Lesniewski, L.A., Muller-Delp, J.M., Majors, A.K., Scalise, D. & Delp, M.D. (2001) Hindlimb unloading induces a collagen isoform shift in the soleus muscle of the rat. *American Journal of Physiology and Regulatory Integrational Comparative Physiology* **281**, R1710–1717.

Miyao, M., Hosoi, T., Emi, M., *et al*. (2000) Association of bone mineral density with a dinucleotide repeat polymorphism at the calcitonin (CT) locus. *Journal of Human Genetics* **45**, 346–350.

Miyao, M., Hosoi, T., Inoue, S., *et al*. (1998) Polymorphism of insulin-like growth factor I gene and bone mineral density. *Calcified Tissue International* **63**, 306–311.

Miyao, M., Morita, H., Hosoi, T., *et al*. (2000) Association of methylenetetrahydrofolate reductase (MTHFR) polymorphism with bone mineral density in postmenopausal Japanese women. *Calcified Tissue International* **66**, 190–194.

Mizuguchi, T., Furuta, I., Watanabe, Y., *et al*. (2004) LRP5, low-density-lipoprotein-receptor-related protein 5, is a determinant for bone mineral density. *Journal of Human Genetics* **49**, 80–86.

Mizunuma, H., Hosoi, T., Okano, H., *et al*. (1997) Estrogen receptor gene polymorphism and bone mineral density at the lumbar spine of pre- and postmenopausal women. *Bone* **21**, 379–383.

Montgomery, H., Clarkson, P., Barnard, M., *et al*. (1999) Angiotensin-converting-enzyme gene insertion/deletion polymorphism and response to physical training. *Lancet* **353**, 541–545.

Montgomery, H. & Dhamrait, S. (2002) ACE genotype and performance. *Journal of Applied Physiology* **92**, 1774–1775; author reply 1776–1777.

Montgomery, H.E., Clarkson, P., Dollery, C.M., *et al*. (1997) Association of angiotensin-converting enzyme gene I/D polymorphism with change in left ventricular mass in response to physical training. *Circulation* **96**, 741–747.

Montgomery, H.E., Marshall, R., Hemingway, H., *et al*. (1998) Human gene for physical performance. *Nature* **393**, 221–222.

Morrison, N.A., Qi, J.C., Tokita, A., *et al*. (1994) Prediction of bone density from vitamin D receptor alleles. *Nature* **367**, 284–287.

Moseley, I.F. (2000) The neuroimaging evidence for chronic brain damage due to boxing. *Neuroradiology* **42**, 1–8.

Murphey, L.J., Gainer, J.V., Vaughan, D.E., & Brown, N.J. (2000) Angiotensin-converting enzyme insertion/deletion polymorphism modulates the human *in vivo* metabolism of bradykinin. *Circulation* **102**, 829–832.

Myerson, S., Hemingway, H., Budget, R., Martin, J., Humphries, S. & Montgomery, H. (1999) Human angiotensin I-converting enzyme gene and endurance performance. *Journal of Applied Physiology* **87**, 1313–1316.

Myerson, S.G., Montgomery, H.E., Whittingham, M., *et al*. (2001) Left ventricular hypertrophy with exercise and ACE gene insertion/deletion polymorphism: a randomized controlled trial with losartan. *Circulation* **103**, 226–230.

Nathan, B.P., Bellosta, S., Sanan, D.A., Weisgraber, K.H., Mahley, R.W. & Pitas, R.E. (1994) Differential effects of apolipoproteins E3 and E4 on neuronal growth *in vitro*. *Science* **264**, 850–852.

Nazarov, I.B., Woods, D.R., Montgomery, H.E., *et al*. (2001) The angiotensin converting enzyme I/D polymorphism in Russian athletes. *European Journal of Human Genetics* **9**, 797–801.

Nordstrom, A., Gerdhem, P., Brandstrom, H., *et al*. (2004) Interleukin-6 promoter polymorphism is associated with bone quality assessed by calcaneus ultrasound and previous fractures in a cohort of 75-year-old women. *Osteoporosis International* **15**, 820–826.

North, K.N., Yang, N., Wattanasirichaigoon, D., Mills, M., Easteal, S. & Beggs, A.H. (1999) A common nonsense mutation results in alpha-actinin-3 deficiency in the general population. *Nature Genetics* **21**, 353–354.

Ogawa, S., Hosoi, T., Shiraki, M., *et al*. (2000) Association of estrogen receptor beta gene polymorphism with bone mineral density. *Biochemical and Biophysical Research Communications* **269**, 537–541.

Ogawa, S., Urano, T., Hosoi, T., *et al*. (1999) Association of bone mineral density with a polymorphism of the peroxisome proliferator-activated receptor gamma gene: PPARgamma expression in osteoblasts. *Biochemical and Biophysical Research Communications* **260**, 122–126.

Orr, R.M. (2001) Technology evaluation: fomivirsen, Isis Pharmaceuticals Inc/CIBA vision. *Current Opinion in Molecular Therapeutics* **3**, 288–294.

Patel, S., Woods, D.R., Macleod, N.J., *et al*. (2003) Angiotensin-converting enzyme genotype and the ventilatory response to exertional hypoxia. *European Respiratory Journal* **22**, 755–760.

Payne, J. & Montgomery, H. (2004) Genetic variation and physical performance. *World Review of Nutrition and Dietetics* **93**, 270–302.

Peeters, R.P., van den Beld, A.W., van Toor, H., *et al*. (2005) A polymorphism in type I deiodinase is associated with circulating free insulin-like growth factor I levels and body composition in humans. *Journal of Clinical Endocrinology and Metabolism* **90**, 256–263.

Peeters, R.P., van Toor, H., Klootwijk, W., *et al*. (2003) Polymorphisms in thyroid hormone pathway genes are associated with plasma TSH and iodothyronine levels in healthy subjects. *Journal of Clinical Endocrinology and Metabolism* **88**, 2880–2888.

Pepe, G. (1993) A highly polymorphic (ACT)n VNTR (variable nucleotide of tandem repeats) locus inside intron 12 of COL1A2, one of the two genes involved in dominant osteogenesis imperfecta. *Human Mutation* **2**, 300–305.

Pluijm, S.M., Dik, M.G., Jonker, C., Deeg, D.J., van Kamp, G.J. & Lips, P. (2002) Effects of gender and age on the association of apolipoprotein E epsilon 4 with bone mineral density, bone turnover and the risk of fractures in older people. *Osteoporosis International* **13**, 701–709.

Pluta, R. (2000) The role of apolipoprotein E in the deposition of beta-amyloid peptide during ischemia-reperfusion brain injury. A model of early Alzheimer's disease. *Annals of the New York Academy of Sciences* **903**, 324–334.

Pluta, R., Kida, E., Lossinsky, A.S., Golabek, A.A., Mossakowski, M.J. & Wisniewski, H.M. (1994) Complete cerebral ischemia with short-term survival in rats induced by cardiac arrest. I. Extracellular accumulation of Alzheimer's beta-amyloid protein precursor in the brain. *Brain Research* **649**, 323–328.

Pocock, N.A., Eisman, J.A., Hopper, J.L., Yeates, M.G., Sambrook, P.N. & Eberl, S. (1987) Genetic determinants of bone mass in adults: A twin study. *Journal of Clinical Investigation* **80**, 706–710.

Poirier, J. (1994) Apolipoprotein E in animal models of CNS injury and in Alzheimer's disease. *Trends in Neurosciences* **17**, 525–530.

Priori, S.G., Napolitano, C., Gasparini, M., et al. (2002) Natural history of Brugada syndrome: Insights for risk stratification and management. *Circulation* **105**, 1342–1347.

Priori, S.G., Napolitano, C., Tiso, N., et al. (2001) Mutations in the cardiac ryanodine receptor gene (hRyR2) underlie catecholaminergic polymorphic ventricular tachycardia. *Circulation* **103**, 196–200.

Priori, S.G., Napolitano, C. & Vicentini, A. (2003) Inherited arrhythmia syndromes: Applying the molecular biology and genetic to the clinical management. *Journal of Interventional Cardiac Electrophysiology* **9**, 93–101.

Quinn, L.S., Haugk, K.L. & Damon, S.E. (1997) Interleukin-15 stimulates C2 skeletal myoblast differentiation. *Biochemical and Biophysical Research Communications* **239**, 6–10.

Quinn, L.S., Haugk, K.L. & Grabstein, K.H. (1995) Interleukin-15: A novel anabolic cytokine for skeletal muscle. *Endocrinology* **136**, 3669–3672.

Ralston, S.H. (2002) Genetic control of susceptibility to osteoporosis. *Journal of Clinical Endocrinology and Metabolism* **87**, 2460–2466.

Rankinen, T., Perusse, L., Borecki, I., et al. (2000a) The Na$^+$-K$^+$-ATPase alpha2 gene and trainability of cardiorespiratory endurance: The HERITAGE family study. *Journal of Applied Physiology* **88**, 346–351.

Rankinen, T., Wolfarth, B., Simoneau, J.A., et al. (2000b) No association between the angiotensin-converting enzyme ID polymorphism and elite endurance athlete status. *Journal of Applied Physiology* **88**, 1571–1575.

Rhee, E.J., Oh, K.W., Lee, W.Y., et al. (2005) The effects of C161→T polymorphisms in exon 6 of peroxisome proliferator-activated receptor-gamma gene on bone mineral metabolism and serum osteoprotegerin levels in healthy middle-aged women. *American Journal of Obstetrics and Gynecology* **192**, 1087–1093.

Riechman, S.E., Balasekaran, G., Roth, S.M. & Ferrell, R.E. (2004) Association of interleukin-15 protein and interleukin-15 receptor genetic variation with resistance exercise training responses. *Journal of Applied Physiology* **97**, 2214–2219.

Rigat, B., Hubert, C., Alhenc-Gelas, F., Cambien, F., Corvol, P. & Soubrier, F. (1990) An insertion/deletion polymorphism in the angiotensin I-converting enzyme gene accounting for half the variance of serum enzyme levels. *Journal of Clinical Investigation* **86**, 1343–1346.

Riggs, B.L., Nguyen, T.V., Melton, L.J. 3rd, et al. (1995) The contribution of vitamin D receptor gene alleles to the determination of bone mineral density in normal and osteoporotic women. *Journal of Bone and Mineral Research* **10**, 991–996.

Rivera, M.A., Dionne, F.T., Simoneau, J.A., et al. (1997) Muscle-specific creatine kinase gene polymorphism and $V_{O_{2max}}$ in the HERITAGE Family Study. *Medicine and Science in Sports and Exercise* **29**, 1311–1317.

Rivera, M.A., Wolfarth, B., Dionne, F.T., et al. (1998) Three mitochondrial DNA restriction polymorphisms in elite endurance athletes and sedentary controls. *Medicine and Science in Sports and Exercise* **30**, 687–690.

Rizzoli, R., Bonjour, J.P. & Ferrari, S.L. (2001) Osteoporosis, genetics and hormones. *Journal of Molecular Endocrinology* **26**, 79–94.

Roth, S.M., Metter, E.J., Lee, M.R., Hurley, B.F. & Ferrell, R.E. (2003a) C174T polymorphism in the CNTF receptor gene is associated with fat-free mass in men and women. *Journal of Applied Physiology* **95**, 1425–1430.

Roth, S.M., Schrager, M.A., Ferrell, R.E., et al. (2001) CNTF genotype is associated with muscular strength and quality in humans across the adult age span. *Journal of Applied Physiology* **90**, 1205–1210.

Roth, S.M., Schrager, M.A., Lee, M.R., Metter, E.J., Hurley, B.F. & Ferrell, R.E. (2003b) Interleukin-6 (IL6) genotype is associated with fat-free mass in men but not women. *Journals of Gerontology Series A, Biological Sciences and Medical Sciences* **58**, B1085–1088.

Rotimi, C.N., Cooper, R.S., Cao, G., et al. (1999) Maximum-likelihood generalized heritability estimate for blood pressure in Nigerian families. *Hypertension* **33**, 874–878.

Rupert, J.L., Kidd, K.K., Norman, L.E., Monsalve, M.V., Hochachka, P.W. & Devine, D.V. (2003) Genetic polymorphisms in the renin-angiotensin system in high-altitude and low-altitude Native American populations. *Annals of Human Genetics* **67**, 17–25.

Sack, M.N., Rader, T.A., Park, S., Bastin, J., McCune, S.A. & Kelly, D.P. (1996) Fatty acid oxidation enzyme gene expression is downregulated in the failing heart. *Circulation* **94**, 2837–2842.

Sainz, J., Van Tornout, J.M., Loro, M.L., Sayre, J., Roe, T.F. & Gilsanz, V. (1997) Vitamin D-receptor gene polymorphisms and bone density in prepubertal American girls of Mexican descent. *New England Journal of Medicine* **337**, 77–82.

Salmen, T., Heikkinen, A.M., Mahonen, A., et al. (2003) Relation of aromatase gene polymorphism and hormone replacement therapy to serum estradiol levels, bone mineral density, and fracture risk in early postmenopausal women. *Annals of Medicine* **35**, 282–288.

Sanada, M., Nakagawa, H., Kodama, I., Sakasita, T. & Ohama, K. (1998) Apolipoprotein E phenotype associations with plasma lipoproteins and bone mass in postmenopausal women. *Climacteric* **1**, 188–195.

Saunders, A.M., Strittmatter, W.J., Schmechel, D., et al. (1993) Association of apolipoprotein E allele epsilon 4 with late-onset familial and sporadic Alzheimer's disease. *Neurology* **43**, 1467–1472.

Sayer, A.A., Syddall, H., O'Dell, S.D., *et al.* (2002) Polymorphism of the IGF2 gene, birth weight and grip strength in adult men. *Age and Ageing* **31**, 468–470.

Schlager, G. (1965) Heritability of blood pressure in mice. *Journal of Heredity* **56**, 278–284.

Schmieder, R.E., Martus, P. & Klingbeil, A. (1996) Reversal of left ventricular hypertrophy in essential hypertension. A meta-analysis of randomized double-blind studies. *Journal of the American Medical Association* **275**, 1507–1513.

Schmieder, R.E., Schlaich, M.P., Klingbeil, A.U. & Martus, P. (1998) Update on reversal of left ventricular hypertrophy in essential hypertension (a meta-analysis of all randomized double-blind studies until December 1996). *Nephrology, Dialysis, Transplantation* **13**, 564–569.

Schrager, M.A., Roth, S.M., Ferrell, R.E., *et al.* (2004) Insulin-like growth factor-2 genotype, fat-free mass, and muscle performance across the adult life span. *Journal of Applied Physiology* **97**, 2176–2183.

Schuelke, M., Wagner, K.R., Stolz, L.E., *et al.* (2004) Myostatin mutation associated with gross muscle hypertrophy in a child. *New England Journal of Medicine* **350**, 2682–2688.

Schunkert, H., Dzau, V.J., Tang, S.S., Hirsch, A.T., Apstein, C.S. & Lorell, B.H. (1990) Increased rat cardiac angiotensin converting enzyme activity and mRNA expression in pressure overload left ventricular hypertrophy. Effects on coronary resistance, contractility, and relaxation. *Journal of Clinical Investigation* **86**, 1913–1920.

Schunkert, H., Hengstenberg, C., Holmer, S.R., *et al.* (1999) Lack of association between a polymorphism of the aldosterone synthase gene and left ventricular structure. *Circulation* **99**, 2255–2260.

Scott, W., Stevens, J. & Binder-Macleod, S.A. (2001) Human skeletal muscle fiber type classifications. *Physical Therapy* **81**, 1810–1816.

Sedlacek, K., Fischer, M., Erdmann, J., *et al.* (2002) Relation of the G protein beta3-subunit polymorphism with left ventricle structure and function. *Hypertension* **40**, 162–167.

Seeman, E. (1994) Reduced bone density in women with fractures: Contribution of low peak bone density and rapid bone loss. *Osteoporosis International* **4** (Supplement 1), 15–25.

Seeman, E., Hopper, J.L., Young, N.R., Formica, C., Goss, P. & Tsalamandris, C. (1996) Do genetic factors explain associations between muscle strength, lean mass, and bone density? A twin study. *American Journal of Physiology* **270**, E320–327.

Seeman, E., Tsalamandris, C., Formica, C., Hopper, J.L. & McKay, J. (1994) Reduced femoral neck bone density in the daughters of women with hip fractures: the role of low peak bone density in the pathogenesis of osteoporosis. *Journal of Bone and Mineral Research* **9**, 739–743.

Seibert, M.J., Xue, Q.L., Fried, L.P. & Walston, J.D. (2001) Polymorphic variation in the human myostatin (GDF-8) gene and association with strength measures in the Women's Health and Aging Study II cohort. *Journal of the American Geriatrics Society* **49**, 1093–1096.

Semplicini, A., Siffert, W., Sartori, M., *et al.* (2001) G protein beta3 subunit gene 825T allele is associated with increased left ventricular mass in young subjects with mild hypertension. *American Journal of Hypertension* **14**, 1191–1195.

Shapiro, L.E., Samuels, H.H. & Yaffe, B.M. (1978) Thyroid and glucocorticoid hormones synergistically control growth hormone mRNA in cultured GH1 cells. *Proceedings of the National Academy of Sciences of the USA* **75**, 45–49.

Shearman, A.M., Karasik, D., Gruenthal, K.M., *et al.* (2004) Estrogen receptor beta polymorphisms are associated with bone mass in women and men: The Framingham Study. *Journal of Bone and Mineral Research* **19**, 773–781.

Shenoy, U. & Cassis, L. (1997) Characterization of renin activity in brown adipose tissue. *American Journal of Physiology* **272**, C989–999.

Shiraki, M., Shiraki, Y., Aoki, C., *et al.* (1997) Association of bone mineral density with apolipoprotein E phenotype. *Journal of Bone and Mineral Research* **12**, 1438–1445.

Shliakhto, E.V., Shwarts, E.I., Sokolova, L.A., *et al.* (2003) [Association of a polymorphic marker C825T of the beta(3) subunit of G-protein with myocardial hypertrophy in patients with hypertensive disease]. *Kardiologiia* **43**, 44–46.

Siegel, S.G., Patton, B. & English, A.W. (2000) Ciliary neurotrophic factor is required for motoneuron sprouting. *Experimental Neurology* **166**, 205–212.

Singh, J.P., Larson, M.G., O'Donnell, C.J., Tsuji, H., Evans, J.C. & Levy, D. (1999) Heritability of heart rate variability: The Framingham Heart Study. *Circulation* **99**, 2251–2254.

Smith, D.M., Nance, W.E., Kang, K.W., Christian, J.C. & Johnston, C.C. Jr. (1973) Genetic factors in determining bone mass. *Journal of Clinical Investigation* **52**, 2800–2808.

Sonna, L.A., Sharp, M.A., Knapik, J.J., *et al.* (2001) Angiotensin-converting enzyme genotype and physical performance during US Army basic training. *Journal of Applied Physiology* **91**, 1355–1363.

Sowers, M., Willing, M., Burns, T., *et al.* (1999) Genetic markers, bone mineral density, and serum osteocalcin levels. *Journal of Bone and Mineral Research* **14**, 1411–1419.

Splawski, I., Shen, J., Timothy, K.W., *et al.* (2000) Spectrum of mutations in long-QT syndrome genes. KVLQT1, HERG, SCN5A, KCNE1, and KCNE2. *Circulation* **102**, 1178–1185.

Splawski, I., Tristani-Firouzi, M., Lehmann, M.H., Sanguinetti, M.C. & Keating, M.T. (1997) Mutations in the hminK gene cause long QT syndrome and suppress IKs function. *Nature Genetics* **17**, 338–340.

Staessen, J.A., Wang, J.G., Ginocchio, G., *et al.* (1997) The deletion/insertion polymorphism of the angiotensin converting enzyme gene and cardiovascular-renal risk. *Journal of Hypertension* **15**, 1579–1592.

Strittmatter, W.J., Saunders, A.M., Goedert, M., *et al.* (1994) Isoform-specific interactions of apolipoprotein E with microtubule-associated protein tau: implications for Alzheimer disease. *Proceedings of the National Academy of Sciences of the USA* **91**, 11183–11186.

Swan, L., Birnie, D.H., Padmanabhan, S., Inglis, G., Connell, J.M. & Hillis, W.S. (2003) The genetic determination of left ventricular mass in healthy adults. *European Heart Journal* **24**, 577–582.

Sweeney, H.L. (2004) Gene doping. *Scientific American* **291**, 62–69.

Szabo, G., Dallmann, G., Muller, G., Patthy, L., Soller, M. & Varga, L. (1998) A deletion in the myostatin gene causes the compact (Cmpt) hypermuscular mutation in mice. *Mammalian Genome* **9**, 671–672.

Taboulet, J., Frenkian, M., Frendo, J.L., Feingold, N., Jullienne, A. & de Vernejoul, M.C. (1998) Calcitonin receptor polymorphism is associated with a decreased fracture risk in postmenopausal women. *Human Molecular Genetics* **7**, 2129–2133.

Taguchi, T., Kishikawa, H., Motoshima, H., *et al.* (2000) Involvement of bradykinin in acute exercise-induced increase of glucose uptake and GLUT-4 translocation in skeletal muscle: Studies in normal and diabetic humans and rats. *Metabolism* **49**, 920–930.

Takala, T.E. & Virtanen, P. (2000) Biochemical composition of muscle extracellular matrix: The effect of loading. *Scandinavian Journal of Medicine and Science in Sports* **10**, 321–325.

Taylor, R.R., Mamotte, C.D., Fallon, K. & van Bockxmeer, F.M. (1999) Elite athletes and the gene for angiotensin-converting enzyme. *Journal of Applied Physiology* **87**, 1035–1037.

Teasdale, G.M., Nicoll, J.A., Murray, G. & Fiddes, M. (1997) Association of apolipoprotein E polymorphism with outcome after head injury. *Lancet* **350**, 1069–1071.

Thakkinstian, A., D'Este, C., Eisman, J., Nguyen, T. & Attia, J. (2004) Meta-analysis of molecular association studies: Vitamin D receptor gene polymorphisms and BMD as a case study. *Journal of Bone and Mineral Research* **19**, 419–428.

Tiainen, K., Sipila, S., Alen, M., *et al.* (2004) Heritability of maximal isometric muscle strength in older female twins. *Journal of Applied Physiology* **96**, 173–180.

Timmermans, P.B. & Smith, R.D. (1994) Angiotensin II receptor subtypes: Selective antagonists and functional correlates. *European Heart Journal* **15** (Supplement D), 79–87.

Torgerson, D.J., Campbell, M.K., Thomas, R.E. & Reid, D.M. (1996) Prediction of perimenopausal fractures by bone mineral density and other risk factors. *Journal of Bone and Mineral Research* **11**, 293–297.

Tremaine, W.J., Newcomer, A.D., Riggs, B.L. & McGill, D.B. (1986) Calcium absorption from milk in lactase-deficient and lactase-sufficient adults. *Digestion Disease and Sciences* **31**, 376–378.

Tsianos, G., Eleftheriou, K.I., Hawe, E., *et al.* (2005) Performance at altitude and angiotensin I-converting enzyme genotype. *European Journal of Applied Physiology and Occupational Physiology* **93**, 630–633.

Tsianos, G., Sanders, J., Dhamrait, S., Humphries, S., Grant, S. & Montgomery, H. (2004) The ACE gene insertion/deletion polymorphism and elite endurance swimming. *European Journal of Applied Physiology and Occupational Physiology* **92**, 360–362.

Tsujinaka, T., Fujita, J., Ebisui, C., *et al.* (1996) Interleukin 6 receptor antibody inhibits muscle atrophy and modulates proteolytic systems in interleukin 6 transgenic mice. *Journal of Clinical Investigation* **97**, 244–249.

Uitterlinden, A.G., Burger, H., Huang, Q., *et al.* (1998). Relation of alleles of the collagen type I alpha1 gene to bone density and the risk of osteoporotic fractures in postmenopausal women. *New England Journal of Medicine* **338**, 1016–1021.

Urano, T., Shiraki, M., Ezura, Y., *et al.* (2004) Association of a single-nucleotide polymorphism in low-density lipoprotein receptor-related protein 5 gene with bone mineral density. *Journal of Bone and Mineral Metabolism* **22**, 341–345.

Vakili, B.A., Okin, P.M. & Devereux, R.B. (2001) Prognostic implications of left ventricular hypertrophy. *American Heart Journal* **141**, 334–341.

Valimaki, V.V., Alfthan, H., Lehmuskallio, E., *et al.* (2005) Risk factors for clinical stress fractures in male military recruits: A prospective cohort study. *Bone* **37**, 267–273.

Van Pottelbergh, I., Goemaere, S. & Kaufman, J.M. (2003) Bioavailable estradiol and an aromatase gene polymorphism are determinants of bone mineral density changes in men over 70 years of age. *Journal of Clinical Endocrinology and Metabolism* **88**, 3075–3081.

Van Pottelbergh, I., Goemaere, S., Nuytinck, L., De Paepe, A. & Kaufman, J.M. (2001) Association of the type I collagen alpha1 Sp1 polymorphism, bone density and upper limb muscle strength in community-dwelling elderly men. *Osteoporosis International* **12**, 895–901.

van Rossum, E.F., Koper, J.W., Huizenga, N.A., *et al.* (2002) A polymorphism in the glucocorticoid receptor gene, which decreases sensitivity to glucocorticoids *in vivo*, is associated with low insulin and cholesterol levels. *Diabetes* **51**, 3128–3134.

van Rossum, E.F., Voorhoeve, P.G., te Velde, S.J., *et al.* (2004) The ER22/23EK polymorphism in the glucocorticoid receptor gene is associated with a beneficial body composition and muscle strength in young adults. *Journal of Clinical Endocrinology and Metabolism* **89**, 4004–4009.

Vergara, C. & Ramirez, B. (2004) CNTF, a pleiotropic cytokine: Emphasis on its myotrophic role. Brain Research. *Brain Research Reviews* **47**, 161–173.

Verhaaren, H.A., Schieken, R.M., Mosteller, M., Hewitt, J.K., Eaves, L.J. & Nance, W.E. (1991) Bivariate genetic analysis of left ventricular mass and weight in pubertal twins (the Medical College of Virginia twin study). *American Journal of Cardiology* **68**, 661–668.

Visser, M., Pahor, M., Taaffe, D.R., *et al.* (2002) Relationship of interleukin-6 and tumor necrosis factor-alpha with muscle mass and muscle strength in elderly men and women: the Health ABC Study. *Journals of Gerontology. Series A, Biological Sciences and Medical Sciences* **57**, M326–332.

World Anti-Doping Agency (WADA) (2003) *The World Anti-Doping Code: International Standard for Testing.* Version 3.0, 1–41.

WADA (2005) *Gene Doping. Play True* **1**, 1–24.

Wang, A.Y., Chan, J.C., Wang, M., *et al.* (2003) Cardiac hypertrophy and remodeling in relation to ACE and angiotensinogen genes genotypes in Chinese dialysis patients. *Kidney International* **63**, 1899–1907.

Wang, Q., Curran, M.E., Splawski, I., *et al.* (1996) Positional cloning of a novel potassium channel gene: KVLQT1 mutations cause cardiac arrhythmias. *Nature Genetics* **12**, 17–23.

Wang, Q., Shen, J., Splawski, I., *et al.* (1995) SCN5A mutations associated with an inherited cardiac arrhythmia, long QT syndrome. *Cell* **80**, 805–811.

Wang, Z.Q., Ouyang, Z., Wang, D.M. & Tang, X.L. (1990) Heritability of blood pressure in 7- to 12-year-old Chinese twins, with special reference to body size effects. *Genetic Epidemiology* **7**, 447–452.

Watanabe, K., Fujii, H., Takahashi, T., *et al.* (2000) Constitutive regulation of cardiac fatty acid metabolism through peroxisome proliferator-activated receptor alpha associated with age-dependent cardiac toxicity. *Journal of Biological Chemistry* **275**, 22293–22299.

Weiss, R.E. & Refetoff, S. (1996) Effect of thyroid hormone on growth. Lessons from the syndrome of resistance to thyroid hormone. *Endocrinology and Metabolism Clinics of North America* **25**, 719–730.

Wicklmayr, M., Dietze, G., Gunther, B., *et al.* (1980) The kallikrein–kinin system and muscle metabolism: clinical aspects. *Agents and Actions* **10**, 339–343.

Wieling, W., Borghols, E.A., Hollander, A.P., Danner, S.A. & Dunning, A.J. (1981) Echocardiographic dimensions and maximal oxygen uptake in oarsmen during training. *British Heart Journal* **46**, 190–195.

Williams, A.G., Dhamrait, S.S., Wootton, P.T., *et al.* (2004) Bradykinin receptor gene variant and human physical performance. *Journal of Applied Physiology* **96**, 938–942.

Williams, A.G., Rayson, M.P., Jubb, M., *et al.* (2000) The ACE gene and muscle performance. *Nature* **403**, 614.

Willing, M., Sowers, M., Aron, D., *et al.* (1998) Bone mineral density and its change in white women: Estrogen and vitamin D receptor genotypes and their interaction. *Journal of Bone and Mineral Research* **13**, 695–705.

Winnicki, M., Somers, V.K., Accurso, V., *et al.* (2002) α-Adducin Gly460Trp polymorphism, left ventricular mass and plasma renin activity. *Journal of Hypertension* **20**, 1771–1777.

Wollert, K.C. & Drexler, H. (1999) The renin-angiotensin system and experimental heart failure. *Cardiovascular Research* **43**, 838–849.

Woods, D., Onambele, G., Woledge, R., *et al.* (2001) Angiotensin-I converting enzyme genotype-dependent benefit from hormone replacement therapy in isometric muscle strength and bone mineral density. *Journal of Clinical Endocrinology and Metabolism* **86**, 2200–2204.

Woods, D.R., Humphries, S.E. & Montgomery, H.E. (2000) The ACE I/D polymorphism and human physical performance. *Trends in Endocrinology and Metabolism* **11**, 416–420.

Woods, D.R., Pollard, A.J., Collier, D.J., *et al.* (2002a) Insertion/deletion polymorphism of the angiotensin I-converting enzyme gene and arterial oxygen saturation at high altitude. *American Journal of Respiratory and Critical Care Medicine* **166**, 362–366.

Woods, D.R., World, M., Rayson, M.P., *et al.* (2002b) Endurance enhancement related to the human angiotensin I-converting enzyme I-D polymorphism is not due to differences in the cardiorespiratory response to training. *European Journal of Applied Physiology and Occupational Physiology* **86**, 240–244.

Wu, S., Hong, J., Li, H., *et al.* (2000) No correlation of polymorphism of angiotensin-converting enzyme genes with left ventricular hypertrophy in essential hypertension. *Hypertension Research* **23**, 261–264.

Yamada, Y., Ando, F., Niino, N. & Shimokata, H. (2003a) Association of polymorphisms of interleukin-6, osteocalcin, and vitamin D receptor genes, alone or in combination, with bone mineral density in community-dwelling Japanese women and men. *Journal of Clinical Endocrinology and Metabolism* **88**, 3372–3378.

Yamada, Y., Ando, F., Niino, N. & Shimokata, H. (2003b) Association of polymorphisms of the osteoprotegerin gene with bone mineral density in Japanese women but not men. *Molecular Genetics and Metabolism* **80**, 344–349.

Yamada, Y., Ando, F. & Shimokata, H. (2005) Association of polymorphisms in CYP17A1, MTP, and VLDLR with bone mineral density in community-dwelling Japanese women and men. *Genomics* **86**, 76–85.

Yamada, Y., Miyauchi, A., Goto, J., *et al.* (1998) Association of a polymorphism of the transforming growth factor-beta1 gene with genetic susceptibility to osteoporosis in postmenopausal Japanese women. *Journal of Bone and Mineral Research* **13**, 1569–1576.

Yang, N., MacArthur, D.G., Gulbin, J.P., *et al.* (2003) ACTN3 genotype is associated with human elite athletic performance. *American Journal of Human Genetics* **73**, 627–631.

Yildiz, A., Akkaya, V., Hatemi, A.C., *et al.* (2000) No association between deletion-type angiotensin-converting enzyme gene polymorphism and left-ventricular hypertrophy in hemodialysis patients. *Nephron* **84**, 130–135.

Yoneya, K., Okamoto, H., Machida, M., *et al.* (1995) Angiotensin-converting enzyme gene polymorphism in Japanese patients with hypertrophic cardiomyopathy. *American Heart Journal* **130**, 1089–1093.

Young, L.E., Rogers. K. & Wood, J.L. (2005) Left ventricular size and systolic function in thoroughbred racehorses and their relationships to race performance. *Journal of Applied Physiology* **99**, 1278–1285.

Zeldis, S.M., Morganroth, J. & Rubler, S. (1978) Cardiac hypertrophy in response to dynamic conditioning in female athletes. *Journal of Applied Physiology* **44**, 849–852.

Zhao, H.Y., Liu, J.M., Ning, G., *et al.* (2003) [Association of calcitonin receptor gene polymorphism with bone mineral density in Shanghai women.] *Zhongguo Yi Xue Ke Xue Yuan Xue Bao* **25**, 258–261.

Zhou, S., Murphy, J.E., Escobedo, J.A. & Dwarki, V.J. (1998) Adeno-associated virus-mediated delivery of erythropoietin leads to sustained elevation of hematocrit in nonhuman primates. *Gene Therapy* **5**, 665–670.

Chapter 20

Sports Nutrition: Practical Guidelines for the Sports Physician

LOUISE M. BURKE

The science of sports nutrition has become so sophisticated that specific eating strategies can be developed to suit each sport and, perhaps, even each event or type of workout undertaken by the athlete. Although the specific nutritional goals and needs of each athlete are unique, there are some common themes that arise across and within sports. The aim of this chapter is to provide an overview of common nutritional issues as they typically present to a sports physician. The chapter covers the background to these issues, strategies for the prevention or management of common nutrition-related problems, and guidelines for optimal nutrition practice by athletes. Finally, the role of the sports physician in identifying and managing nutrition problems, and the interplay with a multidisciplinary team including a sports dietitian, are also discussed.

Issue 1: How can I lose or gain weight to reach an ideal level for performance?

The stereotype of an athlete is of a lean and well-muscled physique. Indeed, in a number of sports, these characteristics have a direct role in performance. For example, a high level of muscularity is favorable for activities based on strength and power. Low body mass and low levels of body fat are of value in sports where an athlete must move their body over a distance (e.g., distance running),

against gravity (e.g., road cycling on a hilly course), or in a small space (e.g., gymnastics or diving). In other sports, athletes compete in weight divisions (e.g., boxing, lightweight rowing, wrestling) or are judged on the aesthetics of their physique (e.g., bodybuilding, gymnastics). Some high-level athletes "naturally" display the physique characteristics that are required for their sport – as a result of the genetic traits that have caused them to gravitate to this activity as well as the conditioning effects of serious training. By contrast, other athletes have to undertake specific programs to manipulate their body mass, muscle mass, and body fat levels. In fact, weight loss is the most popular reason for an athlete to consult a sports dietitian.

Many athletes pursue rigid criteria for the "ideal physique" for their sport, based on the characteristics of successful competitors or, in the case of sports favoring leanness, the attainment of minimum levels of body fat. The pressure to conform to such an ideal comes from coaches, trainers, other athletes, as well as the athlete's own perfectionism and drive to succeed. However, there are several dangers and disadvantages to the establishment of rigid prescriptions for the body weight or body fat levels of individual athletes. It fails to acknowledge that there is considerable variability in the physical characteristics of successful athletes, even between individuals in the same sport. It also fails to take into account that it can take many years of training and maturation for an athlete to achieve their ideal shape and body composition. There are problems when changes in body mass or crude measures of body composition are assumed to be markers of

The Olympic Textbook of Medicine in Sport, 1st edition. Edited by M. Schwellnus. Published 2008 by Blackwell Publishing, ISBN: 978-1-4051-5637-0.

fatness and muscle mass. Unfortunately, many athletes and coaches rely on such crude markers.

There are a number of reliable and valid techniques for the assessment of body fat levels or lean body mass. These range from techniques that are best suited to the laboratory (e.g., hydrodensitometry and dual-energy X-ray absorptiometry [DEXA] scans) to protocols that can be undertaken in the field. In practice, useful information about body composition can be collected from anthropometric data such as measurements of skinfold (subcutaneous) fat, body girths, and circumferences (Kerr 2006). Sports scientists who undertake these assessments on athletes should be appropriately trained to minimize their measurement error and to understand the limitations of their assessments. These techniques can then be used to set a range of acceptable values for body fat and body weight within each sport, and to monitor the health and performance of individual athletes within this range. Longitudinal profiling of an athlete can monitor the development of physical characteristics that are associated with good performance for that individual, as well as identify the changes in physique that can be expected over a season or period of specialized training.

There are situations when an athlete is clearly carrying excess body fat and will improve their health and performance by reducing body fat levels. This may occur because of heredity or lifestyle factors, or because the athlete has been exposed to a sudden change in energy expenditure without a compensatory change in energy intake (e.g., failing to reduce energy intake while injured or during the off-season). Loss of body fat should be achieved through a program of eating and exercise that achieves a sustained and moderate energy deficit, but still allows the athlete to meet their nutritional needs and to enjoy some of the pleasure and social opportunities that food normally provides. Guidelines for such a plan are summarized in Table 20.1.

In many "weight-sensitive" sports, athletes often strive to reduce their body mass and body fat to below levels that seem "healthy" or to achieve these losses in a rapid manner. In the short term, a sudden improvement in the body's "power : weight" ratio may produce an improvement in performance. However, long-term disadvantages arise from the effects of excessive training, chronically low intakes of energy and nutrients, and psychologic distress. These are likely to include illness, injury, reduced well-being, and impaired performance. Additional problems have been noted in "weight-making" sports in which athletes undertake rapid weight loss in the days before competition in order to make their event "weight target." According to surveys of athletes in weight category sports (Steen & Brownell 1990; Moore et al. 2002; Oppliger et al. 2003), strategies used to achieve this weight loss may include fasting, techniques causing dehydration (diuretics, saunas, or exercising in a hot environment), and purging (vomiting, laxatives). Various efforts by sports physicians and sports scientists to educate athletes and change the conditions under which they compete appear to have attenuated but not eliminated such unsafe weight loss practices (Oppliger et al. 1998). In extreme cases, athletes have died as a result of their "weight making" pursuits; in particular, undertaking prolonged and intense training sessions while dehydrated, and following severe energy restriction (Centers for Disease Control and Prevention 1998).

It is important that successful weight control for an individual athlete considers measures of long-term health and performance. Some individuals are naturally light and have low levels of body fat, or can achieve these without paying a substantial penalty. Furthermore, some athletes vary their body fat levels over a season so that very low levels are achieved only for a specific and short time. In general, however, athletes should not undertake strategies to minimize body fat levels unless they can be sure there are no side-effects or disadvantages. Although it is difficult to obtain reliable statistics on the prevalence of eating disorders or disordered eating behavior and body image among athletes, there appears to be a higher risk of problems among female athletes, and among athletes in sports in which success is associated with specific weight targets or low body fat levels (Beals & Manore 1994; Sundgot-Borgen 2000). Even where clinical eating disorders do not exist, many athletes appear to be "restrained eaters," reporting energy intakes that are considerably less than expected

Table 20.1 Guidelines for manipulating energy intake for weight loss and weight gain in athletes. After Burke (2001).

General ideas for weight loss

- Targets for ideal body mass (BM) and body fat should be set on an individual basis. It is often useful to consider an ideal range of BM and body fat that the athlete may achieve at various times of the training and competitive season. Where fat loss is required, this should be achieved gradually and in conjunction with an appropriate exercise program
- Fat loss should be achieved via a moderate energy deficit (e.g., 2–4 MJ or 500–1000 kcal·day^{-1}) achieved by manipulating diet and/or exercise. Excessive restriction of energy intake should be avoided such that energy availability (total intake minus the energy cost of training) is below 30 kcal^{-1}·kg body mass^{-1} (126 kJ·kg^{-1} body mass)
- Although reduced energy intake may reduce total intake of protein and carbohydrate, the athlete should consume these nutrients at strategic times such as immediately after key training sessions. This may be achieved by altering the timetable of meals in relation to training
- There is no evidence to support the long-term success of currently fashionable weight loss diets such as low-carbohydrate, high-protein programs, or the Zone (40:30:30) diet. These diets are nutritionally unbalanced, and inconsistent with guidelines that are scientifically supported to optimize athletic performance
- The athlete should consume a wide variety of nutrient-dense foods, to meet protein and micronutrient requirements from a reduced energy intake. Micronutrient supplementation should be considered where restricted energy intake is a long-term issue
- Meals/snacks should be planned to avoid long periods without food intake and to promote post-exercise recovery
- A high volume of food intake can be achieved by making use of high-fiber, low energy-density foods, such as fruits and vegetables. Carbohydrate-rich foods with a low glycemic index and protein–carbohydrate food matches also help to promote satiety of meals and snacks
- Energy-rich fluids and energy-dense foods should not be consumed in excessive amounts
- A food diary may help to identify the athlete's *actual* intake rather than perceived intake, and note the occasions or situations in which the athlete is unable to adhere to their plan
- Behavior modification can overcome inappropriate eating practices such as eating for comfort or to relieve stress and boredom
- Athletes should seek professional advice from a sports dietitian, especially where nutritional goals are complex, or where previous dieting behaviors have already caused food-related stress

General ideas for eating to support a gain in muscle mass

- The athlete should aim for a pattern of small, frequent meals each day to achieve an adequate energy intake and promote recovery/adaptation to resistance training and other key training sessions
- A snack providing carbohydrate and protein will enhance recovery after key training sessions, as well as contribute to total daily energy intake. Such a snack should also be consumed prior to resistance training sessions. Examples of foods combining these nutrients are provided in Table 20.5
- Carbohydrate should be consumed during prolonged exercise to provide additional fuel as well as contribute to total daily energy intake
- A food diary may help to identify the athlete's *actual* intake rather than perceived intake, and note the occasions or situations in which the athlete is unable to adhere to their plan of frequent meals and snacks
- The athlete is often faced with a chaotic and over-committed lifestyle. Good skills in time management should see the athlete using quieter periods to undertake food shopping and meal preparation activities so that food is available during hectic periods
- The traveling athlete should take a supply of portable and non-perishable snacks that can be easily prepared and eaten (e.g., breakfast cereal and powdered milk, cereal bars, sports bars, liquid meal supplements, dried fruit/nuts and creamed rice)
- Specialized products, such as sports drinks, sports gels and sports bars, provide a practical form of carbohydrate during exercise, while sports bars and liquid meal supplements provide an accessible form of carbohydrate and protein for post-exercise recovery
- Energy-containing drinks, such as liquid meal supplements, flavored milk, fruit smoothies, sports drinks, soft drinks and juices, provide a low-bulk way to consume energy and other important nutrients while meeting fluid needs
- Although fiber intake is important in a healthy diet, excessive intake of high-fiber foods may limit total energy intake or lead to gastrointestinal discomfort. It may be necessary to moderate intake of wholegrain or fiber-enriched versions of foods

energy requirements, and with considerable stress related to food intake (Beals & Manore 1994). There is considerable evidence that a low level of "energy availability," defined as total energy intake minus the energy cost of the athlete's exercise program, has serious consequences on the hormonal, immunologic, and health status of the athlete (Loucks 2004). The "female athlete triad," the coexistence of disordered or restricted eating, menstrual dysfunction, and impaired bone density, has received considerable publicity as a potential outcome of the excessive pursuit of thinness by female athletes (Otis *et al.* 1997; Loucks & Nattiv 2005). Incremental changes in "energy availability" lead to a dose-dependent relationship between energy restriction and metabolic and hormonal function (Loucks & Thuma 2003). The threshold for maintenance of normal menstrual function in females is an energy availability of above 30 kcal·kg^{-1} (125 kJ·kg^{-1}) fat-free mass (FFM) (Table 20.2). It is likely that male athletes also suffer consequences that are not as yet well described. Expert advice from sports medicine professionals, including dietitians, psychologists, and physicians, is important in the early detection and management of problems related to body composition and nutrition. The reader is referred to the excellent textbook by Beals (2004) for more information on the treatment of disordered eating in athletes.

An increase in muscle mass is desired by many athletes whose performance is linked with size, strength, or power. In addition to the increase in muscle mass and strength that occurs during adolescence, particularly in males, many athletes pursue specific muscle hypertrophy through a program of progressive muscle overload. An important nutritional requirement to support such a program is adequate energy. This is required for the manufacture of new muscle tissue, as well as to provide fuel for the training program that supplied the stimulus for this muscle growth. Many athletes do not achieve a sufficiently positive energy balance to optimize muscle gains during a strength-training program. Specialized nutrition advice can help the athlete improve this situation by making energy-dense foods and drinks accessible and easy to consume (Burke 2001). Despite the interest in gaining muscle size and strength, there is little rigorous scientific study of the amount of energy required, the optimal ratio of macronutrients supplying this energy, and the requirements for micronutrients to enhance this process.

It is tempting to hypothesize that an increase in dietary protein will stimulate muscle gain. Indeed, many strength-trained athletes consume very large amounts of protein, in excess of 2–3 g·kg body mass^{-1}·day^{-1} (2–3 times the recommended intakes for protein in most countries), in the belief that this

Table 20.2 Example of energy availability.

Athlete A

Body mass	65 kg
% Body fat	10
Fat free mass (FFM)	65 − 6.5 kg = 58.5 kg
Mean daily energy expenditure in training	1000 kcal/4200 kJ
Mean daily energy intake	3500 kcal/14,700 kJ
Energy availability	3500 − 1000 kcal = 2500 kcal/10,500 kJ = 43 kcal/kg FFM (180 kcal/kg FFM)
Interpretation	This energy intake seems reasonable for this athlete's requirements

Athlete B

Body mass	60 kg
% Body fat	10
FFM	65 − 6 kg = 59 kg
Mean daily energy expenditure in training	1000 kcal/4200 kJ
Mean daily energy intake	2500 kcal/10,500 kJ
Energy availability	2500 − 1000 kcal = 1500 kcal/6300 kJ = 25 kcal/kg FFM (107 kcal/kg FFM)
Interpretation	This energy intake is below the threshold required for optimal body function and is likely to lead to health problems

will enhance the gains from resistance training programs. However, the value of very high protein intakes in optimizing muscle gains remains unsupported by the scientific literature (Tipton & Wolfe 2004). Instead, there is recent evidence that the strategic *timing* of the intake of protein in relation to training may be the important dietary factor in enhancing gains in muscle size and strength. Specifically, consuming protein after or even before a resistance training session has been shown to substantially increase net protein balance compared with the control condition (Rasmussen *et al.* 2000; Tipton *et al.* 2001). There is inadequate information to provide specific details of amount and type of protein to achieve the optimal response in net protein balance. However, it appears that consuming a relatively modest amount of protein (a source providing ~3–6 g essential amino acids or ~20 g of a high biologic value protein) either before or after a resistance workout causes a substantial increase in net protein synthesis (Tipton *et al.* 2001; Borsheim *et al.* 2002; Miller *et al.* 2003). This enhancement is still apparent in the 24 h picture of protein balance (Tipton *et al.* 2003). There may also be some benefits to net protein balance in combining carbohydrate with these protein "recovery" snacks (Borsheim *et al.* 2004a,b). These ideas are incorporated into the guidelines in Table 20.1.

Issue 2: Why am I so tired and unable to train or perform at my best?

According to Brendan Foster, Bronze Medalist in the 10,000 m at the 1976 Olympic Games: "All top international athletes wake up in the morning feeling tired and go to bed feeling very tired." At times, however, many athletes experience an excessive and chronic level of fatigue, which impacts on their health, performance, and emotional well-being. Although illness, overtraining, and an over-committed lifestyle may be implicated in such problems, poor nutritional practices and inadequate nutritional status may also be involved. The most common nutritional causes of fatigue and inability to recovery between training sessions are inadequate carbohydrate intake or fuel depletion, and iron deficiency.

Inadequate carbohydrate intake

According to sports nutrition guidelines, an athlete's carbohydrate intake should meet the fuel requirements of training and competition and the restoration of muscle glycogen content between training sessions (Burke *et al.* 2004). Chronic depletion of muscle glycogen stores because of the failure to consume adequate carbohydrate is likely to lead to a perception of fatigue and an impaired ability to train (Costill *et al.* 1988; Achten *et al.* 2004). Table 20.3 summarizes factors underpinning inadequate carbohydrate intake, noting athletes who are at risk as a result of the presence of one or more of these factors. The muscle content of glycogen can be measured using both invasive (muscle biopsy) and non-invasive (magnetic resonance spectroscopy) techniques. Although these techniques allow the assessment of an athlete's muscle glycogen stores, they have limited value in the diagnosis of inadequate carbohydrate intake and chronic glycogen depletion in an athlete. The muscle biopsy is a medical procedure that can cause discomfort and some degree of medical risk. Both techniques involve reasonable expense, the need for specialized equipment and technical expertise; as such they are confined to the realms of research to monitor changes in muscle glycogen in response to various interventions. If used in a clinical situation they would presumably be able to provide a single "snapshot" of an athlete's glycogen stores which may have little relevance to daily training situations.

A diagnosis of inadequate carbohydrate intake must be made from several pieces of information which together provide support for this diagnosis. An assessment of the training and competition program and the estimated energy and fuel cost of this activity should be undertaken. The usual dietary patterns of the athlete should also be investigated to estimate energy intake, total carbohydrate intake, and the strategic intake of carbohydrate in relation to training and competition (i.e., before, during, and after sessions). Finally, feedback from performance in training and competition should be considered, especially when interventions, such as changes in carbohydrate intake and changes in training, are implemented. The presence of risk

Table 20.3 Risk factors for inadequate carbohydrate intake by athletes.

Causes of inadequate intake of carbohydrate by athletes	Athletes at risk of inadequate carbohydrate intake
1 High training volume, or sudden increase in training volume or intensity, unaccompanied by adequate dietary changes	Athletes during periods of intensive training, especially two-a-day training, daily competition (tournaments, cycle tours)
2 Inadequate energy intake The inadequate energy intake reduces the "budget" available for intake of carbohydrate-rich foods. In addition, it impairs post-exercise refuelling by reducing the dietary substrates available for storage	Female athletes, athletes in "weight division" sports and other athletes who restrict energy intake to achieve their weight/body fat goals
3 Inadequate intake of carbohydrate-rich foods • Food cultures or food environments where carbohydrate-rich foods are not plentiful • Diets promoting avoidance or reduced intake of carbohydrate • Diets promoting avoidance or reduced intake of key carbohydrate-rich foods • Reliance on bulky high-fiber foods that limit total dietary intake • Poor nutrition knowledge	• Young athletes with poor nutrition knowledge and food skills • Groups or environments with focus on protein-rich eating • Athletes following Zone, Atkins, or other carbohydrate-restricted diets • Athletes with coeliac disease or other conditions involving avoidance of wheat- or gluten-containing foods • Natural food eaters, or athletes with obsessive ideas about eating "healthy" high fiber, sugar-free diets • Athletes with poor appetites exacerbated by fatigue or gastrointestinal concerns
4 Poor achievement of strategic timing of intake of carbohydrate-rich foods (before, during, or after training) • Poor nutrition knowledge • Gastrointestinal discomfort associated with consuming food close to intensive exercise • Poor access to food over days or in relation to training sessions	• Athletes following a chaotic lifestyle, especially involving travel away from familiar environment • Athlete with poor finances who cannot afford between-meal snacks, convenience foods, or specialized sports foods • Athletes with gastrointestinal problems exacerbated by consuming food before, during, or after exercise

factors for inadequate intake of carbohydrate and energy intake, and the absence of other problems to explain the fatigue, are also valuable in finalizing the diagnosis.

The main limitations of diagnosing inadequate carbohydrate using these techniques relate to the imprecision in estimating fuel requirements and the athlete's actual dietary intake. A dietary assessment is best undertaken by an expert such as a sports dietitian. The limitations of dietary survey methodology have been well documented (Burke *et al.* 2001) and include errors of how well the dietary survey instrument documents actual intake and how well this intake reflects usual intake. This is the case for

both retrospective methods of dietary assessment (e.g., food frequency questionnaires, dietary history) and prospective methods (e.g., food diaries). The usual bias of self-reported information is to under-report energy intake and, presumably, intake of key nutrients. The results of dietary assessments must be carefully interpreted in light of these problems.

Once a diagnosis of inadequate carbohydrate intake is suspected, the athlete should experiment with their dietary patterns to increase the total amount of carbohydrate consumed and to consume carbohydrate at strategic times in relation to training and competition. The expertise of a sports dietitian is valuable in assisting the athlete to achieve their goals for carbohydrate intake in the light of the challenges of gastrointestinal discomfort, food likes and dislikes, and total energy needs. In the case of the athlete who must restrict their energy intake to achieve a (sensible) target of weight loss or maintenance, there may be need to "periodize" dietary goals. For example, on days or periods of lighter training it may be possible for the athlete to consume less than their theoretical carbohydrate needs in order to prioritize their goal of energy restriction. However, on days when high-intensity training is undertaken, strategic intake of carbohydrate before, during, and after workouts should be undertaken to support training performance and to reduce the immunosuppression that accompanies prolonged training (Gleeson *et al.* 2004). Finally, during competition where optimal performance is desired, the athlete should prioritize the achievement of optimal fuel stores in their overall eating patterns and competition eating strategies (see Issues 3 and 4). Recent guidelines for carbohydrate intake by athletes are provided in Table 20.4.

Inadequate iron status

An inadequate iron status is the most likely micronutrient deficiency among athletic populations, just as it is within the general community. Inadequate iron status can reduce exercise performance via suboptimal levels of hemoglobin, and perhaps also via changes in the muscle, including reduced myoglobin and iron-related enzymes (Hood *et al.* 1992). Exercise itself causes the alteration of many of the measures of iron status, because of changes in plasma volume or the acute phase response to stress. Therefore, it is hard to find the true prevalence of problematic iron deficiency in athletic groups, based on conventional hematologic standards, and it is often difficult to detect the stage of iron deficiency at which impairment of exercise performance is observed. Despite initial conflict in the literature, there is some evidence that iron depletion in the absence of anemia (i.e., reduced serum ferritin concentrations) may impair exercise performance (for review see Deakin 2006). In addition, athletes with reduced iron stores complain of

feeling fatigued and failing to recover between a series of competitions or training sessions. Because low ferritin levels may become progressively lower and eventually lead to iron deficiency anemia, there is merit in monitoring athletes deemed to be at high risk of iron depletion and implementing an intervention as soon as iron status appears to decline substantially or to symptomatic levels. A cost–benefit analysis of routine screening of athletes found little overall benefit in screening all male athletes but justification for screening female athletes, because of the higher prevalence of iron deficiency problems in this population (Fallon 2004).

A diagnosis of iron deficiency requires multiple sources of information that assess the presence of risk factors for low iron status and determine whether this has led to a functional outcome. These include clinical signs and symptoms suggestive of iron deficiency or anemia (e.g., unexplained fatigue, reduced recovery, recurrent infections, pallor), a dietary assessment that indicates an inadequate intake of bioavailable iron, the presence or absence of other factors that may predict an increase in iron requirements or loss, and hematologic and biochemical information suggestive of reduced iron status.

There are various limitations to the assessment and interpretation of such information. For example, problems related to the accuracy and reliability of self-reported information about dietary intake have previously been discussed. In addition, the clinical symptoms and signs described above may be attributed to a number of causes other than iron deficiency. Finally, biochemical and hematologic data can be useful in such an assessment, but must be interpreted in light of known changes to iron status parameters that reflect an acute or chronic response to exercise rather than a true change in iron status, and perhaps what seems normal for the individual athlete.

Iron deficiency anemia is marked by the presence of pale (hypochromic) and small (microcytic) red blood cells on a blood film and a plasma hemoglobin level that is below laboratory reference range (typically 120 g·L^{-1} for females and 140 g·L^{-1} for males). These parameters will remain normal with iron deficiency without anemia. Although iron deficiency in the general population is normally

Table 20.4 Updated guidelines from the IOC consensus on Nutrition for Athletes for the intake of carbohydrate (CHO) in the everyday or training diets of athletes (Burke *et al.* 2004).

Recommendations for:

- Athletes should aim to achieve CHO intakes to meet the fuel requirements of their training program and to optimize restoration of muscle glycogen stores between workouts. General recommendations can be provided, but should be fine-tuned with individual consideration of total energy needs, specific training needs, and feedback from training performance:

  Immediate recovery after exercise (0–4 h): 1–1.2 $g \cdot kg^{-1} \cdot h^{-1}$ consumed at frequent intervals

  Daily recovery: moderate duration/low-intensity training: 5–7 $g \cdot kg^{-1} \cdot day^{-1}$

  Daily recovery: moderate–heavy endurance training: 7–12 $g \cdot kg^{-1} \cdot day^{-1}$

  Daily recovery: extreme exercise program (4–6 h+·day^{-1}): 10–12 $g \cdot kg^{-1} \cdot day^{-1}$

- It is valuable to choose nutrient-rich CHO foods and to add other foods to recovery meals and snacks to provide a good source of protein and other nutrients. These nutrients may assist in other recovery processes, and in the case of protein, may promote additional glycogen recovery when CHO intake is suboptimal or when frequent snacking is not possible

- When the period between exercise sessions is <8 h, the athlete should begin CHO intake as soon as practical after the first workout to maximize the effective recovery time between sessions. There may be some advantages in meeting CHO intake targets as a series of snacks during the early recovery phase

- During longer recovery periods (24 h), the athlete should organize the pattern and timing of CHO-rich meals and snacks according to what is practical and comfortable for their individual situation. There is no difference in glycogen synthesis when liquid or solid forms of CHO are consumed

- CHO-rich foods with a moderate to high glycemic index provide a readily available source of CHO for muscle glycogen synthesis, and should be the major CHO choices in recovery meals

- Adequate energy intake is also important for optimal glycogen recovery; the restrained eating practices of some athletes, particularly females, make it difficult to meet CHO intake targets and to optimize glycogen storage from this intake

Recommendations against

- Guidelines for CHO (or other macronutrients) should not be provided in terms of percentage contributions to total dietary energy intake. Such recommendations are neither user-friendly nor strongly related to the muscle's absolute needs for fuel

- The athlete should not consume excessive amounts of alcohol during the recovery period because it is likely to interfere with their ability or interest to follow guidelines for post-exercise eating. The athlete should follow sensible drinking practices at all times, but particularly in the period after exercise

---

denoted by the reduction in serum ferritin levels below the normal reference range of 12 ng·mL^{-1}, in athletic populations a cut-off mark of 20 ng·mL^{-1} (Nielsen & Nachtigall 1998) or 30 ng·mL^{-1} (Fallon 2004) is often applied in clinical practice. Plasma measurements of soluble transferrin receptors have been described as a new marker of iron status, but may not be a reliable marker of low ferritin levels in athletic populations (Pitsis *et al.* 2004).

Changes to iron status parameters occur with acute or chronic training. These include hemodilution caused by the increase in plasma volume that occurs with onset of endurance training or a chronic period of increased exercise. This effect would dilute key markers, such as blood ferritin and hemoglobin levels, without reflecting a true impact on iron status. The drop in hemoglobin that accompanies

plasma expansion does not impair exercise capacity. Conversely, the acute dehydration associated with exercise may cause hemoconcentration and an increase in blood ferritin and hemoglobin levels without reflecting a true impact on iron status. Finally, an increase in serum ferritin (an acute phase reactant) can be expected in response to a single strenuous bout of exercise, inflammation, or infection. This does not mark a true change in iron status.

Hematological and biochemical tests undertaken in athletes should be administered in a way that standardizes these effects (e.g., carry out all tests in the same laboratory, and after a light training day and before any exercise is undertaken for that day; for review see Deakin 2006). Serial monitoring of an athlete might help to establish the normal range over which such parameters vary for that athlete over the training and competition year, and to differentiate changes that appear to be associated with an impairment of health, function, or performance.

The evaluation and management of iron status in athletes should be undertaken by a sports physician and considered on an individual basis. The publicity during the 1990s surrounding iron deficiency in athletes probably led to an overdiagnosis of the true prevalence of the problem. It is tempting for the fatigued athlete and his or her coach to self-diagnose iron deficiency and to self-medicate with iron supplements which are available as over-the-counter medications. However, there are dangers in self-prescription, or long-term supplementation in the absence of medical follow-up. Iron supplementation is not a replacement for medical and dietary assessment and therapy, because it typically fails to correct underlying problems that have caused iron requirements and losses to exceed iron intake. Chronic supplementation with high doses of iron carries a risk of iron overload, especially in males for whom the genetic traits for hemochromatosis are more prevalent. Finally, iron supplements can also interfere with the absorption of other minerals such as zinc and copper.

Of course, iron supplementation may have a role in the prevention and treatment of iron deficiency. However, the management plan should be based on long-term interventions to reverse iron drain – reducing excessive iron losses and increasing dietary iron. Dietary interventions to improve iron status need not only to increase total iron intake, but also to increase the bioavailability of this iron. The heme form of iron found in meat, fish, and poultry is better absorbed than the organic or non-heme iron found in plant foods, such as fortified and wholegrain cereal foods, legumes, and green leafy vegetables (Hallberg 1981; Monsen 1988). However, iron bioavailability can be manipulated by matching iron-rich foods with dietary factors promoting iron absorption (e.g., vitamin C and other food acids, "meat factor" found in animal flesh) and reducing the interaction with inhibitory factors for iron absorption (e.g., phytates in fiber-rich cereals, tannins in tea) (Hallberg 1981; Monsen 1988). Changes to iron intake should be achieved with eating patterns that are compatible with the athlete's other nutrition goals (e.g., achieving fuel requirements for sport, achieving desired physique). Such education is often a specialized task, requiring the expertise of a sports dietitian.

Issue 3: What can I do to recover between training sessions or repeated competition bouts?

Recovery is a major challenge for the athlete who undertakes two or even three workouts each day during certain phases of the training cycle, with 4–24 h between each session. Many athletes also compete in sports in which the final outcome of competition requires several heats or games. Recovery involves a complex range of processes of restoration and adaptation to physiologic stress of exercise, including:

• Restoration of muscle and liver glycogen stores;
• Replacement of fluid and electrolytes lost in sweat;
• Synthesis of new protein following the catabolic state and damage induced by the exercise; and
• Responses of the immune system.

Detailed information regarding post-exercise refueling (Burke et al. 2004) and rehydration (Shirreffs et al. 2004) strategies is summarized below, while a summary of the recently accumulating information on practices that enhance net protein balance following exercise were summarized under Issue 1.

The major dietary factor involved in post-exercise refueling is the amount of carbohydrate consumed. As long as total energy intake is adequate (Tarnopolsky et al. 2001), increased carbohydrate intake promotes increased muscle glycogen storage until the threshold for glycogen synthesis is reached. Until recently, guidelines for athletes recommended that optimal glycogen storage is achieved when approximately 1–1.5 g carbohydrate is consumed every hour in the early stages of recovery, leading to a total carbohydrate of 6–10 g·kg body mass^{-1} over 24 h (American College of Sports Medicine et al. 2000). However, these guidelines were developed on the basis of maximum glycogen storage during a passive recovery period, and may both overestimate the carbohydrate needs of athletes who do not substantially deplete glycogen stores in their daily training, and underestimate the daily refueling needs of athletes with extremely high training or competition workloads. The revised guidelines for the carbohydrate needs of athletes recognize different carbohydrate needs based on exercise load (Table 20.4).

The type and timing of carbohydrate intake may have some effect on the rate of glycogen restoration, with interest in the hypothesis that strategies to enhance blood glucose availability or insulin levels might enhance glycogen synthesis. For example, moderate and high glycemic index (GI) carbohydrate-rich foods and drinks appear to promote greater glycogen storage than meals based on low GI carbohydrate foods (Burke *et al.* 1993); however, the mechanisms may include additional factors, such as the malabsorption of low GI carbohydrate rather than differences in the glycemic and insulinemic response to such foods alone (Burke *et al.* 1996). The form of the carbohydrate – fluids or solids – does not appear to affect glycogen synthesis (Keizer *et al.* 1986; Reed *et al.* 1989).

Early research indicated that glycogen synthesis was enhanced by the addition of protein to carbohydrate snacks consumed after exercise, an observation that was explained by the protein-stimulated enhancement of the insulin response (Zawadzki *et al.* 1992). However, these findings have been refuted in other studies, especially when the energy content of protein or amino acids included in recovery feedings was matched (for review see Burke *et al.* 2004). The consensus from the literature is that co-ingestion of protein or amino acids with carbohydrate does not clearly enhance glycogen synthesis, with benefits being limited to the first hour of recovery (Ivy *et al.* 2002) or to situations in which the total amount of carbohydrate or pattern of intake is below the threshold for maximal glycogen synthesis and the protein provides an additional energy source. Nevertheless, the combination of protein and carbohydrate in recovery meals may allow the athlete to meet other nutritional goals including the enhancement of net protein balance after exercise. This may be important for the optimization of the goals of a hypertrophy-based training program (Issue 1), but may also be useful for recovery from a strenuous session of endurance exercise because of the potential to enhance protein synthesis underpinning the repair of muscle damage and the desired adaptations to the training stimulus (Levenhagen *et al.* 2001). Examples of food combinations that provide a combination of protein and carbohydrate for a post-exercise recovery snack are shown in Table 20.5.

Athletes have been advised to enhance recovery by consuming carbohydrate as soon as possible after the completion of a workout. The highest rates of muscle glycogen storage occur during the first hour after exercise, and the immediate intake of carbohydrate takes advantage of this effect (Ivy *et al.* 1988). Conversely, the failure to consume carbohydrate during post-exercise recovery leads to very low rates of glycogen restoration until feeding occurs. Therefore, early intake of carbohydrate following strenuous exercise is valuable because it provides an immediate source of substrate to the muscle cell to start effective recovery, as well as taking advantage of a period of moderately enhanced glycogen synthesis. Although early feeding may be important when there is only 4–8 h between exercise sessions (Ivy *et al.* 1988), it may have less impact over a longer recovery period (Parkin *et al.* 1997). Overall, it appears that when the interval between exercise sessions is short, the athlete should maximize the effective recovery time by beginning carbohydrate intake as soon as possible. However, when longer recovery periods are available, athletes can choose their preferred meal schedule as long as total carbohydrate intake goals are achieved. It is not always practical to consume substantial meals or snacks immediately after the finish of a strenuous workout. There is some evidence that refueling during the first hours of recovery is enhanced when carbohydrate intake targets $(1 \text{ g·kg}^{-1}\text{·h}^{-1})$ are met via a series of small snacks every 15–30 min (Van Hall *et al.* 2000; Jentjens *et al.* 2001). Guidelines are summarized in Table 20.3.

Despite drinking fluids during exercise, most athletes can expect to be at least mildly dehydrated at the end of their session and should aim to restore fluid losses before the next workout. This is difficult in situations where moderate to high levels of hypo-hydration have been incurred (e.g., a fluid deficit equivalent to 2–5% body mass or greater) and the

Table 20.5 Risk factors for reduced iron status among athletes.

Risk factors for iron deficiency in athletes	Specific athletes or situations at risk of iron deficiency
Predictors of increased iron requirements	
• Recent growth spurt in adolescents	• Adolescents
• Pregnancy (current or within the past year)	• Female athletes who are currently pregnant or returning to exercise after a pregnancy
Predictors of increased iron loss or malabsorption	
• Sudden increase in heavy training load, particularly running on hard surfaces, causing an increase in intravascular hemolysis	• Runners, triathletes and other "foot contact" athletes who have just resumed training after a lay-off (start of new season or following injury) or increased training volume
• Gastrointestinal bleeding (e.g. some anti-inflammatory drugs, ulcers)	• Athletes with long-term (and unsupervised) use of aspirin and non-steroidal anti-inflammatory drugs (NSAIDs)
• Gastrointestinal malabsorption problems	• Athletes with ulcers or Crohn's disease, ulcerative colitis, parasitic infestations
• Heavy menstrual blood losses	
• Excessive blood losses such as frequent nose bleeds, recent surgery, substantial contact injuries	• Athletes who donate blood frequently
• Frequent blood donation	• Female athletes
Predictors of inadequate intake of bio-available iron	
• Chronic low energy intake (<2000 kcal·day^{-1} or 8 MJ·day^{-1})	• Athletes who restrict energy intake to achieve their weight/body fat goals; especially female athletes and athletes in "weight division" sports
• Vegetarian eating – especially poorly constructed diets in which alternative food sources of iron are ignored (e.g. legumes, nuts, and seeds) and which contain large amounts of inhibitory factors for iron absorption (e.g., phytates)	• Athletes who concentrate on carbohydrate-rich meals to the exclusion of other foods; athletes with poor finances or poor cooking skills who rarely include meat at meals
• Restricted variety of foods in diet, and failure to promote matching of iron-containing foods with dietary factors that promote iron absorption such as ascorbic and other food acids, meat factor	• Athletes who adopt vegetarian eating on a whim
• Overconsumption of micronutrient-poor convenience foods and sports foods (e.g., high carbohydrate powders, gels)	• Picky eaters
	• Athletes following fad diets; compulsive athletes who follow a rigid intake of "allowable" low-fat foods
• Very high carbohydrate diet with high fiber content and infrequent intake of meats/fish/chicken	• Athletes with poor nutrition knowledge and cooking skills following erratic diet
• Natural food diets: failure to consume iron-fortified cereal foods such as commercial breakfast cereals and bread	

interval between sessions is less than 6–8 h. Voluntary intake is enhanced when fluids are flavored (Carter & Gisolfi 1989), kept at a cool temperature (Hubbard *et al.* 1990), and by the addition of sodium to preserve thirst (Nose *et al.* 1988). However, in situations where rapid rehydration of fluid deficits >2% body mass is desired, athletes are advised to follow a plan of fluid intake rather than relying on thirst.

Because sweating and obligatory urine losses continue during the recovery phase, the athlete must replace more than their post-exercise fluid deficit before finally achieving fluid restoration. Typically, a volume of fluid equivalent to approximately 150% of the post-exercise fluid deficit must be consumed over the 4–6 h of recovery to compensate for these ongoing losses and ensure that fluid balance is achieved (Shirreffs *et al.* 1996). However, fluid replacement alone will not guarantee that rehydration goals are achieved. Unless there is simultaneous replacement of the electrolytes lost in sweat, particularly sodium, consumption of large amounts of fluid will simply result in large urine losses (Shirreffs *et al.* 1996). The addition of sodium to rehydration fluids has been shown to better maintain equilibrium between the restoration of plasma volume and plasma osmolality, reduce urine losses, and enhance net fluid balance at the end of 6 h of recovery (Maughan & Leiper 1995; Shirreffs *et al.* 1996). In contrast, with no or little sodium replacement, subjects were still substantially dehydrated at the end of the 6-h recovery period, despite drinking 150% of the volume of their post-exercise fluid deficit. On a practical note, the acute replacement of large amounts of fluid in the absence of sodium may provide false information to the athlete, because they will observe the production of "copious amounts of clear urine" despite being in fluid deficit. Recovery may also be interrupted if such urine production occurs during the night, leading to interrupted sleep.

The optimal sodium level in a rehydration drink appears to be approximately 50–80 mmol·L^{-1} (Maughan & Leiper 1995), as is provided in Oral Rehydration Solutions manufactured for the treatment of diarrhea. This is considerably higher than the concentrations found in commercial carbohydrate-electrolyte drinks or "sports drinks" (typically 10–25 mmol·L^{-1}) and may be unpalatable to many athletes. Sports drinks may confer some rehydration advantages over plain water, in terms of palatability as well as fluid retention (Gonzalez-Alonso *et al.* 1992). Nevertheless, where maximum fluid retention is desired, there may be benefits in increasing the sodium levels of rehydration fluids to levels above those provided in typical sports drinks. Alternatively, sodium may be ingested during post-exercise recovery via everyday foods containing sodium (e.g., bread, breakfast cereal, cheese) or by adding salt to meals.

Because caffeine and alcohol increase urine production, consumption of alcoholic- and caffeine-containing drinks during post-exercise recovery may result in greater fluid losses than other fluids (Gonzalez-Alonso *et al.* 1992; Shirreffs & Maughan 1997). Athletes are often advised that caffeine-containing beverages (e.g., tea, coffee, and cola or "energy" drinks) are not suitable rehydration fluids and should be avoided in situations where there is a risk of developing dehydration, such as during and after exercise or during air travel. However, according to a recent review of caffeine and hydration status, there is little evidence that caffeine intake impairs fluid status (Armstrong 2002). Instead, it appears that the effect of caffeine on diuresis is overstated, and may be minimal in people who are habitual caffeine users. Importantly, the voluntary intake of fluids that are well liked and cemented into normal eating behaviors may more than compensate for small increases in fluid loss. Of course, the intake of large amounts of alcoholic beverages after exercise will interfere with recovery, particularly by distracting the athlete from undertaking their recommended dietary practices and by promoting high-risk behavior (Burke & Maughan 2000).

Issue 4: What should I eat before and during my event?

To achieve optimal competition performance, the coach and athlete should identify nutritional factors that are likely to cause fatigue during their event, and undertake strategies before, during, and after the event that minimize or delay the onset of this fatigue. The nutritional challenges vary according to the length and intensity of the event, the environment, and factors that influence opportunities to eat and drink during the event or in recovery afterwards. Issues include dehydration, depletion of glycogen stores, low blood glucose concentrations and other disturbances of the central nervous system, gastrointestinal distress, and hyponatremia. Of course, competition nutrition strategies need to be undertaken with consideration of practical issues such as the availability of suitable foods or drinks during an event, gastrointestinal challenges to eating or drinking while exercising, and finding access to food supplies when competition takes place away from home.

Pre-event eating

The usual resting glycogen concentrations of the trained athlete (100–120 mol·kg wet weight [ww]$^{-1}$) appear adequate to meet the fuel needs of events lasting up to 60–90 min in duration (Hawley et al. 1997). In the absence of severe muscle damage, such stores can be achieved by 24 h rest and an adequate carbohydrate intake (7–10 g·kg body mass^{-1}·day^{-1}) (Costill et al. 1981). The term "carbohydrate loading" describes practices that aim to maximize muscle glycogen stores prior to longer competitive events. Carbohydrate loading protocols, evolved in the late 1960s with a 6-day strategy that involved glycogen depletion (3 day low carbohydrate diet and training) followed by glycogen supercompensation (3 day tapered training and high carbohydrate intake) (Bergstrom & Hultman 1966). This strategy was shown to elevate muscle glycogen stores to approximately 150–250 mmol·kg ww^{-1}. A modification to this protocol in the 1980s found that well-trained athletes do not need to include a depletion phase prior to carbohydrate loading protocols. Carbohydrate loading strategies were later modified when trained muscle was shown to be able to supercompensate glycogen stores without a severe depletion or "glycogen stripping" phase (Sherman et al. 1981). More recent studies show that maximal glycogen storage can be achieved by well-trained athletes in as little as 36–48 h following the last exercise session, at least when the athlete rests and consumes adequate carbohydrate intake (Bussau et al. 2002). Such preparation of fuel stores may enhance the performance of prolonged events, such as a marathon, but may also be useful for athletes in prolonged intermittent sports, such as tennis or soccer, who may otherwise deplete glycogen reserves.

The meal consumed in the 1–4 h prior to an event should include carbohydrate-rich foods and drinks (see Table 20.6 for suggestions), especially in the case where body carbohydrate stores are suboptimal because of inadequate recovery from the previous workout, or where the event is of sufficient duration and intensity to challenge these stores. Carbohydrate consumed during the hours prior to the event enhances carbohydrate availability by increasing muscle and liver glycogen stores (Coyle et al. 1985), and by storing glucose in the gastrointestinal space for later release. Because liver glycogen stores are labile and may be substantially depleted by an overnight fast, carbohydrate intake on the morning of an event may ensure that hepatic

glucose output is able to maintain blood glucose levels during the latter stages of prolonged exercise. Compared with trials undertaken after an overnight fast, the intake of a substantial amount of carbohydrate (~200–300 g) in the 2–4 h before exercise has been shown to enhance endurance and performance (Neufer et al. 1987; Wright et al. 1991).

There have been claims that meals based on low GI carbohydrates enhance performance of subsequent prolonged exercise compared with high GI carbohydrate sources (Thomas et al. 1991), because of a smaller perturbation of blood glucose and better maintenance of carbohydrate oxidation during exercise. However, not all studies comparing pre-event meals of different GI have found differences in performance outcomes in a range of exercise protocols. More importantly, metabolic and performance differences arising from pre-event meals have been shown to be minimized by the recommended strategy of consuming carbohydrate during the event (Burke et al. 1998). Therefore, the athlete should choose a pre-event meal based on familiar and practical foods rather than strict food guidelines.

In the field it is not always practical to consume a substantial carbohydrate-rich meal or snack in the 4 h before a sporting event. For example, it is unlikely that an athlete will want to sacrifice sleep to eat a large meal before an early morning race start. In this situation, many athletes will settle for a lighter meal or snack before the event, and consume carbohydrate throughout the event to balance missed fuelling opportunities. The size and composition of the pre-event meal may need to be modified for athletes who are at risk of gastrointestinal discomfort or upset during exercise, particularly to reduce the intake of protein, fat, or fiber. The athlete should also be conscious of fluid needs, and consume adequate fluid to ensure that they are well hydrated at the start of the event.

Fluid and food intake during event

Some degree of dehydration is inevitable in most sports because of the mismatch between the athlete's sweat losses and his or her capacity to replace fluids during the event. Sometimes the athlete may

Table 20.6 Carbohydrate-rich choices suitable for special issues in sport. From Burke (2007).

Carbohydrate-rich choices for pre-event meals
Breakfast cereal + low-fat milk + fresh/canned fruit
Muffins or crumpets + jam/honey
Pancakes + syrup
Toast + baked beans (note this is a high fiber choice)
Creamed rice (made with low-fat milk)
Rolls or sandwiches
Fruit salad + low-fat fruit yogurt
Spaghetti with tomato or low-fat sauce
Baked potatoes with low-fat filling
Fruit smoothie (low-fat milk + fruit + yogurt/ice cream)
Liquid meal supplement

Carbohydrate-rich foods suitable for intake during exercise
(50 g carbohydrate portions)
600–800 mL sports drink
2 × sachets sports gel
1.5 sports bars
2 cereal bars or granola bars
Large bread roll filled with jam/honey/cheese
2 bananas/3 medium pieces of other fruit
60 g jelly confectionery
450 mL cola drinks
80 g chocolate bar
100 g fruit bread or cake
80 dried fruit or 120 g trail mix

Recovery snacks – to be eaten post-exercise, or pre-exercise in
the case of resistance training to promote refueling and
protein responses
(Each serve provides 50 g carbohydrate and at least 10 g
protein)

250–350 mL liquid meal supplement or milk shake/fruit
smoothie
500 mL flavored low-fat milk
Sports bar + 200 mL sports drink
60 g (1.5–2 cups) breakfast cereal with 1/2 cup milk
1 round of sandwiches with cheese/meat/chicken filling,
and 1 large piece of fruit or 300 mL sports drink
1 cups of fruit salad with 200 g carton fruit-flavored yogurt
or custard
200 g carton fruit-flavored yogurt or 300 mL flavored milk
and 30–35 cereal bar
2 crumpets or English muffins with thick spread of peanut
butter
250 g tin of baked beans on 2 slices of toast
250 g (large) baked potato with cottage cheese or grated
cheese filling
150 g thick-crust pizza

Portable carbohydrate-rich foods suitable for the traveling athlete
Breakfast cereal (and skim milk powder)
Cereal bars, granola bars
Dried fruit, trail mixes
Rice crackers, dry biscuits plus spreads – jam, honey, etc.
Quick cook noodles and rice
Baked beans
Sports bars
Liquid meal supplements – powder and ready-to-drink tetra
packs
Sports drink

even start competition with a fluid deficit, as a result of the deliberate use of dehydration to reduce body mass or "make weight", or the failure to replace sweat losses arising from an unaccustomed environment or previous exercise. The disadvantages of dehydration are most apparent when prolonged or high-intensity exercise is undertaken in the heat (Sawka & Pandolf 1990). In the laboratory at least, a fluid deficit of ~2% of the athlete's body mass has been shown to reduce exercise capacity and performance by a detectable amount (Walsh et al. 1994). In addition, the degree of thermoregulatory and cardiovascular impairment, and increased perception of effort associated with the exercise, appear to be directly related to the size of fluid deficit (Montain & Coyle 1992). Dehydration may

also reduce skill and decision-making abilities (Gopinathan et al. 1988).

Although it may not be possible, and in some cases even undesirable, to avoid some level of dehydration, the athlete should aim to keep the fluid deficit associated with their event to an acceptable level by developing a plan of pre-, during-, and post-event hydration strategies. During events lasting longer than 30 min there is usually both a need and an opportunity for intake of fluid during the exercise to offset sweat losses. Evaporation of sweat provides a key mechanism for dissipating the heat generated as a byproduct of exercise, and sweat rates vary across and between sports according to factors such as the intensity of exercise, the environmental conditions, the athlete's individual characteristics and level of acclimatization (Sawka & Pandolf 1990). A range of factors influence fluid intake during events, but across a range of sports and exercise activities, athletes typically drink at a rate that offsets only 30–70% of their sweat losses (Noakes *et al.* 1988; Broad *et al.* 1996). It is not always possible, and in some cases even undesirable, to replace all sweat losses during exercise. When sweat rates exceed 800–1000 mL·h^{-1}, it becomes difficult to drink to keep pace with such losses and, in some events, sweat rates exceeding 2 L·h^{-1} are commonly reported. However, there is potential for many athletes to improve their current fluid intake practices and benefit from reducing the fluid deficit that accumulates during exercise.

The past 30 years have produced an evolution in the guidelines for athletes regarding hydration during exercise. There have been changes from the initial focus on fluid needs to the realization that strategies to supply both fluid and fuel needs during exercise can be successfully integrated. Many investigations have demonstrated that the intake of carbohydrate drinks of 4–8% concentration promotes effective rehydration during exercise and provides a useful source of additional fuel for the muscle and central nervous system. As a result, current guidelines on rehydration during exercise support the use of commercially available sports drinks (4–8% carbohydrate, 10–25 mmol·L^{-1} sodium) during a range of prolonged sports and exercise activities (American College of Sports Medicine 1996), although water is still positioned as a suitable choice of beverage for exercise of less than 60 min duration.

The current guidelines have also evolved from the rigid prescription of recommended volumes of fluid intake to the recognition of the variable nature of sport and exercise activities, and individual differences that occur between athletes (American College of Sports Medicine 1996). Issues that must be taken into account include individual sweat rates and fluid needs, sports-specific opportunities for fluid intake, and practical challenges such as making fluid available, preventing gastrointestinal discomfort, and being aware of fluid needs. Each athlete should consider how these issues arise in their sport to develop their own fluid intake plan. According to the sport, an infrastructure of aid stations, a team fluid supply, trainers or handlers taking fluids to the athlete, individual drink bottles or set drink breaks may be needed to put the plan into practice. The plan may also be fine-tuned with the information provided by fluid balance monitoring activities; weight changes over an exercise session, and the volume of fluids and/or foods consumed during the session can be monitored to estimate total sweat losses, success in replacing these during the session, and the residual fluid deficit at the end of the session.

The most recent accommodation to fluid guidelines during exercise is the recognition that some athletes overhydrate during exercise (Noakes 2003). This is not a common occurrence in most sports lasting less than 2–3 h but can occur in certain individuals who are overzealous with their interpretation of hydration guidelines, and drink at a rate that is in excess of their rates of sweat loss (Almond *et al.* 2005). Risk factors for this syndrome, which in severe cases can lead to the potentially fatal condition of symptomatic hyponatremia (low plasma sodium concentrations), include being female, and undertaking endurance and ultra-endurance events at a slow pace, which both reduces the rate of sweat loss and provides opportunity to drink multiple servings of fluid provided at aid stations throughout the event. Some sports scientists have criticized guidelines that promote fluid intake during exercise, claiming that such advice is not necessary and is potentially dangerous (Noakes 2003). While this stance will draw attention to this rare but serious condition, most sports scientists prefer a view that balances the risk of overhydration (low prevalence, serious outcomes) and underhydration (high prevalence, mild–serious outcomes) in most sports and exercise activities. In other words, athletes should be warned against the behaviors that lead to both problems at both ends of the spectrum.

When carbohydrate is consumed during exercise to enhance or maintain otherwise declining body carbohydrate availability, there is clear evidence of an enhancement in endurance and exercise capacity (for review see Hargreaves 1999). There are also some studies that show that carbohydrate intake reduces the decline in the movement patterns and skill levels of complex and unpredictable sports (Vergauwen *et al.* 1998; Ostojic & Mazic 2002; Welsh *et al.* 2002). Even when benefits are not found, carbohydrate intake during exercise does not cause an impairment of exercise performance. Nowadays, during exercise of more than 60–90 min duration, athletes are encouraged to consume a source of carbohydrate to provide an available glucose supply of at least 30–60 g·h^{-1} (American College of Sports Medicine 1996). Sports drinks provide a convenient form of carbohydrate intake during exercise for most athletes. However, the culture and conditions of many sports allow a range of carbohydrate-containing foods and drinks to be consumed to meet fuel needs during the event (Table 20.6).

Of considerable interest are the growing number of studies to report benefits of carbohydrate ingestion during performance of high-intensity exercise lasting about 1 h (Below *et al.* 1995; Jeukendrup *et al.* 1997; Millard-Stafford *et al.* 1997). These findings are puzzling, because muscle carbohydrate stores are not considered to be limiting in events of this duration. Further research is needed to confirm and explain the effects, but it is possible that benefits are via "central performance," involving the brain and nervous system (Carter *et al.* 2004). One study has found that the benefits of carbohydrate ingestion, at least to the performance of 1 h high-intensity cycling, are independent and additive to the effects of fluid ingestion (Below *et al.* 1995). Whatever strategies of fluid and fuel intake during an event are chosen, the athlete should practice in training and minor events to fine-tune a successful competition eating strategy.

Issue 5: What supplements and sports foods are effective and safe to use?

Because the winners of sporting competitions are often separated from their colleagues by milliseconds and millimeters, elite athletes are constantly searching for any product or intervention that might improve performance by even a small margin. Even recreational athletes appear to be bedazzled by the multitude of supplements that promise to enhance speed, increase endurance, improve recovery, reduce body fat levels, increase muscle mass, or whatever it takes to make them a better athlete. The widespread use of supplements and the large range of different types and brands of products is illustrated by the results of a study of 77 elite Australian swimmers (Baylis *et al.* 2001). This sur-

vey found that 94% of the group reported the use of supplements in pill and powder form, and when the use of specialized sports foods, such as sports drinks, was also taken into account, 99% of swimmers reported supplement use, and a total of 207 different products were identified.

Although supplements and sports foods carry many claims that they can enhance an athlete's performance, in reality only a small proportion of the available products are supported by credible scientific support (for review see Burke *et al.* 2006). These include sports foods, such as sports drinks, sports gels, liquid meal supplements, and sports bars, which may be used as a practical alternative to everyday foods to allow athletes to meet their special nutritional goals for training or competition. Other supplements that enjoy considerable scientific support for a potential role in enhancing performance include caffeine, creatine, and bicarbonate/citrate as a buffering agent. Information about these products, including validated protocols of use, a review of studies investigating performance enhancement, and concerns associated with their use can be found in Burke *et al.* (2006), and among the resources underpinning the AIS Sports Supplement Program can be found at www.ais.org.au/nutrition. It is beyond the scope of this chapter to review this information further. It is important that the athlete is aware that it is the appropriate use of the product, as much as the product itself, that leads to the beneficial outcome. Therefore, education about specific situations and strategies for the use of supplements and sports foods is just as important as the formulation of the product. Any decision to use sports supplements or foods should consider the evidence for real or even placebo-driven benefits versus the risk of side-effects or a positive doping outcome. Supplement use, even when it provides a true performance advantage, is an expense that athletes must acknowledge and prioritize appropriately within their total budget.

A number of ingredients that may be found in supplements are considered prohibited substances by the codes of the World Anti-Doping Agency (WADA) and other sports bodies. These include prohormones (steroid-related compounds, such as androstenedione, DHEA, 19-norandrostenedione) and stimulants, such as ephedrine or related substances. In some countries, including the USA, these substances are available in supplements and over-the-counter "medical" preparations. Drug education programs highlight the need for athletes to read the labels of supplements and sports foods carefully to ensure that they do not contain such banned substances. This is a responsibility that athletes must master to prevent inadvertent doping outcomes.

However, inadvertent intake of banned substances from supplement products can still occur even when athletes take such precautions. This is because some supplements contain banned products, not identified on the label, as a result of contamination or poor labeling processes. The prohormone substances seem to provide the greatest risk of inadvertent consumption via supplement use, with a positive test for the steroid nandrolone being one of the possible outcomes. The most striking evidence of these problems was uncovered by a study carried out by a laboratory accredited by the International Olympic Committee (Geyer *et al.* 2004). This study analyzed 634 supplements from 215 suppliers in 13 countries, with products being sourced from retail outlets (91%), the Internet (8%), and telephone sales. None of these supplements declared prohormones as ingredients, and came both from manufacturers who produced other supplements containing prohormones, as well as companies who did not sell these products. Ninety-four of the supplements (15% of the sample) were found to contain hormones or prohormones that were not stated on the product label. A further 10% of samples provided technical difficulties in analysis such that the absence of hormones could not be guaranteed. Of the "positive" supplements, 68% contained prohormones of testosterone, 7% contained prohormones of nandrolone, and 25% contained compounds related to both. Forty-nine of the supplements contained only one steroid, but 45 contained more than one, with eight products containing five or more different steroid products. According to the labels on the products, the countries of *manufacture* of all supplements containing steroids were the USA, the Netherlands, the UK, Italy, and Germany; however, these products were *purchased* in other countries. In fact, 10–20% of products purchased in Spain and Austria were found

to be contaminated. Just over 20% of the products made by companies selling prohormones products were positive for undeclared prohormones, but 10% of products from companies that did not sell steroid-containing supplements were also positive. The brand names of the "positive" products were not provided in the study, but included amino acid supplements, protein powders, and products containing creatine, carnitine, ribose, guarana, zinc, pyruvate, B-hydroxy B-methylbutyrate (HMB), *Tribulus terristris*, herbal extracts, and vitamins and minerals.

This is a major area of concern for serious athletes who compete in competitions that apply anti-doping codes, because many of these codes place liability with the athlete for ingestion of banned substances, regardless of the circumstances and the source of ingestion. As such, full penalties can be expected for a positive doping test arising from the ingestion of a banned substance that is a contaminant or undeclared ingredient of a supplement. Further information on contamination of supplements can be found in a recent review of this topic (Maughan 2005). Athletes should make enquiries at the anti-doping agencies within their countries for advice on the specific risks identified with supplement use, and any initiatives to reduce this risk.

Issue 6: How can I achieve all my nutrition goals when I am traveling for a special training camp or competition?

Most elite athletes are well-seasoned travelers, undertaking trips to training camps or specialized environments (e.g., altitude) and to compete. Athletes must be able to achieve their peak performance at important competitions, such as the Olympic Games or World Championships, in an environment that is often both far away and different from their homebase. In some sports, national or regional competitions require athletes to travel weekly or bi-weekly to compete against the other members of their league. Frequent travel can pose a number of challenges. Table 20.7 summarizes common challenges, along with strategies to cope with these issues to achieve performance goals. Examples of portable sources of carbohydrate, including nutrient-rich fuel supplies are also included in Table 20.6.

Table 20.7 Challenges and solution for the traveling athlete.

Challenges of traveling
Disruptions to the normal training routine and lifestyle while the athlete is en route
Changes in climate and environment that create different nutritional needs
Jet lag
Changes to food availability including absence of important and familiar foods
Reliance on hotels, restaurants, and takeaways instead of home cooking
Exposure to new foods and eating cultures
Temptations of an "all you can eat" dining hall in an athletes' village
Risk of gastrointestinal illnesses due to exposure to food and water with poor hygiene standards
Excitement and distraction of a new environment

Strategies to cope with the challenges of traveling
1 *Planning ahead*
The athlete should investigate food issues on travel routes (e.g., airlines) and at the destination before leaving home.
  Caterers and food organizers should be contacted well ahead of the trip to let them know meal timing and menu needs

2 *Supplies to supplement the local fare*
A supply of portable and non-perishable foods should be taken or sent to the destination to replace important items that
  missing
The athlete should be aware that many catering plans only cover meals. Because the athlete's nutrition goals are likely to
  include well-timed and well-chosen snacks, supplies should be taken to supplement meals en route and at the destination

3 *Eating and drinking well en route*
Many athletes will turn to "boredom eating" when confined. Instead, they should eat according to their real needs, taking
  into account the forced rest while traveling
When moving to a new time zone, the athlete should adopt eating patterns that suit their destination as soon as the trip
  starts. This will help the body clock to adapt
Unseen fluid losses in air-conditioned vehicles and pressurized plane cabins should be recognized; a drinking plan should
  be organized to keep the athlete well hydrated

4 *Taking care with food and water hygiene*
It is important to find out whether the local water supply is safe to drink. Otherwise, the athlete should stick to drinks
  from sealed bottles, or hot drinks made from well-boiled water. Ice added to drinks is often made from tap water and
  may be a problem
In high-risk environments, the athlete should eat only at good hotels or well-known restaurants. Food from local stalls and
  markets should be avoided, however tempting it is to have an "authentic cultural experience"
Food that has been well-cooked is the safest; it is best to avoid salads or unpeeled fruit that has been in contact with local
  water or soil

5 *Adhering to the food plan*
The athlete should choose the best of the local cuisine to meet their nutritional needs, supplementing with their own
  supplies where needed
The athlete should be assertive in asking for what they need at catering outlets – e.g., low-fat cooking styles or an extra
  carbohydrate choice
The challenges of "all you can eat" dining should be recognized. The athlete should resist the temptation to eat "what is
  there" or "what everyone else is eating" in favor of their own meal plan

References

Achten, J., Halson, S.H., Moseley, L., Rayson, M.P., Casey, A. & Jeukendrup, A.E. (2004) Higher dietary carbohydrate content during intensified running training results in better maintenance of performance and mood state. *Journal of Applied Physiology* **96**, 1331–1340.

Almond, C.S.D., Shin, A.Y., Fortescue, E.B., *et al.* (2005) Hyponatremia among runners in the Boston marathon. *New England Journal of Medicine* **352**, 1550–1556.

American College of Sports Medicine (1996) Position stand: exercise and fluid replacement. *Medicine and Science in Sports and Exercise* **28**, i–vii.

American College of Sports Medicine, American Dietetic Association & Dietitians of Canada (2000) Nutrition and athletic performance. *Medicine and Science in Sports and Exercise* **32**, 2130–2145.

Armstrong, L.E. (2002) Caffeine, body fluid–electrolyte balance, and exercise performance. *International Journal of Sport Nutrition and Exercise Metabolism* **12**, 189–206.

Baylis, A., Cameron-Smith, D. & Burke, L.M. (2001) Inadvertent doping though supplement use by athletes: assessment and management of the risk in Australia. *International Journal of Sport Nutrition and Exercise Metabolism* **11**, 365–383.

Beals, K.A. (2004) *Disordered Eating Among Athletes: A Comprehensive Guide for Health Professionals.* Human Kinetics, Champaign, IL.

Beals, K.A. & Manore, M.M. (1994) The prevalence and consequences of subclinical eating disorders in female athletes. *International Journal of Sport Nutrition* **4**, 175–195.

Below, P.R., Mora-Rodriguez, R., Gonzalez-Alonso, J. & Coyle, E.F. (1995) Fluid and carbohydrate ingestion independently improve performance during 1 h of intense exercise. *Medicine and Science in Sports and Exercise* **27**: 200–210.

Bergstrom, J. & Hultman, E. (1966) Muscle glycogen synthesis after exercise: an enhancing factor localized to the muscle cells in man. *Nature* **210**, 309–310.

Borsheim, E., Aarsland, A. & Wolfe, R.R. (2004a) Effect of an amino acid, protein, and carbohydrate mixture on net muscle protein balance after resistance exercise. *International Journal of Sport Nutrition and Exercise Metabolism* **14**, 255–271.

Borsheim, E., Cree, M.G., Tipton, K.D., Elliott, T.A., Aarsland, A. & Wolfe, R.R. (2004b) Effect of carbohydrate intake on net muscle protein synthesis during recovery from resistance exercise. *Journal of Applied Physiology* **96**, 674–678.

Borsheim, E., Tipton, K.D., Wolf, S.E. & Wolfe, R.R. (2002) Essential amino acids and muscle protein recovery from resistance exercise. *American Journal of Physiology. Endocrinology and Metabolism* **283**, E648–E657.

Broad, E.M., Burke, L.M., Cox, G.R., Heeley, P. & Riley, M. (1996) Body weight changes and voluntary fluid intakes during training and competition sessions in team sports. *International Journal of Sport Nutrition* **6**, 307–320.

Burke, L.M. (2001) Energy needs of athletes. *Canadian Journal of Applied Physiology* **26**, S202–S219.

Burke, L.M. (2006) Preparation for competition. In: *Clinical Sports Nutrition*, 3rd edn (Burke, L. & Deakin, V., eds.) McGraw Hill, Sydney.

Burke, L.M. (2007) *Practical Sports Nutrition*. Human Kinetics, Champaign, IL.

Burke, L.M., Claassen, A., Hawley, J.A. & Noakes, T.D. (1998) Carbohydrate intake during prolonged cycling minimizes effect of glycemic index of preexercise meal. *Journal of Applied Physiology* **85**, 2220–2226.

Burke, L.M., Collier, G.R., Davis, P.G., Fricker, P.A., Sanigorski, A.J. & Hargreaves, M. (1996) Muscle glycogen storage after prolonged exercise: effect of the frequency of carbohydrate feedings. *American Journal of Clinical Nutrition* **64**, 115–119.

Burke, L.M., Collier, G.R. & Hargreaves, M. (1993) Muscle glycogen storage after prolonged exercise: the effect of the glycemic index of carbohydrate feedings. *Journal of Applied Physiology* **75**, 1019–1023.

Burke, L.M., Cort, M., Cox, G.R., *et al.* (2006) Supplements and sports foods. In: *Clinical Sports Nutrition*, 3rd edn (Burke, L. & Deakin, V., eds.) McGraw Hill, Sydney.

Burke, L.M., Cox, G.R., Cummings, N.K. & Desbrow, B. (2001) Guidelines for daily CHO intake: do athletes achieve them? *Sports Medicine* **31**, 267–299.

Burke, L.M., Kiens, B. & Ivy, J.L. (2004) Carbohydrates and fat for training and recovery. *Journal of Sports Sciences* **22**, 15–30.

Burke, L.M. & Maughan, R.J. (2000) Alcohol in sport. In: *Nutrition in Sport* (Maughan, R.J., ed.) Blackwell Science, Oxford: 405–414.

Bussau, V.A., Fairchild, T.J., Rao, A., Steele, P.D. & Fournier, P.A. (2002) Carbohydrate loading in human muscle: an improved 1 day protocol. *European Journal of Applied Physiology and Occupational Physiology* **87**, 290–295.

Carter, J.E. & Gisolfi, C.V. (1989) Fluid replacement during and after exercise in the heat. *Medicine and Science in Sports and Exercise* **21**, 532–539.

Carter, J.M., Jeukendrup, A.E. & Jones, D.A. (2004) The effect of carbohydrate mouth rinse on 1-h cycle time trial performance. *Medicine and Science in Sports and Exercise* **36**, 2107–2111.

Centers for Disease Control and Prevention (1998) Hyperthermia and dehydration-related deaths associated with intentional rapid weight loss in three collegiate wrestlers, North Carolina, Wisconsin, and Michigan, November–December 1998. *Journal of the American Medical Association* **279**, 824–825.

Costill, D.L., Flynn, M.G., Kirwan, J.P., *et al.* (1988) Effects of repeated days of intensified training on muscle glycogen and swimming performance. *Medicine and Science in Sports and Exercise* **20**, 249–254.

Costill, D.L., Sherman, W.M., Fink, W.J., Maresh, C., Witten, M. & Miller, J.M. (1981) The role of dietary carbohydrates in muscle glycogen resynthesis after strenuous running. *American Journal of Clinical Nutrition* **34**, 1831–1836.

Coyle, E.F., Coggan, A.R., Hemmert, M.K., Lowe, R.C. & Walters, T.J. (1985) Substrate usage during prolonged exercise following a preexercise meal. *Journal of Applied Physiology* **59**, 429–433.

Deakin, V. (2006) Iron depletion in athletes. In: *Clinical Sports Nutrition*, 3rd edn (Burke, L. & Deakin, V., eds.) McGraw Hill, Sydney.

Fallon, K.E. (2004) Utility of hematological and iron-related screening in elite athletes. *Clinical Journal of Sports Medicine* **14**, 145–152.

Geyer, H., Parr, M.K., Reinhart, U., Schrader, Y., Mareck, U. & Schanzer, W. (2004) Analysis of non-hormonal nutritional supplements for anabolic-androgenic steroids: results of an international study. *International Journal of Sports Medicine* **25**, 124–129.

Gleeson, M., Nieman, D.C. & Pedersen, B.K. (2004) Exercise, nutrition and immune function. *Journal of Sports Sciences* **22**, 115–122.

Gonzalez-Alonso, J., Heaps, C.L. & Coyle, E.F. (1992) Rehydration after exercise with common beverages and water. *International Journal of Sports Medicine* **13**, 399–406.

Gopinathan, P.M., Pichan, G. & Sharma, V.M. (1988) Role of dehydration in heat stess-induced variations in mental performance. *Archives of Environmental Health* **43**, 15–17.

Hallberg, L. (1981) Bioavailability of dietary iron in man. *Annual Review of Nutrition* **1**, 123–147.

Hargreaves, M. (1999) Metabolic responses to carbohydrate ingestion: effects on exercise performance. In: *Perspectives in Exercise Science and Sports Medicine*

(Lamb, D.R. & Murray, R., eds.) Cooper, Carmel, IN: 93–124,

Hawley, J.A., Schabort, E.J., Noakes, T.D. & Dennis, S.C. (1997) Carbohydrate-loading and exercise performance: An update. *Sports Medicine* **24**, 73–81.

Hood, D.A., Kelton, R. & Nishio, M.L. (1992) Mitochondrial adaptations to chronic muscle use: effect of iron deficiency. *Comparative Biochemistry and Physiology* **101A**, 597–605.

Hubbard, R.W., Szlyk, P.C. & Armstrong, L.E. (1990) Influence of thirst and fluid palatability on fluid ingestion during exercise. In: *Perspectives in Exercise Science and Sports Medicine* (Gisolfi, C.V. & Lamb, D.R., eds.) Benchmark Press, Carmel, IN: 39–95.

Ivy, J.L., Goforth, H.W., Damon, B.D., McCauley, T.R., Parsons, E.C. & Price, T.B. (2002) Early post-exercise muscle glycogen recovery is enhanced with a carbohydrate-protein supplement. *Journal of Applied Physiology* **93**, 1337–1344.

Ivy, J.L., Katz, A.L., Cutler, C.L., Sherman, W.M. & Coyle, E.F. (1988) Muscle glycogen synthesis after exercise: effect of time of carbohydrate ingestion. *Journal of Applied Physiology* **64**, 1480–1485.

Jentjens, R.L., van Loon, L.J.C., Mann, C.H., Wagenmakers, A.J.M. & Jeukendrup, A.E. (2001) Addition of protein and amino acids to carbohydrates does not enhance postexercise muscle glycogen synthesis. *Journal of Applied Physiology* **91**, 839–846.

Jeukendrup, A., Brouns, F., Wagenmakers, A.J.M. & Saris, W.H.M. (1997) Carbohydrate-electrolyte feedings improve 1 h time trial cycling performance. *International Journal of Sports Medicine* **18**, 125–129.

Keizer, H.A., Kuipers, H., Van Kranenburg, G. & Guerten, P. (1986) Influence of liquid and solid meals on muscle glycogen resynthesis, plasma fuel hormone response, and maximal physical working capacity. *International Journal of Sports Medicine* **8**, 99–104.

Kerr, D. (2006) Kinanthropometry: physique assessment of the athlete. In: *Clinical Sports Nutrition*, 3rd edn (Burke, L. & Deakin, V., eds.) McGraw Hill, Sydney.

Levenhagen, D.K., Gresham, J.D., Carlson, M.G., Maron, D.J., Borel, M.J. & Flakoll, P.J. (2001) Postexercise nutrient intake timing in humans is critical to recovery of leg glucose and protein homeostasis.

American Journal of Physiology* **280**, E982–E993.

Loucks, A.B. (2004) Energy balance and body composition in sports and exercise. *Journal of Sports Sciences* **22**, 1–14.

Loucks, A.B. & Nattiv, A. (2005) The female athlete triad. *Lancet* **366**, S49–50.

Loucks, A.B. & Thuma, J.R. (2003) Luteinizing hormone pulsatility is disrupted at a threshold of energy availability in regularly menstruating women. *Journal of Clinical Endocrinology and Metabolism* **88**, 297–311.

Maughan, R.J. (2005) Contamination of dietary supplements and positive drug tests in sport. *Journal of Sports Sciences* **23**, 883–889.

Maughan, R.J. & Leiper, J.B. (1995) Sodium intake and post-exercise rehydration in man. *European Journal of Applied Physiology and Occupational Physiology* **71**, 311–319.

Millard-Stafford, M., Rosskopf, L.B., Snow, T.K. & Hinson, B.T. (1997) Water versus carbohydrate-electrolyte ingestion before and during a 15-km run in the heat. *International Journal of Sport Nutrition* **7**, 26–38.

Miller, S.L., Tipton, K.D., Chinkes, D.L., Wolf, S.E. & Wolfe, R.R. (2003) Independent and combined effects of amino acids and glucose after resistance exercise. *Medicine and Science in Sports and Exercise* **35**, 449–455.

Monsen, E.R. (1988) Iron nutrition and absorption: dietary factors which impact iron bioavailability. *Journal of the American Dietetic Association* **88**, 786–790.

Montain, S.J. & Coyle, E.F. (1992) Influence of graded dehydration on hyperthermia and cardiovascular drift during exercise. *Journal of Applied Physiology* **73**, 1340–1350.

Moore, J.M., Timperio, A.F., Crawford, D.A., Burns, C.M. & Cameron-Smith, D. (2002) Weight management and weight loss strategies of professional jockeys. *International Journal of Sport Nutrition and Exercise Metabolism* **12**, 1–13.

Neufer, P.D., Costill, D.L., Flynn, M.G., Kirwan, J.P., Mitchell, J.B. & Houmard, J. (1987) Improvements in exercise performance: effects of carbohydrate feedings and diet. *Journal of Applied Physiology* **62**, 983–988.

Nielsen, P. & Nachtigall, D. (1998) Iron supplementation in athletes: current recommendations. *Sports Medicine* **26**, 207–216.

Noakes, T.D. (2003) Overconsumption of fluid by athletes. *British Medical Journal* **327**, 113–114.

Noakes, T.D., Adams, B.A., Myburgh, K.H., Greeff, C., Lotz, T. & Nathan, M. (1988) The danger of an inadequate water intake during prolonged exercise. *European Journal of Applied Physiology* **57**, 210–219.

Nose, H., Mack, G.W., Shi, X.R. & Nadel, E.R. (1988) Role of osmolality and plasma volume during rehydration in humans. *Journal of Applied Physiology* **61**, 325–331.

Oppliger, R.A., Landry, G.L., Foster, S.W. & Lambrecht, A.C. (1998) Wisconsin minimum weight program reduces weight-cutting practices of high school wrestlers. *Clinical Journal of Sports Medicine* **8**, 26–31.

Oppliger, R.A., Steen, S.N. & Scott, J.R. (2003) Weight loss practices of college wrestlers. *International Journal of Sport Nutrition and Exercise Metabolism* **13**, 29–46.

Ostojic, S.M. & Mazic, S. (2002) Effects of a carbohydrate-electrolyte drink on specific soccer tests and performance. *Journal of Sports Science and Medicine* **1**, 47–53.

Otis, C.L., Drinkwater, B., Johnson, M., Loucks, A. & Wilmore, J. (1997) American College of Sports Medicine position stand. The female athlete triad. *Medicine and Science in Sports and Exercise* **29**, i–ix.

Parkin, J.A.M., Carey, M.F., Martin, I.K., Stojanovska, L. & Febbraio, M.A. (1997) Muscle glycogen storage following prolonged exercise: effect of timing of ingestion of high glycemic index food. *Medicine and Science in Sports and Exercise* **29**, 220–224.

Pitsis, G.C., Fallon, K.E., Fallon, S.K. & Fazakerley, R. (2004) Response of soluble transferrin receptor and iron-related parameters to iron supplementation in elite, iron-depleted, non-anaemic female athletes. *Clinical Journal of Sports Medicine* **14**, 300–304.

Rasmussen, B.B., Tipton, K.D., Miller, S.L., Wolf, S.E. & Wolfe, R.R. (2000) An oral essential amino acid-carbohydrate supplement enhances muscle protein anabolism after resistance exercise. *Journal of Applied Physiology* **88**, 386–392.

Reed, M.J., Brozinick, J.T., Lee, M.C. & Ivy, J.L. (1989) Muscle glycogen storage postexercise: effect of mode of carbohydrate administration. *Journal of Applied Physiology* **66**, 720–726.

Sawka, M.N. & Pandolf, K.B. (1990) Effects of body water loss on physiological function and exercise performance. In: *Perspectives in Exercise Science and Sports Medicine* (Gisolfi, C.V. & Lamb, D.R., eds.) Benchmark Press, Carmel, IN: 1–38.

Sherman, W.M., Costill, D.L., Fink, W.J. & Miller, J.M. (1981) Effect of exercise-diet manipulation on muscle glycogen and its subsequent utilisation during performance. *International Journal of Sports Medicine* **2**, 114–118.

Shirreffs, S.M., Armstrong, L.E. & Cheuvront, S.N. (2004) Fluid and electrolyte needs for preparation and recovery from training and competition. *Journal of Sports Sciences* **22**, 57–63.

Shirreffs, S.M. & Maughan, R.J. (1997) Restoration of fluid balance after exercise-induced dehydration: effects of alcohol consumption. *Journal of Applied Physiology* **83**, 1152–1158.

Shirreffs, S.M., Taylor, A.J., Leiper, J.B. & Maughan, R.J. (1996) Post-exercise rehydration in man: effects of volume consumed and drink sodium content. *Medicine and Science in Sports and Exercise* **28**, 1260–1271.

Steen, S.N., & Brownell, K.D. (1990) Patterns of weight loss and regain in wrestlers: has the tradition changed? *Medicine and Science in Sports and Exercise* **22**, 762–768.

Sundgot-Borgen, J. (2000) Eating disorders in athletes. In: *Nutrition in Sport* (Maughan R.J., ed.) Blackwell Science, Oxford: 510–522.

Tarnopolsky, M.A., Zawada, C., Richmond, L.B., *et al.* (2001) Gender differences in carbohydrate loading are related to energy intake. *Journal of Applied Physiology* **91**, 225–230.

Thomas, D.E., Brotherhood, J.R. & Brand, J.C. (1991) Carbohydrate feeding before exercise: effect of glycemic index. *International Journal of Sports Medicine* **12**, 180–186.

Tipton, K.D., Borsheim, E., Wolf, S.E., Sanford, A.P. & Wolfe, R.R. (2003) Acute response of net muscle protein balance reflects 24-h balance after exercise and amino acid ingestion. *American Journal of Physiology. Endocrinology and Metabolism* **284**, E76–E89.

Tipton, K.D., Rasmussen, B.B., Miller, S.L., *et al.* (2001) Timing of amino acid-carbohydrate ingestion alters anabolic response of muscle to resistance exercise. *American Journal of Physiology. Endocrinology and Metabolism* **281**, E197–E206.

Tipton, K.D. & Wolfe, R.R. (2004) Protein and amino acids for athletes. *Journal of Sports Sciences* **22**, 65–79.

Van Hall, G., Shirreffs, S.M. & Calbert, J.A.L. (2000) Muscle glycogen resynthesis during recovery from cycle exercise: no effect of additional protein ingestion. *Journal of Applied Physiology* **88**, 1631–1636.

Vergauwen, L., Brouns, F. & Hespel, P. (1998) Carbohydrate supplementation improves stroke performance in tennis. *Medicine and Science in Sports and Exercise* **30**, 1289–1295.

Walsh, R.M., Noakes, T.D., Hawley, J.A. & Dennis, S.C. (1994) Impaired high-intensity cycling performance time at low levels of dehydration. *International Journal of Sports Medicine* **15**, 392–398.

Welsh, R.S., Davis, J.M., Burke, J.R. & Williams, H.G. (2002) Carbohydrates and physical/mental performance during intermittent exercise to fatigue. *Medicine and Science in Sports and Exercise* **34**, 723–731.

Wright, D.A., Sherman, W.M. & Dernbach, A.R. (1991) Carbohydrate feedings before, during, or in combination improve cycling endurance performance. *Journal of Applied Physiology* **71**, 1082–1088.

Zawadzki, K.M., Yaspelkis, B.B. & Ivy, J.L. (1992) Carbohydrate–protein complex increases the rate of muscle glycogen storage after exercise. *Journal of Applied Physiology* **72**, 1854–1859.

Index